CLINICAL ANATOMY

Principles

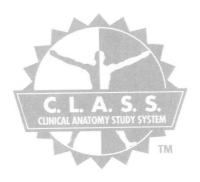

OTHER PRODUCTS IN THE
CLINICAL ANATOMY STUDY SYSTEM

Clinical Anatomy Atlas
Clinical Anatomy Dissections
Clinical Anatomy Interactive Lesson
Clinical Anatomy Interactive Lab Practical

CLINICAL ANATOMY
Principles

LAWRENCE H. MATHERS, JR., M.D., PH.D.
Chief, Division of Human Anatomy
Associate Professor of Pediatrics and Surgery (Human Anatomy)
Stanford University School of Medicine
Stanford, California

ROBERT A. CHASE, M.D.
Emile Holman Professor Emeritus
Department of Surgery
Division of Human Anatomy
Stanford University School of Medicine
Stanford, California

JOHN DOLPH, M.A.
Lecturer, Division of Human Anatomy
Stanford University School of Medicine
Stanford, California

ERIC F. GLASGOW, M.D.
Professor, Division of Human Anatomy
Stanford University School of Medicine
Stanford, California
Honorary Professorial Fellow, Department of Anatomy
Monash University
Melbourne, Australia

JOHN A. GOSLING, M.D.
Professor, Division of Human Anatomy
Stanford University School of Medicine
Stanford, California
Professor and Chairman, Department of Anatomy
The Chinese University of Hong Kong
Hong Kong, China

with 625 illustrations
by C.W. Hoffman and Nadine B. Sokol

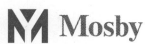

St. Louis Baltimore Boston Carlsbad Chicago Naples New York Philadelphia Portland
London Madrid Mexico City Singapore Sydney Tokyo Toronto Wiesbaden

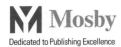

Mosby
Dedicated to Publishing Excellence

A Times Mirror Company

Editor: Emma D. Underdown
Editorial Assistant: Alicia E. Moten
Project Manager: John Rogers
Senior Production Editors: Helen Hudlin, Kathleen Teal
Designer: Dave Zielinski
Design Coordinator: Renée Duenow
Manufacturing Supervisor: Theresa Fuchs
Artists: C.W. Hoffman, Nadine B. Sokol
Section Opener Photography: John Phelan

Printed in the United States of America
Composition by Black Dot
Printing/binding by Von Hoffmann Press

Mosby–Year Book, Inc.
11830 Westline Industrial Drive
St. Louis, Missouri 63146

Library of Congress Cataloging in Publication Data

Clinical anatomy principles / Lawrence H. Mathers, Jr. . . . [et al.].
    p.   cm.
    "Clinical anatomy study system, C.L.A.S.S."—P. i.
    Includes index.
    ISBN 0-8016-6356-3 (hardcover). — ISBN 0-8151-1749-3
    (package)
    1. Human anatomy.   I. Mathers, Lawrence H., 1945-   . II. Title:
Clinical anatomy study system.
    [DNLM: 1. Anatomy.]
QM23.2.C585 1995
611—dc20
DNLM/DLC
for Library of Congress

95 96 97 98 99 / 9 8 7 6 5 4 3 2 1

Preface

Why a new anatomy book? Admittedly, many good books are already available. The fundamental knowledge base that defines anatomy has been stable for decades, and little new research on the basic structure of the human body has been produced in recent years. What *has* changed recently, however, is (1) the explosion of new information in molecular biology and genetics rightfully competing with anatomy for space and time in the crowded medical curriculum, (2) the fall-off in knowledge of vertebrate biology and development possessed by the typical student entering medical school, and (3) the increasing anatomic knowledge needed to use intelligently the clinico-anatomic information produced by computed tomography, ultrasound, and magnetic resonance imaging technologies.

Curriculum committees have reduced the amount of time devoted to teaching anatomy in a great many medical schools, yet the central importance of anatomy in medicine cannot be denied. Today's student, no less than those decades ago, knows instinctively that a working knowledge of anatomy is the first sure sign that his or her medical career truly has begun.

The study of anatomy resembles the study of *language*. Literally thousands of new words must be learned. Successful anatomy students learn the art of accurate, concise description and will find this to be a valuable skill throughout their medical careers. However, a real understanding of anatomy requires *three-dimensional visualization*—because anatomic structures are always related to other anatomic structures, and a true comprehension of these relationships allows a student to understand and even anticipate many pathologic processes. To learn anatomy well requires a dual approach: the *regional* description of structures and their relationships to each other and an understanding of the major *systems* of the body—vascular, muscular, skeletal, nervous, and lymphatic. This text is organized around a regional approach to anatomy, but time is taken in each section to review information from the standpoint of systems because true understanding requires that both approaches be used.

We believe that anatomy is best learned by emphasizing its connection to *clinical medicine.* However, other valid approaches attempt to define the structure of human anatomy in terms of embryologic development or link anatomic concepts to vertebrate structure comparing human structure to that of other primates and mammals. This text makes use of all three approaches, but its fundamental organization is built around the relationship of anatomy to clinical medicine. Clinical cases are presented throughout the text; however, the subject of anatomy is far too detailed and intricate to be learned in this fashion alone. What the text, therefore, does is to present a basic *core* of anatomic knowledge necessary to comprehend the structure and workings of the body and adds to that anatomic information that has real pertinence to the everyday practice of medicine.

An anatomy text is only as good as its illustrations, and we have endeavored to provide figures that "speak a thousand words" and truly help to improve comprehension. *Clinical Anatomy Principles* can be used to great advantage when combined with its companions, the *Clinical Anatomy Atlas*, *Clinical Anatomy Dissections*, and with the multimedia-based depiction of anatomy available on the *Clinical Anatomy Interactive Lesson*, a CD-ROM also created by this author team.

Those studying anatomy in the 1990s will be the medical practitioners of the first half of the 21st century. Their education must include reference to the new technologies that continually renew the need for competent physicians to know and understand anatomy. We believe that to know the structure of the body is to know not only its appearance and the location of its regions but also its function. This book attempts to explain anatomy in terms of *both* structure and function.

v

Approaching the study of the body in this fashion elevates the study of anatomy above the level of memorization to the realm of comprehension and even wonder.

For those of us who have labored to produce this book, our fascination with the human body and its intricacies grows with every passing year. We hope to pass that enthusiasm along to our students and are confident that, if we can succeed in this hope, future generations of health care providers will derive great professional pride and pleasure from their understanding of the human body, that most remarkable of nature's creations.

Lawrence H. Mathers, Jr., M.D., Ph.D.
Robert A. Chase, M.D.
John Dolph, M.A.
Eric F. Glasgow, M.D.
John A. Gosling, M.D.

Stanford, California

Acknowledgments

The authors of this text represent well over a 100 years of experience in teaching anatomy on four continents. We have tried to apply to the creation of this book not only our familiarity with the factual knowledge of anatomy but also our experience in effective ways to present and explain complex information. **Charles Hoffman** and **Nadine Sokol,** the medical illustrators whose artistic renderings of anatomy are a major asset of this text, displayed both artistic creativity and considerable knowledge of anatomy in producing these superlative illustrations.

We would also like to acknowledge and thank many people who made constructive suggestions to the design of the text and helped ensure its accuracy and clarity. Mosby–Year Book Publishing, Inc., was unfailingly supportive in seeing this project through to its completion. In the early stages of our work, **Emma Underdown** labored tirelessly, making valuable suggestions about the structure of the text and rearranging our prose to make it clearer and more readable. On assuming her position as Acquisitions Editor, Emma continued to guide the project through its completion. **Helen Hudlin** has provided invaluable direction throughout the production phase. We also thank our anonymous colleagues who, in reviewing early drafts of the text, pointed out many strengths and weaknesses and made suggestions that have led to its betterment.

Many individuals contribute to the successful completion of a project such as this. We want to thank **Johnella Stevick,** administrator in the Anatomy Division at Stanford, for organizing the correspondence between us and Mosby, coordinating our schedules, planning meetings, and, in general, anticipating our needs.

Dr. Pavarti Dev, of *SUMMIT,* the computer/multimedia facility at Stanford, worked with us not only on this text but on the CD-ROM tutorial that accompanies the text. **Dr. Steve Daane, Ramon Felciano,** and **Philip Constantinou,** also of *SUMMIT,* made many valuable suggestions as well. Medical students, **David Kim** and **Matt Lewis,** among many others, were especially good at providing the student perspective.

Any project of this magnitude requires long hours of work on the part of the authors and inevitably produces disruptions in their personal and family lives. We want **Mil, Ann, Kate,** and **Roz** to know that their patience and forbearance is much appreciated and that without their support the project could have never succeeded. We dedicate this text to them and to all that have added to our lives.

Lastly, and most importantly, we want the text to be useful for **students of human structure,** and we want to thank them for the inspiration they have provided us. Seeing talented young people go through the monumental transition from students to health care professionals is a source of professional and personal satisfaction. We are certain that, in the future, they will bring continued honor to the field of anatomy and confirm its place as a keystone in the education of health care professionals.

Lawrence H. Mathers, Jr., M.D., Ph.D.
Robert A. Chase, M.D.
John Dolph, M.A.
Eric F. Glasgow, M.D.
John A. Gosling, M.D.
Stanford, California

Contents

Introduction

Basic Anatomic Terminology, 3
Fabric of the Human Body, 8
Introduction to the Body Systems, 20
Techniques for Imaging the Human Body, 36

SECTION ONE

Thorax

1.1 Introduction to the Thorax, 49
1.2 Chest Wall, 54
1.3 Pleural Spaces, Tracheobronchial Tree, and Lungs, 74
1.4 Heart, 86
1.5 Mediastinum, 109
1.6 Systems Review and Surface Anatomy of the Thorax, 120
1.7 Case Studies: Thorax, 125

SECTION TWO

Head and Neck

2.1 Skull, 133
2.2 Brain and Central Nervous System, 145
2.3 Cranial Nerves, 164
2.4 Pharyngeal Arches, 170
2.5 Scalp and Face, 174
2.6 Temporal and Infratemporal Fossae, 187
2.7 Posterior Triangle of the Neck, 198
2.8 Anterolateral Neck, 206
2.9 Ear, 224
2.10 Eye and Orbit, 234
2.11 Nasal Cavity, 253
2.12 Mouth and Palate, 263
2.13 Pharynx, 276
2.14 Larynx, 284
2.15 Systems Review and Surface Anatomy of the Head and Neck, 291
2.16 Case Studies: Head and Neck, 297

SECTION THREE

Upper Limb

3.1 Shoulder, 309
3.2 Axilla, 330
3.3 Brachial Plexus, 336
3.4 Arm, 342
3.5 Forearm, 348
3.6 Wrist, 369
3.7 Hand, 378
3.8 Systems Review and Surface Anatomy of the Upper Limb, 394
3.9 Case Studies: Upper Limb, 401

SECTION FOUR

Back and Spinal Cord

4.1 Back and Vertebral Column, 409
4.2 Spinal Cord, 434
4.3 Systems Review and Surface Anatomy of the Back and Spinal Cord, 448
4.4 Case Studies: Back and Spinal Cord, 451

SECTION FIVE

Abdomen

5.1 Abdominal Wall, 457
5.2 Inguinal Canal and Descent of the Testes, 464
5.3 Peritoneal Membranes and Development of the Gut, 473
5.4 Liver, Gallbladder, Spleen, and Pancreas, 484
5.5 Esophagus, Stomach, and Lesser Sac, 499
5.6 Small Intestine, 507
5.7 Colon and Anorectal Region, 515
5.8 Kidneys and Suprarenal Glands, 522
5.9 Posterior Wall and Diaphragm, 529
5.10 Systems Review and Surface Anatomy of the Abdomen, 536
5.11 Case Studies: Abdomen, 539

SECTION SIX

Pelvis and Perineum

6.1   Bony Pelvis, 549
6.2   Perineum, 561
6.3   Pelvic Vasculature and Nerve Supply, 586
6.4   Urinary System, 594
6.5   Pelvic Viscera in the Female, 604
6.6   Pelvic Viscera in the Male, 613
6.7   Systems Review and Surface Anatomy of the Pelvis and Perineum, 622
6.8   Case Studies: Pelvis and Perineum, 628

SECTION SEVEN

Lower Limb

7.1   Anteromedial Thigh, 637
7.2   Gluteal Region, 663
7.3   Posterior Thigh and Knee, 672
7.4   Leg and Ankle Joint, 688
7.5   Foot, 705
7.6   Systems Review and Surface Anatomy of the Lower Limb, 722
7.7   Case Studies: Lower Limb, 728

CLINICAL ANATOMY

Principles

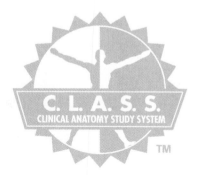

C.L.A.S.S.
CLINICAL ANATOMY STUDY SYSTEM
TM

Introduction

▶   Basic Anatomic
    Terminology

▶   Fabric of the Human Body

▶   Introduction to the Body
    Systems

▶   Techniques for Imaging
    the Human Body

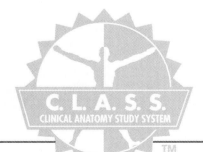

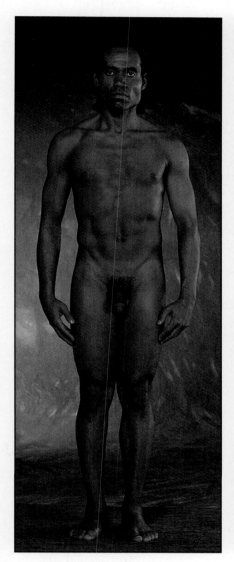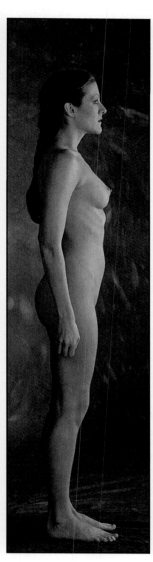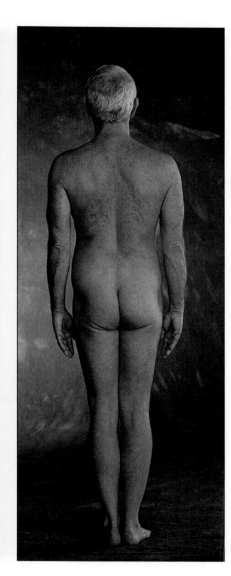

Introduction

▶ Basic Anatomic Terminology

▶ Fabric of the Human Body

▶ Introduction to the Body Systems

▶ Techniques for Imaging the Human Body

BASIC ANATOMIC TERMINOLOGY

Anatomists and physicians have agreed to use a standardized terminology to ensure accurate description and clear communication.

Anatomic Position and Body Regions

To ensure consistency, it is agreed to describe body structures and their positions with reference to a person standing upright, facing forward, feet slightly spread on the floor, with the arms hanging at the sides and the palms facing forward. This is known as **the anatomic position** (Figure I-1). When the person is lying on the back, the position is said to be **supine;** when lying face down the position is said to be **prone.**

The **head** includes the brain, the cranial bones surrounding it, the base of the skull, and the facial structures. The **upper limb** includes everything from the shoulder to the fingertips: the segment from the shoulder to the elbow is the *arm,* from the elbow to the wrist the *forearm,* and the wrist bones are also known as the *carpal bones.* The armpit is known as the *axilla.* The **thorax** and **abdomen** comprise the *trunk.* The **pelvis** region includes the lower part of the abdominal wall, commencing at the level of the brim of the hip bones. The **lower limb** extends from the hip to the toes: the segment from hip to knee is the *thigh,* from knee to ankle is the *leg.* The ankle bones are also known as the *tarsal bones.*

Relationship of Structures to Each Other

It is frequently necessary to describe the position of one anatomic structure *in relation to another.* A group of terms has been developed to make such descriptions clear and precise. **Medial** means closer to the midline and **lateral** means further from it. A given structure may be lateral to one structure but medial to another; thus the middle finger is *medial* to the thumb (in the anatomic position) but is *lateral* to the little finger. Describing the limbs, the terms *proximal* and *distal* are often used. A structure is **proximal** if it is nearer its point of origin (or of the attachment of the limb to the trunk) and **distal** if it is further from its point of origin (or attachment of the limb to the trunk). Thus the elbow is *distal* to the shoulder but *proximal* to the wrist. The terms **deep** and **superficial** are used when describing layers of muscle or other tissue in relation to the surface of the body; thus, in the chest wall, the skin is superficial to the ribs. **Anterior** means on or toward the front of the body (see next section), and **posterior** refers to the back surface of the body. A structure is anterior to another structure if it lies nearer to the anterior surface of the body. **Internal** and **external** are used to describe something that is nearer the center or nearer the surface. Remember that no structure is *absolutely* medial, lateral, anterior, posterior, etc.—these terms always *compare* the position of structures (Figure I-2).

Planes of the Body

The standard or cardinal planes of the body are coronal, sagittal, and transverse (horizontal). Viewing the body in the anatomic position, the **coronal plane** passes from left to right through the body, dividing it into an anterior and posterior part. The **sagittal planes** pass from anterior to posterior, dividing the body into a left and right side. When the plane is precisely in the midline, it is said to be in the **median sagittal** or **midsagittal** plane; all other parallel planes are **parasagittal.** **Transverse planes** are parallel to the ground and divide the body into an upper and lower portion (Figure I-3).

Anterior (ventral) means in front of the coronal plane through the middle of the body; **posterior** or **dor-**

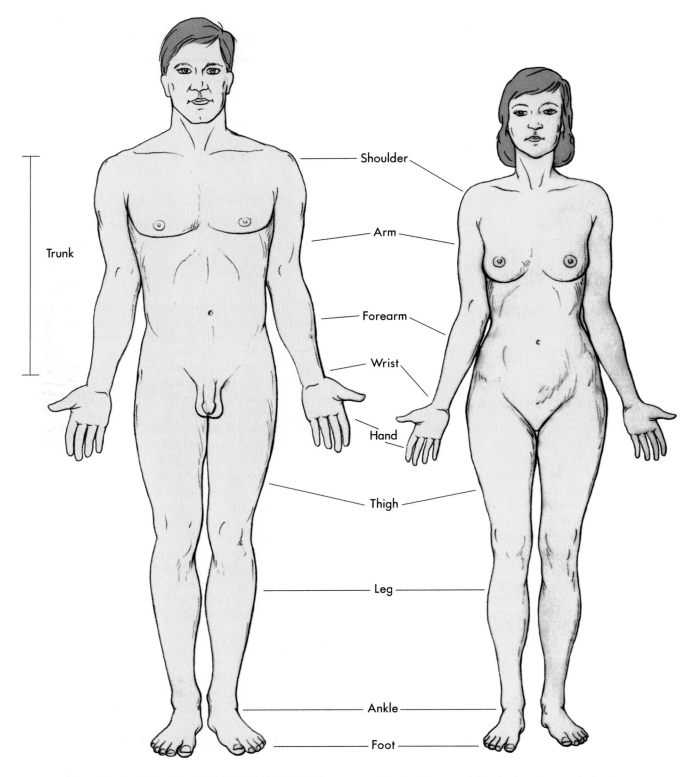

Figure I-1   ANATOMIC POSITION. The person is standing upright, facing forward, feet slightly separated, arms hanging to the side with palms facing forward. Structures are named and their positions described in this standard position.

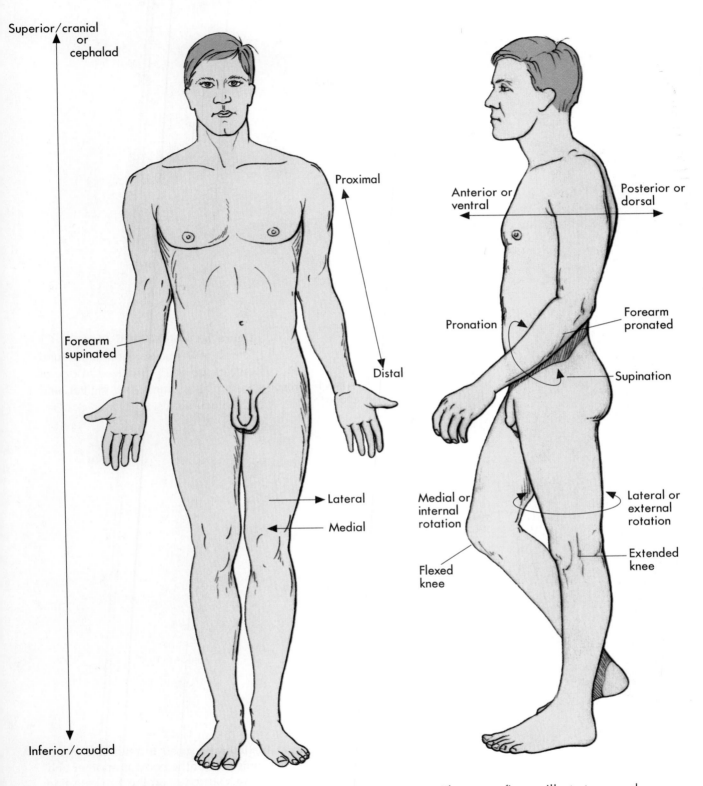

Figure I-2 TERMS OF POSITION AND MOVEMENT. These two figures illustrate several types of positional terms and movements.

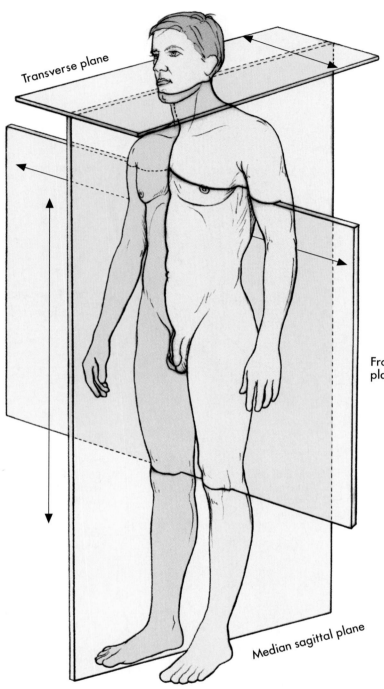

Transverse plane

Frontal/coronal plane

Median sagittal plane

Figure I-3   ANATOMIC PLANES. CT scans, MRI images, and ultrasound images are often displayed in one of these planes: transverse, sagittal, and frontal (coronal).

sal means behind the midcoronal plane. **Superior** means above a transverse plane, and **inferior** means below it.

Many regions of the body are described by terms that apply nowhere else. In the *hand* the anterior surface (in the anatomic position) is **palmar;** the anterior surface of the forearm is also **volar;** the opposite side is the **posterior** or **dorsal** surface. For the *foot,* the portion contacting the ground is the **plantar** surface; the opposite is called **dorsal.** Many structures in the body are

paired; the term **ipsilateral** is used to refer to a structure that is on the same side of the body as another and **contralateral** to refer to a structure on the opposite side of the body; thus the left median nerve innervates muscles in the *ipsilateral* (i.e., left) upper limb.

Terms Describing Movement

In general, when the angle of a joint such as the elbow or the knee is narrowed, the movement is de-

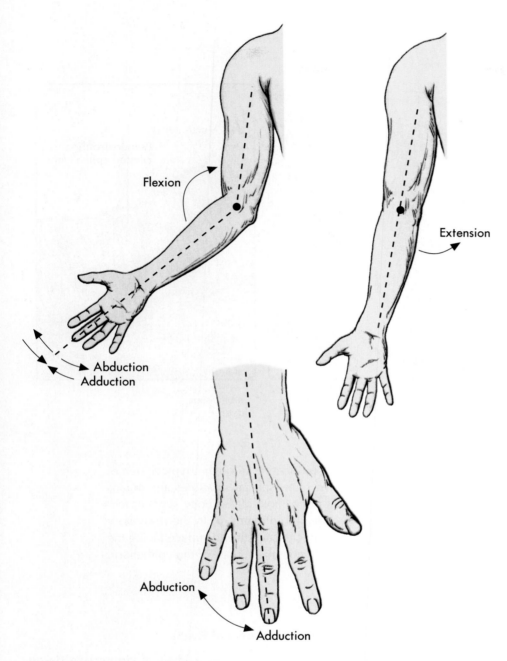

Figure I-4 UPPER LIMB MOVE-MENTS. This figure illustrates some of the movements of the upper limb.

scribed as **flexion.** The opening up of such joints, increasing the size of the angle, is **extension** (Figure I-4). Another way to describe flexion is to say that the "fetal position" involves flexion of most joints, while extension is the opposite. **Abduction** means moving away from the midline, and **adduction** means moving toward it. For example, pulling the upper limb downward in a plane parallel to the anterior surface of the body so that it lies snugly alongside the chest wall is *adduction* of the shoulder joint. Moving the upper limb downward in a plane perpendicular to the anterior surface of the body is, however, extension of the shoulder joint. Elongated structures such as the limbs can often *rotate* around their long axes. When the rotation results

in the anterior surface of a limb rotating toward the midline, it is **medial rotation;** the opposite is **lateral rotation.**

Special Terms

Supination is the act of turning the palm so that it faces forward (in the anatomic position); **pronation** is the opposite. These movements involve special interactions between the two long bones of the forearm, the *ulna* and *radius.* Turning the sole of the foot to face medially is **inversion** and the opposite **eversion;** these movements are *not* comparable to supination/pronation in the forearm, however.

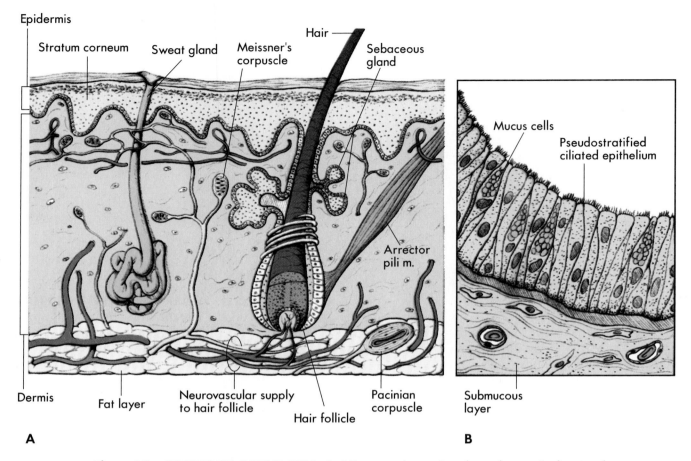

Epidermis
Stratum corneum
Sweat gland
Meissner's corpuscle
Hair
Sebaceous gland
Mucus cells
Pseudostratified ciliated epithelium
Arrector pili m.
Dermis
Fat layer
Neurovascular supply to hair follicle
Hair follicle
Pacinian corpuscle
Submucous layer

A   **B**

Figure I-5   STRUCTURE OF THE SKIN. A, Microscopic section through a typical area of skin shows the dermal and epidermal layers and the many special structures and organs found within. Stratified squamous epithelium, found on most of the body surface, features a thickened layer of degenerated cells, the stratum corneum. **B,** In the respiratory system, the lining epithelium is columnar, with a characteristic ciliated surface facing the lumen of the airway. Numerous cells secrete mucus to coat the surface of the epithelium. (Structures are not drawn to scale.)

FABRIC OF THE HUMAN BODY

Skin

Skin covers the entire surface of the body and provides protection, preservation of moisture, and regulation of temperature. The **epidermis** is most superficial and the **dermis** lies just deep to it (Figure I-5, *A*); much of the upper segment of the epidermis is dead cells and is continuously sloughed off and renewed from deeper layers. The dermis contains *connective tissue, sweat glands, sebaceous glands, hair follicles, nerve endings,* and *capillaries* (see Figure I-5, *A*). The ducts of the glands and the hairs growing from the follicles extend upward through the epidermis to reach the surface. The hairs and glands are present or absent in different regions of the body. **Nails** are special modifications of the epidermis found at the tips of the digits.

Connective Tissue and Fascia

Deep to the skin lies a layer of **connective tissue,** which shows tremendous variety in different regions of the body. It is made up of a variety of *cells* (fibroblasts, fat cells, macrophages, plasma cells, etc.) and a large amount of *extracellular material* or *matrix,* secreted primarily by the fibroblasts. The matrix is made up of *proteoglycan molecules* (protein core plus glycosaminoglycans)—a material formerly known as *mucopolysaccharide.* In addition to the secreted matrix there is one or more of the 10 to 12 varieties of *collagen fibers,* or *elastic fibers,* and other specialized molecules secreted by the connective tissue cells (Figure I-6, *A*). The relative proportions of these structural substances determines the stiffness or flexibility of connective tissue in different regions of the body—for example, the connective tissue

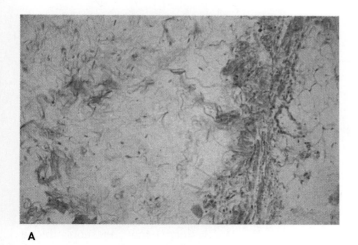

A

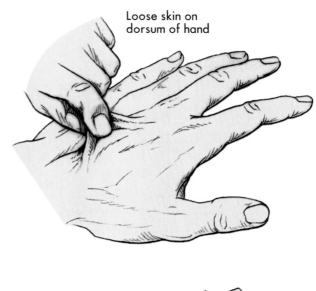

Loose skin on
dorsum of hand

Figure I-6 CONNECTIVE TISSUE, LIGHT MICRO-GRAPH. A, Connective tissue is made up of cells and a considerable amount of intercellular material, consisting of a proteoglycan ground substance and a variety of fibers. It serves as the interface or packing substance between all other tissues or organs in the body. (See "Connective Tissue" in Section One for further details.) **B,** This figure shows the mobility of connective tissue and fascia on the dorsum of the hand (*top*) and the relatively small number of transverse fibers that anchor the skin of the hand to the underlying bones (*bottom*). (**A,** From Erlandsen S, Magney J: *Color atlas of histology,* St Louis, 1992, Mosby.)

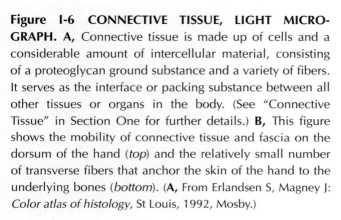

Skin incised,
collagen fibers
exposed

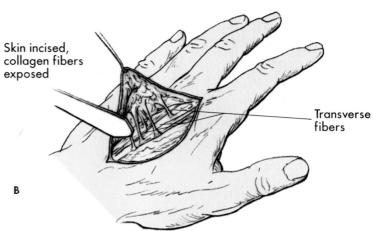

Transverse
fibers

B

on the sole of the foot needs to be thick and durable, while that of the eyelids needs to be softer and more malleable.

When connective tissue is sufficiently organized that it may be distinguished as a distinct layer it is known as **fascia.** It usually exists as a layer of **superficial fascia** and a layer of **deep fascia,** although one of these may be absent in particular areas of the body. The superficial fascia is also known as *subcutaneous tissue* and contains a mixture of connective tissue and *adipose* (fatty) tissue. It may be very loose and mobile, as on the surface of the face or the dorsum of the hand (Figure I-6, *B*); in other areas, such as the palm of the hand, it is very tight and allows little movement of the overlying skin. The deep fascia covers the large muscles, forms layers that create fascial compartments, and may extend deeply to attach to underlying bones. In many areas (the limbs, the neck) it condenses into thickened sheets or layers that help to support structures contained within. Fascia serves as a "filling material" be-

tween large structures, such as muscles and bones, but it is also a very *metabolically active tissue,* which plays a vital role in immunologic activities, wound healing, and growth.

Very dense and strong connective tissue structures called **ligaments,** with tightly packed and highly ordered bundles of collagen molecules, characteristically connect bones to other bones or cartilages and often reinforce joints (see following discussion and Figure I-11).

Bone and Cartilage

Bones are living tissues, made up of a proteoglycan matrix (ground substance) onto which calcium salts are deposited, producing a very rigid and solid entity. Bone is a highly specialized form of connective tissue. In the center of most bones is a reticulated marrow cavity, containing important *hematopoietic* (blood-forming) cells (Figure I-7). Living cells are scattered in a highly organized fashion throughout the substance of bone,

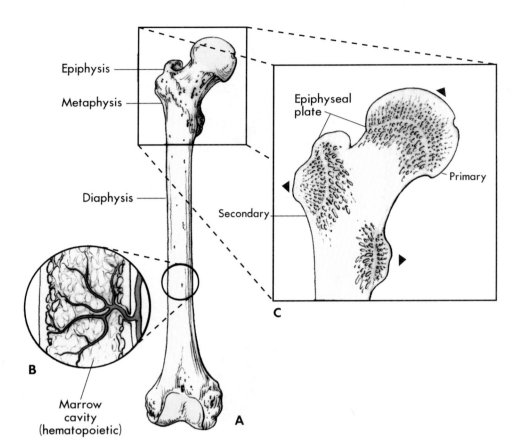

Figure I-7 BONE STRUCTURE. A, Typical long bone (the femur). It has a central shaft, the diaphysis, and an epiphysis at each end. The metaphysis is the zone of transition between the epiphysis and diaphysis. **B,** Typical nutrient foramen, through which blood vessels reach the interior of a long bone and supply blood to its internal marrow cavity. **C,** Two epiphyseal plates at the upper end of the femur. At these plates new bone is formed, laid down in an orderly fashion that leads to the elongation or change in shape of the bone (*arrowheads*).

and, moreover, both the living cells and the ground substance undergo a continuous process of destruction and replacement. This normal process of destruction and replacement also makes it possible for fractured or otherwise injured bones to repair themselves.

The great majority of bones form when calcium salts are deposited onto cartilaginous *anlage* (embryonic precursors) formed in the same general shape as the bone that will ultimately replace it. This process is known as **endochondral ossification** (see Figure I-7) and occurs in the long bones of the limbs and trunk as well as the vertebral column and parts of the head. Individual bones have one or more **ossification centers** where the true bone cells are generated. Any childhood injury involving the ossification centers is threatening to the continued normal growth of the bone.

Other bones, primarily those of the cranium, form when calcium salts are deposited directly into embryonic mesenchyme, bypassing the formation of cartilaginous anlage. This is known as **intramembranous ossification.**

Bones take many years to mature. For example, the timing and sequence of bone maturation in the upper limb is shown in Table I-1. When children suffer fractures, the clinician must be concerned about the degree of growth lying ahead for the injured bone, and whether or not the trauma will disturb this growth. Assessment of bone age can also be useful in forensic

medicine, or in anthropology, to determine the age of deceased specimens.

Bone is highly dependent on an intact blood supply, and various arteries and veins reach the interior of bones through **nutrient foramina** on the surface of the bone. Any disease process or trauma that affects these vessels adversely might also threaten the continued growth and health of the bone (see Figure I-7, *B*).

Cartilage makes up a significant fraction of the skeleton. It is formed from a mucopolysaccharide matrix that has *not* undergone deposition of calcium. Like bone, it consists of living cells scattered within the matrix, but the organization of cells characteristic of bone is lacking in cartilage (Figure I-8). Cartilage has no internal vascular system, and its size is limited by the ability of nutrients and oxygen to diffuse into the center of a cartilaginous mass. Cartilage is less strong than bone but can provide some support to structures and is more flexible than bone. Cartilage is often found in parts of the skeleton where motion is involved (e.g., the attachment of the ribs to the sternum, see Figure I-9) and covers the surfaces of bone that face each other in joints (see following and Figure I-11). It is also found at some points where bones attach firmly to each other and an immobile joint is involved (e.g., the union of individual bones at the base of the skull [see Figure I-10] or the union of the two hip bones in the *pubic symphysis*).

Table I-1   Bone Growth and Maturation in the Upper Limb

Bone	Ossification Centers	Ossification Begins	Ossification Complete
Clavicle	Matures lateral to medial	Week 7	~25 years
Scapula	Independent ossification centers in coracoid, acromion	Week 8	~20 years
Humerus	Ossification centers in head, tubercles, epicondyles	Week 8	~20 years
Radius/ulna	Matures proximal to distal	Week 8	13 to 15 years
Carpals	Each carpal bone has one ossification center	From week 4 to several years postnatally	10 to 12 years
Metacarpals	For fingers, ossification center in head end of metacarpal; for thumb, metacarpal ossification center is in base	Week 9	15 to 18 years
Phalanges	Ossification centers in bases of all phalanges; matures proximal to distal	Week 11 to 12	14 to 17 years

Skeleton

The skeleton is the assembled set of bones and cartilages (Figure I-9). The **appendicular skeleton** (that of the upper and lower limbs) is usually distinguished from the **axial skeleton** (the skull, thorax, and vertebral column). The appendicular skeleton generally allows for considerable *mobility,* and the axial skeleton provides *strength* and serves as a reference point for movements of the rest of the body.

Joints. Bones are joined to other bones (and some times to cartilages) by **joints.** Joints always provide a combination of strength and mobility, sometimes emphasizing strength and other times mobility. The joints along which bones of the cranial vault are joined to each other, known as *sutures,* are examples of the former, because when mature they allow little or no movement between adjacent bones. The knee joint is a classic example of the latter, and its mobility makes it one of the joints most often involved in traumatic injury.

Classification of joints can be confusing, and several systems for differentiating them have evolved. Table I-2 describes a relatively simple method for describing joints. *Fibrous joints* (Figure I-10) are strong but nearly immobile. Examples include the sutures of the skull, the intervertebral disks, and the attachment between the teeth and the mandible or maxilla. *Cartilaginous joints* are of two principal types: those represented by the epiphyseal cartilage in growing long bones and those consisting of fibrocartilage and located in the midline of the body.

Other joints, known as *synovial joints* (Figure I-11), consist of two bones in proximity with their facing (articular) surfaces covered by cartilage, an interior cavity lined by a thin and delicate synovial membrane, and an external covering layer of fibrous tissue and sometimes ligaments. Synovial joints are sometimes very mobile but may be so at the expense of strength.

Muscles

Striated muscle. Striated muscle is made up of individual muscle cells or **fibers** (Figure I-12). It is also known as *skeletal* or *voluntary muscle.* It usually connects one bone to another and crosses over the joint at which adjacent bones articulate. Striated muscle cells (fibers) are multinucleate and represent a syncitium, packed with highly organized contractile filaments,

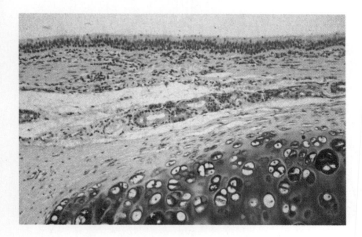

Figure I-8   HYALINE CARTILAGE. Hyaline cartilage consists of a homogeneous matrix and chondrocytes, each in a spherical lacunar cavity. The matrix consists largely of type II collagen and provides considerable tensile strength to hyaline cartilage. Other types of cartilage include **elastic** (in certain nasal cartilages and cartilages of the ear) and **fibrocartilage** (found in the intervertebral disks and the pubic symphysis). (From Erlandsen S, Magney J: *Color atlas of histology,* St Louis, 1992, Mosby.)

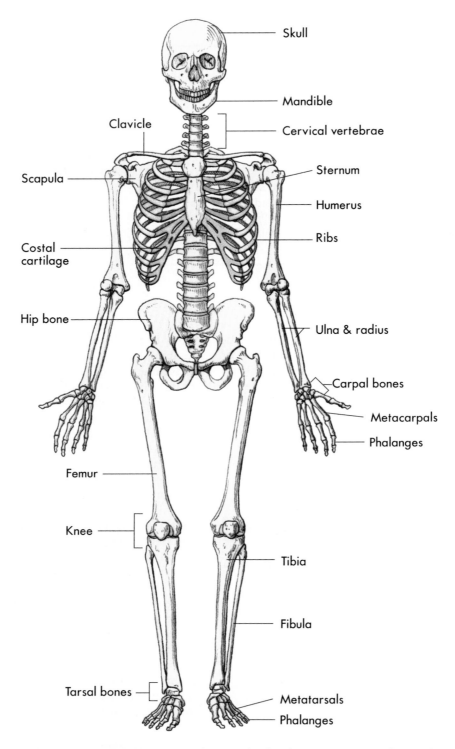

Figure I-9   SKELETON, ANTERIOR VIEW. The vertebral column, cranium, ribs, and sternum comprise the **axial skeleton;** the limb girdles and limb bones make up the **appendicular skeleton.**

Table I-2   Classification of Joints

Type of Joint	Structural Characteristics	Examples	Comments
Fibrous joint (see Figure I-10)	Consists of *fibrous tissue* connecting two adjacent bones	Distal tibiofibular joint (a *syndemosis*) Cranial *sutures* (of calvarium) Attachment of teeth to jaws	May have *zero mobility* (sutures) or *slight mobility* (e.g., teeth in jaws)
Cartilaginous joint (primary) (see Figure I-7)	Composed of *hyaline cartilage* Derived from cartilaginous anlage, which ossify everywhere but the region of this "joint" Allow little or no movement	Epiphyseal cartilages of developing long bones (a *synchondrosis*) Selected sutures in base of skull Manubriosternal joint	When bone growth is completed, these joints are replaced with ordinary bone tissue
Cartilaginous joint (secondary)	Composed of fibrocartilage Allow much more movement than primary cartilaginous joints	Intervertebral disks Pubic symphysis	Most examples are in midline of body
Synovial joint (diarthroses) (see Figure I-11)	*Synovial cavity,* lined by *synovial membrane,* separates the bones *Articular cartilage* (hyaline) on facing surfaces of bones *Capsule* and *capsular ligaments* surround joint Certain synovial joints have cartilaginous disks within (e.g., sternoclavicular ulno-carpal)	Comprise majority of joints in body—elbow, knee, hip, wrist, etc. Subdivided thus: 1. *Sliding* (intercarpal, intertarsal, acromioclavicular) 2. *Ball and socket* (hip) 3. *Hinge* (knee) 4. *Rotary* (atlantoaxial) 5. *Multiple axes* (thumb, metacarpal-phalangeal)	Allow considerable mobility but very vulnerable to traumatic and/or degenerative disease Many joints have *bursal sac* external to areas of much movement

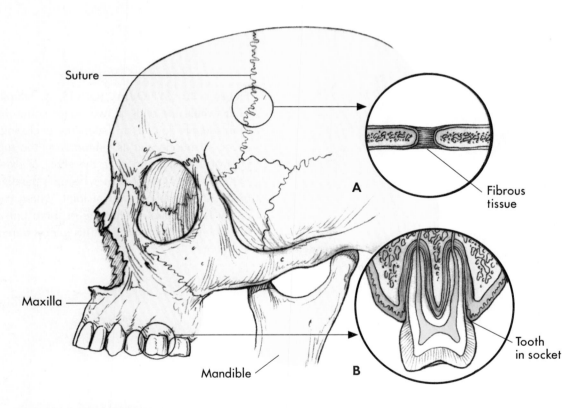

Figure I-10   EXAMPLES OF FIBROUS JOINTS. Illustrated is a suture between adjacent bones of the skull (**A**) and a tooth (**B**) in its socket in the maxilla. Both are secured by fibrous tissue connecting the adjacent structures. See Table I-2 for details.

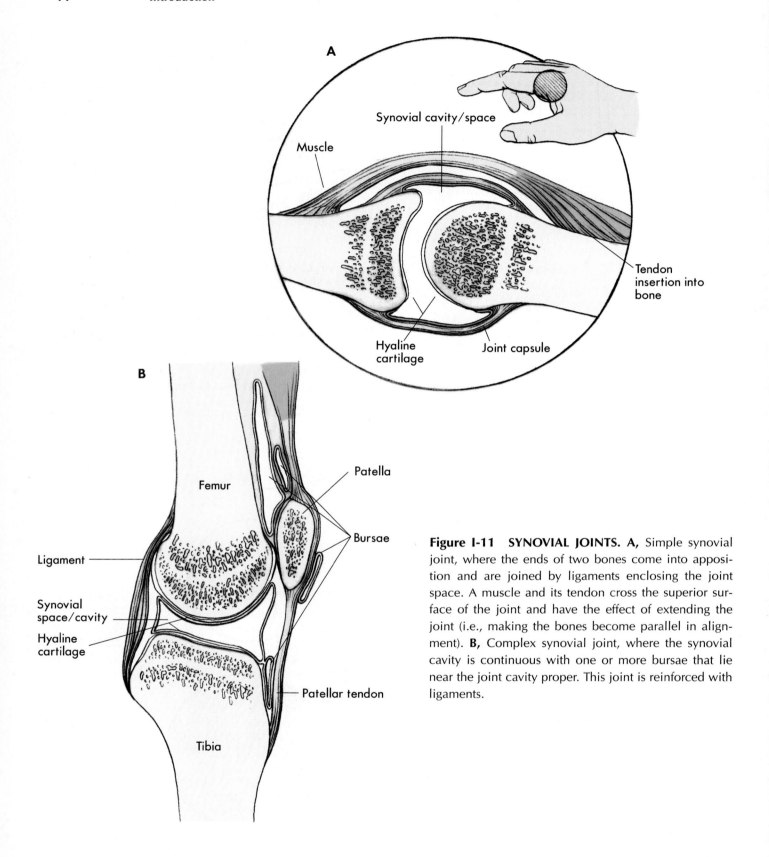

A

Synovial cavity/space

Muscle

Tendon insertion into bone

Hyaline cartilage

Joint capsule

B

Femur

Patella

Bursae

Ligament

Synovial space/cavity

Hyaline cartilage

Patellar tendon

Tibia

Figure I-11 SYNOVIAL JOINTS. A, Simple synovial joint, where the ends of two bones come into apposition and are joined by ligaments enclosing the joint space. A muscle and its tendon cross the superior surface of the joint and have the effect of extending the joint (i.e., making the bones become parallel in alignment). **B,** Complex synovial joint, where the synovial cavity is continuous with one or more bursae that lie near the joint cavity proper. This joint is reinforced with ligaments.

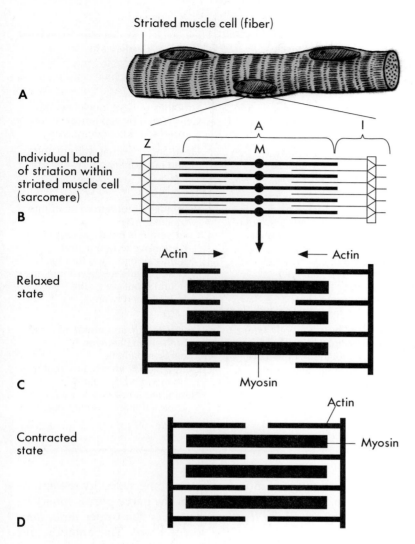

Striated muscle cell (fiber)

A

Individual band
of striation within
striated muscle cell
(sarcomere)

B

Actin →   ← Actin

Relaxed
state

Myosin

C

Contracted
state

Actin

Myosin

D

Figure I-12 STRIATED MUSCLE. A, Part of a single muscle cell or fiber, with its multiple nuclei located peripherally. Vertical striations are evident within the cell. The repeating unit of this striation is the **sarcomere** (**B**). Its major constituents are the proteins, actin and myosin, which slide with relation to each other to produce relaxation or elongation (**C**) or contraction (**D**). Neural signals stimulate the movement of calcium ions within the muscle fiber, and these calcium ions stimulate the sliding movement of the actin and myosin proteins.

which represent the molecular mechanisms by which individual muscle cells shorten during contraction (see Figure I-12 and Table I-3). Striated muscles have little intrinsic contractility and depend on neural input to produce changes in muscle length. When striated muscles are "at rest," they are really in a midrange state of contraction, and neural input may increase or decrease the state of contraction. In this manner, a single source of neural input to a muscle can *either increase or decrease* the state of contraction of that muscle. The health and integrity of striated muscles cells also depends on regular and frequent neural stimulation. Nerves innervating striated muscle enter the muscle on its deep surface, with few exceptions.

Striated muscles usually form **tendons** near where they attach to bones (see Figures I-11, I-13). A tendon is a cylindrical mass of connective tissue; when a tendon is flattened into a thin broad sheath, it is called an **aponeurosis.**

Control of striated muscle contraction occurs in both voluntary and involuntary fashion, often in the same muscle. A nerve innervating a striated muscle—for example, the phrenic nerve innervating the diaphragm—may be controlled *voluntarily* (as when you wish to draw in a deep breath) or just as efficiently *involuntarily* (as when your diaphragm continues to contract to ensure regular breathing while you sleep).

Striated muscles act on joints and often work in combination with other nearby striated muscles. Muscles that carry out a given action (e.g., flexion of the elbow) are referred to as **agonists;** those that carry out the opposing action (e.g., extension of the elbow) are known as **antagonists.**

Contraction of striated muscle may be **isotonic,** which means that there is actual *movement* at the joint involved (e.g., the arm moves with respect to the shoulder joint when you do a "push-up"), or **isometric,** where there is contraction of muscle but no actual movement at a joint (as when squeezing your fingers around a rigid sphere). Isometric contraction is important in most actual movements because it is usually necessary to **stabilize** a part of the body against which

Table I-3   Classification of Muscles

Feature	Striated Muscle	Smooth Muscle	Cardiac Muscle
Cell type	Very elongated cells, up to 50 mm (³/₁₆″)	Elongated cells, up to 250 μ in length	Elongated branching cells, up to 500 μ long
Histology	Striations present Multinucleate; nuclei located peripherally in myocytes	Striations absent (but contractile proteins similar to striated muscles)	Striations present; nuclei central Cells joined by gap junctions for rapid spread of contraction
Location	Most are attached to bones or other skeletal structures; a few are subcutaneous	Walls of gut, lung, skin, reproductive organs, eyes, glands, blood vessels, bronchioles	Heart and proximal walls of aorta and pulmonary artery
Function(s)	Movement of trunk, limbs, head, and neck Capable of rapid, highly controlled, and precise movements	Hair erection; sweat glands Movement of materials through hollow viscera (gut, urinary tract, etc.). Regulation of blood vessel and bronchiolar diameter Regulation of pupil size Movements are slower, less precise, less well regulated	Pumping of blood from heart into vascular tree Contraction is rapid, quickly responsive to neural and humoral regulation (but heart can beat efficiently without any neural input—e.g., the transplanted heart)
Neural input	Innervated by somatic motor nerves Requires neural input to maintain histologic integrity Voluntary and involuntary contraction Neural input needed for contraction (i.e., no intrinsic contraction)	Innervated by autonomic nerves: both sympathetic and parasympathetic in certain muscles, one only in other muscles Nearly all contraction is involuntary	Innervated by autonomic nerves: both sympathetic and parasympathetic Contraction is involuntary (but may be modified by volition) Neural input not necessary for contraction or muscle integrity

the actual motion of another part occurs. For example, when the elbow joint is flexed, muscles around the shoulder contract isometrically to stabilize the shoulder joint. This and other examples underscore the point that when a given muscle or muscles is described as being responsible for a given movement, a much larger group of fixating and stabilizing muscles actually must contract to make the movement possible.

Striated muscle is found in virtually every area of the body wall, upper limbs, lower limbs, and neck, scalp, and face. In the region of the head and neck, special groupings of striated muscle surround the mouth, nose, ears, eyes, and form the tongue and upper portion of the pharynx. It exists in a variety of shapes and sizes, and the direction in which the muscle fibers run has much to do with the kind of force they exert on the structures to which they are attached (Figure I-13).

The striated muscles of the upper and lower limbs develop from masses of mesoderm lying anterior and posterior to an **axial line** (Figure I-14) through the limb bud, in the coronal plane (i.e., left-to-right plane). Both sets of limb buds later go through complex rotations (see the sections on the upper and lower limbs), but the muscles and their innervations retain identities as pre- and postaxial muscle groups. This embryologic pattern of innervation explains the sometimes confusing groupings of muscles that are innervated by the anterior and posterior divisions of the nerve plexus innervating the limbs (*brachial plexus* for the upper limb; *lumbosacral plexus* for the lower limb). The anterior and posterior divisions are simply those groups of axons innervating preaxial (usually flexor) or postaxial (usually extensor) muscle groups, respectively.

Smooth muscle. Smooth muscle (Figure I-15) is made up of individual cells and often forms a layer in the wall of a hollow organ such as the stomach or the oviduct. While smooth muscle contains the same variety of contractile filaments as found in striated muscle and the contractile mechanisms are quite similar, they are not organized into the discrete intracellular bundles that give striated muscle its characteristic appearance and name. Smooth muscle is also found in the walls of many blood vessels, in the walls of the thoracic, intestinal, genitourinary, and pulmonary systems, and in selected other areas such as the eye. Smooth muscle usually lacks *tendons* or *aponeuroses* because it is most often *embedded* in a structure rather than being attached to it, as with striated muscle. Smooth muscle is *regulated* by neural input (sympathetic and/or parasympathetic), but it does not depend on this innervation for its structural integrity, as is the case with striated muscle. It also lacks special structures whose purpose it is to

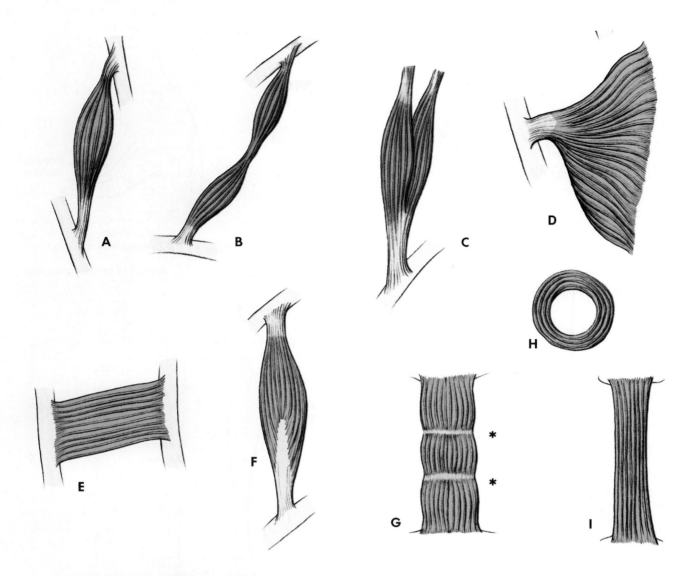

Figure I-13 SHAPES OF STRIATED MUSCLES. The shape of a muscle has much to do with the kind of force it can generate. **A,** Simple elongated muscle (e.g., brachialis). **B,** Digastric muscle (e.g., digastric of neck). **C,** Muscle with two heads (e.g., biceps brachii). **D,** Triangular muscle (e.g., pectoralis major). **E,** Quadrangular muscle (e.g., quadratus femoris). **F,** Bipennate muscle (e.g., vastus medialis). **G,** Tendinous inscriptions (∗) (e.g., rectus abdominis). **H,** Sphincter muscle (e.g., external anal sphincter). **I,** "Strap" muscle (e.g., sternohyoid).

sense and help regulate the resting muscle tone (such as is the case with *muscle spindles* in striated muscle).

Smooth muscle has a great deal of intrinsic contractility and can function successfully in the absence of neural input. But neural input can and does regulate smooth muscle contraction, especially in the gut and reproductive tracts. There is a sizeable body of knowledge about neural inputs from the *parasympathetic* (vagus and pelvic splanchnic) and *sympathetic* nerves. In addition, there is an intricate and poorly understood network of neurons and axons embedded in the walls

of the gastrointestinal tract, an entity often referred to as the *enteric nervous system.* For the most part, smooth muscle is not subject to voluntary regulation although in certain individuals training and practice can control some movements mediated by smooth muscle.

The principal organs and tissues in which smooth muscle plays an important role are the *digestive system* (where smooth muscle provides the propulsive force for peristalsis), the *respiratory system* (where smooth muscle in the walls of bronchioles helps increase or decrease the diameter of the air passages), in the *female re-*

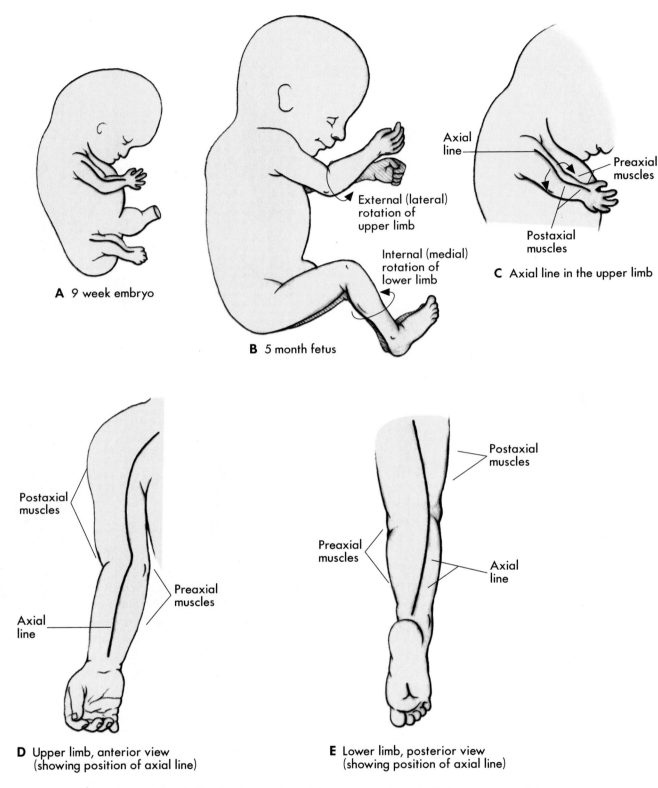

A 9 week embryo

B 5 month fetus

External (lateral) rotation of upper limb

Internal (medial) rotation of lower limb

Axial line

Preaxial muscles

Postaxial muscles

C Axial line in the upper limb

Postaxial muscles

Preaxial muscles

Axial line

D Upper limb, anterior view (showing position of axial line)

Postaxial muscles

Preaxial muscles

Axial line

E Lower limb, posterior view (showing position of axial line)

Figure I-14   AXIAL LINES. A, Position of the upper and lower limb buds in the third month of gestation. **B,** By 5 months the upper and lower limbs have rotated, the former laterally and the latter medially. **C,** More detailed view of the pre- and postaxial musculature in the upper limb bud. **D** and **E,** Fully developed limbs and the positions of the axial lines after limb rotation and development are complete. See Figure I-24 for a more detailed view of limb bud development and axial lines.

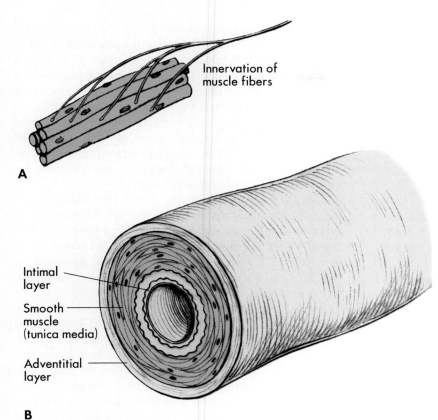

A

Innervation of
muscle fibers

Intimal
layer

Smooth
muscle
(tunica media)

Adventitial
layer

B

Figure I-15 SMOOTH MUSCLE. A, Smooth muscle cells are multinucleate with contractile proteins not organized into the characteristic banding of striated and cardiac muscle cells. Autonomic nerves modify smooth muscle contraction, but, unlike the situation with striated muscle and somatic nerves, smooth muscle can function independently of neural input. **B,** Cross-section of a typical arteriole in which there is a prominent layer of smooth muscle.

productive system (where the smooth muscle of the uterus produces the contractions that lead to childbirth), in the *male reproductive system* (where the smooth muscle in the walls of the genital ducts propels semen toward the penis), in the *urinary system* (where the ureters and wall of the bladder are made up of smooth muscle), in *blood vessels* (where smooth muscle in the walls of smaller arteries and veins regulates the diameter of the vessels and influences the ease of blood flow and the blood pressure), in the *eye* (where smooth muscle influences pupillary size and the focusing mechanism in the eye), and in association with the *hairs* of the skin (where smooth muscle contraction leads to elevation of the hairs away from the skin).

Cardiac muscle. Cardiac muscle is found in the heart and to a small degree in the walls of the roots of the aorta and pulmonary artery. It is a hybrid of appearance and properties that are found in striated and smooth muscle. It has the look of striated muscle, with highly organized contractile filaments and a distinct "banded" appearance under the microscope (Figure I-16). However, the individual cells of cardiac muscles have single centrally placed nuclei, unlike their striated muscle counterparts. Individual myocytes are linked by low-electrical resistance **gap junctions.** These junctions allow rapid spread of electrical signals throughout the heart and help ensure a synchronous contraction. The structural integrity of cardiac muscle does not depend on intact and functioning innervation, whereas such

denervation leads to structural deterioration of striated muscle. Cardiac muscle has a great capacity for spontaneous contraction, without any input from extrinsic

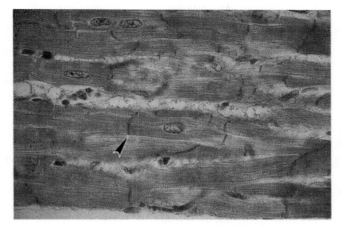

Figure I-16 CARDIAC MUSCLE. Cardiac muscle cells, shown here in longitudinal section, are also striated but have centrally located nuclei. The cells are linked to each other by low-resistance gap junctions, which facilitate the spread of a depolarization across adjacent cells as rapidly as possible. The gap junctions are known as intercalated disks, and one is shown by the *arrowhead.* This facilitates coordinated contraction of the entire heart muscle. (From Erlandsen S, Magney J: *Color atlas of histology,* St Louis, 1992, Mosby.)

nerves (as the success of heart transplantation attests).

Sympathetic input generally accelerates the rate and strength of cardiac contraction, while *parasympathetic input* decelerates and lessens the strength of the heartbeat.

INTRODUCTION TO THE BODY SYSTEMS

Viscera are the various organs and organ systems of the body. Familiar structures like the heart or liver are easily understood to be organs. Less obvious but no less accurately described as organs are entities such as the vascular system and the skin even though they are spread widely through the body. Although the study of anatomy is primarily organized around body regions, a knowledge of these systems is crucial to a full and complete understanding of the body.

Nervous System

There are two major regions of the nervous system: (1) the **central nervous system** or **CNS,** consisting of the brain and spinal cord, lying within the cranial vault and vertebral canal and (2) the **peripheral nervous system,** or **PNS,** lying in the periphery (i.e., outside the cranial vault and vertebral canal). The CNS is the *brain* and *spinal cord,* while the PNS is the collection of *peripheral nerves* and *ganglia* (see following discussion) that lie outside the cranial cavity or vertebral canal.

Cellular components of the nervous system. The entire nervous system is made up of *neurons* (Figure I-17), the functioning cellular elements, *glial cells* (in the CNS), and *Schwann* and *satellite cells* (in the PNS) that ensheath axons and occupy space between the neural elements, *connective tissue* interspersed with the neural tissue itself, and discrete membranous connective tissue layers—the *dura mater, arachnoid mater,* and *pia mater*—known collectively as the **meninges.** Clusters of neurons located in the PNS are called **ganglia.**

The **neuron** is a unique cell, which comes in many shapes and sizes (Figure I-18). The portion of the neuron's cytoplasm located near the cell nucleus is called the *cell body* or *perikaryon* (see Figure I-17), the numerous short processes extending away from the cell body are *dendrites,* and the usually elongated single process extending a significant distance away from the cell body is the *axon* (see Figure I-18). Neurons have the special ability to receive a chemical signal from incoming axons, usually on their dendrites, undergo an electrical depolarization themselves, and propagate that electrical change (called an *action potential*) over long distances—sometimes a distance of many meters. There are many billions of neurons in the entire nervous system, and the axonal connections between them are highly ordered, specific, and immensely complex.

In the PNS, groups of axons traveling toward or returning from a common area are collected into discrete bundles called **peripheral nerves** (see Figure I-19 and I-21). Schwann cell sheaths surround individual axons of the PNS; when multiple concentric layers of Schwann cell membrane encircle an axon, they form **myelin** (Figure I-20, *A*), an important phospholipid coating of larger axons, which enhances the speed of axonal conduction. Myelin forms as individual PNS axons become encircled with layers of Schwann cell cytoplasm (Figure I-20, *B*). CNS axons become myelinated as they are encircled with layers of cytoplasm of *oligodendroglial cells* (see Figure I-21 and Section 2).

Just external to myelin are connective tissue coverings of individual axons called the *endoneurium.* Small bundles of axons are called *fascicles,* and the connective tissue sheath surrounding each fascicle is known as the *perineurium.* Layers of connective tissue surrounding the many fascicles forming the complete peripheral nerve are called the *epineurium* (Figure I-21).

Neurons with many dendrites and an axon are termed *multipolar* (see Figures I-17, *B,* and I-18); **motor neurons** and those of sympathetic and parasympathetic ganglia are multipolar in structure. There is one important subclass of neurons that is distinctly different— the **sensory neuron.** Sensory neurons are described as *pseudounipolar neurons* because they have a cell body, *no* dendrites, and originally two processes extending away from the cell body region—(1) a *peripheral process,* which extends away from the cell body out into the periphery, and (2) a *central process,* which travels into the spinal cord or brainstem. As development proceeds, the two processes appear to fuse and emanate from a single stalk—hence the name "pseudounipolar." The cell bodies of sensory neurons are located in **sensory ganglia** arrayed alongside the brainstem and spinal cord (Figure I-22).

A second important type of ganglion is the **autonomic ganglion,** which consists of larger *motor neurons* and many smaller *interneurons.* Autonomic ganglia are either *sympathetic* or *parasympathetic* and serve as a relay point between the pre- and postganglionic neurons that comprise the obligatory two-neuron pathway by which sympathetic and parasympathetic input is delivered to peripheral target tissues. The multipolar ganglionic neurons receive preganglionic axonal input and generate a signal in the postganglionic axon that leaves the ganglion to innervate smooth muscle or glandular tissue in the periphery.

Functional groups of neurons. Neurons and axons of the PNS are either *sensory* or *motor.* Almost every spinal nerve and some cranial nerves have some sensory axons. All spinal nerves and most cranial nerves contain motor axons. Motor nerves of the PNS are more complex and varied than sensory neurons, structurally and functionally. The simplest are **somatic motor neurons** (Figure I-23), whose axons innervate striated muscle. Cell bodies for these neurons are in the gray matter of the spinal cord or brain, and their axons extend pe-

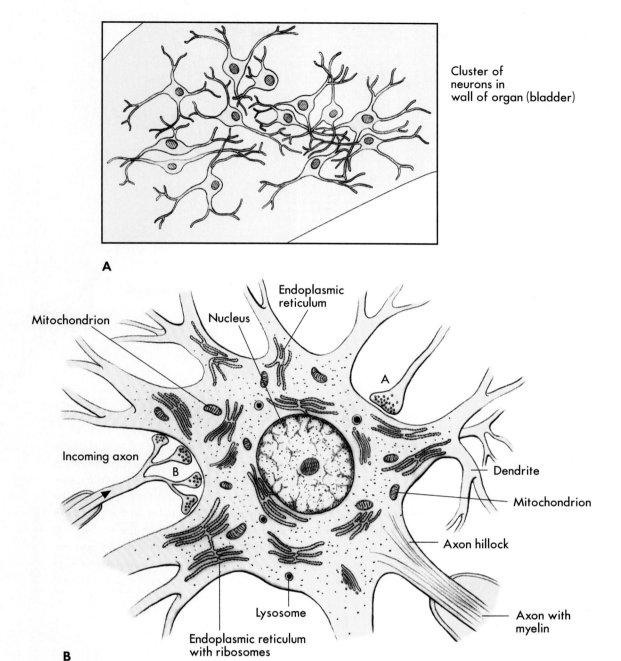

Cluster of
neurons in
wall of organ (bladder)

A

B

Figure I-17 NEURONS. A, Cluster of multipolar neurons, in the wall of the urinary bladder. Each neuron displays the characteristic central perikaryal area, nucleus, and surrounding dendrites. The single axon emanating from each neuron cannot be differentiated from the multiple dendrites with this technique of staining. (The neurons are drawn far larger than they would be in relation to bladder wall thickness.) **B,** Typical internal structure of a neuron. The axon hillock (origin of the axon) is distinguished from dendrites by its lack of endoplasmic reticulum and ribosomes, and the abundant intracellular filaments found there. *A,* Axosomatic (on cell body) synapse; *B,* axodendritic (on dendrite) synapses. Commonly, a single neuron receives thousands of individual synaptic inputs.

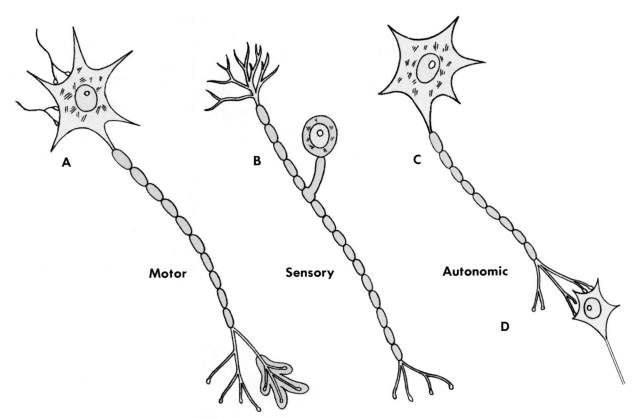

Figure I-18   VARIETIES OF NEURONS. A, Typical multipolar motor neuron, with multiple dendrites, an elongated myelinated axon, and synaptic terminals ending either on a striated muscle cell or another neuron. **B,** Typical peripheral sensory neuron. It has a nucleus located midway between a central process and a peripheral process. The central process enters the spinal cord or brain and synapses there. The peripheral process terminates in the periphery (e.g., skin, muscle, or fascia), where it can respond to sensory stimuli. Both the central and peripheral process conduct electrical signals rapidly, as is typical for axons. These neurons have no typical dendrites. **C** and **D,** Arrangement typical of autonomic (sympathetic and parasympathetic) neurons, where a pregnaglionic neuron (**C**) synapses upon a postganglionic neuron (**D**).

ripherally, as components of spinal nerves, directly to the muscle being innervated.

Autonomic motor neurons and networks are more elaborate (see Figure I-23). The innervation of smooth muscle, cardiac muscle, or certain glands (the targets of the autonomic neurons) always involves two neurons, the first called the *preganglionic* and the second the *postganglionic*. The connections and locations of autonomic neurons are detailed in Table I-4.

Organization of the nervous system. The CNS and PNS both demonstrate *topographic organization*—that is, regions of the CNS and PNS are devoted to nerve supply for certain regions of the body. For example, much of the surface of the cerebral cortex of the brain is topographically related to regions of the body, so that a part

of the cortex that provides innervation to the hand, the ear, or the knee may be identified. In a similar fashion, regions of the body that are innervated by given segments of the spinal cord or brain can be identified. All of the body surface, excluding the face and upper anterior neck, receives sensory innervation from the spinal cord (the face and upper anterior neck receive innervation from the fifth cranial nerve—the trigeminal). The specific skin areas of innervation related to individual segments of the spinal cord or brainstem are known as **dermatomes** (Figure I-24). For example, the top of the shoulder is innervated by the fourth and fifth cervical segments (C4 and C5) of the spinal cord.

It is also possible to group the muscles of the body according to the spinal cord segments from which they

Figure I-19 UNMYELINATED AXONS. Electron micrograph showing numerous small axons in cross-section. Each axon is embedded in Schwann cell cytoplasm, but only one is encircled multiply truly forming myelin (see Figure 1-20, *B*). *ma*, myelinated axon; *Sc*, Schwann cell nucleus; *∗*, examples of individual unmyelinated axons. (From Erlandsen S, Magney J: *Color atlas of histology*, St Louis, 1992, Mosby.)

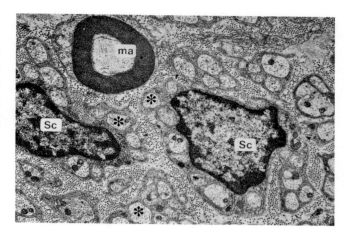

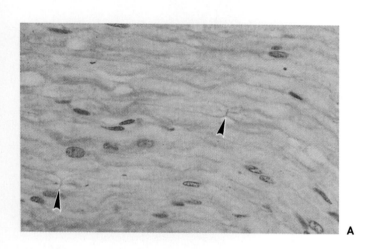

A

Figure I-20 COVERINGS OF AXONS. A, Peripheral nerves in longitudinal section. The *arrowheads* indicate nodes of Ranvier, a small discontinuity where the cytoplasm of one Schwann cell ends and the next begins. Small flattened nuclei of fibroblasts and endothelial cells and large vesicular nuclei of Schwann cells are also visible. **B,** On the left, the cytoplasm of one Schwann cell of the PNS wraps around a single axon several times, forming myelin. In the CNS, multiple axons may be enclosed within the cytoplasm of one oligodendrocyte. In this illustration, no axon has multiple layers of covering, and so none is truly myelinated. (**A,** From Erlandsen S, Magney J: *Color atlas of histology*, St Louis, 1992, Mosby.)

Peripheral nervous system

Central nervous system

Schwann cell

Axon

Oligodendrocyte

Axon

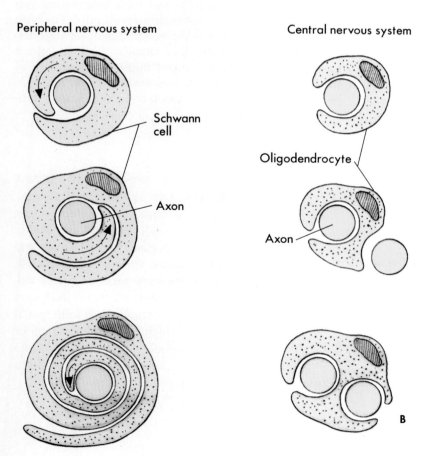

B

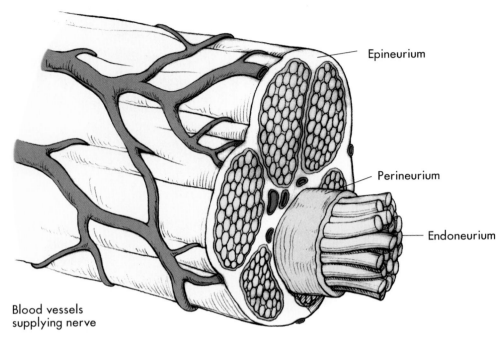

Figure I-21   CONNECTIVE TISSUE AND AXONS. A peripheral nerve visible to the naked eye consists of the connective tissue endoneurium surrounding individual axons, the perineurium surrounding bundles of axons, and the epineurium surrounding the entire peripheral nerve. Blood vessels supplying the nerve are embedded in the epineurium.

derive their motor innervation. The muscles sharing innervation from a given spinal cord or brainstem segment are known as **myotomes** (Table I-5). In many cases, myotomes (groups of muscles sharing innervation from a certain cord segment) work cooperatively to produce a certain movement (e.g., flexion of the elbow, extension of the hip). Knowledge of these func-

tional groupings of muscle and their innervation can also provide clues to segmental nerve injury. For both dermatomes and myotomes, recognition of sensory disturbance (in a skin area) or muscle weakness (in a group of muscles) can suggest injury to a segment of the spinal cord and the nerves originating in it. A patient who has no patellar tendon reflex (i.e., knee exten-

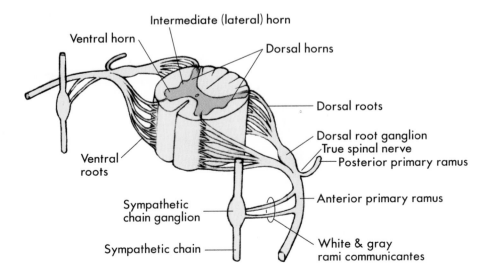

Figure I-22   SPINAL CORD, SPINAL NERVES, AND SYMPATHETIC CHAIN. This is a cross-section through the thoracic spinal cord. The gray matter contains dorsal, intermediate, and ventral horns. The surrounding white matter contains ascending and descending axon tracts. Dorsal and ventral roots combine to form spinal nerves, which divide into anterior and posterior primary rami. White and gray rami link spinal nerves to the sympathetic ganglia.

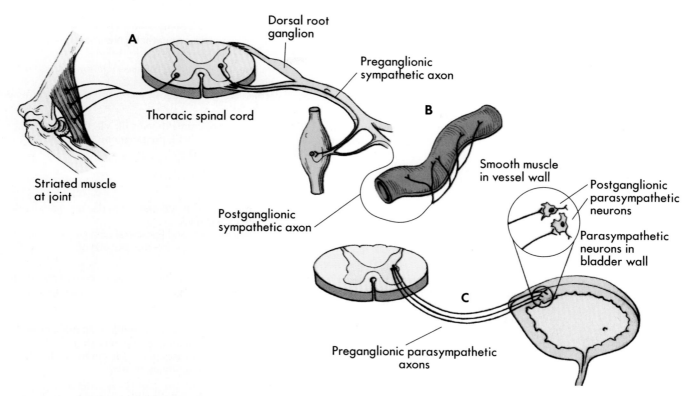

Figure I-23 SOMATIC MOTOR AND AUTONOMIC NERVES. A, Example of a somatic motor neuron with its axon leaving the ventral horn of the spinal cord and directly innervating a striated muscle. **B,** Example of a sympathetic connection with its preganglionic axon traveling from the spinal cord to the sympathetic chain ganglion and the postganglionic axon traveling from the sympathetic chain ganglion to the smooth muscle in the wall of a blood vessel. **C,** Parasympathetic innervation, where the preganglionic axon travels from spinal cord to the target organ and synapses upon postganglionic neurons there. These neurons have short axons, ramifying locally.

sion), for example, may have injury to the L3 and L4 spinal cord segments or the nerves that arise in them.

Cardiovascular System

The cardiovascular system consists of the **heart** and **blood vessels.** The heart in reality produces a left- and right-sided circulation, the former dedicated to perfusing blood through the body (except the lungs), and the latter dedicated to perfusing the lungs (Figure I-25, *A*). In both cases the arterial blood leaves the heart (through the *aorta* and *pulmonary artery*), passes through a series of *arterial branches,* and then passes through a series of successively smaller vessels known as *arterioles.* Next the blood enters the *capillary beds* (Figure I-25, *B*), a series of very small vessels (the diameter of the capillaries is often less than the diameter of a red blood cell) whose walls are thin. Molecules and flu-

ids can be exchanged across the thin endothelial cells lining the capillaries. Additionally, endothelial cells are in some places very loosely bound to each other or "leaky" (e.g., the kidneys), the result of which is that the liquid phase of blood and even some of the low molecular weight molecules can leave the bloodstream and enter other extracellular compartments in these tissues. In other parts of the body (e.g., the brain), the endothelial cells are tightly bound to each other, and substances in the blood have a very difficult time diffusing from the blood into the brain tissue.

The arterioles just proximal to the capillary beds are known as *precapillary arterioles.* Smooth muscle *sphincters* ("precapillary sphincters") in the walls of such vessels are important in directing the blood flow in the body toward certain capillary beds and away from others (Figure I-25, *C*). For example, the precapillary sphincters in the digestive system relax and allow

Table I-4   Anatomy of Autonomic Neurons in the PNS

Type	Sympathetic Neurons	Parasympathetic Neurons
Location of preganglionic cell body	In lateral horn of spinal cord gray matter, only in segments T1 to L2	From interior of brainstem, in association with cranial nerves III, VII, IX, X Intermediate gray matter in sacral spinal cord segments S2 to S4
Location of preganglionic axon(s)	In white rami communicans, branching only from spinal nerves T1 to L2; some synapse in adjacent sympathetic ganglion; others ascend or descend in sympathetic chain Some continue past sympathetic chain as splanchnic nerves	Travel as part of cranial nerves III, VII, IX, and X Sacral parasympathetic preganglionics separate as "pelvic nerve"
Location of postganglionic cell body(s)	In ganglia ("paravertebral ganglia") of the sympathetic chain In paraaortic "prevertebral" ganglia along abdominal aorta (receive splanchnic nerves)	For cranial nerves III, VII and IX: in discrete ganglia of the head and neck For cranial nerve X and the sacral parasympathetic nerves: in ganglia scattered in walls of target organs
Location of postganglionic axon(s)	*For paravertebral ganglia*: in gray rami communicantes, which distribute in spinal nerves (very small number ascend or descend within sympathetic chain) *For prevertebral ganglia*: axons distribute along abdominal arteries	Postganglionic axons from ganglia of cranial nerves III, VII, and IX are longer, extending from ganglia to innervated glands Postganglionic axons from ganglia of cranial nerve X and sacral parasympathetics are very short, originating from clusters of neurons in the walls of target organs and ramifying nearby
Part(s) of body innervated	Virtually every part of the body	By cranial nerves III, VII, and IX constrictor of pupil, muscle of lens; lacrimal gland; salivary glands By cranial nerve X and sacral parasympathetics: heart, lungs, digestive tract, genitourinary tract
General effect on body	Increase heart rate and blood pressure; dilate airways; slow digestive activity; sweating	Decrease heart rate; constrict small airways; increase digestive activity

increased blood flow to the digestive tract when food has been ingested, but similar sphincters associated with capillaries in the large muscles of the lower limbs simultaneously contract and reduce blood flow to these muscles. Conversely, during vigorous exercise, the pre-capillary sphincters in the lower limb relax and increase blood flow to the limbs, while sphincters in the digestive system contract and reduce blood flow to the intestinal tract.

Beyond the capillary beds, blood collects into a series of progressively larger vessels, beginning with *venules* and ending in the larger structures named *veins*. Ultimately these deliver blood back to the right atrium of the heart. Postcapillary venules are known as *capacitance vessels* (see Figure I-25, C) because they are most active in contracting and relaxing the smooth muscle in their walls (Figure I-26) as a means of regulating the blood pressure within the vascular tree. Two important determinants of blood pressure are the *volume of blood* and the *capacity within the vascular system*. Relaxation and contraction of postcapillary venules is of prime importance in increasing or decreasing the

Table I-5   Examples of Myotomes

Movement	Spinal Cord Segment(s)
Shoulder extension	C6, C7
Shoulder flexion	C5, C6
Elbow extension	C6, C7
Elbow flexion	C5, C6, C7
Wrist extension	C7, C8
Wrist flexion	C6, C7, C8
Hand, intrinsic muscles	C8, T1
Hip extension	L4, L5
Hip flexion	L3, L4
Knee extension	L3, L4
Knee flexion	L4, L5
Ankle extension	L4, L5
Ankle flexion	L5, S1
Foot inversion	L4, L5
Foot eversion	L5, S1

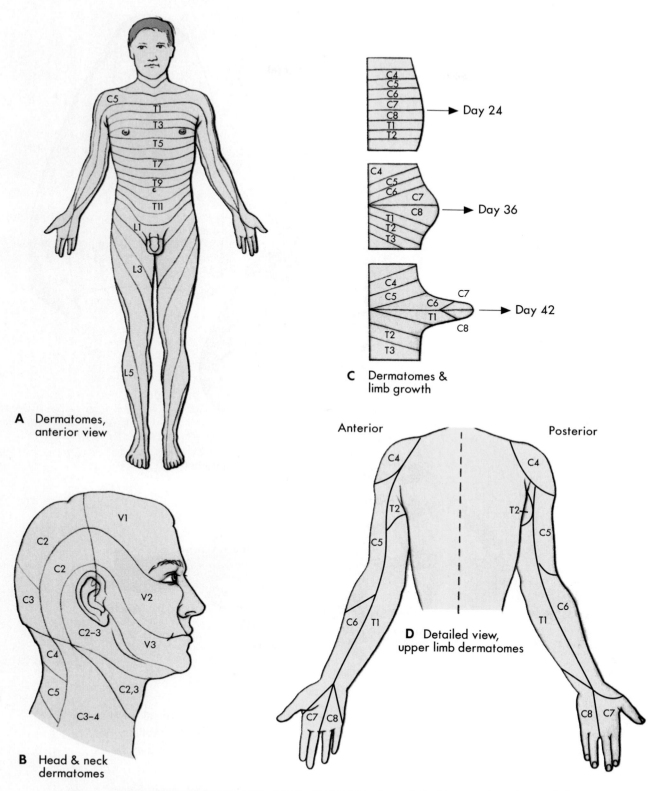

A Dermatomes, anterior view

B Head & neck dermatomes

C Dermatomes & limb growth

Day 24

Day 36

Day 42

D Detailed view, upper limb dermatomes

Anterior   Posterior

Figure I-24 DERMATOMES AND LIMB GROWTH. A and **B,** Views of regions of the body with the skin innervated by specific segments of the spinal cord and brainstem (dermatomes). **C** and **D,** The fate of individual dermatomes in the upper limb bud as the limb elongates and rotates. Note that in the proximal arm (**D**) dermatomes of C5 and T2 come to lie adjacent to each other because the intervening dermatomes (C6, C7, C8, and T1) extend outward as the limb elongates.

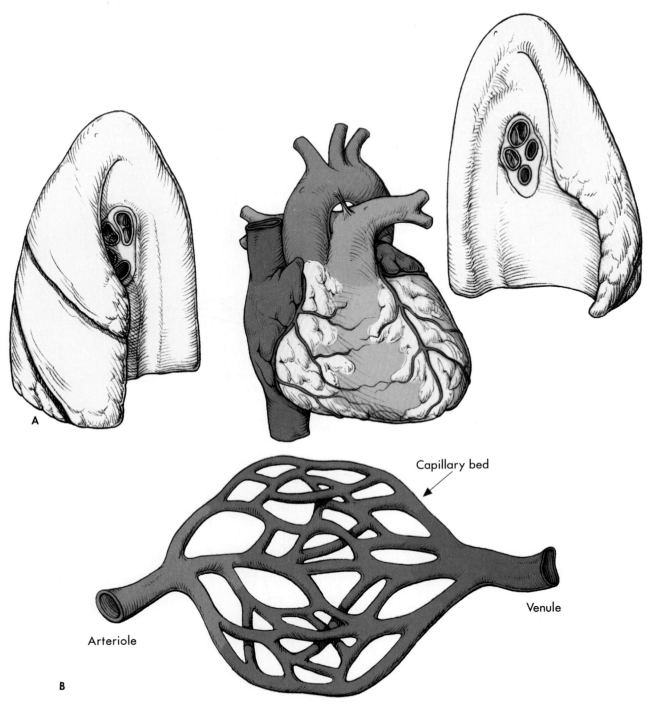

Figure I-25   CARDIOVASCULAR SYSTEM. A, Heart and lungs. **B,** In a typical capillary bed, arteriolar blood flows into a complex network of very small vessels, the capillary bed, and is drained from the capillary bed through small venules. It is at this level that the exchange of oxygen, carbon dioxide, and metabolites takes place.

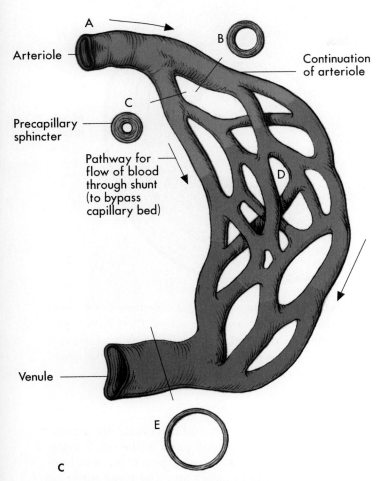

Arteriole

B

Continuation
of arteriole

C

Precapillary
sphincter

Pathway for
flow of blood
through shunt
(to bypass
capillary bed)

D

Venule

E

C

Figure I-25 (Continued). C, Regulation of blood flow and vascular shunts. Arteriolar blood flows toward a capillary bed and most often flows along vessel *B,* into the capillary bed (*D*). If, however, it should be necessary to bypass the capillary bed, then the muscular sphincter at *B* may close, the musculature in vessel *C* will relax, and blood will flow from *A* to *C* to *E,* bypassing most of the capillary bed (*D*). Vessel *C* is sometimes called a "shunt vessel."

capacity of the vascular tree, which directly affects blood pressure.

On the venous side of the circulation, blood must return to the heart without benefit of a pump to propel it along its course (arterial blood, of course, is pumped through arteries by the action of the heart). Venous blood must flow to the heart even if flowing against gravity (e.g., in the lower limbs, while a person is in the upright position). To aid in this process, many venous vessels have *valves* (see Figure I-26). These valves are crescentic folds of tissue that protrude into the lumen of the vessel. They "trap" blood within the vessels and reduce the amount of blood that flows in a retrograde direction. These valves, along with the "squeezing" ac-

tion of large muscles in the trunk and limbs, make it possible for blood to return to the heart even if the direction of that flow is against gravity (e.g., the return of venous blood from the lower limb to the inferior vena cava). Arteries, in which blood flows at higher pressures, and where the pumping action of the heart is quite important, do not possess valves.

Lymphatic System

The lymphatic system is an extensive collection of small vessels that drain extracellular fluid from most of the tissues of the body and return that fluid to the venous side of the blood vascular system. The brain and spinal cord lack lymphatic drainage, but essentially all other body regions are drained by lymphatic vessels. Lymph first collects in small capillaries, which drain into successively larger vessels that ultimately empty into the large **thoracic duct** (Figure I-27), which drains all of the body below the diaphragm and the left side of the upper body and empties into the veins in the base of the neck. A smaller similar vessel draining the right side of the thorax and upper body is known as the *right lymphatic duct.* Along their course, lymph vessels pass through clusters of lymphatic tissue known as **lymph nodes** (Figure I-28). At these nodes, particulate matter is filtered from the lymph, and lymphocytic cells are added to the lymph. Lymph nodes may become enlarged in various infectious and malignant diseases, and infectious organisms or malignant cells may spread through the body by way of the lymphatic vessels. Although nearly all lymphatic vessels are too small to be seen by the naked eye, the thoracic duct and a few larger vessels can be seen (see Figure I-27). When a contrast material is injected into a patient, and the lymphatic vessels are allowed to take it up, an x-ray dramatically demonstrates the extent of the lymphatic vasculature (Figure I-29).

Respiratory System

The lungs are collections of millions of tiny air sacs known as **alveoli** (Figure I-30). These alveoli are the final point in a complex series of branching pathways (the *tracheobronchial tree*), which convey fresh inhaled air to the alveoli. The alveoli are surrounded by networks of *pulmonary capillaries.* Only a very thin layer of tissue separates the interior of the capillaries from the interior of the alveoli, and so gas exchange occurs across this thin layer of tissue. CO_2 is here allowed to diffuse from the blood into the alveolar gas, and O_2 is allowed to diffuse from the alveolar gas into the blood.

The lungs themselves consist of the complex branching of the tracheobronchial tree and the aforementioned alveoli, supported in a connective tissue meshwork. The lung is covered by a thin capsule and a

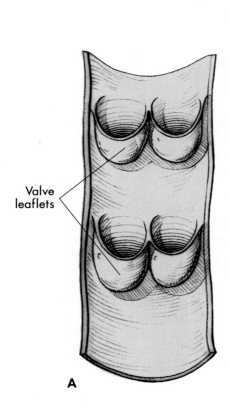

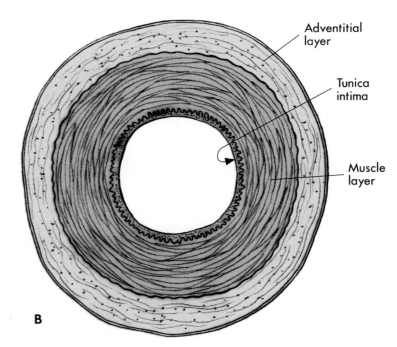

Adventitial layer

Tunica intima

Muscle layer

Valve leaflets

B

A

Figure I-26   VEINS AND VALVES. A, Many veins, especially those in the lower limb, have scallop-shaped leaflets protruding inward as valves. These have the effect of minimizing the retrograde flow of blood, even when the flow of blood is against gravity (e.g., the return of venous blood in the lower limbs to the heart). **B,** Cross-section through the wall of a muscular vein.

smooth *pleural membrane.* Since the lung must enlarge and diminish in size with each cycle of inspiration and expiration, its tissues must be pliant. In addition, the lung is suspended within a cavity known as the **pleural sac,** the smooth lining of which helps to minimize the friction that such repetitive movements of the lung might produce. The lungs originate as an outgrowth of the digestive system, with which they share certain structural similarities.

Gastrointestinal System

The *intestinal tract* begins as an elongated cylinder extending from the mouth to the anus. Throughout development it undergoes increased growth in certain areas and a very complex pattern of rotation, resulting in the series of intestinal coils found in the abdominal cavity. Actually, the digestive system includes the mouth and pharynx in the head and neck area, the esophagus in the thorax, and the stomach, small intestine, and large intestine in the abdominopelvic cavity. The *mouth* and *pharynx* are designed to soften and grind ingested food into small pieces soft enough to be swallowed. The *esophagus* pushes the ingested material downward into the stomach, where both chemical and mechanical forces further soften and break down the ingested food. In the first and shortest part of the small intestine, the *duodenum,* powerful digestive enzymes are added (by the liver and pancreas), and the chemical

breakdown of fats, proteins, and carbohydrates is maximized. In the remaining long parts of the small intestine, the *jejunum* and *ileum,* food products are selectively absorbed into the bloodstream. The large intestine receives unabsorbed material from the small intestine and propels it toward the rectum and anal canal. Within the large intestine, much water is reabsorbed from the feces.

The entire gastrointestinal tract from the stomach to the rectum consists of a *mucosa* or lining layer of cells, surrounded by concentric layers of connective tissue and smooth muscle (Figure I-31). Groups of neurons and axons are interspersed in the layers of the intestinal tract. The mucosa is responsible for secreting many digestive enzymes and for allowing the absorption of desired food material to take place. The smooth muscle wall is important for the peristaltic muscular waves that propel food material from proximal to distal. The neural networks in the walls of the intestine are the most important means by which peristaltic activity can be regulated by autonomic input. However, the intestine has a very considerable amount of intrinsic contractility (see preceding section on smooth muscle) not dependent on any external neural input.

Urinary System

The urinary system consists of the *kidneys, ureters, urinary bladder,* and *urethra* (Figure I-32). Part of it de-

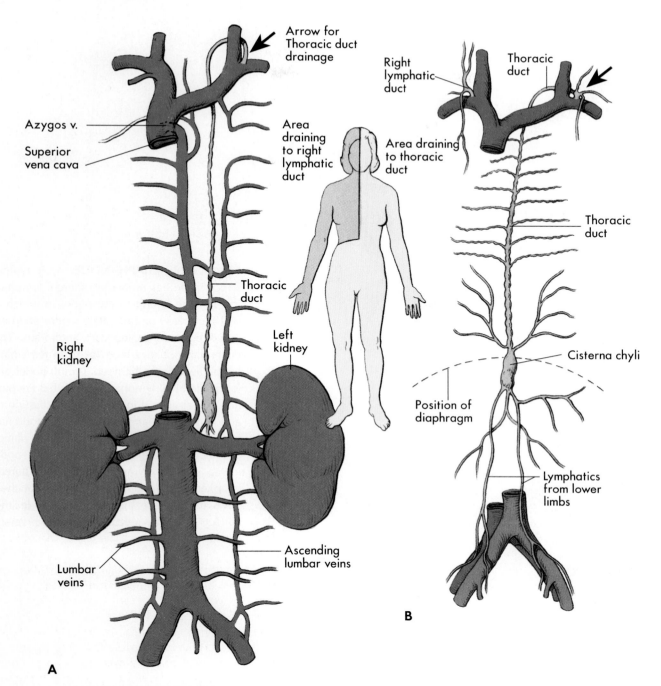

Arrow for
Thoracic duct
drainage

Azygos v.

Superior
vena cava

Area
draining
to right
lymphatic
duct

Thoracic
duct

Right
kidney

Left
kidney

Lumbar
veins

Ascending
lumbar veins

A

Right
lymphatic
duct

Thoracic
duct

Area draining
to thoracic
duct

Thoracic
duct

Cisterna chyli

Position of
diaphragm

Lymphatics
from lower
limbs

B

Figure I-27 THORACIC DUCT. A, The venous system of the posterior abdominal and
thoracic walls and the thoracic duct draining into the junction of the left subclavian and internal jugular veins (*arrow*). **B,** Tributaries of the thoracic duct and its partial counterpart on the
right, the right lymphatic duct. The shaded area on the *inset* is that part of the body drained of
lymph by the right lymphatic duct. All the rest of the body drains lymph to the thoracic duct.

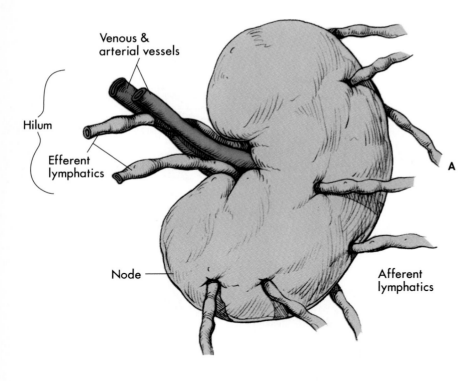

Venous &
arterial vessels

Hilum

Efferent
lymphatics

Node

Afferent
lymphatics

A

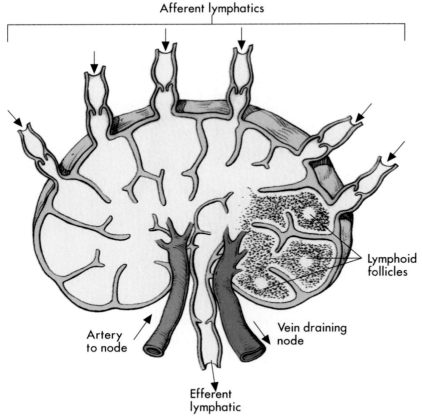

Afferent lymphatics

Lymphoid
follicles

Artery
to node

Vein draining
node

Efferent
lymphatic

B

Figure I-28   LYMPH NODE. A, A typical lymph node has numerous afferent lymphatics bringing lymph to the node, in which it will be filtered of particulate matter and certain substances coated with antibodies. The efferent lymphatics then take the remaining lymph away from the node. Lymph nodes are found along all lymphatic vessels but are particularly abundant in the neck, mediastinum, abdominal wall, and groin. **B,** This node has been sectioned in the midsagittal plane. Connective tissue septa separate the node into a series of lymphoid follicles. Afferent lymphatics bring lymph to the node; it then flows through the interior of the node and collects into the efferent lymphatic vessel leaving the node.

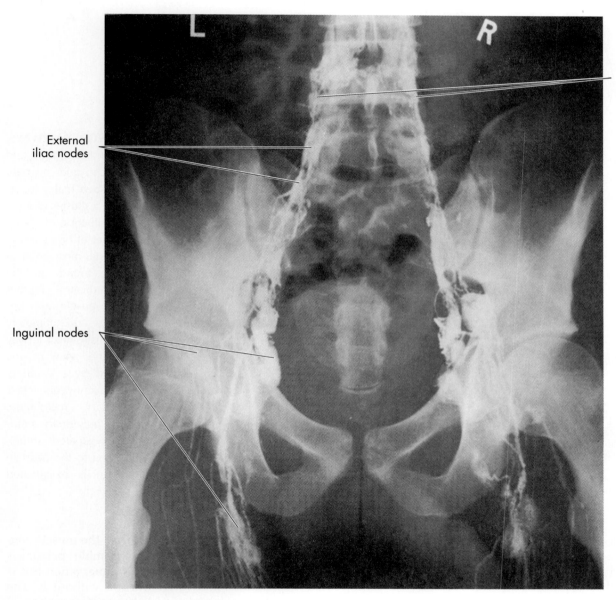

Figure I-29 LYMPHANGIOGRAM. Dye material has been injected into the soft tissues on the dorsum of each foot, and several hours later an x-ray of the pelvic region taken. The dye material has been taken up by the lymphatics and transported upward toward the cisterna chyli and eventually to the thoracic duct. (From Weir J, Abrahams PJ: *An imaging atlas of human anatomy*, London, 1992, Mosby.)

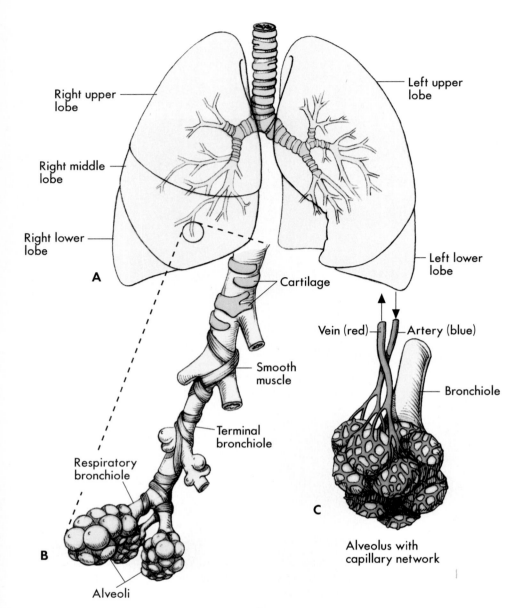

A

Right upper lobe

Right middle lobe

Right lower lobe

Cartilage

Smooth muscle

Terminal bronchiole

Respiratory bronchiole

B

Alveoli

Left upper lobe

Left lower lobe

Vein (red)   Artery (blue)

Bronchiole

C

Alveolus with capillary network

Figure I-30 LUNGS, AIRWAYS, AND ALVEOLI. A Trachea, right and left mainstem bronchi, and the right and left lungs with their major lobes. **B,** Detailed view of a cluster of alveoli, lying at the termination of a successively narrower set of bronchi and bronchioles. The distal-most point at which cartilage is found on the bronchial tree is indicated. Further distally, the smooth muscle layer becomes discontinuous and ultimately is absent from the distal-most airway branches. **C,** Magnified view of one alveolus, surrounded by a capillary network. Gas exchange occurs across the alveolar-capillary membrane. Note that incoming *pulmonary arterial* blood is deoxygenated (blue), while blood returning to the heart in the pulmonary vein is oxygenated (red).

velops as an outgrowth of the lower end of the primitive digestive system (i.e., the ureters and parts of the kidney), and another part of the kidney develops from mesoderm that condenses around the ureteric outgrowths. The *urinary bladder* is a large muscular sac positioned in the lower pelvis, which serves as a reservoir for urine until such time that it may be emptied from the body. The *urethra* leads from the bladder to the exterior, in the upper vaginal region in the female and along the penis in the male. In the male, the urethra is also used as a *genital duct,* through which semen is passed as well.

Both the ureter and the bladder are lined with smooth muscle, the contractions of which are responsible for moving the urine (and semen in the male) for-

ward through the system. In the *ureter,* the muscle contracts in an organized fashion that resembles peristalsis in the gut. Ureteric muscle receives innervation but is quite capable of effective contraction without it. The *bladder* wall is composed of thick layers of smooth muscle, which are innervated by sympathetic and parasympathetic nerves. Unlike the ureter, the innervation of the bladder is very important in its normal function.

Reproductive System

In both sexes, the genital system consists of a pair of *gonads* (the ovaries or testes), which produce the gametes, and a system of *ducts* through which the gametes pass as they move away from the gonads (Figure

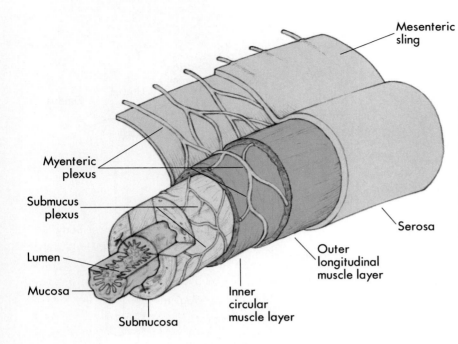

Mesenteric sling

Myenteric plexus

Submucus plexus

Lumen

Mucosa

Submucosa

Inner circular muscle layer

Outer longitudinal muscle layer

Serosa

Figure I-31   LAYERS OF THE GUT WALL. In the stomach, small intestine, and large intestine, certain layers are much enlarged or diminished in size. A neural plexus (myenteric) is found between the outer smooth muscle layer and another plexus is found deep to the muscle layers (the submucus plexus).

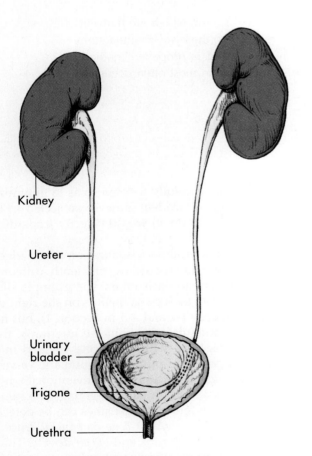

Kidney

Ureter

Urinary bladder

Trigone

Urethra

Figure I-32   URINARY SYSTEM. The lining of the ureter and bladder wall is a characteristic transitional epithelium, which can stretch and change form to accommodate accumulated urine.

I-33). In the male, the *sperm* (the gametes) are conducted from the testis (in the scrotum) through the ductus deferens and urethra to reach the distal end of the penis, from which, during sexual intercourse, they are expelled and deposited into the vagina. In the female, the *ovum* (the gamete) from the ovary in the pelvis is conducted through the *oviduct* (where it normally is fertilized), and deposited into the interior of the *uterus*, a thick-walled hollow muscular organ.

Endocrine System

An *endocrine organ* is defined by its ability to manufacture a product (often called a hormone) and release it into the bloodstream for circulation to other parts of the body. By contrast, an *exocrine gland* manufactures a product and deposits it into a space, such as the deposition of digestive enzymes into the lumen of the gut by the salivary glands. The major endocrine organs are the anterior lobe of the *pituitary gland*, the *thyroid gland*, the *parathyroid glands*, the *islets of the pancreas*, the *adrenal glands*, and the *gonads*. In addition to these major endocrine glands, there are many other small collections of tissue that function as endocrine glands.

Many hormones manufactured in the anterior lobe of the pituitary control hormone production by other endocrine glands.

The pituitary gland (Figure I-34) is located in the cranial cavity, attached to the basal surface of the brain. Other endocrine glands are in the neck (thyroid and parathyroid glands), abdomen (pancreas, adrenal glands) and pelvis (ovary or testis).

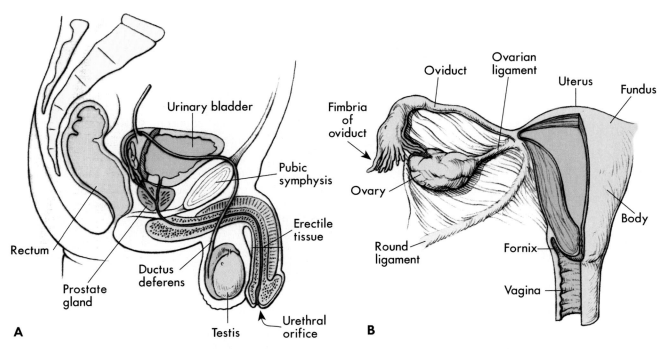

Figure I-33 **GENITALIA.** In the male (**A**), the testis produces sperm, which are transmitted through the ductus deferens to the urethra. In the female (**B**), the ovary manufactures an ovum, which is ovulated from the surface of the ovary and is propelled medially through the oviduct to reach the lumen of the uterus. Implantation most often occurs on the upper posterior wall of the uterus.

TECHNIQUES FOR IMAGING THE HUMAN BODY

Especially in the last 20 years, a variety of techniques for observing body structure in the living human being has been developed. Conventional x-rays are still in frequent use, but there is a growing trend to employ powerful newer techniques such as computed tomography (CT), ultrasound imaging, and magnetic resonance imaging (MRI). Physicians of the future will have expanding opportunities to visualize the structure of the human body through these and even more sophisticated technologies.

Conventional X-Ray Imaging

With x-ray technique, the image is created by positioning the part of the body to be studied between a source of x-rays and a sheet of photographic film (Figure I-35). Tissues of different densities absorb x-rays to different degrees, and, when x-rays are passed through the body, a "shadow" of the structures within the body is cast on the film (Figure I-36). Every effort is taken to minimize the dose of x-rays delivered to the body, and they are carefully focused so as to minimize "scatter." A pregnant woman is never subjected to x-rays, unless to fail to do so would directly jeopardize her health.

Conventional x-rays allow visualization of the edges of structures only when tissues of sufficiently different density are adjacent to each other. For example, the edge of the heart can be seen as it abuts on the right or left lung (see Figures 1-4 and 1-5 in Section 1), but no details can be distinguished within the interior of the heart, though it is filled with blood and divided into four chambers by a dense muscular septum and valves. None of these is visible because in a conventional x-ray blood and muscle appear to have essentially the same density. In fact, only four basic densities can be detected in a conventional x-ray: (1) *bone* or *mineral density*, (2) *tissue density*, (3) *fat density*, and (4) *air density*. Thus in the previous example, the heart border can be seen because the muscle of the heart lies against the air-filled lung; the septum in the interior of the heart cannot be seen because the blood within the heart and the heart muscle against which it lies are in the same category of density.

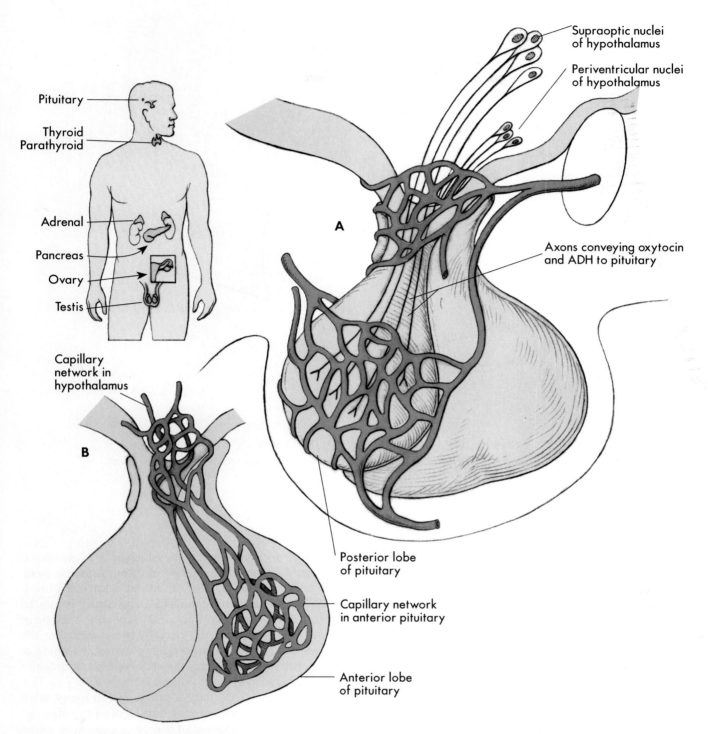

Figure I-34 PITUITARY GLAND AND ENDOCRINE SYSTEM. The *inset* shows the location of the pituitary gland, thyroid gland, parathyroid glands, pancreas, adrenal glands, and gonads, the major constituents of the endocrine system. **A,** Pituitary gland has a distinct anterior lobe (adenohypophysis) and posterior lobe (neurohypophysis). The supraoptic and periventricular nuclei of the hypothalamus manufacture oxytocin and antidiuretic hormone and convey them downward along axons into the posterior lobe of the pituitary, where the hormones are released into the bloodstream. **B,** Hypophyseal portal system—a system of capillaries that take up trophic hormones from the hypothalamus and convey them to a second set of capillaries in the anterior lobe of the pituitary, where these trophic hormones act on cells and cause them to secrete a variety of hormones into the general circulation.

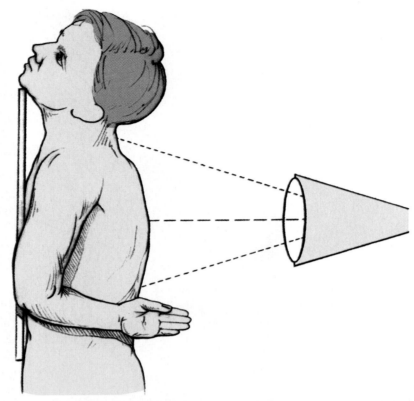

Figure I-35   POSITION FOR POSTEROANTERIOR (PA) X-RAY OF CHEST. The source of x-rays is positioned posterior to the patient, who presses the chest wall against a film cassette containing the x-ray film.

Conventional x-rays are still widely employed because they are technically simpler than cross-sectional technologies, have been in use for decades, and involve comparatively small expense. By injecting a highly dense material into the bloodstream, a body cavity, or any region in which there is a special interest, an x-ray shows a much greater degree of detail about the structure of interest. In Figure I-37, contrast material has been injected into the renal artery and its many fine branches made visible.

Computed Tomography (CT)

Computed tomography (CT) employs x-rays, but its images are created by computer reconstructions of data when x-rays are passed through a single segment of the body repeated at several angles. The reconstructed image looks like a "slice" through the body—a slice that the computer can reconstruct in literally any plane. The technique requires the patient to lie within the cen-

ter of a large circular gantry in which an x-ray source is positioned on one side, and a collecting sensor is positioned 180 degrees opposite the x-ray source (Figure I-38). While the patient remains still, the gantry is rotated through 360 degrees and an x-ray exposure is made at several points around the circle. After integrating the information derived from the x-ray exposures made at each point around the arc, the cross-sectional image of the body is reconstructed (Figure I-39).

The reconstructed image is composed of many small squares or pixels, each of which has a density value derived from the integration of the x-ray exposures taken at various angles. The extraordinary power of the CT scan is in what the computer can do with these pixels. The computer can display the image in a variety of density ranges (called "windows"), which have the effect of greatly increasing the resolution of the image in comparison to a conventional x-ray. That is, whereas the conventional x-ray can distinguish only four cardinal densities (see preceding section), the CT scanner

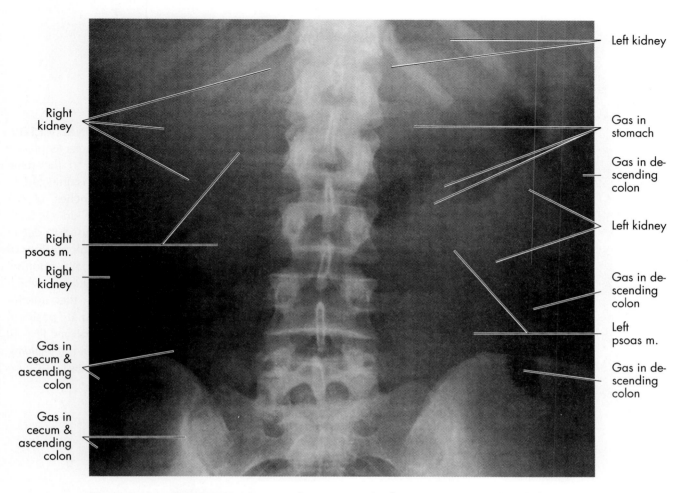

Figure I-36   ABDOMINAL X-RAY. This is a standard anterior view of the abdomen and would be used to evaluate patients with abdominal pain, abnormal urination, or complaints related to the lumbar spine. (From Weir J, Abrahams PH: *An imaging atlas of human anatomy,* London, 1992, Mosby.)

can bring out subtle differences in density between adjacent tissues. Thus with the CT scanner, the ventricular septum within the heart *can* be seen, and tumors *can* be distinguished within the brain or liver that would be invisible on a conventional x-ray—invisible because the difference in density of such tumors in comparison to surrounding normal tissue is below the threshold of density difference that the conventional x-ray can detect.

Magnetic Resonance Imaging

Magnetic Resonance Imaging (MRI) is a technique developed in the physical chemistry laboratory, which has now been transferred with great success to medicine. It produces cross-sectional images of the body and has the great advantage of requiring the use of no radiation. The technique involves placing the body in a magnetic field (Figure I-40) and, upon release of that magnetic field, collecting the radio frequency energy that is produced as molecules in the body move out of the artificial alignment imposed on them by the magnetic field. The technical complexities of the technique are far beyond the scope of this book, but the information gathered is processed by a computer in a manner similar to that in CT scanning, and a reconstructed image of the body is produced. The MRI technique is superior to the CT technique in imaging certain types

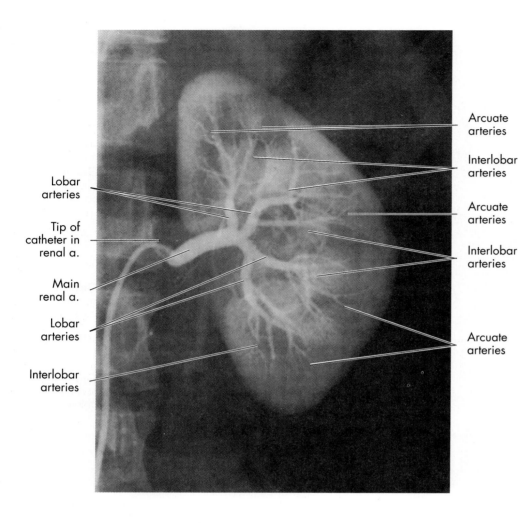

Lobar
arteries

Tip of
catheter in
renal a.

Main
renal a.

Lobar
arteries

Interlobar
arteries

Arcuate
arteries

Interlobar
arteries

Arcuate
arteries

Interlobar
arteries

Arcuate
arteries

Figure I-37 RENAL ARTERI-OGRAM. A catheter is placed in the entrance to the renal artery, and dye is injected to outline the branches of the artery within the kidney. Such studies may be used to detect interruptions in blood flow or the presence of an abnormal mass in the kidney, which would displace the arteries from their normal position. (From Weir J, Abrahams PH: *An imaging atlas of human anatomy,* London, 1992, Mosby.)

of tissues (Figure I-41), and the CT superior for other types of tissues. The MRI scan requires that the patient be as still as possible for several minutes while the scan is being completed, whereas the CT scan requires the patient to hold still only for brief periods while each x-ray exposure is made. This makes MRI imaging more difficult for children. MRI imaging is also not possible for individuals with ferromagnetic clips in their bodies or with certain types of pacemakers since the imposition of a magnetic field on such patients can put them at risk.

Figure I-42 shows, respectively, a CT scan set to display soft tissues (*A*), a scan set to show bony tissues (*B*), and an MRI of approximately the same area of the chest (*C*). Note the difference in I-42, *A*, and I-42, *B*, especially in the midline mediastinum and heart. In *A* there is a good deal of detail in this area but virtually no detail in the area of the lungs. In *B* there is a good deal of detail in the lung fields but virtually none in the

mediastinum and heart. The MRI scan (*C*) shows much more detail in the soft tissues, including the mediastinum, heart, and muscles surrounding the chest cavity, but yields very little information about bones. A clinician needs to understand the strengths and weaknesses of the techniques available and should choose the form of test that will yield the most useful information—always bearing in mind the risks that such procedures may pose to the patient.

Ultrasonagraphy

Another method of imaging body structure is to pass sonic waves into the body and collect the reflected waves as they bounce off reflective surfaces within the body (Figure I-43). This technique has increasingly broad application and is especially useful in imaging the intracranial cavity (in newborns, see Figure I-44), the abdominal cavity, the reproductive organs, the

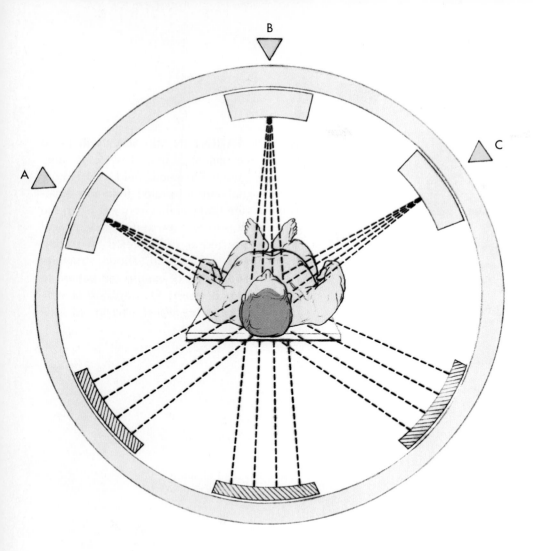

Figure I-38   TECHNIQUE FOR CT SCAN. In this technique, x-rays are passed through the patient from a variety of angles (*A, B,* and *C*). Sensors are positioned opposite each of these source positions, and the data from each angle stored. A computer is required to reconstruct the final image from the various individual scans.

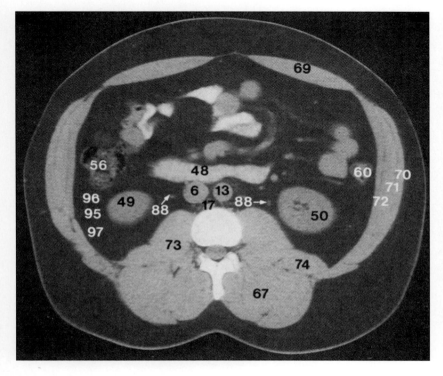

Figure I-39   ABDOMINAL CT SCAN. This scan is at the level of the pancreas, in the upper abdomen. This is a good example of the level of detail that can be discerned with the technique, in comparison to conventional x-rays. (From Weir J, Abrahams PH: *An imaging atlas of human anatomy,* London, 1992, Mosby.)

6 Inferior vena cava	70 External oblique
13 Aorta	muscle
17 Right crus of di-	71 Internal oblique
aphragm	muscle
48 Horizontal part of	72 Transversus abdo-
duodenum	minis muscle
49 Right kidney	73 Psoas major mus-
50 Left kidney	cle
56 Ascending colon	74 Quadratus lumbo-
60 Descending colon	rum muscle
67 Erector spinae	88 Ureter
muscle	95 Renal fascia
69 Rectus abdominis	96 Perirenal fat
muscle	97 Pararenal fat

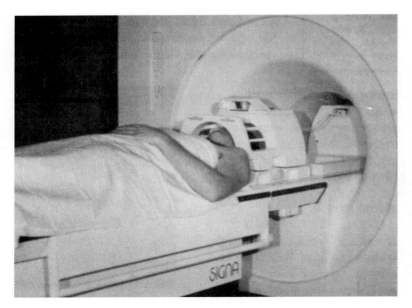

Figure I-40   PATIENT IN MRI SCANNER. In an MRI scan, the patient is placed within a large ring magnet, and the magnetic field is turned on. Electrical signals are generated from the molecules within the body as they reorient when the magnetic field is turned off, and these electrical signals are detected and interpreted by a computer to yield information about structure. MRI examinations do not expose the patient to radiation. (From Bontrager KL: *Textbook of radiographic positioning and related anatomy,* ed 3, St Louis, 1993, Mosby.)

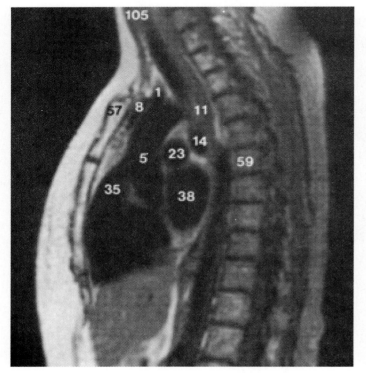

Figure I-41   THORAX MRI. This sagittal MRI view reveals many details of the internal structure of the heart and vertebral column. (From Weir J, Abrahams PH: *An imaging atlas of human anatomy,* London, 1992, Mosby.)

1 Brachiocephalic trunk	**35** Pulmonary artery
5 Ascending aorta	**38** Left atrium
8 Left brachiocephalic vein	**57** Manubrium
11 Esophagus	**59** Body of vertebra
14 Left main bronchus	**105** Thyroid lobe
23 Right pulmonary artery	

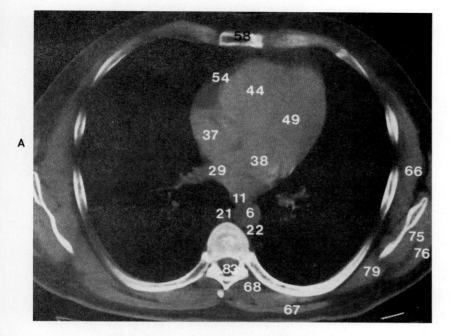

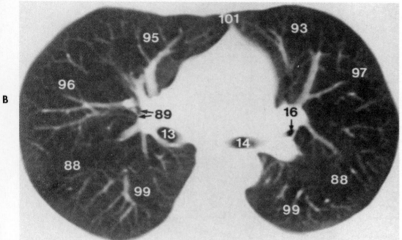

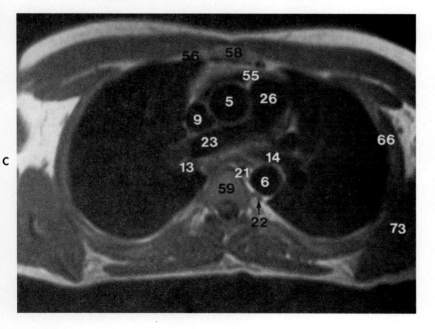

Figure I-42 THORACIC CT SCAN AND MRI. A, The CT scanner can be instructed to display tissues in a given range of densities to reveal the maximum detail of structures within that range of tissue densities. Section of the thorax shows detail of the tissue within the heart and mediastinum ("tissue window"). **B,** Same cross-sectional CT image as in **A** can be displayed differently to emphasize details of the lungs and their vasculature ("lung window"). **C,** Transverse MRI scan through the same area of the chest as in **A** and **B** showing the power of MRI to display finer details of structure, particularly in the muscle layers of the anterior chest wall and the scapular region. (From Weir J, Abrahams PH: *An imaging atlas of human anatomy,* London, 1992, Mosby.)

5 Ascending aorta	muscle
6 Descending aorta	**67** Trapezius muscle
9 Superior vena cava	**68** Erector spinae muscle
11 Esophagus	**73** Subscapularis muscle
13 Right main bronchus	**75** Infraspinatus muscle
14 Left main bronchus	**76** Latissimus dorsi muscle
16 Left superior lobe bronchus	**79** Rhomboid major muscle
21 Azygos vein	**83** Vertebral foramen
22 Hemiazygos vein	**88** Plane of oblique fissure
23 Right pulmonary artery	**89** Middle lobe of segmental bronchus
26 Pulmonary trunk	
29 Right inferior pulmonary vein	**93** Anterior segment of superior lobe
37 Right atrium	**95** Medial segment of middle lobe
38 Left atrium	
44 Right ventricular cavity	**96** Lateral segment of middle lobe
49 Left ventricular cavity	**97** Superior lingular segment
54 Pericardium	**99** Apical segment of inferior lobe
55 Pericardial recess	
56 Internal thoracii artery and vein	**101** Right and left parietal pleura
58 Body of sternum	
59 Body of vertebra	
66 Serratus anterior	

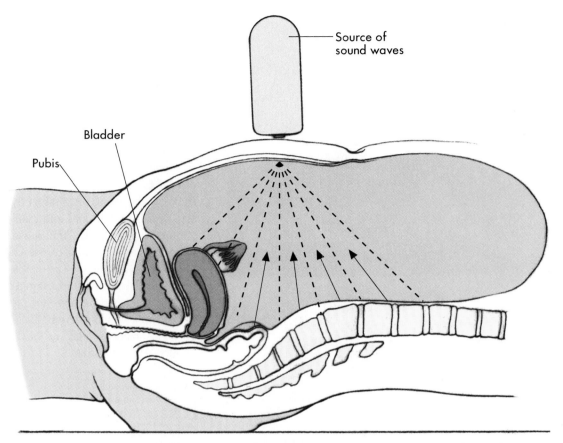

Source of
sound waves

Bladder

Pubis

Figure I-43   TECHNIQUE FOR ABDOMINAL ULTRASOUND. The source of sound waves also includes a sensing device, and, when the sound waves reflect off internal body structures, they are sensed and an image of the body displayed on a cathode-ray tube.

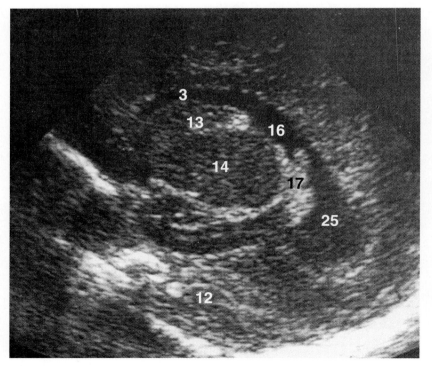

Figure I-44   ULTRASOUND OF THE HEAD, INFANT. Ultrasound images rely on the reflection of sound waves off structures of different densities. By placing the ultrasound transducer on the fontanelle of the infant, the examiner can detect the shape and size of the ventricles and other components of the brain in a noninvasive and convenient manner. Compare to Figure 2-14. (From Weir J, Abrahams, PH: *An imaging atlas of human anatomy,* London, 1992, Mosby.)

3	Anterior horn of left ventricle	**16**	Body of left lateral ventricle
12	Cerebellum	**17**	Choroid plexus in left lateral ventricle
13	Left caudate nucleus	**25**	Posterior horn of left lateral ventricle
14	Thalamus		

heart, and the limbs. It has become a standard technique in evaluating the growth and development of the fetus *in utero*. It has the distinct advantage of being technically simpler than the cross-sectional techniques described previously, relatively inexpensive, and requiring no ionizing radiation. It can be performed by use of portable machines at the patient's bedside or in the physician's office.

Currently, the general physician is expected to have a working knowledge only of certain types of commonly used conventional x-rays (chest x-rays, x-rays of the limbs, etc.). The interpretation of CT scans, MRI images, and ultrasonograms is the province of special branches of medicine and requires specialized training and experience.

SECTION ONE

Thorax

▶ **1.1** Introduction to the Thorax

▶ **1.2** Chest Wall

▶ **1.3** Pleural Spaces,
Tracheobronchial Tree,
and Lungs

▶ **1.4** Heart

▶ **1.5** Mediastinum

▶ **1.6** Systems Review and
Surface Anatomy of the
Thorax

▶ **1.7** Case Studies: Thorax

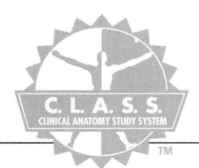

C. L. A. S. S.
CLINICAL ANATOMY STUDY SYSTEM
™

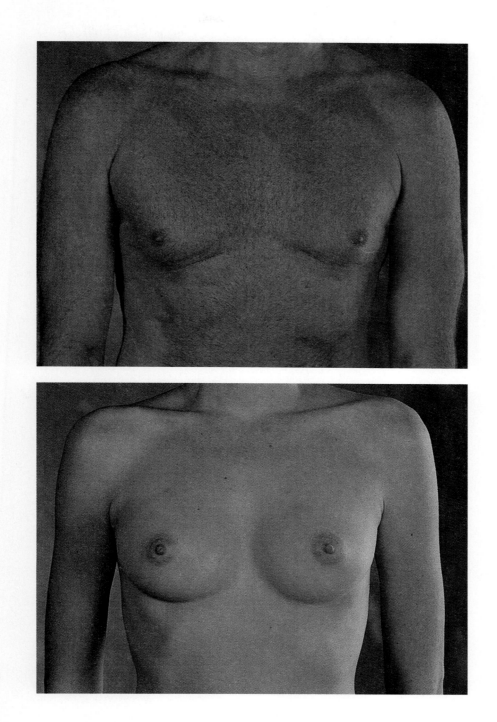

Introduction to the Thorax

▶ Thoracic Wall and Thoracic Cavity

▶ Serous Cavities, Pleurae, and Pericardium

▶ Mediastinum

THORACIC WALL AND THORACIC CAVITY

The thoracic vertebral column, 12 pairs of ribs, and sternum comprise the **thoracic wall.** The costal cartilages of the upper seven ribs articulate directly along the lateral border of the sternum. Anterolaterally, the costal cartilages of ribs 8 to 10 turn upward to attach to the costal cartilage above, forming the **costal margin** (Figure 1-1). The **diaphragm,** a domed muscle, is attached to the upper two to three lumbar vertebrae, the inferior margins of the twelfth ribs, the costal angle, and the xiphoid process at the inferior end of the sternum. The diaphragm represents the lower limit of the thoracic cavity. Superiorly, the thoracic cavity is limited by a roughly horizontal plane passing through the pair of first ribs and the body of T1 (first thoracic vertebra).

The thoracic viscera are contained within the thoracic cavity although portions of the lungs and pleurae extend into the neck as well. The **thoracic viscera** include the heart, lungs, the great vessels (aorta, pulmonary artery, pulmonary veins, and venae cavae), the esophagus, the trachea, the thoracic duct, the sympathetic chains, the phrenic nerves, and vagus nerves. Because the diaphragm is a domed muscle, the upper parts of certain abdominal viscera are enclosed within the lower ribs and are said to be protected by the **thoracic cage,** although they are not in the thoracic cavity since they lie inferior to the diaphragm.

SEROUS CAVITIES, PLEURAE, AND PERICARDIUM

The **pleural cavities** are two enclosed sacs, lying on each side of the **mediastinum.** They are examples of **serous cavities,** which are also found in association with the heart (the **pericardium**), the abdominal organs (the **peritoneum**), and many of the tendons in the fingers and toes (the **mesotendons**).

The arrangement of visceral and parietal pleurae may be better understood by imaging a balloon, partially inflated with air (Figure 1-2). As you press inward on the surface of the balloon with your fist, one layer of the balloon becomes tightly applied to the skin of your hand (this represents the *visceral pleural layer*). As you press your fist further in, it literally disappears into the balloon. There is now a second layer of the balloon, mimicking the shape and position of the visceral pleural layer but lying external to it. This is analogous to the **parietal pleura.** Where the two pleurae are continuous, as the balloon folds back on itself around your wrist, is the **hilum** of the organ. Although your fist is now well covered by balloon material, it is *not* within the pleural cavity, because the **pleural cavity** is the space *between* the visceral and parietal pleural layers, and contains nothing but a little air and fluid.* Thus we

---

*Although this analogy may be illuminating, it is *not* the actual method by which serous membranes and cavities form. Consult your embryology textbook.

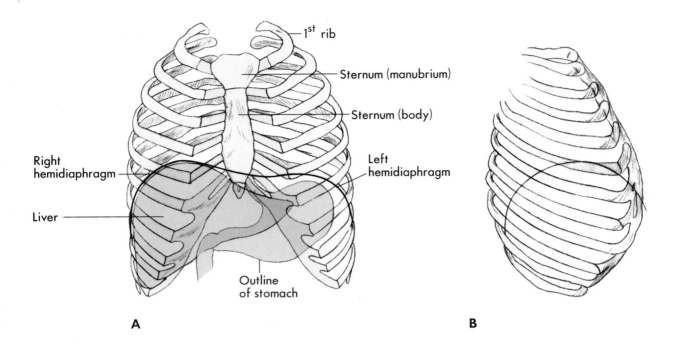

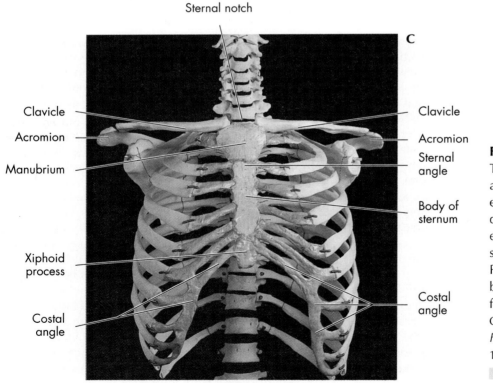

Figure 1-1 THORACIC CAGE. The thoracic cage is shown in anterior view (**A**) and in right lateral view (**B**). The position of the diaphragm is shown in black (at expiration), and the liver and stomach are outlined in red. **C,** Photograph of the articulated bony thoracic cage is included for comparison. (**C** from Chumbley CC, Hutchings RT: *Color atlas of human dissection,* ed 2, London, 1992, Mosby.)

See Atlas, Figs. 1-1, 1-5

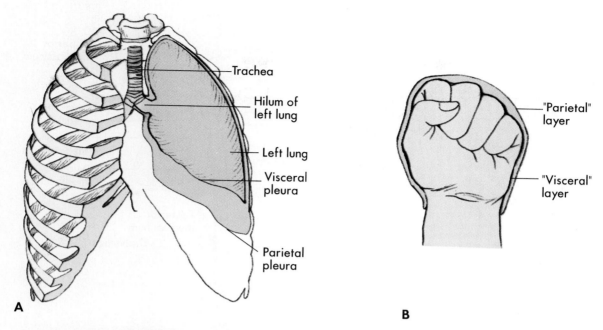

Figure 1-2 FORMATION OF A SEROUS CAVITY. A, Serous cavities feature a visceral layer, covering most of the organ itself; a parietal layer, lining most of the cavity in which the organ is suspended; and a collar at which the two are continuous. **B,** The arrangements of the serous membranes may be clarified by imaging a clenched fist being pushed into a partially inflated balloon. The layer of material closely covering the fist itself is the visceral layer; the more external layer of balloon is the parietal layer. The visceral and parietal layers are continuous at the hilum of the organ. The space between the two is a thin serous cavity. SEE ATLAS, FIG. 1-2

SEROUS MEMBRANES AND SPACES

Serous membranes are thin smooth layers that line several important body cavities. The spaces surrounded by serous membranes are called **serous cavities.** Serous cavities meet a very important need for several organs and tissues of the body. They are found wherever an organ or other structure must move, change shape, or contract and expand. Serous membranes allow these things to be done with a minimum of friction or resistance from surrounding tissues. For example, the lungs must enlarge and shrink repeatedly, as air enters and leaves them. In order to avoid injury to the surface of such an expanding and contracting organ, serous cavities have formed (known as the **pleural cavities** in the case of the lung). The serous membrane not only lines the cavity in which an organ such as the lung is suspended (the **parietal** layer) but covers the organ suspended within the cavity as well (the **visceral** layer).

may say that the lung is within the chest, but *not* truly within the pleural cavity. When fluid, blood, or air does occupy the pleural cavity, the situation is by definition pathologic, and in most cases steps are taken to evacuate the pleural space of these materials.

The hilum of the lung may be thought of as a "stalk" by which the lung is attached to the mediastinum and through which nerves, blood vessels, lymphatics, and branches of the airways reach the lungs. For the heart, abdominal viscera, and even for tendons, a similar stalk exists by which these organs are attached to surrounding tissues, though in each of these cases the shape of this stalk is far more complex than that for the lung. For example, the heart really has two pedicles or stalks—one for arterial vessels and one for venous vessels. As in the case of the lungs, it is through these pedicles that nerves, vessels, and lymphatics reach the heart. The heart has a **visceral serous pericardium** applied to the heart itself and a reflected **parietal serous pericardium,** in turn, lining the **fibrous pericardial sac** in which the heart is suspended (see Chapter 1.4, p. 87).

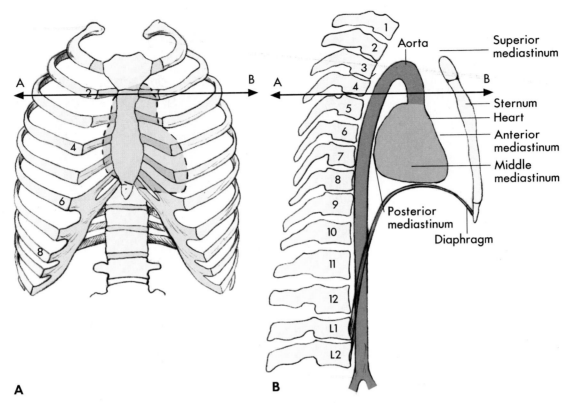

Figure 1-3   BOUNDARIES OF THE MEDIASTINUM. A, Anterior view of the thoracic cage with the position of the heart shown in dotted lines. Line A↔B separates the superior and inferior mediastinum. **B,** Lateral view of a cutaway drawing of the thorax. Line A↔B defines the boundary of the superior and inferior mediastinum. The position of the heart defines the middle mediastinum; the space anterior to it is the anterior mediastinum, ending at the sternum. The space posterior to the heart is the posterior mediastinum, limited by the vertebral column. The superior mediastinum is not subdivided into anterior, middle, and posterior. The diaphragm is the lower limit of the mediastinum, and superiorly the neck blends with the mediastinum.

MEDIASTINUM

The **mediastinum** (L. *mediastinus,* a helper, assistant; or *mediastinum,* being in the middle) is that region that lies between the two pleural sacs. It has no easily identifiable boundaries (Figure 1-3; see also Figure 1-24, *B*) and is best considered as a region in which many crucial structures lie (the heart, thymus, etc.), and through which other very important structures pass (esophagus, aorta, trachea, thoracic duct, etc.). The medi-

astinum is divided into regions by a plane through the sternal angle and the lower part of the body of the T4 vertebra—the **inferior mediastinum,** with its **anterior, middle,** and **posterior divisions,** and the **superior mediastinum**—and is described more fully in Chapters 1.3, 1.4, and 1.5.

Figures 1-4 and 1-5 show radiographs of the thorax in two views commonly used clinically.

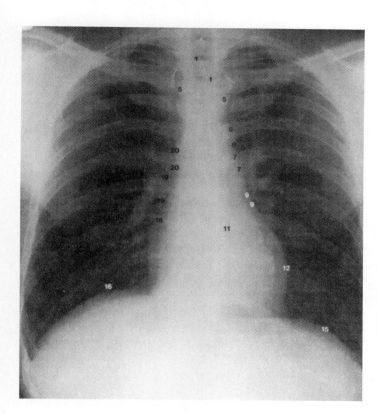

Figure 1-4 POSTEROANTERIOR CHEST X-RAY. In this technique, the x-ray beams pass through the patient from posterior to anterior and then fall on a film plate held up against the patient's anterior chest wall. (From Weir J, Abrahams PH: *An imaging atlas of human anatomy,* London, 1992, Mosby.)

1 Trachea	**12** Left ventricle
5 Sternum	**15** Left diaphragm
6 Aortic knob or knuckle	**16** Right diaphragm
7 Lateral margin of pulmonary trunk	**18** Right atrial border
	19 Right pulmonary artery
9 Edge of left atrial appendage	**20** Superior vena cava
11 Left edge of descending aorta	

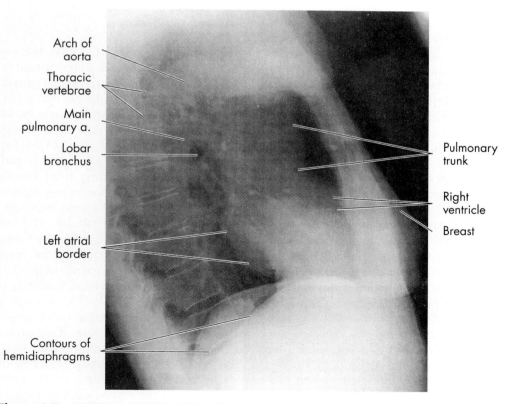

Arch of aorta

Thoracic vertebrae

Main pulmonary a.

Lobar bronchus

Left atrial border

Contours of hemidiaphragms

Pulmonary trunk

Right ventricle

Breast

Figure 1-5 LATERAL CHEST X-RAY. X-rays pass from side-to-side through the patient. (From Weir J, Abrahams PH: *An imaging atlas of human anatomy,* London, 1992, Mosby.)

1.2

Chest Wall

▶ Breast

▶ Structure of the Chest Wall

▶ Thoracic Vertebrae

▶ Ribs and Costal Cartilages

▶ Clavicle and Scapula

▶ Sternum

▶ Muscles of the Chest Wall

▶ Blood Vessels of the Chest Wall

▶ Intercostal Nerves

▶ Intercostal Space

*T*he vertebral column, ribs, and sternum comprise a bony frame, the **thoracic cage,** to which many muscles of the chest, upper limb, and neck are attached, forming the **chest wall.** The chest wall is covered by skin, deep to which is the **superficial fascia.** Deep to this is a layer of **deep fascia** in which the major chest wall muscles are embedded. Often an especially thickened component of the deep fascia forms an external covering or *investing layer* over these major chest wall muscles. Deep to the major muscles are the bony elements of the chest wall—the **ribs, sternum,** and thoracic **vertebrae.** In the chest wall can be seen the clearest evidence of the segmental organization of the human body—that is, a pair of ribs and their associated soft tissues are "stacked" upon each other, forming an elongated cylinder composed of structurally repetitive elements. In other parts of the body, such as the limbs, the segmental pattern is still present but is much more difficult to discern. The chest wall and its associated soft tissues comprise the upper half of the **trunk.**

The thoracic cage is significant as a framework for the muscles of the trunk, neck, and upper limb. It plays an important role in respiration and encloses and protects the internal organs of the thoracic cavity (and those of the upper abdominal cavity as well) from traumatic injury.

BREAST

The **breast** is located within the superficial fascia (Figure 1-6). In the male, very little fat is present in the breast, and the glandular system normally does not develop. When abnormal levels of steroid hormones are present in the male, as at puberty, the breast can begin to develop (gynecomastia). Breast development in the pubertal male is almost always transient. The postpubertal female breast is made up of **connective tissue** sheets or **septa,** extending from the investing fascial layer to the superficial fascia (see Figure 1-6, *A* and *B*). These septa divide the breast into ~20 lobes, each of which contains several lobules. The lobules are composed of (1) a large amount of *fat* (comprising 85% to 90% of the breast mass) and (2) the compound tubuloalveolar *glands,* which produce milk.

The breast lobules contain hundreds of thousands of spherical **alveoli** (L. *alveolus,* a small cavity), which drain into a series of progressively larger ducts and ultimately into 15 to 20 large **lactiferous ducts.** These ducts converge on the region just deep to the nipple. The lactiferous ducts end by emptying through a series of tiny apertures on the apex of the nipple. Just deep to the surface of the nipple, each of these 15 to 20 lactiferous ducts expands into a saclike **lactiferous sinus.**

The breast is shaped like a thickened disk and is po-

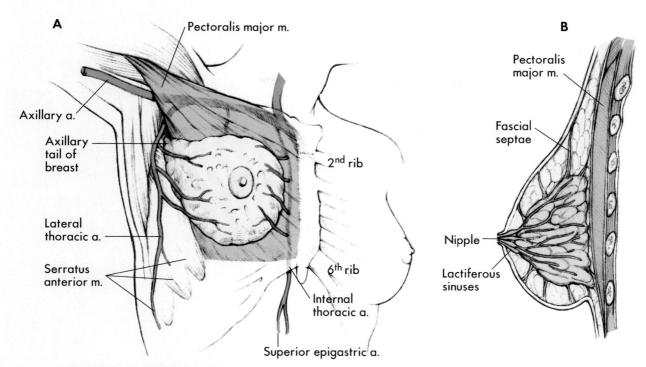

A

Pectoralis major m.

Axillary a.

Axillary tail of breast

Lateral thoracic a.

Serratus anterior m.

2nd rib

6th rib

Internal thoracic a.

Superior epigastric a.

B

Pectoralis major m.

Fascial septae

Nipple

Lactiferous sinuses

Figure 1-6   FEMALE BREAST.   A, The breast shown as a thickened circular disk of tissue positioned on the anterior chest wall. **B,** A sagittal section of the breast showing the lactiferous sinuses (just deep to the nipple) and the fatty lobes and septae that make up most of the substance of the breast. See Atlas, Figs. 1-8, 1-9

sitioned on the anterior surface of the *pectoralis major* muscle, centered on the fourth or fifth rib of the underlying ribcage. A prominent lateral extension of tissue, the **axillary tail** of the breast, crosses over the inferolateral edge of the pectoralis major muscle to reach the axilla. The axillary tail is important because it contains the largest share of the breast's glandular tissue, and a great percentage of breast tumors occurs there.

The **nipple** is positioned on the anterior surface of the breast and is surrounded by a roughly circular hyperpigmented region, the **areola.** In the areola are small sebaceous glands (glands of Montgomery), which enlarge to form swollen tubercles during pregnancy, as the areola becomes darker. Small collections of smooth muscle located at the base of the nipple may cause erection of the nipple during nursing or sexual arousal. Humans normally have one nipple on each side of the anterior chest wall. However, during early embryonic development, a **milk line** of multiple nipples extends on each side from the upper thigh and groin region superiorly to the axilla. In many mammals (cats, dogs, etc.), these persist as fully formed mammary glands, but in humans only one breast on each side develops. Occasionally, however, a supernumerary (i.e., extra) nipple or breast may develop along this milk line in humans.

Blood is supplied to the breast from the segmental arteries and veins (i.e., intercostal vessels coursing from posterior to anterior around the chest wall; see Figures 1-20 and 1-21). In addition, the large **lateral thoracic, internal thoracic, thoracoacromial,** and **superior epigastric arteries** have branches supplying the breast. Venous drainage is to the **intercostal, internal thoracic,** and **axillary veins.** The breast is innervated by branches of the **intercostal nerves** from T2 to T7. However, the important physiologic changes in the breast are mediated not by nerves but by circulating hormones (e.g., oxytocin causes milk "letdown"; high levels of estrogen lead to growth of milk glands; prolactin produces overall breast growth).

STRUCTURE OF THE CHEST WALL

The skeleton of the chest wall is composed of thoracic **vertebrae, ribs,** and the **sternum** (see Figure 1-1). The upper limb is attached to the chest wall through the **clavicle** and indirectly the **scapula, which together comprise the shoulder girdle** (see Figure 1-13). These structural elements form the framework of the chest and upper limb and are involved in movements of the chest and upper limb as well.

The chest wall has many important functions. First,

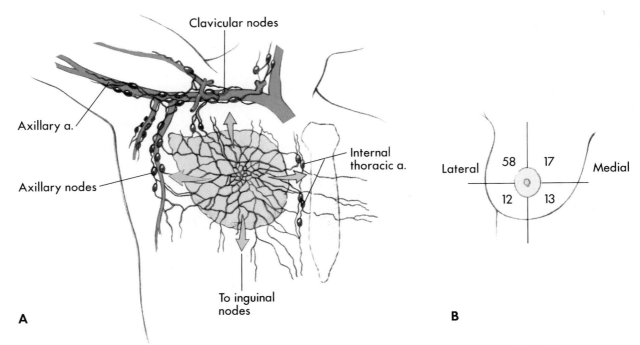

Figure 1-7 LYMPHATIC DRAINAGE OF THE BREAST. A, Several routes of lymphatic drainage of the breast. **B,** The percentage incidence of female breast cancers in the four quadrants of the breast. The quadrants are designated upper outer, upper inner, lower outer, and lower inner.

it serves as a protective shield for the thoracic organs. Second, because the diaphragm extends superiorly as far as the T5-T6 vertebral level, *upper abdominal organs are also protected by the lower part of the ribcage* (see Figure 1-1). Third, the articulations of the ribs, sternum, and vertebral column are central to respiration, because the movements of the ribs result in a cyclic increase and decrease in the volume of air in the lungs (see Figure 1-18

CLINICAL ANATOMY OF

THE BREAST

BREAST CANCER AND LYMPHATIC SPREAD

Because breast tumors metastasize (or spread) through the lymphatic channels that drain the breast, it is especially important to learn the routes of this lymphatic drainage (Figure 1-7). Lymph vessels transfer extracellular fluid from most of the tissues of the body (except for the central nervous system) through a series of tiny channels back, ultimately, to the venous system. The biggest share (~70%) of breast lymphatic drainage is to the axilla, but important drainage also occurs from the breast to the tissues near the clavicle, along the internal thoracic vessels, across the sternum to the opposite breast, and even to distant sites like the anterior abdominal wall and the inguinal region. Surgeons removing breast tumors must explore these adjacent tissues carefully (especially the axilla), to ensure that all lymph nodes containing malignant breast tumor tissue are removed as

well. The normally smooth contour of the breast may be interrupted by breast tumors, which can cause a "dimpling" or "puckering" of the smooth surface of the normal breast, due to fibrosis of ligaments extending from the deep fascia to the skin.

INCIDENCE OF BREAST CANCER

Breast **cancer** will afflict one in every thirteen white females at some time during their lives, with a lower incidence for black and Asian women. **Mammograms** (x-rays of the breast) have revolutionized the detection and early treatment of breast tumors (Figure 1-8). Tumors can be detected even when very small, and the least invasive surgical or medical option utilized for treatment. No other medical or surgical treatment to date can rival the use of mammograms in the detection and treatment of breast cancer.

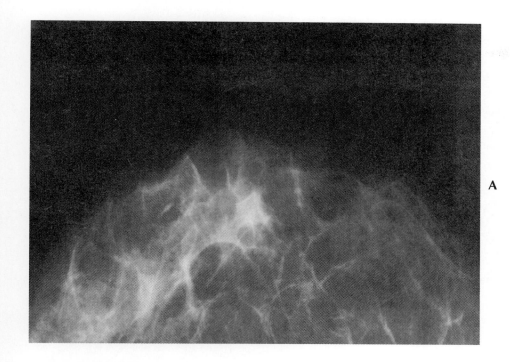

A

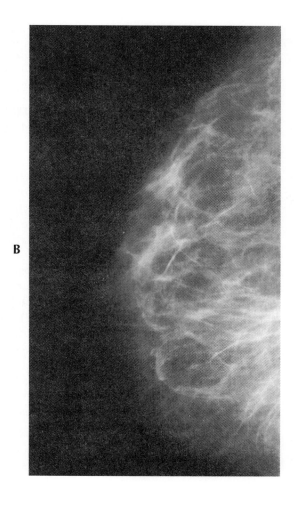

B

Figure 1-8 MAMMOGRAM. Craniocaudal (**A**) and lateral (**B**) mammograms. Normal densities in the breast and the fatty lobules that they delineate should be mentally subtracted so that the underlying connective and glandular structures can be analyzed. (From LeTreut A, Dilhujdy MH: *Mammography: a guide to interpretation,* St. Louis, 1991, Mosby.)

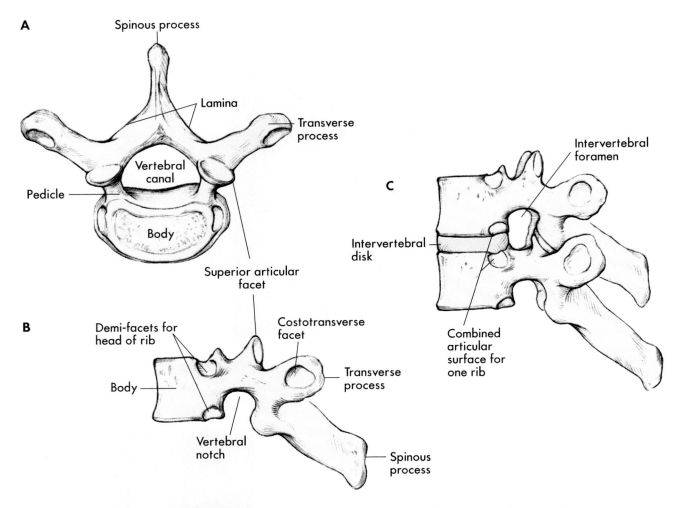

Figure 1-9   THORACIC VERTEBRAE. Typical thoracic vertebrae, viewed superiorly (**A**), laterally (**B**), and as two articulated vertebrae viewed laterally (**C**).

for further details). Movements of the head, neck, upper limbs, and vertebral column all involve muscles with attachments to the chest wall. The chest wall is important for students of anatomy because it is the region where the segmental organization of the body is best illustrated.

The T1 vertebra, the two first ribs, and the manubrium of the sternum surround an aperture, known to anatomists as the **thoracic inlet** (but, paradoxically, to clinicians as the *thoracic outlet*). This aperture is roughly oval but is indented posteriorly by the body of the T1 vertebra (Figures 1-9 and 1-10). A similar but much larger aperture is located inferiorly, bounded by the T12 vertebra, ribs 11 and 12, the costal cartilages of ribs 7 to 10, and the xiphoid process. This, at least in anatomic terminology, is the *thoracic outlet.*

THORACIC VERTEBRAE

Vertebrae are discussed in more detail in Section Four, The Back; here only the thoracic vertebrae are

described briefly. A vertebra consists of a solid cylindrical **body** and a posterior semicircular **arch** of bone that encloses the **vertebral canal** (see Figure 1-9). Adjacent vertebral bodies are separated by an **intevertebral disk,** which is strong yet flexible enough to allow considerable mobility of the vertebral column. The posterior arch of bone is composed of a pair of **pedicles,** a pair of **laminae,** and a posterior midline **spinous process.** Thoracic vertebrae are characterized by their slender and downswept spinous processes. The bony transverse processes of thoracic vertebrae are short and protrude laterally and somewhat posteriorly (at about a 30° degree angle). On the transverse processes of thoracic vertebrae 1-10 is a roughly circular **facet,** a slightly depressed surface intended for articulation with the tubercle of the corresponding rib. This articulation is the **costotransverse joint,** and it is a typical synovial joint (Figure 1-11). Ribs 11 and 12 lack costotransverse articulations; thus there are no articular facets on the tubercles of these two ribs nor on the transverse processes of vertebrae T11 and T12.

Anterior

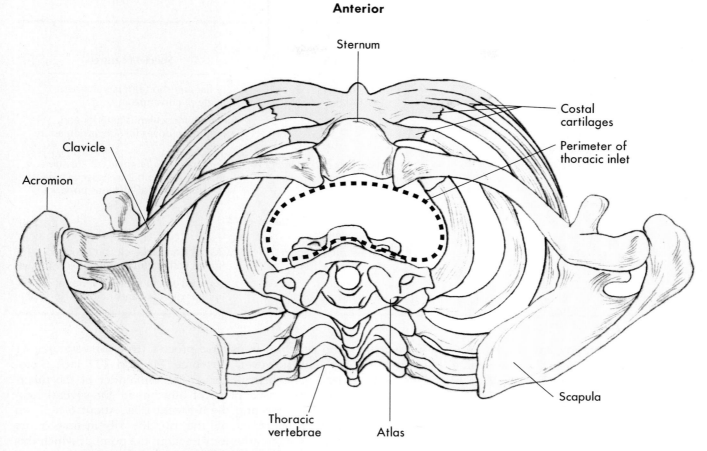

Figure 1-10 THORACIC INLET. The clavicles, sternum, first ribs, and vertebral column surround a narrow aperture known as the thoracic inlet (or "thoracic outlet," in clinical terminology).

The bodies of all 12 thoracic vertebrae have small articular facets, at which the **heads** of the ribs articulate with the vertebral bodies (costovertebral joints; see Figure 1-11). The pattern of articulation, however, is not always a simple "one rib–one vertebra" arrangement (Table 1-1). While the heads of ribs 1, 10, 11, and 12 do articulate solely with the body of the vertebra to which they correspond numerically, the heads of ribs 2 to 9 articulate with two adjacent vertebral bodies: (1) the body of the vertebra with which the rib shares a

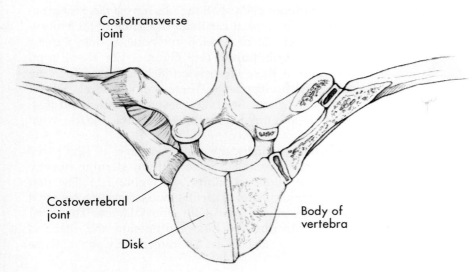

Figure 1-11 JOINTS BETWEEN THE RIBS AND VERTEBRAE. On the left are shown the intact costovertebral and costotransverse joints, reinforced by ligaments. On the right the joints have been opened, revealing the synovial spaces within.

Table 1-1   Costovertebral Articulations

Rib Number	Head of Rib Articulates With	Neck and Tubercle of Rib Articulate With	Special Feature(s)
1	Body of T1 only	Transverse process of 1st vertebra	Very flat and short rib; has sharpest angle of curvature
			Tubercles for scalenus anterior and medius; grooves for subclavian artery and vein
2-9	Body of vertebra with same number plus the body of the vertebra above and the intervening intervertebral disk	Transverse process of vertebra of same number	Progressively wider angles of curvature than for rib 1; rib 2 has special area for attachment of scalenus posterior
10	Body of T10 only	Transverse process of vertebra of same number	—
11	Body of T11 only	Lacks a neck/tubercle; no costotransverse joint	Lacks neck and tubercle; anterior end tipped with cartilage; incomplete groove
12	Body of T12 only	Lacks a neck/tubercle; no costotransverse joint	Lacks neck and tubercle; anterior end tipped with cartilage; no costal groove

numerical designation and (2) the vertebra just superior to it, in addition to the intervening intervertebral disk (e.g., rib 3 with the bodies of the T2 and T3 vertebrae and the intervening disk). The **costovertebral articular surfaces** (see Figures 1-9 and 1-11) are roughly circular, and the portion of the surface on an individual vertebra is known as a **demifacet.** See Section 4, The Back, for a more thorough discussion of vertebral structure and the many common pathologic changes in vertebrae and their disks.

RIBS AND COSTAL CARTILAGES

Ribs provide structural reinforcement of the thoracic cage so that the chest wall does not collapse as a result of the subatmospheric pressure within the trachea and airways. Most individuals have 12 pairs of ribs, though not uncommonly an extra rib is present or one is missing. Each rib is an elongated curved bone (Figure 1-12), extending from its vertebral attachments posteriorly around the chest wall to its attachment anteriorly to the costal cartilages. Ribs 3 to 9 share common structural features and are called **typical ribs;** ribs 1, 2, 10, 11, and 12 have unique structural features and are called **atypical ribs.**

A typical rib (ribs 3 to 9) is in the shape of a half-circle. The shaft of the rib is smoothly curved and contributes to the formation of the lateral thoracic wall. Posteriorly, the **head** of the rib has two articular facets, meant to articulate with the facets on the two adjacent vertebral bodies (see Table 1-1). The **tubercle** of the rib lies about 3 to 4 cm lateral to the head. The tubercle forms a roughened posterior protrusion on the rib, and part of it is specialized as a facet for articulation with

the vertebral transverse process (true for vertebrae T1 to T10; however, vertebrae T11 and T12 lack costotransverse articulations). The remainder of the tubercle serves as a point of attachment for several ligaments connecting the adjacent ribs. About 6 to 7 cm further lateral along the rib, the rib inclines more sharply in an anterior direction; the point at which this change in the angle of curvature occurs is the *posterior angle* of the rib. Beyond this, the rib curves much more sharply in an anterior direction. It then sweeps around the lateral body wall, in such a way that the anterior end of the rib lies lower (i.e., more inferior) than its head.

Supernumerary ribs are unusual because they occur on cervical or lumbar vertebrae not because their shape is always unusual for a rib. They are often incomplete, however, and may not extend all the way from the vertebral column to the anterior chest.

The anterior ends of all the ribs have a facet for articulation with a **costal cartilage,** a portion of the embryonic rib that fails to develop into bone, as does the rest of the rib primordium (see Figure 1-12). There is no true joint at these costochondral junctions, which are reinforced by ligaments. These costochondral "joints" allow only minor flexibility. Several muscles and ligaments of both the chest and the neck attach to the costal cartilages.

Further, medially, the costal cartilages of ribs 1 to 7 (and sometimes 8) articulate with the sternum directly (the **sternochondral joints;** see Figure 1-1). The first sternochondral joint is cartilaginous, lacking a synovial cavity. The others are usually synovial joints. The costal cartilages of ribs 8 to 10 sweep upward and attach to the costal cartilage of the rib immediately above; those

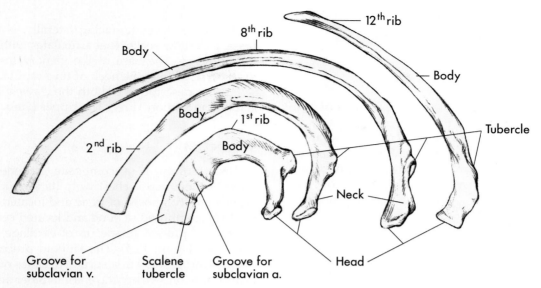

Figure 1-12 RIBS. Four different ribs: the first, second, eighth, and twelfth. Each has a head, neck, tubercle and body, although they are of different sizes and shapes.
SEE ATLAS, FIG. 1-6

of ribs 11 and 12 are very small and do not attach to the sternum or the adjacent costal cartilages.

CLAVICLE AND SCAPULA

The **clavicle** is a curved bony strut in the shape of an S, with its medial two thirds convex in the anterior di-

rection and its lateral one third convex in the posterior direction (Figure 1-13; see also Figure 1-10). The *medial end* of the clavicle is cylindrical, with specialized surfaces for articulation with the *manubrium* of the sternum and the *first costal cartilage* (see Figure 1-14). The *lateral end* of the clavicle is flattened and has a specialized flattened surface for articulation with the *acromion*

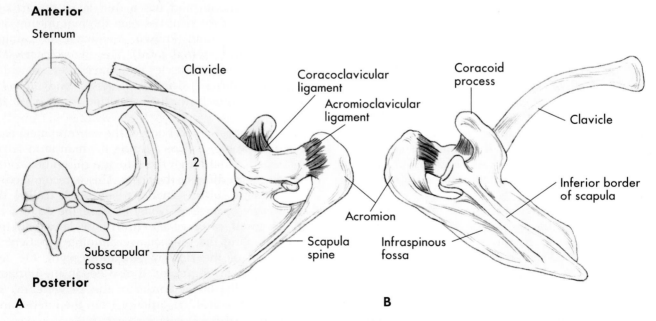

Figure 1-13 ARTICULATIONS OF THE SCAPULA AND CLAVICLE. Superior (**A**) and inferior (**B**) views. The clavicle and scapula constitute the shoulder girdle and bridge the gap between the humerus and the chest wall. The shoulder girdle is mobile and allows for a great range of movement. Two important joints, the coracoclavicular and acromioclavicular, join the two together.

THE RIBS

EXTRA RIBS

Cervical ribs are found in a small number of individuals. They arise from the *costal element* of a cervical vertebra, which normally does nothing more than complete the enclosure of the foramen transversarium. Cervical ribs may cause no symptoms but are likely to obstruct further the already narrow thoracic inlet and impede the flow of blood through one of the major vessels, or produce paresthesias (abnormal sensations) by compressing components of the brachial plexus. Even more rarely, there may be small ribs associated with the first lumbar vertebrae (**lumbar ribs**). These have little or no clinical significance.

INFLAMMATION OF THORACIC CAGE

Tietze's syndrome is a condition of inflammation in the costal cartilages, resulting in chest pain, which, when localized to the upper ribs, may be confused with the anterior chest pain resulting from a myocardial infarction ("heart attack"). When evaluating a patient complaining of chest pain, tenderness in the chest wall might lead to consideration of this syndrome as the cause for the chest pain.

of the scapula (the flattened bony prominence at the lateral end of the scapular spine) (see Figure 1-13). The medial one half of the clavicle has elongated attachments for the *pectoralis major* and the *sternocleidomastoid* muscles and a small area for attachment of the *sternohyoid* muscle. On its lateral third are surfaces for attachment of the *trapezius* and the *deltoid* muscles. The *subclavius* muscle has a narrow elongated attachment on the inferior surface of the middle third of the clavicle.

The scapula and clavicle comprise the **shoulder girdle,** the role of which is to connect the upper limb to the trunk and to take part in maximizing the mobility of the upper limb. The **scapula** is a bone of complex shape (see Figure 1-13). Part of the scapula is a thin inverted triangle positioned on the posterior thoracic wall. In its "resting" position, it extends from the second to the seventh rib, but it is quite mobile and can slide anteriorly (protraction) and posteriorly (retraction), be elevated or depressed, and rotate as well. The scapula has two angles, an **inferior angle** (located at the apex of this inverted triangle) and a **superior angle** (really better described as superomedial). At the third

corner of the triangle, facing laterally, is the **glenoid fossa,** a shallow socket that articulates with the head of the humerus. The base of the glenoid fossa is sometimes referred to as the **neck of the scapula.**

Further description of both the clavicle and scapula is found in Section Three, The Upper Limb.

STERNUM

The **sternum** is a composite flattened bone located in the anterior chest wall. Its three parts are the *manubrium* (composed of bone and located superiorly), the *body* (composed of bone and located centrally), and the *xiphoid* process (made up of cartilage and located inferiorly; Figure 1-14). The xiphoid process generally calcifies through the first several decades of life and appears dense on x-ray of the chest in older adults.

Along the superior margin of the **manubrium** is a midline **jugular (sternal) notch,** flanked on each side by a curved articular facet for the *clavicle.* The manubrium has a smooth **clavicular articular facet** facing directly lateral on each side, into which the medial end of each clavicle fits. While the other joints between the costal cartilages and the sternum are generally synovial, the first sternochondral joint is cartilaginous. Just inferior to the first rib facet, the *second costal cartilage* articulates with a facet beginning on the inferior margin of the manubrium and extending across to the superolateral margin of the adjacent *body* of the sternum. The inferior margin of the manubrium is horizontal and smooth and has a thin layer of cartilage forming part of the joint between the manubrium and body of the sternum (known, somewhat confusingly, as the **manubriosternal joint**). The *sternocleidomastoid* and *pectoralis major* muscles both have fibers attaching to the manubrium. The *sternothyroid* and *sternohyoid* muscles attach to the posterior surface of the manubrium.

The manubrium and body of the sternum meet each other at an angle, and, as a result, the manubriosternal joint is palpable through the skin as a raised horizontal ridge in the midline of the chest. This is recognized as an important surface anatomy landmark (called the *sternal angle* or *angle of Louis*) because the second rib and its costal cartilage are invariably lateral to this ridge, enabling the physician examining a patient to identify all of the ribs by palpation, using the second rib as a starting point. It also lies in the horizontal plane of the lower border of the T4 vertebra, the plane that separates the superior from the inferior mediastinum.

The **body** of the sternum is an elongated plate, which actually forms from the fusion of four different segments or *sternebrae.* Some evidence of its segmentation may persist as horizontal ridges between the adjacent segments. Its superior margin is horizontal and

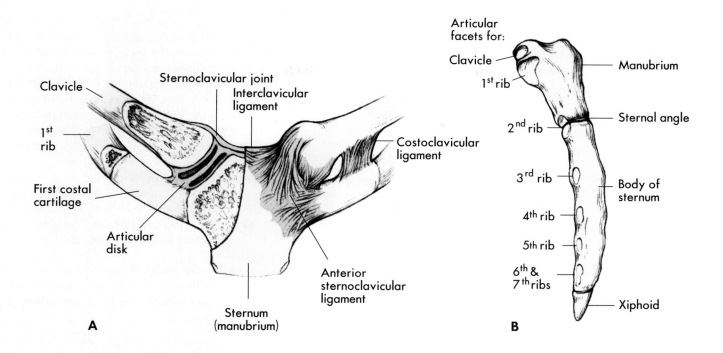

Figure 1-14 STERNUM AND STERNOCLAVICULAR JOINT. A, Longitudinal section through the sternoclavicular joint. **B,** Entire sternum viewed from an oblique lateral perspective. **SEE ATLAS, FIG. 1-7**

smooth, forming part of the manubriosternal joint. At the junction of its lateral and superior edges is a small facet which, along with a similar structure on the manubrium, forms an articulation with the second costal cartilage. Shallow facets for costal cartilages 3 to 6 are present along the margins of the body of the sternum. The *pectoralis major* muscle attaches to the anterior surface of the sternal body and the *transversus thoracis* muscle to the posterior surface.

The **xiphoid process** articulates with the lower margin of the sternal body. The xiphoid is variable in shape. The seventh costal cartilage articulates with the sternum at the joint between the body and xiphoid. The **linea alba** (a thickened vertical cord of connective tissue in the midline of the abdominal wall) attaches to the xiphoid process, as do small portions of many large and important muscles—the *diaphragm,* the *rectus abdominis,* and the *external* and *internal oblique* muscles.

CLINICAL ANATOMY OF

THE STERNUM

ANOMALIES OF THE STERNUM

If the sternum is depressed, the anterior chest wall appears "sunken" and the condition is termed **pectus excavatum.** This condition can be mainly a cosmetic and self-image problem (especially in adolescents) but may also compromise respiration by limiting the vital capacity of the chest. The opposite condition, where the sternum protrudes abnormally, is known as **pectus carinatum** (L. *carina,* the keel of a ship).

MEDIAN STERNOTOMY INCISION

Many cardiac surgeries are carried out through a

median sternotomy incision, allowing the surgeon access to the mediastinum without having to enter the pleural cavities (which prolongs recovery from surgery). After the sternum is split longitudinally and the surgery completed, the two halves of the sternum are reapproximated using strong wire sutures.

STERNUM AND BONE MARROW SAMPLING

The body of the sternum contains a significant amount of **bone marrow** and is used as a site for the collection of diagnostic samples.

MUSCLES OF THE CHEST WALL

Several groups of muscles are found in the chest wall (Table 1-2). Some of these muscles attach ribs to other ribs, while others join ribs and sternum or vertebrae. The function common to all of these muscles is that they can move the ribs, in addition to whatever other movements they produce. Movement of the ribs is the fundamental action producing respiration, as detailed following (pp. 65-66).

The space between adjacent ribs is filled with a set of **intercostal muscles,** of which there are three layers—the **external, internal,** and **innermost intercostal muscles** (Figure 1-15). These muscle groups differ from each other in the direction in which their muscle fibers are arrayed and the degree to which they are present at all points around the full curvature of the chest wall, from the vertebral column posteriorly to the costal cartilages anteriorly. At points where an intercostal muscle itself is not present, it is represented by a **membrane** (e.g., the external intercostal muscle is not continuous all the way anterior to the costal cartilages, and, anteriorly, the *anterior intercostal membrane* is found in its place). Also a separate and distinct muscle may be found in the plane of the innermost intercostal muscles and may be thought of as a continuation of that layer of intercostal musculature (e.g., the **transversus thoracis** and **subcostal** muscles).

Apart from the intercostal muscles, the chest wall is an attachment for many important muscles of the upper limb and neck (Figures 1-16 and 1-17). Movement of the ribs is an essential part of changing the shape and volume of the chest and is essential for respiration.

There is no agreement about the activity of specific intercostal muscles in the various phases of respiration. Most agree that the external intercostals are elevators of

Table 1-2 Muscles of the Chest Wall

Muscle	Attachments	Comments	Innervation
External intercostal	Present from rib tubercles forward to costochondral junction; replaced anteriorly by anterior intercostal membrane Joins ribs to adjacent ribs	Fibers run inferomedially; active in forced inspiration, especially in lower five to six segments; has only small role in relaxed breathing	Intercostal nerves for each segment
Internal intercostal	Present from sternum posterior to the rib angles; replaced posteriorly by the posterior intercostal membrane Joins ribs to adjacent ribs	Fibers run inferolaterally; neurovascular bundle for intercostal space, lies just deep to internal intercostal	Intercostal nerves for each segment
Innermost intercostal	Similar to that of internal intercostal; replaced anteriorly by transversus thoracis and posteriorly by subcostalis Joins ribs to adjacent ribs	Often absent at higher thoracic levels	Intercostal nerves for each segment
Transversus thoracis	On interior of thorax, slips of muscle from surfaces of ribs 5 to 8 pass superolaterally and attach to ribs 2 to 6 Joins ribs to distant ribs	In reality specialized anterior portion of the innermost intercostal—i.e., in the same muscle plane; acts to depress the costal cartilages	Intercostal nerves for each segment
Subcostal muscles	From angles of ribs, fibers pass inferiorly to ribs one to three segments below, on internal surface of ribs Joins ribs to distant ribs	In reality a specialized posterior portion of the innermost intercostal—i.e., in the same muscle plane; depresses ribs	Intercostal nerves for each segment
Levatores costarum	From transverse processes of C7-T11 to external upper surface of rib below, near tubercle; muscles from T8-T11 also attach to second rib below Joins ribs to vertebrae	In plane of external intercostals (which are also represented by posterior intercostal membrane); the levatores costarum act to elevate the ribs and also act in vertebral rotation	By dorsal primary rami of segmental nerves
Subclavius	From rib 1 at junction with costal cartilage to middle one third of clavicle Joins first rib to clavicle	Lies in plane of chest wall; can be accessory respiratory muscle	Nerve to subclavius, from upper trunk brachial plexus
Serratus posterior superior	From spines of C7-T3 to external surface of ribs 2 to 5 near their angle Joins ribs to vertebrae	Muscle fibers inclined downward and laterally; does not correspond to an intercostal muscle; elevates the ribs	Branches of intercostal nerves 2 to 5
Serratus posterior inferior	From spines of T10-L3 to external surface of ribs 9 to 12 near angles Joins ribs to vertebrae	Muscle fibers inclined upward and laterally; does not correspond to an intercostal muscle; depresses the ribs	Branches of intercostal nerves 8 to 12

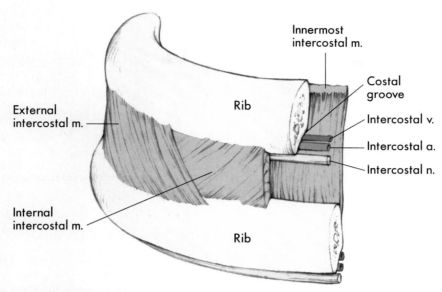

Figure 1-15   TYPICAL INTERCOSTAL SPACE. Note that the neurovascular bundle travels in the space between the internal and innermost intercostal muscles. **SEE ATLAS, FIG. 1-13**

the ribs (and therefore active in inspiration), but the role of the internal and the innermost intercostals is unclear. The actions of the **diaphragm,** a muscle more important to respiration than any other single muscle, are discussed on pp. 66-67.

Movements of the Chest Wall and Respiration

The vertebral column serves as a fixed immobile rod against which the ribs and sternum move during respiration. Respiration consists of inspiration and expiration. Quiet inspiration usually lasts about 1 second, and

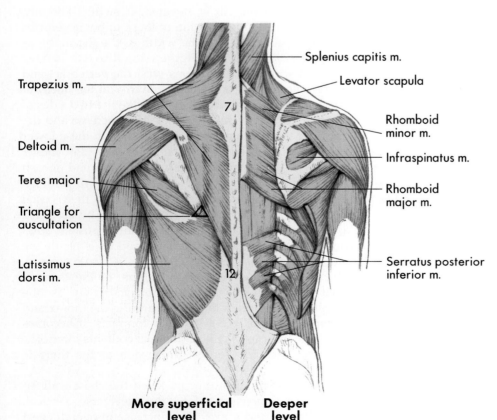

Figure 1-16 POSTERIOR TRUNK MUSCLES. On the left are shown the more superficial muscles of the posterior chest wall—trapezius, deltoid, and latissimus dorsi. On the right are shown the deeper muscles—splenius capitis, rhomboid major and minor, serratus posterior inferior, and the infraspinatus.

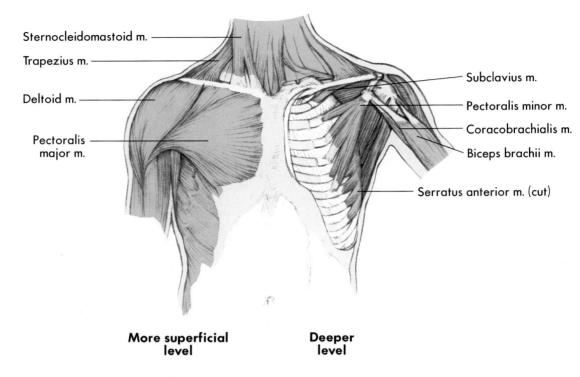

Sternocleidomastoid m.

Trapezius m.

Deltoid m.

Pectoralis major m.

Subclavius m.

Pectoralis minor m.

Coracobrachialis m.

Biceps brachii m.

Serratus anterior m. (cut)

More superficial level

Deeper level

Figure 1-17   ANTERIOR TRUNK MUSCLES. On the right are shown the superficial muscles of the anterior chest wall—sternocleidomastoid, trapezius, deltoid, and pectoralis major. On the left are shown the deeper muscles—pectoralis minor, biceps brachii, and the serratus anterior. See ATLAS, Figs. 1-11, 1-12

quiet expiration about 3 seconds. During **inspiration,** the volume of the thoracic cavity increases, the lung remains adherent to the inner surface of the chest wall, and for a brief instant the pressure within the airways becomes subatmospheric. This draws air into the trachea and bronchial tree, leading to gas exchange at the alveolar level. During **expiration,** air exits the tracheobronchial tree, and the volume of the thoracic cavity decreases back to baseline. Inspiration is active, requiring the coordinated contraction of several muscles; expiration during quiet breathing is passive, relying on the elastic recoil of the chest wall and lungs. Forced expiration (e.g., blowing up a balloon), however, is an active process, requiring muscle contraction.

The structure of the chest wall permits the changes in volume that are necessary for respiration. Various muscles exert an upward pull on the ribs, and, when this occurs, the overall dimensions of the chest wall increase, drawing air into the lungs. The first seven ribs have direct attachments to the sternum (through their costal cartilages), and an imaginary axis exists along a line drawn from the sternochondral joint posterior to a point just lateral to the tubercle of the rib (Figure 1-18).

The first seven ribs can rotate along this imaginary axis, much as a bucket handle may move through an arc while its two ends remain attached to the side of a bucket. When the rib is elevated, it swings laterally, and collectively the elevation of these upper seven ribs results in an increase of the width of the thorax by as much as 12% to 15% (see Figure 1-18). Ribs 8 to 10 have different sorts of articulations with the vertebrae, and as a result their movement is primarily in the horizontal plane, "opening" and "closing" like the two sides of a pincer. This movement results in an increase and decrease of the width of the lower ribcage. In these lower ribs, there is a minimum of the "bucket handle" movement of the upper ribs. At rest, the anterior end of each rib is inferior to the posterior end, but during forced inspiration, the anterior ends of the ribs, their costal cartilages, and the sternum itself elevate by as much as 2 to 3 cm. In addition, the sternum is pushed anterior during elevation of the ribs, and as a result the anteroposterior dimension of the ribs is also increased, further increasing the overall volume of the thoracic cavity. The "floor" of the thoracic cavity is the **diaphragm,** a domed muscle separating the thorax and abdomen (Figure 1-19). When it contracts, it becomes flattened and pushes the abdominal contents inferiorly. This increases the vertical dimension of the thoracic cavity.

In sum, **inspiration** begins when the chest wall increases its dimensions along the transverse, vertical, and anteroposterior axes. This increase in overall chest

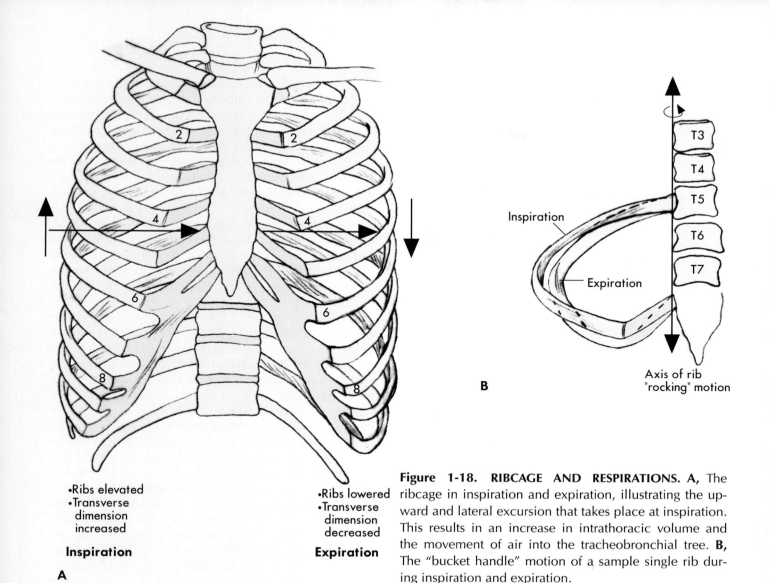

- Ribs elevated
- Transverse dimension increased

Inspiration

A

- Ribs lowered
- Transverse dimension decreased

Expiration

Axis of rib "rocking" motion

B

Inspiration

Expiration

T3
T4
T5
T6
T7

Figure 1-18. RIBCAGE AND RESPIRATIONS. A, The ribcage in inspiration and expiration, illustrating the upward and lateral excursion that takes place at inspiration. This results in an increase in intrathoracic volume and the movement of air into the tracheobronchial tree. **B,** The "bucket handle" motion of a sample single rib during inspiration and expiration.

Figure 1-19 DIAPHRAGM. Superior surface. The eighth rib is shown posteriorly, and the costal margin is left intact anteriorly to show the attachment of the diaphragm to it. The inferior vena cava traverses the diaphragm at vertebral level T8. Posteriorly, the esophageal hiatus and the aortic hiatus are shown. They traverse the diaphragm at vertebral levels T10 and T12, respectively.

SEE ATLAS, FIG. 1-34

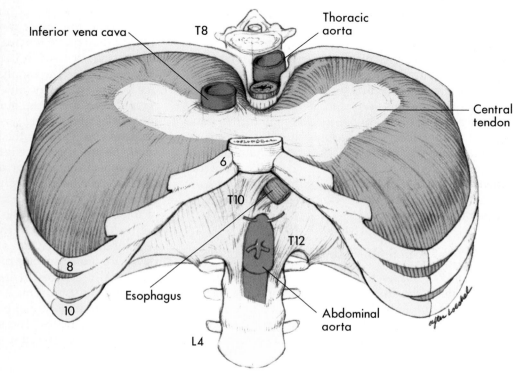

Inferior vena cava

T8

Thoracic aorta

Central tendon

Esophagus

Abdominal aorta

L4

PRINCIPLES

■ *HOW DOES AIR ENTER THE LUNGS?*

The musculoskeletal anatomy of the thoracic cage makes it possible for the dimensions of the ribcage to increase. Momentarily, this creates a subatmospheric pressure within the trachea and proximal bronchial tree. Almost immediately, air is "sucked" into the large airways and ultimately into the lungs. Because subatmospheric pressure draws air into the lungs, the cells and tissues lining the airways are not subjected to high pressures during respiration. This lessens the chance that any pressure-related injury to the lining of the airway might occur. In the great majority of respirators, however, the air is delivered by positive pressure (like air being pushed into the lungs with a bellows), and the incidence of pressure-related injury is high. This risk is one of the major limitations to the use of positive pressure ventilation in patients with serious lung disease.

capacity draws air into the lungs. Normal *quiet inspiration* is carried out largely by the diaphragm. If *forceful inspiration* is required, the intercostal muscles are recruited, starting with those in the inferior four to six intercostal spaces and adding those more superior with increasing degrees of effort. Any other muscle that elevates the ribcage can function as an **"accessory" muscle of respiration.** The *sternocleidomastoid, scalene, pectoralis minor,* and upper fibers of the *pectoralis major* muscles fall into this category. **Expiration** is normally passive, relying on elastic recoil of all the tissues that were moved as part of the inspiration. *Forceful expiration* is abetted by any muscle that depresses the ribs, thereby reducing the intrathoracic volume, or by any increase in intrathoracic pressure. The *internal intercostals* accomplish this by exerting a downward pull on the ribs. The *latissimus dorsi* muscle assists by exerting a downward pull on the humerus, which in turn is transmitted to the ribcage by various muscles linking the humerus and the chest wall. The abdominal wall muscles aid in forced expiration by (1) pulling the ribs downward and (2) increasing *intrabdominal pressure,* which in turn elevates the diaphragm and raises intrathoracic pressure.

BLOOD VESSELS OF THE CHEST WALL

The *arterial supply* to the chest wall arises in two main sources: the **intercostal vessels** and the various branches of the **subclavian** and **axillary arteries** that reach the chest. Each **intercostal artery** runs a roughly semicircular course, arising posteriorly (from different

sources; see following) and coursing around the chest wall to unite with the internal thoracic artery anteriorly (Figures 1-20 and 1-21). The component originating from the aorta (or other posterior source) is called the **posterior intercostal artery** and the component branching from the internal thoracic artery is known as the **anterior intercostal artery,** although in fact they form one single continuous vessel. Along its course each artery gives off several branches, supplying nearby muscles, connective tissues, bones, and skin. The *collateral supply* between intercostal spaces is so extensive that to produce ischemic injury to just one intercostal space, blood flow to that space and to several intercostal spaces superior and inferior to it would have to be obstructed.

The **origins** of the 12 intercostal arteries are subject to considerable variation. The **upper two intercostal arteries,** on both sides, usually arise from the left and right **superior intercostal arteries,** themselves branches of the **costocervical trunk** of the subclavian artery (Figure 1-22). These upper intercostal arteries arch posteriorly, drape over the apex of each lung, and then turn inferiorly to lie just anterior to the necks of ribs 1 and 2. Here vessels assume a position just inferior to the rib and course anteriorly around the chest wall as the **first** and **second intercostal arteries.** The second intercostal artery forms collateral connections with the **third intercostal artery.** Segmental arteries for the next nine intercostal spaces (i.e., *intercostal arteries 3 to 11*) arise from the thoracic (descending) aorta in pairs (one each for left and right side of the chest wall). The 12th intercostal artery lying inferior to the 12th rib, also arises from the aorta and is known as the **subcostal artery.** Because the aorta lies on the left side of the posterior thoracic wall, the lower nine *right intercostal arteries* are longer than the lower nine intercostal arteries on the left. As they move toward the right side, the right side intercostal arteries 3 to 12 pass anterior to the vertebrae but posterior to the esophagus, thoracic duct, and azygos veins. The lower nine *left intercostal arteries,* originating from the aorta, simply move laterally into the intercostal space, lying posterior to the hemiazygos and azygos veins. On both the left and right, the *sympathetic trunks* lie anterior to the intercostal arteries at all levels.

Moving from anterior to posterior, a series of separate arteries helps supply the chest wall. Each also forms anastomoses with intercostal arteries in the area of the chest supplied. The **internal thoracic artery** (see Figure 1-22) arises from the inferior surface of the first part of the subclavian artery and travels inferiorly down the inner surface of the chest wall, just deep to the costal cartilages. It lies about 1 cm lateral to the margin of the sternum. At the level of the sixth rib, it divides into its terminal **musculophrenic** and **superior epigastric** branches. The **superior thoracic artery** is a small branch of the first part of the axillary artery. It

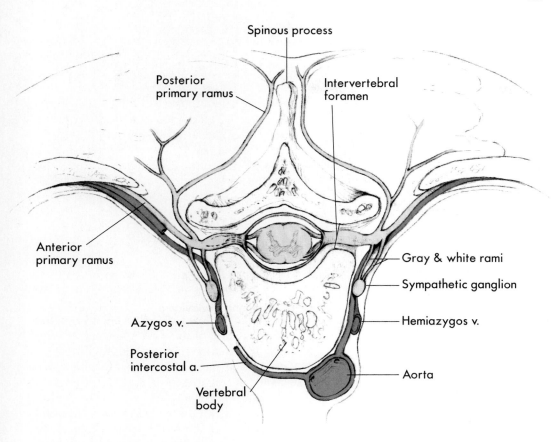

Spinous process

Posterior primary ramus

Intervertebral foramen

Anterior primary ramus

Gray & white rami

Sympathetic ganglion

Azygos v.

Hemiazygos v.

Posterior intercostal a.

Aorta

Vertebral body

Figure 1-20 TYPICAL THORACIC SPINAL CORD SEGMENT. Cross-section through a midthoracic segment of the vertebral column and spinal cord. Illustrated are the aorta, giving rise to posterior intercostal arteries for both sides of the chest wall; the azygos and hemiazygos veins, draining venous blood on each side of the chest wall; the paired sympathetic ganglia, from which arise communicating rami that supply axons to the segmental spinal nerves; and the spinal cord itself, illustrating its meningeal coverings and its protected location in the vertebral canal.

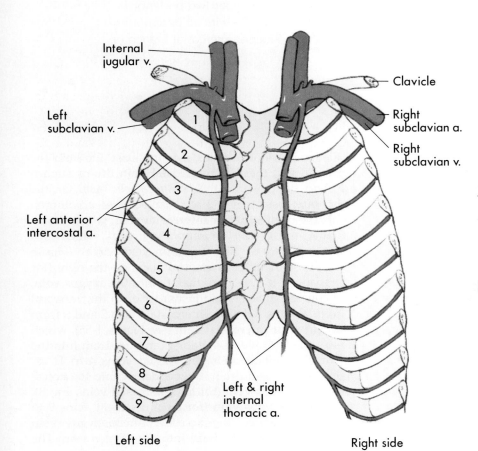

Internal jugular v.

Clavicle

Left subclavian v.

Right subclavian a.

Right subclavian v.

Left anterior intercostal a.

Left & right internal thoracic a.

Left side

Right side

Figure 1-21 INTERNAL THORACIC ARTERIES. Deep (interior) surface of the anterior thoracic wall. Descending along the lateral borders of the sternum are the internal thoracic arteries with anterior intercostal branches.

Sᴇᴇ Aᴛʟᴀs, Fɪɢs. 1-19, 1-20

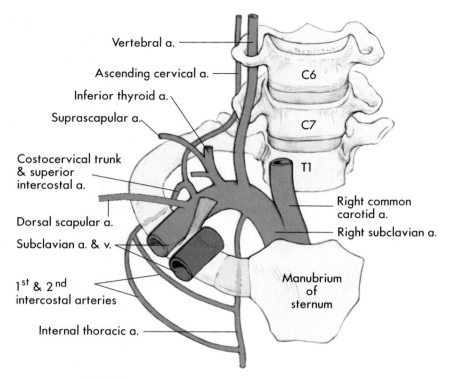

Vertebral a.

Ascending cervical a.

Inferior thyroid a.

Suprascapular a.

Costocervical trunk
& superior
intercostal a.

Dorsal scapular a.

Subclavian a. & v.

1ˢᵗ & 2ⁿᵈ
intercostal arteries

Internal thoracic a.

C6

C7

T1

Right common
carotid a.

Right subclavian a.

Manubrium
of
sternum

Figure 1-22   UPPER INTERCOSTAL ARTERIES. The origin of the upper two posterior intercostal arteries from the costocervical trunk is illustrated. As is true with all posterior intercostal arteries, there is an anterior anastomosis with the anterior intercostal branch of
the internal thoracic artery.

passes medial to the pectoralis minor and anastomoses
with the upper two to three intercostal arteries. The **lateral thoracic artery** is another branch of the axillary
artery, from its second part. It descends along the lateral border of the pectoralis minor and supplies many
muscles on the anterolateral chest wall. The lateral thoracic artery anastomoses with the internal thoracic,
subscapular, and intercostal arteries. In the female it
has an especially large branch supplying the breast.
The **subscapular artery,** arising from the third part of
the axillary artery, descends along the posterior axillary
wall parallel to the inferior border of the latissimus
dorsi. It anastomoses with many other arteries around
the scapula and with the lateral thoracic and intercostal
vessels as well. The **dorsal scapular artery** arises from
the subclavian artery, passes to the posterior side of the
trunk, and descends along the medial border of the
scapula, deep to the rhomboid muscles. It anastomoses
with the upper posterior intercostal arteries.

Eleven pairs of **intercostal veins** exist. On both the
right and left, the **first intercostal vein** drains superiorly and directly into the *brachiocephalic vein.* On the
right, intercostal veins 2 to 4 collect into a common
trunk, the **right superior intercostal vein,** which drains
into the *azygos vein* (an important vein, which is a
major tributary of the superior vena cava) (Figure
1-23). The remaining intercostal veins on the right (for
interspaces 5 to 11) drain directly into the **azygos vein,**
as it courses superior and just anterior to the vertebral
column. On the left side, intercostal veins 2 and 3 form
a **left superior intercostal vein** (see Figure 1-55), which
crosses the left side of the aortic arch to drain into the
left brachiocephalic vein. Intercostal veins 4 to 11 remain separate and drain independently into the **accessory hemiazygos vein** (for left intercostal veins 4 to 8),
or the **hemiazygos vein** (for left intercostal veins 9 to
11). In midthorax, the accessory hemiazygos vein
crosses the midline to drain into the azygos vein. The

CONNECTIONS BETWEEN ARTERIES

In many areas of the body, anastomoses exist when small branches of one artery allow blood flow into similar small branches of an adjacent but separate artery. If, for example, one artery is obstructed, its distal branches would receive no blood flow if it were not for the anastomotic branches of another artery, which are connected to the distal parts of the obstructed vessel and restore blood flow to it. Where anastomatic branches are numerous, the blood flow to vital organs is protected especially well, and injury to these organs resulting from obstruction to blood flow is rare. In other areas, however, where the anastomotic flow is not as abundant, obstruction of the principal blood flow to an organ is more likely to injure that organ. This is one of the factors in the high incidence of vascular injury to the heart and brain (heart attack, stroke), where anastomotic connections are unfortunately poor.

crosses the midline to drain into the azygos vein. The hemiazygos vein also crosses the midline to drain into the azygos vein or may instead first join the accessory hemiazygos vein. In this fashion, most of the venous drainage of both sides of the chest wall ultimately empties into the azygos vein.

INTERCOSTAL NERVES

Eleven pairs of **intercostal nerves** course between adjacent ribs, and the **subcostal nerves** course below each 12th rib. These nerves are the continuation of the ventral primary rami of thoracic segments of the spinal cord (see Figure 1-20). The intercostal nerves travel just inferior to the inferior margin of the rib, in the **costal groove** (see following and Figure 1-15). Each intercostal nerve contains somatic **sensory** and **motor axons** as well as **sympathetic axons** that innervate sweat glands, arrector pili muscles (for the elevation of hairs), and vascular smooth muscle. Each intercostal nerve innervates *deep* structures, such as the intercostal muscles, the lateral rim of the diaphragm, and the parietal pleura, and has *cutaneous branches* innervating the skin and superficial fasciae. Intercostal nerves 7 to 12 continue inferomedially to innervate the abdominal wall.

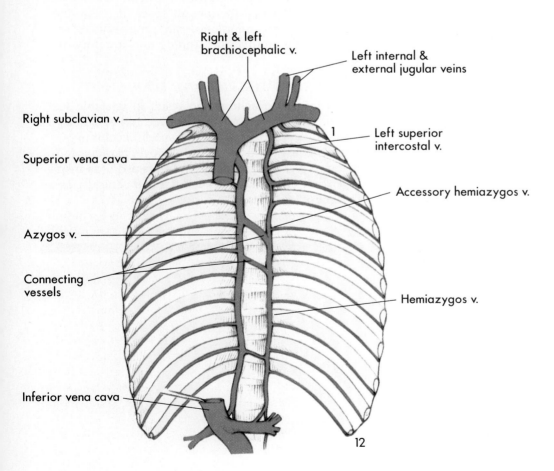

Right & left
brachiocephalic v.

Left internal &
external jugular veins

Right subclavian v.

Superior vena cava

1

Left superior
intercostal v.

Accessory hemiazygos v.

Azygos v.

Connecting
vessels

Hemiazygos v.

Inferior vena cava

12

Figure   1-23 AZYGOS AND HEMIAZYGOS VEINS. Most right intercostal veins drain into the azygos vein, which ascends just lateral to the midline to drain into the superior vena cava. Most of the left intercostal veins drain into the hemiazygos and accessory hemiazygos veins, which cross the midline and drain into the azygos vein.

THE CHEST WALL

DERMATOMES AND THE CHEST WALL

The area of the skin innervated by an individual intercostal nerve is known as the **dermatome** of that nerve. Each intercostal nerve innervates its own intercostal space but also supplies collateral branches to one to two intercostal spaces both above and below. Therefore complete local anesthesia of one intercostal space may require the injection of anesthetic into two to three intercostal spaces on each side of the space intended for anesthesia.

HERPES ZOSTER AND THE INTERCOSTAL SPACE

Shingles (herpes zoster) is an inflammatory disease producing a series of painful raised vesicles on the skin. The viruses causing this condition migrate to the skin along the small branches of peripheral nerves, and the pattern of skin vesicles recreates the dermatome of the particular nerve infected.

INTERCOSTAL NERVE BLOCKS

Intercostal block is intended to anesthetize intercostal nerves, in anticipation of performing minor surgery on some part of the thoracic wall (e.g., removal of a skin tag, sewing a laceration, or relief of pain in a rib fracture). The posterior angle of the rib is palpated, and the anesthetic introduced along the lower edge of the rib(s) selected. The aim is to bathe the intercostal nerve with the local anesthetic and eliminate sensation in the intercostal space anterior to this point. Remember that several intercostal nerves must be blocked to achieve real anesthesia in just one segment because of the presence of collateral branches.

REMOVING FLUID/AIR FROM THE PLEURAL SPACE

Thoracentesis is the placement of a needle or flexible tube through the chest wall and into the pleural space to remove air or fluid. The proper insertion of the needle or tube depends heavily on knowledge of the anatomy of the intercostal space, in order to minimize risk of injury to the intercostal nerves or vessels.

RIBS AND COLLATERAL BLOOD FLOW

Rib notching, which occurs because of the proximity of the ribs and the intercostal arteries, is underscored in conditions where blood flow through the aorta is diminished, and blood is shunted through various pathways of collateral flow, so that intended tissues are well perfused. Important among these collateral paths are the intercostal arteries, which in this situation experience much higher volumes of blood flow than normal. When this occurs, the vessels enlarge, so much so that they erode the bony structure of the ribs. On a chest x-ray, the smooth contour of the ribs is altered, and their edges appear irregular—an appearance known as "rib notching."

PNEUMOTHORAX

Fracture of the ribs can lead to **pneumothorax,** accumulation of air in the pleural space. If it is under pressure, the pneumothorax can progressively collapse the lung on that side, leading to respiratory distress.

FRACTURE OF THE RIBS AND FLAIL CHEST

Multiple rib fractures can result in unstable sections of one or more ribs, which are not attached to the sternum anteriorly or to the vertebral column posteriorly. These sections of ribs move paradoxically during respiration (i.e., they move inward with inspiration) and create a situation described clinically as a "flail chest."

CATEGORIZING PERIPHERAL NERVES

Peripheral nerves such as the intercostal nerves divide into branches, some of which innervate muscle (e.g., the intercostal muscles), while other branches innervate the skin and subcutaneous tissues. A common mistake is to refer to the former as "motor branches" and the latter as "sensory branches." In fact, both of the branches described contain **both motor** and **sensory axons.** A nerve branch to a muscle contains axons that innervate the muscle's fibers and cause their contraction (motor axons). The branch also contains sensory axons to receptors in the muscle tissue itself. The receptors are an important part of regulating the tone of the muscles. Better terms for the two types of nerves mentioned would be **muscular branches** and **cutaneous branches.**

INTERCOSTAL SPACE

The **intercostal space** is bounded by two ribs, a superior and an inferior. The external surface of the *superior rib* extends downward as a lip or ridge, just posterior to which is the **costal groove,** into which the intercostal nerve is settled (see Figure 1-15). The superior surface of the *inferior rib* is rounded and smooth, with no grooves or other specializations. In the intercostal space, the neurovascular bundle (intercostal vein, artery, and nerve) is positioned between the innermost and the internal intercostal muscle layers. The *intercostal nerve* is in the most inferior position in the costal groove, the *intercostal artery* is immediately superior to the nerve, and the *intercostal vein* is superior to the artery (see Figure 1-15). All three structures have *lateral cutaneous branches,* which emerge into the superficial fascia in approximately the midaxillary line. Further anterior is an *anterior cutaneous branch,* which reaches the superficial fascia just lateral to the sternum. These cutaneous vascular branches anastomose with each other and afford protection for the intercostal arteries and veins against the interruption of flow should there be any trauma or other injury to an individual vessel along its course. Lymphatics are present in each intercostal space and drain anteriorly to the internal thoracic chain of nodes, communicating with the breast and axilla, or posteriorly to the posterior mediastinal nodes.

Pleural Spaces, Tracheobronchial Tree, and Lungs

▶ Serous Cavities and Pleural Spaces of the Lung

▶ Trachea

▶ Lungs

▶ Blood Vessels and Lymphatics of the Lungs

▶ Innervation of the Lungs and Pleurae

*T*he respiratory system begins at the nose and extends downward to the deepest recesses of the lungs. Those portions of the respiratory tract lying above the level of the vocal cords are said to comprise the *upper respiratory tract;* those below the cords comprise the *lower respiratory tract.* Parts of the respiratory tract (e.g., the pharynx) are *aerodigestive* because they are also involved in digestive functions. Important muscular mechanisms exist to ensure that ingested solids and liquids do not enter the lower respiratory tract and that inspired and exhaled air do not enter the esophagus. The close relationship of the digestive and respiratory tracts is underscored by the common embryologic origins of many of their organs.

SEROUS CAVITIES AND PLEURAL SPACES OF THE LUNG

The lung is covered, over most of its surface, by a thin and smooth membrane, the **visceral pleura.** On the medial surface of the lung, at the **hilum** (L., a little thing) this smooth membrane reflects away from the surface of the lung and folds back to line the internal surface of the cavity in which the lung is suspended (Figure 1-24; see also Figure 1-2). This latter layer is known as the **parietal pleura** and covers the inner surface of the chest wall, the superior surface of the diaphragm, and the lateral surface of the mediastinum. Specialized regions of the **parietal pleural** membrane are named for the structures they cover. The **mediastinal pleura** covers the lateral surface of the mediastinum. The **diaphragmatic pleura** covers the superior surface of the diaphragm. The **costal pleura** lines the internal surface of the ribcage. The most superior portion of the pleural membrane, the **cervical pleura,** or dome of the pleura, extends 1 to 2 cm into the neck above the level of the clavicle and first rib. All of these portions of the parietal pleura are, of course, continuous with each other (see Figure 1-2).

The visceral and parietal pleurae are continuous with each other at the hilum, where a slightly elongated "collar" of pleura forms. Encircled by this collar are the structures that connect the lung to the mediastinum: the pulmonary and bronchial vessels, the air-

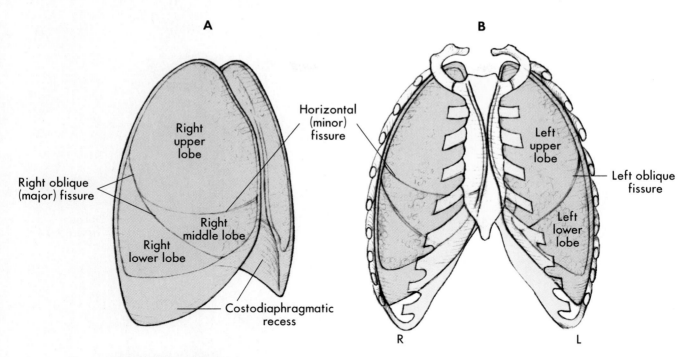

Figure 1-24 LUNGS AND PLEURAL SACS. A, Right anterior oblique view, in which the pleural sacs are represented as transparent membranes through which can be seen the lungs (shown in pink). **B,** Pleural sacs and lungs viewed anteriorly, with the sternum and parts of the ribs shown.

ways, nerves, lymphatics, and the connective tissue (Figure 1-25). A small inferior extension of this pleural collar is known as the **pulmonary ligament,** and, in the living, it may be palpated during surgery as a firm shelf of tissue on the medial surface of the lung. The **pleural cavity** is the potential space between the visceral and parietal pleurae.

Inferolaterally on each side of the chest, where the lateral edge of the diaphragm meets the chest wall, is the **costodiaphragmatic (costophrenic) recess** (Figure 1-26). This recess is very lucent (i.e., dark) on an x-ray when the lung expands fully to fill it; at expiration, however, the lung recedes upward and the diaphragm and chest wall move near to each other once again, and the lucency disappears. If, however, a patient has blood or inflammatory fluid in the pleural cavity, the fluid flows down into this recess, and in such a patient's x-ray at inspiration the angle is "blunted" by the accumulated fluid. There is another normally widened area of the pleural cavity anterior to the heart, on the left side, known as the **costomediastinal recess** (see Figure 1-26). It becomes lucent at inspiration when the *lingula* of the left lung expands into it.

THE PLEURAL SPACE

SUBSTANCES ABNORMALLY FILLING THE PLEURAL SPACE

When air accumulates in the pleural cavity it is known as **pneumothorax,** and the air can compress portions of the lung and impair respiration. When blood accumulates the condition is known as **hemothorax,** and when lymph accumulates (usually as the result of injury to the thoracic duct), it is known as a **chylothorax.** In each of these cases, a tube often must be inserted through the chest wall into the pleural space to evacuate the accumulated material.

PLEURITIS

Inflammation of the pleural membranes is known as **pleuritis.** When it involves the visceral pleural layer alone, it may cause little pain, but if the costal or diaphragmatic pleurae are involved, the patient experiences sharp pain. Pleuritis may be detected with the stethoscope as a rough grating sound (a "pleural rub") heard when the inflamed pleural membranes scrape against each other during inspiration-expiration.

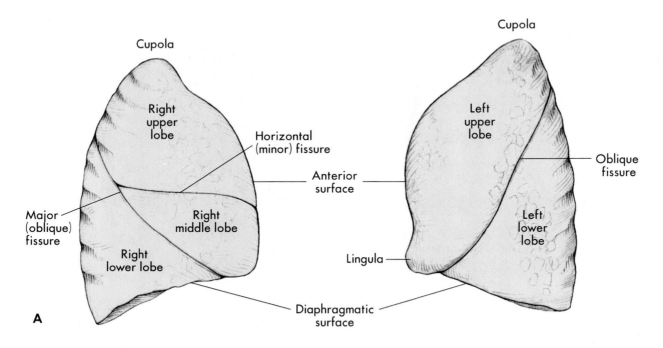

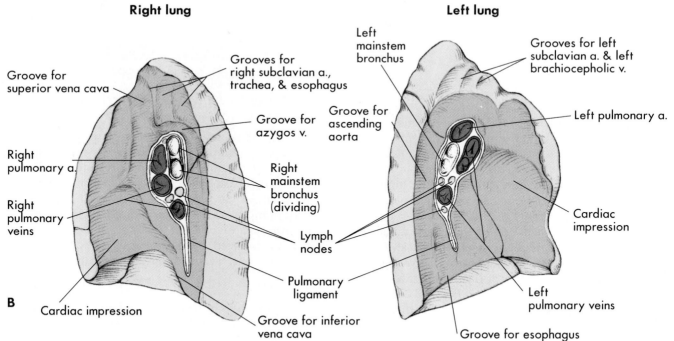

Figure 1-25   RIGHT AND LEFT LUNGS. A, Lateral views of the right and left lungs. **B,** Medial views of the same. The medial views of each lung illustrate the pulmonary ligament, a downwardly extending double fold of pleura. SEE ATLAS, FIGS. 1-23 TO 1-28

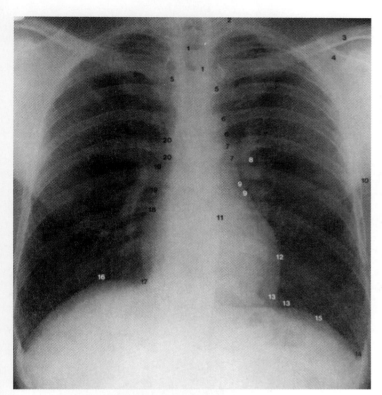

Figure 1-26   RADIOGRAPHIC ANATOMY OF THE LUNGS. Note the costodiaphragmatic (costophrenic) recess and costomediastinal recess. (From Weir J, Abrahams PH: *An imaging atlas of human anatomy,* London, 1992, Mosby.)

1	Trachea	12	Left ventricle
5	Sternum	13	Costomediastinal recess
6	Aortic knob or knuckle	14	Costodiaphragmatic
7	Lateral margin of pul-		(costophrenic) angle
	monary trunk	15	Left diaphragm
9	Edge of left atrial ap-	16	Right diaphragm
	pendage	18	Right atrial border
11	Left edge of descending	19	Right pulmonary artery
	aorta	20	Superior vena cava

TRACHEA

The **trachea** commences in the neck just inferior to the **cricoid cartilage,** usually opposite the C6 vertebra, and descends inferiorly through the thoracic inlet into the superior mediastinum. At the level of the inferior border of the T4 vertebra, it divides into the left and right mainstem bronchi (Figure 1-27; see also Figure 1-28).

The trachea is capable of elongation, as must occur when the larynx is elevated as part of swallowing or changes in the pitch of the voice. It is almost perfectly vertical as it descends into the chest. The trachea is composed of a series of U-shaped cartilages, open posteriorly. These posterior gaps in the tracheal cartilages are filled by the **trachealis** muscle, making the trachea a closed cylinder, flattened posteriorly. Most of the muscle fibers of the trachealis are transverse, so that its contraction diminishes the cross-sectional area of the trachea. Some striated fibers are present in the upper trachea, but the majority of the trachealis muscle is made up of smooth muscle cells. The trachealis muscle is innervated by the *vagus nerve* through its recurrent laryngeal branch.

The entire trachea is lined by **pseudostratified ciliated columnar epithelium** and **goblet cells,** typical of the respiratory system. Cilia on the surface of the epithelial cells are important in transporting mucus upward toward the mouth, where it may be swallowed or expectorated. The upper 2 to 3 cm of the trachea lie just beneath the skin and are easily palpable. In the lower neck and upper mediastinum, the **thyroid gland** lies anterior to the trachea. Posterior to the trachea is the esophagus, and lateral to it are the recurrent laryngeal nerves and the lateral lobes of the thyroid gland. Deeper in the thorax, in the superior mediastinum, the trachea lies posterior to the sternum and remains anterior to the esophagus; to its left is the aortic arch and to its right is the azygos vein. Just superior to these, the apex of each lung and surrounding pleurae lie posterolateral to the trachea.

The **bifurcation of the trachea** occurs opposite the lower margin of the T4 vertebra. Looking down the lumen of the trachea from above, the **carina** (L. keel) a raised ridge of tissue in the sagittal plane, marking the bifurcation of the trachea into the right and left mainstem bronchi can be seen. The right and left mainstem bronchi enter the hila (roots) of their respective lungs and divide into **lobar bronchi,** which in turn divide into **segmental bronchi.** The segmental bronchi, which represent the third order of branching from the trachea, aerate regions of the lungs referred to as the **bronchopulmonary segments** (Table 1-3).

The **right mainstem bronchus** is shorter than the **left mainstem bronchus.** It also turns to the right at a shallower angle (see Figure 1-27) than the left mainstem bronchus, which turns more sharply to the left.

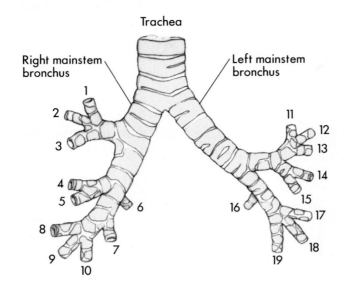

A

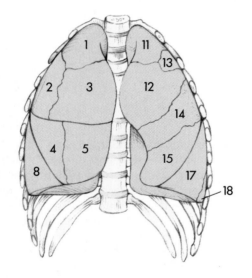

B

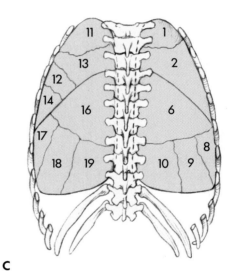

C

Figure 1-27 TRACHEA AND BRONCHOPULMONARY SEGMENTS. Bronchopulmonary segments are defined as those regions of lung tissue aerated by a tertiary bronchus (i.e., a third-generation branch of the trachea). **A,** Third-order branches of the tracheobronchial tree and anterior (**B**) and posterior (**C**) views of the lungs with the borders of the bronchopulmonary segments sketched in.

SEE ATLAS, FIG. 1-29

1 Apical segment, right upper lobe
2 Posterior segment, right upper lobe
3 Anterior segment, right upper lobe
4 Lateral segment, right middle lobe
5 Medial segment, right middle lobe
6 Superior segment, right lower lobe
7 Medial basal segment, right lower lobe (not seen)
8 Anterior basal segment, right lower lobe
9 Lateral basal segment, right lower lobe
10 Posterior basal segment, right lower lobe

11 Apical segment, left upper lobe
12 Anterior segment, left upper lobe
13 Posterior segment, left upper lobe
14 Superior lingular segment, left upper lobe
15 Inferior lingular segment, left upper lobe
16 Superior segment, left lower lobe
17 Anterior basal segment, left lower lobe
18 Medial basal segment, left lower lobe
19 Lateral basal and posterior basal segments, left lower lobe

THE AIRWAYS

OBSTRUCTION OF THE LARGE AND SMALL AIRWAYS

Different pathologic conditions affect the large (trachea, proximal bronchi) vs. the small (distal bronchi, bronchioles) airways. The larger airways are subject to obstruction by aspirated objects or by lesions that grow within the lumen of the airway (tumor, hemangioma, etc.). The small airways are more commonly obstructed by mucus or are narrowed by contraction of smooth muscle.

ASTHMA OR "REACTIVE AIRWAYS DISEASE (RAD)"

One of the most common varieties of respiratory disturbance is narrowing of the small airways, by either mucus plugging, smooth muscle contraction, or both. Relief is sought by patients by either aerosolized fluids to loosen the mucus, or a variety of medications that relax the bronchiolar smooth muscle, increasing airway diameter and allowing easier airflow.

VASCULAR SHUNTING WITHIN THE LUNGS

When segments of the lung are diseased and alveoli are filled with inflammatory fluid or otherwise dysfunctional, the alveolar capillary beds are often closed or at least resistant to normal blood flow. In these conditions, the degree of **intrapulmonary shunting** increases. This accounts, in part, for a patient's need for increased amounts of oxygen when suffering from such pulmonary diseases (because a certain increased fraction of the blood flowing to the lungs returns to the left atrium without being oxygenated). If such shunts did not exist, however, then blood pumped from the right ventricle could not flow easily through the lungs, and might "back-up" in the pulmonary arteries or the heart itself.

PERFORMING A TRACHEOTOMY

Tracheotomy may be performed through the anterior surface of the upper trachea, between the first and second or second and third tracheal rings, between the upper margin of the thyroid isthmus and the larynx. Further inferior, the great veins lie just anterior to the trachea. The successful and safe performance of an emergency tracheotomy depends on understanding the proximity of both the thyroid gland and the great veins and avoiding the catastrophic hemorrhage that would result if they were lacerated.

Table 1-3   Bronchopulmonary Segments

Lung	Upper Lobe	Middle Lobe	Lower Lobe
Right lung	Apical Posterior Anterior	Medial Lateral	Superior Medial basal Anterior basal Lateral basal Posterior basal
Left lung	Apical Posterior Anterior Superior lingular Inferior lingular	(No middle lobe; equivalent bronchi in lingula of upper lobe)	Superior Medial basal Anterior basal Lateral basal Posterior basal

Because the right mainstem bronchus is more nearly parallel to the trachea than is the left mainstem bronchus, it is often said that foreign objects aspirated into the trachea are more likely to lodge in the right mainstem bronchus than in the left, but in practice aspirated objects may lodge literally anywhere in the proximal tracheobronchial tree.

The **right upper lobe bronchus** is found about 2 cm from the origin of the right mainstem bronchus and turns superolaterally at a sharp angle. The **azygos vein** arches over it, from posterior to anterior, and the **right pulmonary artery** lies anterior to it and parallels the course of the bronchus. It divides, in turn, into the *apical, anterior,* and *posterior* segmental bronchi. The right mainstem bronchus continues on past the takeoff of the right upper lobe bronchus and is often called the **bronchus intermedius** at this point. The **right middle lobe bronchus** arises on the anterior surface of the bronchus intermedius and extends in a lateral direction, where it soon divides into *lateral* and *medial segmental bronchi.* Continuing inferolaterally is the *right lower lobe bronchus,* which ends by dividing into five segmental bronchi—the *superior,* the *medial basal,* the *anterior basal,* the *lateral basal,* and the *posterior basal.* Particularly in the case of the right lower lobe bronchus, variability in the pattern of segmental branching is considerable (see Figure 1-27).

The **left mainstem bronchus** is somewhat narrower and a good deal longer (5 to 6 cm) than the right mainstem bronchus. It slopes laterally at a slightly sharper angle than does the right. The *pulmonary trunk* lies anterior to the origin of the left mainstem bronchus. The *left pulmonary artery* arches over the bronchus as it moves laterally. The *esophagus* lies posterior to the origin of the left mainstem bronchus, and the *descending aorta* is posterior to the middle portion of the left mainstem bronchus. The *left upper lobe bronchus* arises about 4 to 5 cm distal to the origin of the left mainstem bronchus. It turns superolaterally at a sharp angle and soon divides into its segmental branches—the apical-posterior (sometimes recognized as two separate bronchi), the anterior, the superior lingular, and the inferior lingular. The *left lower lobe bronchus* continues inferolaterally past the origin of the left upper lobe bronchus, for a total length of 4 to 5 cm. About midway along its course, the *superior segmental bronchus* arises from the medial surface of the left lower lobe bronchus. The bronchus then travels the remaining 2 to 3 cm of its total length before terminating as the *medial basal,* the *anterior basal,* the *lateral basal,* and the *posterior basal* segmental bronchi. As on the right, the branching of the left lower lobe segmental bronchi is particularly subject to variation.

LUNGS

Each lung is shaped roughly like a cone, with a concave inferior surface facing the upper surface of the diaphragm, an **apex** (protruding above the level of the first rib and clavicle into the base of the neck), a semicircular **costal surface** facing the inner surface of the ribcage, and a **mediastinal surface** facing medially. Each lung also has a **hilum** where branches of the tracheobronchial tree and vascular, lymphatic, neural, and other tissues enter and leave the lung (see Figure 1-25). The lung is covered by the visceral pleura, (continuous at the hilum with the parietal pleura), which lines the pleural cavity in which each lung is suspended. On full expansion, the lungs fill the **costodiaphragmatic recesses** in both pleural spaces and the **costomediastinal recess** (found on the left side only).

The functional unit of the lung is the **alveolus;** each adult lung contains many millions of alveoli. The alveolus is a tiny saccule to which inspired air is delivered, after traversing the many branches of the tracheobronchial tree. The wall of the alveolus is very thin and permits the exchange of gases between its lumen and nearby capillaries. In the spaces between alveoli are blood vessels, nerves, lymphatics, lymph nodes, and connective tissue.

Pulmonary Hilum

All of the vascular, neural, and other connective tissue elements reaching the lung do so by traveling through the *pulmonary hilum,* a roughly circular region on the medial surface of the lung surrounded by a collar of pleura (see Figure 1-25). At the hilum the visceral pleura is continuous with the parietal pleura (see preceding discussion). The pulmonary hilum is usually located opposite the bodies of vertebrae T5 to T7. In general, at the hilum, the *pulmonary artery* and its branches are most superior, the *bronchi* and its branches are intermediate and posterior, and the *pulmonary veins* are inferior. The hilum also contains autonomic nerves, lymphatics, tracheobronchial lymph nodes, and the bronchial vessels.

Right Lung

The right lung is slightly larger than the left lung and has three lobes, whereas the left lung has two (see Figure 1-25). Fissures incompletely separate the three lobes and are lined by extensions of the visceral pleura covering the lung. The **oblique (major) fissure** of the right lung is a deep, flat, and narrow cleft, originating at the level of the T3 vertebra posteriorly and extending anterolaterally along a line just deep to the fifth intercostal space. Thus the "upper" lobe of the right lung is in fact superior and anterior, and the "lower" lobe is in fact inferior and posterior. The plane of the major fissure passes through the pulmonary hilum. In the right lung but not the left is a smaller **horizontal (minor) fissure,** beginning at the level of the hilum on the medial side of the lung and extending across the lung to intersect the oblique fissure at the lateral margin of the lung. Just inferior to the horizontal fissure is the right middle lobe, bounded superiorly by the horizontal fissure and inferiorly by the anterior limb of the major fissure.

The **surfaces** of the right lung are closely related to various structures, which cause impressions on the lung of the preserved cadaver. On the **costal surface** are found impressions of the ribs, on the **diaphragmatic surface** an impression of the dome of the diaphragm, on the medial surface of the **apex** impressions for the superior vena cava, subclavian artery, trachea, and upper esophagus from anterior to posterior). On the **medial surface** are impressions of the azygos vein (superior to the hilum), central part of the esophagus (posterior), the cardiac impression (anterior), and the inferior vena cava (inferior and just anterior to the pulmonary ligament) (see Figure 1-25).

Left Lung

The **left lung** has only an **oblique fissure,** similar to the right lung, but lacks a horizontal fissure and, therefore, a middle lobe (see Figure 1-25). The oblique fissure of the left lung is more nearly vertical than the oblique fissure of the right lung, and, as on the right, is an incomplete fissure lined by visceral pleura. Like the right lung, the left lung's *upper lobe* is anterosuperior and its *lower lobe* posteroinferior. The upper lobe, at the inferior end of its anteromedial edge, has a small semicircular *cardiac notch* representing the point where the lateral border of the left ventricle and its pericardial covering abut the left lung and its pleural covering. Just inferior to the cardiac notch is a small process, the **lingula,** extending medially in front of the heart. The lingula represents two segments of the left upper lobe and is comparable embryologically to the middle lobe of the right lung.

In the preserved cadaver, the **costal** and **diaphragmatic** surfaces of the left lung show impressions similar to these surfaces on the right lung, and on its medial apical surface are impressions for the left common carotid and left subclavian arteries. On its **medial** surface, the preserved left lung shows a large concave *cardiac impression* anteroinferior to the hilum, a small impression for the *thymus* anterosuperiorly, and a groove for the *aortic arch* just superior to the hilum. It also shows a long and deep groove for the *desending aorta* posterior to a hilum and a small groove for the distal *esophagus* inferiorly, just posterior to the pulmonary ligament (see Figure 1-25).

BLOOD VESSELS AND LYMPHATICS OF THE LUNGS

The **arterial vascular supply** bringing blood to the lungs is of two varieties: (1) the **pulmonary arteries,** which deliver blood to the alveoli, where exchange of O_2 and CO_2 can occur (Figure 1-28) and (2) several small branches of the aorta, the **bronchial arteries** (Figure 1-29). The blood of the **bronchial arteries** is delivered to capillary beds surrounding the tracheobronchial tree, the connective tissue septae, and the tissue at or near the hilum of the lung (Figure 1-29). The bronchial arteries are two to five in number, arise from the anterior surface of the descending aorta, and enter the pulmonary hila directly.

By far the largest fraction of the blood flow, the *deoxygenated pulmonary arterial blood,* is delivered through the **pulmonary arteries** (Figure 1-30; see also Figure 1-28) and their numerous branches to the capillary beds surrounding the alveoli. The structure of the *pulmonary trunk* and *main pulmonary arteries* is described on pp. 96-97. In the pulmonary hilum, the pulmonary arteries lie in an anterior and superior position. Once within the substance of the lung, the pattern of branching for the pulmonary arteries closely follows that of the right and left bronchi.

Figure 1-28 BRANCHES OF THE PULMONARY ARTERY. The pulmonary artery (*PA*) divides, within the concavity of the aortic arch, into the right and left pulmonary arteries (*RPA, LPA*). The left pulmonary artery is draped over the left mainstem bronchus, and the right pulmonary artery is anterior to the right mainstem bronchus. Subsequent branches of the pulmonary artery mimic those of the tracheobronchial tree.

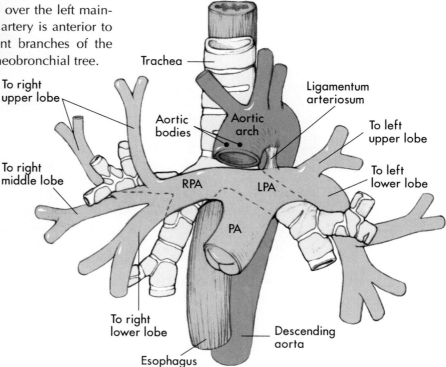

Figure 1-29 ESOPHAGEAL AND BRONCHIAL ARTERIES. The upper part of the descending aorta gives rise to a small number of individual arteries supplying the bronchial tree and the esophagus.

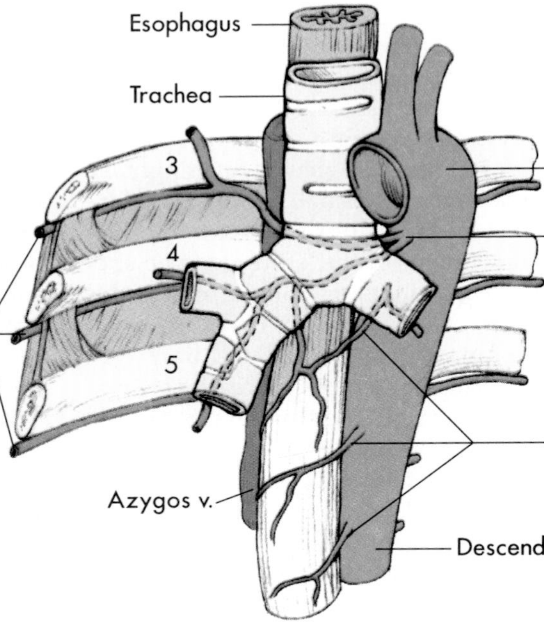

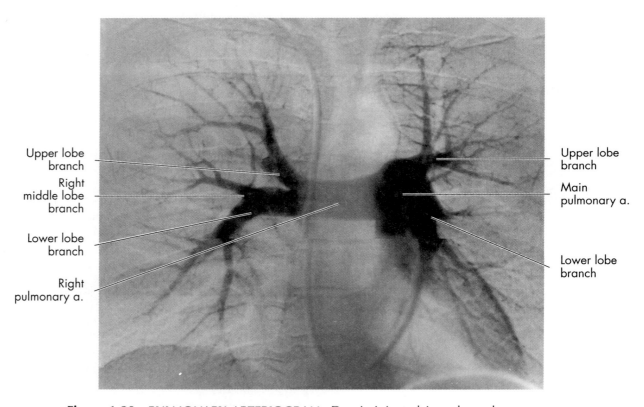

Figure 1-30 PULMONARY ARTERIOGRAM. Dye is injected into the pulmonary artery by passing a catheter through the great veins and into the right atrium, right ventricle, and out past the pulmonary valve into the proximal pulmonary artery. An x-ray exposure is then made just after the dye is injected, and the pulmonary vascular tree is imaged. With this technique, clinicians can discover if any major branches of the pulmonary artery are obstructed. (From Weir J. Abrahams PH: *An imaging atlas of human anatomy,* London, 1992, Mosby.)

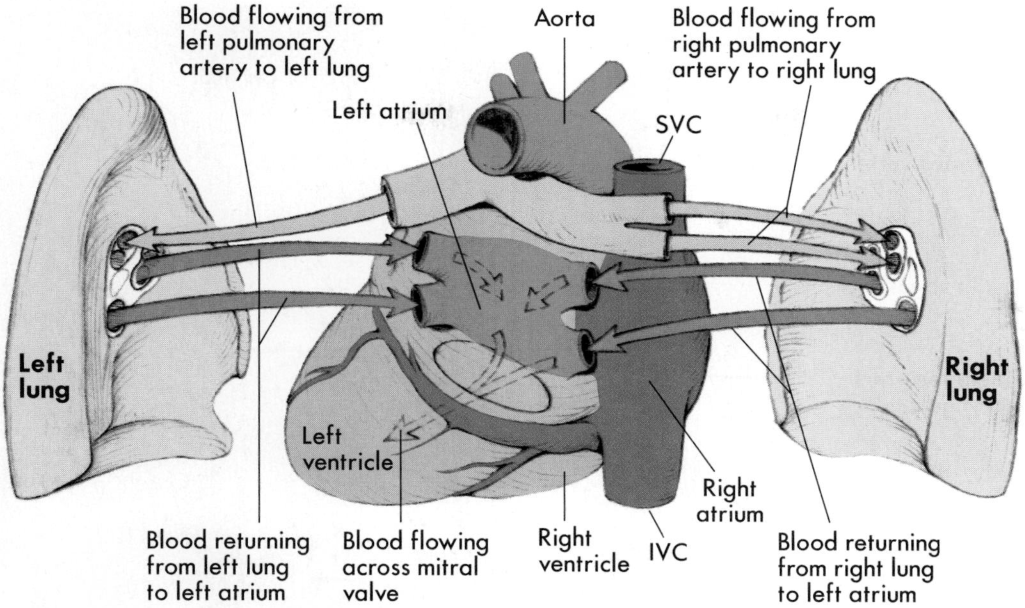

Figure 1-31   BLOOD FLOW BETWEEN THE LUNGS AND HEART, POSTERIOR VIEW. The pulmonary artery delivers deoxygenated blood to the lungs (*blue arrows*). It is returned to the heart via the four pulmonary veins (*red arrows*). Once in the left atrium, the blood traverses the mitral valve to enter the left ventricle (*dashed arrows*).

Pulmonary venous flow returns oxygenated blood to the heart through the four **pulmonary veins** (see Figures 1-31, 1-35, 1-39). The pulmonary veins, in contrast to the pulmonary arteries, do *not* follow the branching of the airways faithfully, and veins may even cross between bronchopulmonary segments. One pulmonary vein drains each of the five lobes of the lungs, but the veins from the right upper and middle lobes usually unite so that there are two pulmonary veins from each lung entering the left atrium (see Figure 1-31). In the pulmonary hilum, the pulmonary veins lie in an anterior and inferior position.

CLINICAL ANATOMY OF

THE PULMONARY VASCULATURE

HIGH PRESSURE IN THE PULMONARY VASCULATURE

Several pathologic conditions can lead to **pulmonary hypertension,** a situation of abnormally high resistance in the pulmonary artery and arterioles and subsequent inadequate oxygenation of blood. A pulmonary embolism in the main pulmonary artery produces major obstruction to blood flow and is often fatal.

PRINCIPLES

VASCULAR SHUNTING WITHIN THE LUNGS

A substantial number of **arteriovenous shunts** are present within the lungs, especially near the terminal and respiratory bronchioles. These small "shunt vessels" directly connect branches of the pulmonary artery and tributaries of the pulmonary veins. The shunt vessels have in their walls a layer of smooth muscle which, by contracting or relaxing, regulates the amount of blood flowing through these shunt vessels. When segments of the lung are diseased, and alveoli are filled with inflammatory fluid or otherwise are dysfunctional, blood flow to these areas does not result in gas exchange. Through local release of vasoactive substances, the alveolar capillary beds are often closed or at least resistant to normal blood flow. In such disease states, the shunt vessels in these areas relax, allowing a large fraction of the blood to bypass the diseased alveoli. This accounts, in part, for a patient's need for increased amounts of oxygen when suffering from such pulmonary diseases (because an increased fraction of the blood flowing to the lungs bypasses the alveoli and returns to the left atrium without being oxygenated).

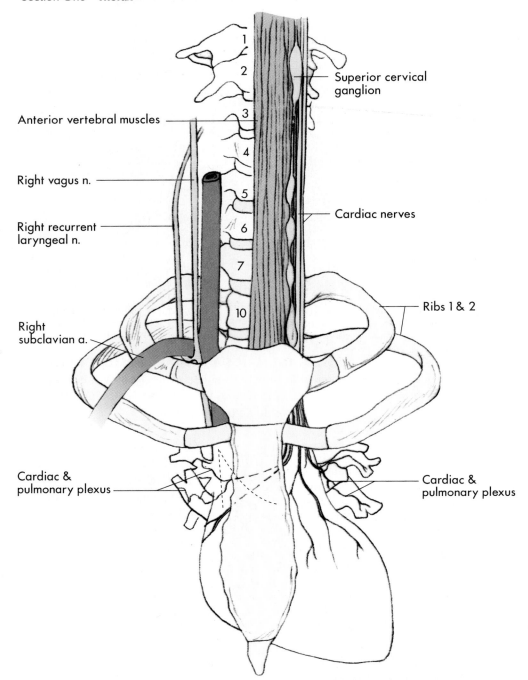

Anterior vertebral muscles

Right vagus n.

Right recurrent
laryngeal n.

Right
subclavian a.

Cardiac &
pulmonary plexus

Superior cervical
ganglion

Cardiac nerves

Ribs 1 & 2

Cardiac &
pulmonary plexus

Figure 1-32 AUTONOMIC INNERVATION OF THE LUNGS AND HEART. On the right
side is the vagus nerve, descending through the neck to enter the thorax. Its recurrent laryngeal branch loops under the right subclavian artery. Branches also descend from the
neck into the mediastinum and become part of the pulmonary and cardiac plexuses. On
the left, the cervical sympathetic chain is shown descending on the surface of the anterior vertebral muscles. Branches of these ganglia, or cardiac nerves, enter the chest and
also become part of the pulmonary and cardiac plexuses.

Some arterial blood from the **bronchial arteries** (see
Figure 1-29), especially that destined for tissues deep
within the lung, is returned to the heart through the
pulmonary veins; thus there is a slight diminution in the
overall degree of oxygenation of pulmonary venous

blood. The remainder of blood taken to the lung by the
bronchial arteries drains, through **bronchial veins,**
back to the azygos, superior intercostal, or accessory
hemiazygos veins.

Pulmonary **lymphatics** are of two main varieties.

THE LUNGS AND PLEURAE

ALVEOLAR DISEASE

Pulmonary diseases affect primarily the alveoli causing the exudation of inflamatory fluid into the alveoli, making gas exchange impossible. Such diseases are **pneumonia** or **pneumonitis.**

BRONCHOGENIC CYST

Bronchogenic cyst is a cavity, not continuous with the airways, found within the lung. It is subject to infection and, when it enlarges, can cause collapse of nearby healthy lung tissue. Such a cyst is usually removed surgically.

TRACHEOESOPHAGEAL FISTULA

Tracheoesophageal fistula is a developmental abnormality producing improper separation of the trachea and esophagus (which have a common embryologic origin). There are many specific types; they can result in the spilling of esophageal and gastric contents into the trachea and lungs. In addition, there may form an obstruction preventing food and liquid from passing from mouth and pharynx to the stomach.

PULMONARY SEQUESTRATION

Pulmonary sequestration is a mass of tissue within the lung (or sometimes just adjacent to it), usually in one of the lower lobes, which receives its blood supply from a branch of the aorta, not from the pulmonary or bronchial arteries. In addition, the sequestered segment is usually not connected to the tracheobronchial tree.

BRONCHOSCOPY

Bronchoscopy is a technique of inserting a hollow, cylindrical instrument down through the trachea and out into the larger bronchi. If a flexible instrument is used, even more distal parts of the airway can be viewed. Tissue biopsies, removal of foreign objects, viewing anatomic abnormalities, and removal of mucus samples for diagnosis are just some of the uses of bronchoscopy.

ATELECTASIS

Atelectasis is the collapse of alveolar sacs so that they may not be inflated during inspiration. This often results from an inflammation of the alveoli, leading to a deficiency in **surfactant,** the "soapy" surface active material that makes inflation of alveoli much easier than in its absence.

The *superficial network* of lymphatics located just beneath the visceral pleura creates a reticulated appearance to the lung when inhaled carbon particles are trapped within them. Both this system and a *deeper system* of lung lymphatic channels drain to the **tracheobronchial nodes** and **hilar lymph nodes.**

INNERVATION OF THE LUNGS AND PLEURAE

Nerve supply to the lung is *autonomic* and is mainly devoted to the regulation of mucus secretion and to the regulation of the diameter of bronchioles by contraction or relaxation of smooth muscle in their walls. The lungs are supplied with both **sympathetic** and **parasympathetic** nerves. The postganglionic *sympathetic nerves* have their cell bodies in the superior cervical ganglion. Axons from these neurons, the **cardiac nerves,** descend through the neck and mediastinum and enter the hilum of the lung (Figure 1-32). *Parasympathetic nerves* arise from small ganglia within the substance of the lungs. The vagus nerves are the source of preganglionic parasympathetic input to these small ganglia. All of these axons take part in the formation of the anterior and posterior *pulmonary plexuses* at the hilum of the lung. The sympathetic innervation produces *dilation* of the bronchioles. In fact, many drugs used to treat asthma are designed to mimic or stimulate the sympathetic nerves supplying the lungs, thus opening the small airways and improving breathing. The parasympathetic nerves have the effect of constricting the bronchioles and increasing the amount of airway mucus. Drugs blocking the parasympathetic effect are also used to treat asthma.

1.4

Heart

▶ Pericardial Sac

▶ Position and Orientation of the Heart

▶ Fibrous Skeleton of the Heart

▶ Blood Vessels of the Heart

▶ Right Atrium

▶ Tricuspid Valve

▶ Right Ventricle

▶ Pulmonary Valve

▶ Pulmonary Artery

▶ Pulmonary Veins

▶ Left Atrium

▶ Mitral Valve

▶ Left Ventricle

▶ Aortic Valve

▶ Ascending Aorta

▶ Blood Flow Through the Heart

▶ Cardiac Conduction System

▶ Innervation of the Heart

▶ Fetal Circulation

*T*he **heart** is a muscular organ whose role is to circulate blood throughout the body. The heart is responsible for two pathways of circulation, which are in series with each other. The **right side of the heart** (right atrium, right ventricle, and pulmonary arteries) is responsible for delivering systemic venous blood to the lungs, where the blood releases CO_2 to the exhaled air and is replenished with O_2. The **left side of the heart** (the left atrium, left ventricle, and aorta) is responsible for delivering oxygenated blood to the remainder of the body (except the lungs). The function of the heart depends on the **coronary circulation,** through which the heart muscle itself is supplied with blood. It is no surprise that diagnosis and treatment of coronary artery disease is a major focus of the entire field of medicine. The *rhythmic contraction* of the heart is regulated by autonomic nerves, but the heart is quite capable of contracting efficiently without any neural input (as illustrated most dramatically by the transplanted heart). Like the lungs, the heart is suspended within a serous cavity, the *pericardial sac.* The heart and pericardial sac lie in the middle compartment of the inferior mediastinum, known as the **middle mediastinum.**

PERICARDIAL SAC

The surface of the heart itself is covered by a thin membrane, the **epicardium.** The epicardium is the *visceral* layer of the serous pericardium (Figures 1-33 and 1-34). At the roots of the *great vessels* (the aorta, pulmonary artery, pulmonary veins, and venae cavae), this visceral pericardium folds back on itself as the parietal layer of the serous pericardium and lines the interior of the fibrous pericardium. The thin space between the visceral and the parietal serous pericardium is the **pericardial cavity** and normally contains only a small

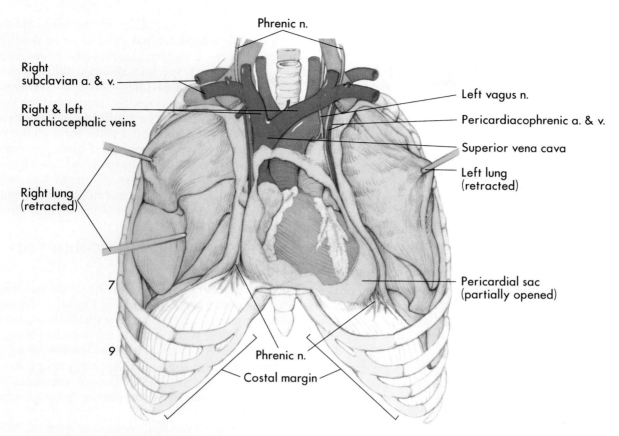

Phrenic n.

Right subclavian a. & v.

Right & left brachiocephalic veins

Right lung (retracted)

Left vagus n.

Pericardiacophrenic a. & v.

Superior vena cava

Left lung (retracted)

Pericardial sac (partially opened)

7

9

Phrenic n.

Costal margin

Figure 1-33 PERICARDIAL AND PLEURAL SACS. Anterior portions of both pleural sacs and the pericardial sac have been removed. The lungs have also been gently pulled laterally. Note that the initial few centimeters of the aorta and pulmonary artery are covered by fibrous pericardium. At that point the serous pericardium reflects back inferiorly from the heart to line the fibrous pericardium. The phrenic nerves and pericardiacophrenic vessels lie in a plane between the pericardial and pleural sacs on each side of the mediastinum. SEE ATLAS, FIG. 1-32

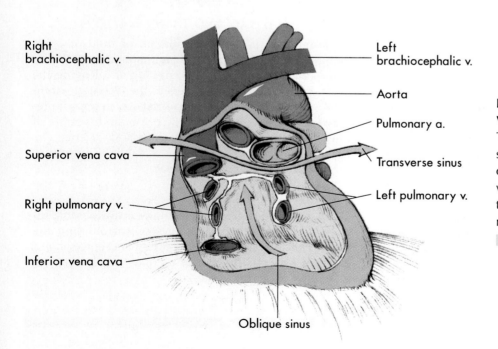

Right brachiocephalic v.

Left brachiocephalic v.

Aorta

Pulmonary a.

Transverse sinus

Superior vena cava

Left pulmonary v.

Right pulmonary v.

Inferior vena cava

Oblique sinus

Figure 1-34 OBLIQUE AND TRANS-VERSE PERICARDIAL SINUSES. These two sinuses test our understanding of the spatial relationships of the great vessels and the heart with respect to the pericardium. In this figure, the heart has been removed from the pericardial sac.

SEE ATLAS, FIG. 1-69

amount of fluid to minimize friction as the pericardial layers slide against each other with the filling and emptying of the heart.

The parietal serous pericardium is covered externally with a thick and firm layer of connective tissue, the **fibrous pericardium.** The fibrous pericardium fuses superiorly with the adventitia of the great vessels, inferiorly with the central tendon of the diaphragm, and is attached anteriorly to the sternum by **sternopericardial ligaments.** The **phrenic nerve** travels in the space between the mediastinal layer of the pleura and the external (fibrous) layer of the pericardium. Accompanied by the **pericardiacophrenic artery,** the phrenic nerve traverses the mediastinum to innervate the diaphragm below. Along the way, it provides sensory innervation to the pericardium.

The heart is suspended within the pericardial cavity, but, just as with the lung, connection between the heart and the surrounding mediastinum is needed, so that nerves, blood vessels, and lymphatics can reach the heart. For the heart there are two such areas or "roots"—one for the arterial vessels leaving the heart (aorta and pulmonary artery) and one for the venous vessels delivering blood to the heart (inferior vena cava, superior vena cava, and pulmonary veins). Each set of vessels is accompanied by nerves and lymphatics and is surrounded by an individual "collar" of serous pericardium, in a manner similar to the "collar" of pleura surrounding the hilum of the lung. However, these cardiac collars are not circular or as readily apparent as in the lung (see Figure 1-34). These arrangements produce two special recesses within the pericardial sac. The first compartment is the **transverse sinus,** a horizontal tunnel between the arterial and the venous roots of the heart. A probe can be passed posterior to the heart, from one side to the other, through the transverse sinus. The second specialized space is created by the pulmonary veins of the heart, which are arrayed in the shape of a semicircle, open inferiorly. This semicircle is closed superiorly, and the *cul-de-sac* surrounded by the venous vessels is known as the **oblique sinus.**

POSITION AND ORIENTATION OF THE HEART

The left and right sides of the heart are not truly on the left and right; the rotation of the heart during development results in the right ventricle being anterior as well as to the right, and the left ventricle being posterior and to the left (Figure 1-35, see also Figure 1-38). Furthermore, the ventricular septum, passing superior to inferior between the left and right ventricles, is not vertical but instead is inclined to the left at about a 35-degree angle.

The position of the four major chambers of the heart can be discerned by a series of grooves and sulci on the

---

THE PERICARDIUM

PERICARDITIS

Inflammation of the pericardial sac can cause the production of an exudate, which accumulates within the pericardial sac. This fluid can prove toxic to the heart muscle or even mechanically impede its motion. It is often necessary to insert a thin needle into the pericardial sac to remove such fluid for diagnosis and/or for therapy (see following).

CARDIAC SURGERY AND THE PHRENIC NERVES

The **phrenic nerves,** source of the main sensory and motor innervation of the diaphragm, descend through the chest just lateral to the pericardial sac on the left and right (see Figure 1-33). Any surgery that involves incision of the pericardial membrane poses a theoretic risk to the phrenic nerves, without which the diaphragm loses its contractile ability.

PERICARDIAL SAC AND TAMPONADE

Tamponade is the accumulation of fluid or other material in the pericardial sac and subsequent limitation of the amount of blood entering and leaving the heart. **Pericardiocentesis** refers to the technique of inserting a needle into the pericardial sac, in order to remove fluid causing tamponade or obtain a sample of fluid for detection of possible infectious agents, etc. Usually a subxiphoid approach is taken to introduce the needle into the pericardial sac.

PNEUMOPERICARDIUM

Air can accumulate within the pericardial sac, producing an abnormal dark shadow surrounding the heart. This air can impede the filling and emptying of the heart, as can fluid. The air may need to be removed by pericardiocentesis.

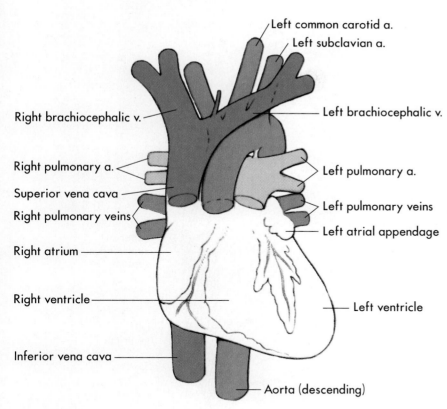

Left common carotid a.
Left subclavian a.
Right brachiocephalic v.
Left brachiocephalic v.
Right pulmonary a.
Left pulmonary a.
Superior vena cava
Left pulmonary veins
Right pulmonary veins
Left atrial appendage
Right atrium
Right ventricle
Left ventricle
Inferior vena cava
Aorta (descending)

Figure 1-35   HEART AND GREAT VESSELS. Anterior view. Note the close proximity of the aorta, superior vena cava, and pulmonary artery as they ascend into the superior mediastinum.   SEE ATLAS, FIGS. 1-37, 1-64

external surface of the heart. The **atrioventricular groove** (coronary sulcus) encircles the upper portion of the heart and shows the line where the atria are separated from the ventricles internally. The position of the ventricular septum is indicated by the **anterior** and **posterior interventricular sulci.** The anterior interventricular sulcus (see Figures 1-38 and 1-39) is an oblique elongated channel, usually fat-filled, in which the **anterior interventricular coronary artery** lies. The **base** of the heart is that part that faces posterior and includes much of the posterior wall of the left atrium and a small part of the wall of the right atrium. The base of the heart is also the anterior wall of the oblique sinus (see preceding). It lies anterior to vertebral bodies T5 to T8. The **apex** of the heart is the inferolateral tip of the left ventricle and, to a lesser extent, the tip of the right ventricle. It is positioned at the fifth left interspace in the midclavicular line. The embryonic rotation and inclination of the heart mean that the *anterior* or *sternal surface* is predominantly the right ventricular wall, with a small portion of the left ventricle and right atrium. The *posterior surface* is predominatly left atrium, with smaller parts of left ventricle and right atrium. The *inferior* or *diaphragmatic surface* is nearly all right ventricle, and the *superior border* is represented by the roots of the aorta, pulmonary artery, and superior vena cava.

FIBROUS SKELETON OF THE HEART

The walls of the heart consist mostly of **myocardial muscle.** Especially in the ventricles, the muscle is quite thick. When the ventricular muscles contract, they produce a "wringing" motion, because of the spiral orientation of the muscle fibers (Figure 1-36). This propels blood forcibly across the aortic and pulmonary valve

CLINICAL ANATOMY OF

THE HEART

ABNORMALITIES IN HEART POSITION

The position of the heart is usually slightly to the left of the midline, and the strongest heart sounds are to the left of the sternum. In **dextrocardia,** however, the heart is on the right side of the chest and the strongest cardiac impulse is to the right of the sternum. In the purest form of dextrocardia, the ventricle pumping into the aorta forms the **right** cardiac border, and the **apex** of the heart is directed laterally and to the right. When other organs in the chest and even the abdomen are similarly reversed in orientation, **situs inversus** exists. Often such a condition produces no symptoms and is undiscovered until death, or when surgery for other reasons is performed.

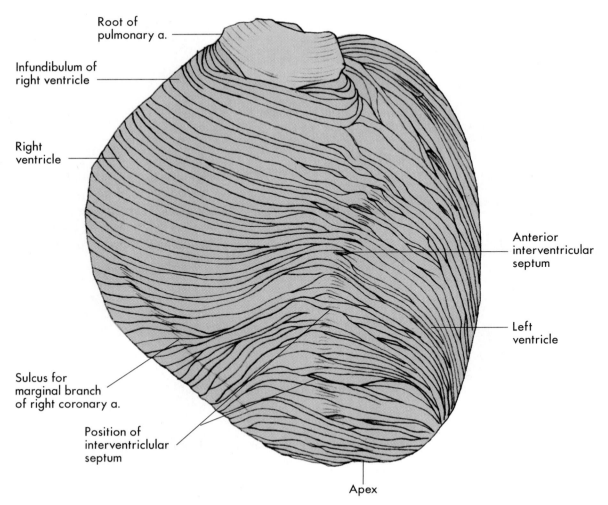

Root of
pulmonary a.

Infundibulum of
right ventricle

Right
ventricle

Sulcus for
marginal branch
of right coronary a.

Position of
interventriclular
septum

Anterior
interventricular
septum

Left
ventricle

Apex

Figure 1-36 MUSCULATURE OF THE HEART. Here the coronary vessels and fat have been stripped off the surface of the heart to show the pattern of its muscle fibers. The muscle is attached to the fibrous skeleton of the heart, in which the root of the pulmonary artery is embedded, and swirls inferiorly toward the apex of the heart.

SEE ATLAS, FIG. 1-61

orifices. The muscle of the heart is anchored in the **fibrous skeleton of the heart,** a thick connective tissue plate (Figure 1-37) in which the aortic, tricuspid, and mitral valves are embedded (the pulmonary valve is also attached but is somewhat distant from the other three). Within this fibrous skeleton there is a **central fibrous body,** between the mitral and tricuspid valves, from which connective tissue processes, anchoring the three valves, originate (see Figure 1-37). The **atrioventricular (A-V) node** (see p. 103) of the conduction system is also embedded in this fibrous skeleton.

BLOOD VESSELS OF THE HEART

The blood vessels of the heart comprise the coronary arteries and cardiac veins, carrying blood to and away from most of the heart muscle. Some subendocardial tissue lying just external to the endocardium receives

nourishment via direct diffusion of oxygen and nutrients from blood within the cardiac chambers. The coronary arteries and cardiac veins travel across the surface of the heart just deep to the **epicardium** (visceral serious pericardium), embedded in fat, although in the atrioventricular sulcus they are sometimes embedded in the myocardium. The arteries generally lie deeper than the veins.

The *coronary arteries* originate at the base of the aorta, from two of the three sinuses found in the wall of the proximal aorta (the sinuses above the *right anterior* and *left anterior* leaflets of the aortic valve). The **right coronary artery (RCA)** (Figures 1-38 to 1-40) is responsible for arterial supply to parts of the right atrium and ventricle and to the sinu-atrial (SA) node in most individuals. The proximal portion of the right coronary artery travels posterior to the right atrial appendage, in the coronary sulcus, to reach the right cardiac border.

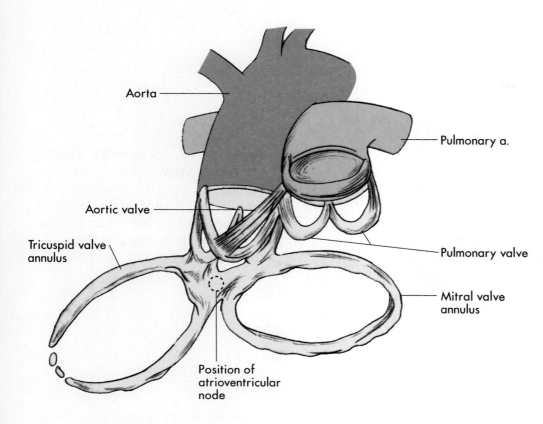

Aorta

Aortic valve

Tricuspid valve
annulus

Pulmonary a.

Pulmonary valve

Mitral valve
annulus

Position of
atrioventricular
node

**Figure   1-37   FIBROUS
"SKELETON" OF THE HEART.**
This figure is drawn as
though all of the muscle tissue of the heart had been removed and all that remains
is the firm connective tissue
framework of the heart valves.
The aortic, mitral, and triscu-
pid valves are closely linked
to each other, while the
pulmonary valve is located
superior to the others and is
not as firmly anchored in the
common fibrous skeleton.

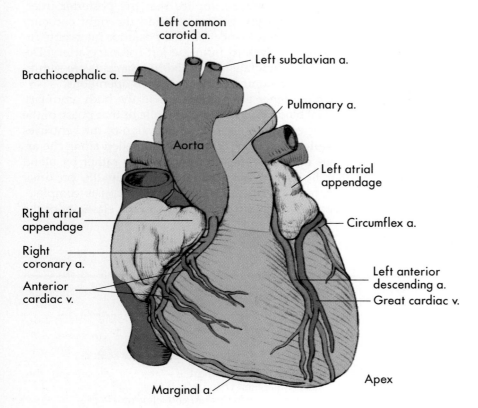

Left common
carotid a.

Brachiocephalic a.

Left subclavian a.

Pulmonary a.

Aorta

Left atrial
appendage

Right atrial
appendage

Circumflex a.

Right
coronary a.

Anterior
cardiac v.

Left anterior
descending a.

Great cardiac v.

Marginal a.

Apex

**Figure 1-38 CORONARY VESSELS,
ANTERIOR VIEW.** Anterior view showing the major anterior branches of
both the left and right coronary arteries
and the accompanying cardiac veins.

SEE ATLAS, FIG. 1-57

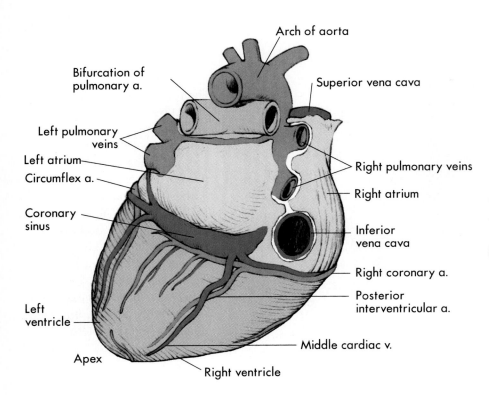

Arch of aorta

Bifurcation of
pulmonary a.

Superior vena cava

Left pulmonary
veins

Left atrium

Circumflex a.

Coronary
sinus

Right pulmonary veins

Right atrium

Inferior
vena cava

Left
ventricle

Right coronary a.

Posterior
interventricular a.

Middle cardiac v.

Apex

Right ventricle

**Figure 1-39   CORONARY VESSELS,
POSTERIOR VIEW.** Posterior view showing the large coronary sinus, into which
drains blood from most cardiac veins.
Also illustrated are the posterior
branches of the coronary arteries.

SEE ATLAS, FIGS. 1-39, 1-58

Along the way it gives rise to the **nodal artery** (in ~70% of individuals) and a **right marginal artery** descending along the right cardiac border. It then continues posteriorly in the coronary sulcus to reach the posterior interventricular groove. Its terminal branch is the **posterior interventricular artery** (in the majority of individuals), which descends in this groove.

The **left coronary artery (LCA)** (see Figures 1-38 to 1-40) supplies much of the left ventricle, a smaller part of the right ventricle, the ventricular septum, and some of the left atrium. It arises from the aorta and passes leftward and posterior to the pulmonary trunk. On reaching the coronary sulcus, it divides into a **circumflex** and **left anterior descending artery** (*anterior interventricular artery*). The circumflex artery continues in the coronary sulcus, gives rise to the **left marginal artery,** and then continues to the posterior aspect of the heart. Here it anastomoses with branches of the right coronary artery, where one or the other parent vessel

(or sometimes both) is the source of the posterior interventricular artery. Importantly, the interventricular septum is supplied principally by branches of the *left coronary artery*. Individual branches of the coronary arteries are listed in Table 1-4.

Right dominance implies that the posterior interventricular artery is derived from the right coronary artery; **left dominance** that the posterior interventricular artery is derived from the left coronary artery. Details of the circulation in individual patients are significant when planning coronary bypass operations.

Unlike other arterial systems in the body, coronary arterial blood flows during **diastole** or that phase of the cardiac cycle just after the contraction of the ventricles (**systole**). Coronary flow is not propelled along the arteries by the force of contraction but rather by blood that flows in a retrograde direction in the proximal aorta after a forceful systolic contraction is complete. Coronary arterial flow depends on the elasticity of the

Table 1-4   Coronary Arteries and Their Branches

	Coronary Artery Branch	Area of Heart Supplied
Branches of right coronary artery	Nodal branch	Right atrium and sinu-atrial node
	Right marginal	Anterior wall of right ventricle
	Posterior interventricular	Posterior wall of right ventricle, posterior septum
Branches of left coronary artery	Left anterior descending [LAD]	Anterior left ventricle, most of ventricular septum, and apex
	Left marginal	Lateral wall of left ventricle
	Circumflex	Posterior wall of left atrium and left ventricle

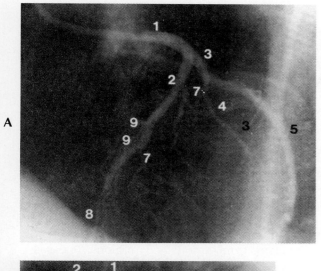

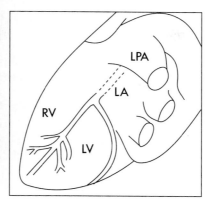

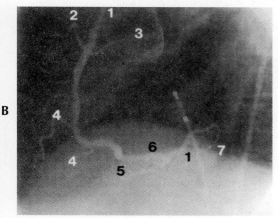

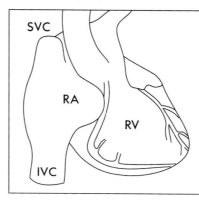

Figure 1-40 CORONARY ARTERIOGRAMS. A, the left coronary artery has been injected with dye and an x-ray taken, outlining the position of the left coronary artery and its branches. **B,** A similar injection has been made into the orifice of the right coronary artery. The accompanying diagrams show the position of the heart for each injection. Such studies are used to define obstructions in the coronary arteries. (From Weir J. Abrahams PH: *An imaging atlas of human anatomy,* London, 1992, Mosby.)

A	B
1 Left mainstem coronary artery	**1** Right coronary artery
2 Left anterior interventricular branch (left anterior descending)	**2** Conus artery
3 Circumflex artery	**3** Sinu-atrial nodal artery
4 First ⎱ obtuse marginal branch	**4** Right marginal arteries
5 Second ⎰ of circumflex artery	**5** Posterior interventricular septal artery (posterior descending artery)
6 Diagonal arteries	
7 Left anterior interventricular artery (also termed LAD) curving round apex of heart	**6** Atrioventricular nodal artery
	7 Lateral ventricular branch to left ventricle
8 Septal arteries	

aorta to "push" blood into the coronary arteries at diastole. Very rapid heart rates (>120 beats per minute in an adult) can diminish coronary flow simply because time between the rapid heartbeats is not sufficient to permit adequate coronary artery filling.

The **cardiac veins** are distributed over the surface of the heart in correspondence with the major coronary arteries (see Figures 1-38 and 1-39). Accompanying the anterior interventricular artery (or left anterior descending artery, LAD) is the **great cardiac vein.** It drains both ventricles and parts of the left atrium. The **middle cardiac vein** lies in the posterior interventricular groove and drains the posterior ventricular surface. The **small cardiac vein** travels in the atrioventricular groove on the right and drains the posterior right atrium and ventricle. The **posterior vein of the left ventricle** lies on the posterior surface of the left ventricle and drains to the coronary sinus (see following). **Anterior cardiac veins** span the atrioventricular groove and, in so doing, drain blood from the upper surface of the right ventricle to the right atrium directly. Within the walls of the heart are irregular small vascular chan-

CLINICAL ANATOMY OF

THE CORONARY VESSELS

CORONARY ARTERY DISEASE

Insufficient coronary blood flow, or outright occlusion of coronary vessels leads to **ischemia** (inadequate blood supply to an organ). If moderate, this may produce **angina pectoris** (chest pain). If severe, the heart may experience dysrhythmias or even cardiac arrest. **Infarction** is an extreme degree of ischemia and implies some permanent injury resulting from ischemia. The most common cause of coronary occlusion is arteriosclerosis, in which fatty deposits and smooth muscle hypertrophy gradually obstruct a coronary artery.

"HEART ATTACKS" AND MYOCARDIAL INJURY

Patients with "mild" **heart attacks,** or even those in whom such attacks go unnoticed (so-called silent attacks), may suffer ischemia in some areas of the ventricular wall. Eventually these areas may scar and be subject to gradual dilatation (aneurysm) and eventual rupture of the wall, causing sudden death.

REFERRED PAIN AND THE HEART

Referred pain is a painful sensation in a part of the body other than the actual location of the pathologic process—inflammation, infection, infarction, etc. The pain is referred to another part of the body, probably as a result of interconnections within the spinal cord of sensory axons from various body regions. One classic example is that of the pain produced by a myocardial infarction ("heart attack"). The direct painful sensations from the ischemic insult to the heart itself are usually described as tightening or "crushing" chest pains. Referred painful sensations may be felt in the arm, neck, or even perceived as dental pain.

---

nels or **sinusoids.** Through these, some coronary blood (especially in the right atrium) can drain through the heart wall and be deposited directly into the interior of the heart (through the **venae cordis minimae**), without having to pass through a cardiac vein. Most coronary blood, however, does drain back to the right atrium by traversing cardiac veins and entering the coronary sinus.

Most of the cardiac venous blood converges on the **coronary sinus,** a large elongated venous channel located in the posterior atrioventricular sulcus (see Figure 1-39). The coronary sinus receives drainage of the great cardiac vein, middle cardiac vein, small cardiac vein, and posterior vein of the left ventricle. The coronary sinus empties into the right atrium through a small orifice adjacent to the orifice of the inferior vena cava. There is usually a small crescent-shaped fold of tissue serving as a *valve* in the orifice of the coronary sinus (valve of the coronary sinus) (see Figure 1-41).

RIGHT ATRIUM

The **right atrium (RA)** has a sharp right-side *border* abutting the right middle lobe of the lung, and extends anteriorly and toward the left as an *atrial appendage.* Much of the right atrium faces the posterior surface of the sternum. The **atrial appendage** (auricle) has its base on the anterior surface and its tip medially, lying just in front of the root of the aorta (see Figures 1-38 and 1-42).

The smooth-walled *posterior part* of the right atrium, into which the inferior and superior vena cava (IVC and SVC) empty, is the **sinus venarum.** It is derived embryologically from the right horn of the sinus venosus. The rough-walled *anterior part,* derived embryologically from the atrium proper, is continuous with the interior of the atrial appendage. The **crista terminalis,** a raised ridge on the atrial interior, demarcates its anterior and posterior parts. The position of the crista is often visible as a groove, the **sulcus terminalis,** on the exterior surface of the right atrium. The rough features of the interior of the atrial appendage are called **musculi pectinati** (the same term applies to the interior of the left atrial appendage) (Figure 1-41).

The right atrium has large openings for the SVC and IVC. These vessels are positioned so that they almost seem to be continuations of each other, along a superior-inferior line. The orifice for the SVC is positioned superiorly, and where the crista terminalis meets the perimeter of the SVC orifice is found the **sinu-atrial (SA) node.** The orifice for the IVC is incompletely guarded by a semilunar crescent of tissue serving as a **valve of the IVC** (the SVC has no comparable valve). The valve of the IVC consists of two layers of endocardium and a little intervening connective tissue. In fetal life this valve helps divert IVC blood toward the patent foramen ovale, to reach the left atrium (across the patent foramen ovale). The **valve of the coronary sinus** is guarded by a crescent-shaped fold of tissue partially covering its entrance. The orifice for the coronary sinus lies between the septal leaflet of the tricuspid valve and the orifice of the IVC.

The **septal wall** of the right atrium, due to the rota-

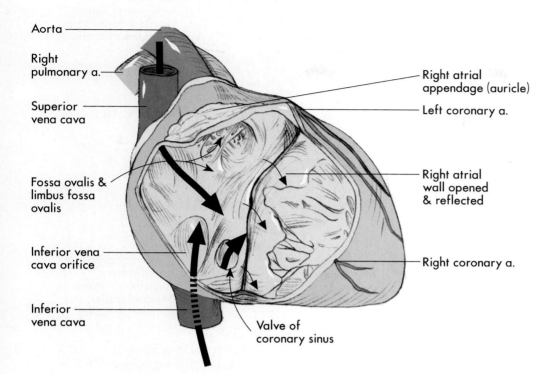

Aorta

Right
pulmonary a.

Superior
vena cava

Fossa ovalis &
limbus fossa
ovalis

Inferior vena
cava orifice

Inferior
vena cava

Right atrial
appendage (auricle)

Left coronary a.

Right atrial
wall opened
& reflected

Right coronary a.

Valve of
coronary sinus

**Figure 1-41   INTERIOR OF
THE RIGHT ATRIUM.** Ante-
rior view of an exposure of
the right atrium, showing
the entrances of the inferior
vena cava, superior vena
cava, and coronary sinus.
Also visible are the fossa
ovalis on the septal wall of
the right atrium and the location of the atrioventricular node near the septal
leaflet of the tricuspid
valve. See ATLAS, Fig. 1-40

tion of the heart, is arrayed at a 45-degree angle rather than being in the sagittal plane. The right atrium is thus anterior, to the right, and slightly inferior to the left atrium. The septal wall of the right atrium has a central depression, the **fossa ovalis,** site of the fetal *foramen ovale.* The anterior part of the margin of this fossa is raised and forms the **limbus fossae ovalis.** It is a rem-nant of the embryonic *septum secundum.* In the medial and superior wall of the right atrium is found an in-ward bulging, caused by the presence of the proximal ascending aorta just beyond the aortic valve.

TRICUSPID VALVE

The **tricuspid valve** is in the anteroinferior portion of the right atrial wall; it is typically the largest of the four heart valves (Figure 1-42; see also Figure 1-37). It has *three leaflets*—the *septal, anterior,* and *posterior.* In fact these three leaflets may be considered as a continuous "curtain" originating from the inner perimeter of the valve annulus. The **commissures** are the gaps separat-ing the adjacent leaflets. The valve orifice is vertical but "faces" ~45 degrees out of the sagittal plane, rotated so that it faces leftward and slightly inferiorly.

Each valve leaflet has a **rough zone** along its free edge on both the superior and inferior surfaces. The *su-perior surface* of the rough zone is that part of the leaflet that touches the other leaflets during full valve closure. Attaching to the *inferior surface* of the rough zones are the **chordae tendineae,** slender strands of connective tissue. Inferiorly, chordae tendineae attach to either the **anterior** or **posterior papillary muscles,** peglike exten-

sions of ventricular muscle on the wall of the right ven-tricle. Small numbers of chordae tendineae arise from other areas of the RV wall as well or from a variably present septal papillary muscle.

Chordae tendineae tether the valve leaflets of the tri-cuspid and mitral valves to the ventricular wall and help keep the valve leaflets closely approximated dur-ing **systole,** when pressures within the ventricular chambers are at their highest. Without the chordae tendineae, blood would leak from the ventricle back into the atrial chamber, rather than leaving the ventri-cle and entering the aorta (from the left ventricle) or pulmonary artery (from the right ventricle).

RIGHT VENTRICLE

The wall thickness of the **right ventricle (RV)** is typi-cally less than that of the left ventricle (Figure 1-43). The interior of the right ventricle is crescent shaped be-cause the ventricular septum actually "bows" into the right ventricle. The *inflow tract of the right ventricle* is that part of the wall just inferior to the tricuspid valve. The inflow area is rough surfaced, having many **trabec-ulae carneae** (raised ridges or bands of myocardium) protruding inwardly. The right ventricular lining typi-cally has an *anterior* and *posterior papillary muscle.* The **septomarginal fasciculus (moderator band)** is a thick band of myocardium passing from the inferior portion of the septal wall to the base of the anterior papillary muscle (on the lateral ventricular wall). It contains the continuation of an important part of the conduction system, the **right bundle branch** (see p. 104).

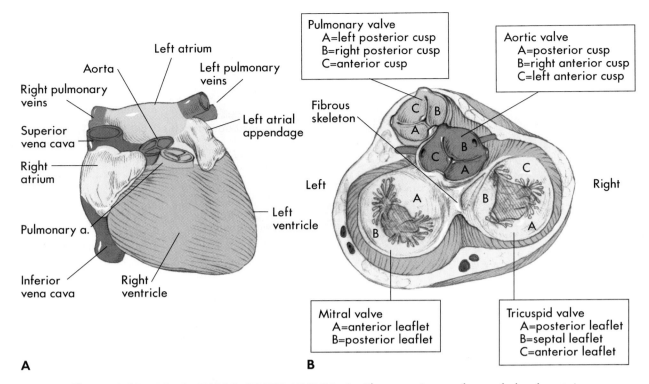

Figure 1-42 FOUR MAJOR HEART VALVES. A, The anterior surface of the heart is shown to illustrate the relationship of the pulmonary valve to the aortic valve. **B,** Superior view of the heart transected at the level of the four major valves—the aortic, pulmonary, tricuspid, and mitral. SEE ATLAS, FIGS. 1-4, 1-44, 1-53

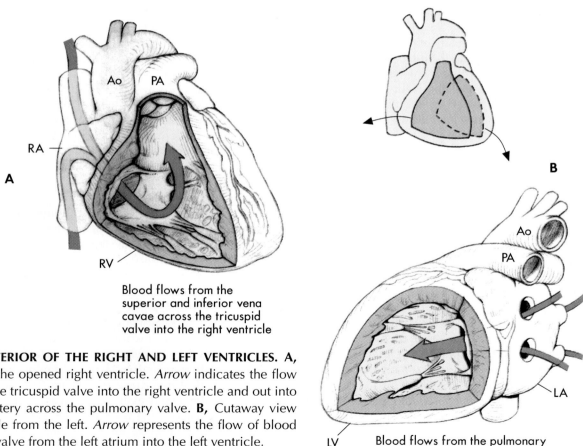

Blood flows from the superior and inferior vena cavae across the tricuspid valve into the right ventricle

Figure 1-43 INTERIOR OF THE RIGHT AND LEFT VENTRICLES. A, Anterior view of the opened right ventricle. *Arrow* indicates the flow of blood across the tricuspid valve into the right ventricle and out into the pulmonary artery across the pulmonary valve. **B,** Cutaway view of the left ventricle from the left. *Arrow* represents the flow of blood across the mitral valve from the left atrium into the left ventricle.

SEE ATLAS, FIG. 1-46

Blood flows from the pulmonary veins into the left atrium and across the mitral valve into the left ventricle

The *outflow tract* or **infundibulum of the right ventricle** is smooth-walled and ends at the pulmonary valve. The thick **supraventricular crest** is a raised portion of myocardium marking the transition from trabeculae carneae to infundibulum. It has been postulated that the smooth walls of the infundibulum help to decrease turbulence as blood is ejected from the right ventricle across the pulmonary valve.

PULMONARY VALVE

The **pulmonary valve (PV)** faces superiorly, slightly to the left and posterior (see Figures 1-42 and 1-43). The *fibrous ring* forming the perimeter of the pulmonary valve (the valve **annulus**) is to some degree separate from similar fibrous rings of the aortic, mitral, and tricuspid valves, which are closely bound to each other (see Figure 1-37). The pulmonary valve has three *leaflets* or *cusps*—the *left posterior, right posterior,* and *anterior.*

Just distal to the attachment of the leaflets to the valve annulus are small, thinned, and outwardly dilated areas of the pulmonary artery wall known as **sinuses;** these are smaller than those of the aorta (see pp. 92; 98) and of course do not give rise to any vessels as they do in the aorta. During diastole (the period of relaxation following forceful ventricular contraction), the inner margins of the valve leaflets of the pulmonary (and aortic) valves meet and prevent retrograde blood flow across the valve. Each leaflet has a collagenous **nodule** in the middle of its free margin (see Figure 1-44 for similar structures in the **aortic valve**); the three nodules come into apposition during valve closure and strengthen the seal created. In diastole the valve leaflets distend and expand inward from the pressure of the column of blood above them. This increases further the strength of the seal between the valve leaflets and prevents regurgitation of blood from the pulmonary artery backward into the right ventricle.

PULMONARY ARTERY

The **pulmonary artery** or **trunk (PA)** runs superiorly and posteriorly from the pulmonary valve and usually is 5 to 6 cm in length before branching into the right and left pulmonary arteries (see Figure 1-28). In clinical practice the pulmonary artery is often called the **main pulmonary artery.** The pulmonary artery is wholly contained within pericardium. At its base the pulmonary artery is anterior to the ascending aorta; higher up the aorta passes from anterior to posterior in arching over the pulmonary artery, as it divides into its left and right branches. Part of the **cardiac plexus,** a mesh of autonomic axons supplying the heart and lungs, lies between the pulmonary artery and the aorta, as does the **ligamentum arteriosum,** a fibrous remnant of the fetal vessel conveying blood from the pulmonary artery to the aorta (the *ductus arteriosus*).

The **right pulmonary artery (RPA)** passes rightward, posterior to the ascending aorta and the SVC. It is anterior to the esophagus and the right mainstem bronchus. It enters the pulmonary hilum and divides into a superior branch to the upper lobe and an inferior branch to the middle and lower lobes. The **left pulmonary artery (LPA)** passes leftward anterior to the left mainstem bronchus and the descending aorta. It divides into an upper and lower branch, which supply the upper and lower lobes. The right and left pulmonary arteries lie outside the pericardium (see Figure 1-33).

PULMONARY VEINS

Generally there are *four main pulmonary veins*—one draining the lower lobe of each lung, one from the left upper lobe, and one from the right middle and upper lobes—although considerable variation exists (see Figures 1-31 and 1-43). The veins usually enter the left atrium separately; they have no valves.

LEFT ATRIUM

Musculi pectinati are present only in the atrial appendage; the remainder of the left atrial wall is smooth. Much of the wall is originally derived from embryonic pulmonary veins, not the true embryonic atrium. The **left atrium (LA)** lies posterior and to the left of the right atrium, but predominantly **posterior** (see Figure 1-39). The left and right atria are separated by the interatrial septum. The **left atrial appendage** is narrower than the right; its tip overlaps the origin of the pulmonary artery.

MITRAL VALVE (LEFT ATRIOVENTRICULAR VALVE)

The **mitral valve** faces anterolaterally and to the left, with a slight inferior inclination. Like the tricuspid valve, the mitral valve has a foundation of two *subendocardial fibrous rings,* although in reality the "rings" are not quite complete circles (see Figures 1-37 and 1-42). Classically the mitral valve is described as having a *posterior* and *anterior* leaflet and is, therefore, *bicuspid;* however, only the anterior is a true single leaflet, while the posterior leaflet is a composite of two to three smaller subleaflets. Some authors refer to a *posterior valve leaflet complex* or *area* rather than to a specific posterior leaflet. The positions of the anterior and posterior leaflets are defined by the *commissures,* which separate them. The large fissure between the anterior and posterior leaflets is at right angles to the long axis of the septal leaflet of the tricuspid valve. The mitral valve leaflets have a peripheral *rough zone* onto which attach the various **chordae tendineae** of the left ventricle

(Figure 1-44). The mitral valve leaflets are otherwise very smooth. This smoothness helps direct left atrial blood deep into the left ventricle, toward its apex.

The anterior leaflet has *chordae tendineae* from both the anterior and posterior **papillary muscles** of the left ventricle. The anterior leaflet is also to some degree anchored in the subendocardial fibrous tissue supporting the *aortic valve*. The posterior leaflet complex also is attached to chordae tendineae from both *anterior* and *posterior papillary muscles*. There are also minor or "false" chordae tendineae arising from other areas of the left ventricular wall. As with the tricuspid valve, chordae tendineae of the mitral valve tether the valve leaflets to the papillary muscles and help prevent mitral regurgitation during systole.

LEFT VENTRICLE

The **left ventricle (LV)** is longer and narrower than the right ventricle, but the left ventricle walls are about 3 to 4 times thicker than the right ventricle wall (see Figure 1-47). The left ventricle constitutes more of the ventricular apex than does the right ventricle. The **inflow tract** for the left ventricle (i.e., path of blood flow from left atrium to left ventricle) and the **outflow tract** (path of blood flow from left ventricle to aorta) are very near to each other. The ventricular endocardium just inferior to the aortic valve is smooth and is referred to as the **aortic vestibule;** it is less extensive, however, than the comparable region of the right ventricle (the *infundibulum*). As with the right ventricle infundibulum, the smooth walls of the aortic vestibule are assumed to help increase laminar blood flow across the aortic valve.

AORTIC VALVE

The **aortic valve,** at the origin of the ascending aorta, faces superiorly, slightly anterior, and rightward. The underlying framework of the **aortic annulus** is in reality three semilunar arcs of connective tissue, one corresponding to each of the aortic valve leaflets (see Figures 1-37 and 1-42). The aortic annulus is firmly attached to the trigonal fibrous tissue of the mitral valve, and the fibrous rings of the mitral, tricuspid, and aortic valves are closely interlocked, while that of the pulmonary valve is set somewhat apart. As with the pulmonary valve, the leaflets of the aortic valve have marginal **nodules,** which help enhance the seal of the valves during diastole, preventing aortic regurgitation (see Figure 1-44).

The three valve leaflets are named differently by anatomists and clinicians. In anatomical science the leaflets may be named in one of two ways: (1) according to their embryonic position (prior to heart rotation)—**right anterior, left anterior,** and **posterior**
leaflets,** or (2) according to their adult position—**right posterior, left posterior,** and **anterior leaflets.** In clinical medicine (cardiology, cardiac surgery, etc.), the practice is to name the leaflets for the aortic sinus and coronary artery with which they are associated. Thus in clinical parlance there is a **right** (for the sinus from which arises the right coronary artery), a **left,** and a **noncoronary leaflet.**

Each aortic valve leaflet has a **nodule** on its free margin. The free edge of tissue radiating away from the nodule to the commissure is called the **lunule.** The **aortic sinuses** (of Valsalva) are three small dilations of the aortic wall (see Figure 1-44) positioned just above the attachment of valve leaflets to the valve annulus. Like the valve leaflets, the sinuses may be named in at least three ways; they are most directly described as **left coronary, right coronary,** and **noncoronary.** The aortic sinuses are larger than those of the pulmonary valve.

As with the pulmonary valve, the pressure of blood in the proximal aorta during diastole fills each sinus, causing the adjacent leaflet to "fall" inward and abut the free margins of the other leaflets. This effects a closure of the valve. During systole, the pressure of blood being ejected from the left ventricle not only deflects the leaflets upward but also distends the aortic valve annulus, so that its circumference is increased by 15% to 20%. Additionally, it is thought that a small amount of aortic blood swirls and forms a vortex between each valve leaflet and the lining of the aorta (i.e., in the sinus), so that the valve leaflets are not tightly compressed against the endothelium of the aorta. The vortex currents in the sinuses also produce smooth blood flow into the coronary orifices during diastole.

ASCENDING AORTA

The **ascending aorta** is about 5 to 6 cm in length; beginning at the aortic valve, it passes upward and slightly to the right, with the PA lying slightly anterior and to its left (see Figure 1-35). Both are covered with a collar of fibrous pericardium, and a superior extension of the serous pericardial sac. The ascending aorta ends at the sternal angle, where it is continuous with the aortic arch. To the right of the ascending aorta are the RCA, RA, and SVC; to its left are the LCA, LA, and part of the PA (see Figure 1-38). Posterior to it are the right mainstem bronchus and right pulmonary artery (RPA), and anterior to it are contents of the anterior mediastinum and the sternum (Figure 1-3).

Two chemoreceptors, the **aortic bodies** or **aorticopulmonary bodies,** are located in the wall of the ascending aorta. Structurally, these resemble the carotid body in the neck. Evidence indicates that these structures can monitor the pH, Pco_2 and/or Po_2 of the blood and release catecholamines or other hormones to affect the rate of respiration (which can modify pH, Pco_2 and/or Po_2).

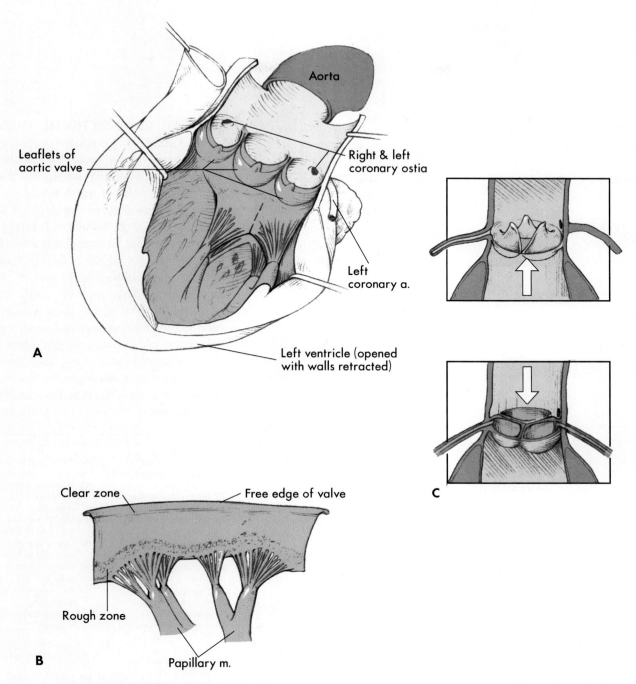

A

Aorta

Leaflets of
aortic valve

Right & left
coronary ostia

Left
coronary a.

Left ventricle (opened
with walls retracted)

C

B

Clear zone

Free edge of valve

Rough zone

Papillary m.

Figure 1-44   MITRAL AND AORTIC VALVES. An exposure of the left ventricle and proximal aorta (**A**) and a detailed view of the chordae tendineae of the mitral valve (**B**). **C,** The aortic valve leaflets shown during systole (*above*) and diastole (*below*). At diastole the sinuses are distended and blood is allowed to flow into the two coronary arteries.

SEE ATLAS, FIGS. 1-45, 1-50

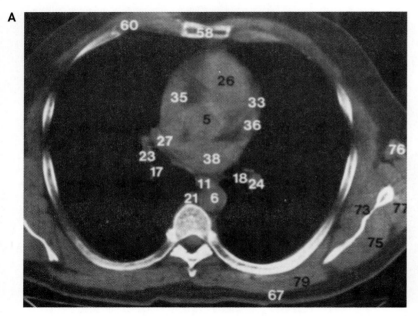

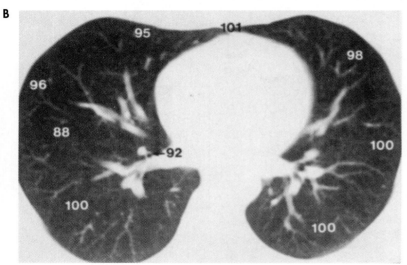

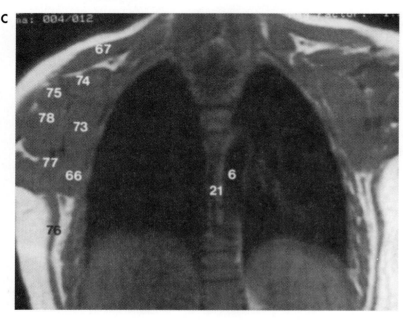

Figure 1-45 CROSS-SECTIONAL IMAGING OF THE CHEST. A, Computed tomographic (CT) transverse image through the midchest. It is displayed at settings that emphasize the details of the structure of the heart and mediastinum but show little of the detailed structure of the lungs. **B,** Similar CT image but displayed at settings that emphasize the detail of the lungs, sacrificing the detail of structures within the mediastinum and heart. **C,** Magnetic resonance imaging (MRI) study of the chest in the coronal plane. Displayed in this fashion, this technique does not provide good detail of the bony structures but gives high quality images of muscle, lung, and other soft tissues. (From Weir J. Abrahams PH: *An imaging atlas of human anatomy,* London, 1992, Mosby.)

SEE ATLAS, FIG. 1-35

A	B
5 Ascending aorta	**88** Plane of oblique fissure
6 Descending aorta	
11 Esophagus	**92** Basal segment bronchus, right upper lobe
17 Right inferior lobe bronchus	
18 Left inferior lobe bronchus	**95** Medial segment, right middle lobe
23 Right pulmonary artery	**96** Lateral segment, right middle lobe
24 Left pulmonary artery	**98** Inferior segment, lingula
26 Pulmonary trunk	**100** Basal segment, right lower lobe
27 Right superior pulmonary vein	**101** Junction of anterior pleurae
33 Anterior interventricular branch of left coronary artery	**C**
35 Right atrial appendage	**6** Descending aorta
36 Left atrial appendage	**21** Azygos vein
38 Left atrium	**66** Serratus anterior muscle
58 Body of sternum	**67** Trapezius muscle
60 Pectoralis major muscle	**73** Subscapularis muscle
67 Trapezius muscle	**74** Supraspinatus muscle
73 Subscapularis muscle	**75** Infraspinatus muscle
75 Infraspinatus muscle	**76** Latissimus dorsi muscle
76 Latissimus dorsi muscle	**77** Teres major muscle
77 Teres major muscle	**78** Teres minor muscle
79 Rhomboid major muscleT	

THE HEART

INJURY TO CARDIAC VALVES

Valves may be permanently scarred following infections (especially rheumatic fever) and become narrowed (**stenosis**) or allow retrograde leakage (**incompetence** or **insufficiency**) as a result. If, for example, the mitral valve is incompetent, then the heart beats more rapidly and forcefully to compensate for that fixed fraction of the LV blood being regurgitated back into the LA with each beat of the heart.

ATRIAL AND VENTRICULAR SEPTAL DEFECTS IN CHILDREN

Concerning **septal defects in atrium and ventricle:** if blood shunts from right to left (e.g., RV to LV, or RA to LA), then the lungs will be undercirculated. As a result, systemic blood will be poorly oxygenated and the patient will look cyanotic (blue). Inadequate blood oxygen content, if chronic, produces major injury to a wide range of organ systems. If the shunt is LV to RV, or LA to RA, then the patient will not look cyanotic, but the lungs will be overcirculated and the pulmonary vessels will suffer structural damage (**pulmonary hypertension**).

MITRAL VALVE PROLAPSE

Mitral valve prolapse is usually a benign condition of incompetency of the leaflets of the mitral valve. Up to 10% of the population may have this condition, and there is a strong female predominance. When serious, it produces chest pain, shortness of breath, and may lead to serious disturbances of cardiac rhythm.

ANOMALOUS PULMONARY VENOUS RETURN

When pulmonary veins drain into structures other than the LA (e.g., the RA, the SVC, the hepatic veins), it is described as **anomalous pulmonary venous return.** The general result of this abnormality is resistance to pulmonary venous flow and resultant pulmonary congestion.

The **coronary arteries** originate in two of the three **aortic sinuses** (the **right anterior and left anterior**). These two vessels are the aorta's first branches. The major branches of the aortic arch are the **brachiocephalic artery,** the **left common carotid artery,** and the **left subclavian artery.**

BLOOD FLOW THROUGH THE HEART

Systemic venous blood (i.e., traveling to the heart from all of the body except the lungs) returns to the heart through the IVC and SVC, each of which delivers blood to the *right atrium.* The *coronary sinus* also empties into the right atrium, delivering blood that has traveled through the coronary circulation and supplied the heart itself. Coronary venous return represents about 5% of the total systemic venous blood returned to the heart. At the same time, **pulmonary venous blood** is delivered to the *left atrium* through the four pulmonary veins (Figure 1-46).

The **cardiac cycle** consists of **diastole** (ventricular filling) and **systole** (ventricular emptying) (Figure 1-47). Diastole begins with the closure of the aortic and pulmonary valves, marking the end of the previous cardiac cycle and the beginning of the next. During diastole, blood flows from the right atrium across the tricuspid valve into the right ventricle and from the left atrium across the mitral valve into the left ventricle. When the ventricles are filled, systole begins, as the ventricular muscle begins to contract. The early stage of ventricular contraction is **isometric,** during which time pressure builds in the ventricle but its volume does not decrease (i.e., no blood flows across the aortic and pulmonary valves). The growing intraventricular pressure quickly forces the mitral and tricuspid valves to close. When the ventricular pressure exceeds the resting pressure in the aorta and pulmonary arteries, blood flows across the aortic and pulmonary valves and the period of **isotonic** ventricular contraction begins (ventricles contract and ventricular volume falls as blood exits). Throughout systole, meanwhile, blood flows into the atria, preparing them for the next diastole. When the ventricles have emptied, the ventricular muscle relaxes and the pulmonary and aortic valves close, marking the beginning of a new cycle.

Systole and **diastole** are usually defined with reference to the contraction or relaxation of *ventricular* muscle. Late in diastole the atria contract forcibly, helping to propel blood from the atria to the ventricles. Some refer to this as "atrial systole," or the "atrial kick" (see following). At more rapid heart rates, when the duration of diastole is shortened, the atrial kick becomes more important to successful ventricular filling.

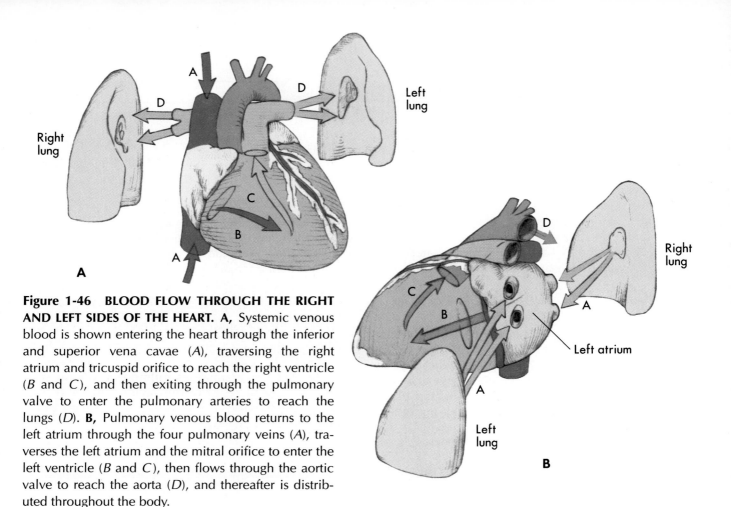

Figure 1-46 BLOOD FLOW THROUGH THE RIGHT AND LEFT SIDES OF THE HEART. A, Systemic venous blood is shown entering the heart through the inferior and superior vena cavae (*A*), traversing the right atrium and tricuspid orifice to reach the right ventricle (*B* and *C*), and then exiting through the pulmonary valve to enter the pulmonary arteries to reach the lungs (*D*). **B,** Pulmonary venous blood returns to the left atrium through the four pulmonary veins (*A*), traverses the left atrium and the mitral orifice to enter the left ventricle (*B* and *C*), then flows through the aortic valve to reach the aorta (*D*), and thereafter is distributed throughout the body.

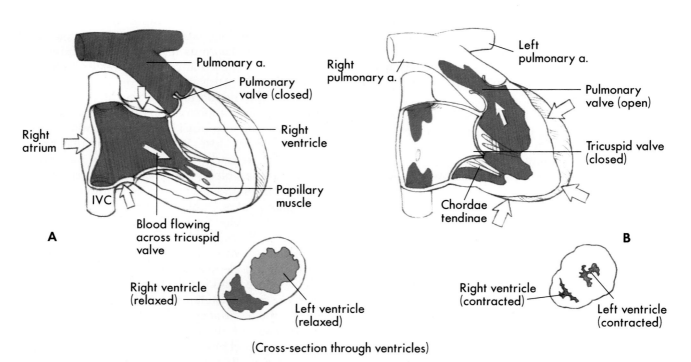

(Cross-section through ventricles)

Figure 1-47 CARDIAC CYCLE. A, Diastole, when the atria contract and expel blood across the atrioventricular valves to enter the ventricles. **B,** Systole, when the ventricles contract and the pulmonary and aortic valves open, permitting blood to flow into the pulmonary artery and aorta, respectively. SEE ATLAS, FIG. 1-47

CARDIAC CONDUCTION SYSTEM

The vertebrate heartbeat is **intrinsic** to the cardiac myocytes and is only *regulated* by neural and hormonal influences (the successful functioning of a transplanted heart, which is denervated, proves this point dramatically). Vertebrate cardiac myocytes are connected by **gap junctions,** which speed the spread of polarization changes among the cardiac myocytes. All cardiac myocytes are capable of **spontaneous depolarization-repolarization** but do so at different rates; therefore, the group of cells with the fastest intrinsic rate "drives" the overall rate of the heart. If the entire conduction system is defective, ventricular myocytes beat at a rate of 25 to 40 bpm. This is usually insufficient to sustain life. Intrinsic atrial frequency is 40 to 60 bpm, and this rate can sustain life. The conduction system (Figure 1-48) consists of certain very specialized groups of cardiac myocytes (**nodal cells, transitional cells,** and the **subendocardial Purkinje fibers**), almost devoid of contractile filaments and given over entirely to impulse transmission. Cells of the conduction system have variable velocities of conduction. The total time required for one cardiac beat (the *cardiac cycle*) is determined by the sum of these conduction velocities, plus the aggregated delays at the SA node and AV node.

The **sinu-atrial or SA node** (at junction of SVC and crista terminalis in the right atrial wall) is normally the pacemaker (see Figure 1-48). It generates a heartbeat of 65 to 80/minute at rest. Its name comes from its embryonic origin from tissues at the junction of the *sinus venosus* and the true *atrium*. This elongated mass lies closer to the epicardial than to the endocardial surface of the atrial wall. The **nodal artery,** of unusually large diameter, runs directly through the SA node. This vessel may be a branch of the *right* or *left coronary artery* (~65% vs. ~35% incidence). Within the SA node, myocytes directly adjacent to the nodal artery are probably the true pacemakers; myocytes placed more peripherally in the node are transitional and have somewhat slower conduction velocities than the myocytes surrounding the nodal artery.

The **atrioventricular** or **AV Node** (see Figure 1-48) is stimulated by depolarizations traveling from the SA node diffusely through the atrial wall (although some argue that there are specialized paths for SA to AV nodal conduction in the atrial wall). The AV node lies beneath the endocardium of the right atrium, near the

Figure 1-48 CARDIAC CONDUCTION SYSTEM. The conduction system begins at the sinu-atrial (SA) node, located in the junction of the superior vena cava and the right atrial wall. From the SA node, conduction pathways in the atrial myocardium extend downward to the atrioventricular (AV) node, located in the upper posterior interventricular septum. The bundle of His (atrioventricular bundle) extends away from the AV node and soon divides into the right and left bundle branches, which descend through the interventricular septum. The important moderator band or septomarginal fasciculus is also shown. SEE ATLAS, FIG. 1-60

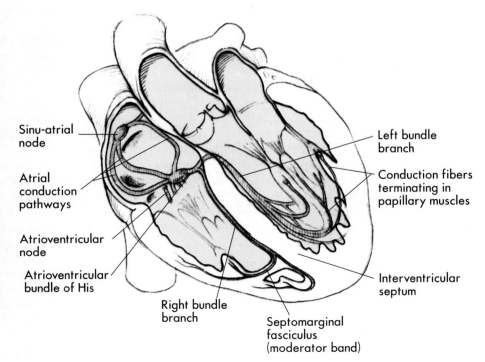

Sinu-atrial node

Atrial conduction pathways

Atrioventricular node

Atrioventricular bundle of His

Right bundle branch

Septomarginal fasciculus (moderator band)

Interventricular septum

Conduction fibers terminating in papillary muscles

Left bundle branch

THE HEART

HEART VALVES AND HEART SOUNDS

With the stethoscope can be heard two **heart sounds**—the "lub" and the "dub". These sounds usually are best heard in the left fifth interspace in the midclavicular line. The **first heart sound,** or "lub," is thought to be caused by the vibration of blood in the ventricular chambers as systole begins and the A-V valves close (with mitral slightly preceding tricuspid). The **second heart sound,** or "dub," is the result of similar vibrations in ventricular blood caused by closure of the aortic and pulmonary valves at the end of systole (with aortic valve closure slightly preceding pulmonary valve closure).

CATEGORIES OF CONGENITAL HEART DISEASE

Congenital cardiac lesions are varied and complex, but the majority of them produce one of two major abnormal physiologic situations: **increased flow of blood to the lungs** (as in ventricular septal defect, patent ductus arteriosus, truncus arteriosus, etc.) or **decreased circulation to the lungs** (pulmonic valve stenosis, atresia of the tricuspid valve, etc.). The timing of surgery (in general, the surgeon would prefer the child to be > 1 yr old and weigh > 15 to 20 lbs) is often based on concern about the permanent injury that the lungs may suffer if the abnormal circulatory arrangement is left untreated (especially **overcirculation**). In the past 10 to 15 years, great strides have been made in the techniques of surgery, so that the size of the patient is less likely to delay surgery than was true in the past.

base of the interatrial septum, alongside the orifice of the coronary sinus, and adjacent to the septal leaflet of the tricuspid valve. A large **posterior septal artery,** derived from the right coronary artery, most often provides the blood supply to the AV node. The myocytes of the AV node have a slow conduction velocity and produce the **AV conduction delay,** which allows complete atrial emptying into the ventricles before ventricular systole.

The **atrioventricular bundle** (of His) leaves the AV node and travels anteroinferiorly through the central fibrous body of the heart (see Figure 1-37). It passes anteriorly in the upper membranous part of the interventricular septum and then divides into the right and left bundle branches.

The **right bundle branch (RBB)** travels inferiorly in the muscular part of the ventricular septum toward the ventricular apex, entering the **septomarginal fasciculus (moderator band)** and terminating in the base of the *anterior papillary muscle* of the right ventricle (see Figure 1-48). The RBB gives off numerous side branches in the ventricular wall, which comprise the **subendocardial plexus of Purkinje fibers.**

The **left bundle branch (LBB)** also travels in the interventricular septum and quickly breaks up into a major *anterior* and *posterior limb,* each of which terminates in the base of a papillary muscle of the left ventricle. As with the RBB, the terminal branches form a subendocardial plexus, which courses from the apex toward the base of the left ventricle. Because conducted impulses reach the papillary muscles first, these muscles contract first, minimizing the risk of ventricular reflux through the A-V valves (because contraction of the papillary muscles puts tension on the chordae tendineae, preventing the leaflets of the A-V valves from "flipping" superiorly and allowing A-V reflux). Contraction always proceeds from the apex toward the base of the ventricles. Impulses also travel from the endocardium outward toward the subepicardial region, because the conducting plexus is subendocardial.

INNERVATION OF THE HEART

The heart receives both **sympathetic** and **parasympathetic** innervation as well as visceral sensory innervation. The *sympathetic preganglionic* cells are in the lateral horn of the spinal cord at segments T1 to T6. The *postganglionic* neurons are located in the cervical and upper one or two thoracic sympathetic ganglia (see Figure 1-32). The *parasympathetic preganglionic* neurons are in the nuclei of the **vagus nerve;** the *postganglionic* cell bodies are located in the *cardiac plexus* and in the walls of the heart, particularly those of the atrium near the SA node (Figure 1-49). The **cardiac plexus** is usually described as divided into a *superficial* (between aortic arch and pulmonary artery) and *deep* (between aorta and tracheal bifurcation) component. This plexus is diffuse and quite variable in size. It contains sympathetic postganglionic, parasympathetic pre- and postganglionic, and sensory axons. These axons innervate the heart, lungs, and mediastinum. From the cardiac plexus, *adrenergic* (sympathetic) axons are distributed to both atria and ventricles, but the *cholinergic* (parasympathetic) axons are largely distributed to the atria. The termination of autonomic axons (in particular parasympathetic) is especially dense around the SA and AV nodes. Sympathetic innervation increases the strength and rate of cardiac contraction; parasympathetic innervation decreases the strength and rate of contraction.

Sensory axons travel along with both the sympa-

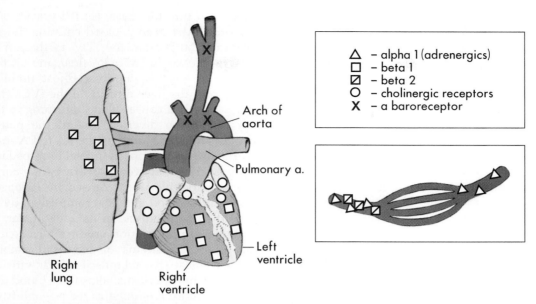

Figure 1-49 LOCATION OF RECEPTORS INFLUENCING BLOOD PRESSURE. Several important types of receptors are found in the lungs, heart, and vascular system. When appropriate hormones or drugs bind to these receptors, they affect heart rate and blood pressure. Stimulation of alpha-1 receptors causes vasoconstriction and an increase in blood pressure. Stimulation of beta-1 receptors causes increase in heart rate and strength of heart contraction. Stimulation of beta-2 receptors causes dilation of bronchioles within the lungs. Stimulation of cholinergic receptors slows the heart and weakens its contraction. Stimulation of baroreceptors (pressure), brought about by an increase in blood pressure, causes a reflex slowing of the heart rate. *Inset* shows the typical location of alpha-1 and beta-2 receptors near capillary beds.

CLINICAL ANATOMY OF

THE HEART

ARTIFICIAL PACING OF THE HEART

If the **cardiac conduction system** fails, an artificial pacemaker may be employed. Through a small incision in the lower chest wall, thin wires may be guided to the heart and implanted in the wall of the heart. Rhythmic electrical pulses then are delivered directly to ventricular or atrial muscle, producing rhythmic contractions. A long-lasting battery pack is placed beneath the skin. Recently, pacemakers became available that can sense the onset of a serious dysrhythmia and turn themselves on only when the patient's condition requires it (a "demand" pacemaker). Still other implantable devices can monitor the heart's rhythm and deliver a defibrillation electrical pulse in those suffering the initial stages of a life-threatening dysrhythmia.

TRANSVENOUS PACEMAKERS

In urgent circumstances, **temporary pacemakers** also may be inserted transvenously (i.e., through one of the large veins—subclavian, jugular, femoral) and will enter the heart through the IVC or SVC. The tips of these venous catheters are then positioned so that they are in contact with the ventricular endocardium. Pulsed electrical charges are delivered, and rhythmic cardiac contractions result.

ANATOMY OF CARDIAC TRANSPLANTATION

In performing a **heart transplant,** parts of recipient atria are left in place and the donor ventricles and parts of the atria of the donor heart are implanted. The donor heart has intact coronary circulation but lacks innervation, although some nerves may grow from recipient to donor tissues over time.

thetic and parasympathetic nerves; their cell bodies are in the dorsal root ganglia of cord segments T1 to T6. Sensory axons to the heart are important in the process that leads to the referred chest pain of angina pectoris (usually indicative of a heart attack). See pp. 119 for a fuller explanation of referred pain.

FETAL CIRCULATION

In the fetus, there is no need to send large quantities of blood to the lungs since they are not inflated with air and are not functioning as organs of respiration. Blood entering the right side of the fetal heart is diverted away from the lungs at two levels: (1) in the atrium, where a **foramen ovale** in the atrial septum allows oxygenated blood (remember that in the fetus, right atrial blood is highly oxygenated) to cross from the right atrium directly into the left atrium and (2) at the **ductus arteriosus,** a vessel that shunts blood from pulmonary artery to the aorta (Figure 1-50). Also, the fetus depends on the placenta of the mother for exchange of O_2 and CO_2, the delivery of nutrients, and removal of waste. This set of challenges is met by the **two umbilical arteries** and single **umbilical vein** (Figures 1-51 and 1-52). These vessels are embedded within the umbilical cord. Blood returning from the placenta to the fetus passes through an intrahepatic shunt vessel called the **ductus venosus.** This delivers placental blood to the fetal heart without having to pass through the liver's capillary beds. Following are detailed descriptions of these and other structures unique to the fetal circulation.

The **fetal circulation** depends on (1) the *patency of the ductus arteriosus* to divert PA blood away from the lungs and into the aorta, (2) the *patency of the foramen ovale* to divert venous blood entering the right atrium (especially that from the IVC) to the left atrium, by-passing the RA to RV to PA flow, and (3) the *patency of the ductus venosus,* to divert most umbilical venous blood past the liver directly to the IVC. The crescentic *valve of the IVC* causes blood returning to the heart via the IVC to be diverted toward the patent foramen ovale, further encouraging the RA to LA shunt.

The **ductus arteriosus** in fetal life (see Figure 1-50) is a large vessel that even may exceed the aorta in diameter. Its initial closure is caused by rising oxygen tensions in the blood and is accomplished by the contraction of smooth muscle in its walls. Later, intimal and endothelial proliferation produce a true closure. In the laboratory, conditions of increased ambient oxygen cause increased ductal muscle tone in vitro. The closure of the ductus arteriosus helps force blood to flow to the lungs (because it eliminates the possibility of a right to left shunt of blood). After birth, closure of the ductus arteriosus may be pharmacologically encouraged (by giving indomethacin) or discouraged (by giving prostaglandin E_1). In certain newborn patients, especially those with congenital heart lesions, the degree of ductal blood flow is a key physiologic feature. Blood supplying the carotid arteries is the most highly oxygenated blood in the fetus since it departs the arch of the aorta proximal to the point where the deoxygenated blood of the ductus arteriosus enters the aorta and lowers the net oxygen saturation of aortic blood distal to that point. Proximal to the entrance of the ductus, aortic blood is derived from the left ventricle alone and is maximally oxygenated. This arrangement ensures especially good O_2 supply to the developing

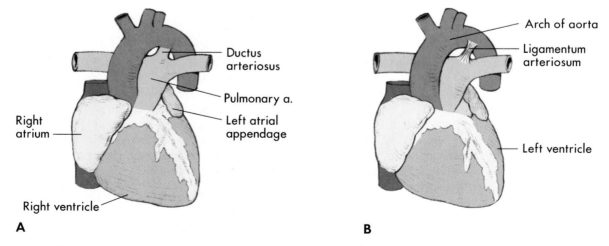

A   **B**

Figure 1-50   FORMATION OF THE LIGAMENTUM ARTERIOSUM. A, The prenatal condition of the ductus arteriosus, where the vessel is open and shunts a large fraction of pulmonary arterial blood away from the lungs and directly into the aorta. **B,** The postnatal state, the ductus arteriosus has closed and the lungs now receive a full blood supply. The ductus arteriosus persists as a solid cord of tissue, the ligamentum arteriosum.

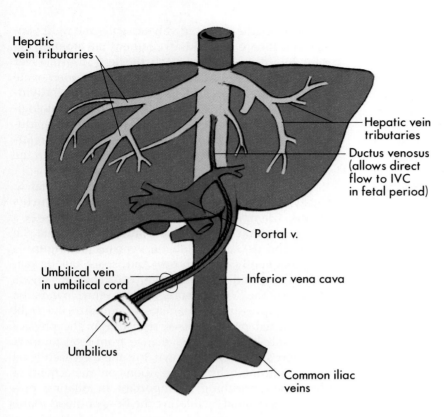

Hepatic
vein tributaries

Hepatic vein
tributaries

Ductus venosus
(allows direct
flow to IVC
in fetal period)

Portal v.

Inferior vena cava

Umbilical vein
in umbilical cord

Umbilicus

Common iliac
veins

Figure 1-51 DUCTUS VENOSUS. During fetal life, the ductus venosus shunts the majority of umbilical venous blood directly into the inferior vena cava, bypassing the liver. This provides high oxygenated blood directly to the heart.

brain. After ductal closure, the level of oxygenation should be nearly identical in all of the numerous branches of the aorta.

A second and equally important postnatal change is the **closure of the foramen ovale.** The most important result of this closure is a marked increase in the pulmonary blood flow (from RA to RV to PA and branches) and subsequently the increased filling of the left atrium. In fetal life, the patency of the foramen ovale depends upon right atrial pressure being much higher than that in the left atrium (forcing blood across the foramen ovale). With increased pulmonary flow, the left atrial pressure equals that of the right atrial pressure, causing the margins of the *septum primum* and *septum secundum* to become apposed and sealing off the atrial septum. This means that all right atrial blood

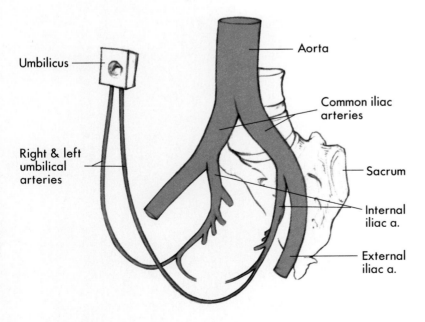

Umbilicus

Aorta

Common iliac
arteries

Right & left
umbilical
arteries

Sacrum

Internal
iliac a.

External
iliac a.

Figure 1-52 UMBILICAL ARTERIES. The two fetal umbilical arteries arise from the internal iliac arterial system and leave the fetal body at the umbiilicus, traveling from there through the umbilical cord to the placenta. After birth, the umbilical vessels are severed, and the portion of them remaining within the body deteriorate, except for small persisting arteries supplying the bladder.

CLINICAL ANATOMY OF

THE FETAL CIRCULATION

PATENT DUCTUS ARTERIOSUS

If there is a persistently **patent ductus arteriosus,** blood will flow from the aorta into the pulmonary artery because of the considerable pressure difference between the two vessels. The lungs will then receive a dangerously large amount of blood flow and can suffer irreversible damage as a result. Surgical closure is often necessary.

PERSISTENCE OF FETAL CIRCULATION (PFC)

Persistence of fetal circulation refers to a situation that occurs in the postnatal period when the blood flow to the lungs remains minimal (thus mimicking the fetal situation). As a result, the baby's postductal aortic oxygenation is inadequate (because venous blood from the right ventricle continues to be shunted into the aorta via the pathologically patent ductus arteriosus).

now traverses the tricuspid valve to enter the right ventricle (and thence to the lungs), rather than crossing the patent foramen ovale to reach the left atrium. Over time, in most people, the closure of the foramen ovale becomes anatomically permanent, but in some individuals the closure of the foramen ovale, while physiologically complete, never closes physically. Such individuals are said to have a *"probe-patent" foramen ovale* (referring to the ease with which a probe passes between the leaflets of this foramen when the heart is dissected).

A third major step in the transition from fetal to adult-type circulation is the **closure of the ductus venosus.** Clamping of the umbilical cord results in a drastic reduction in blood flow into the IVC (via the ductus venosus), and the ductus venosus (see Figure 1-51) subsequently thromboses and seals off permanently. This sudden interruption of umbilical venous flow lowers the IVC pressure, which in turn lowers the right atrial pressure. This helps to equalize the right and left atrial pressures (see preceding). The physiologic signals leading to the change from fetal to adult circulation are not fully known, but the increased level of oxygen in the baby's blood upon commencement of independent breathing is important in dilating pulmonary vessels and facilitating the flow of blood to the lungs.

Mediastinum

▶ Superior Mediastinum

▶ Posterior Mediastinum

▶ Anterior Mediastinum

*T*he **mediastinum** (L. *mediastinus,* a helper, assistant, or *mediastinum,* being in the middle) is that region that lies between the two pleural sacs. It has no easily identifiable boundaries (Figure 1-53); it is best considered as a region in which many crucial structures lie (the heart, thymus, etc.) and through which other very important structures pass (esophagus, aorta, trachea, thoracic duct, etc.). The mediastinum is divided into regions— the **inferior mediastinum,** with its anterior, middle, and posterior divisions, and the **superior mediastinum** (see Figure 1-3). The middle mediastinum is essentially synonymous with the heart and pericardial sac, which were described in Chapter 1.4.

SUPERIOR MEDIASTINUM

The leftward and rightward limits of the superior mediastinum are the pleural sacs on the left and right sides of the chest. Its *inferior limit* is approximated by a horizontal line drawn between the sternal angle and the lower part of the body of vertebra T4. The bifurcation of the trachea lies at this level (see Figures 1-3 and 1-33). The *superior limit* of the superior mediastinum is the **thoracic inlet** (the space surrounded by the T1 vertebra, first ribs, and manubrium; see Figure 1-10). The *superior mediastinum* contains, from anterior to posterior, the thymic remnants, brachiocephalic veins, superior vena cava, arch of the aorta and its branches, the lower trachea, the phrenic, vagus, and left recurrent laryngeal nerves, the sympathetic chains, cardiac nerves, and other descending autonomic nerves destined for the mediastinum, the esophagus, the thoracic duct, and numerous lymph nodes.

Arch of the Aorta and Great Vessels

The **aorta arch** begins at the level of the sternal angle and passes posterior and leftward as it rises to form an arch to the left of the bifurcation of the trachea. The aortic arch ends posteriorly where it is continuous with the descending aorta at vertebral level T4. The bifurcation of the pulmonary artery lies opposite the concavity of the aortic arch (Figure 1-54). Along the left side of the aortic arch are, from anterior to posterior, the **left phrenic nerve,** the **vagal** and **sympathetic** branches to the heart, and the **left vagus nerve** itself, giving rise to its **recurrent laryngeal branch.** Also on the left is the **left superior intercostal vein,** crossing the arch and traveling superficial to the vagus but deep to the phrenic nerve. In the preserved cadaver, the aortic arch makes an impression on the medial surface of the left lung. On the right side of the aortic arch are the **cardiac plexus, left recurrent laryngeal nerve,** and, from anterior to posterior, the **SVC,** the **bifurcation of the trachea,** the **thoracic duct,** and the **esophagus.**

From the undersurface of the arch itself originates the **ligamentum arteriosum,** connecting the aortic arch to the pulmonary artery. It represents the remnant of the fetal ductus arteriosus. The point of attachment for the ligamentum arteriosum to the aorta is approximately opposite the origin or "takeoff" of the left subclavian artery. The **left recurrent laryngeal nerve,** a branch of the left vagus nerve, loops under the aorta and around the left side of the ligamentum arteriosum.

The aortic arch, lying at the level of T4 to T5, gives rise to three large vessels: the **brachiocephalic artery**

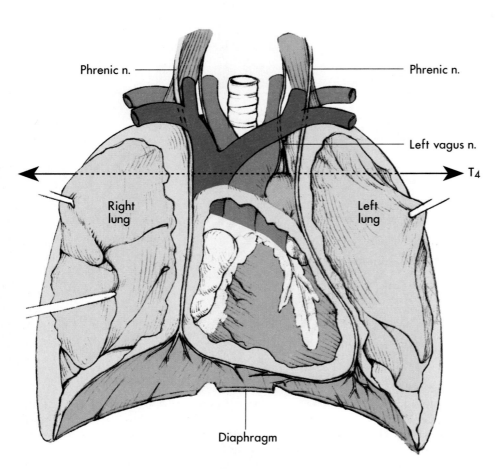

Phrenic n.

Phrenic n.

Left vagus n.

T4

Right lung

Left lung

Diaphragm

Figure 1-53 PHRENIC NERVES AND THE MEDIASTINUM. The mediastinum is the region between the two pleural sacs and includes a superior and inferior division. The inferior division is further divided into anterior, middle, and posterior regions. SEE ATLAS, FIG. 1-67

on the right and the **left common carotid** and **left subclavian arteries** on the left. The unpaired **brachiocephalic artery** passes obliquely upwards and backwards, toward the right, and eventually lies just to the right of the trachea. Just behind the right sternoclavicular joint it divides into the **right subclavian** and **right common carotid arteries.** The brachiocephalic artery normally gives off no other branches, except for an occasional small *thyroidea ima* branch (this may also arise directly from the aortic arch).

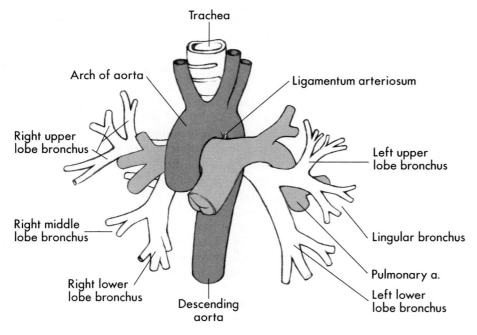

Trachea

Arch of aorta

Ligamentum arteriosum

Right upper lobe bronchus

Left upper lobe bronchus

Right middle lobe bronchus

Lingular bronchus

Right lower lobe bronchus

Pulmonary a.

Descending aorta

Left lower lobe bronchus

Figure 1-54 AORTA, PULMONARY ARTERIES, AND BRONCHI. The arch of the aorta, bifurcation of the pulmonary arteries, and the bifurcation of the trachea occur in a very confined space in the superior mediastinum. Branches of the pulmonary artery and bronchi follow each other closely in the substance of the lungs. SEE ATLAS, FIG. 1-66

PRINCIPLES

STRUCTURES AND SPACES

Many named areas within the body are regions rather than precise structures, and the two concepts must be kept separate. The **mediastinum** is a region or space, defined by the structures that surround it (the pleural membranes, sternum, and vertebral column, for example). Another region is the **gluteal region,** or buttocks, which contains a number of discrete structures, such as the gluteus maximus muscle and the superior gluteal artery.

The study of human anatomy involves frequent reference to spaces or regions, sometimes defined as distinct regions because they contain structures that work together to perform a function (for example, the muscles of the posterior forearm). Regions or spaces often contain structures that are supplied by a common artery or innervated by a common nerve. In clinical medicine, pathologic processes (infection, hemorrhage, expansion of a malignancy, etc.) often confine themselves to these regions or spaces.

The **left common carotid artery** has a small *thoracic portion,* ending as the vessel passes behind the left sternoclavicular joint, where the *cervical portion* of the vessel begins. The left common carotid arises directly to the left of the brachiocephalic and inclines to the left side of the trachea. Because the arch of the aorta at this point is nearly in an anteroposterior plane, the **left subclavian artery** may be said to arise more posterior to the left common carotid than to its left. It arches laterally, posterior to the scalenus anterior and then becomes the axillary artery as it passes over the lateral border of the first rib.

Brachiocephalic Veins and Superior Vena Cava

On both sides, the internal jugular and subclavian veins converge on the superior mediastinum. These combine to form a **brachiocephalic vein** on each side, anterior to the arch of the aorta and posterior to the medial end of the clavicle (see Figure 1-35).

The **left brachiocephalic vein** runs a longer course than does the right brachiocephalic vein (~6 cm vs. 2 to 3 cm). It commences as the left internal jugular and subclavian veins unite. It then passes posterior to the manubrium, rightward, and somewhat inferiorly. Behind the first chondrosternal joint on the right it unites with the right brachiocephalic vein to form the **superior vena cava (SVC).** In crossing posterior to the manubrium, it lies anterior to the left subclavian, left common carotid, and brachiocephalic arteries as well as the phrenic and vagus nerves.

The **right brachiocephalic vein** begins behind the medial end of the right clavicle, as the right internal jugular and subclavian veins unite. Unlike the left brachiocephalic, it then travels more vertically downward to unite with its partner from the other side (see preceding) behind the first chondrosternal joint on the right. Here it lies anterior and to the right of the brachiocephalic artery. The superior vena cava forms from the two brachiocephalic veins, receives the azygos vein, and sometimes receives directly the right vertebral and internal thoracic veins, plus occasional others.

Phrenic Nerves

The **phrenic nerves** arise in the neck from anterior primary rami of nerves C3 to C5 (C4 is the most constant and most important segment of origin). The nerve descends on the anterior surface of *scalenus anterior* muscle, embedded within the prevertebral fascia covering that muscle. It lies posterior to the inferior belly of omohyoid, the internal jugular vein, and the suprascapular artery. It next enters the superior mediastinum (see Figure 1-33) traveling between the subclavian artery and vein, anterior to the proximal part of the internal thoracic artery, and ultimately passes anterior to the root of the lung (Figure 1-55). As it descends through the chest it lies between the pericardial and pleural membranes.

On the left side the nerve crosses the left side of the aortic arch laterally. On the right it descends to the right of the SVC and reaches the diaphragm just to the right of the aperture for the inferior vena cava (see Figure 1-55). It finally ramifies in the substance of the diaphragm, which it innervates with somatic motor, sensory, and visceral motor axons. It also provides sensory innervation to the peritoneum and pleura covering the superior and inferior surfaces of the diaphragm, and pericardium, and mediastinal pleura.

Vagus and Recurrent Laryngeal Nerves

The paired **vagus nerves** are large cranial nerves, (#10), which arise in the cranial cavity, descend through the neck and enter the chest. They enter the superior mediastinum just posterolateral to the great arterial vessels on each side (see Figure 1-55). On the right, the vagus nerve descends alongside the trachea and passes posterior to the hilum of the right lung. It contributes axons to the cardiac plexus and continues posteriorly to reach the esophagus, on which it ramifies to form a plexus. On the left, the vagus nerve crosses the arch of the aorta on its left side, posterior to the phrenic nerve, and is crossed by the left superior intercostal vein. At the lower border of the aortic arch, the left vagus gives off the **left recurrent laryngeal nerve,** which passes around the left side of the ligamentum arteriosum and

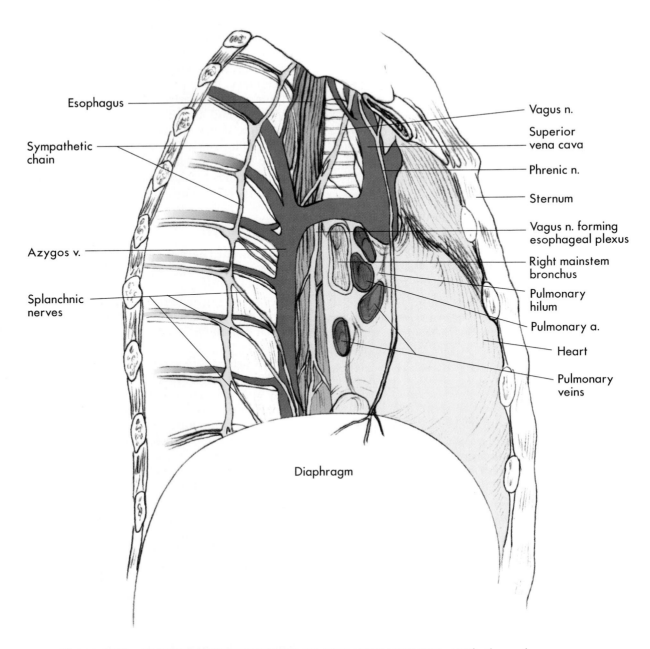

Esophagus

Sympathetic
chain

Azygos v.

Splanchnic
nerves

Vagus n.

Superior
vena cava

Phrenic n.

Sternum

Vagus n. forming
esophageal plexus

Right mainstem
bronchus

Pulmonary
hilum

Pulmonary a.

Heart

Pulmonary
veins

Diaphragm

Figure 1-55   RIGHT LATERAL SURFACE OF THE MEDIASTINUM. With the pulmonary hilum as a reference, note that the phrenic nerve lies anterior and the vagus nerve and sympathetic chain lie posterior to the mediastinum. Many of the structures depicted here make impressions on the medial surfaces of the lungs in the dissecting room specimen (see Figure 1-25).

loops under the arch of the aorta (the recurrent laryngeal nerve on the right does not descend into the mediastinum but instead loops under the right subclavian artery in the base of the neck). Both recurrent laryngeal nerves ascend in the neck toward the larynx, occupying a groove between the trachea and esophagus. The left vagus nerve ends by contributing to the plexus on the esophagus. Both right and left vagal axons accom-

pany the esophagus into the abdomen and supply much of the digestive tract with parasympathetic innervation.

Sympathetic Chains

The paired **sympathetic chains** (see Figure 1-55) are two series of ganglia linked by connecting axons, lying

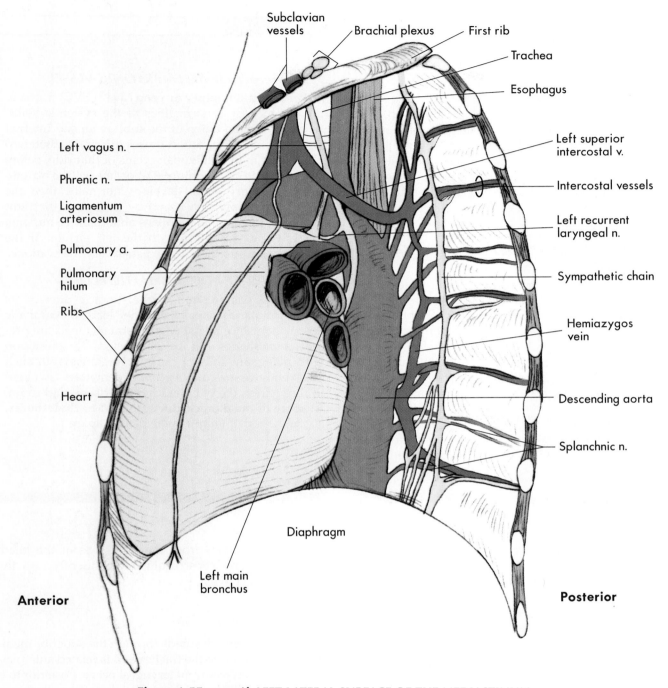

Subclavian vessels

Brachial plexus

First rib

Trachea

Esophagus

Left vagus n.

Phrenic n.

Ligamentum arteriosum

Pulmonary a.

Pulmonary hilum

Ribs

Heart

Left superior intercostal v.

Intercostal vessels

Left recurrent laryngeal n.

Sympathetic chain

Hemiazygos vein

Descending aorta

Splanchnic n.

Diaphragm

Left main bronchus

Anterior

Posterior

Figure 1-55—cont'd LEFT LATERAL SURFACE OF THE MEDIASTINUM

SEE ATLAS, FIGS. 1-65, 1-76, 1-77

to the left and right of the vertebral column. In the thoracic region, the vertically oriented chains lie anterior to the necks of the ribs and extend upward into the neck and downward into the lumbosacral region. Early in development there is one sympathetic ganglion for each spinal segment, but in the adult several of the ganglia fuse to make a total of 22 or 23 ganglia (whereas there are 34 spinal nerve segments). In the superior mediastinum are located the upper four thoracic sympathetic ganglia. The **cervicothoracic or stellate ganglion** is formed by the fusion of sympathetic ganglia for segments C7, C8, and T1. It is situated between the neck of the first rib (posteriorly) and the vertebral artery (anteriorly). Numerous important **cardiac**

THE MEDIASTINUM

RIGHT-SIDED AORTIC ARCH

The arch of aorta may pass to the right side of trachea, rather than its normal position to the left of the trachea, but nonetheless produce no symptoms or functional abnormality. The presence of a right-sided arch, however, increases the risk statistically that other abnormalities of the great vessels and/or other neck structures might be present. A right-sided aortic arch is often present in people with trisomy 21 (Down's syndrome).

TRAUMATIC INJURY AND THE SUPERIOR MEDIASTINUM

Trauma to the upper chest can result in aortic arch injury. A tear of the aorta will often lead to mediastinal widening due to hemorrhage (because of bleeding "compressed" within the mediastinum) or perhaps a pseudoaneurysm developing in the wall of the aorta itself. X-rays are mandatory for the evaluation of trauma in this area, and an overall widening of the mediastinum strongly suggests aortic injury.

SUPERIOR VENA CAVA SYNDROME

Superior vena cava syndrome results from obstruction of the SVC, leading to fluid accumulation and edema in the head, neck, and upper limbs.

PERSISTENCE OF AN EMBRYONIC VESSEL

Persistent left superior vena cava (LSVC) is one of the commonest abnormalities of the systemic veins. Arising from the union of the subclavian and internal jugular veins on the left, it passes inferiorly, often tangling itself in the pulmonary veins of that side, before emptying into the right (>90%) or left (<10%) atrium. If the coronary sinus develops normally, then the LSVC will empty into it and by extension, the right atrium. If the coronary sinus is abnormal, or missing, the LSVC drains directly to the left atrium. If the LSVC drains into the LA, the patient may be cyanotic.

INTERRUPTION OF LYMPHATIC FLOW

External compression of the thoracic duct or its major tributaries usually will not lead to lymphatic obstruction since so many collateral channels are present. Lymphatics can be obstructed by infestation with malignant cells or parasitic organisms. In such cases body tissues may become edematous (swollen) in those areas the lymphatics otherwise would drain. **Rupture** of the thoracic duct can lead to **chylothorax,** accumulation of lymph in the pleural space.

---

branches arise in the cervical sympathetic ganglia (and not from the thoracic ganglia) and descend into the mediastinum where they contribute to the **cardiac plexuses.** Within these sympathetic nerves are axons—which regulate heart rate, vascular tone, bronchial muscle tone, and airway mucus secretion—and numerous sensory axons.

Thoracic Duct

The **thoracic duct** begins at the aortic hiatus of the diaphragm, anterior to vertebra T12 (Figure 1-56). It ascends in the posterior mediastinum, lying between the azygos vein and the descending aorta. It passes through the superior mediastinum and enters the neck, where it arches forward between the vertebral artery and subclavian artery, to empty into the venous system at the junction of the left internal jugular and left subclavian veins. The comparable **right lymphatic duct,** draining the upper chest, right side of head, and right upper limb, empties into the junction of the internal jugular and subclavian veins on the right. It is often incomplete, or missing altogether, in which case

lymphatic channels from the right side of the head, upper limb, and chest drain independently into the right subclavian vein.

Esophagus and Trachea

The **esophagus** descends through the superior mediastinum posterior to the trachea and is related anterolaterally to the left recurrent laryngeal nerve. Posterior to it is the vertebral column; the medial surfaces of the lungs are lateral to it. The esophagus receives direct blood supply from the **esophageal arteries** (see Figure 1-29), branches of the descending aorta, and branches of the inferior thyroid arteries in the superior mediastinum.

In the superior mediastinum, the **trachea** extends from the thoracic inlet to the level of the T4 vertebra, with the esophagus posterior to it. As it bifurcates, the arch of the aorta lies to its left (see Figure 1-28).

POSTERIOR MEDIASTINUM

The **posterior mediastinum** is that space located between the vertebral column posteriorly and the poste-

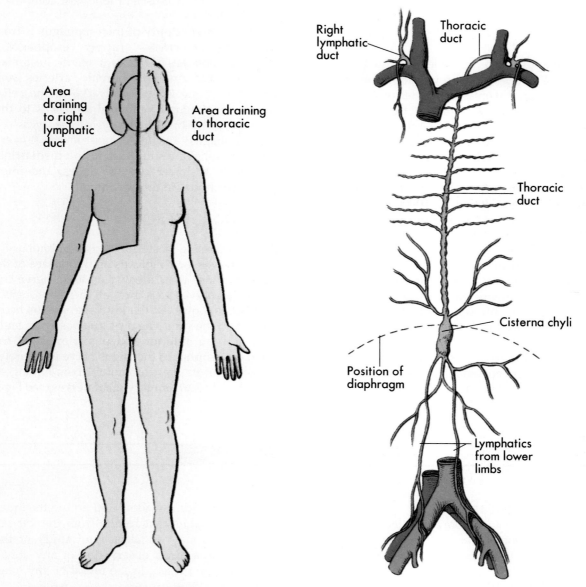

Figure 1-56 MAJOR LYMPHATIC VESSELS IN THE CHEST AND ABDOMEN. Abdominal and lower limb lymphatic drainage converges on the cisterna chyli. The thoracic duct ascends in the posterior mediastinum to drain to the left internal jugular/subclavian vein junction. The right lymphatic duct drains the right upper limb, the head and neck on the right, and drains into the right internal jugular/right subclavian vein junction.

rior surface of the pericardial sac anteriorly. The superior border is at vertebral level T4, and its lower limit is the diaphragm. The contents include the esophagus and vagal plexus, descending aorta and its branches, the thoracic duct, the azygos/hemiazygos system of veins, the sympathetic chains and splanchnic nerves, along with numerous lymph nodes.

Esophagus

The **esophagus** begins at the level of the cricoid cartilage (about C6), descends through the superior mediastinum, and then traverses the posterior mediastinum to penetrate the diaphragm opposite the body of vertebra T10. The esophagus lies against the anterior surface of the vertebral column except near its termination, where it moves somewhat anterior and leftward to penetrate the diaphragm. As it moves to the left, it passes anterior to the descending aorta. The esophagus is about 28 to 30 cm long (in the ~70 kg adult male) and undergoes a gradual transition from proximal striated to distal smooth musculature in its walls. The esophagus narrows in three places: (1) superiorly, where it blends with the cricopharyngeus muscle of the pharynx, (2) at its midpoint, where it is constricted by the aortic arch and left mainstem bronchus, and (3) inferiorly, where it passes through the diaphragm. Posterior to the esophagus are the thoracic duct, right intercostal arteries and the hemiazygos/accessory hemiazygos connection to the azygos vein. The distal one third of the esophagus lies posterior to the *left atrium*. The esophagus is not contained within a serous membrane

casing, and, therefore, esophageal neoplasms can expand unimpeded to nearby tissues.

The lower part of the esophagus functions as a **gastroesophageal sphincter,** though histologically such a sphincter is not evident. A true histological sphincter is present at the upper end of the esophagus as the **cricopharyngeus** muscle, the lowest component of the laryngopharynx.

The **arterial supply** of the esophagus is from the *inferior thyroid arteries* (upper esophagus), direct *esophageal branches* of the aorta (central esophagus), the superior and inferior phrenic arteries and small branches of the *left gastric branch* of the celiac artery (lower esophagus). **Venous drainage** is to the *thyroid veins* (upper esophagus), *azygos/hemiazygos veins* (central esophagus) and the *left gastric vein* (lower esophagus). Lymphatic drainage is to the mediastinal nodes, superiorly to lower cervical nodes, and inferiorly to paraaortic nodes in the abdomen.

Vagus Nerves

After passing posterior to the pulmonary hila, the **vagus nerves** form a plexus on the surface of the esophagus and lose their identity as large nerve trunks. As the vagus nerves pass through the diaphragm with the esophagus, however, the left vagal plexus becomes anterior and the right vagal plexus posterior, and they reform into an **anterior** and **posterior vagal trunk.** Beyond the esophagus the vagus nerve is a purely visceral nerve, all of its branchiomotor fibers having separated to form the **recurrent laryngeal nerves** (see Figure 1-55).

CLINICAL ANATOMY OF

THE ESOPHAGUS

GASTROESOPHAGEAL REFLUX

The esophagus can become irritated with the frequent **reflux** of stomach acid in an upward direction (often interpreted as heartburn).

ABNORMAL INNERVATION OF THE ESOPHAGUS

Dysfunction of the normal motility of the distal esophagus (**achalasia**) leads to obstruction, with dilation of the esophagus above the obstruction.

ESOPHAGUS AND IMAGING OF THE HEART

Before the era of ultrasound or cross-sectional imaging, left atrial enlargement (usually a consequence of rheumatic fever) was diagnosed by per-

forming a barium swallow and noting the indentation of the esophagus that results from the left atrial enlargement. Today, an ultrasound study of the heart can provide a direct observation of any abnormality that might be present in the mitral or any other heart valve.

ESOPHAGUS AND LIVER DISEASE

The lower part of the esophagus has **venous drainage** anastomosing with that of the stomach, an important consideration in the development of **esophageal varices** (dilated vessels in the mucosa, vulnerable to hemorrhage) in **portal hypertension** (high blood pressure in the portal vein) secondary to liver disease.

Descending Aorta and its Branches

The **descending aorta** extends from the plane of the sternal angle superiorly to the aortic hiatus of the diaphragm inferiorly, at the level of T12. Posterior to the aorta are the midthoracic vertebral bodies, the hemiazygos/accessory hemiazygos veins, and the posteromedial portion of the left lung. To its left is the medial surface of the left lung. The esophagus and thoracic duct lie to the right of the upper and middle portions of the aorta, but near the diaphragm the esophagus passes anterior to the aorta. Anterior to the upper and middle portions of the descending aorta are the left pulmonary veins.

Branches of the aorta (see Figure 1-29) are: (1) pairs of **posterior intercostal arteries** (for intercostal spaces 3 to 12—see following), (2) several **bronchial arteries** supplying the lung hilus on both sides, (3) several **esophageal branches,** and (4) a few minor branches to the posterior surface of the **pericardium.** Remember that the *first and second intercostal arteries* are branches of the *superior intercostal artery,* itself a branch of the costocervical trunk from the subclavian artery.

Thoracic Duct (and Right Lymphatic Duct)

The **thoracic duct** drains lymph from both sides of the body below the diaphragm, and the entire left side of the body including upper limb and head and neck above the diaphragm (the right upper limb and head and neck are drained by **right lymphatic duct**). The thoracic duct originates at the **cisterna chyli,** a dilation

---

CLINICAL ANATOMY OF

THE AORTA

ANEURYSMS OF THE THORACIC AORTA

The thoracic aorta is prone to **aneurysm** development (the dilation and "ballooning" of parts of the vessel wall) and sudden life-threatening rupture. With large aneurysms in the aortic arch, the left recurrent laryngeal nerve may be compressed and cause the patient's voice to be hoarse.

COARCTATION OF THE AORTA AND COLLATERAL CIRCULATION

In cases of **coarctation** (congenital narrowing) of the aorta, the proximal thoracic aorta beyond the ductus arteriosus is most commonly involved in the narrowing. It is this postductal coarctation in which extensive **collateral circulation** may develop, including **rib notching** from hypertrophic intercostal arteries.

---

and confluence of lymphatic channels in the posterior abdominal wall (see Figure 1-56). The cisterna is positioned posterior to the aorta and anterior to the bodies of vertebrae L1 and L2, at the level of the crura of the diaphragm. It receives lymphatic drainage from both lower limbs, the pelvic and abdominal walls, the testis or ovary, and the retroperitoneal viscera. The cisterna chyli passes through the aortic hiatus along with the azygos vein. Many individuals lack a single cisterna chyli, and multiple channels take its place.

The thoracic duct is positioned between the azygos vein and aorta, anterior to the vertebral column. Above the level of the sternal angle it deviates to the left. The thoracic duct then drains into the *left subclavian vein,* at its junction with the internal jugular vein. Its counterpart on the right, the **right lymphatic duct,** empties into the junction of the right subclavian and internal jugular veins. It forms in the neck from the confluence of lymphatic channels from the right upper limb, right side of head and neck, and the right side of the chest and mediastinum. It is sometimes absent.

Azygos/Hemiazygos Veins

The veins of the **azygos/hemiazygos/accessory hemiazygos** system (see Figure 1-23) are subject to considerable variation, and many different patterns should be anticipated from individual to individual. What follows should be viewed as the commonest arrangement.

The **azygos vein** lies on the right side of the vertebral column, along the posterior body wall. The azygos vein commences at the aortic hiatus or may pass directly through the right crus of the diaphragm as it originates. It represents a continuation of the segmental chain of lumbar veins from the posterior abdominal wall. The azygos vein ascends along the posterior abdominal wall, lying just anterior to the thoracic vertebral bodies. It empties into the *superior vena cava,* by arching over the right mainstem bronchus in a posterior to anterior direction, at the T4 vertebral level. The number of intercostal spaces it drains varies. The *first posterior intercostal vein* on the right drains directly to the brachiocephalic vein. The second to fourth intercostal spaces drain into the *right superior intercostal vein,* which is simply a common trunk draining blood from these three spaces into the azygos vein. Below this level, veins from intercostal spaces 5 to 12 on the right simply drain directly to the azygos vein.

The **hemiazygos vein** commences at the level of the diaphragm on the left. Like the azygos vein, it receives blood from the segmental lumbar veins of the posterior abdominal wall (but on the left). It ascends, collecting blood from posterior intercostal veins in segments T8 to T12. Next, the hemiazygos vein turns rightward and crosses the vertebral column to drain into the azygos vein. It often receives a bridging vessel from the accessory hemiazygos vein, draining more superior intercostal spaces on the left (see following).

The **accessory hemiazygos vein** descends on the left side of the vertebral column from the third to fourth intercostal space to the level of the seventh or eighth intercostal space. It receives the fourth to eighth intercostal veins (as on the right, there is a *first posterior intercostal vein* and a *superior intercostal vein* draining segments above this, the latter draining to the left brachiocephalic vein). The accessory hemiazygos turns rightward and crosses anterior to the vertebral column at ~T7. There is often a bridging vein connecting it to the hemiazygos vein at the next segment below.

Sympathetic Chain and Splanchnic Nerves

The **sympathetic chains** (Figure 1-57; see also Figure 1-55) are paired sets of **ganglia** (where nerve cell bodies and axons are found) united by **connectives** (bundles of axons and connective tissue coverings). Each chain lies alongside the vertebral column, anterior to the heads of the ribs, just external to the parietal pleura.

Each sympathetic ganglion is linked to the spinal nerve of the same segment by a **gray ramus** or **rami** (containing *postganglionic sympathetic* axons). In the case of **ganglia at T1 to L2,** an additional **white ramus** or **rami** (containing *preganglionic sympathetic* axons) unites the ganglion to its spinal nerve. These white rami are not present in sympathetic ganglia above T1 and below L2 because above T1 and below L2 there are no preganglionic sympathetic neurons in the spinal cord. Sympathetic ganglia above T1 and below L2 rely on the vertical sympathetic chains to bring preganglionic sympathetic axons to them. At the gross level, the gray and white rami are not obviously different, but microscopically they are distinct. The axons in gray rami are mostly unmyelinated, while those in white rami are myelinated.

Each sympathetic ganglion gives off small groups of postganglionic axons directed medially to viscera. The **greater, lesser,** and **least splanchnic nerves** are **preganglionic axons** which travel medially and inferiorly along the posterior thoracic wall toward the abdominal cavity. They arise from thoracic sympathetic chain ganglia ~T5 to T12 and are absent in other ganglia of the sympathetic chain. In the abdominal cavity they synapse in *prevertebral ganglia* along the abdominal aorta (see section on spinal nerves). Those branches from ganglia at T5 to T9 collect into the **greater splanchnic nerve,** those from T10 to T11 into the **lesser splanchnic nerve,** and those from T12 into the **least splanchnic nerve.** After these nerves synapse in abdominal prevertebral ganglia, postganglionic axons arising in these ganglia innervate large areas of the intestinal tract.

ANTERIOR MEDIASTINUM

The anterior mediastinum contains far fewer structures than the superior mediastinum. Included are **fat, sternopericardial ligaments, lymph nodes,** and **internal thoracic vessels.** The internal thoracic arteries originate as early branches of the subclavian artery (see Figure 1-21). As they descend posterior to the sternum, they give off **anterior intercostal branches** (for the upper five to seven intercostal segments), which anastomose with the posterior intercostal arteries arising from the descending aorta and coursing around the curvature of the thoracic wall. The **pericardiacophrenic artery,** a significant branch of the internal thoracic, joins the phrenic nerve to descend through the chest between the pleural and pericardial membranes. The internal thoracic arteries terminate by dividing at the level of the sixth intercostal space into the **musculophrenic** and **superior epigastric arteries.** The **internal thoracic veins** ascend to drain into the left and right brachiocephalic veins. Internal thoracic lymph nodes drain the anterior chest wall and breast.

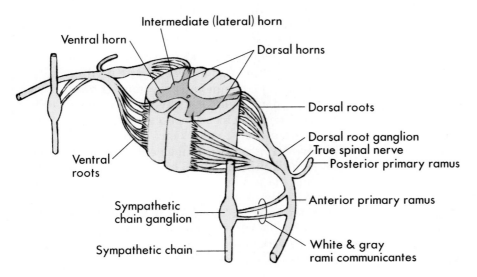

Ventral horn

Intermediate (lateral) horn

Dorsal horns

Dorsal roots

Dorsal root ganglion

True spinal nerve

Posterior primary ramus

Ventral roots

Anterior primary ramus

Sympathetic chain ganglion

Sympathetic chain

White & gray rami communicantes

Figure 1-57 SPINAL CORD, SPINAL NERVES, AND SYMPATHETIC CHAIN. Section typical of the thoracic and upper lumbar sections of the spinal cord. In cervical, lower lumbar, and sacral portions of the spinal cord, there would be only gray rami communicants connecting the sympathetic chain to the spinal nerve at those levels.

THE MEDIASTINUM

REMNANTS OF THYMIC TISSUE

Remnants of thymic tissue may also be found in the adult; these may be the source of tumors developing from germinal cell tissues.

SURGICAL APPROACHES THROUGH THE ANTERIOR MEDIASTINUM

A **sternotomy** (or longitudinal splitting of the sternum and dissection through the anterior mediastinum) is a commonly used surgical approach to the heart and other structures in the middle mediastinum.

REFERRED PAIN AND THE MEDIASTINUM

Referred pain—irritative or inflammatory processes in the upper abdomen, involving the liver and its covering peritoneum—may cause irritation of the phrenic nerve (because it provides sensory as well as motor innervation to the diaphragm). Through a mechanism poorly understood, spinal cord sensory pathways at C3 to C5 (where the phrenic nerve originates) can become activated, and the nerves of ordinary sensation for the C3 to C5 dermatomes are stimulated. The result of this is the experience of pain in the shoulder and upper arm, although the pathology is really in the abdomen. The pain is said to be **referred** to the shoulder.

VARIATIONS IN THE GREAT VESSELS

The **great vessels** are subject to frequent variations in structure (right-sided aorta, aberrent subclavian arteries, double superior vena cava, etc.) Most of these variations are the result of abnormal persistence of what are supposed to be transient embryonic and fetal vessels. Some of these variants may compress the trachea and impair breathing (so aortic abnormalities always should be considered as a possible cause for some types of abnormal breathing).

CATHETERS IN THE GREAT VEINS OF THE HEAD AND NECK

Placement of **catheters** in subclavian or internal jugular veins is often necessary for accurate assessment of blood pressure and cardiac function. Such catheters are often placed through the skin, aiming the tip of the needle where the vein is known to be, based on knowledge of anatomic arrangements.

AORTA AND THE RECURRENT LARYNGEAL NERVES

Compression of the left recurrent laryngeal nerve may result from aortic aneurysms or from an abnormal arrangement of the aortic arch and its branches. Hoarseness is a common symptom of such compression of the left recurrent laryngeal nerve.

SYMPATHETIC NERVES AND HORNER'S SYNDROME

The dilator pupillae muscle is innervated by postganglionic sympathetic axons arising in the superior cervical ganglion and reaching the eye via the branches of the internal carotid artery. Injury to these nerves leads to excessive constriction of the pupil, along with absence of sweat on one side of the face, and a drooping of the upper eyelid on the same side (known as Horner's syndrome). All of these functions are supported by sympathetic innervation. Pathology in the upper chest, affecting the thoracic portion of the sympathetic chains, can lead to this syndrome. The clinical importance of this situation is that an abnormality in the size of the pupil can result from pathology in distant sites.

STELLATE GANGLION BLOCK

The stellate ganglion is the fusion of the T1 ganglion and the lowest 1-2 cervical ganglia. Using anatomic landmarks as a guide, it is relatively easy to place the tip of a needle near the neck of the first rib and bathe the stellate ganglion in local anesthetic (a stellate "block"). This produces a temporary interruption of sympathetic function, which is very useful when trying to decide if a permanent (i.e., surgical) resection or removal in the stellate ganglion would benefit a patient with excess vasoconstriction in the upper limb on that side.

THYMUS GLAND AND MYASTHENIA GRAVIS

Although normally the thymus gland is a remnant in the adult, we find that 25% to 50% of those suffering from **myasthenia gravis** have thymic hyperplasia (excess growth). Circulating antibodies to the acetylcholine (ACh) receptor in the blood of those with myasthenia also may be associated with thymic hyperplasia.

VISUAL INSPECTION OF THE MEDIASTINUM

In **mediastinoscopy,** a fiberoptic flexible tube may be inserted into the mediastinum through a small skin incision on the upper chest. The mediastinoscope is then passed over the jugular notch and directed inferiorly into the mediastinum, and direct exploration and/or biopsy of structures in the mediastinum is carried out.

1.6 Systems Review and Surface Anatomy of the Thorax

▶ Musculoskeletal Anatomy of the Thorax

▶ Vascular Supply of the Thorax

▶ Lymphatic Drainage of the Thorax

▶ Innervation of the Thorax

▶ Surface Anatomy and Physical Examination of the Thorax

MUSCULOSKELETAL ANATOMY OF THE THORAX

The skeletal framework of the thorax consists of the **vertebral column, ribs, sternum,** and certain elements of the **shoulder girdle.** The thorax must serve as a protective cage for the thoracic and upper abdominal viscera but at the same time must be mobile and flexible to accommodate motions of the upper limb and trunk. The 12 pairs of ribs are suspended between the thoracic vertebrae posteriorly and the sternum anteriorly although only the first seven ribs articulate directly with the sternum). The ribs articulate through synovial joints, posteriorly with the vertebrae themselves and anteriorly with the costal cartilages, which in turn articulate with the sternum. Rib motion has been likened to the movement of a bucket handle through an arc, resulting in important changes in the volume of the thoracic cavity. Accordingly, muscles that elevate the ribs (external intercostals, pectoralis minor, sternocleidomastoid, etc.) can be described as **muscles of inspiration.** Muscles that depress the ribs (internal intercostals, serratus posterior inferior, etc.) can be described as **muscles of expiration.** Respiration, then, is a repetitive cycle in which air is drawn into the tracheobronchial tree by the expansion of the chest cavity and passively exhaled as the chest wall relaxes and thoracic volume decreases. Note that the normal mechanism of breathing never involves increasing pressure inside the tracheobronchial tree and lungs, thus avoiding injury that would inevitably result.

Chest wall musculature takes part in the important **Valsalva maneuver.** This complex action involves the tight apposition of the two vocal cords, so that no air can escape from the lungs and trachea, and the simultaneous contraction of various muscles in the thoracic and abdominal wall. This produces an increase in pressure inside the thorax and especially the abdomen and is an integral part of such activities as urination, defecation, and childbirth (parturition).

The thorax also serves as a foundation for movements of the upper limb. The **shoulder girdle** (the clavicle and scapula) permits the upper limb to be projected away from the chest wall, greatly increasing the range of motion. There are chest wall muscles that move the shoulder girdle anteriorly (e.g., pectoralis major and minor) and others that move it posteriorly (e.g., the rhomboids, serratus posterior, latissimus dorsi). Still others elevate the scapulae (e.g., levator scapula) and clavicle (e.g., sternocleidomastoid), and all of these muscles in combination result in a wide variety of possible motions for the shoulder girdle.

The arrangement of ribs and muscles in the thoracic wall vividly illustrates the **segmental** nature of the human body. This organizational scheme expresses itself in the vascular and nervous system anatomy of the chest wall as well as the musculoskeletal structure. Each rib and the intercostal musculature accompanying it are supplied by an individual intercostal nerve and artery (although there is considerable overlap between segments). An understanding of this segmental arrangement in the thorax facilitates study of the remainder of the trunk, the limbs, and the head and neck, where the segmental arrangements are considerably distorted.

VASCULAR SUPPLY OF THE THORAX

The chest wall is supplied with blood by a series of **intercostal arteries.** Most of these vessels are supplied with blood by *posterior intercostal branches,* arising mainly from the **aorta,** and *anterior intercostal branches,* arising from the left and right **internal thoracic arteries.** The intercostal arteries course along the inferior surface of each rib and supply not only the interspace in which they lie but also one or two interspaces on each side. Additionally, there are posterior, lateral, and anterior **cutaneous branches** of the intercostal arteries, whcih penetrate upward into the superficial fascia of the chest wall. Intercostal arteries for the upper two (or sometimes three) interspaces arise from the subclavian artery and costocervical trunk. The chest wall also receives blood from several branches derived from the subclavian-axillary system of arteries—the **pectoral, lateral thoracic,** and **subscapular arteries,** among others. The overall arterial supply to the chest wall is richly anastomotic.

The thoracic viscera, consisting of the heart, lungs, and mediastinal structures, have a unique arterial supply. The heart and lungs have their own arterial inputs—the **coronary arteries** for the heart, and the **pulmonary** and **bronchial arteries** for the lungs (the pulmonary arteries carry deoxygenated blood). The structures within the mediastinum generally receive arterial input from branches of the descending aorta or, in the upper mediastinum, from branches of the subclavian or external carotid arteries.

Venous drainage of the chest wall is via the **intercostal veins,** which converge on a vertical collecting vein on the posterior thoracic wall (**azygos vein** on the right; **hemiazygos/accessory hemiazygos veins** on the left). The azygos/hemiazygos veins return blood primarily to the superior vena cava and thence to the heart. Again, **thoracic viscera** have unique venous drainage. The heart is drained by several **cardiac veins,** which deliver blood to the **coronary sinus.** The lungs are drained of conventional venous blood mainly by the **bronchial veins** and of oxygenated blood by the **pulmonary veins.** Draining of bronchial venous blood into the pulmonary veins slightly diminishes the oxygen content of the otherwise fully oxygenated pulmonary venous blood. The remaining mediastinal structures return their venous blood to the azygos, subclavian, and brachiocephalic veins.

LYMPHATIC DRAINAGE OF THE THORAX

The lymphatic drainage of the chest wall is directed at **lymph nodes** in the clavicular, axillary, and even the inguinal regions. The most important structure in this region is the **breast** since spread of breast tumors occurs through lymphatic channels. Lymphatic drainage of the heart and lungs is directed at the posterior mediastinum and the nodes at the **pulmonary hilum,** respectively. Lung tumors and serious infections such as tuberculosis spread first via lymph nodes in the pulmonary hilum. The remaining mediastinal structures also direct their lymphatic drainage to nodes near the pulmonary hila and in the mediastinum.

INNERVATION OF THE THORAX

The **chest wall** is innervated by **intercostal nerves.** These nerves supply the deep tissues within the intercostal space and have **posterior, lateral** and **anterior cutaneous branches,** which pass into the superficial fascia, along with similarly named vessels. Innervation of both the deep and superficial parts of the chest wall involves striated muscle control, ordinary sensory innervation, and autonomic innervation of arrector pili muscles and sweat glands.

The important **phrenic nerves** traverse the chest as they pass from the neck to innervate the diaphragm. They course along the anterior surface of the scalenus anterior muscles, pass posterior to the clavicle and first rib, and descend in the plane between the pleural and pericardial sacs, accompanied by the periocardiacophrenic vessels. Upon reaching the lower part of the thorax, they ramify and provide all of the motor and most of the sensory innervation of the diaphragm. The mediastinal pleura and pericardium are also innervated by the phrenic nerve.

The **heart** is innervated by **sympathetic nerves** via the cardiac nerves, descending from the upper neck, through the mediastinum and into the heart. They accelerate and increase the force of the heartbeat. **Parasympathetic nerves,** branches of the **vagus,** also innervate the heart and slow its rate of contraction. The **lungs** receive sympathetic and parasympathetic input from the same sources as innervate the heart. In the lungs, sympathetic input helps relax small airway smooth muscle and dilate the airways, while parasympathetic input narrows the airways and increases mucus secretion. Autonomic innervation of the remainder of the **mediastinum** is principally involved with *vasomotor tone*—the control of blood pressure by constricting or relaxing smooth muscle in the walls of vessels.

SURFACE ANATOMY AND PHYSICAL EXAMINATION OF THE THORAX

For the physician, the thorax provides an opportunity to collect a great deal of information about the status of the patient's health. Palpation and inspection of the **breast** are of paramount importance for the female patient. Each woman should be skilled at examining her own breasts since subtle changes may be evident to her long before they become evident to a physician. An examination of the breast should always include thorough palpation of the axillary region since the axillary tail of the breast extends well into the axilla. The examiner should always be conscious of palpable lymph nodes, especially in the axilla, since they may be harbingers of a malignancy in the breast.

Certain inflammatory diseases of the chest wall reveal the **dermatomal** pattern of the thorax, as displayed in herpes zoster (shingles). Palpation of the chest wall is important to assess for tenderness, suggesting a fractured rib or inflammation at one of the joints involving the ribs. The patient's respirations should be observed since a frequent sign of respiratory distress is **retractions**—the visualization of ribs through the chest wall due to the forceful muscle contractions necessary to draw breath into the lungs when inflammation of the lungs and/or airways is present.

Several **surface landmarks** help the examiner visualize the position of structures within the chest. The **jugular** or **sternal notch,** a semicircular depression in the upper edge of the sternum, should be located in all examinations (Figure 1-58). Next, the examiner should locate the **sternal angle**—the articulation of the manubrium and body of the sternum—since it localizes the second rib and allows numbering of all ribs using rib two as a reference. The **xiphoid process** should be located because it defines the lower end of the sternum and also because it localizes the T7 dermatome. When palpating the inferior margin of the **costal angle**—the collected costal cartilages of ribs 8 to 10, meeting in the midline at the xiphoid process—it can be appreciated how near the lower margin of the thoracic cage comes to the upper surface of the ilium of the pelvis. The nipple marks the location of the T4 dermatome. Next the examiner can palpate laterally along the superior surface of the **clavicle,** appreciating its S-shaped configuration and the lateral articulation with the acromion in

the **acromioclavicular joint.** When palpating the **axilla,** the **anterior** and **posterior axillary folds** (raised vertical ridges of skin that cover the inferior edges of the pectoralis major and latissimus dorsi muscles, respectively) should be observed. Clinicians often refer to a set of vertical lines on the chest when describing the location of various structures. The **midclavicular line** is an imaginary vertical line drawn from the midclavicle downward on the anterior chest wall. The **anterior axillary line** is a similar vertical line drawn from the anterior axillary fold downward. The **posterior axillary line** is an imaginary line drawn from the posterior axillary fold downward. The **midaxillary line** is an imaginary vertical line midway between the anterior and posterior axillary lines (Figure 1-58, B).

An imaginary horizontal line drawn from the sternal angle posteriorly will intersect the lower margin of the T4 vertebral body. This line passes through the level of the bifurcation of the trachea and demarcates the inferior border of the **superior mediastinum** (see Figure 1-3). The lower border of the inferior mediastinum is, of course, the diaphragm. It should be appreciated that during deep expirations, the diaphragm may rise as high as the level of the fourth or fifth rib anteriorly.

Percussion (gentle tapping on the surface of the chest, to detect the presence of solid organs or air-filled spaces beneath the surface) can be employed to define the upper and lower limits of a solid organ like the liver, and it will be clear to the examiner that the upper edge of the liver is often two to three rib interspaces above the costal margin and its lower margin well below the costal margin.

The position of both the heart and lungs should be visualized on the chest wall (see Figure 1-58). The **heart** is positioned so that most of its forward-facing surface is actually the wall of the right ventricle. The **left border** of the heart is actually a crescent of the left ventricle, and the **right border** is the lateral wall of the right atrium. Additionally, the heart is tipped to the left so that the **apex** of the heart lies to the left, in the midclavicular line at the fifth intercostal space. The lower part of the right atrial wall and the wall of the right ventricle face inferiorly, toward the diaphragm. This tipping of the heart means that when blood flows through the atrioventricular valves it is flowing in a nearly horizontal direction, rather than vertical, as one might expect. The **mitral** and **tricuspid valves** are positioned at the level of the fourth and fifth ribs. The **pulmonary** and **aortic valves** are located superior to the atrioventricular valves, deep to the sternum opposite the third and fourth ribs. The **right cardiac border** is nearly vertical and extends from the level of the second intercostal space to the fifth intercostal space, just lateral to the chondrosternal junction. The **left cardiac border** also extends from the second to the fifth intercostal spaces, on the left, but lies at a 45 degree angle (Figure 1-58, B).

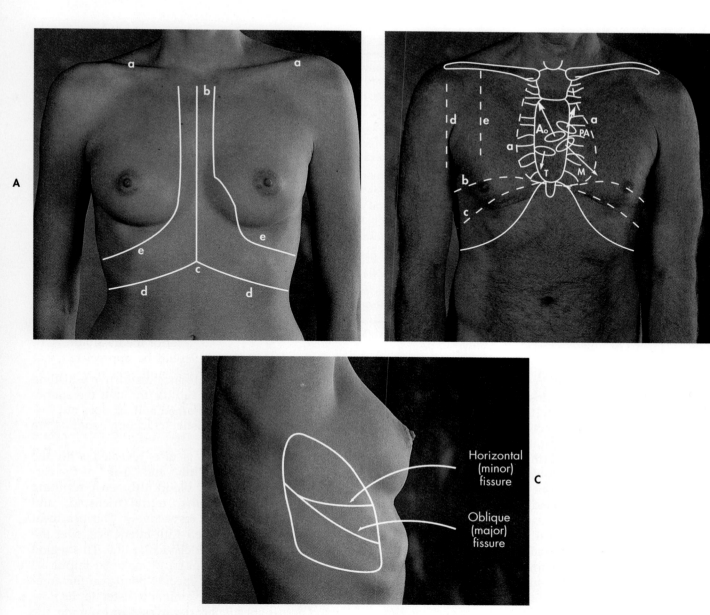

Figure 1-58   SURFACE ANATOMY OF THE CHEST WALL. A, Female anterior chest wall with lines indicating the position of the clavicles (*a*), sternal notch (*b*), midsagittal line (*c*), costal angle (*d*), and the medial borders of the two pleural sacs (*e*). **B,** Outlines of the sternum, ribs, costal angle, and clavicles are superimposed on the male anterior chest wall. *Ovoid dashed line* (*a*) indicates the position of the heart. *Ao,* aortic valve; *PA,* pulmonary valve; *T,* tricuspid valve; *M,* mitral valve. *Arrows* indicate the point on the chest where the sound of blood crossing each valve is best heard. The position of the diaphragm at expiration (*b*) and inspiration (*c*) is also shown. The anterior axillary fold (*d*) and the midclavicular line (*e*) are also shown. **C,** Position of the right lung is projected on a lateral view of the chest wall.

Table 1-5   Surface Projections of Thoracic Structures

Anterior Landmark	Structure(s)	Posterior Landmark
Above medial clavicle	Apex of the lung(s)	Body of T1
First chondrosternal joint	Aortic arch	
Second chondrosternal joint (at sternal angle)	Tracheal bifurcation	Body of T3
	Arch of azygos vein	
	Bifurcation of pulmonary artery	Lower body of T4
Third chondrosternal joint	Pulmonary valve (on left)	Body of T7
	Junction of SVC and RA	
Fourth chondrosternal joint	Mitral valve (on left)	Disk at T7 to T8
	Aortic valve (in midline)	
Fifth chondrosternal joint	Tricuspid valve (on right)	Body of T8
Seventh chondrosternal joint	IVC passing through diaphragm	Body of T8 to T9
Xiphoid process	Esophageal hiatus	Body of T10
Left fifth intercostal space, midclavicular line	Apex of heart (in midclavicular line)	Body of T11
	Gastroesophageal junction	

The **lungs** change position with the degree of inspiration or expiration. At full inspiration the **apex** of each lung and its covering pleura (the cupola) protrudes 2 to 3 cm above the first rib and clavicle into the base of the neck. Inferiorly, at full inspiration, the lungs extend inferiorly to the level of the 11th rib. The **oblique fissure,** separating the upper and lower lobes of each lung, can be visualized on the posterior chest wall as a line commencing at the third thoracic vertebra posteriorly and lying deep to the fifth intercostal space as it courses anterolaterally around the chest wall (Figure 1-58, C). For the right lung, the **horizontal (minor) fissure** may be visualized as a line on the anterior chest wall paralleling the lower border of the fourth costal cartilage.

In the superior mediastinum, the **aortic arch** is located in the midline, at the level of the second anterior rib. The **superior vena cava** begins with the union of the two brachiocephalic veins, just posterior to the first chondrosternal joint on the right. The bifurcation of the **pulmonary trunk** occurs slightly to the left of the midline, posterior to the sternum at the level of the third rib. Table 1-5 is a summary of *positional relationships* between deep thoracic structures and landmarks on the chest wall.

Use of the **stethoscope** for **auscultation** is an important part of physical examination of the chest. The movement of air in and out of the **lungs** can be assessed in this way. When major regions of the lung are not properly aerated, the examiner will note the absence of "breath sounds" in those areas. Obstruction of the smaller airways may produce distinctive whistling noises such as **wheezing,** audible through the stethoscope. When alveoli are inflamed and air does not easily inflate them, characteristic "crackling" sounds are heard (**rales**).

Much about the **heart** is also revealed with the stethoscope. The normal **"lub"** and **"dub"** of the cardiac cycle are produced by blood turbulence resulting from the closing of the mitral/tricuspid and aortic/pulmonary valves, respectively. The heartbeat is usually loudest in the left fifth interspace, over the apex, at the level of the midclavicular line. This region is known as the **PMI** or "point of maximal impulse." Placing the stethoscope at specific points on the anterior chest wall allows the examiner to listen to the flow of blood across specific heart valves—for example, the blood crossing the mitral valve is heard best with the stethoscope positioned over the apex of the heart, and blood crossing the aortic valve is heard best along the upper right sternal border. Abnormally turbulent movement of blood produces **murmurs** ("whooshing" sounds, heard between the normal lub and dub). The flow of blood through congenital holes (**septal defects**) in the atrial or ventricular septae may also produce murmurs. Inflammation within the **pericardial sac** produces a grinding grating sound (a "friction rub"). Much of the art of interpretation of heart sounds is increasingly being supplanted by the frequent use of ultrasound imaging techniques to define abnormalities in heart structure.

1.7 ◀ Thorax

■ CASE 1

CHEST WALL

A 51-year-old woman, Ms. R.M., reports to her physician that she has felt very fatigued for the past 2 to 3 weeks. She has been in general good health and has not visited a physician for many years. She tells her physician that she has lost 7 to 10 pounds over the past month not because of dieting but because of a general lack of interest in food. After taking a thorough history, the physician undertakes a physical examination of Ms. R.M. She discovers that in Ms. R.M.'s left breast there is a firm nodular density, seemingly about 3 to 4 cm in diameter, that is anchored in tissue several centimeters beneath the skin.

Questions

1. To which additional areas of this woman's body should the physician direct special attention during the physical examination and why?
2. If the lesion in this patient's breast is malignant and the goal were surgically to remove the entire breast alone, could this procedure be performed without having to make an incision in the deep fascia of the thorax?
3. What are the surgical options for Ms. R.M.'s condition, and what are the anatomic components of each surgical option?

■ CASE 2

PLEURAL SPACES AND SEROUS CAVITIES

A 27-year-old man was seriously injured in a motorcycle accident. He was brought to an Intensive Care Unit where his physicians decided he would benefit from placement of a central venous catheter, specifically in his right subclavian vein. The catheter is placed successfully, but, approximately 30 minutes after catheter placement, the patient begins to breathe rapidly, requires more oxygen, and is generally distressed. Physical examination is significant for a shift of the heartbeat to the far left side of the chest and very poor breath sounds on the right side of the chest by stethoscope. A chest x-ray shows dense "white-out" of much of the right side of the patient's chest.

Questions

1. What anatomic landmarks guide the placement of the central venous catheter?
2. What might cause the right side of the patient's chest to be poorly aerated, and cause the heart to shift to the left side of the chest?
3. What procedure might be undertaken to remedy this problem, and what anatomic landmarks might guide the procedure?

■ *CASE 3*

TRACHEOBRONCHIAL TREE AND LUNGS

A 67-year-old man developed a worsening cough over several months, and, when the sputum began to show streaks of blood, he consulted a physician. The patient's medical history was significant for 40 years of smoking cigarettes. An x-ray of the chest revealed an irregularly shaped density in the lower right chest and loss of definition of the right cardiac border. Surgical removal of the affected area was scheduled.

Questions

1. What lobe of the right lung is likely involved, and how does the x-ray confirm this?
2. How can it be determined whether the cancer is confined to the area seen on the x-ray or has spread to other areas of the body?
3. How will knowledge of the pattern of pulmonary arterial and pulmonary venous blood supply to the lung figure in the surgeon's planning for this operation?

■ *CASE 4*

HEART

A 74-year-old man was playing golf, and, while walking from one tee to the green, felt a tingling and weakness in his left arm. He continued to play but some 10 minutes later began to have difficulty breathing and became dizzy. He sat down on a nearby bench but soon complained of a heavy weight on his chest and then lapsed into unconsciousness. He was rushed to a nearby emergency room where an electrocardiogram showed irregular heart electrical activity and pulse. Some minutes later he deteriorated markedly, and his blood pressure dropped dramatically. He

lapsed into a deep coma. An echocardiogram showed that his mitral valve was now nonfunctional, and blood was regurgitating freely from the left ventricle to the left atrium. He died several minutes later. An autopsy showed total obstruction of the left coronary artery and near complete obstruction of the right coronary artery due to atherosclerosis.

Questions

1. How does coronary artery obstruction cause arm tingling and weakness?
2. How does coronary artery disease cause irregularities in the heartbeat?
3. How did the dysfunction in his mitral valve drop his blood pressure?

■ *CASE 5*

MEDIASTINUM

An 8-year-old male was found to have high blood pressure on a school physical examination. He was referred to his physician, who verified the high blood pressure and noted that his femoral pulses were weak in comparison to the radial or carotid pulses. His feet seemed cool to the touch, and the patient said he always had to wear warm socks even in summer. A chest x-ray was remarkable for irregular lower borders on several of the ribs on both sides of his chest. The diagnosis was then made, and plans for treatment discussed with the patient and his parents.

Questions

1. What explains the different pulses in upper and lower limbs?
2. What important anatomic principle is illustrated by the irregularity in the rib borders ("rib notching")?
3. Why did the patient have high blood pressure?

■ CASE 1

1. The physical examination should be directed at the (1) **axilla,** (2) **opposite breast,** (3) **supra- and infraclavicular regions,** and (4) the **parasternal** region. Malignancies of the breast commonly spread to these areas.
2. Since the breast lies within the superficial fascia, it is possible in theory to remove the breast without having to dissect into the deep fascia. In practice, however, breast malignancies usually are treated surgically by removal of the breast and varying but substantial amounts of the deep chest wall tissues (pectoralis major, minor, etc.).
3. Several surgical therapies are available for breast tumors. The larger the tumor, the more likely it will have spread. In addition, the time that elapses between the actual appearance of the tumor and its detection are important predictors of the degree of surgical invasiveness that will be required.
   - Lumpectomy: Removal of the breast tumor and the adjacent breast tissue and superficial fascia but no entry into the deep fascia.
   - Modified radical mastectomy: Removal of the entire breast, including the axillary tail, plus the pectoralis major and adjacent lymph nodes.
   - Radical mastectomy: Removal of the entire breast, including the axillary tail, plus the pectoralis major and pectoralis minor muscles, and the adjacent lymph nodes and connective tissue.

■ CASE 2

1. The catheter is placed in the right **subclavian vein** by introducing a needle along the inferior surface of the midclavicle and directing the needle toward the jugular notch of the sternum. When the needle enters the subclavian vein, a soft flexible catheter is introduced using the needle as a guide. By keeping the needle as close to the posterior surface of the clavicle as possible while inserting it further medially, it should enter the subclavian vein since the vein lies immediately posterior to the clavicle. If the needle is allowed to pass even a few centimeters posterior to the clavicle, instead of moving along its posterior surface, the needle might enter the subclavian artery (remember it lies posterior to the subclavian vein and is separated from it medially by the **scalenus anterior** muscle).
2. In this patient, the insertion of a catheter apparently caused a tear in the wall of the subclavian vein, leading to hemorrhage into the pleural space. The subclavian artery might be similarly torn and, in fact, would lead to more rapid accumulation of blood in the pleural space. The accumulation of blood in the right pleural space (a **hemothorax**) eventually causes partial collapse of the right lung and puts pressure on the mediastinum, shifting it (and the heart) to the left.
3. The next step would be to remove the blood from the **pleural space.** This is accomplished by a **thoracentesis,** where a catheter or tube is inserted into the pleural space. Such tubes are inserted by creating a small incision in the chest wall and directing the tube or catheter over the superior border of a rib and into the pleural space.

▎ *CASE 3*

1. The **right middle lobe** is likely involved. Because the lung cancer has caused the right middle lobe not to fill with air at inspiration, the right cardiac border cannot be seen clearly (because normally the air-filled right middle lobe lies just lateral to the right heart border, and the air in the lung makes the solid tissue of the heart border stand out).
2. A malignancy arising in the lungs likely will spread first to the lymph nodes at the **pulmonary hilum.** These might be detected on x-ray, by CT scan or MRI, or by direct visualization at surgery.
3. Pulmonary arterial blood follows the pattern of bronchial branching closely, so that the **bronchopulmonary segments** are defined by the **tertiary branches** of both the bronchial tree and the pulmonary artery. Thus if a surgeon wished to remove the right middle lobe, she/he would need to find and tie off the segmental bronchial and arterial branches for the lateral and medial segments of the right middle lobe, before removing the lung tissue. The pulmonary veins, however, do not respect these bronchopulmonary segmental boundaries, and more care would be necessary to prevent venous bleeding once the lung tissue is removed.

▎ *CASE 4*

1. Arteriosclerosis in the coronary arteries ultimately causes interruption of blood flow to the heart muscle itself (a **myocardial infarction**). This leads to the production of lactic acid (from anaerobic metabolism in the heart muscle), causing irritation of the heart muscle. Sensory nerves in the heart, traveling with the sympathetic and parasympathetic nerves, carry this sensation back to the spinal cord. In the spinal cord, it is believed that the incoming sensory volley from the heart somehow activates sensory neurons, which also receive input from somatic sensory nerves (in this case from the upper limb). No one knows how this "cross-talk" between sets of neurons works. Since any activation of a neuron in the "circuit" for normal innervation of a structure produces a sensation in that structure, the patient whose pathology is really in the heart experiences a sensation in the upper limb. The jaw and neck may also be involved in this process, known as **referred pain.** This term is apt because the sensation actually occurring in one structure (the heart) is referred to another area of the body (the upper limb).
2. Obstruction of blood flow to the heart may affect not only the heart muscle but the **conduction system** of the heart. In this case, branches of the left anterior descending artery are especially important in supplying the ventricular septum, where the **left** and **right bundle branches** are found. Abnormalities in the conduction system appear as an abnormal electrocardiogram (ECG).
3. Interruption of blood flow to the heart muscle often has a dramatic effect on the **papillary muscles,** where the chordae tendineae are anchored. If the papillary muscles rupture, the chordae tendineae are released, and the mitral valve leaflets flip upward into the atrium, failing to seal off the mitral valve orifice during ventricular systole. Blood now regurgitates into the atrium, drastically dropping aortic pressure.

■ *CASE 5*

1. This patient suffers from a **coarctation of the aorta,** probably occurring in the middescending aorta in the posterior thoracic wall. A coarctation is a narrowing in the aorta, and so, below the level of the coarctation, the amount of aortic blood flow (and the pulse) is diminished.

2. The rib borders are "notched" because the intercostal arteries are significantly enlarged and have become tortuous in shape, literally eroding into the substance of the rib. This occurs because the blood that can no longer easily flow down the descending aorta is directed through the important process of **collateral anastomotic flow** into the various intercostal arteries. This means that the posterior intercostal arteries arising from the aorta above the coarctation are forced to accept a very high volume of blood, and they enlarge in size as a result. The body is equipped with numerous normal collateral vascular connections in most regions, and more can form in response to the obstruction of a vessel.

3. Patients with coarctations deliver less blood down the aorta distal to the coarctation. This includes the **kidney,** which responds to this diminished blood flow as though it were a sign of diminished blood volume throughout the body. The kidney then produces a hormone, **renin,** which leads to the production of other substances that elevate the blood pressure. The kidney is one of the most important sites at which the blood flow/pressure in the body are monitored, so that the body's natural assortment of hormones can be adjusted to bring the blood pressure back toward normal.

SECTION TWO

Head and Neck

▶ **2.1** Skull

▶ **2.2** Brain and Central Nervous System

▶ **2.3** Cranial Nerves

▶ **2.4** Pharyngeal Arches

▶ **2.5** Scalp and Face

▶ **2.6** Temporal and Infratemporal Fossae

▶ **2.7** Posterior Triangle of the Neck

▶ **2.8** Anterolateral Neck

▶ **2.9** Ear

▶ **2.10** Eye and Orbit

▶ **2.11** Nasal Cavity

▶ **2.12** Mouth and Palate

▶ **2.13** Pharynx

▶ **2.14** Larynx

▶ **2.15** Systems Review and Surface Anatomy of the Head and Neck

▶ **2.16** Case Studies: Head and Neck

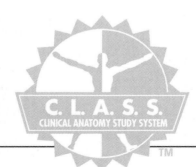

C. L. A. S. S.
CLINICAL ANATOMY STUDY SYSTEM

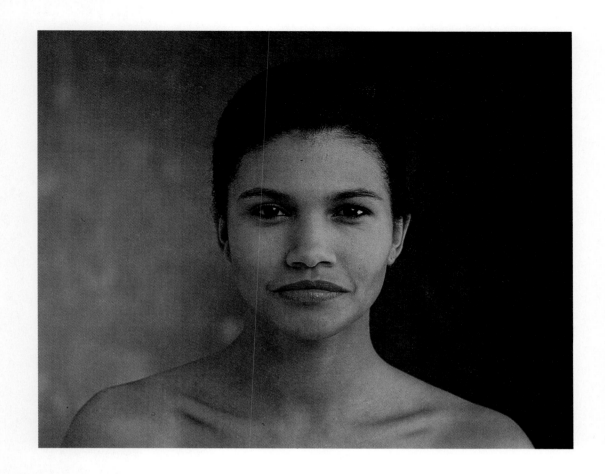
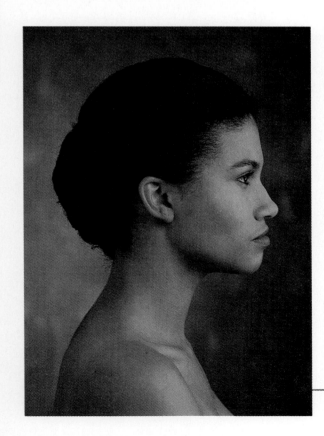

Skull

▶ Introduction

▶ Cranial Vault

▶ Sutures of the Skull

▶ Skull of the Child

▶ Landmarks on the Surface of the Skull

▶ Floor of the Cranial Cavity

▶ Base of the Skull

▶ Skeletal Components of the Face

▶ Air Sinuses Within the Skull

INTRODUCTION

The anatomy of the head and neck poses a particular challenge for the student. The relationships of adjacent anatomic structures are especially difficult, and an ability to visualize in three dimensions is absolutely essential to success in studying this area of the body. Though the area contains literally dozens of **bones,** only the mandible, hyoid bone, ossicles, and cervical vertebrae are movable. The remaining bones compose the skull and face and are firmly attached to each other at **synchondroses** (cartilaginous joints), allowing little or no motion. Many of these synchondroses ossify (become bony due to deposition of calcium salts) in later decades of life.

The **muscles** of the head and neck range from the delicate stapedius of the middle ear to the thick masseter muscle of the jaw. Several organs of special sense (vision, hearing, taste, smell, and balance) are housed in unique and intricate anatomic structures (the orbit, middle and inner ear, semicircular canals, and nose). There are examples of somatic, sympathetic, and parasympathetic nerves in the head and neck. The skull—with its hollow cranial vault, orbits, and intricate face—is the essential starting point for study of the head and neck.

Arterial blood flow for the head and neck arises from two pairs of large vessels—the common carotid and vertebral arteries. The brain requires a nearly-constant flow of arterial blood for normal function, and a special mechanism (autoregulation) exists to ensure this steady flow, even when accelerations or gravitational forces might produce major changes in flow. **Venous drainage** from the head and neck converges in the jugular veins, with a small additional component leaving the intracranial compartment through the vertebral veins. Because the skull is a nondistensible space, disturbances in the normal inflow and outflow of blood can produce very serious increases in intracranial pressure and subsequent disturbance to normal brain function.

Lymphatic drainage varies throughout the head and neck. The brain and spinal cord themselves *lack* lymphatic vessels and nodes. The function of circulating and exchanging extracellular fluid, an important role for the lymphatic system elsewhere in the body, is probably carried out by the steady production and flow of cerebrospinal fluid in the central nervous system (CNS). Lymphatic drainage of the face and scalp converges in the deep or superficial lymph nodes. Lymph nodes are especially plentiful around the lower margin of the mandible, ear, and mastoid process, and along the internal jugular vein of the neck. Deep structures in the head and neck (that is, the nose, mouth, pharynx, and larynx) drain to the deep cervical nodes. The globe lacks lymphatic drainage, because much of the globe is really a part of the CNS, but the tissues of the lids and orbit drain along with the remainder of the face.

The skull has several major functions. First, it forms a cranial vault and base, providing protection and support for the brain. Second, it forms the skeletal framework of the face. Other bony structures in the head and neck are derived from the *pharyngeal* or *brachial arch* apparatus, the evolutionary remnant of the gill mechanism; in humans, it forms embryologically and gives rise to tissues that migrate widely over the head and neck region, forming certain bones, cartilages, muscles, and blood vessels.

Many special organs and tissues of the region (e.g., the **eyes,** suspended within a protective orbit; the organs of **hearing** and **balance;** the **nasal** and **oral apertures;** and the **masticatory** (chewing) **structures,** including the jaws, tongue, pharynx, and facial muscles) are anchored in the bones of the skull. Third, the strength and rigidity of the skull help to protect the complex pattern of arteries and veins through which the brain receives the continuous blood supply on which it is particularly dependent. (Of all organs and tissues in the body, the brain is the least tolerant of interruptions to blood flow.)

CRANIAL VAULT

The walls and roof of the cranial vault are a composite of several individual bones, including the **frontal bone, occipital bone,** and the paired **temporal** and **parietal bones** (Figure 2-1). In the adult, the margins of these platelike bones of the cranial vault are firmly bound to each other at fibrous joints, also known as *sutures.*

Certain blood vessels (especially the *sigmoid* and *transverse venous sinuses* and the *middle meningeal artery*) lie against the inner surface of the cranial vault and make *inscriptions* on its surface. These are visible in the skull specimens we study in the laboratory. The close proximity of these and other vessels to the surface of the skull explains the frequency of hemorrhage of these vessels when the skull is fractured.

The floor of the cranial vault or **floor of the skull** (see Figure 2-7) is formed by the articulation of parts of four separate bones of the skull—the *ethmoid, sphenoid, temporal,* and *occipital bones* (see following section).

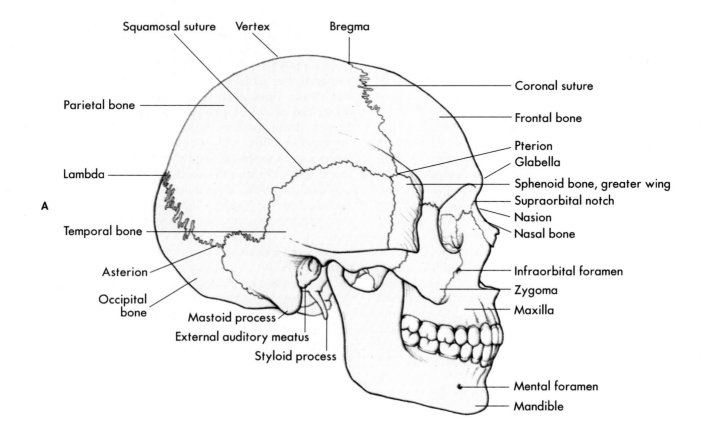

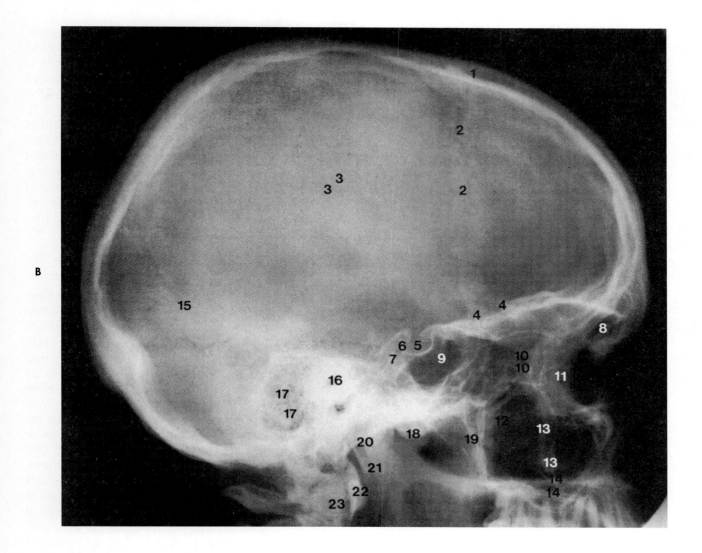

B

Figure 2-1 LATERAL VIEW OF SKULL. A, Schematic drawing (see opposite page). **B,** X-ray image. This view makes possible visualization of the maxillary sinuses, sphenoid sinus, and frontal sinuses. The pituitary is also clearly visible. (**B** from Weir J, Abrahams PH: *An imaging atlas of human anatomy,* London, 1992, Mosby.) **SEE ATLAS, FIG. 2-21**

1 Diploë	**14** Palatine process of maxilla
2 Coronal suture	**15** Lambdoid suture
3 Grooves for middle	**16** External acoustic meatus
meningeal vessels	**17** Mastoid air cells
4 Greater wing of sphenoid	**18** Articular tubercle for tem-
5 Pituitary fossa (sella turcica)	poromandibular joint
6 Dorsum sellae	**19** Coronoid process
7 Clivus	**20** Condyle of mandible
8 Frontal sinus	**21** Ramus of mandible
9 Sphenoidal sinus	**22** Anterior arch of atlas (C1
10 Ethmoidal air cells	vertebra)
11 Frontal process	**23** Odontoid process (dens) of
12 Arch of zygoma	axis (C2 vertebra)
13 Maxillary sinus	

The skull consists of three main regions—a **neurocranium,** a **dermatocranium,** and a **visceral skeleton** (structures derived from the pharyngeal arch apparatus).

The *neurocranium* develops from a set of cartilages that eventually ossify and form the floor of the skull, including parts of the occipital, temporal, sphenoid, and ethmoid bones. Also included are cartilages that condense around the developing nasal epithelium and middle ear and become incorporated into the floor of the skull. The *dermatocranium* includes "roofing bones" that encase the brain (frontal and parietal bones), certain bones of the upper jaw, palate, and most of the bones forming the medial and inferior walls of the orbits. The *pharyngeal arches* contribute parts of the upper jaws, lower jaws (mandibles), middle ear bones, and several cartilages and bones of the anterior neck.

The *floor of the skull* is composed of parts of the frontal, ethmoid, sphenoid, temporal, and occipital bones. All of the major apertures in the floor of the skull, in fact, are apertures in the ethmoid, sphenoid, temporal, or occipital bones, or apertures that lie along the borders where these bones meet. The important vessels and nerves entering and leaving the interior of the skull pass through these apertures.

The number of individual bones in the skull and facial region of the "higher" vertebrates is in general less than that found in the "lower" vertebrates. Also, the importance of the pharyngeal arch region changes dramatically when comparing those vertebrates that use the region for feeding and respiration (through gills) with those in which the pharyngeal arches are modified for use in vocalization, for the attachment of tongue muscles, and for swallowing (for example, in mammals and birds).

The bewildering complexity of skull and facial bones can be understood more clearly with some reference to the evolution of these structures through the progression of vertebrates.

SUTURES OF THE SKULL

Once complete ossification has occurred, the edges of adjacent bones of the cranial vault are represented by narrow tortuous lines known as **sutures.** The line between the posterior margin of the frontal bone and the anterior edges of the two parietal bones is the **coronal suture** (Figures 2-1, *A,* and 2-2). That between the posterior edges of the two parietal bones and the ante-

rior edge of the occipital bone is the **lambdoidal suture** (Figures 2-1, *A,* and 2-3). Running along the sagittal midline of the skull, between the two parietal bones, is the **sagittal suture** (Figure 2-3). On the lateral surface of the skull, the **squamosal suture** marks the apposition of the temporal and parietal bones (see Figure 2-1). Occasionally, there are additional sutures in the skull of certain individuals, surrounding areas known as "independent" or "Wormian" bones. One of these, located at the junction of the sagittal and lambdoidal sutures, was particularly frequent in the skulls of the Inca Indians of South America and is known as the "os incae." It is also present in the skulls of *Homo erectus,* an important precursor species to modern humans.

SKULL OF THE CHILD

The human infant is born with a cranial vault whose component bones are not tightly attached to each other. The larger gaps between the adjacent edges of the parietal, temporal, frontal, and occipital bones of the child are joined by soft fibrous tissue, which later ossify and become rigid. This process generally takes 14 to 24 months, after which time the skull is a firmer and more resistant protective encasement for the brain. Particularly wide gaps between adjacent skull bones are known as **fontanelles.** The most well-known of these are the *anterior fontanelle* and *posterior fontanelle* (the "soft spots" of the baby's head; Figure 2-4). The anterior fontanelle lies at the junction of the frontal bone and the two parietal bones; the posterior fontanelle lies at the junction of the two parietal bones and the occipital bone. The presence of large fontanelles in the baby permits the continued growth of the brain to take place in an expansible compartment and assists in molding (temporary distortion in the shape of the skull) during birth. Premature sutural closure can have adverse effects on brain development.

At birth and through the first and second years of life, the size ratio of cranial vault/face is much greater than in the older child and adult (Figure 2-5). The proportionate size of the face increases through childhood, as the air sinuses enlarge within the bones of the face itself.

LANDMARKS ON THE SURFACE OF THE SKULL

The intact skull may be viewed from a number of different vantage points—the lateral view (see Figure 2-1, *A*), the frontal or anterior view (see Figure 2-2), and the posterior view (see Figure 2-3). In addition, the base of the skull or inferior view (see Figure 2-9) should be compared with the view of the floor of the skull, seen from the interior (Figures 2-6 and 2-7).

We recognize a set of landmarks on the surface of

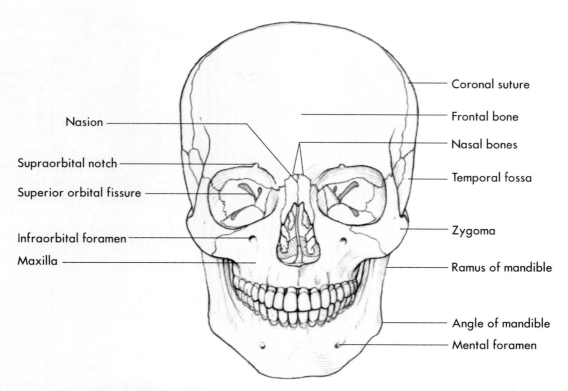

Coronal suture

Frontal bone

Nasal bones

Temporal fossa

Zygoma

Ramus of mandible

Angle of mandible

Mental foramen

Nasion

Supraorbital notch

Superior orbital fissure

Infraorbital foramen

Maxilla

Figure 2-2   ANTERIOR, OR FRONTAL VIEW OF SKULL.   See Atlas, Figs. 2-20, 2-22, 2-97

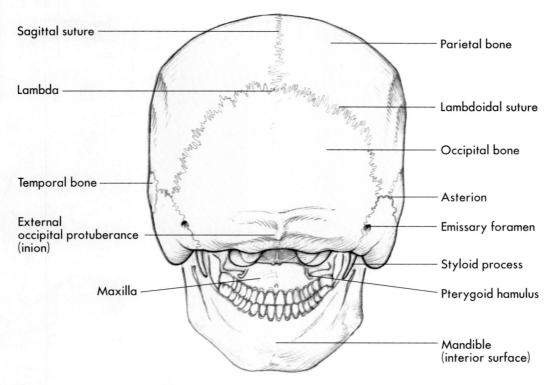

Sagittal suture

Lambda

Temporal bone

External
occipital protuberance
(inion)

Maxilla

Parietal bone

Lambdoidal suture

Occipital bone

Asterion

Emissary foramen

Styloid process

Pterygoid hamulus

Mandible
(interior surface)

Figure 2-3   POSTERIOR VIEW OF SKULL.

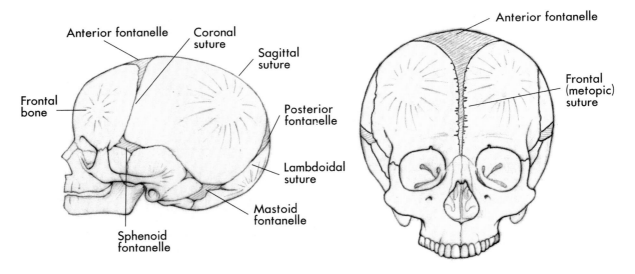

Figure 2-4   FETAL SKULL. The skull of the newborn has a smaller proportion devoted to facial structures and has several fontanelles (gaps where cranial vault bones are not closely attached to each other).

Figure 2-5   SKULL OF THE CHILD AND THE SKULL OF THE ADULT. The facial structures of the skull of the child compose a much smaller fraction of the overall size of the head, presumably because air sinuses are lacking.

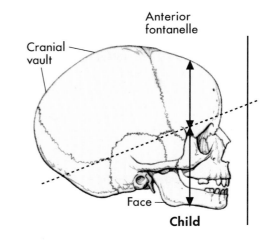

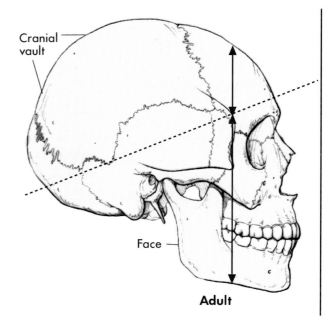

the skull, most of them located at the points where sutural lines intersect. The most important of the sutures are the coronal suture, the sagittal suture, and the lambdoidal suture. An occasional specimen has a frontal or metopic suture, running vertically in the midline on the anterior surface of the frontal bone. Figures 2-1, 2-2, and 2-3 show the most important of these landmarks. They are described in Table 2-1.

FLOOR OF THE CRANIAL CAVITY

The floor of the skull is divided into three major fossae (see Figures 2-6 and 2-7). The **anterior fossa** is bounded posteriorly by the lesser wing of the sphenoid bone, and its perimeter is formed by parts of the ethmoid, frontal, and sphenoid bones. The anterior fossa supports the frontal lobes of the brain. The **middle fossa** lies between the lesser wing of the sphenoid bone anteriorly and the petrous ridge of the temporal bone posteriorly. The sphenoid, petrous temporal, and squamous temporal bones form its perimeter. It supports the temporal lobes of the brain. The **posterior fossa** (see Figure 2-10, *B*) extends from the petrous ridges of the temporal bones anteriorly to the occipital bone posteriorly. The occipital and petrous temporal bones de-

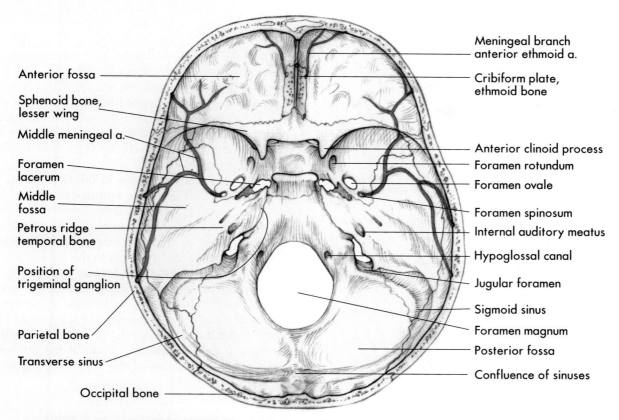

Figure 2-6   FLOOR OF SKULL. The brain and meninges have been removed to reveal the bony surface of the floor of the skull.   See ATLAS, Figs. 2-92, 2-93

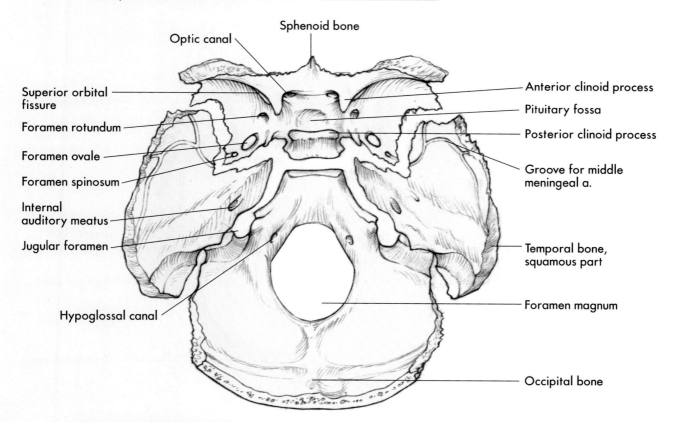

Figure 2-7   DETAILED VIEW OF BASE OF SKULL. The sphenoid, occipital, and temporal bones are shown here slightly separated, to reveal how many of the important apertures traversing the floor of the skull are found within one of these bones or along their mutual borders.

Table 2-1   Landmarks of the Skull

Skull Landmark	Location
Bregma	At the junction of the coronal and sagittal sutures
Lambda	At the junction of the lambdoidal and sagittal sutures
Pterion	At the junction of the frontal, parietal, temporal, and sphenoid (greater wing) bones
Asterion	At the junction of the temporal, parietal, and occipital bones
Inion	The external occipital protuberance, just superior to the foramen magnum
Nasion	At the junction of the frontal and the two nasal bones
Glabella	A prominence on the frontal bone, just superior to the nasion
Vertex	The most superior part of the skull, located along the superior sagittal suture

fine its outline. The occipital lobes and the cerebellum are supported by the posterior fossa.

The floor of the anterior fossa is formed by parts of the frontal, ethmoid, and sphenoid bones. The floor of the middle fossa comprises parts of the sphenoid and temporal bones, while the floor of the posterior fossa is made up of the occipital bone (with its large and important foramen magnum).

All of the important *apertures* in the floor of the skull (Figures 2-6 and 2-8) lie either within one of four bones (the *sphenoid, ethmoid, temporal,* and *occipital*), or along a line of apposition between these bones (see Figure 2-7). These four bones, as a unit, compose the floor of the skull. In life, most of the apertures in the floor of the skull are partially occupied with cartilage or other dense connective tissue. This closes any gaps remaining where the nerves or vessels traverse the individual apertures. The cranial vault usually has a number of irregularly placed **emissary foramina,** small apertures through which pass small *emissary veins* connecting some of the intracranial venous sinuses with veins of the scalp (see Figure 2-3).

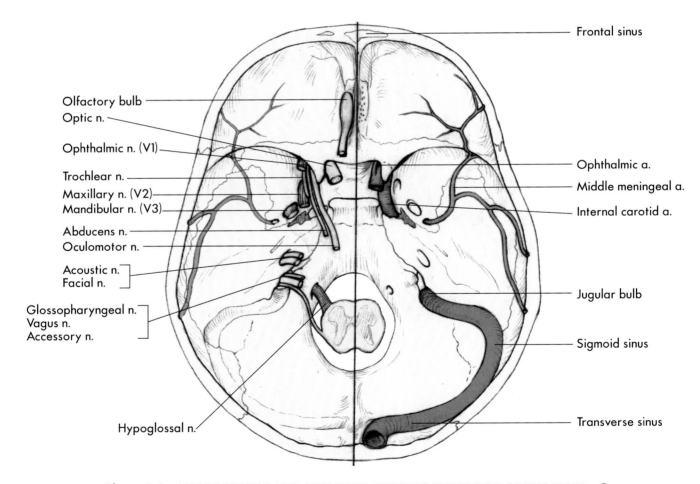

Figure 2-8   MAJOR VESSELS AND NERVES TRAVERSING THE FLOOR OF THE SKULL. On the left are shown all of the cranial nerves and the apertures through which they traverse the floor of the skull. On the right are shown major arteries and veins and the apertures they traverse.

Some of these emissary foramina are large, especially in the parietal and occipital bones (Table 2-2). When scalp infections are present, infectious organisms may pass through these veins and reach the interior of the skull, threatening the patient with meningitis.

Table 2-2   Major Apertures in the Skull

Aperture	In Bone(s)	What Traverses It
Cribriform plate (floor)	Ethmoid	Olfactory fila (part of cranial nerve I*)
Optic canal (floor)	Sphenoid	Optic nerve (II), ophthalmic artery
Superior orbital fissure (floor)	Sphenoid	Ophthalmic vein, III, IV, V1 (ophthalmic nerve), VI
Foramen rotundum (floor)	Sphenoid	V2 (maxillary nerve)
Foramen ovale (floor)	Sphenoid	V3 (mandibular nerve), accessory meningeal artery, lesser petrosal nerve
Foramen spinosum (floor)	Sphenoid	Middle meningeal artery, meningeal branch of V3
"Foramen" lacerum† (floor)	Sphenoid, temporal, occipital	Contains internal carotid artery
Carotid canal (base)	Temporal	Internal carotid artery, sympathetic plexus
Internal auditory meatus (floor)	Temporal (petrous part)	VII, VIII, labyrinthine artery
Stylomastoid foramen (base)	Temporal	Muscular portion of VII
Jugular foramen (floor)	Temporal, occipital	Internal jugular vein, IX, X, XI
Hypoglossal canal (floor)	Occipital	XII nerve
Foramen magnum (base and floor)	Occipital	Spinal cord, vertebral vessels, spinal root of XI

*Cranial nerves are conventionally identified by Roman numerals, as well as by their names; see p. 165 for a listing of the cranial nerves.
†Not a true foramen, because it is a *gap* between adjacent bones and filled in with cartilage in life.

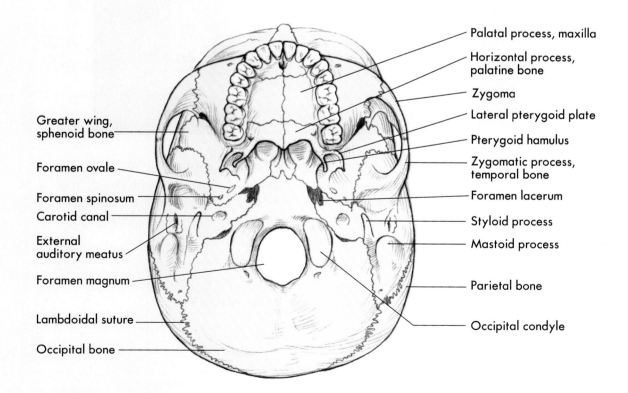

Figure 2-9   BASAL VIEW OF SKULL. This view reveals several of the important foramina conveying nerves and vessels in and out of the cranial cavity.   SEE ATLAS, FIG. 2-96

BASE OF THE SKULL

Viewed from the inferior aspect, the inferior surface or **base of the skull** presents a complex array of bony prominences and apertures (Figure 2-9). These apertures are the "opposite side" of the apertures described in the section "Floor of the Cranial Cavity" and are of particular importance, because through them travel various nerves and vessels entering and leaving the skull. Modern imaging techniques permit us to see many of these apertures with considerable clarity (Figure 2-10).

SKELETAL COMPONENTS OF THE FACE

The bones of the cranial vault contribute little to the shape of the face, but parts of the frontal and temporal bones, in particular, *do* contribute importantly (see Figure 2-2). The frontal bones forms much of the perimeter of the orbits, giving shape to the bony ridges above the eyes. The temporal bones forms part of the zygomatic arch ("cheekbone") on each side of the face. The nasal and maxillary bones give shape to the center of the face and the mandible to the lower third of the face.

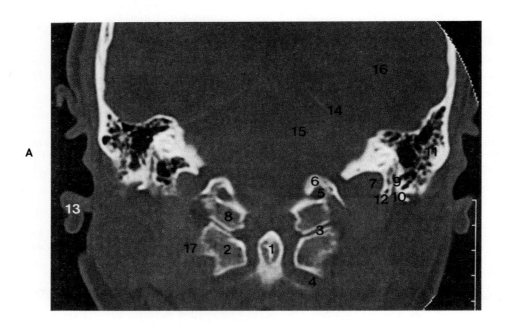

Figure 2-10   CT IMAGE OF BASE OF SKULL ("BONE WINDOWS"). By displaying the image in such a way that bony anatomy is presented in maximal detail, the detection of subtle fractures or other derangements in an area—such as the base of the skull—are made possible. (From Weir J, Abrahams PH: *An imaging atlas of human anatomy,* London, 1992, Mosby.)

A	
1 Odontoid process (dens)	**9** Descending segment of canal for facial nerve
2 Lateral mass of atlas (C1 vertebra)	**10** Stylomastoid foramen
3 Atlantooccipital joint	**11** Mastoid air cells
4 Atlantoaxial joint	**12** Styloid process
5 Hypoglossal canal	**13** Pinna of ear
6 Jugular tubercle	**14** Tentorium cerebelli
7 Jugular fossa	**15** Posterior fossa
8 Occipital condyle	**16** Cerebral hemisphere
	17 Transverse process of atlas

AIR SINUSES WITHIN THE SKULL

Several of the bones in the cranial vault and base of the skull contain cavities, or **air sinuses.** These sinuses are lined with a mucus-rich respiratory-ciliated epithelium, and ultimately they all drain into the nasal cavity. The sinuses are located in the *frontal, ethmoid,* and *sphe-*noid bones, and there is an additional large one in each *maxillary bone.* They are discussed in more detail in Chapter 2.11; also see Figure 2-114. In humans, these sinuses may contribute to the unique qualities of sound that we recognize as each other's characteristic voices. Some believe that in flying vertebrates, such as birds, they also help to minimize the weight of the skull.

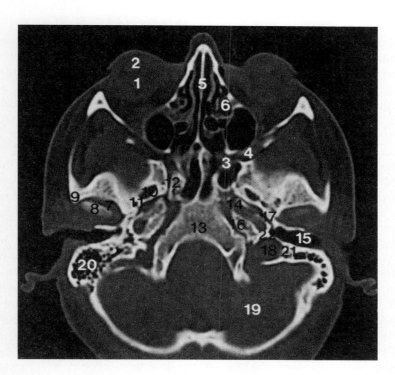

B

B	**12** Pterygoid (vidian) canal
1 Globe	**13** Basisphenoid
2 Lens	**14** Foramen lacerum
3 Pterygopalatine fossa	**15** External acoustic meatus
4 Pterygomaxillary fissure	**16** Petrooccipital fissure
5 Nasal septum	**17** Auditory (Eustachian) tube
6 Ethmoidal air cells	**18** Jugular foramen
7 Mandibular fossa	**19** Cerebellar hemisphere
8 Mandibular condyle	**20** Mastoid air cells
9 Articular condyle	**21** Facial nerve canal
10 Foramen ovale	**22** Caroticojugular spine
11 Foramen spinosum	

THE SKULL

FRACTURES OF THE SKULL

Simple fractures of the skull rarely need treatment, because no portion of the skull is displaced downward to threaten the brain. Such fractures usually heal spontaneously. When the fractured segment of the skull is depressed, however, the risk of hemorrhagic brain injury and/or infection is much greater, and the brain itself may be injured from the pressure of the depressed skull fragment.

THE FRONTAL SUTURE

About 5% to 6% of humans have a frontal or metopic suture, produced when the two embryonic frontal bones fail to fuse completely. It appears as an anterior continuation of the superior sagittal suture and is of little or no clinical significance.

VARIATIONS IN SKULL SHAPE

The overall shape of the skull may be elongated (scaphocephaly), when the sagittal suture fuses prematurely, or flattened, when the coronal suture fuses prematurely. These variations may occur as isolated instances of premature sutural closure, may be a part of larger syndromes, or in their mildest forms may simply be normal variations.

THE SKULL AND CHILDBIRTH

This pliability of the skull serves the very useful purpose of allowing it to mold itself to the proportions of the mother's pelvis, to permit successful passage of the head during birth. Indeed, many children born by such a vaginal delivery emerge with their heads elongated, a condition that invariably resolves in a few days, much to the relief of the concerned parents. When the size of the baby's head and the dimensions of the mother's pelvis simply are not compatible with a successful vaginal delivery, then a Caesarian section (delivery of the baby through an abdominal incision and surgical opening of the uterus) is often elected.

STEREOTAXIC SURGERY

The skull landmarks are used as points of reference for stereotaxic triangulation when determining the three-dimensional coordinates of various structures deep within the brain. Using such coordinates, a surgeon may guide an instrument through a small hole in the skull and place the tip of the instrument directly into a desired region of the brain. Small samples of tissue may then be removed for diagnostic purposes, or lesions may be placed in the brain for the purpose of destroying small brain areas (sometimes used to try to destroy the sources of frequent epileptic activity, when drugs fail to control it).

X-RAYS OF THE SKULL

X-rays of the skull may be used to evaluate patients for possible skull fracture. Especially in children, care must be taken not to confuse the normal sutural lines (which appear as thin lucent stripes on the x-rays) with actual fractures (see Figure 2-1, B).

Brain and Central Nervous System

▶ General Anatomic Features of the Brain

▶ Major Regions of the Brain

▶ Functional Areas of the Cerebral Cortex

▶ Deep Structures of the Forebrain

▶ Ventricular System

▶ Meninges

▶ Arterial Circulation of the Brain

▶ Venous Circulation of the Brain

The brain has a self-evident importance in a wide range of body functions and is afforded extraordinary protection by the cranial vault. In addition to this bony encasement, the brain is suspended in **cerebrospinal fluid,** which provides further protection from traumatic injury. The cerebrospinal fluid flows through a set of complex cavities within the brain—the **ventricles**—and also covers the outside surface of the brain. A set of membranes, the **meninges,** covers the surface of the brain and is also attached to the inner surface of the skull, providing further stability to the brain. The **cranial nerves,** a set of 10 pairs of true peripheral nerves and two tracts of the CNS emanating from the posterior area of the brain, leave the cranial vault through various skull apertures discussed in a previous section. The important blood vessels supplying the brain also traverse large apertures in the skull. Our focus is the general anatomy of the brain, its blood supply, the meninges, and the ventricular system. The spinal cord is the second major component of the CNS.

GENERAL ANATOMIC FEATURES OF THE BRAIN

The brain is made up of **neurons** (the functional brain cells; Figure 2-11), **glial cells** (supportive and nutritive cells that form myelin coverings over axons and vastly outnumber the neurons; Figures 2-11 and 2-12), a relatively small amount of **connective tissue** (less than 5% of the total volume of the brain), and **axons** (the conducting processes of neurons). The larger axons are myelinated (covered with multiple concentric layers of glial cell tissue), whereas the smaller ones are either completely uncovered or encircled with only one layer of glial cell tissue (nonmyelinated axons).

Gray matter is found in many areas of the brain. It is a mixture of neurons, glial cells, and axons, and has a grayish color in the fresh (i.e., unembalmed) state (Figure 2-13). Areas of **white matter** contain abundant myelinated axons and are relatively poor in neurons. The "whiteness" of the white matter in the fresh state results from the large amount of phospholipid present in the myelin. Deeper still within the brain are masses of gray matter referred to as **nuclei,** whereas in the peripheral nervous system, masses of gray matter are known as **ganglia.**

The **cerebral cortex** is formed from superficial gray matter and deeper white matter. The much thinner raised strips of gray matter found on the cerebellum are known as **folia.** In the cerebellum, the gray matter is also external and the white matter internal, but the histologic organization and neuronal "circuitry" is vastly different than in the cerebral cortex.

Compared with other body tissues, the brain has very little extracellular space. It does not have lymphat-

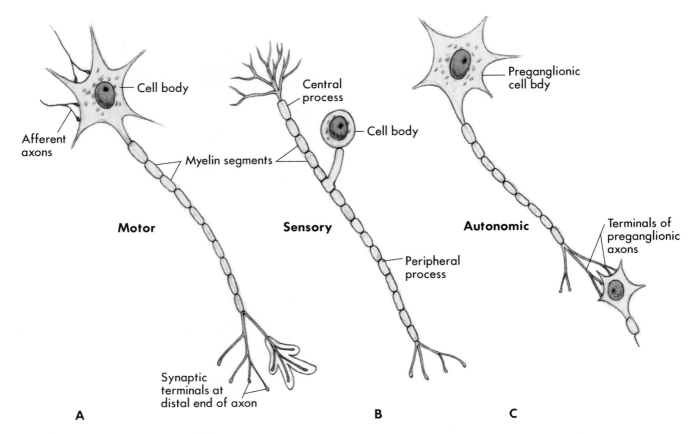

Figure 2-11   VARIETIES OF NEURONS. A, Typical *peripheral motor* neuron, extending from the spinal cord or brain into the periphery to innervate a muscle. **B,** Typical *peripheral sensory neuron,* whose cell body is in a ganglion, whose peripheral process extends outward to where the sensations are detected, and whose central process conveys that information to the CNS. **C,** Typical two-neuron *autonomic circuit.* The cell body of the second neuron in the circuit is often located in a peripheral ganglion or in the wall of the target organ or tissue.

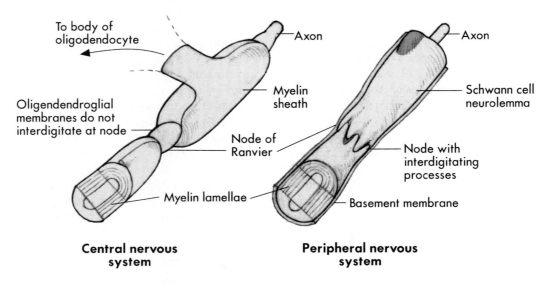

Figure 2-12   MYELIN AND THE NODE OF RANVIER. Typical peripheral nerve node of Ranvier and a typical central nervous system node of Ranvier.

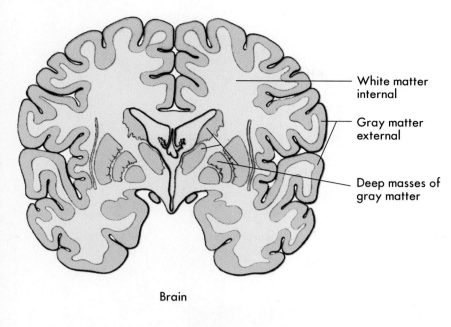

White matter
internal

Gray matter
external

Deep masses of
gray matter

Brain

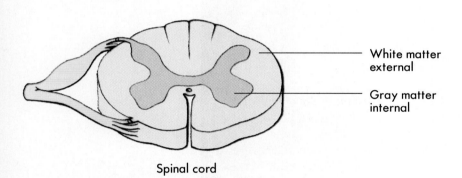

White matter
external

Gray matter
internal

Spinal cord

Figure 2-13   GRAY MATTER AND WHITE MATTER IN THE SPINAL CORD AND BRAIN. In the brain, the gray matter coats the exterior of the brain and also is found in discrete aggregations (nuclei) deep within the brain. The white matter lies in between. In the spinal cord, the gray matter is internal, surrounded by a mantle of white matter.

ics, and the small amount of extracellular fluid present is returned to the venous system by becoming part of the cerebrospinal fluid. Paradoxically, brain tissue itself is not innervated (supplied with nerves), so that cutting or stretching the brain tissue itself causes little sensation or pain. The dura mater, by contrast, is richly innervated with sensory axons.

MAJOR REGIONS OF THE BRAIN

Moving from posterior to anterior, the major regions of the brain are the *medulla, pons, cerebellum, mesencephalon, diencephalon,* and *telencephalon* (Figure 2-14). The diencephalon consists of the thalamus and hypothalamus, and the telencephalon includes the basal ganglia and cerebral cortex. The *brainstem* is a widely-used term that refers to the medulla, pons, and midbrain. The brainstem is concealed by the overlying cerebral cortex, but a midsagittal section through the brain more clearly shows the central position of the thalamus and mesencephalon (Figure 2-14, *B*). The cerebellum is a spherical mass positioned on the dorsal

surface of the brainstem. The term *hindbrain* refers to both the medulla and pons. The mesencephalon is also called the *midbrain,* and the diencephalon and telencephalon together compose the *forebrain.* These terms are derived from study of the comparative anatomy of the brain in vertebrates and from a study of brain development (Table 2-3).

The subdivisions listed here are defined by certain anatomic characteristics (sulci, fissures, gyri, and so on). From the clinical standpoint, however, more useful ways of identifying divisions of the brain are with reference to (1) the brain's regional blood supply, and (2) certain subdivisions of the space enclosed by the skull (known as fossae).

Considering first the *regional blood supply,* areas of the brain that share a common vascular supply may or may not correspond to anatomically defined areas. Damage to a given artery, for example, might cause injury to both the pons and the cerebellum, even though these structures are certainly distinct by purely anatomic criteria. Groups of structures supplied by branches of a common artery are often injured in cere-

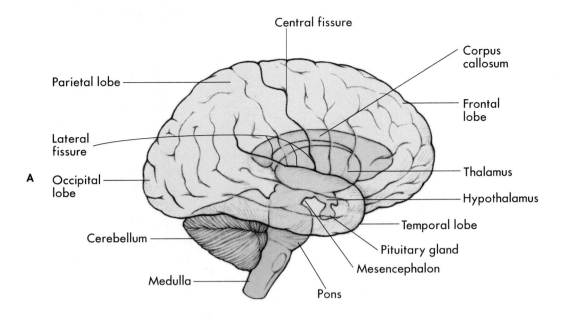

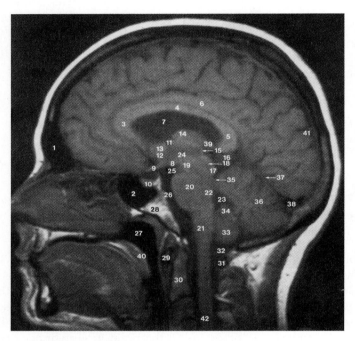

Figure 2-14 LATERAL VIEW OF THE BRAIN. A, Schematic drawing. **B,** Midsagittal MRI.
(From Weir J, Abrahams PH: *An imaging atlas of human anatomy,* London, 1992, Mosby.)

SEE ATLAS, FIGS. 2-23, 2-60, 2-89

1 Frontal sinus	**16** Quadrigeminal cistern	**29** Anterior arch of atlas (C1 vertebra)
2 Sphenoidal sinus	**17** Quadrigeminal plate of mid-brain	**30** Odontoid process (dens)
3 Genu of corpus callosum	**18** Aqueduct of Sylvius	**31** Posterior arch of atlas
4 Body of corpus callosum	**19** Cerebral peduncles of mid-brain	**32** Cisterna magna (cerebellomedullary cistern)
5 Splenium of corpus callosum	**20** Pons	**33** Cerebellar tonsil
6 Cingulate gyrus	**21** Medulla oblongata	**34** Nodule of cerebellum
7 Lateral ventricle	**22** Tegmentum of pons	**35** Superior medullary velum
8 Mammillary body	**23** Fourth ventricle	**36** Cerebellum
9 Optic chiasma in suprasellar cistern	**24** Third ventricle	**37** Tentorium cerebelli
10 Pituitary gland	**25** Oculomotor nerve in interpeduncular cistern	**38** Transverse sinus
11 Interventricular foramen of Monro	**26** Prepontine cistern	**39** Fornix
12 Lamina terminalis	**27** Nasopharynx	**40** Uvula
13 Anterior commissure	**28** Fat in marrow of clivus	**41** Parietooccipital fissure
14 Massa intermedia		**42** Cervical spinal cord
15 Posterior commissure		

Table 2-3 Nomenclature Describing the Brain

Region of Brain	Anatomic Term	Embryologic Term	Associated Ventricular Space
Forebrain	Cerebral cortex	Telencephalon	Lateral ventricle
	Thalamus	Diencephalon	Third ventricle
	Hypothalamus	Diencephalon	Third ventricle
Midbrain	Midbrain	Mesencephalon	Cerebral aqueduct
	Cerebellum	Metencephalon	Fourth ventricle
Hindbrain	Pons	Metencephalon	Fourth ventricle
	Medulla	Myelencephalon	Fourth ventricle

bral vascular accidents (CVAs, or strokes). Knowledge of the targets of individual arteries may allow you to match the symptoms in a given patient with the probable location of a vascular injury.

Second, the extent and localization of brain injury is often dictated by grouping of structures in the *fossae*, or *compartments*, of the cranial cavity (see Figure 2-6). When trauma to the head occurs, structures that lie within the anterior, middle, or posterior fossae of the skull (see "Floor of the Cranial Cavity") may be injured together. Another widely applied terminology in clinical medicine distinguishes injuries to those structures that lie *above* the tentorium cerebelli (so-called *"supratentorial"* structures [see Figure 2-20]—the parietal, occipital, temporal, and frontal lobes) from those parts of

the brain lying *below* the tentorium cerebelli (the so-called *"infratentorial"* structures—the cerebellum and brainstem [Figure 2-14]).

FUNCTIONAL AREAS OF THE CEREBRAL CORTEX

The cerebral cortex is the external mantle of tissue of the surface of the telencephalon. It comprises a complex series of raised elongated "strips" of gray matter that cover most of the surface of the cerebral cortex, with white matter located deep to the gray matter. Numerous grooves are also found on the surface of the cerebral cortex (Figure 2-15). The largest of these are referred to as **fissures,** whereas the far more numerous

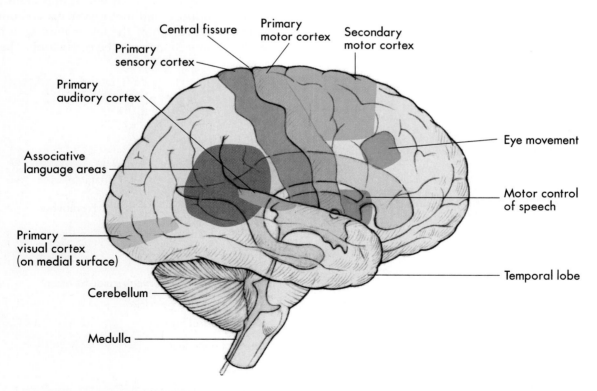

Figure 2-15 DIAGRAM OF BRAIN SHOWING BRODMANN AREAS. (See also Table 2-4.) SEE ATLAS, FIG. 2-86

Table 2-4   Important Brodmann Areas of the Cerebral Cortex

Cortical Area	Landmark/Location	Function
Area 1, 2, 3—primary sensory cortex	Just posterior to the central (Sylvian) fissure	Receives afferent axons for general sensation (touch, pressure, pain, etc.)
Area 4, 6—primary motor cortex	Just anterior to the central (Sylvian) fissure	Origin for axons regulating voluntary movements
Area 44—motor speech area	Small circular area anterior to base of central fissure	Essential for voluntary expressive language (e.g., speech)
Area 17—primary visual cortex	On medial surface of occipital lobe, actually deep in a fissure	Receives axons excited by visual stimuli; necessary for visual perception
Area 41, 44—primary auditory cortex	On anterolateral surface of temporal lobe, just inferior to the lateral fissure	Receives axons excited by auditory stimuli
Area 39, 40—receptive speech cortex	At posterior end of lateral fissure	Necessary for comprehension of speech or other language-based input
Area 23, 24—cingulate gyrus	On medial brain, just above corpus callosum	Plays a role in unconscious autonomic regulation

smaller ones are known as **sulci.** The raised areas of cortical tissue between the sulci and fissures are called **gyri.**

The cerebral cortex has been described as consisting of nearly 100 distinct "functional areas," called **Brodmann areas** (see Figure 2-15). These areas are defined by their position, gross anatomic appearance, and histologic characteristics. There is great clinical importance to some of these areas, because even small injuries to them may cause serious motor and/or sensory deficits. Some important areas of the cerebral cortex are shown in Figure 2-15 and Table 2-4.

DEEP STRUCTURES OF THE FOREBRAIN

There are several masses of gray matter deep within the forebrain, including the *basal ganglia, thalamus,* and *hypothalamus* (see Figure 2-14). Axons passing between the spinal cord and cerebral cortex frequently synapse in the *thalamus* and *basal ganglia.* The *hypothalamus* receives neural input from many regions of the brain but directs most of its output to the pituitary gland. The *midbrain* is a small region in which important parts of the visual, auditory, and motor systems are found. The *pons* is a small region of the lower brainstem that has numerous connections with the cerebellum. The *cerebel-*

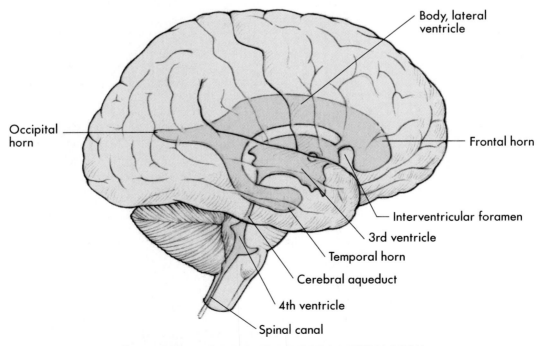

Figure 2-16   VENTRICULAR SYSTEM, LATERAL VIEW.

Occipital horn

Body, lateral ventricle

Frontal horn

Interventricular foramen

3rd ventricle

Temporal horn

Cerebral aqueduct

4th ventricle

Spinal canal

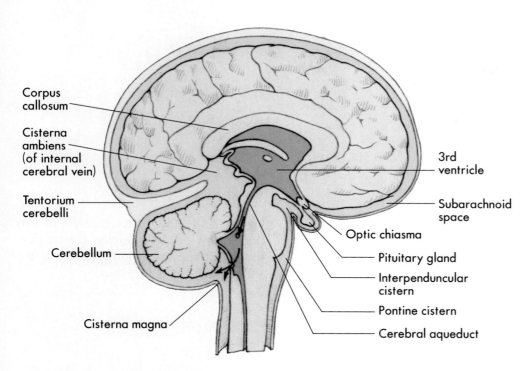

Corpus callosum

Cisterna ambiens (of internal cerebral vein)

Tentorium cerebelli

Cerebellum

Cisterna magna

3rd ventricle

Subarachnoid space

Optic chiasma

Pituitary gland

Interpenduncular cistern

Pontine cistern

Cerebral aqueduct

Figure 2-17 INTERIOR OF THE VENTRICULAR SYSTEM. Midsagittal section through the brain illustrates the flow of cerebrospinal fluid (CSF) from the third to the fourth ventricles and thence outward into the subarachnoid space. CSF leaves the ventricular system to enter the subarachnoid space in the lower medulla (*double-headed arrow*).

CLINICAL ANATOMY OF

THE BRAIN AND CENTRAL NERVOUS SYSTEM

STROKES AND THE BRAIN

"Strokes" are injuries to regions of the brain produced by an insufficiency of blood supply to that area. They can result from (1) the blockage of an artery supplying an area, producing ischemia or (2) a hemorrhage, preventing adequate blood flow beyond the hemorrhage.

DISEASES OF WHITE MATTER

Pathologic conditions affect white matter far more often than they affect gray matter (that is, neurons themselves). Such diseases as multiple sclerosis (MS) and amyotrophic lateral sclerosis (ALS) cause progressive deterioration of myelin and ultimately lead to disturbance of normal conduction between neurons and muscle.

INTRACRANIAL HEMATOMAS

Hemorrhages inside the skull can lead to accumulation of blood in the subdural or subarachnoid spaces, thereby producing pressure on the underlying brain tissue. These are known as subdural or subarachnoid hematomas and frequently require surgical evacuation.

FUNCTIONAL REGIONS OF THE BRAIN

Knowledge of the functional localizations within the cerebral cortex can be used to infer the location of brain injury. For example, if a patient has seizures (epileptic activity) confined to the lower limb on the right side, we can presume that the seizure "focus" is located in the most superior part of areas 4 and 6 on the left side of the brain (because the motor cortex on one side regulates activity on the opposite ("contralateral") side of the body.

CRITICAL REGIONS WITHIN THE BRAIN

Knowledge of the proximity of certain structures within the cranial cavity can explain sometimes perplexing combinations of symptoms. For example, even a small tumor in the vicinity of the optic chiasma can lead to partial or complete blindness (from pressure on the optic nerves), hormonal imbalance (from effect on the nearby pituitary gland), and electrolyte disorders (from injury to the nearby basal portions of the hypothalamus).

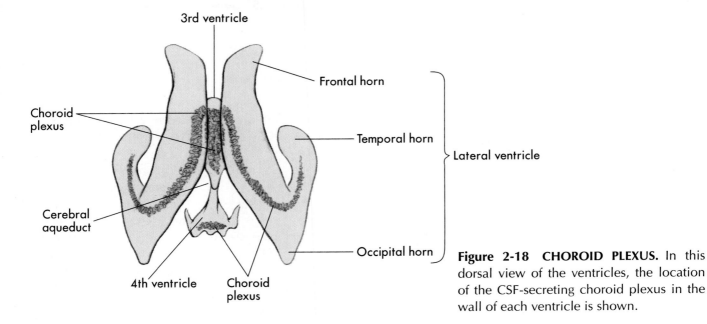

Figure 2-18 CHOROID PLEXUS. In this dorsal view of the ventricles, the location of the CSF-secreting choroid plexus in the wall of each ventricle is shown.

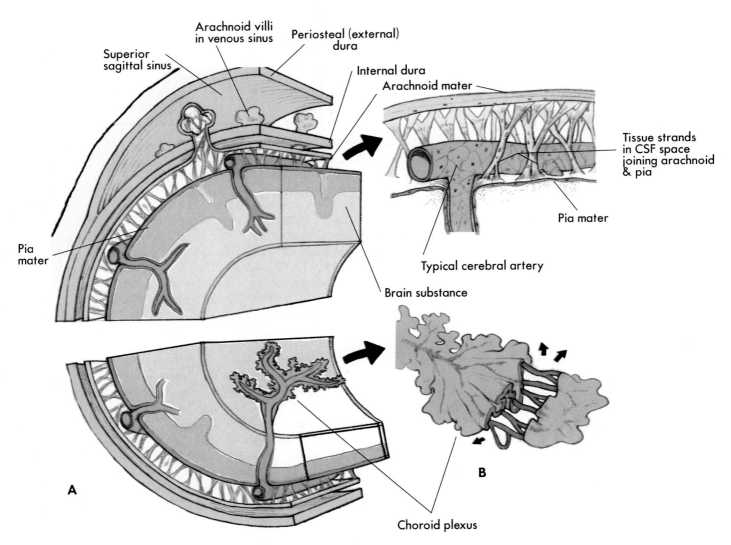

Figure 2-19 CHOROID PLEXUS AND ARACHNOID GRANULATIONS. A, Choroid plexus, from which cerebrospinal fluid originates, and the subarachnoid space, in which it flows before being deposited back into the bloodstream through the arachnoid granulations. **B,** More detailed views of the subarachnoid space and structure of the choroid plexus.

THE VENTRICULAR SYSTEM AND CEREBROSPINAL FLUID

MENINGITIS

Disease processes that cause inflammation of the arachnoid membrane (meningitis) or produce elevations of the pressure within the venous system (congestive heart failure) tend to retard the normal flow of cerebrospinal fluid.

AQUEDUCTAL STENOSIS

Anatomic blockages to the flow of cerebrospinal fluid can occur at various points in the ventricular system but occur most commonly at the cerebral aqueduct (aqueduct of Sylvius), between the third and fourth ventricles.

HYDROCEPHALUS

Increases of the amount and/or pressure of cerebrospinal fluid within the ventricular system lead to dilation of the ventricles (hydrocephalus) and subsequent destruction of the surrounding brain tissue. In a small child, hydrocephalus can force the separation of the not-yet-ossified sutures of the skull and increase the size of the child's head.

TREATMENTS FOR HYDROCEPHALUS

When hydrocephalus is chronic, neurosurgeons may place a ventriculoperitoneal (VP) shunt. This slender catheter is placed into the lateral ventricle and drains cerebrospinal fluid downward into the abdominal cavity or into the superior vena cava.

THE LUMBAR PUNCTURE (SPINAL TAP)

Cerebrospinal fluid can be removed (for diagnostic purposes) from any portion of the ventricular system or from the subarachnoid space. By far the most frequently chosen site is the lumbar puncture in the subarachnoid space in the lower lumbar part of the vertebral column below the level of the spinal cord. Cerebrospinal fluid can be removed from the lateral ventricles or from the cisternal magna as well, but these should be attempted only by those expert in these procedures.

---

lum is a large globular mass of neural tissue attached to the dorsal surface of the brainstem; it plays an important role in the control of motion. The *medulla* links brain and spinal cord. Most of the 12 pairs of cranial nerves exit the brain from points along the midbrain, pons, and medulla.

VENTRICULAR SYSTEM

The ventricular system is a complex series of interconnected chambers (**ventricles**) within the brain (Figure 2-16). These chambers are derived from the initially simple hollow cylinder in the interior of the neural tube. As the brain grows and adopts an increasingly convoluted shape, the ventricles also become more complex in shape. In the adult, the ventricular system consists of four major ventricles (the two lateral ventricles, the single third ventricle, and single fourth ventricle) (Figure 2-16; see also Figure 2-18).

The **left and right lateral ventricles** lie deep to the surface of the cerebral hemispheres. They are elongated, curved cylinders, beginning in the frontal lobe and extending posteriorly and inferiorly into the parietal, occipital, and temporal lobes. The components of the lateral ventricle lying deep to these areas of the brain are, respectively, the frontal horn, body, occipital horn, and temporal horn (Figures 2-16 and 2-18). Each of the

lateral ventricles empties into the single midline third ventricle. The narrow **third ventricle,** positioned in the midline between the two thalamuses, is a slitlike space that receives cerebrospinal fluid from the lateral ventricles.

Cerebrospinal fluid (CSF) is a clear liquid produced within the ventricles. These chambers are connected with each other, and the cerebrospinal fluid flows between them. At the base of the brain, cerebrospinal fluid passes through some small foramina to reach the external surface of the brain. The cerebrospinal fluid eventually drains back into the venous system. This fluid is drained from the intercellular spaces of the brain and spinal cord.

Cerebrospinal fluid leaves the third ventricle posteriorly and enters a long narrow passage running through the interior of the brainstem and emptying into the fourth ventricle. This passage, the **cerebral aqueduct (aqueduct of Sylvius)** (Figure 2-17), is one of the more common sites of obstruction to the flow of cerebrospinal fluid and consequent hydrocephalus. The **fourth ventricle** is a broad triangular space located between the cerebellum and the superior surface of the pons and medulla (see Figure 2-16).

Cerebrospinal fluid leaves the interior of the ventricular system through three small apertures in the posterior aspect of the fourth ventricle. These are the midline

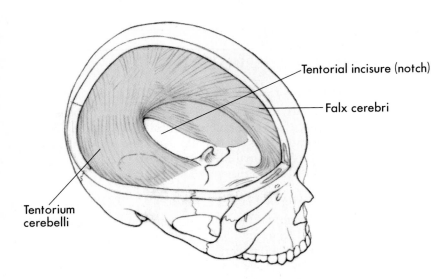

Tentorial incisure (notch)

Falx cerebri

Tentorium cerebelli

Figure 2-20 REFLECTIONS OF THE DURA MATER. SEE ATLAS, FIG. 2-90

foramen of Magendie and the two lateral **foramina of Luschka.** Having traversed these small apertures, the cerebrospinal fluid spreads out in the subarachnoid space to form a thin fluid jacket around the surface of the brain and spinal cord (see Figure 2-17). Here it serves as a shock absorber and insulates the brain and may also function to convey chemical messengers from one part of the brain to another. Also, because the brain has no lymphatic drainage, it is widely believed that cerebrospinal fluid serves as a means to remove extracellular fluid from brain tissue. In most places this layer is thin, but in selected areas it is wider, and it is in these

areas that a needle or catheter may be inserted to remove cerebrospinal fluid. The subarachnoid space extends to the inferior portion of the sacrum, whereas the spinal cord itself ends at vertebral level L1 to L2. Thus, below L2 the subarachnoid space is widened and accessible for the insertion of a needle. This is the most frequent site for the removal of cerebrospinal fluid. Within the skull, just inferior to the lower margin of the cerebellum, there is a widened area of cerebrospinal fluid known as the **cisterna magna** (see Figure 2-17). Other cisterns are located near the optic chiasma and the base of the brainstem. Only the cisterna magna is accessible

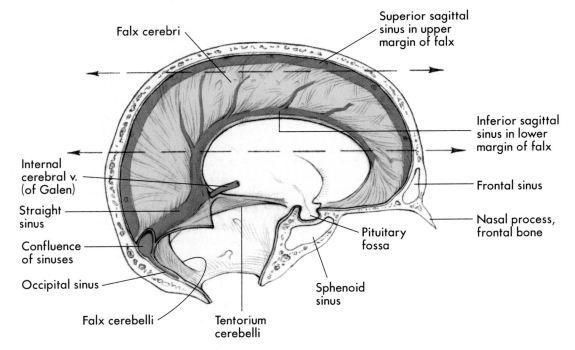

Falx cerebri

Superior sagittal sinus in upper margin of falx

Inferior sagittal sinus in lower margin of falx

Frontal sinus

Nasal process, frontal bone

Pituitary fossa

Sphenoid sinus

Tentorium cerebelli

Falx cerebelli

Occipital sinus

Confluence of sinuses

Straight sinus

Internal cerebral v. (of Galen)

Figure 2-21 FALX CEREBRI AND SAGITTAL SINUSES. Shown here is the falx cerebri and the inferior and superior sagittal sinuses, the former lying in its upper margin and the latter lying in its lower free margin. The straight sinus forms from the union of the inferior sagittal sinus and the internal cerebral vein.

to the physician, and aspiration of cerebrospinal fluid from it should only be attempted by someone highly trained in this procedure.

Small cuboidal epithelial cells, known as **ependyma,** line the ventricles. In certain areas these ependymal cells interact with underlying connective tissue and blood vessels to form the **choroid plexus,** an elongated tuft of tissue protruding into the lumen of the lateral, third, and fourth ventricles (Figures 2-18 and 2-19). The choroid plexus produces the vast majority of the cerebrospinal fluid made each day (600 to 700 cc/day in an adult).

The cerebrospinal fluid in the subarachnoid space is slowly reabsorbed into certain parts of the cerebral venous system by the **arachnoid villi,** small tufts of arachnoid membrane that protrude into the lumina of large venous sinuses near the brain (see Figure 2-19). Cerebrospinal fluid flow is a passive process, depending on the small pressure gradient within the subarachnoid space to cause the cerebrospinal fluid to be transported back into the venous system. Obstructions to the normal flow of cerebrospinal fluid cause it to accumulate in the ventricles and/or subarachnoid space, ul-

timately leading to increases of pressure inside the skull and the considerable risk of injury to the brain. Samples of cerebrospinal fluid may be removed from the subarachnoid space (usually as part of a procedure known as a *lumbar puncture,* or *spinal tap*) or directly from the ventricle by passing a narrow needle through the overlying brain tissue to enter the ventricle.

MENINGES

The meninges are three roughly concentric layers of connective tissue that surround the brain and spinal cord and separate it from the surrounding bony skull and vertebral column (see Figure 2-19). These are called the **dura mater, arachnoid mater,** and **pia mater.** The meninges provide a protective covering for the brain but also serve a variety of other functions: They enclose the cerebrospinal fluid, help to maintain the delicate balance of extracellular fluid in the parenchyma of the brain, support the arterial and venous vessels supplying the brain and spinal cord, and form large septae separating important regions of the brain (Figures 2-19, 2-20, and 2-21).

CLINICAL ANATOMY OF

THE MENINGES

THE TENTORIAL INCISURE ("TENTORIAL NOTCH") (FIGURE 2-20)

The curved margin of dura mater surrounding the upper brainstem as it passes from the posterior to the middle cranial fossa is known as the tentorial incisure. When intracranial pressure increases, the brain can herniate through this incisure. An early sign of this herniation is often a lateral deviation of the eye, because the oculomotor nerve, lying against the medial surface of the temporal lobe, is compressed against the edge of the tentorial incisure, and the innervation of the lateral rectus muscle by the abducens nerve is unbalanced.

COMMUNICATING OR "EXTERNAL" HYDROCEPHALUS

While the most common forms of hydrocephalus involve obstruction to the flow of cerebrospinal fluid at the aqueduct of Sylvius or the interventricular foramen (forms of "internal hydrocephalus"), it is also possible to block the reabsorption of cerebrospinal fluid at the level of the arachnoid villi. This is usually the result of meningitis and is known as "external hydrocephalus," because the blockage to flow does not involve the ventricles or the passages between them.

MENINGITIS

Meningitis is the inflammation of the meninges surrounding the brain and/or spinal cord. It may be caused by bacterial, viral, or fungal organisms, or even by noninfectious irritating substances. In infectious meningitis, the production of toxins by the infective agent disrupts the normal function of the nearby brain tissue, which is usually involved in the infection as well (so that the proper name for the condition would be "meningoencephalitis"). Because the inflammation involves the meninges, it produces movement-associated pain and stiffness in the neck.

MENINGIOMAS

The large majority of tumors of the brain are in reality tumors of meningeal tissue, which cause damage by the pressure they exert on adjacent brain tissue. True tumors of neural tissue occur most often as abnormal collections of very primitive neuroectodermal tissue. This underscores the fact that true neural tissue is highly differentiated, is less likely to become malignant, and for the same reason is incapable of regeneration.

The Pia Mater

The pia mater (see Figure 2-19) is the innermost and most delicate of the three meningeal layers. It is tightly applied to the surface of the brain and spinal cord and conforms to the surface even downward into their sulci and fissures. The pia contains many fine blood vessels whose branches extend inward into the tissue of the brain and spinal cord. In the skull, folds of pia are invaginated inward to take part in the formation of the choroid plexus for the lateral, third, and fourth ventricles. Cranial and spinal nerves traveling away from the brain and spinal cord take with them a short envelopment of pia mater. Further laterally, it blends with the connective tissue coverings of these peripheral nerves.

In the cervical and thoracic regions, a vertical "shelf" of pia mater in the frontal plane extends from each side of the spinal cord laterally to blend with the dura mater (Figure 2-10 and see Chapter 2.1 on spinal cord and vertebrae). These membranes blend with the dura in an interrupted fashion, forming a serrated lateral edge. This shelf of pia, positioned between the dorsal and ventral roots exiting from the spinal cord, is known as the **denticulate ligament.** In the upper cervical region, the spinal root of the accessory nerve lies on the dorsal surface of the denticulate ligament. There is a similar vertical shelf of pia, the **subarachnoid septum** (see Figure 1-11), extending from the posterior midline surface of the spinal cord to the surrounding dura mater in the thoracic region.

At the inferior end of the spinal cord, the pia mater narrows into a slender filament, the **filum terminale.** The filum extends from the level of the L2 vertebra, where the spinal cord ends as the **conus medullaris,** to an attachment opposite the second coccygeal vertebra in the lower end of the vertebral column. From the level of L2 to approximately S2, the filum is surrounded by a wide region of cerebrospinal fluid, in turn surrounded by the arachnoid membrane (plastered against the inner surface of the vertebral canal). It is in this relatively safe portion of the subarachnoid space that the needle is inserted in the ordinary lumbar puncture (the region is "safe" because the cerebrospinal fluid is in a wide space at this level, and the spinal cord itself has ended at L1 to L2). Below the level of S2, the filum is closely surrounded by remnants of dura and arachnoid membrane, obliterating any potential subarachnoid space.

The Arachnoid Mater

The arachnoid mater lies external to the pia, and in most areas is separated from it by a layer of cerebrospinal fluid. The arachnoid does not descend into any but the largest of the fissures and sulci of the brain but instead "bridges" across most of them. The major arterial vessels supplying the brain and spinal cord form a network on the inner surface of the arachnoid membrane, before individual branches descend into the brain or spinal cord tissue itself (see Figure 2-19). In addition to containing cerebrospinal fluid, the space between the arachnoid and dura is bridged by a reticular network of connective tissue filaments, loosely attaching the arachnoid to the pia. These filaments are the source of the name "arachnoid" (Gr. *arachne,* a spider) for this membrane.

The Dura Mater

The dura mater is the thickest and most external of the three meningeal layers. In some areas of the cranium, the dura consists of two layers. Where the dura is bilayered, the *external layer* is synonymous with the inner periosteum of the cranial bones. This layer is closely applied to the cranial bones and ends at the perimeter of the foramen magnum, to which it is tightly attached. The *internal layer* of the cranial dura (and the single layer of spinal dura) is closely applied to the external surface of the arachnoid membrane. The internal layer of cranial dura is continuous through the foramen magnum with the single layer of dura surrounding the spinal cord.

Two very important extensions of the inner layer of cranial dura, the falx cerebri and tentorium cerebelli, protrude inward between major regions of the brain (Figures 2-20, 2-21, and 2-23, *B*). The **falx cerebri** (Figure 2-21) is a vertical "blade" of dura in the midsagittal plane, extending downward from the inferior surface of the dura beneath the sagittal suture to occupy the space between the two cerebral hemispheres. It attaches anteriorly to the crista galli (a specialized part of the ethmoid bone) and posteriorly to the tentorium cerebelli at the internal occipital protruberance. It has a free lower margin, in which the inferior sagittal sinus is enclosed. The **tentorium cerebelli** is a horizontal sheet of dura, shaped like a broad triangle with a curved base (see Figures 2-21 and 2-23, *B*). The curved base ("attached border") is attached along a elongated ridge of bone extending horizontally to the right and left from the internal occipital protruberance on the interior surface of the occipital bone. The two lateral sides of the tentorium cerebelli extend anteriorly and are tightly attached along the margin of the petrous ridge on each side. Within the two leaflets of the tentorium, in the midline, is the straight sinus, running in an anterior-posterior plane. A small vertical ridge of dura, the falx cerebelli, extends in the sagittal plane inferiorly from the tentorium and partially separates the two cerebellar lobes (see Figure 2-21). Anteriorly, there is a large curved aperture where the apex of this triangle would be, to permit the brainstem to pass through, ensuring continuity of brain structures in the posterior fossa with those in the middle and anterior fossae. This aperture is

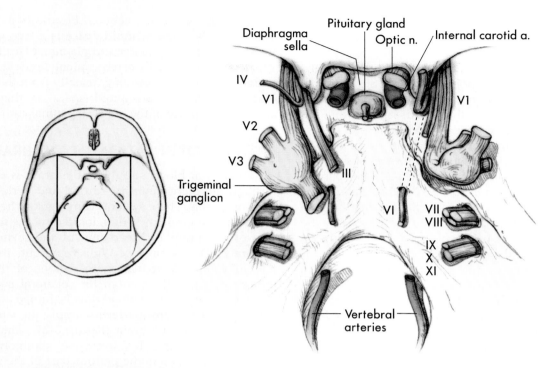

Figure 2-22 PITUITARY GLAND AND DIAPHRAGMA SELLA. Shown here is the area of the pituitary fossa and surrounding nerves and vessels related to the orbit. The diaphragma sella (membrane) is in place, covering most of the pituitary gland. SEE ATLAS, FIG. 2-95

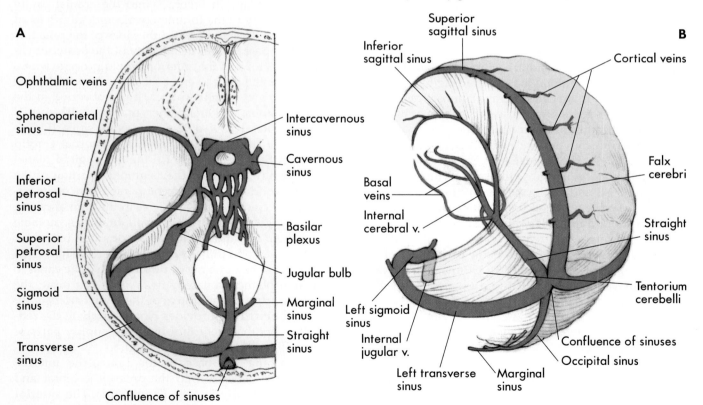

Figure 2-23 CEREBRAL VENOUS SINUSES. A, Superior view. Note the position of the cavernous sinus in relation to the pituitary fossa. **B,** Oblique posterior view. Note the convergence of the several individual sinuses on the internal jugular vein, forming at the jugular bulb. SEE ATLAS, FIG. 2-93

known as the **tentorial notch** or **tentorial incisure** (see Figures 2-20, 2-21). Blood vessels passing between the posterior and middle fossae also traverse the tentorial notch. Laterally, the tentorial notch is attached to the anterior and posterior clinoid processes. Structures in the posterior fossa are sometimes referred to collectively as *infratentorial,* whereas those in the middle and anterior fossae are referred to as *supratentorial.*

The third specialized region of the dura, the **diaphragma sellae,** is a small horizontal sheet of dura positioned over the sella turcica (Figure 2-22). It separates the pituitary gland from the base of the brain and helps hold the pituitary securely in the sella. The diaphragma has a small central aperture through which passes the infundibulum or **stalk of the pituitary gland,** connecting it to the hypothalamus (Figure 2-22).

In the space between the two layers of cranial dura are found several **venous sinuses,** valveless vessels conveying intracranial venous blood. Venous sinuses are distinguished from veins because the former have rigid walls without smooth muscle, whereas veins have flexible walls with smooth muscle layers. The arachnoid membrane lies just interior to the dural layer, and in the region of the venous sinuses, tufts of arachnoid membrane protrude through the dural tissue and project themselves into the lumen of the sinuses. It is at these **arachnoid granulations,** or **villi,** that cerebrospinal fluid is "filtered" back into the blood stream (see Figure 2-19).

The **superior sagittal sinus** (Figures 2-21 and 2-23, *B*) lies along the line of intersection between the falx cerebri and the dura along the superior sagittal sinus; it is especially rich in arachnoid granulations. The **inferior sagittal sinus** lies in the free lower margin of the falx cerebri. The **straight sinus** connects the posterior ends of the superior and inferior sagittal sinuses (Figures 2-21 and 2-23, *A*). The **transverse** and **sigmoid sinuses** lie along the lateral margins of the tentorium cerebelli (see Figures 2-8 and 2-23, *A*). The **petrous sinuses** lie along the upper margin of the petrous ridges. Many of the sinuses found in the lateral and superior regions of the dura converge on a region lying over the internal occipital protruberance, known as the **confluence of sinuses** (see Figures 2-21 and 2-23). Ultimately, the vast majority of venous blood in these sinuses leaves the skull through the internal jugular veins.

The **epidural space,** in the cranial cavity, is only a potential space between the outer layer of cranial dura and the skull itself. When there is bleeding from the middle meningeal artery, or another similar artery in the anterior or posterior fossa, then this potential space may be widened dramatically (see Figure 2-59). The **subdural space** lies between the dura mater and the arachnoid mater (see Figure 2-19), and is also a potential space where the dura and arachnoid are attached loosely by connective tissue. It becomes widened most often as a result of venous bleeding—a *subdural hematoma.* The **subarachnoid space** is a true space between the arachnoid mater and pia mater (see Figure 2-19), and is filled with cerebrospinal fluid. It may be widened by arterial bleeding, usually from the arteries that lie in the subarachnoid space as they course around the surface of the brain and spinal cord.

ARTERIAL CIRCULATION OF THE BRAIN

The arterial blood supply to the brain is delivered through the paired internal carotid and vertebral systems of vessels. These systems converge on the **circulus arteriosus,** or **circle of Willis,** located on the undersurface of the brain in the region of the diencephalon (Figure 2-24). The circle of Willis represents the potential for collateral circulation to regions of the brain, though the overall potential for collateral support of brain areas deprived of blood flow is limited.

The **internal carotid arteries** supply the largest volume of blood to the brain (Figure 2-25). The internal carotid artery separates from the common carotid artery and next enters the petrous part of the temporal bone through the **carotid canal.** As it ascends in the canal, it inclines forward and passes over the **foramen lacerum,** which in life is filled inferiorly to the vessel with fibrocartilage. It emerges into the cranial cavity posteromedially to the foramen ovale and travels in an anteromedial direction toward the sides of the sella turcica. It then passes from the vicinity of the posterior clinoid process toward the anterior clinoid process, where it penetrates the dura to enter the cranial cavity. Where it lies alongside the sella turcica, it is embedded in the cavernous sinus, and cranial nerves V1, V2, III, and IV lie in the lateral wall of the cavernous sinus (Figure 2-26). While traversing this area, the internal carotid follows an S-shaped course (in the parasagittal plane) and is often described as the "sigmoid" portion of the internal carotid artery. It is accompanied here on its lateral side by cranial nerve VI. Once in the cranial cavity, the artery gives off several small branches, notable among them the **ophthalmic artery,** the first branch of the internal carotid (it has none in the neck). This vessel accompanies the optic nerve through the optic canal to the inside of the orbital cavity. Within the orbit, the opthalmic artery is the source of the *central artery of the retina* and ultimately provides blood supply to the retina. Other ophthalmic artery branches supply parts of the eyeball, orbit, nose, and forehead.

On reaching the base of the brain, the internal carotid artery divides into the anterior cerebral and middle cerebral arteries (see Figure 2-24). The **anterior cerebral artery** courses forward along the base of the brain, then turns superiorly to enter the longitudinal fissure (between the two hemispheres), and runs an arching course posteriorly, along the superior surface

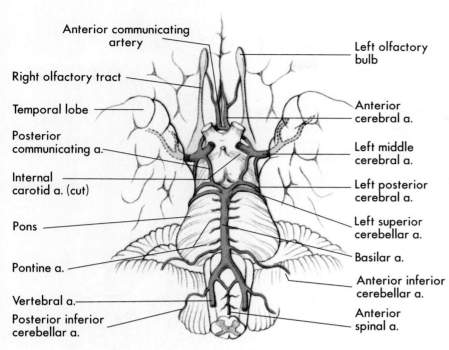

Anterior communicating artery

Right olfactory tract

Temporal lobe

Posterior communicating a.

Internal carotid a. (cut)

Pons

Pontine a.

Vertebral a.

Posterior inferior cerebellar a.

Left olfactory bulb

Anterior cerebral a.

Left middle cerebral a.

Left posterior cerebral a.

Left superior cerebellar a.

Basilar a.

Anterior inferior cerebellar a.

Anterior spinal a.

Figure 2-24 CIRCULUS ARTERIOSUS (OF WILLIS) AND ARTERIAL SUPPLY TO THE UNDERSURFACE OF THE BRAIN.

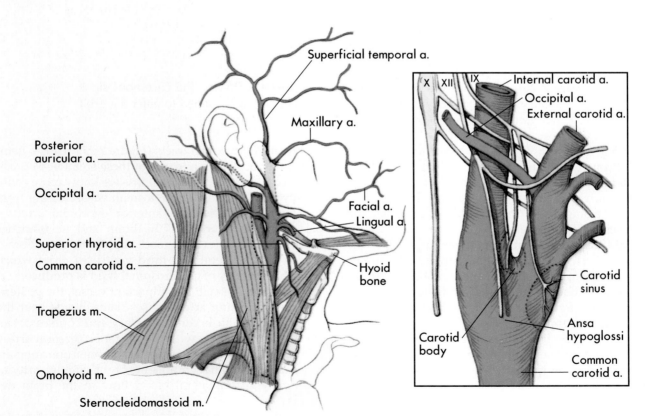

Superficial temporal a.

Maxillary a.

Posterior auricular a.

Occipital a.

Superior thyroid a.

Common carotid a.

Trapezius m.

Omohyoid m.

Sternocleidomastoid m.

Facial a.

Lingual a.

Hyoid bone

Internal carotid a.

Occipital a.

External carotid a.

Carotid sinus

Ansa hypoglossi

Common carotid a.

Carotid body

Figure 2-25   BRANCHES OF EXTERNAL CAROTID ARTERY. The *inset* shows the detailed grouping of the nerves and vessels found in the vicinity of the bifurcation of the common carotid artery. On the left is shown the relationship of the external carotid to important neck muscles.

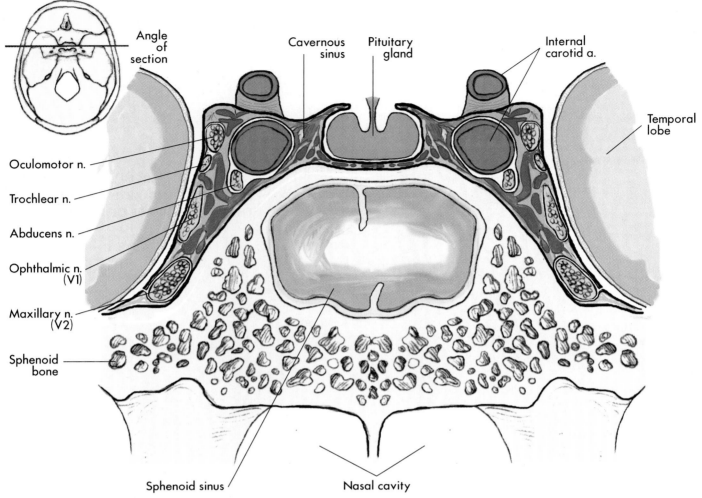

Angle
of
section

Cavernous
sinus

Pituitary
gland

Internal
carotid a.

Temporal
lobe

Oculomotor n.

Trochlear n.

Abducens n.

Ophthalmic n.
(V1)

Maxillary n.
(V2)

Sphenoid
bone

Sphenoid sinus

Nasal cavity

Figure 2-26   DETAILED CROSS-SECTION OF CAVERNOUS SINUS. The cavernous sinus
is intimately related to many of the vessels and nerves that are destined to enter the orbit
just anterior to the cavernous sinus.

of the corpus callosum. It supplies blood to the medial
surface of much of the frontal and parietal lobes. At its
most anterior point on the base of the brain, the anteri-
or cerebral artery is linked to its partner on the opposite side by a single short midline bridging vessel, the
anterior communicating artery.

The **middle cerebral artery** is much larger than the
anterior cerebral. It passes upward between the anteri-
or end of the temporal lobe and the insula and then divides into a number of branches, a few supplying the
insula and most fanning out over the lateral surface of
the hemisphere, supplying parts of the frontal, parietal,
and temporal lobes. It supplies nearly all of the lateral
surface of the entire hemisphere, save for a ~1-cm–wide
strip around the periphery (this area is supplied by
branches of the anterior and posterior cerebral arteries).
Second, although they are small, some of the most important branches of the middle cerebral artery arise just
after its separation from the anterior cerebral artery.
These are the *striate* and *thalamostriate arteries,* and their
importance derives from the fact that they pierce the
undersurface of the brain and supply large and impor-

tant nuclei and axonal tracts (Figure 2-27). Thus a hemorrhage or obstruction in one of these small vessels can
produce the severe functional loss we know more collo-
quially as a "stroke." Third, a small vessel arising from
the internal carotid—the anterior choroidal artery—
passes to the interior of the brain and its branches
eventually become the blood supply to the choroid
plexus of the lateral and third ventricles, from which
the great majority of cerebrospinal fluid is produced.

Last, another small but important vessel, the **posteri-
or communicating artery,** arises on each side near the
origin of the middle cerebral artery and courses posteriorly to anastomose with the posterior cerebral artery
on the same side. The two posterior communicating arteries are important components of the circulus arteriosus, on which collateral blood flow to the brain depends.

Nearly all of the remaining cerebral circulation derives form the **vertebral-basilar artery** and its branches. The two vertebral arteries arise from the first part of
the subclavian artery and move posteriorly and superiorly to ascend through the transverse foramina of cer-

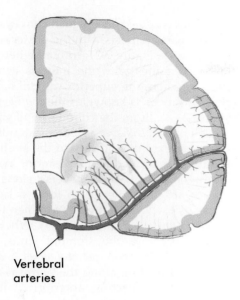

Vertebral
arteries

Figure 2-27 OBLIQUE VIEW OF THE BASAL VES-SELS OF THE BRAIN. The numerous small vessels that penetrate upward from the vessels shown here are often small in size but supply exceedingly important brain areas. In such cases, a relatively small injury to a vessel may have widespread functional impact. SEE ATLAS, FIG. 2-94

vical vertebrae C6 to C1 (there is a foramen in the C7 vertebra, but the vertebral artery does not usually traverse it). The vessel then passes posteriorly to the lateral mass of the atlas, penetrating the lower margin of the atlantooccipital membrane. The vertebral arteries enter the cranial cavity through the foramen magnum and soon unite to form the **basilar artery.** From here the basilar artery ascends along the anteromedial border of the medulla, giving off a medial branch that unites with a similar branch from the other side to form the **anterior spinal artery.** This important vessel runs inferiorly along the anterior median fissure of the spinal cord. Further inferiorly, each vertebral artery gives off a large **posterior inferior cerebellar artery,** supplying the cerebellum.

It then inclines medially to meet and unite, at the inferior end of the pons, with its partner from the opposite side. The two vertebral arteries thus unite to form the single basilar artery (see Figure 2-24). This artery ascends in a shallow groove on the ventral surface of

the brainstem to the level of the mesencephalon, where it divides into the left and right **posterior cerebral arteries.** Each of these follows an arching course laterally around the side of the brainstem to provide a number of branches to the inferolateral surfaces of the occipital and temporal lobes. Before forming this pair of terminal branches, the basilar artery gives off several paired branches. Important among these are the **labyrinthine artery** (entering the internal auditory meatus and supplying the inner ear), the **anterior inferior cerebellar arteries,** and the **superior cerebellar arteries.** The oculomotor nerve emerges from the ventral surface of the mesencephalon between the superior cerebellar and posterior cerebral arteries. The posterior cerebral arteries anastomose with the posterior communicating artery on their side, completing two of the important linkages of the circulus arteriosus.

The circulus arteriosus (**circle of Willis**) is formed from branches of the internal carotid and vertebral systems. On each side, the internal carotid gives rise to the

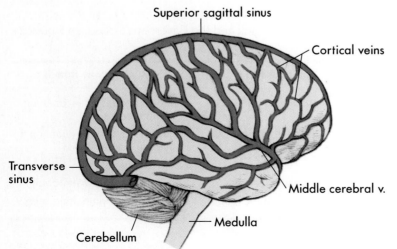

Superior sagittal sinus

Cortical veins

Transverse sinus

Middle cerebral v.

Medulla

Cerebellum

Figure 2-28 CEREBRAL VEINS. These veins, draining the surface of the cerebral cortex, drain into the superior sagittal sinus and transverse sinus. They cross the subarachnoid space and can be torn in traumatic injuries to the head.

middle and anterior cerebral arteries, and the basilar system gives rise to the posterior cerebral artery. The posterior communicating arteries on each side and the single midline anterior communicating artery complete the circular anastomosis. As many as 50% of people have abnormalities in the structure of the circle, including hypoplastic or missing branches. Several important structures are intimately associated with the circle. The *optic nerve (II)* lies just medial to the internal carotid arteries as they enter the circle. The *oculomotor nerve (III)* emerges from the brainstem between the posterior cerebral and superior cerebellar arteries. The *abducens nerve (IV)* emerges from the ventral surface of the pons just superior to the anterior inferior cerebellar artery.

VENOUS CIRCULATION OF THE BRAIN

The **venous sinuses** are encased between the two layers of the dura mater and are found opposite the superior, lateral, and inferior regions of the brain. Sinuses differ from ordinary veins in having no smooth muscle in their walls and maintain their patency, because their walls are held in the open position by attachments to surrounding connective tissue. Important sinuses located opposite the base of the brain are the *cavernous sinus,* the *superior* and *inferior petrosal sinuses,* and the *occipital sinus.* Important sinuses embedded in the dura lining the remainder of the cranial vault are the *superior sagittal sinus, inferior sagittal sinus, straight sinus, confluence of sinuses, transverse sinus,* and *sigmoid sinus* (see Figures 2-21 and 2-23). Drainage from the majority of these sinuses converges on the **jugular bulb,** a dilation at the origin of the internal jugular vein (see Figures 2-6 and 2-23, *A*). The jugular bulb is located in the jugular foramen, an aperture located between the temporal and occipital bones of the floor of the skull. Venous blood, especially that from the anterior base of the brain, may drain not to the jugular vessels, but through the cavernous sinus anteriorly to the veins of the face. Detailed descriptions of the individual sinuses follow.

Blood from the deep central portions of the brain, especially on the medial surfaces of the hemispheres, collects into the **internal cerebral vein** (great vein of Galen) and meets with the inferior sagittal sinus posteriorly to form the **straight sinus** (see Figure 2-23, *B*). The inferior sagittal sinus is positioned in the lower free margin of the falx cerebri, and the straight sinus runs from anterior to posterior between the dural layers in the midline of the tentorium cerebelli.

Blood draining from the superolateral surfaces of the brain collects into **cortical veins,** which extend across the subarachnoid space to drain into the venous sinuses (Figure 2-28). These cortical veins are subject to tears when strong shearing forces are applied, as during head trauma. Blood from these cortical veins converges

on the *superior sagittal sinus,* which conveys blood posteriorly to an anastomosis with the posterior end of the *straight sinus* (see Figure 2-21, formed when the inferior sagittal sinus unites with the internal cerebral vein). This region, where the superior sagittal sinus and the straight sinus meet, is known as the *confluence of sinuses* (see Figure 2-23). From the confluence of sinuses, there originates a pair of *transverse sinuses,* extending laterally in grooves on the inner surface of the skull. The transverse sinuses are located in the posterior margins of the tentorium cerebelli. Each transverse sinus then turns sharply toward the anterior to form a *sigmoid sinus,* which travels toward the jugular foramen to drain into the jugular bulb (see Figure 2-23, *A*). Where the transverse sinus becomes the sigmoid sinus, it receives drainage from the *superior petrosal sinus,* a diagonal venous channel traveling along the petrosal ridge of the temporal bone, connecting anteriorly with the cavernous sinus.

The **cavernous sinuses** (see Figure 2-26) are blood-filled spaces between the two layers of dura mater located on each side of the central portion of the sphenoid bone, surrounding the sphenoid sinus and the sella turcica. The interior is criss-crossed by lacy connective tissue filaments, and blood flow through the cavernous sinuses is slow and prone to thrombus formation. In the center of the cavernous sinus are found the *internal carotid artery* and the *abducens nerve (VI).* Lateral to the cavernous sinus are found, from superior to inferior, the *oculomotor (III), trochlear (IV), ophthalmic (V1)* and *maxillary (V2) nerves.* All of these structures appear to be embedded in the cavernous sinus but are outside the vascular endothelium and not truly within the cavernous sinus (Table 2-5).

The venous sinuses in the superolateral parts of the dura mater, especially the superior sagittal sinus, are invaginated by tufts of the nearby layers of arachnoid mater. These tufts of arachnoid membrane, called **arachnoid granulations,** actually protrude into the center of the lumen of the sagittal sinus, and it is at these

Table 2-5   Veins and the Cavernous Sinus (see Figure 2-23)

Draining into it	Draining away from it
Ophthalmic veins	Superior petrosal sinus (draining to transverse sinus)
Middle cerebral vein	Inferior petrosal sinus (draining to internal jugular veins)
Inferior cerebral veins	Pterygoid plexus
Sphenoparietal sinus	Facial vein via ophthalmic veins
Central vein of the retina	Facial vein via ophthalmic veins

THE CEREBRAL BLOOD FLOW

THE CIRCULUS ARTERIOSUS (CIRCLE OF WILLIS)

Although the circulus arteriosus appears to be an elaborate anastomotic circuit, in fact its efficiency in protecting against ischemia (poor blood flow) to the brain is only fair. In many individuals, one or more portions of the circle is very small or incompletely formed.

ANEURYSMS AND THE CIRCULUS ARTERIOSUS

The fact that many vessels of the circle intersect with each other at sharp angles predisposes to the formation of aneurysms at those sites of intersection. Ruptured aneurysms in the circle of Willis are a frequent cause of sudden death in young and middle-aged individuals.

CEREBRAL BLOOD FLOW

Blood flow into the cranial cavity would be subject to great increases and decreases in blood volume and pressure (with the effects of gravity, head position changes, and so on) were it not for the phenomenon of autoregulation. Using sensors in the carotid sinus and other parts of the cerebral arterial tree, the CNS can influence the heart rate and muscle tone in the vascular tree to maintain a consistent flow and pressure of blood to the brain. Because the brain is completely dependent on its blood supply for oxygen and glucose supply, we would be subject to dangerous increases and decreases in cerebral blood pressure without this autoregulatory mechanism

sites that cerebrospinal fluid from the subarachnoid space diffuses back into the venous circulation (see Figure 2-19). Sinuses in the superolateral part of the cranial cavity have connections through small **emissary veins** with the vascular spaces between the two layers of the skull, and thence to the scalp. The importance of these veins is that infections in the scalp can potentially spread to the venous sinuses inside the cranial cavity and lead to meningitis. Infections of the scalp should always be treated aggressively to avoid this potential complication.

2.3

Cranial Nerves

▶ Components of the Cranial Nerves

▶ Functional Categories of Axons

▶ Sensory Ganglia of the Cranial Nerves

▶ Sympathetic Innervation of the Head and Neck

▶ Parasympathetic Innervation of the Head and Neck

COMPONENTS OF THE CRANIAL NERVES

Spinal nerves, with a few exceptions, are stereotypical replicas of each other. There is at each cord level two paired groups of nerve rootlets, one attached to the dorsolateral aspects of the spinal cord and the other to the ventrolateral aspects of the cord. At each spinal cord segment, these dorsolateral rootlets on each side collect into a single trunk, known as the *dorsal root,* for that spinal cord segment. The *dorsal root ganglion,* attached to the dorsal root, contains the cell bodies from which dorsal root axons arise. Each of these axons is in fact divided into two branches—a *central process,* extending medially into the spinal cord, and a *lateral process,* extending laterally to join and become part of the spinal nerve (see Figure 2-11). The ventrolateral group of rootlets at each segment collects on each side into a single bundle, known as the *ventral root,* which also courses laterally to join the corresponding dorsal root and become part of the spinal nerve.

Cranial nerves, in contrast to spinal nerves, are often not similar to each other and do not fit into a stereotypical plan. There are no structures in cranial nerves equivalent to the dorsal and ventral roots of spinal nerves. Some cranial nerves are wholly sensory, some wholly motor, and still others are mixed (containing both sensory and motor axons). Whereas all spinal nerves contain sympathetic axons, there are no sympathetic axons in any cranial nerve as it emerges from the brainstem (see following). Parasympathetic axons are found only in spinal nerves S2, S3, and S4 (that is, sacral nerves 2 to 4) and are confined to nerves III, VII, IX, and X among the cranial nerves.

FUNCTIONAL CATEGORIES OF AXONS

There is a wide variety of axon functional types in cranial nerves. They are sometimes classed in relation to what they innervate and other times on the basis of embryologic origin (Table 2-6). **Somatic motor axons** innervate striated muscle not of pharyngeal arch origin. **Branchiomotor axons** innervate striated muscles which are of pharyngeal (branchial) arch origin. **Visceral motor axons** innervate certain smooth muscles and glands. **Special sensory axons** supply organs of special sense, unique to the head and neck region. **General sensory axons** mediate ordinary sensation (touch, pressure, heat, cold, and so on), and the sensations may or may not be experienced consciously. They innervate the skin and subcutaneous tissues of the head and neck, as well as certain deeper receptor structures, such as muscle spindles. **Visceral sensory axons** innervate the endodermally lined portions of the middle ear and auditory tube, pharynx, and larynx, as well as providing sensory innervation of such deeply-placed structures as blood vessels and glands. This sensory information generally does not reach consciousness.

SENSORY GANGLIA OF THE CRANIAL NERVES

By reviewing Table 2-6, we see that cranial nerves V and VII to X carry true sensory axons and therefore must have sensory ganglia associated with them. (Recall that cranial nerves I and II, though they are sensory nerves, are really tracts of the CNS, not true pe-

Table 2-6   Classification of Cranial Nerve Axons

Cranial Nerve	Somatic Motor	Branchiomotor	Visceral Motor	Special Sensory	General Sensory	Visceral Sensory
I—Olfactory*	—	—	—	(X)*	—	—
II—Optic*	—	—	—	(X)*	—	—
III—Oculomotor	X	—	X	—	—	—
IV—Trochlear	X	—	—	—	—	—
V—Trigeminal	—	X	—	—	X	—
VI—Abducens	X	—	—	—	—	—
VII—Facial	—	X	X	X	—	—
VIII—Vestibulocochlear (Acoustic)	—	—	—	X	—	—
IX—Glossopharyngeal	—	X	X	X	—	X
X—Vagus	—	X	X	X	—	X
XI—Accessory	—	X	—	—	—	—
XII—Hypoglossal	X	—	—	—	—	—

*The olfactory and optic nerves (nerves I and II) are not true cranial nerves but rather tracts of the central nervous system, positioned so that they resemble nerves and so named many decades ago (see Figure 2-29).

ripheral nerves, and thus lack the peripheral ganglia that typify the sensory axons found in true cranial and spinal nerves [Figure 2-29]).

The large **trigeminal ganglion** (see Figure 2-29), containing the cell bodies for sensory neurons, lies a short distance from the pons, encased in two layers of dura

and positioned in a shallow depression (the *cavum trigeminale*) on the anterior side of the petrous temporal ridge. Accompanying the sensory axons of the trigeminal nerve is a smaller *motor root*, whose axons will distribute exclusively with the mandibular branch of the trigeminal nerve. The large trunk entering the ganglion

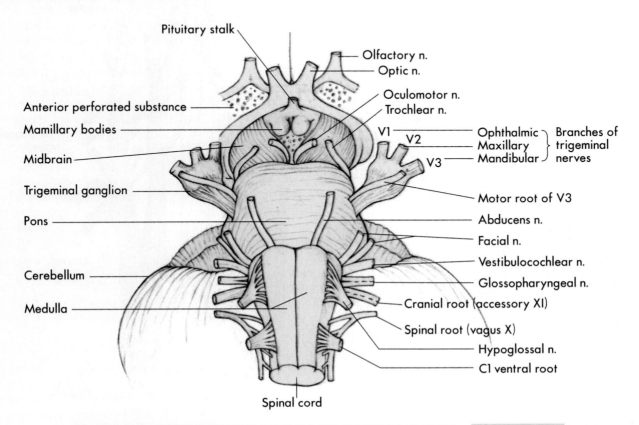

Figure 2-29   CRANIAL NERVES ON THE BASE OF THE BRAINSTEM.   SEE ATLAS, FIG. 2-87

posteromedially represents the central processes of the sensory neurons whose cell bodies lie in the ganglion. Emerging from the anterolateral margin of the ganglion are three separate trunks, containing the peripheral processes of the *three divisions of the trigeminal nerve*— the ophthalmic (V1), maxillary (V2), and mandibular (V3) nerves. These three divisions travel forward and enter the superior orbital fissure, foramen rotundum, and foramen ovale, respectively. They provide general sensory innervation to the superior portion of the orbit, forehead, and anterior scalp (V1); inferior portion of the orbit, central face, and skin superior and anterior to the ear (V2); and the region of the mandible and area just inferior to the ear (V3). The mandibular nerve also contains a small fascicle of motor axons (the brachiomotor component) innervating the muscles of mastication and several other muscles in the lower face and mouth.

The special sensory function of the *facial nerve (VII)* is represented by the taste axons innervating the anterior two thirds of the tongue. The cell bodies for these axons are located in the **geniculate ganglion,** a small cluster of neurons located along the course of the facial nerve as it passes posteriorly to the middle ear cavity,

enclosed within the temporal bone. Other axons sometimes pass very near to the geniculate ganglion or seem to be partially embedded in it, but only the taste axons have their cell bodies in it.

The *glossopharyngeal nerve (IX)* provides special sensory (taste) innervation to the posterior third of the tongue and visceral sensory innervation to the mucosa of the posterior third of the tongue, epiglottis, oropharynx, laryngopharynx, middle ear cavity, and the interior of the mastoid air cells. It has two ganglia, a very small **superior** and a larger **inferior ganglion**—see Figure 2-71 (nodose ganglion). Both are attached to the glossopharyngeal nerve as it traverses the jugular foramen. The cell bodies for the neurons providing all the sensory functions listed in Table 2-6 are found in these ganglia, predominantly in the inferior ganglion.

Though the *vagus nerve (X)* is usually discussed primarily as a motor nerve, in fact the large majority of its axons are sensory (Figure 2-30). It provides special sensory innervation to a few taste buds located on the epiglottis and visceral sensory innervation to the laryngeal mucosa, heart, lungs, and digestive tract, as far distal as the transverse colon. The vagus nerve also conveys a small number of general sensory axons that

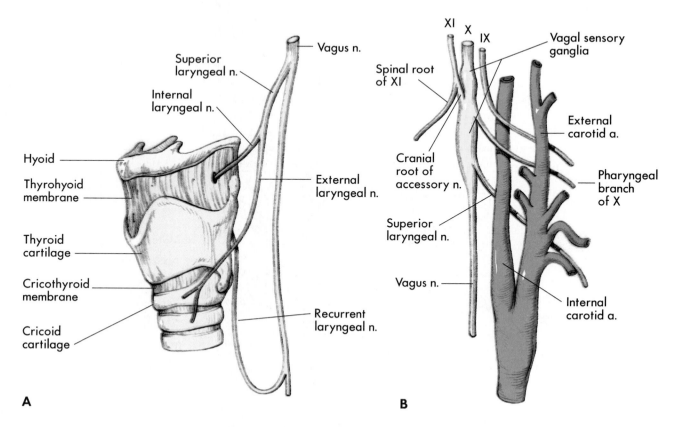

Figure 2-30   BRANCHES OF CRANIAL NERVES IX, X, AND XI. A, Vagal innervation of the larynx. **B,** Note the complex branching of these nerves in the vicinity of the carotid bifurcation. *IX,* Glossopharyngeal; *X,* vagus; *XI,* accessory.

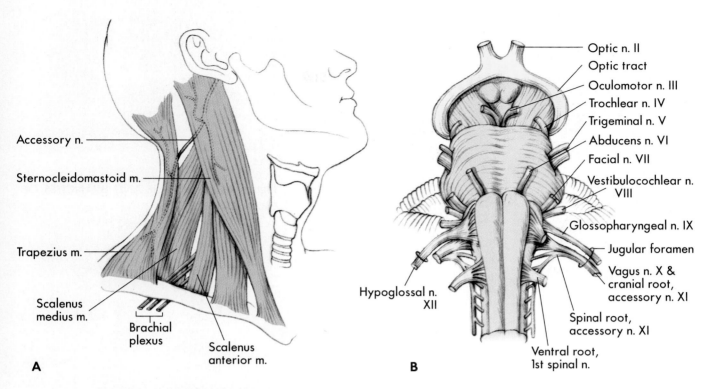

Figure 2-31 THE ACCESSORY NERVE (XI). A, The accessory nerve and the posterior triangle. **B,** Origins and apertures through which cranial nerves IX, X, XI, and XII exit the skull.

innervate a portion of the external surface of the tympanic membrane. When these axons from the tympanic membrane enter the brainstem, they form connections with regions that also receive many incoming sensory axons from the 5th nerve. It is as though this small group of vagal axons was somehow displaced from being a part of the trigeminal nerve but retains the central connections appropriate for nerve V.

Like nerve IX, the vagus has two sensory ganglia. The smaller **superior ganglion** (Figure 2-30) is located just proximal to the jugular foramen and contains the cell bodies of those axons which innervated the tympanic membrane. The larger **inferior ganglion** is suspended from the vagus nerve just after it exits the cranium through the jugular foramen. Its axons provide the visceral sensory laryngeal, pulmonary, cardiac, and digestive tract innervation.

The *accessory nerve (XI)* is a pure motor nerve (Figure 2-31). It has a *cranial root,* the axons of which actually join the vagus nerve and become incorporated into it shortly after the vagus nerve leaves the brainstem. Accessory nerve axons, as branches of the vagus, innervate the larynx and parts of the pharynx. The *spinal root* of the accessory nerve arises in the upper five or six cervical spinal cord segments. Its axons collect into trunks that ascend through the foramen magnum and immediately turn laterally to reexit the skull through the jugular foramen. Axons of the spinal root of the accessory nerve innervate the sternocleidomastoid and trapezius muscles.

The *hypoglossal nerve (XII)* arises in the lower medulla and exits the skull through the hypoglossal canal to innervate the tongue. Similar to the accessory, it is a pure motor nerve (Figure 2-32).

SYMPATHETIC INNERVATION OF THE HEAD AND NECK

Structures and tissues of the head and neck are supplied with **postganglionic sympathetic axons** through the dense plexus of axons found on the internal and external carotid arteries and all of their branches. For example, tissues of the nose receive sympathetic input by way of axons traveling on the sphenopalatine artery and its branches, and the frontal lobe of the brain receives sympathetic input through the plexus on the middle and anterior cerebral arteries. These postganglionic nerves have their cell bodies in the superior cervical ganglion (Figure 2-33; see Figure 2-76). As the carotid arteries pass near this ganglion in the upper neck, multiple small postganglionic nerve branches extend from the ganglion to the vessels. It is here that the carotid arteries acquire a covering sympathetic plexus. As the various branches of the carotid arteries reach the

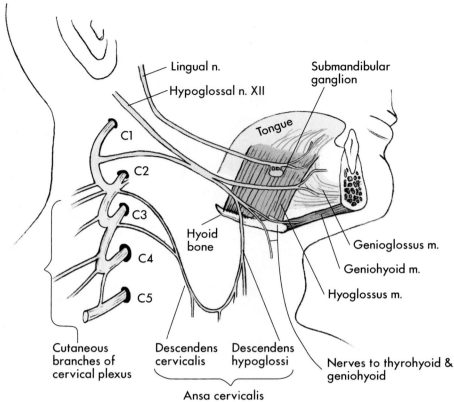

Figure 2-32 **COURSE AND BRANCHES OF CRANIAL NERVE XII.**

areas they innervate, the axons depart from the arterial plexus. In certain areas, these postganglionic sympathetic axons join with distal branches of trigeminal nerve that are supplying that same area of the head and neck. For example, sympathetic axons intended to in-

nervate the lacrimal gland travel on the ophthalmic artery to reach the orbit. Here, they leave the ophthalmic artery and join the *lacrimal nerve*, a distal branch of V1, on the final part of their journey to the lacrimal gland. Sympathetic axons of the head and

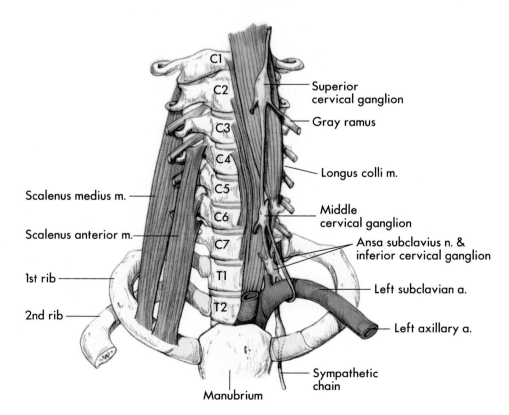

Figure 2-33 **CERVICAL SYMPATHETIC CHAIN.** The sympathetic chain lies on the anterior surface of the longus colli muscles, just posterior to the carotid sheath (not shown).

PRINCIPLES ■

Cranial nerves III, IV, VI, and XII resemble the ventral roots of spinal nerves, in that they are entirely motor (though they lack the sympathetic axons found in some ventral roots). Cranial nerves V, VII, IX, and X provide sensory innervation to pharyngeal arches 1, 2, 3, and 4 to 6, respectively (though they each carry many additional motor axons as well). Remember that cranial "nerves" I and II are in reality tracts of the CNS and as such are not strictly comparable to spinal nerves.

Cranial nerves in fact represent phylogenetically older nerves than spinal nerves. The twelve pairs of human cranial nerves enter and leave the cranial cavity through apertures in or between the four bones of the floor of the skull—the ethmoid, sphenoid, temporal, and occipital bones.

neck regulate the tone of musculature in blood vessels, sweat gland secretion, and hair arrector muscles, and in addition can dilate the pupil.

PARASYMPATHETIC INNERVATION OF THE HEAD AND NECK

Four of the cranial nerves contain **preganglionic parasympathetic axons** as they emerge from the brainstem. They are the *oculomotor, facial, glossopharyngeal,* and *vagus nerves.* The parasympathetic axons in these nerves synapse on postganglionic parasympathetic neurons in a peripheral ganglion or, in the case of the vagus nerve, on small clusters of postganglionic parasympathetic neurons scattered in the wall of the target organ or tissue (the heart, digestive tract, and so on).

The ganglion in which the preganglionic parasympathetic axons of the oculomotor nerve synapse is the **ciliary ganglion** in the orbit. Axons arising from neurons in the ciliary ganglion innervate the ciliaris muscle

and sphincter of the pupil. For the facial nerve, there are two target ganglia—the **pterygopalatine ganglion** and the **submandibular ganglion.** Postganglionic parasympathetic axons arising from neurons in the pterygopalatine ganglion innervate the lacrimal gland and the minor salivary glands of the soft palate. Postganglionic parasympathetic axons arising from neurons in the submandibular ganglion innervate the submandibular and sublingual salivary glands. Preganglionic parasympathetic axons in the glossopharyngeal nerve synapse in the **otic ganglion.** Postganglionic parasympathetic axons arising in the otic ganglion innervate the parotid gland.

In the vagus nerve, preganglionic parasympathetic axons descend through the neck and into the thorax and abdomen. These axons are destined to synapse on neurons grouped in small clusters throughout the walls of the heart, the interior of the lungs, and the submucosal muscular layers of the digestive tract as far distal as the midtransverse colon. These small groups of neurons give rise to postganglionic parasympathetic axons that generally travel only a short distance before terminating on muscular or glandular structures in the walls of these organs and tissues.

A major role played by the parasympathetic axons in the facial, glossopharyngeal, and vagus nerves is to stimulate activities associated with digestion. The stimulation of the parotid, submandibular, and sublingual glands promotes the secretion of saliva. Vagal innervation of intramural ganglia in the gut promotes peristalsis and secretion of gastric acid and mucus and relaxes the pyloric sphincter, all of which are part of the digestive process. In addition to its effect on the digestive process, the vagus nerve also produces slowing of the heart and narrowing of the bronchiolar air passages. The parasympathetic function of the oculomotor nerve does not involve the digestive process. The oculomotor nerve produces constriction of the pupil and changes the shape of the lens to allow focusing on nearby objects.

section two.four

Pharyngeal Arches

▶ Structure and Position of the
   Pharyngeal Arches

▶ Components of the Individual
   Arches

▶ Pharyngeal Pouches and Clefts

STRUCTURE AND POSITION OF THE PHARYNGEAL ARCHES

The pharyngeal arches (branchial arches) are paired masses of mesenchyme located opposite each other in the lateral walls of the foregut in the developing neck (Figure 2-34). In many lower vertebrates, there are vertical gaps between the arches (gills), but in mammals, true gills never form and the individual masses on each side are connected by thin membranes covering what would be the gill opening. In the human there are six pairs of branchial arches, numbered 1 to 6 from cranial to caudal. The more cranial arches develop earlier than do the posterior ones, and at no point are all six present at once. The arches are separated from each other by infoldings of ectoderm (*clefts*) situated opposite outpouchings of endoderm (*pouches*).

Each pharyngeal arch is covered exteriorly by **ectoderm** and internally by **endoderm.** Between these two layers in each arch is a mass of **mesoderm** (the actual "arch") that gives rise to certain striated muscles, bones, ligaments, and connective tissue elements (Figure 2-35). The tissues that originate in these separate arches may be distributed over a wide area of the head and neck, so that seemingly very different structures may have a common early origin in one of the pharyngeal arches.

COMPONENTS OF THE INDIVIDUAL ARCHES

Tissues that originate in a given pharyngeal arch may migrate to seemingly unrelated regions of the head and neck. When developmental errors involving

the pharyngeal arches occur, the set of structures that are abnormally formed may not seem to "make sense," unless their common origin is appreciated. Table 2-7 lists the individual bones, cartilages, muscles, nerves, vessels, and special structures that derive from the pharyngeal arches. Certain syndromes occur in clinical medicine that are best understood with reference to the concept of pharyngeal arch derivatives. For example, the first arch syndromes typically involve hypoplasia of the mandible, recession of the maxilla, and malformation of the external ear and sometimes the palate.

During early development, each arch has a major arterial vessel coursing through it. These are "bridging" vessels, extending from the ventral aortic sac, lying just in front of the heart, to the dorsal aortal on either side of the dorsal midline of the neck (Figure 2-36). Particularly in the case of the lower arches, these vessels go on to form important components of the great vessels of the upper thorax and neck.

Pharyngeal arches 1 to 3 are considered to have a *primary nerve* of their own, plus a smaller branch (known as the *pretrematic branch*) that extends into it from the arch immediately posterior. As an example, the *chorda tympani*—a pretrematic branch of the facial nerve—is distributed to first arch structures by traveling with the *lingual nerve,* and both nerves innervate the anterior two thirds of the tongue. The facial nerve (VII) is the primary nerve of the second arch, but within the second arch is found a small pretrematic branch of the *glossopharyngeal nerve* (the primary nerve of the third arch). This small branch of nerve IX is the *tympanic nerve,* which innervates tissues derived from the second pharyngeal arch (for example, the middle ear cavi-

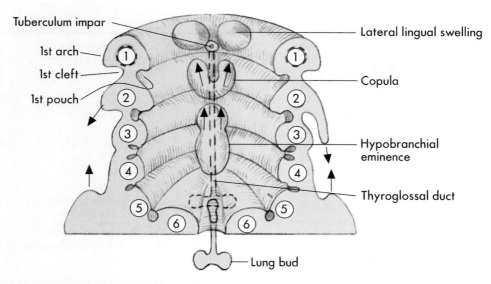

Figure 2-34 HORIZONTAL SECTION THROUGH THE EMBRYONIC PHARYNGEAL ARCHES. Here is shown the interior of the pharyngeal arch region, viewing the floor of the area and the paired pharyngeal (branchial is a synonym for pharyngeal in this case) arches that forms its walls. Much of the tongue develops from the floor of the pharynx, and a wide variety of structures develop from the individual pharyngeal arches. The tracheal bud evaginates from the floor of the most caudal part of the pharyngeal region and proliferates extensively to form the lungs.

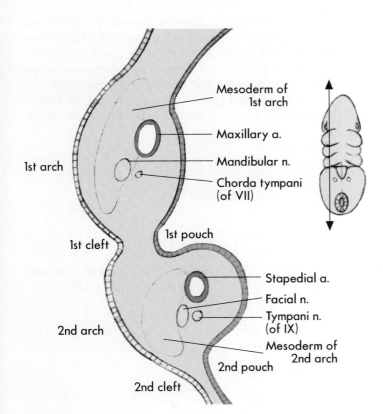

Figure 2-35 SCHEMATIC OF "TYPICAL" PHARYNGEAL ARCH. This is a horizontal section through one side of the pharyngeal arch region, showing the positions of the clefts and pouches and the interior contents of a typical arch.

Table 2-7   Derivatives of the Pharyngeal Arches

Arch	Skeletal	Muscular, Ligamentous	Neural	Vascular	Glands, etc.
First arch	Mandible, maxilla, malleus, incus	Muscles of mastication, tensor tympani, tensor palatini, anterior digastric, mylohyoid, malleus, sphenomandiblar ligament	CN V (V3), plus chorda tympani from nerve VII and part of V2	Maxillary artery	External auditory canal (1st cleft), auditory tube (1st pouch)
Second arch	Stapes, part of incus and hyoid bone	Facial muscles; stapedius, stylohyoid, posterior digastric, stylohyoid ligaments	CN VII and tympanic branch of nerve IX	Stapedial artery	Palatine tonsil (2nd pouch)
Third arch	Lower hyoid bone	Stylopharyngeus	CN IX	Proximal internal carotid artery	Thymus, inferior parathyroids
Fourth arch	Laryngeal cartilages	Pharyngeal and laryngeal constrictors	CN X (superior laryngeal nerve)	Part of aortic arch and right subclavian artery	Thymus, superior parathyroids, ultimobranchial body
Sixth arch*	Laryngeal cartilages	Intrinsic laryngeal muscles	CN X (recurrent laryngeal nerve)	Right pulmonary artery, ductus arteriosus (L)	

*The fifth arch is usually rudimentary and disappears early in development.

ty). Along with the vertebrae, the pharyngeal arches provide the best evidence of segmentation of the human body in the cervical region.

PHARYNGEAL POUCHES AND CLEFTS

Shallow grooves separating the pharyngeal arches (see Figure 2-34) can be visualized on both the exterior surface of the neck (where they are known as pharyngeal or branchial clefts) and on the interior surface of the neck (where they are known as pharyngeal or branchial pouches).

The **pharyngeal clefts** appear on the external surface of the developing neck only between arches 1 and 2, 2 and 3, 3 and 4, and 4 and 5. The *1st pharyngeal cleft,* which is caudal to the first arch and thus between arches 1 and 2, deepens inward and meets the first pharyngeal pouch, invaginating outward from the interior of the developing pharynx. The two cavities almost meet, and eventually only a thin bilayered membrane separates them. This bilayered membrane is the tympanic membrane. The first cleft later forms the *external auditory meatus.*

From the external surface of the *second pharyngeal arch,* there grows outward and downward a large mass of mesodermal tissue. This extension overlaps the second to fourth pharyngeal clefts (that is, between arches 2 and 3, 3 and 4, and 4 and 5). The large space between the outgrowing part of the second arch and the rest of the pharynx is the cervical sinus. Normally, the down-

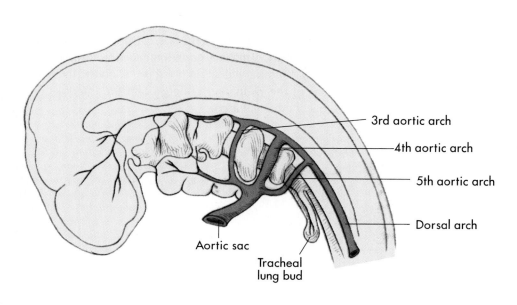

3rd aortic arch

4th aortic arch

5th aortic arch

Dorsal arch

Aortic sac

Tracheal lung bud

Figure 2-36   AORTIC ARCHES AND PHARYNGEAL ARCHES.

PRINCIPLES

The pharyngeal (branchial) arches are the embryonic forerunners of what forms much of the gill apparatus in lower vertebrates and the neck structures in higher vertebrates. In those vertebrates with gills, this area of the body is central to respiration and the ingestion of food. In higher, nonaquatic vertebrates, the respiratory function of the pharyngeal arches is absent because a mechanism for drawing air into the body has developed. In these animals, the pharyngeal arch contributes to the digestive system (as the pharynx) and to the process of vocalization and speech (as the larynx).

wardly growing part of the second arch meets and fuses with the surface of the pharynx further inferior on the neck. Usually, no space remains, and the cervical sinus disappears. The *third, fourth,* and *fifth pharyngeal* *clefts* normally do not develop into any recognizable adult structure.

The inner endodermal **pharyngeal pouches** develop into many specialized structures. The *first pouch,* between arches 1 and 2, begins as an outward evagination from the upper interior wall of the pharynx on each side. It extends laterally and helps form the lining of the auditory tube, the interior of the middle ear cavity (where it almost meets the first pharyngeal cleft), the mastoid air cells, and the inner layer of the tympanic membrane. The *second pouch* does not invaginate as greatly as the first and forms the bed for the palatine tonsil. The *third pouch* invaginates laterally into two partially separate limbs, and they go on to form the inferior parathyroid glands and the thymus gland. The *fourth pouch* gives rise to the superior parathyroid glands, and the *fifth pouch,* the calcitonin-secreting cells of the thyroid gland (known as the ultimobranchial body).

CLINICAL ANATOMY OF

PHARYNGEAL ARCH DERIVATIVES

FIRST-ARCH SYNDROMES

Specific first-arch syndromes include the Treacher-Collins syndrome and the Pierre Robin syndrome. The former is an autosomal dominant trait and includes a small lower jaw (micrognathia), middle ear anomalies, a malformed external ear, and abnormalities of the lower eyelid and upper jaw. The Pierre Robin syndrome involves micrognathia and cleft palate, plus ear anomalies.

DI GEORGE SYNDROME

Referring to the principle that separate and seemingly unrelated tissues can share a pharyngeal arch origin, there is a condition—the Di George syndrome—that involves the malformation or absence of the thymus gland (derived from the third arch), along with an abnormally formed aorta and brachiocephalic and carotid arteries (derived from the fourth and sixth arches). Patients afflicted with this condition may have the combination of abnormal blood flow through the great vessels and recurrent infections (the latter a result of inadequate T-cell development, owing to the absent thymus).

LATERAL NECK MASSES

Lateral masses in the neck are most often enlarged lymph nodes; less often than that, they result from a neoplastic growth in a lymph node; and more rarely, they may result from an enlarged cervical cyst.

PHARYNGEAL CYSTS

If the lateral wall of the neck does not close and the space beneath the surface of the skin (the cervical sinus) persists, the resultant pharyngeal or branchial cyst may become inflamed and filled with fluid. If the cervical sinus remains open to the outside, it is known as a lateral cervical fistula.

PHARYNGEAL FISTULAS

Rarely, the second pharyngeal cleft and pouch become confluent with each other and remain open at both ends, forming a pharyngeal fistula. In this case, there is an external opening in the lateral aspect of the neck and an internal opening in the vicinity of the palatine tonsillar bed.

MIGRATION OF THE THYMUS GLAND

The thymus gland normally descends into the upper part of the anterior mediastinum. It may fail to descend this far, however, and be found in the base of the neck or anywhere along the path of migration.

THE PARATHYROID GLANDS

The parathyroid glands are also subject to variations in their migration. Normally, they are found on the posterior surface of the thyroid gland, but they may descend only partway, to be found superior to the thyroid gland, or descend further than they should, to reside in the upper thorax.

2.5

section two.five

Scalp and Face

▶ Layers of the Scalp

▶ Blood Supply and Innervation of the Scalp

▶ Introduction to the Face

▶ Skeletal Framework of the Face

▶ Cutaneous Innervation of the Face and Scalp

▶ Muscles of Facial Expression

▶ Innervation of the Facial Muscles

▶ Vascular Supply of the Face

▶ Parotid Gland

LAYERS OF THE SCALP

The scalp is composed of five layers (Figure 2-37), whose names form an acronym for "scalp":

*S*kin, the dermis and epidermis of typical skin

*C*onnective tissue, a dense layer closely adherent to the underlying aponeurosis

*A*poneurosis, the broad flat sheet connecting the frontalis and occipitalis muscles

*L*oose areolar tissue, very vascular, but only loosely attached to the layers above

*P*eriosteum, the outer covering layer of the skull bones (also called pericranium)

The aponeurotic third layer of the scalp is also known as the **galea aponeurotica,** connecting the frontalis and occipitalis muscles (known together as the **epicranius muscle**). This muscle is innervated by branches of cranial nerve VII. The frontalis muscle is instrumental in movements of the eyebrows and forehead and is an important muscle of facial expression.

BLOOD SUPPLY AND INNERVATION OF THE SCALP

The upper three layers of the scalp are firmly attached to each other and behave as a single unit in cases of scalp injury. The fourth layer is very loosely organized and accounts for the mobility of the scalp with respect to the underlying skull. It is also highly vascular, supplied by branches of the **superficial temporal, posterior auricular, occipital,** and **supraorbital/supratrochlear arteries** (Figure 2-38).

The posterior half of the scalp is innervated by branches of the **cervical plexus,** principally derived from C2 and C3; the anterior half of the scalp is innervated by the **supraorbital** and **supratrochlear nerves,** derived from the ophthalmic branch of the trigeminal nerve (V1) (Figure 2-38). Laterally, the scalp is innervated by branches of the second and third divisions of the trigeminal nerve (the **zygomaticotemporal** and **auriculotemporal nerves,** respectively).

INTRODUCTION TO THE FACE

The face is the anterior part of the head. It consists of (1) a complex bony framework derived from parts of the frontal, nasal, zygomatic, maxillary, and mandibular bones, (2) a collection of thin muscles, known collectively as the muscles of facial expression, and (3) cutaneous nerve supply derived from branches of cranial nerve V and muscular innervation from branches of cranial nerves V and VII. The shape of the face is determined to a significant degree by the size of several air sinuses, especially those located in the frontal and maxillary bones.

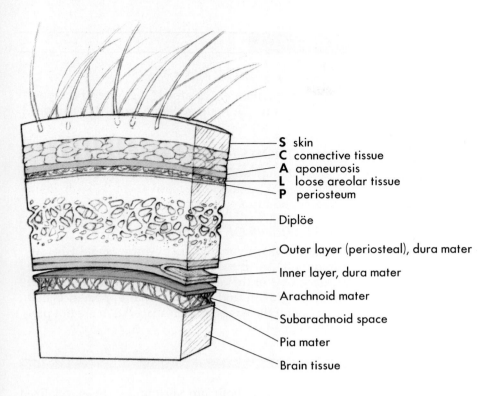

S skin
C connective tissue
A aponeurosis
L loose areolar tissue
P periosteum

Diplöe

Outer layer (periosteal), dura mater

Inner layer, dura mater

Arachnoid mater

Subarachnoid space

Pia mater

Brain tissue

Figure 2-37 LAYERS OF THE SCALP. The acronym "S C A L P" describes the five layers of the scalp. Deep to the scalp is the two-layered bone of the skull, whose interior cavity is known as the diploë. Interior to the skull are the two layers of cranial dura mater, arachnoid mater, subarachnoid space, pia mater, and brain tissue proper. SEE ATLAS, FIG. 2-30

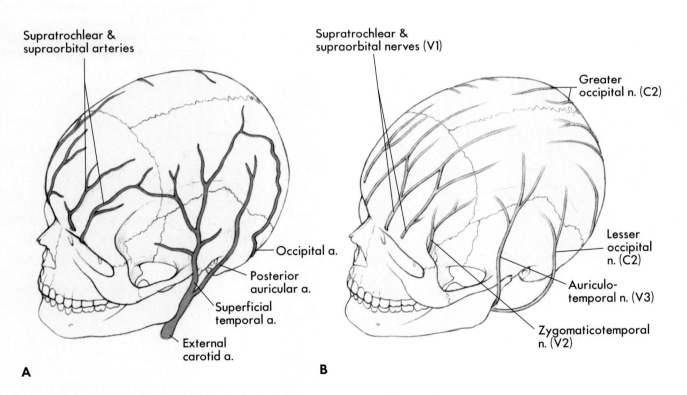

Supratrochlear & supraorbital arteries

Supratrochlear & supraorbital nerves (V1)

Greater occipital n. (C2)

Occipital a.

Posterior auricular a.

Superficial temporal a.

External carotid a.

Lesser occipital n. (C2)

Auriculo-temporal n. (V3)

Zygomaticotemporal n. (V2)

A   B

Figure 2-38   NERVES AND ARTERIES OF THE SCALP. A, The superficial temporal artery supplies the lateral side of the head and the supraorbital and supratrochlear arteries, terminal branches of the ophthalmic artery, supply the anterior forehead and scalp. **B,** Terminal branches of the ophthalmic nerve (supraorbital/supratrochlear nerves), maxillary nerve (zygomatic branches), mandibular nerve (auriculotemporal nerve), and the upper cervical segments of C2 (greater occipital nerve). SEE ATLAS, FIG. 2-30

THE SCALP

THE GALEA APONEUROTICA

The upper three layers of the scalp are closely adherent, and when the scalp is injured, these layers often separate from those below. The aponeurotic layer is under some tension, because of its attachment to the frontalis muscle of the forehead and the occipitalis muscle of the posterior skull. So, when lacerated, the edges of the aponeurosis tend to retract from each other, making spontaneous closure of the wound difficult and prolonging the bleeding that inevitably occurs.

"SCALPING"

The scalp is frequently injured badly when those with long hair have their hair trapped in machinery. When severe tearing forces are applied by such acci-

dents, the patient is "scalped" because the upper three layers of the scalp separate from those underneath.

ANASTOMOSES IN THE SCALP

Even though scalp injuries may be severe, successful healing is possible because there is such good anastomotic supply.

LACERATIONS OF THE EYEBROW

Lacerations involving the eyebrow should be sutured only by those experienced in reconstructive surgery. One of the reasons for this is the obliquity of eyebrow growth and the abnormal appearance that will result if the edges of such a laceration are not precisely aligned.

The structure of the face can best be understood by considering how it serves the purpose of protecting several important apertures that lead to cavities deeper within the head. The paired **orbital cavities** are bounded by roughly circular apertures (the *orbital rims*) in the upper face, and both are surrounded by specialized sets of muscles that can open or close the eyelids, protecting the anterior surface of the eyes and maintaining their lubrication. The midline **nasal cavity** opens anteriorly by two external apertures (*nostrils*, or *nares*), and

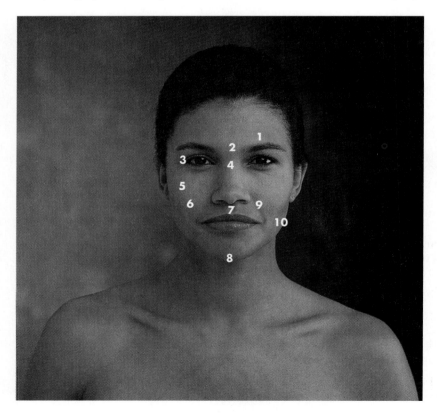

Figure 2-39 SURFACE ANATOMY OF THE FACE. *1,* Supraciliary ridge; *2,* glabella; *3,* lateral canthal fold; *4,* nasal bridge; *5,* zygomatic arch; *6,* buccal fat pad; *7,* philtrum; *8,* mental symphysis; *9,* nasolacrimal groove; *10,* angle of mandible.

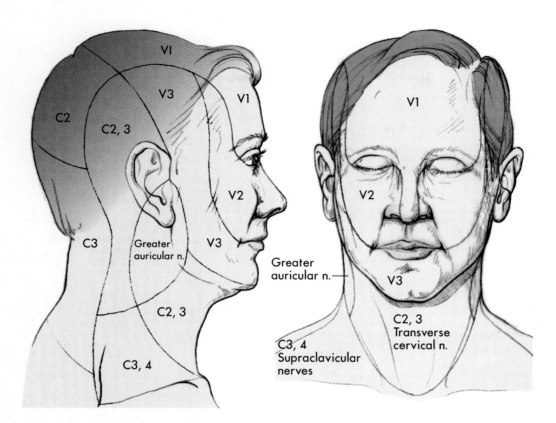

Figure 2-40   SEGMENTAL INNERVATION OF THE HEAD AND NECK. The three branches of the trigeminal nerve and the upper three cervical spinal segments provide cutaneous innervation to the head and neck.   SEE ATLAS, FIGS. 2-3, 2-29

these too have surrounding muscles that can regulate their size and shape. Control of the nares is an important element in the control of respiration. Last, the single **oral cavity** opens anteriorly through the *mouth,* and the shape and position of the lips surrounding the mouth are regulated by several significant muscles. The size and position of the oral opening is important in both respiration and the intake of food, and the muscles controlling the lips also play a role in mastication (chewing).

SKELETAL FRAMEWORK OF THE FACE

The face is bilaterally symmetric, and its unique shape in each of us is derived from a number of bony and soft tissue characteristics (Figure 2-39). The forehead is composed of the anterior surface of the frontal bone and overlying muscle and soft tissue. Especially prominent bulges on each side of the upper forehead are known as "frontal bossing" and when extreme are indicative of certain inherited syndromes. The **supraciliary ridges** are the upper rims of the orbits, and they too can be excessively broad and prominent in those with certain syndromes of growth hormone excess. The

nose is built of a combination of bone and cartilage. The **nasal bone** underlies the "bridge" of the nose, and the bony base of the lateral wall on each side is formed by part of the **maxilla.** Most of the rest of the nose is composed of **cartilage**—in particular, the lateral nasal cartilage, the alar cartilages (forming the perimeter of the nares), and the septal cartilage, which forms the most anterior third of the nasal septum. The "cheekbones," or **zygomatic arches,** are formed by a combination of the zygomatic processes of the maxilla and temporal bone and part of the zygoma, an independent facial bone. A small mass of fat, known as the **buccal fat pad,** is positioned inferomedially to the zygomatic arch, and when this fat pad is small, then the contour of the zygoma is easily visible and a person is said to have "high cheekbones." The central part of the maxilla and its attached teeth form the **upper jaw,** and the mandible and its attached teeth form the **lower jaw.** The posterior and inferior part of the mandible (the angle) may be hypertrophied in those with syndromes of excess growth hormone and give the appearance of a very "prominent jaw." Both the maxilla and mandible change shape when teeth are lost in old age. The mandible becomes considerably thinned in old age.

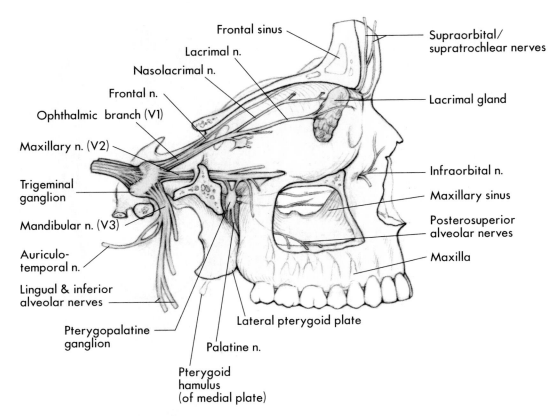

Figure 2-41   THREE DIVISIONS OF THE TRIGEMINAL NERVE. See text for details of individual branches.   **See Atlas, Fig. 2-2**

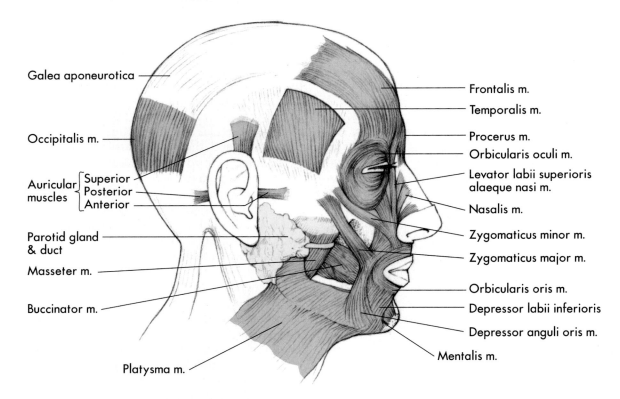

Figure 2-42   FACIAL MUSCLES, LATERAL VIEW. Shown here are the major superficial muscles of the face and scalp and the parotid gland and its duct.   **See Atlas, Figs. 2-24, 2-25, 2-26, 2-27**

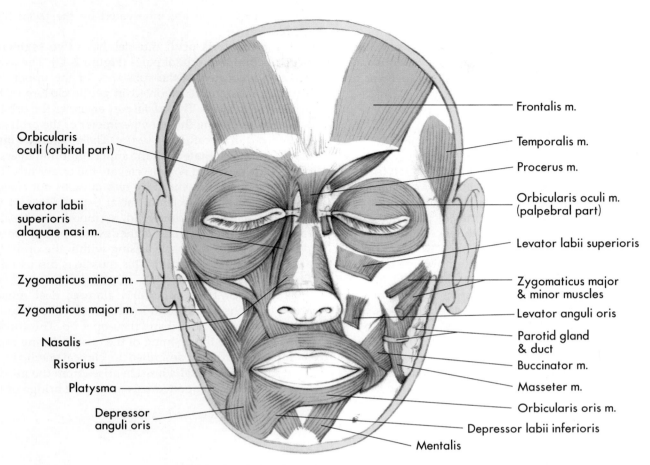

Frontalis m.

Temporalis m.

Procerus m.

Orbicularis oculi m.
(palpebral part)

Levator labii superioris

Zygomaticus major
& minor muscles

Levator anguli oris

Parotid gland
& duct

Buccinator m.

Masseter m.

Orbicularis oris m.

Depressor labii inferioris

Mentalis

Orbicularis
oculi (orbital part)

Levator labii
superioris
alaquae nasi m.

Zygomaticus minor m.

Zygomaticus major m.

Nasalis

Risorius

Platysma

Depressor
anguli oris

Figure 2-43   FACIAL MUSCLES, ANTERIOR VIEW.

CUTANEOUS INNERVATION OF THE FACE AND SCALP

The face is innervated by the three branches of the trigeminal nerve—the ophthalmic (V1), maxillary (V2), and mandibular (V3) nerves (Figures 2-40, 2-41, 2-45, and 2-56). The **ophthalmic nerve** innervates the skin on a narrow midline strip of the nose, both upper eyelids, the forehead, and the anterior half of the scalp. Its domain extends laterally on each side to that part of the anterior half of the scalp covering the frontal and parietal bones, but not over the squamous temporal bone

or the greater wing of the sphenoid (see Figure 2-1). The **maxillary nerve** innervates the lateral side of the nose, the upper lip, the skin over the maxilla, and the skin over the lateral surface of the face as far posterior as the root of the zygoma. The **mandibular nerve** provides cutaneous innervation of the lower lip, chin, body and ramus of the mandible (except the skin over the angle of the mandible), and a strip of skin covering the posterior half of the squamous temporal bone (Figure 2-40). Whereas the ophthalmic and maxillary nerves are wholly devoted to cutaneous innervation of

Table 2-8   The Muscles of Facial Expression

Related to Eye and Orbit	Related to Nasal Cavity	Related to Oral Cavity	
Orbicularis oculi	Levator labii superioris alaquae nasi	Orbicularis oris	Depressor labii inferioris
Occipitofrontalis (epicranius)	Nasalis	Levator labii superioris	Mentalis
	Procerus	Zygomaticus major	Risorius
		Zygomaticus minor	Buccinator
		Levator anguli oris	Platysma
		Depressor anguli oris	

the face, the mandibular nerve is responsible for cutaneous innervation and innervation of several important striated muscles of the face and jaw. The *greater auricular nerve of the cervical plexus* provides cutaneous innervation to the angle of the mandible and the lower portion of the external ear.

MUSCLES OF FACIAL EXPRESSION

The muscles of facial expression are a set of paired superficial muscles (Figures 2-42 and 2-43) that can produce a large variety of facial expressions that we associate with both verbal and nonverbal forms of communication. The facial muscles may also be seen as regulating the major apertures of the face—the two eyes, two nostrils, and the mouth. In fact, we shall present these muscles in groupings that emphasize their control of these apertures (Table 2-8).

The muscles of facial expression differ from other striated muscles by being anchored into the skin. Some are attached to bones or ligaments as well. Most of them are anchored in connective tissue, in the superficial fascia, and are the human species' representative of such muscles as those of cattle or horses that constantly "twitch" the skin of the back and neck. All the muscles

of facial expression are innervated by the facial (7th) nerve.

The **orbicularis oculi** muscles have two segments, the palpebral and orbital parts (Figure 2-43). The *palpebral part* is located in the substance of the upper and lower eyelids and is involved in gentle closure of the eyelids, as in sleep. The *orbital part* encircles the orbit in the fascia overlying the bony perimeter of the orbit and is involved in forceful lid closure. The **epicranius muscle** fibers interdigitate with the superior orbital fibers of orbicularis oculi and so help elevate the upper lids. The eyelids are also influenced by two muscles not considered part of the muscles of facial expression—(1) the **tarsal muscle** of the upper lid, a smooth muscle that helps elevate the lid and (2) the **levator palpebrae superioris,** a striated muscle arising within the orbit that also elevates the upper lid. This muscle is discussed in the section on the orbit.

The **levator labii superioris alaquae nasi muscle** arises from the maxilla and inserts in two slips into the lateral wall of the nostril and the upper lip. This muscle helps to enlarge the opening of the nostril during rapid or forced breathing, described in clinical medicine as *nasal flaring.* The **nasalis muscle** arises from the maxilla and extends by an aponeurosis across the bridge of the

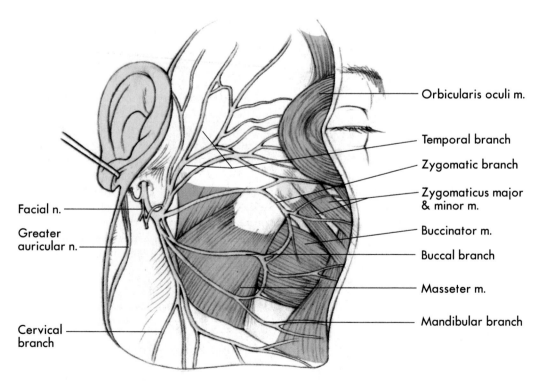

Figure 2-44 BRANCHES OF THE FACIAL NERVE. The temporal, zygomatic, buccal, mandibular, and cervical branches of the facial nerve emerge from superior to inferior along the anterior border of the parotid gland. SEE ATLAS, FIG. 2-28

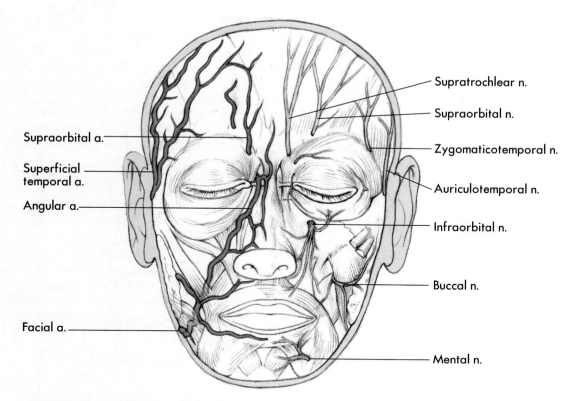

Figure 2-45 **CUTANEOUS VESSELS AND NERVES OF THE FACE.** On the right are the superficial arterial vessels supplying the face and scalp, and on the left are the superficial nerves.

nose to connect to the same muscle on the other side of the face. Contraction of nasalis results in partial closure of the aperture of the nostril.

Orbicularis oris is a circular muscle that surrounds the oral cavity, and its contraction results in a narrowing of the oral aperture, or "pursing" of the lips (Figures 2-42 and 2-43). The muscles fibers are located subcutaneously in the upper and lower lip, just peripheral to the pigmented epithelium of the lips.

INNERVATION OF THE FACIAL MUSCLES

The terminal branches of the **facial nerve** fan out like the five fingers of a hand over the lateral surface of the face (Figures 2-44 and 2-48). The portion of facial nerve passing through the parotid gland is purely motor (branchiomotor). It emerges from stylomastoid foramen, gives small branches to muscles near the ear, and then divides into the following terminal branches within parotid gland (from superior to inferior): temporal, zygomatic, buccal, mandibular, and cervical. Muscles of facial expression receive sensory innervation from the trigeminal nerve.

VASCULAR SUPPLY OF THE FACE

The **superficial temporal, ophthalmic,** and **facial arteries** and their branches provide blood supply to almost all of the face (Figure 2-46, *A*; see also Figure 2-48). The *facial artery* originates from the external carotid artery in the midneck and winds around the lateral surface of the body of the mandible, before coursing diago-

PRINCIPLES

In various regions of the body, there are superficial striated muscles, embedded within the superficial fascia. In certain cases they are wholly contained within the superficial layer but, in other cases, may be attached to a bone or cartilage. In some mammals, these muscles may be used to produce sudden twitching movements of the skin (as when a horse or cow attempts to shake the skin of its back to discourage flies from landing). In man these muscles are confined to the face and neck, where they play a very important role in producing facial expressions. These muscles also participate in vocalization, respiration, and chewing movements.

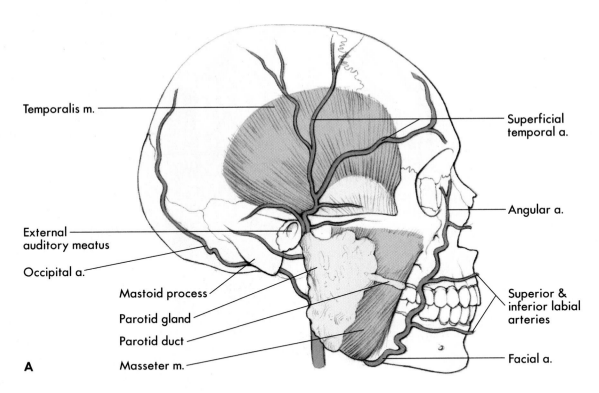

Temporalis m.

Superficial temporal a.

Angular a.

External auditory meatus

Occipital a.

Mastoid process

Parotid gland

Parotid duct

Masseter m.

Superior & inferior labial arteries

Facial a.

A

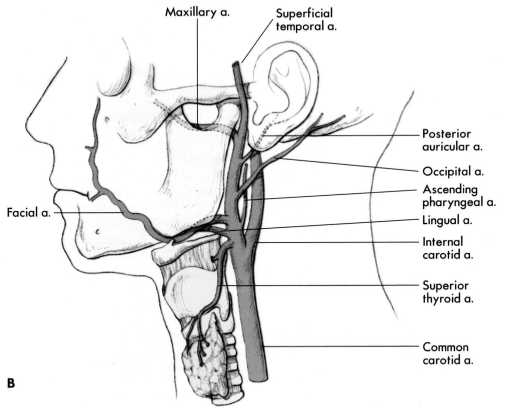

Maxillary a.   Superficial temporal a.

Facial a.

Posterior auricular a.

Occipital a.

Ascending pharyngeal a.

Lingual a.

Internal carotid a.

Superior thyroid a.

Common carotid a.

B

Figure 2-46   VASCULAR SUPPLY OF THE FACE. A, Branches of the external carotid artery.
B, Further branches of the external carotid and the carotid bifurcation.
S<small>EE</small> A<small>TLAS</small>, F<small>IGS</small>. **2-4, 2-34, 2-35, 2-36**

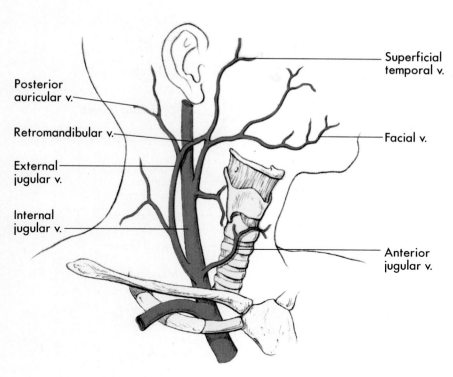

Posterior
auricular v.

Retromandibular v.

External
jugular v.

Internal
jugular v.

Superficial
temporal v.

Facial v.

Anterior
jugular v.

Figure 2-47. EXTERNAL AND INTER-NAL JUGULAR VEINS.
SEE ATLAS, FIGS. 2-4, 2-33

nally toward the corners of the mouth (Figure 2-46, *B*). From here, it ascends along the side of the nose and terminates near the medial angle of the eye. Its terminal branch is sometimes called the *angular artery,* the pulse of which is palpable in the space between the upper nose and the medial angle of the eye. Important branches along the way are the *inferior labial, superior labial,* and *lateral nasal arteries.* **Venous drainage of the face** travels principally through the facial, superficial temporal, and maxillary veins, all of which converge on the external and internal jugular veins.

Blood supply to the scalp (see Figures 2-38, 2-45, and 2-48) derives from three distinct sources: (1) The anterior part of the scalp receives blood from the *supratrochlear* and *supraorbital arteries,* both branches of the *ophthalmic artery,* (2) the lateral side of the scalp is supplied by the *superficial temporal artery,* one of the two terminal branches of the *external carotid artery,* and (3) the scalp posterior to the ear is supplied by branches of the *occipital* and *posterior auricular arteries,* both branches of the *external carotid.* There are numerous anastomoses between terminal branches of all of these vessels. Vascular supply to the scalp is especially rich in the fourth layer (see pp. 174–175), and these vessels are the source of the robust bleeding that often accompanies scalp injury.

Venous drainage of the scalp (*supraorbital, supratrochlear, superficial temporal, occipital,* and *posterior auricular veins*) also converges on the *external* and *internal jugular veins* (Figure 2-47). There are also important

anastomoses between these external veins and intracranial venous systems, through small vessels that pass through the substance of the skull (*diploic veins,* so called because the bilaminar bone of the skull is called the diplöe). Infections on the surface of the scalp can spread to the interior of the skull through these anastomoses. *Emissary veins,* especially in the parietal and occipital regions, pass through foramina in the skull and connect the veins of the scalp with intracranial venous sinuses. Such emissary veins also connect intracranial venous sinuses with important extracranial veins, such as the pterygoid plexus (see Figure 2-58).

PAROTID GLAND

The parotid gland is shaped roughly like an inverted triangle, lying anterior to the external ear, filling the space between the anterior edge of the sternocleidomastoid muscle and the posterior edge of the mandible (Figures 2-46 and 2-48). The gland is covered by a dense fascia, attached superiorly to the zygomatic process and continuous inferiorly with the deep cervical fascia. From the midpoint of the anterior edge of the parotid gland originates the **parotid duct.** This duct travels anteriorly across the surface of the masseter muscle and eventually empties into the oral cavity, on the inner surface of the upper cheek opposite the second upper molar tooth. This represents the place from where, early in development, the parotid gland first forms, as an outgrowth of the oral cavity. Often

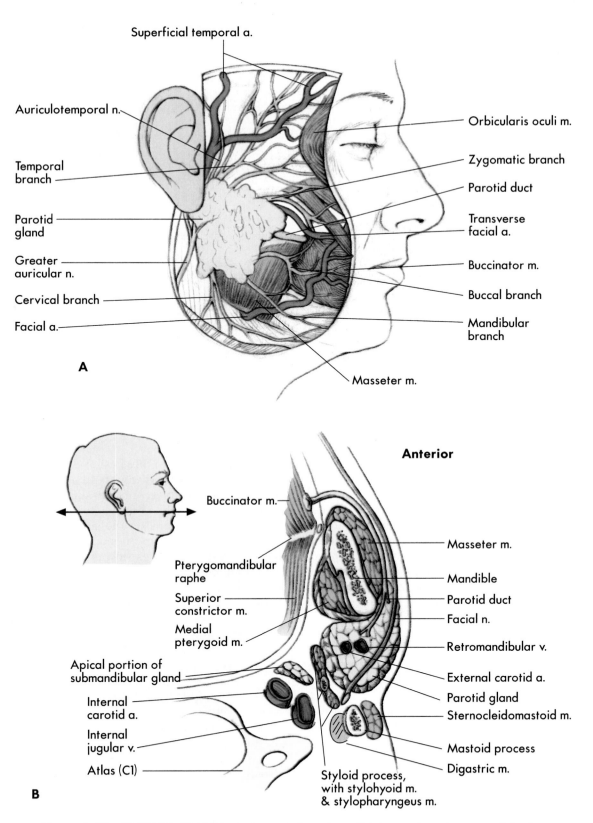

Superficial temporal a.

Auriculotemporal n.

Temporal branch

Parotid gland

Greater auricular n.

Cervical branch

Facial a.

Orbicularis oculi m.

Zygomatic branch

Parotid duct

Transverse facial a.

Buccinator m.

Buccal branch

Mandibular branch

Masseter m.

A

Anterior

Buccinator m.

Pterygomandibular raphe

Superior constrictor m.

Medial pterygoid m.

Apical portion of submandibular gland

Internal carotid a.

Internal jugular v.

Atlas (C1)

Masseter m.

Mandible

Parotid duct

Facial n.

Retromandibular v.

External carotid a.

Parotid gland

Sternocleidomastoid m.

Mastoid process

Digastric m.

Styloid process, with stylohyoid m. & stylopharyngeus m.

B

Figure 2-48 PAROTID GLAND. A, Lateral view. Superficial vessels and nerves of the face and scalp are shown in relation to the parotid gland and its duct. **B,** Horizontal section through the parotid gland. The parotid gland is shown in relation to the many nerves and vessels among which it lies. The facial nerve is the most superficial structure traversing the gland. SEE ATLAS, FIGS. 2-31, 2-32

there is an extension of glandular tissue along the proximal part of the duct. Viewed in horizontal section (Figure 2-48, *B*), the parotid gland is wedge shaped. Posterior to it lie the mastoid process and parts of the sternocleidomastoid and posterior belly of the digastric muscle. Anterior to it are the ramus of the mandible and its attached masseter and medial pterygoid muscles. Deep to it are the styloid process, internal jugular vein, and carotid artery. The posterior surface of the gland is molded to the cartilaginous portion of the external auditory meatus and the temporomandibular joint.

The parotid gland is also important for the three major structures that are found within its substance (Figure 2-48, *B*). Most superficial is the **facial nerve.**

After emerging from the stylomastoid foramen, the facial nerve enters the gland along its posterior surface. Traveling forward within the gland, it emerges from the anterior edge of the gland as two major trunks, which subsequently divide into the five major branches of the facial nerve—the *temporal, zygomatic, buccal, mandibular,* and *cervical.*

The superficial temporal and maxillary veins join to form the **retromandibular vein,** deeper within the gland. The vein emerges from the inferior border of the gland and joins posteriorly with the posterior auricular vein to form the *external jugular vein.* The retromandibular vein also provides an anterior, or communicating, branch to the *facial vein,* which runs at a level deeper than the retromandibular vein and eventually

---

CLINICAL ANATOMY OF

THE FACE

THE PAROTID GLAND

Mumps is a viral infection—inflammation of the parotid gland causing pain caused by swelling within the tight cervical fascial covering of the gland. Swallowing also causes pressure on the inflamed gland and subsequent pain. The parotid duct may become obstructed with stones (calculi) and cause painful swelling.

INNERVATION AND PHARYNGEAL ARCHES

The muscles of facial expression (along with other structures) are derived from the second pharyngeal arch and therefore share innervation by the major nerve of that arch (nerve VII).

CORNEAL LUBRICATION

Failure to properly *lubricate the cornea* leads to drying and eventual ulceration, with serious effects on vision. Thus the small branches of V1 (which innervate the cornea and stimulate blinking) are of tremendous functional importance. Remember that whenever a patient of yours is not able to blink normally (paralyzed during anesthesia for surgery, profoundly ill in the critical care unit, and so on), you must carry out this function for him/her (usually with lubricant drops applied periodically to the cornea), or permanent visual loss may result.

FACIAL NERVE INJURIES

Lesions to the terminal branches of the facial nerve produce loss of function to the muscles on that side—usually a drooping of the angles of the mouth, difficulty in blinking, loss of definition in the nasolabial fold, or weakness of the face as a whole. Lesions paralyzing the orbicularis oculi may lead to corneal ulceration (because the patient cannot maintain corneal lubrication). Inflammation of the facial nerve within the temporal bone leads to Bell's palsy, involving muscular paralysis and disturbance of taste mediated through the chorda tympani (special branch of nerve VII—see following section). The facial nerve is often injured in trauma to the side of the face or in malignant processes involving the parotid gland.

INJURIES TO THE SCALP

Scalp lacerations are common. Bleeding is profuse, because scalp arteries do not retract (that is, go into a spasm) as readily as do those in other areas of the body. Also, the simple number of arteries in the scalp is greater than in other areas. When scalp lacerations are sutured before complete cleansing of the wound, very serious abscesses may develop and spread readily to the brain. Hair transplants, when done improperly, can produce scalp infections. Newborns often have impressive swellings and distortion of their heads; these almost always resolve spontaneously. Two of the most common processes leading to this swelling are (1) cephalohematoma, which is subperiosteal bleeding in the frontal, parietal, temporal, or occipital bones and (2) caput succadaneum, which is a generalized swelling of the connective tissues of the scalp (not the skull bones) extending over part or all of the top of the head. Cephalohematomas, because they are subperiosteal, do not spread beyond the borders of the individual skull bone.

drains into the *internal jugular vein.* Located deepest within the parotid gland is the **external carotid artery.** It enters the gland on its inferior surface and, within the gland, divides into the *superficial temporal* and *maxillary arteries.* Both of these emerge from the anterosuperior surface of the gland and continue on to provide blood supply to the temporal fossa and scalp (superficial temporal artery) and the deep structures of the face and nose (maxillary artery). The parotid gland receives its blood supply largely from the external carotid and maxillary arteries, and its venous drainage is primarily to the retromandibular vein.

The secretory cells of the parotid gland are capable of secreting saliva autonomously, but in fact both sympathetic and parasympathetic nerves innervate the gland. *Postganglionic sympathetic axons* reach the gland by traveling on the plexus found on the external carotid artery and its several branches, as they reach the gland. The cell bodies of these neurons are in the **superior and middle cervical ganglia.** *Preganglionic sympathetic neurons* are found in the upper thoracic spinal cord and send their axons upward through the sympathetic chain to synapse in the superior and middle cervical ganglia. Sympathetic axons can influence secretion both directly and by means of increasing or decreasing the blood flow into the parotid gland.

Postganglionic parasympathetic axons originate in the **otic ganglion** (see Figure 2-57) and travel with the auriculotemporal branch of the mandibular nerve to reach the vicinity of the gland. The secretomotor parasympathetic axons here depart the auriculotemporal nerve and enter the substance of the parotid gland. The *preganglionic parasympathetic axons,* which synapse on the neurons in the otic ganglion, are part of the glossopharyngeal nerve and reach the ganglion in the **lesser petrosal nerve,** which emerges into the floor of the skull after a long and tortuous journey through the middle ear. The lesser petrosal nerve travels across the floor of the middle cranial fossa and turns inferiorly to enter the foramen ovale, where it encounters the otic ganglion.

Temporal and Infratemporal Fossae

▶ Temporal and Infratemporal Fossae

▶ Mandible

▶ Temporomandibular Joint (TMJ)

▶ Muscles of Mastication

▶ Maxillary Artery

▶ Mandibular Branch of the Trigeminal Nerve

▶ Otic Ganglion

▶ Pterygoid Venous Plexus

TEMPORAL AND INFRATEMPORAL FOSSAE

The **temporal fossa** (Figure 2-49) is the area lying immediately lateral and adjacent to the exterior surface of the squamous part of the temporal bone, above the plane of the zygoma. It is covered by the temporalis muscle and its overlying fascia, and the pterion lies deep to it. The **infratemporal fossa** (Figure 2-49) is the region inferior to the squamous part of the temporal bone. It lies between the lateral pterygoid plate and the ramus of the mandible, is bounded anteriorly by the maxilla and posteriorly by the styloid process, and is roofed by the greater wing of the sphenoid bone medially. Within the boundaries of this region lie the *muscles of mastication,* the major branches of the third division of the *trigeminal nerve* and the *maxillary artery.* The infratemporal fossa is directly connected to the interior of the nasal cavity and, by several small apertures, to the interior of the skull. Within this area, we also see the *otic ganglion* (see Figure 2-57), one of four cranial parasympathetic ganglia, and the *chorda tympani,* a small but important nerve that originates as part of nerve VII but distributes itself ultimately by joining branches of nerve V.

MANDIBLE

The mandible (Figure 2-50) consists of a horizontal **body,** which supports the lower teeth, and a pair of vertical platelike **rami,** oriented approximately in the sagittal plane. Where the ramus meets the body is found the angle of the mandible. The mandible changes shape markedly throughout life. As we become edentulous (toothless) in later life, the body of the mandible is partially reabsorbed, making it much thinner. Changes in the shape of the face result from this change in the mandible.

External Mandibular Surface

On the external surface of the body (Figure 2-50) are seen the *mental foramina* and, in the anterior midline, the *mental symphysis* (L., chin), representing the fusion of the two mandibular bodies. The *mental branch of V3* and accompanying vessels pass through the mental foramen. The symphysis represents the line of fusion for the two fetal mandibles. The *mental tubercle* is a raised prominence at the base of the mental symphysis and serves as a point of muscular attachment (see below). The external surface of the ramus is almost entirely covered by the attachment of the masseter muscle.

Internal Mandibular Surface

On the inner surface of the body of the mandible (Figure 2-50), there runs a horizontal *mylohyoid line,* to

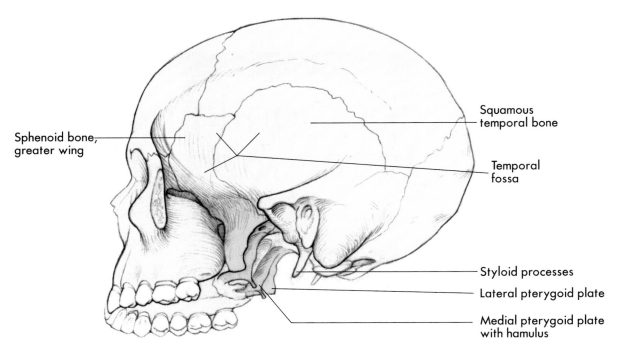

Figure 2-49   INFRATEMPORAL FOSSA. This fossa lies inferior to the squamous temporal bone, bounded superiorly by the zygoma.   SEE ATLAS, FIG. 2-52

which is attached the mylohyoid muscle. Above the mylohyoid line, there is a shallow depression for the *sublingual salivary gland* and below the line a deeper depression posteriorly for the *submandibular gland.* The *pterygomandibular raphe,* descending from the hamulus of the medial pterygoid plate, attaches to the posterior end of the mylohyoid line. At the anterior ends of the

mylohyoid lines and superior to them, near the symphysis, there is a group of prominences referred to collectively as the *genial tubercles.* Muscles attach here also (for example, the geniohyoid).

The inner surface of the *mandibular ramus* is roughened posteriorly, where the medial pterygoid muscle attaches, opposite the superficial attachment of the

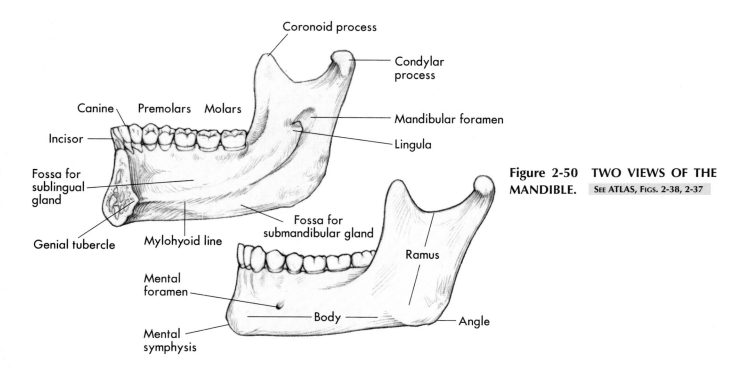

Figure 2-50   TWO VIEWS OF THE MANDIBLE.   SEE ATLAS, FIGS. 2-38, 2-37

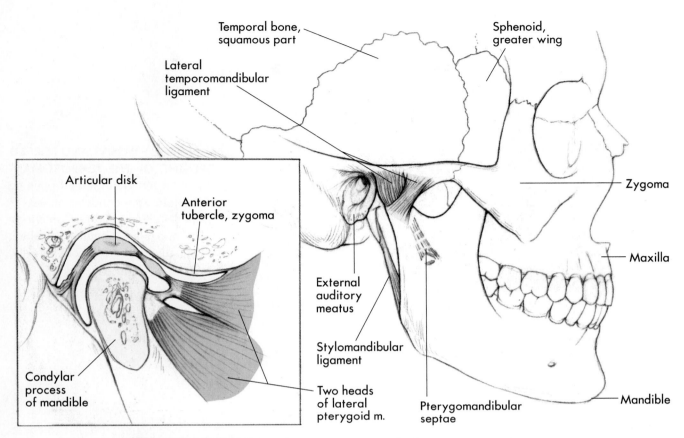

Figure 2-51 TEMPOROMANDIBULAR JOINT/INSET OF ARTICULAR DISK.

masseter. In the center of the internal surface of the ramus is the *mandibular foramen,* where the inferior alveolar vessels and nerve enter the interior of the mandible (see Figures 2-55 and 2-56). The *lingula,* a small bony spur, partially covers the medial aspect of the mandibular foramen. The *sphenomandibular ligament* (Figure 2-51) attaches to the lingula (and superiorly to the sphenoid spine). It passes just medial to the temporomandibular joint. The *stylomandibular ligament* (Figure 2-51) attaches to the posterior margin of the ramus (and superiorly to the styloid process). As it descends, it passes between the parotid from the submandibular glands.

Coronoid and Condylar Processes

The *coronoid process* (see Figure 2-50) is a triangular protruberance from the anterosuperior surface of the ramus. The temporalis muscle attaches here, predominantly on the deep surface. The *condylar process* arises from the posterosuperior aspect of the ramus. It consists of a neck and an expanded head, which articulates with the articular fossa of the temporal bone to form the **temporomandibular joint.** The condylar process is one of the important attachments for the lateral pterygoid muscle.

TEMPOROMANDIBULAR JOINT

The temporomandibular joint (TMJ) joins the mandible to the rigid skull (Figures 2-51 and 2-52). It consists of the head of the **condylar process** of the mandible and the articular fossa and adjacent **articular tubercle** of the temporal bone, plus an intervening fibrocartilaginous **articular disk.** Lying closest to the joint is its fibrous capsule, which surrounds the entire joint. The *lateral TMJ ligament* lies lateral to the joint capsule, which it reinforces, and is connected to the zygomatic arch above and to the neck of the condylar process of the mandible below. The *lateral pterygoid muscle* inserts on the lateral surface of the TMJ joint capsule, the articular disk, and the neck of the mandible. The other muscles of mastication do not serve to reinforce the TMJ. The *sphenomandibular ligament* passes just medial to the joint and may also reinforce it.

Articular Disk of the TMJ

The fibrous disk of the TMJ is ovoid (Figure 2-51), and concave on the side facing the condylar head of the mandible. From its circumference, a ligament attaches it to the inner surface of the fibrous capsule of the TMJ; it is also attached anteriorly to fibers of the lateral

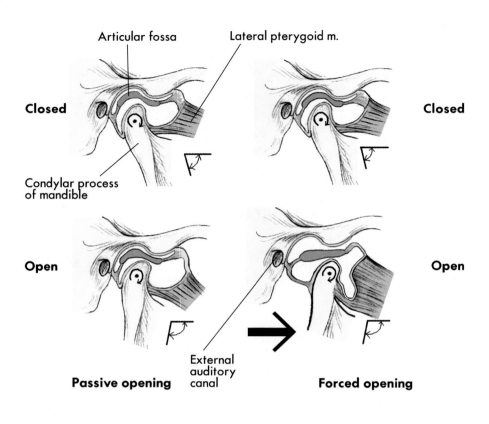

Closed

Articular fossa   Lateral pterygoid m.

Closed

Condylar process
of mandible

Open

Open

Passive opening

External
auditory
canal

Forced opening

Figure 2-52   PASSIVE AND FORCED OPENING OF THE TEMPOROMAN-DIBULAR JOINT. In forced opening of the joint, the condylar process is "pulled" much farther anteriorly than in passive opening, resulting principally from the effect of gravity.

pterygoid muscle. The presence of the articular disk divides the interior of the TMJ into two compartments, in a fashion similar to that found in the sternoclavicular joint.

Nerve Supply of the TMJ

The TMJ is innervated by branches of V3 and is the source of much pain for many who grind their teeth while asleep or have other malalignment conditions. Branches of the auriculotemporal nerve, as well as other direct branches of V3, innervate the joint.

Mechanisms of the TMJ

During the first stage of jaw opening, the condylar process slides forward (protraction) in the articular fossa and abuts the articular tubercle of the temporal bone (see Figure 2-52). As it does, the articular disk also moves forward, so that it remains interposed between the two. In the second stage the jaw opens further, because the mandible rotates around an imaginary axis passing near the lingula of the mandible, and the condylar process slides further forward on to the articular tubercle. The upper synovial cavity of the joint is a complex gliding joint, with the disk flexible enough to adopt to the concave surface of the articular fossa and the convex surface of the articular tubercle. The lower cavity permits rotation in depression or elevation of the mandible. It is possible for the condylar process and

disk to slide too far forward, beyond the articular tubercle, "locking" the jaw in an opened position.

The TMJ joint allows side-to-side sliding, depression/elevation, and protrusion/retraction. Grinding and sliding motions of the TMJ, essential for softening food, are accomplished when the muscles are contracted in an asymmetric fashion.

MUSCLES OF MASTICATION

Mastication (L. *mastic,* from the practice of chewing the resin of the Mediterranean mastic tree) is the formal term for the chewing of food. All of the muscles of mastication are innervated by the *mandibular nerve* (V3). The "official" muscles (Figure 2-53) of mastication (masseter [see Figure 2-44], temporalis, medial, and lateral pterygoid) are aided by others involved in the act of chewing (muscles of the tongue, buccinator, digastric muscles, and so on) (Table 2-9). Many of the motor axons in V3 are destined to innervate these muscles of mastication. The medial pterygoid muscle is innervated by a branch directly from V3, whereas the lateral pterygoid, masseter, and temporalis are innervated by branches of the anterior division of V3.

Special Actions of the Muscles of Mastication

Alternating action of the lateral and/or medial pterygoid muscle allows sliding of the mandible in the left-to-right plane, essential for chewing and grinding.

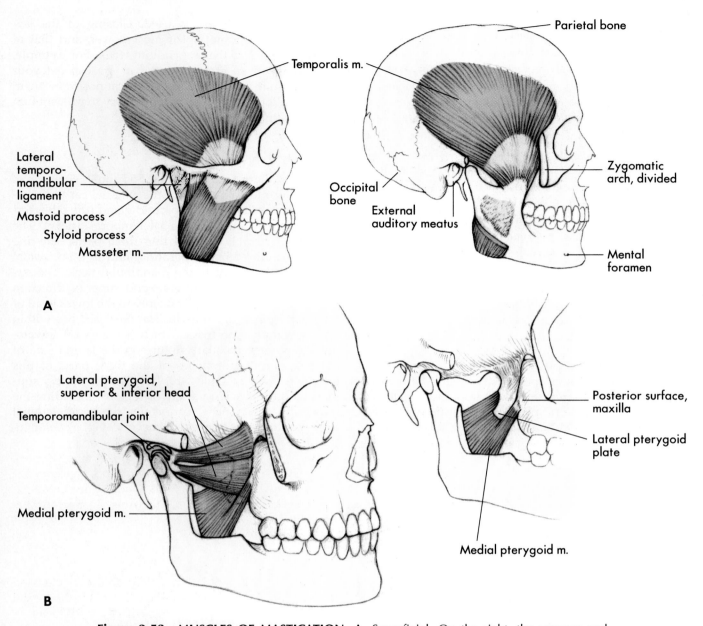

Figure 2-53 **MUSCLES OF MASTICATION. A,** Superficial. On the right, the zygoma and part of the masseter have been removed. **B,** Deep. On the left, the ramus and coronoid process of the mandible have been removed to better show the lateral and medial pterygoid muscles. On the right, the lateral pterygoid has been removed to reveal the attachment of the medial pterygoid to the medial surface of the lateral pterygoid plate. SEE ATLAS, FIGS. 2-36, 2-41

Table 2-9   The Muscles of Mastication

Muscle	Origin	Insertion	Actions
Masseter	Zygomatic arch	Lateral side of mandibular ramus	Elevates mandible; closes jaw
Temporalis	Temporal fascia in temporal fossa	Coronoid process; anteromedial border of mandible	Elevates mandible; retracts mandible (with different subsets of fibers)
Lateral pterygoid	Lateral pterygoid plate; base of sphenoid	Mandibular neck; articular capsule	Protrudes mandible; opens mouth
Medial pterygoid	Medial surface of lateral pterygoid plate; maxilla	Medial surface of angle of mandible	Elevates mandible; protrudes mandible

In man and other mammals, the mandible is the only mobile portion of the chewing apparatus. In other vertebrates, especially reptiles and some birds, both the mandibular and maxillary complexes are mobile, allowing such animals as snakes to open their mouths very wide to ingest their prey. In these animals the maxilla and its associated bones have articulations with the frontal bones. Interestingly, in an animal like a woodpecker, the maxilla and its associated bones are fused to the skull, in a manner similar to a mammal, presumably because the forceful blows the woodpecker strikes with his beak are made more efficiently when the maxilla and skull are a rigid unit.

The temporomandibular joint (TMJ) is the subject of a great deal of mechanical stress during chewing. Similar to joints in the hands, back, and other parts of the body, the TMJ is subject to inflammatory disease and may be the source of considerable pain.

Carnivores (for example, cats and dogs) do not have this ability as well developed as in humans, who share it with herbivorous animals. The temporalis muscle has fibers running in several planes and can retract or elevate the mandible and thus close the jaw, depending on which subset of fibers is used. Closing of the jaw (clenching) is the motion of most power, and that of forced opening of the jaw is quite weak. For example, in fighting off an attacking dog, if you can get your hands around his closed jaws, he cannot force them open; you'll fail, however, when you try to prevent him from closing his jaws on your hand!

MAXILLARY ARTERY

The maxillary artery (Figures 2-54 and 2-55) is one of the two terminal branches of the external carotid, arising in the substance of the parotid gland (the other terminal branch is the superficial temporal artery). The maxillary artery is divided into three parts. The *first part* runs initially in the parotid gland in a horizontal plane and then deep to the mandibular neck. The *second part* courses in an anterior and superior direction and may lie superficially or deeply to the lower head of the lateral pterygoid muscle. The *third part* lies within the pterygopalatine fossa, which it enters by traversing the pterygomaxillary fissure on the lateral side of the face. Various branches of the three parts of this artery are listed in Table 2-10. The maxillary artery supplies blood to a wide variety of regions, including the upper jaw, palate, nose, dura mater, the middle cranial fossa, and muscles of mastication.

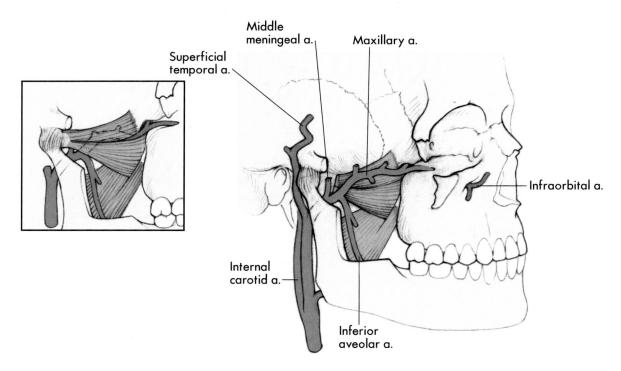

Figure 2-54   BRANCHES AND COURSE OF THE MAXILLARY ARTERY. The *inset* shows a common variant in the course of the maxillary artery, where it passes between the two heads of the lateral pterygoid muscle, not superficial to them.

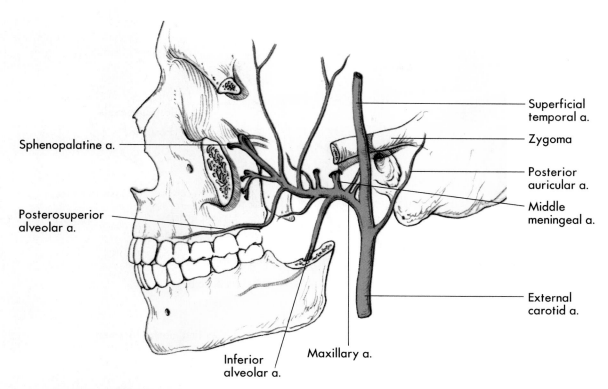

Figure 2-55   BRANCHES OF MAXILLARY ARTERY. Branches of this artery supply the area near the ear, temporal fossa, nose, infratemporal fossa, and the maxilla and the mandible.
SEE ATLAS, FIG. 2-42

MANDIBULAR BRANCH OF THE TRIGEMINAL NERVE (V3)

The **mandibular nerve** component of the trigeminal nerve originates from the trigeminal ganglion, just lateral to the pons. Consisting of a larger sensory branch and the smaller motor branch, the mandibular nerve (V3) separates from the parent trigeminal nerve distal to the trigeminal ganglion and exits the skull at the foramen ovale (Figures 2-56 and 2-57; see also Figure 2-41).

After traversing the foramen ovale (accompanied by the lesser petrosal nerve and often the accessory mid-dle meningeal artery), the mandibular nerve enters the upper infratemporal fossa, passing between the lateral pterygoid muscle and the tensor palatini. Before branching into its major anterior and posterior trunk (Table 2-11), the "undivided trunk" of the mandibular nerve gives off the *nerve to medial pterygoid* (which runs through the otic ganglion), *meningeal nerve,* and *nerves to tensor palatini* and *tensor tympani* (the nerve to medial pterygoid may give rise to the nerves supplying the tensor muscles). The meningeal nerve reenters the skull through the foramen spinosum, along with the middle meningeal artery.

The *anterior* and *posterior trunks* then separate and give rise to the branches, as indicated in Table 2-11. The anterior trunk is predominantly motor, distributing axons to the muscles of mastication and other nearby muscles (see Table 2-11). It has a single important sensory branch, the buccal nerve. The posterior branch is almost entirely sensory. The mandibular nerve carries all of the motor axons of the trigeminal nerve; the ophthalmic (V1) and maxillary (V2) divisions are entirely sensory.

OTIC GANGLION

The otic ganglion (Figure 2-57) is the one of the four *parasympathetic ganglia* found in the head and neck re-

Table 2-10   Branches of the Maxillary Artery

Behind Mandible (First Part)	Infratemporal (Second Part)	Distal Branches (Third Part)
Deep auricular	Deep temporal*	Sphenopalatine*
Anterior tympanic	Pterygoid	Posterosuperior alveolar*
Middle meningeal*	Masseteric	Palatine*
Inferior alveolar*	Artery to pterygoid canal*	Infraorbital*

*Branches of most importance.

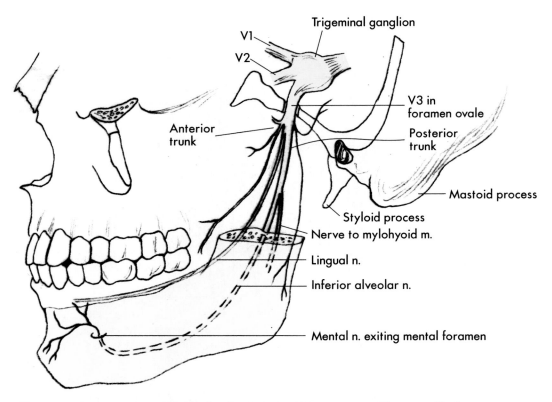

Figure 2-56   DETAILED DIAGRAM OF MANDIBULAR NERVE. The mandibular nerve traverses the foramen ovale and divides into an anterior trunk (mostly motor branches) and a posterior trunk (nearly all sensory branches). Several posterior trunk branches are shown here.   SEE ATLAS, FIGS. 2-42, 2-43, 2-44

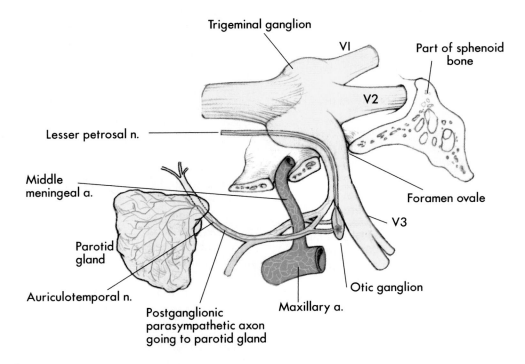

Figure 2-57   CONNECTIONS AND RELATIONS OF THE OTIC GANGLION. Postganglionic axons arising in the otic ganglion travel with the auriculotemporal nerve to innervate the parotid gland.

Table 2-11 Branches of the Mandibular Nerve

Anterior Trunk (most of motor root here and sensory also)	Posterior Trunk (mostly sensory, few motor)
Nerve to lateral pterygoid (muscular)	Lingual nerve (sensory)*
Buccal nerve (sensory)	Inferior alveolar nerve (sensory)†
Masseteric nerve (muscular)	Auriculotemporal nerve (sensory)‡
Deep temporal nerves (muscular)	

*Joined by chorda tympani, after which it contains special sensory and secretomotor axons.
†Contains motor axons of the nerve to mylohyoid, which depart the inferior alveolar nerve before it enters the mandible.
‡The auriculotemporal nerve may arise before the anterior and posterior trunks separate.

gion (the others are the *ciliary, submandibular,* and *pterygopalatine ganglia*). It lies deep to the undivided trunk of V3, after it traverses the foramen ovale. For each, there are preganglionic axons (traveling on various branches of cranial nerve III, VII, or IX), which will synapse in the appropriate parasympathetic ganglion. From each

of these ganglia, there then emerge postganglionic axons, which distribute to their target glands or muscle by traveling with various branches of the trigeminal nerve.

The otic ganglion receives its **preganglionic axons** from cranial nerve IX *(the glossopharyngeal nerve).* These preganglionic axons penetrate the floor of the middle ear cavity and enter it as part of the *tympanic nerve.* Most of this nerve is sensory (to the middle ear, mastoid air cells, and auditory tube) and distributes many branches within those areas. The preganglionic parasympathetic motor axons in the tympanic nerve do not distribute within the middle ear, however, but leave the middle ear cavity thorough its roof and are known thereafter as the *lesser petrosal nerve.* As it passes through the roof of the middle ear cavity, the lesser petrosal nerve "grazes" the geniculate ganglion of the nerve VII and appears grossly to be a branch of it, but in fact it and the geniculate ganglion are related only by their proximity to each other. After emerging onto the superior surface of the petrous ridge, the lesser petrosal nerve travels anteromedially to enter the foramen ovale and synapses below it to the otic ganglion.

From neurons in the otic ganglion, there arise **postganglionic axons** that join and travel with the *auriculotemporal nerve,* a branch of the posterior division of V3. The auriculotemporal nerve usually (but not al-

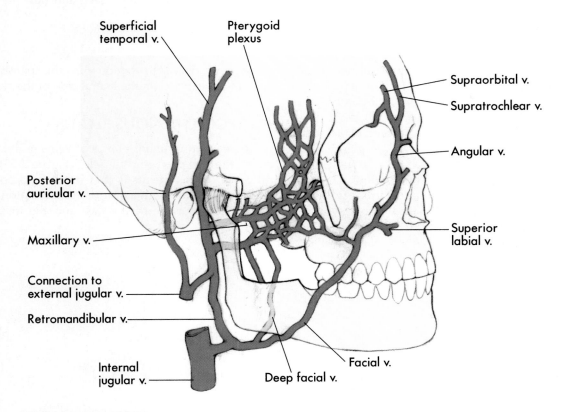

Figure 2-58 PTERYGOID VENOUS PLEXUS. This plexus lies between the pterygoid muscles and connects both to superficial and deep groups of veins in the face and inside the cranial vault.

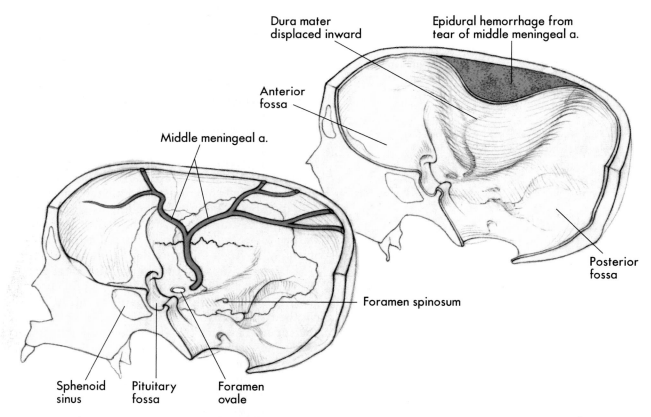

Figure 2-59 MIDDLE MENINGEAL ARTERY AND AN EPIDURAL HEMATOMA. Arterial bleeding from the middle meningeal artery can dissect a wide epidural space and put pressure on the brain, leading rapidly to unconsciousness and death.

ways) forms an encirclement of the middle meningeal artery as the vessel heads toward the foramen spinosum to enter the cranium. As the nerve passes near the parotid gland, the postganglionic axons depart the auriculotemporal nerve, enter the parotid gland, and synapse on myoepithelial cells within the gland. This innervation regulates parotid salivation, though it is not essential for the parotid to be operational. The otic ganglion is also traversed by *sympathetic axons* from the plexus on the maxillary artery. These will not synapse in the ganglion but will distribute with the auriculotemporal nerve to regions in the parotid gland, around the ear and on the lateral side of the skull.

PTERYGOID VENOUS PLEXUS

There is a prominent plexus of veins in the plane between the two pterygoid muscles (Figure 2-58). The significance of this plexus is that it can be a conduit for vascular spread of infection or inflammation between the external surface of the face and the inside of the skull.

THE TEMPORAL AND INFRATEMPORAL REGIONS

DISLOCATION OF THE TMJ

Dislocation of the TMJ is always anterior, as the condylar process slides forward too far past the articular tubercle and cannot return to the articular fossa. It must be depressed before it can be replaced.

JAW MOVEMENTS

Unilateral injury to V3 will produce asymmetric protrusion of the jaw, and this fact may be used in clinical testing for nerve injury.

VASCULAR HEADACHES

Migraine headaches are poorly understood abnormalities of vascular smooth muscle tone (probably vasodilation), the pain of which is transmitted through axons of V3, particularly the auriculotemporal nerve.

LOCAL ANESTHESIA

Local anesthesia of lower jaw structures may be accomplished by infusion of anesthetic around the inferior alveolar nerve just before it enters the mandible (safe in experienced hands) or infusion of local anesthetic around V3 as it emerges from the foramen ovale (difficult, more risky).

SKULL FRACTURES

The middle meningeal artery, arising in the infratemporal fossa, is often injured in trauma involving the lateral surface of the skull. The resultant epidural arterial hemorrhage may accumulate and cause great injury to the brain (Figure 2-59). Rapid surgical removal of the blood and clot is often necessary.

FRACTURES OF THE MANDIBLE

The mandible is frequently fractured. As a result of such trauma, the TMJ may also be disrupted. Displacement of bony fragments often necessitates "wiring" of the mandible, to stabilize it during healing. Fractures in children may disrupt the arrangement of tooth primordia, which lie deep within the mandible.

DEVELOPMENTAL CHANGES OF THE MANDIBLE

At birth, the mandible is not yet joined at the chin. By the second year, the formation of the mental symphysis is usually complete. In the first two decades of life, the angle between the body and neck of the mandible is less acute than it is in later life. In old age, most teeth of the mandible are lost, the body of the mandible becomes much thinner, and the angle between neck and body once again becomes more oblique.

2.7

Posterior Triangle of the Neck

▶ Organization of the Neck

▶ Cervical Fasciae

▶ Neck Triangles

▶ Scalenus Anterior Muscle

▶ Nerve Supply to the Neck

▶ Divisions of the Subclavian Artery

▶ Venous Drainage of the Posterior Triangle

▶ Root of the Neck

▶ Suprapleural Membrane

ORGANIZATION OF THE NECK

The neck is a transitional zone, joining the head to the trunk and upper limb. Its skeletal axis is the column of **seven cervical vertebrae,** placed posteriorly. It has a posterior mass of striated musculature, innervated by posterior or dorsal primary rami, and anterolateral striated musculature, innervated by anterior or ventral primary rami. Many of these anterolateral muscles can be considered analogs to the more familiar muscles of the chest and abdominal wall. A thin sheet of muscle, **platysma,** is located in the superficial fascial space of the neck (Figure 2-60). It sweeps from the lower margin of the mandible inferiorly over the clavicle, and its contraction leads to tightening of the skin of the neck. In the center of the neck are two important tubes—one a part of the digestive system, positioned more posteriorly (the **esophagus**) and the second a part of the respiratory system, positioned more anteriorly (the **trachea**). Lying to either side of these midline viscera is a group of important **carotid/jugular blood vessels,** some of which convey blood to the head region and others that return it to the thorax. Most of the very important **brachial plexus** branches first appear in the neck and move inferolaterally to enter the axilla and continue into the upper limb. The neck contains some unique and important glands—such as the **thyroid, parathyroid,** and **thymus glands**—and many **lymph nodes.**

CERVICAL FASCIAE

Structures in the neck are compartmentalized by discontinuous, concentric layers of fascia. These are defined broadly as the **superficial fascia** and the **deep fascia,** with several separate sublayers, as listed in Table 2-12 and shown in Figure 2-60. The fascial anatomy of the neck can determine the direction in which infection in the neck may spread. In particular, such infections often spread laterally, rather than toward the anterior surface of the neck (where their presence will be evident earlier to the clinician and the patient herself/himself).

NECK TRIANGLES

The triangles of the neck are defined by anatomists and physicians and serve the purpose of dividing this complex region into smaller subcompartments, helping us to comprehend more easily the multiple structures and functions of the neck. The sternocleidomastoid muscle is the key structure, sweeping from posterosuperior to anteroinferior. It divides the neck into a large **posterior triangle** and **anterior triangle.** The posterior triangle is further subdivided by the omohyoid muscle into a **subclavian** and **occipital triangle.** The anterior triangle is subdivided by three structures—another part of the omohyoid muscle, the hyoid bone, and the digastric muscle—into a **submandibular, carotid, submental,** and **muscular triangle** (Figure 2-61).

Table 2-12 The Cervical Fasciae

Fascial Layer	Position	Attachments	Structures Enclosed
SUPERFICIAL FASCIA			
Superficial fascia has no sublayers	In superficial tissue	Attached to platysma; bound mainly to deep fascia and dermis	Platysma; elsewhere, the fascia is scarcely visible
DEEP FASCIA			
Investing layer of fascia	Forms superficial layer of deep fascia	From cervical spines and ligamentum nuchae to midline of neck anteriorly; superiorly, to mandible, mastoid, and nuchal line; inferiorly, to sternum and clavicles	Dorsal paravertebral muscles, trapezius, sternocleidomastoid, submandibular gland; superiorly, extensions of this fascia form the parotid sheath and attach firmly to the zygomatic arch, superior to parotid gland
			Thickened extension forms stylomandibular ligament
Middle cervical fascia	Deep to the investing layer	Hyoid bone, clavicle, and sternum; also to carotid sheath	Infrahyoid muscles, by individual septae; forms pulley for omohyoid
Pretracheal fascia	Deep to investing layer, in anterior part of neck	To deep surface of investing fascia	Pharynx, larynx, esophagus, trachea, thyroid, and parathyroids
Carotid sheath(s)	Paired, in anterolateral neck	Just deep to investing fascia	Common and internal carotid arteries, internal jugular vein, vagus nerve; ansa cervicalis embedded in sheath
Prevertebral fascia	Forms fascial floor for posterior triangle; extends outwardly as axillary sheath	Cervical spines, anterior fascia of trapezius; forms thick anterior sheath across prevertebral muscles	Scalene muscles, levator scapulae, anterior neck muscles

This chapter focuses on the posterior triangle; see Chapter 2.8 for a discussion of the anterior neck.

The posterior triangle, with its apex pointed superiorly, is bounded by the sternocleidomastoid (SCM), trapezius, and the middle third of the clavicle (Figure 2-61). The trunks of the brachial plexus, accessory nerve, phrenic nerve, and several branches of the subclavian artery cross the posterior triangle. The inferior belly of the omohyoid muscle crosses the posterior triangle and subdivides it into the **occipital** and **subclavian triangles.**

The "floor" of the posterior triangle is formed by the muscles shown in Table 2-13. The investing fascial layer of the neck spans the interval between the posterior border of the sternocleidomastoid muscle and the anterior border of the trapezius muscle, creating a tough fascial layer that covers over the structures contained within the triangle. Among the important structures lying within the posterior triangle are the trunks of the brachial plexus, the phrenic nerve, the accessory nerve, lymph nodes, and several branches of the subclavian artery.

SCALENUS ANTERIOR MUSCLE

The scalenus anterior muscle (Figure 2-62) attaches inferiorly to a tubercle on the first rib and superiorly to the transverse processes of cervical vertebrae C3 to C6. Just above the first rib, it is crossed anteriorly by the subclavian vein, and just posterior to the scalenus anterior is the subclavian artery (see above). The scalenus anterior is one of many *accessory muscles of respiration.* It can serve this purpose because it can elevate the ribcage (by exerting upward pull on the first rib). Other muscles with similar capabilities (for example, sternocleidomastoid) also qualify as accessory respiratory muscles and may become important for breathing when the major respiratory muscles (diaphragm, intercostal muscles, and so on) are not functioning properly.

NERVE SUPPLY TO THE NECK
Brachial Plexus in the Neck

The *roots of the brachial plexus* emerge into the neck between the middle and anterior scalene muscles (see

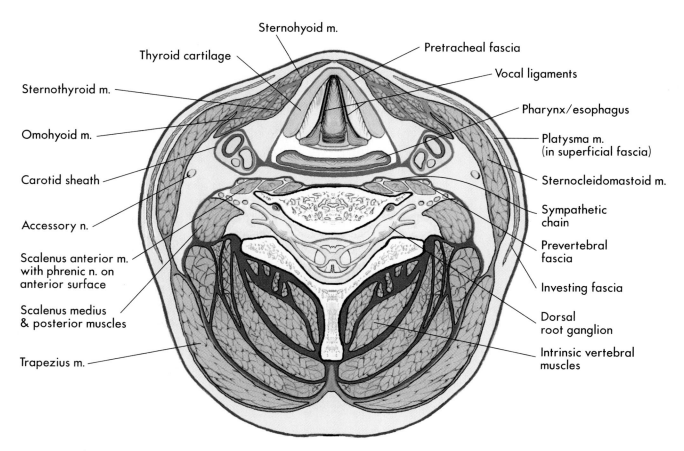

Figure 2-60   CROSS-SECTION OF NECK, WITH FASCIAL LAYERS. The neck may be considered to consist of several fascial compartments, enclosed by the superficial, investigating, pretracheal, and the prevertebral fascia and carotid sheath. These fascial spaces can determine the spread of infection or hemorrhage in the neck.   **SEE ATLAS, FIG. 2-5**

Figure 2-62 and Chapter 2.3). The plexus then passes between the first rib and the clavicle, gaining entrance to the axilla. Within the posterior triangle, the roots recombine to form the *superior, middle, and inferior trunks,* and then each trunk divides into an *anterior and posterior division.* As they leave the posterior triangle and enter the axilla, the anterior and posterior divisions unite to form the *lateral, posterior, and medial cords of the brachial plexus.*

Phrenic Nerve

The phrenic nerve arises from spinal cord levels C3 to C5 (predominantly C4) and travels inferiorly on the anterior surface of the anterior scalene muscle to reach the thorax (see Figure 2-63). It is crossed anteriorly by the transverse cervical and suprascapular arteries. It passes inferiorly into the chest by traveling between the subclavian artery and vein.

Cervical Plexus

The cervical plexus is a set of **cutaneous branches** (Figure 2-63) of the anterior primary rami of C1 to C4. The *muscular branches* of the cervical plexus innervate muscles and deeper structures in the neck and compose the *ansa cervicalis* (see Figure 2-32; see section on carotid triangle). The cervical plexus emerges along the posterior border of the sternocleidomastoid (SCM) at its midpoint and breaks up into several branches—the *supraclavicular, lesser occipital, great auricular,* and *transverse cervical nerves.*

Spinal Accessory Nerve

The spinal accessory nerve (cranial nerve XI) emerges from the posterior border of sternocleidomastoid (which it innervates) and travels posteriorly across the posterior triangle to innervate trapezius (Figure

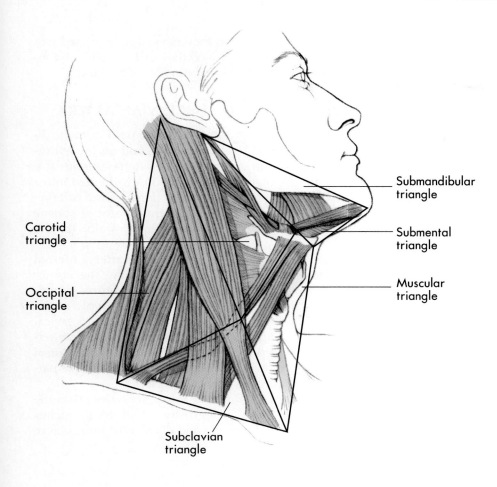

Carotid
triangle

Occipital
triangle

Submandibular
triangle

Submental
triangle

Muscular
triangle

Subclavian
triangle

Figure 2-61 SCHEMATIC OF NECK TRIANGLES, SHOWING BORDERS AND FLOOR. The posterior triangle of the neck includes the occipital and subclavian triangles; the anterior triangle includes the carotid, muscular, submental, and submandibular triangles.

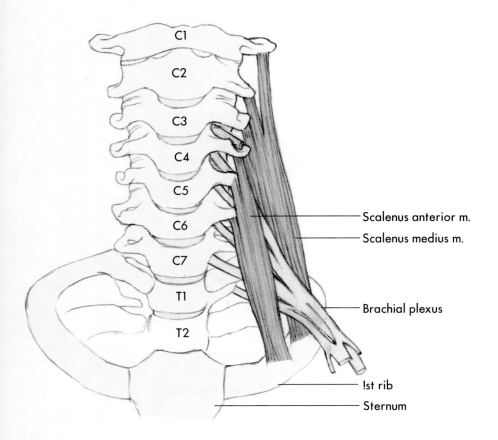

C1

C2

C3

C4

C5

C6

C7

T1

T2

Scalenus anterior m.

Scalenus medius m.

Brachial plexus

!st rib

Sternum

Figure 2-62 SCALENE MUSCLES. The scalene muscles attach the transverse processes of cervical vertebrae to the first and second ribs. They serve as stabilizers of the neck and even as accessory respiratory muscles. The roots of the brachial plexus and the subclavian artery emerge between the anterior and middle scalene muscles.

Table 2-13   The Floor of the Posterior Triangle

Muscle	Attachments
Splenius capitis	Mastoid process to spines of C5-T1
Levator scapulae	Transverse processes C1-C4 to superior angle of scapula
Scalenus posterior	Transverse processes C5-C7 to rib 2
Scalenus medius	Transverse processes C5-C7 to rib 1
Scalenus anterior	Transverse processes C4-C6 to rib 1

2-63). The *spinal root* of the accessory nerve is that part which originates from the upper three to five cervical spinal cord segment neurons. Axons from these neurons travel superiorly along the lateral side of the spinal cord and enter the cranium through the foramen magnum. They leave the skull once again via the jugular foramen, where we recognize them as the spinal accessory nerve. Function is tested by shoulder shrug (trapezius) or head turning (sternocleidomastoid). Within the skull, the cranial root of the accessory nerve joins the spinal root briefly, forming the complete accessory nerve. Sensory axons for these muscles reach the spinal cord through the cervical plexus. Cranial root axons

quickly leave the spinal root axons, however, and join the vagus nerve, with which they exit the skull and innervate many of the striated muscles of the larynx.

DIVISIONS OF THE SUBCLAVIAN ARTERY

The subclavian artery arises on the right from the division of the brachiocephalic artery and on the left directly from the aorta. It travels deep to the anterior scalene, and—by that muscle's position—is divided into a *first part* (medial to the anterior scalene), *second part* (behind it), and *third part* (from lateral border of scalene muscle to the lateral border of the first rib) (Figure 2-64).

From the *first part* arise the **vertebral artery, internal thoracic artery,** and **thyrocervical trunk.** The *inferior thyroid branch* of the thyrocervical trunk courses superiorly into the neck as the major arterial supply of the thyroid gland. The other branches of the thyrocervical trunk are the *suprascapular artery* and the *superficial cervical artery* (but see the following section on the dorsal scapular artery for a discussion of variations in the pattern of the superficial cervical artery).

From the *second part of the subclavian artery* arises the **costocervical trunk.** The costocervical trunk arches posteriorly over the pleura and apex of the lung, before

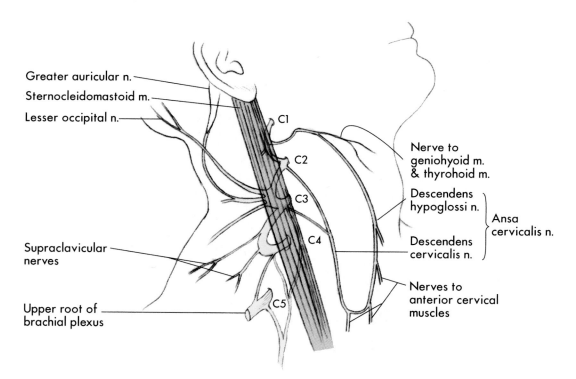

Figure 2-63 SCHEMATIC OF CERVICAL PLEXUS. The anterior branches of the cervical plexus comprise the ansa cervicalis, providing muscle innervation of the anterior neck muscles. The posterior branches of the plexus provide cutaneous innervation to the anterolateral neck and clavicular area.

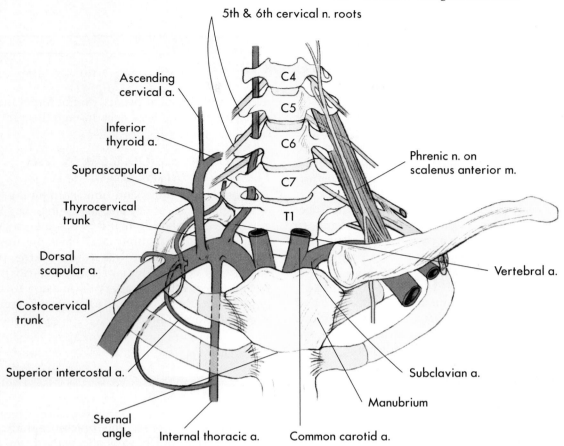

Figure 2-64 BRANCHES OF THE SUBCLAVIAN ARTERY. Branches of this important vessel distribute widely, to the brainstem and spinal cord, neck, upper limb, chest wall, and diaphragm.

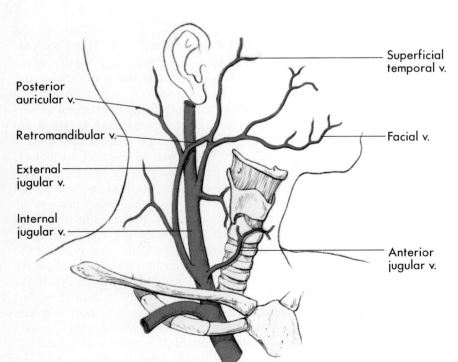

Figure 2-65 VENOUS DRAINAGE OF THE POSTERIOR TRIANGLE OF THE NECK.

THE POSTERIOR TRIANGLE

VULNERABLE STRUCTURES IN THE POSTERIOR TRIANGLE

The accessory nerve is one of the more vulnerable structures during any surgery involving the posterior triangle. Careful isolation and protection of this structure during surgery is essential. One should never forget that the apex of the lung protrudes above the clavicle into the base of the posterior triangle. When needles are being inserted into this area, in an attempt to get a blood sample or place a catheter, the pleura and lung may be injured and a pneumothorax produced.

INJURIES TO THE BRACHIAL PLEXUS

Traumatic injury to this area may produce lethal hemorrhage from the subclavian artery or do serious harm to the roots of the brachial plexus. When a patient is complaining of symptoms indicating a nerve injury to the brachial plexus, do not forget that the lesion may be in the neck even though the pain is in the hand.

COLLATERAL BLOOD FLOW IN THE POSTERIOR TRIANGLE

Though you will spend time learning the branches of the subclavian artery and the course they follow, it is worth remembering that it is possible to tie off the subclavian artery entirely and have the upper limb suffer no injury (this was formerly the preferred surgery for certain kinds of congenital heart lesions, where the subclavian artery is anastomosed to the pulmonary artery). There is a lot of collateral circulation for the upper limb.

---

dividing into the *deep cervical* and the *superior intercostal arteries.* The first two intercostal arteries arise from the superior intercostal (the others arise from the aorta).

The *dorsal scapular artery* arises from the **third part of the subclavian artery.** It passes laterally through the brachial plexus and accompanies the dorsal scapular nerve along the medial border of the scapula, on the deep surface of the rhomboid muscles. Occasionally, the dorsal scapular artery arises from the second part of the subclavian artery, and in still other cases it is absent altogether. When the dorsal scapular artery is absent, the thyrocervical trunk lacks its normal superficial cervical artery and instead gives rise to a *transverse cervical artery.* The deep branch of this transverse cervical artery then supplies structures normally supplied by the dorsal scapular artery. Conversely, when the dorsal scapular artery is present, there is no transverse cervical artery (there is, however, in such cases, the normal superficial cervical branch of the thyrocervical trunk). In any event, the dorsal scapular/deep branch of transverse cervical travels in front of the scalenus medius across the posterior triangle and then descends on the back deeply to the rhomboid muscles (along with the dorsal scapular nerve).

VENOUS DRAINAGE OF THE POSTERIOR TRIANGLE

The **internal jugular** and **subclavian veins** converge and meet in the base of the posterior triangle, where they are joined by the **external jugular vein** (Figure 2-65). From this arises the **brachiocephalic vein** on each side. The brachiocephalic veins from each side unite slightly to the right of the midline, posterior to the sternoclavicular joint on that side, to form the **superior vena cava.**

ROOT OF THE NECK

Boundaries of the root of the neck are (1) the manubrium of the sternum anteriorly, (2) the body of the first thoracic vertebra posteriorly, and (3) the curvature of the first ribs, connecting the manubrium and vertebral body (see Figure 2-64).

The root of the neck is the passage for several important vessels, nerves, and other structures between the neck and the thorax and the neck and the upper limb. There is asymmetry in the root of the neck in that (1) *the major arteries* are represented by the brachiocephalic on the right and by the common carotid and subclavian on the left, (2) the level at which the *vagus nerve* gives off the recurrent branch is unequal on the two sides (passing beneath the junction of the subclavian and common carotid arteries on the right, and beneath the ligamentum arteriosum, deep in the chest, on the left), and (3) *major venous drainage* from both upper limbs and both sides of the neck is directed to the right-sided superior vena cava. In embryologic life, there is a left-sided superior vena cava, which occasionally persists in the fully developed infant. It is just one of a great variety of embryologic veins near the heart, most of which normally disappear before birth.

SUPRAPLEURAL MEMBRANE

A suprapleural membrane, attaching to the medial border of the first rib, effectively separates the thoracic cavity from the neck and forms a floor to the root of the neck. The **dome** or **cupola of the lung** and its covering pleural membrane extend upward into a space limited superiorly by this membrane. This space is well above the plane of the clavicle. Those performing surgical procedures in the root of the neck must always be aware that they may inadvertently enter the pleural cavity and cause a pneumo- or hemothorax.

2.8

Anterolateral Neck

▶ Carotid Triangle

▶ Muscular Triangle

▶ Submandibular Triangle

▶ Submental Triangle

For descriptive purposes, the neck is divided into several triangles, the boundaries of which are formed by several important muscles (see Figure 2-61). In this chapter, we discuss the anterior triangle; for a discussion of the posterior triangle, see Chapter 2.7.

CAROTID TRIANGLE

This triangle is bounded by the sternocleidomastoid, posterior belly of digastric, and superior belly of omohyoid. The latter two muscles are joined at the hyoid bone, and the sternocleidomastoid and posterior belly of digastric approach each other posteriorly in the vicinity of the mastoid process (see Figure 2-61).

The floor of the carotid triangle is composed of parts of the middle and inferior constrictors, the thyrohyoid muscle, and part of the longus capitis muscle of the deep anterior neck. The important structures of the carotid triangle are positioned on the external surface of this muscular floor of the carotid triangle.

The contents of the carotid triangle include the ansa cervicalis, common carotid artery and its bifurcation into the internal and external carotid arteries, branches of the external carotid, internal jugular vein, vagus nerve, superior cervical sympathetic ganglion, and sympathetic trunk.

Carotid Arteries

The *common carotid arteries*, as well and the *internal jugular vein* and the *vagus nerve*, are enclosed within the **carotid sheath** (Figures 2-66 and 2-67). This fascial envelope, an extension of the deep cervical fascia, extends from the apex of the thorax to the base of the skull

(Figure 2-66). Though the common carotid artery is enclosed in the carotid sheath and the internal carotid artery remains within it as it travels upward to the base of the skull, the *external carotid artery* leaves the sheath when the common carotid artery bifurcates at vertebral level ~C4.

The common carotid artery arises on the right as a branch of the *brachiocephalic (innominate) artery* and on the left as a direct branch of the *aortic arch* (subject to some variation, as always). The internal carotid artery has no branches in the neck, whereas the external carotid gives off a number of important branches in the neck (see following).

Special Sensory Structures in the Carotid Arteries

The *carotid sinus* (a baroreceptor sensing blood pressure) and the *carotid body* (a chemoreceptor sensing acid-base status in the blood) lie at the bifurcation of the common carotid artery (Figure 2-68). Both are innervated by the glossopharyngeal nerve.

The **carotid sinus** is an important part of the autoregulation of blood flow to the brain—keeping blood flow near constant despite changes in head position, gravitational forces, and so on. It consists of a dilation in the wall of the carotid at its bifurcation. In its wall are specialized cells that presumably are responsive to pressure within the lumen of the vessel. Carotid sinus massage (rubbing or applying pressure to the anterior neck over the carotid bifurcation) stimulates nerves innervating the carotid sinus and results in a slowing of the heart rate. This technique is often used as part of an attempt to slow excessively rapid heart rates.

The **carotid body** consists of a specialized set of chemoreceptive cells in the wall of the carotid bifurca-

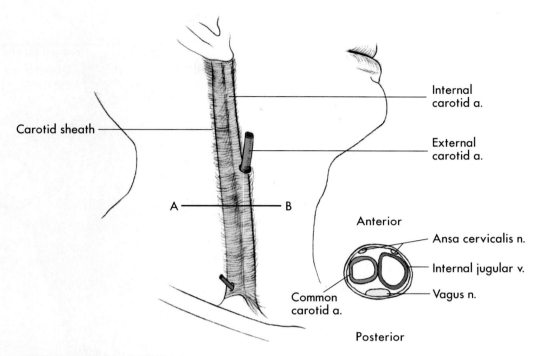

Figure 2-66   CAROTID SHEATH AND CONTENTS. The ansa cervicalis and vagus nerve are embedded in the wall of the carotid sheath, and the internal jugular vein and common carotid/internal carotid artery are contained within. The external carotid artery leaves the interior of the carotid sheath as it separates from the common carotid artery. *Line A-B* represents the level of cross-section shown in the *inset.*

tion. When the blood pH level becomes too acidic, the carotid body senses this and the brain responds by accelerating the rate of respiration, which reduces the amount of CO_2 in the blood and raises the blood pH level. The response of the carotid body to the blood pH level also includes a reduction of blood flow into the inside of the skull. This effect is used in the treatment of head injury, where hyperventilation (that is, low P_{CO_2}

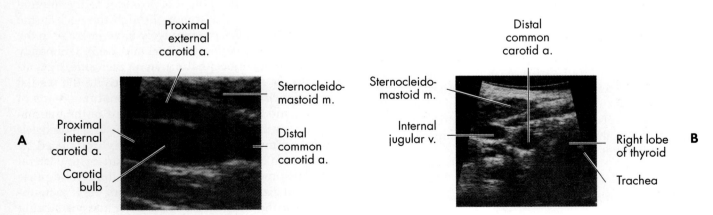

Figure 2-67   ULTRASOUND IMAGES OF THE CAROTID BIFURCATION. A, Longitudinal section. **B,** Transverse section. These techniques make noninvasive early diagnosis of arterial obstruction or the growth of tumors possible. (From Weir J, Abrahams PH: *An imaging atlas of human anatomy,* London, 1992, Mosby.)

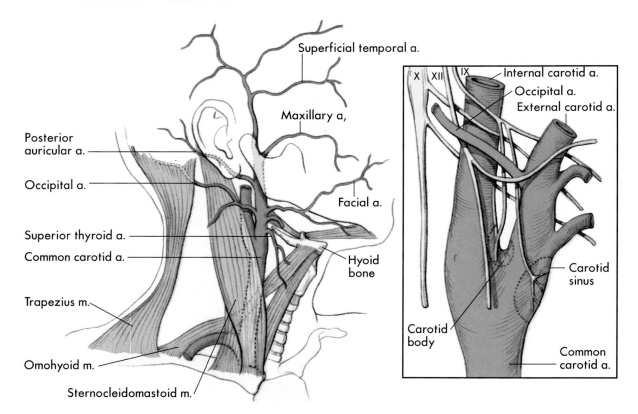

Figure 2-68   BRANCHES OF THE EXTERNAL CAROTID ARTERY. *Inset* shows detailed grouping of the nerves and vessels found in the vicinity of the common carotid artery bifurcation.   SEE ATLAS, FIGS. 2-6, 2-8, 2-18

level and subsequent higher blood pH level) reduces flow of blood to the brain and minimizes edema. The carotid body occasionally becomes neoplastic.

Internal Carotid Artery

Each internal carotid artery (Figure 2-68) separates from the parent common carotid artery at the upper border of the thyroid cartilage, opposite the disk between the C3 and C4 vertebrae. As the internal carotid artery ascends toward the base of the skull, it lies anterior to the upper three cervical transverse processes and lateral to the pharyngeal wall. The superior cervical ganglion lies directly posterior to it.

External Carotid Artery and its Branches

The external carotid and its branches (Table 2-14) supply most of the scalp, anterior and lateral face, oral and nasal cavities, and much of the neck (see Figures 2-46 and 2-68). Some of its terminal branches anastomose with similar terminal branches of the internal carotid system, especially those that supply the nose and the orbital region.

Internal Jugular Vein

The internal jugular vein (IJ) commences just distally to the **jugular bulb,** a dilated sac positioned in the jugular foramen of the floor of the skull. On emergence from the base of the skull, it is posterior to the internal carotid artery. As it descends through the neck in the carotid sheath, it lies progressively more laterally to the carotid arteries (see Figures 2-60 and 2-65). Ultimately it forms the **brachiocephalic vein** on each side, by uniting with the subclavian vein posteriorly to the medial end of the clavicle. It drains blood from brain, parts of the face, and the neck. The inferior part of the internal jugular vein is covered by the digastric and sternocleidomastoid muscles. The IJ is frequently cannulated by insertion of a needle through the skin of the lateral neck. The procedure uses palpation of the carotid pulse and a visualization of the relationship of the IJ to it, underscoring the importance of learning and visualizing anatomic landmarks.

External Jugular Vein

The external jugular vein (EJ) forms at the angle of mandible from the confluence of the posterior division of the **retromandibular vein** and the **posterior auricu-**

Table 2-14 Branches of the External Carotid Artery

Branch	Origin and Course	Branches
Ascending pharyngeal artery	Arises near bifurcation of common carotid, on deep surface; ascends on exterior of pharynx; and is crossed externally by stylopharyngeus and styloglossus	Divides into series of small branches and supplies the pharynx, tympanic membrane, and meninges
Superior thyroid artery	Arises just above carotid bifurcation, then runs on lateral border of thyroid gland deep to strap muscles; meets the inferior thyroid artery from thyrocervical trunk	Major branch is superior laryngeal, which accompanies the internal laryngeal nerve through thyrohyoid membrane to supply the larynx
Lingual artery	Arises from external carotid, above the superior thyroid; runs anteriorly on middle pharyngeal constrictor; then runs deep to hyoglossus	Terminal branches supply the substance of the tongue and the floor of the mouth
Facial artery	Arises from external carotid just deep to the tendon uniting the two bellies of the digastric; then passes deep to the ramus of the mandible and reappears near the midpoint of the lower edge of the mandibular body, where it can be palpated easily; then crosses the external surface of the mandibular body, lies superficial to buccinator, and ascends along the lateral border of the nose to terminate as the angular artery near the medial canthus	Gives off terminal branches to the soft palate, palatine tonsillar bed, upper and lower lips, lateral nasal wall, and lacrimal sac; characteristically, the facial artery is twisted or coiled along its course, while the facial vein is straight
Occipital artery	Arises on posterior surface of external carotid, then travels posterosuperiorly deep to posterior digastric; sternomastoid branch arises early, and passes posteroinferiorly, crossing over the hypoglossal nerve as it does	Terminal occipital artery branches lie between the scalp and occipitofrontalis muscle, and supply posterior scalp; other branches along the way supply sternocleidomastoid, external ear, mastoid air cells, and nearby muscles
Posterior auricular artery	Arises from posterior surface of external carotid, superior to origin of occipital; travels along superior surface of posterior digastric	Supplies styloid process and muscles, external ear, and scalp (anastomoses with occipital)
Superficial temporal artery	Smaller of the two terminal branches of external carotid; passes anterior to ear to anterolateral scalp; runs with auriculotemporal nerve	Major branches are transverse facial, zygomaticoorbital, and various branches to scalp
Maxillary artery	Larger of two terminal branches of external carotid; has three major divisions, based on position as the vessel passes through the infratemporal fossa	Supplies infratemporal, nasal, pharyngeal, meningeal, and palatine areas; may pass deep or superficial to lateral pterygoid muscle

lar vein. It travels external to sternocleidomastoid, generally coursing across it perpendicular to the long axis of the muscle. In the base of the neck, it drains into the subclavian vein. When intrathoracic pressure is increased (for example, by holding one's breath), the EJ distends and can often be seen prominently, crossing the sternocleidomastoid muscle from anterior to posterior. The EJ, similar to the internal jugular vein, is a suitable vein for insertion of a catheter for delivery of medications and monitoring of venous pressures.

Lymphatic Drainage in the Neck

Lymphatic chains follow both the internal and external jugular venous systems (Figure 2-69). The lymphatic network placed most deeply in the neck tends to receive lymphatic drainage from structures deepest in the head and neck—the interior of the mouth and nose and the pharynx. The more superficial lymphatics connect with more superficial scalp and facial structures. Certain patterns of lymphatic drainage give valuable clinical clues—for example, enlargement of lymph nodes in the submental region (just beneath the chin) should alert the physician to the possibility of inflammation or malignancy in the tip of the tongue. On each side, the lymphatics of the neck form a deep jugular trunk that joins the thoracic duct (on the left) or the right lymphatic duct (on the right) to empty into the subclavian vein.

Glossopharyngeal Nerve (IX)

Cranial nerves IX to XII and their branches are intertwined with the internal and external carotid vessels in the upper part of the neck. The foramina through which these nerves pass from the interior of the skull

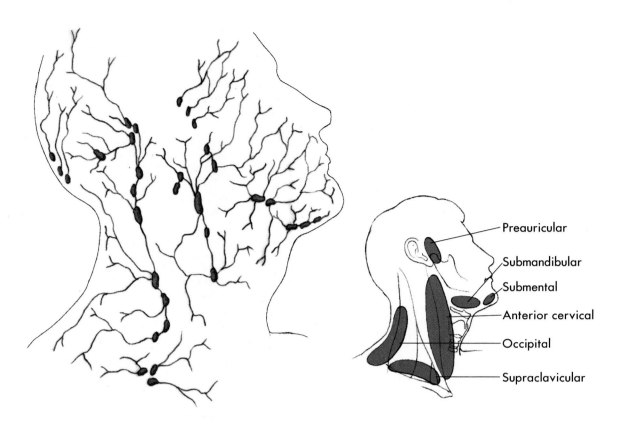

Figure 2-69   LYMPHATICS OF THE HEAD AND NECK. *Inset* shows the major groups of lymph nodes in the neck.

into the neck are very close together, near the styloid process. The individual nerves are described in the following paragraphs.

The **glossopharyngeal nerve** exits the skull through the jugular foramen (Figures 2-68 and 2-70) and, on entering the neck, passes between the external and internal carotid arteries and along the deep surface of styloid process. It then travels along the upper edge of the stylopharyngeus, the only striated muscle that it innervates (Figure 2-71). Next the nerve enters the wall of the oropharynx and laryngopharynx, between the superior and middle constrictors, the mucosal lining of which it also innervates (for sensory but not motor innervation).

Another small branch of the nerve IX supplies general and special sensory innervation (for example, taste) to the posterior third of the tongue (see Figure 2-125). The general sensory innervation of the posterior third of the tongue is much less dense and precisely localized than is the general sensory innervation of the anterior two thirds of the tongue, which is highly localized and exquisitely sensitive. Sensations on the posterior third of the tongue must be considerably more powerful to produce a conscious sensation than those on the anterior two thirds of the tongue. This contrast

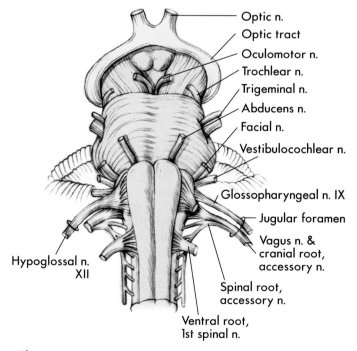

Figure 2-70   LOWER CRANIAL NERVES. Shown are the origins and apertures through which the cranial nerves IX to XII exit the skull.

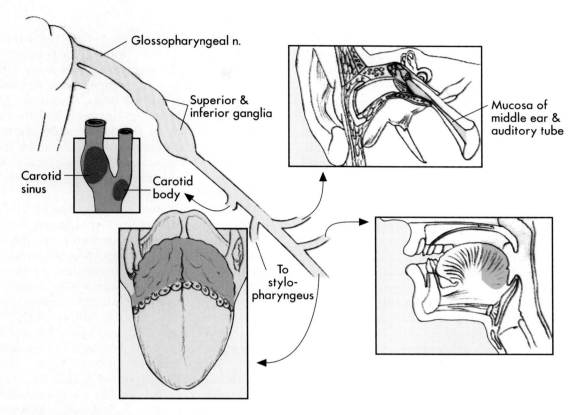

Figure 2-71   DISTRIBUTION OF THE GLOSSOPHARYNGEAL NERVE. The glossopharyngeal nerve provides sensory innervation to the carotid sinus, carotid body, auditory tube, and posterior third of the tongue.

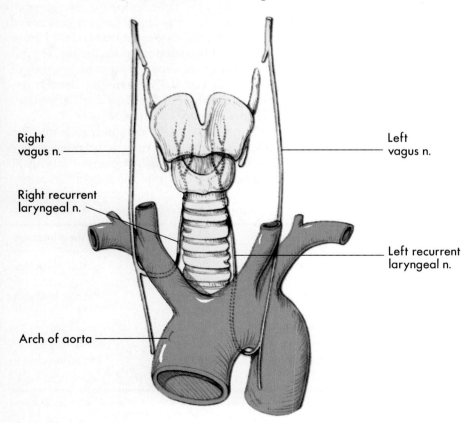

Figure 2-72 RECURRENT LARYNGEAL NERVES. On the right the recurrent laryngeal nerve loops around the distal end of the brachiocephalic artery, while on the left, it loops under the ligamentum arteriosum and aortic arch.

is a good illustration of the physiologic difference between *somatic sensory innervation* (anterior two thirds of tongue) and *visceral sensory innervation* (posterior third of tongue), even though anatomically the sensory neurons that innervate these two areas are quite similar.

Nerve IX innervates the mucosa of the tympanic cavity, mastoid air cells, and auditory tube through its **tympanic nerve,** which traverses a small canal in the base of the skull to reach the middle ear cavity. While in the middle ear cavity, it forms the **tympanic plexus,** lying on the medial wall of the middle ear cavity (see Figure 2-86).

The parasympathetic portion of IX is the **lesser petrosal nerve.** These axons accompany the tympanic nerve but do not distribute within the middle ear cavity, rather penetrating the anterior wall of the middle ear cavity to enter the middle cranial fossa. This group of axons, known as the **lesser petrosal nerve** once it enters the cranial cavity, travels anteromedially across the floor of the skull to enter the foramen ovale and synapse in the otic ganglion (see Figure 2-57). The lesser petrosal nerve consists of preganglionic parasympathetic axons. They participate in the production of saliva from the parotid gland by synapsing on neurons of the otic ganglion, from which new axons arise that accompany the auriculotemporal branch of nerve V to reach the parotid gland (see Figure 2-57).

There are two *sensory ganglia* for the glossopharyngeal nerve (the **superior and inferior ganglia**), whose peripheral processes provide general sensory innervation of the posterior third of the tongue, oropharynx and laryngopharynx, palatine tonsillar bed, lining of the tympanic cavity and auditory tube, and taste to the posterior third of the tongue.

Vagus Nerve (X)

The vagus is the largest of the cranial nerves, and innervates structures in the head and neck, chest abdomen, and pelvis. It is aptly named the "wanderer"—from the same Latin word root as "vagrant." It innervates most of the striated muscles of the lower pharynx, larynx, and the upper esophagus and trachea. It also innervates the smooth muscle of the bronchial passages and the lining of the gut, as far distal as the midtransverse colon. It directly influences heart rate (by slowing it).

In addition to the striated muscle (branchiomotor) innervations mentioned previously, the vagus innervates smooth muscle and glands in much of the respiratory and gastrointestinal tract. This is the parasympathetic component of the vagus. The parasympathetic axons of the vagus are preganglionic axons. The second neuron (of the obligatory two-neuron circuit found in all autonomic neurons) resides in the wall of the organ to be innervated (for example, heart, lung, stomach,

and so on).

Despite these diverse motor functions, however, by far *the majority of axons in the vagus is sensory.* Beyond the point where the recurrent nerves leave it, the vagus contains no further axons innervating striated muscle. The sensory axons of the vagus supply the mucosa of the epiglottis, larynx, tracheobronchial tree, and gastrointestinal tract as far distal as the midtransverse colon. The vagus nerve also provides some taste innervation to the epiglottis and a few axons to the outer surface of the tympanic membrane, as well as the floor of the external auditory meatus.

The vagus has two sensory ganglia, the **superior (jugular)** and **inferior (nodose) ganglia.** The neurons of the superior ganglion probably are the source of those few vagal axons innervating the tympanic membrane. Those of the inferior ganglion are the source of vagal axons providing the extensive sensory innervation to the thoracic and abdominal viscera.

The vagus nerve exits the skull through the jugular foramen (see Figure 2-70) and enters the carotid sheath in the upper neck, lying between and posterior to the carotid vessels and the internal jugular vein. In the neck, the vagus first gives rise to an *auricular branch,* innervating part of the tympanic membrane and external auditory meatus (Table 2-15). Distal to this are the *pharyngeal branches,* the motor component of the pharyngeal plexus, branches to the carotid body, and the superior laryngeal nerve. Each of these three appears to be branches arising from the superior or inferior ganglia. Opposite the hyoid bone, the superior laryngeal nerve divides into an internal and external branch (see Figure 2-30, *A*). The **internal branch** penetrates the thyrohyoid membrane, along with the superior laryngeal branch of the superior thyroid artery. The **external branch** descends alongside the thyroid cartilage and terminates by innervating the cricothyroid muscle.

On the right, the vagus nerve then descends into the chest, passing anterior to the right subclavian artery (Figure 2-72). The important **right recurrent laryngeal nerve** loops beneath the origin of the subclavian artery

Table 2-15   Branches of the Vagus Nerve, Arising

In the Neck	In the Thorax	In the Abdomen
Auricular pharyngeal	Left recurrent laryngeal	Gastric branches
To carotid body	Pulmonary branches	Hepatic branches
Cardiac branches		
Superior laryngeal	Esophageal	Biliary branches
Recurrent laryngeal*	Left recurrent laryngeal	Renal branches

*Could as well be considered to branch in the thorax because the nerve loops beneath the right subclavian artery.

and then ascends into the base of the neck, traveling in the shallow groove between the esophagus and trachea. It innervates the trachealis muscle and most of the muscles of the larynx. As the remainder of the right vagus passes into the superior mediastinum, a group of its axons passes anterior to the right mainstem bronchus, becoming part of the **pulmonary** and **venous plexuses.** The posterior group of axons courses on to the surface of the esophagus and continues to the abdomen.

On the left, the vagus nerve enters the chest by descending within the carotid sheath and then passing between the left brachiocephalic vein and artery. Passing through the superior mediastinum, it crosses along the left side of the aortic arch (Figure 2-72). The left vagus also divides into a posterior group of axons destined for the esophagus and an anterior group contributing to the pulmonary and cardiac plexuses. The **left recurrent laryngeal nerve** loops beneath the ligamentum arteriosum before it begins to ascend into the neck. It too innervates the trachealis muscle and all but one of the intrinsic muscles of the larynx.

Accessory Nerve (XI)

The accessory nerve is formed by the union of two roots, a cranial and a spinal (see Figure 2-70). The entire nerve exists as a single entity only for a short distance within the cranium (see Figure 2-70). The two roots may be distinguished as follows: The cranial root of XI is more logically viewed as a part of the vagus. Axons of the cranial root of XI do join the vagus, just as both nerves traverse the jugular foramen. More distally, axons

of the cranial root of XI separate again, and we recognize these as parts of the pharyngeal plexus and the recurrent laryngeal nerve (though the recurrent laryngeal nerve is generally described as a branch of the vagus).

The **spinal root** axons arise from an elongated cluster of neurons in the spinal cord gray matter of levels C1 to C5. Axons arising in these segments coalesce into a single trunk, which lies alongside the spinal cord dorsally to the denticulate ligament. It ascends to enter the cranium through the foramen magnum. It courses across the floor of the skull to join IX, X, and the cranial root of XI (at which point all components of nerve XI are united, though briefly) as they exit the skull through the jugular foramen. The spinal root of the accessory nerve quickly separates once again, and from this point onward, it is regarded simply as the "accessory" nerve (remember that the cranial root of XI has now joined the vagus nerve). It crosses the floor of the anterior triangle, most often superficial to the internal jugular vein, becoming adherent to the anterior edge of sternocleidomastoid, which it innervates (Figure 2-73). It then continues posteriorly across the floor of the posterior triangle to pass deep to the anterior edge of trapezius, which it also innervates (the sensory innervation of these two muscles, however, is most likely the responsibility of small axons from C3 to C4, which appear as small branches of the cervical plexus).

Hypoglossal Nerve (XII)

The hypoglossal nerve forms from a series of rootlets emerging from the ventrolateral medulla (see Figure

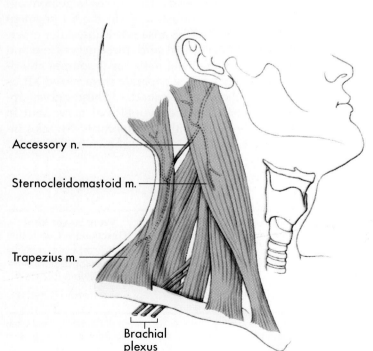

Accessory n.

Sternocleidomastoid m.

Trapezius m.

Brachial plexus

Figure 2-73   THE ACCESSORY NERVE.
SEE ATLAS, FIG. 2-8

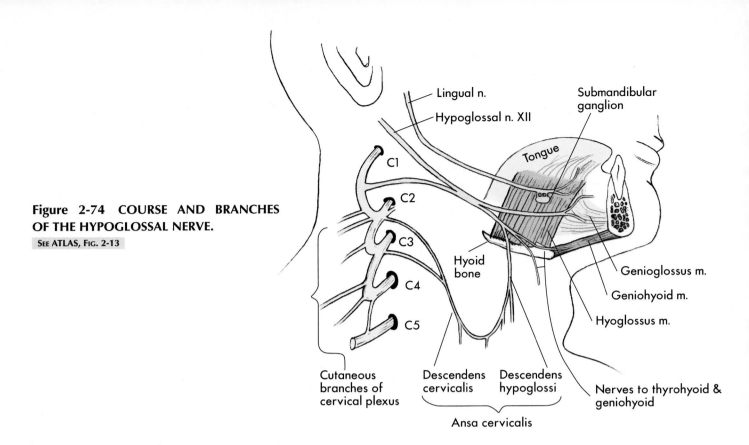

Figure 2-74 COURSE AND BRANCHES OF THE HYPOGLOSSAL NERVE.
SEE ATLAS, FIG. 2-13

Labels in figure: Lingual n.; Hypoglossal n. XII; Submandibular ganglion; Tongue; C1; C2; C3; C4; C5; Hyoid bone; Genioglossus m.; Geniohyoid m.; Hyoglossus m.; Cutaneous branches of cervical plexus; Descendens cervicalis; Descendens hypoglossi; Nerves to thyrohyoid & geniohyoid; Ansa cervicalis

2-70), then exits through the hypoglossal canal (see Figure 2-8). In the upper neck, it assumes a position between the internal carotid and internal jugular vessels. As it descends in the neck, it becomes more superficial, so that when it turns anteriorly to head in the direction of the tongue, it loops underneath the sternomastoid branch of the occipital artery. As it travels anteriorly, it crosses the loop of the lingual artery, then continues on the lateral surface of the hyoglossus muscle (Figure 2-74). It is motor to all the muscles of the tongue, except palatoglossus (innervated by the pharyngeal plexus-vagus nerve).

About 1 or 2 cm inferior to the hypoglossal canal, the hypoglossal nerve is joined by a group of axons arising from spinal cord level C1. For a time, these axons travel with the hypoglossal nerve and appear to have fused with it completely. After the hypoglossal nerve passes anterior and external to the lingual artery, certain of these C1 axons once again leave the hypoglossal nerve and form the **upper root of the ansa cervicalis** (or descendens hypoglossi—see Figure 2-74). Still other C1 axons continue somewhat farther with the hypoglossal nerve, before they too separate from it and form the individual **nerves to the geniohyoid and thyrohyoid.** Thus these latter two muscles may appear to be innervated by a branch of the hypoglossal nerve, but in reality, these "branches" of the hypoglossal arose in C1 in the first place.

Ansa Cervicalis

The **ansa cervicalis** (or ansa hypoglossi; Gr. *ansa*, handle) is a set of nerves arising from spinal cord seg-

ments C1 to C3. The **upper (C1)** and **lower (C2 to C3) roots** of the ansa unite inferiorly in the tissue of the carotid sheath (Table 2-16), and in so doing form a loop in front of the internal jugular vein (Figure 2-75). All of its branches are muscular nerves (by contrast, the cutaneous branches of cervical segments 1 to 4 originate from along the posterior border of sternocleidomastoid and form the **cervical plexus**). The ansa cervicalis innervates three of the infrahyoid or "strap," muscles (see Figure 2-77) of the anterior neck (sternothyroid, sternohyoid, and omohyoid). The nerves to geniohyoid and thyrohyoid, by contrast, arise in the C1 segment but are not branches of the ansa cervicalis. After emergence from the upper spinal cord, these nerves join and accompany the hypoglossal nerve as it courses anteriorly across the neck. They separate from nerve XII as they approach their target muscles. These nerves appear to be branches of the hypoglossal nerve, but in fact they merely travel with it temporarily. Muscles innervated by the ansa cervicalis are shown in Table 2-16.

Table 2-16 The Ansa Cervicalis

From Upper Root (Descendens Hypoglossi)	From Lower Root (Descendens Cervicalis)
Superior belly of omohyoid (C1)*	Inferior (posterior) belly omohyoid (C2-C3)*
Sternohyoid (C1-C3)*	Sternothyroid (C1-C3)

*There is much variability to the exact pattern of branching, and often all of the individual muscular branches arise from a common stem formed by the union of the two roots.

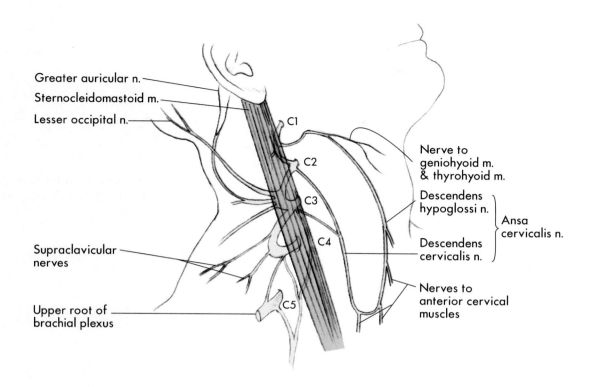

Figure 2-75   THE ANSA CERVICALIS AND CERVICAL PLEXUS.   SEE ATLAS, FIG. 2-13

Cervical Sympathetic Chain

Deep to the carotid sheath is the cervical sympathetic chain (Figure 2-76; see also Figure 2-33), with its prominent **superior cervical ganglion** lying anteriorly to the anterior neck muscles at the level of C2 to C3. A **middle cervical ganglion** lies opposite cervical vertebrae C4 to C5, and an inferior cervical ganglion lies in the base of the neck. The **inferior cervical ganglion** is often fused with the first thoracic ganglion (in which case, the combination of these two is known as the **stellate ganglion**). *Preganglionic sympathetic axons* reach these ganglia by ascending in the sympathetic chain. From these ganglia, *postganglionic sympathetic axons* emerge and are distributed to a variety of targets. Some descend through the neck into the thorax (the cardiac nerves) to supply the heart, lungs, and other chest structures.

CLINICAL ANATOMY OF

THE CAROTID REGION

CAROTID ARTERY THROMBOSIS AND EMBOLISM

The internal carotid artery is a common site for the formation of thrombi, especially at the bifurcation of the common carotid, where arteriosclerotic changes are frequent. From such clots, small emboli can break loose and cause infarctions in the brain.

THE CERVICAL FASCIAE

The various layers of cervical fascia have clinical significance because they constitute confined spaces with strong fascial coverings. Any of several types of fluid (blood, pus, and so on) can accumulate in these spaces. In the case of thyroid surgery, for example, it is not unusual for postoperative bleeding to be confined by the pretracheal fascia and put potentially life-threatening pressure on the trachea.

THE EXTERNAL CAROTID ARTERY

The external carotid artery is responsible for nearly all of the blood supply to extracranial structures in the head. Its maxillary branch ultimately supplies the nose and nasopharynx. The mouth interior is supplied by branches of the facial, maxillary, and lingual arteries. Only the orbit and small areas of the nose are supplied by vessels, not from the external carotid artery (these are supplied by branches of the internal carotid artery).

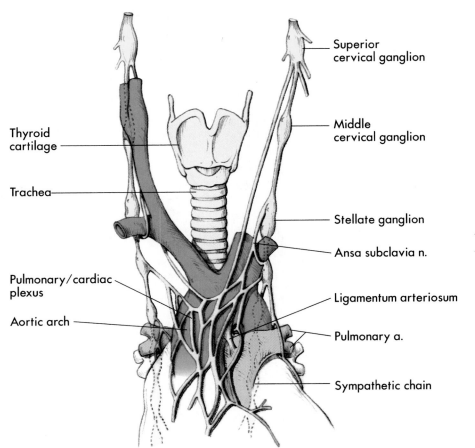

Superior cervical ganglion

Middle cervical ganglion

Thyroid cartilage

Trachea

Stellate ganglion

Ansa subclavia n.

Pulmonary/cardiac plexus

Aortic arch

Ligamentum arteriosum

Pulmonary a.

Sympathetic chain

Figure 2-76   SYMPATHETIC CHAINS AND INNERVATION OF THE MEDIASTINUM.

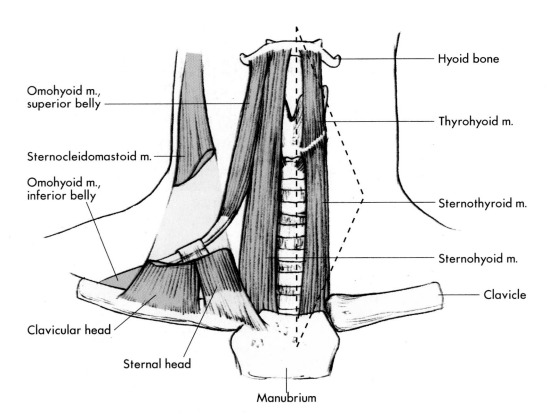

Omohyoid m., superior belly

Sternocleidomastoid m.

Omohyoid m., inferior belly

Clavicular head

Sternal head

Manubrium

Hyoid bone

Thyrohyoid m.

Sternothyroid m.

Sternohyoid m.

Clavicle

Figure 2-77   ANTERIOR NECK MUSCLES. The omohyoid passes through a fibrous sling that is attached to the posterior surface of the sternocleidomastoid. Sternothyroid, thyrohyoid, and sternohyoid muscles are also shown The *dashed lines* outline the muscular triangle. <small>See ATLAS, Fig. 2-12</small>

Sympathetic innervation of the head and neck is represented by the **carotid plexus,** which is formed by contribution of sympathetic axons, especially from the superior and middle cervical sympathetic ganglia and a few additional axons derived from the upper cervical nerve roots themselves. Motor fibers of the carotid plexus are all postganglionic sympathetic and reach all of their targets in the head and neck by traveling on the vascular system and its many branches.

MUSCULAR TRIANGLE

The boundaries of the muscular triangle are the midline of the neck, superior belly of the omohyoid, and lower portion of the anterior border of sternocleidomastoid (Figure 2-77). Because the superior belly of the omohyoid ends at the hyoid bone, by definition the muscular triangle does not extend above the hyoid bone. The region contains the infrahyoid muscles, thyroid and parathyroid glands, and their vessels and nerves. The thyroid and parathyroid glands regulate growth, metabolism, and calcium balance within the body. This region is also of great importance in emergency medical procedures, because it is often necessary to produce an opening in the anterior wall of the trachea just above the thyroid gland to ensure a patent airway (a *tracheostomy*).

Muscles in the Infrahyoid Region

The infrahyoid muscles as a group are sometimes called the **strap muscles,** because many of them are thin, elongated, rectangular muscles, extending between the hyoid bone and the sternum/clavicle. The muscles are **sternothyroid, sternohyoid, thyrohyoid,** and **omohyoid** (Table 2-17). The omohyoid muscle is complex, attaching by its inferior belly to the suprascapular notch of the scapula and by its superior belly to the hyoid bone (Figure 2-77). The midsection of the muscle passes beneath the midsection of the sternocleidomastoid, and it passes through a sling of its deep fas-

cia. It is a muscle of little strength, and its major importance is as a cervical landmark.

The infrahyoid muscles are innervated (Figure 2-75) by the **ansa cervicalis** (C1 to C3). The ansa arises from most of the same cervical roots as the cervical plexus. Branches of both the ansa and the cervical plexus contain both sensory and motor axons. (In the case of the cutaneous nerves of the cervical plexus, the majority of the axons are sensory, but there are sympathetic motor axons to such autonomic structures as smooth muscle, sweat glands, and arrector pili muscles. In the case of the muscular axons of the ansa cervicalis, the majority of the axons are motor, but there are also sensory proprioceptive axons innervating the muscles and ordinary sensory nerves to their surrounding connective tissues.)

The infrahyoid muscles depress the hyoid bone and/or larynx and protect the thyroid gland, larynx, and upper trachea. Movements of the larynx and hyoid bone are central to swallowing and the production of speech. Though normally weak, the infrahyoid muscles can hypertrophy and become accessory muscles of respiration pulling the sternum upward in a person whose major respiratory muscles (for example, the diaphragm) are injured.

Thyroid Gland

The thyroid gland lies adjacent to the upper two or three tracheal rings, covered anteriorly by the infrahyoid muscles (Figure 2-78). It is an endocrine gland, producing thyroxine and thyrocalcitonin (also called calcitonin). The gland consists of **two lateral lobes** with an **isthmus** of tissue between them. The pear-shaped lobes extend from the thyroid lamina down to the level of the sixth tracheal ring. The thyroid gland is tightly bound by the pretracheal fascia to the underlying trachea (see Figure 2-60).

The thyroid is a highly vascular organ, supplied by the *superior and inferior thyroid arteries* (Figure 2-78). The majority of arterial supply is from the inferior thyroid

Table 2-17 The Infrahyoid Muscles

Muscle	Attachments	Innervation	Action(s)
Sternohyoid	Medial clavicle and sternoclavicular joint to body of hyoid bone	Ansa cervicalis (C1-C3), descendens hypoglossi	Depresses hyoid bone
Sternothyroid	Manubrium and first rib cartilage to oblique line of thyroid cartilage	Ansa cervicalis (C1-C3), descendens cervicalis	Depresses thyroid cartilage
Thyrohyoid	Oblique line of thyroid cartilage to greater cornu (horn) of hyoid	C1 (via hypoglossal nerve)	Depresses hyoid or elevates thyroid cartilage
Omohyoid (inferior belly)	Superior border of scapula to medial surface of sternocleidomastoid	Ansa cervicalis (C1-C3), descendens cervicalis	Depresses hyoid bone
Omohyoid (superior belly)	Medial surface of sternocleidomastoid to hyoid bone	Ansa cervicalis (C1-C3), descendens hypoglossi	Depresses hyoid bone

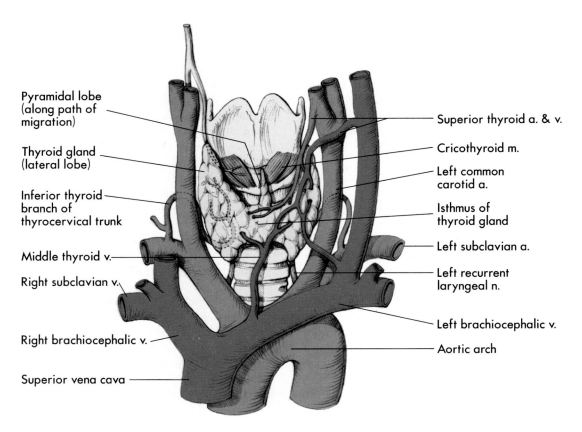

Pyramidal lobe
(along path of
migration)

Thyroid gland
(lateral lobe)

Inferior thyroid
branch of
thyrocervical trunk

Middle thyroid v.

Right subclavian v.

Right brachiocephalic v.

Superior vena cava

Superior thyroid a. & v.

Cricothyroid m.

Left common
carotid a.

Isthmus of
thyroid gland

Left subclavian a.

Left recurrent
laryngeal n.

Left brachiocephalic v.

Aortic arch

Figure 2-78   THYROID GLAND.   Sᴇᴇ Aᴛʟᴀs, Fɪɢs. 2-10, 2-14, 2-15

artery (a branch of thyrocervical trunk). Branches of the superior thyroid arteries anastomose at the isthmus. Venous drainage is through the *superior, middle, and inferior thyroid veins*.

The *superior laryngeal nerve* accompanies the superior thyroid artery as it approaches the upper pole of the gland (see Figure 2-30, *A*). The nerve divides into an internal laryngeal nerve, which pierces the thyrohyoid membrane to provide sensory innervation to the laryngeal mucosa above the level of the vocal cords, and the external branch, which descends to innervate cricothyroideus. The recurrent laryngeal nerve (see Figure 2-72) ascends in the chest and neck between the trachea and the esophagus (in the tracheoesophageal groove). At the level of the thyroid gland, the nerve is embedded in the fascia on the posterior surface of the thyroid gland. If injured during thyroid surgery, there may be temporary or permanent alteration to the voice. The axons making up the recurrent laryngeal nerves were originally part of the cranial roots of the accessory (XI) nerve; see pp. 213.

The embryologic origin of the thyroid gland is from the base of the tongue, and there can be remnant thyroid tissue along the course of the gland's descent in the anterior neck (see Figure 2-78) (*thyroglossal duct cysts* may form from remnants of this migrating tissue).

Parathyroid Glands

The parathyroids secrete parathormone (PTH), mobilizing bone calcium and increasing gut and kidney calcium absorption. The parathyroids are usually four in number (two pairs), located on the posterior surface of thyroid (Figure 2-79). The superior and inferior parathyroids are derived from the fourth and third pharyngeal pouches, respectively.

The parathyroids are usually ~0.5 × 0.8 cm ovoids. Small branches of the superior and inferior thyroid arteries are the usual blood supply. The parathyroids sometimes may be located in other parts of neck or in mediastinum (abnormally-placed, or "ectopic," parathyroid tissue).

SUBMANDIBULAR TRIANGLE

The submandibular and submental triangles are small regions of the neck, just inferior to the lower margin of the mandible (see Figure 2-61). The muscles that form the boundaries and the floors of these two neck triangles are known collectively as the **suprahyoid muscles** (digastric, mylohyoid, geniohyoid, and stylohyoid). The submandibular triangle contains the submandibular gland, as well as several muscles that form the base of the tongue and the floor of the mouth.

CLINICAL ANATOMY OF
THE ANTEROLATERAL NECK

RISKS OF SURGERY ON THE THYROID GLAND

Thyroid surgery is often necessitated by neoplastic growths in the gland. Risk is posed to recurrent laryngeal nerve (leads to hoarseness). Also, great care is necessary to preserve the parathyroid glands. Inadvertent removal can lead to a life-threatening emergency based on the fall in the serum calcium level that follows injury to the parathyroids.

GOITER

A goiter is an enlarged thyroid gland; with a goiter, the patient's thyroid hormone status may be underactive (hypothyroid), overactive (hyperthyroid), or normal (euthyroid), and size of the gland alone does not predict this.

ESTABLISHING EMERGENCY AIRWAY ACCESS

Tracheotomy is performed to provide airway patency on an emergency basis or electively for patients in whom breathing through nose/mouth is unreliable (patients with neurologic injury, growths in the oropharynx, and so on). Emergency tracheotomy is usually performed between the cricoid and first two or three tracheal rings. Risk of thyroid laceration and hemorrhage is considerable. Cricothyrotomy is the creation of an opening in the cricothyroid membrane. This site for establishing airway access involves more risk to the vocal cords and larynx.

THYROID SURGERY AND THE PRETRACHEAL FASCIA

Postoperative hemorrhage after thyroid surgery can compress the trachea and cause suffocation, because the hemorrhage will be confined within the space surrounded by the pretracheal fascia.

SURGERY AND THE PARATHYROID GLANDS

Tendency for accessory parathyroid tissue to be ectopic sometimes necessitates a careful surgical search, especially if the purpose of the surgery is removal of the parathyroids (for example, because of tumor or metabolic overactivity). When thyroidectomy is being performed, care must be taken not to remove the parathyroids inadvertently, along with the thyroid.

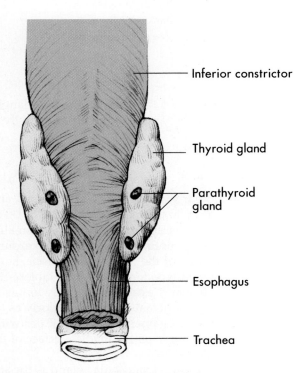

Inferior constrictor

Thyroid gland

Parathyroid gland

Esophagus

Trachea

Figure 2-79 POSTERIOR PHARYNX, THYROID, AND PARATHYROID GLANDS.

Vessels and nerves destined for the interior of the mouth pass from the neck through the submandibular triangle to reach the mouth.

The submandibular triangle is bounded by the ramus of the mandible, anterior belly of the digastric, and posterior belly of the digastric. The anterior belly of the digastric extends from a central tendon (attaching by a sling to the hyoid bone) to the mandibular symphysis. The posterior belly of the digastric extends from the hyoid bone posteriorly to a groove on the medial surface of the mastoid process. Though the two bellies are considered part of one muscle, they have separate innervations—the anterior belly by the nerve to mylohyoid (a branch of V3) and the posterior belly by a branch of the facial nerve (VII).

The anterior part of the floor of the submandibular triangle is formed by mylohyoid muscle (Figure 2-80, *B*), joined in the midline to the mylohyoid muscle of the other side at a *midline raphe.* Each mylohyoid is attached to the hyoid bone and the mylohyoid line on the interior surface of the mandible. The mylohyoid muscle has a free posterolateral edge, or margin, around which is wrapped the *submandibular salivary gland.* Deep to the mylohyoid muscles in the anterior midline is a pair of geniohyoid muscles, extending from the hyoid bone to the genial tubercles on the interior surface of the mandibles.

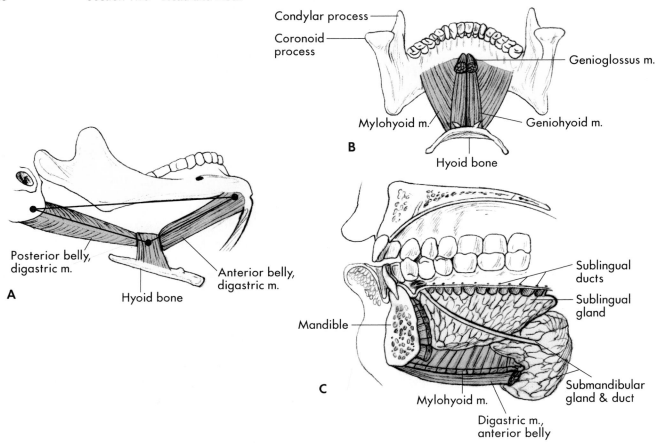

Figure 2-80   SUBMANDIBULAR TRIANGLE. A, Inferolateral view of lower margin of the submandibular triangle comprises the anterior and posterior bellies of the digastric muscle. **B,** Mylohyoid muscle seen from inside the mouth. The geniohyoid and genioglossus muscles are also seen superior to the mylohyoid. **C,** Sublingual gland and submandibular duct. The submandibular duct courses along the medial side of the sublingual gland and exits through the sublingual papilla at the base of the frenulum of the tongue.

Posterior to the mylohyoid, the floor of the submandibular triangle is formed by the hyoglossus muscle and, variably, a small portion of the pharyngeal superior constrictor muscle. The more anterior portion of hyoglossus lies deep to the mylohyoid. The space between these two muscles is known as the **mylohyoid cleft**. The hyoglossus muscle extends from hyoid bone upward and medially into the base of the tongue. In the tongue, it intermingles with fibers of the intrinsic tongue muscles. The superior constrictor muscle extends from the posterior median raphe to the pterygomandibular raphe and is the uppermost of the three concentric muscles forming the pharynx. The *pterygomandibular raphe* is a thick cord of tissue extending from the pterygoid hamulus of the medial pterygoid plate to the mylohyoid line on the interior of the mandible. The superior constrictor approaches this raphe posteriorly and attaches to it. The buccinator muscle originates from this same raphe and extends anteriorly into the substance of the cheek. The stylohyoid muscle extends along the back margin of the submandibular triangle, just external and nearly parallel to the posterior belly of the digastric.

Submandibular Gland

The submandibular gland is irregularly shaped and about $2 \times 3 \times 3$ cm in size (Figures 2-81 and 2-82). The gland consists of a larger superficial part and a smaller deep part. The two are continuous as they wrap around the posterior free edge of the mylohyoid muscle, similar to an old-fashioned wooden clothespin (Table 2-18). The submandibular gland extends anteriorly as far as the anterior belly of the digastric and posteriorly as far as the stylomandibular ligament. Laterally, it lies within the submandibular fossa on the medial surface of the mandible (see Figure 2-50).

Lying medial to the submandibular gland is the *stylomandibular ligament*. It is a broad thickened part of the deep fascia, connecting the styloid process to the

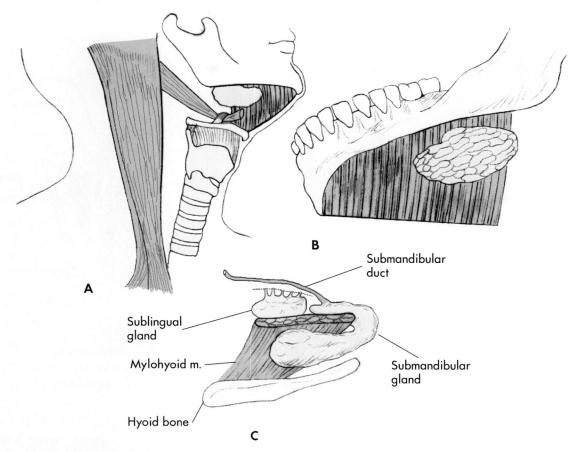

Figure 2-81 POSITION OF THE SUBMANDIBULAR GLAND. A, External portion of the gland is seen along the posterior margin of mylohyoid. **B,** Closer oblique view of the gland. **C,** A coronal section through the lower jaw; the two lobes of the gland are seen on either side of the mylohyoid. See Atlas, Fig. 2-17

medial surface of the mandibular angle. Along its course, the ligament passes between the adjacent surfaces of the submandibular and parotid salivary glands.

The *submandibular (Wharton's) duct* is 4 to 5 cm long. It leaves the deep part of the gland, runs anteriorly on the surface of hyoglossus (and deep to the mylohyoid), and terminates at the *sublingual papilla* in the floor of the mouth. The submandibular duct is accompanied by the lingual nerve along the external surface of hyoglossus. The two sublingual papillae lie side by side in the midline of the floor of the mouth, at the base of the

Table 2-18 Structures Related to the Submandibular Gland

Relationship	Muscles	Vessels	Nerves and Other
Superior	Mylohyoid muscle	Facial artery	Lower margin of mandible
Inferior	Platysma muscle, anterior belly, digastric muscle	Facial vein	Cervical branch of VII, deep fascia
Anterior	Anterior belly, digastric muscle		Lymph nodes
Posterior	Medial pterygoid muscle	Facial artery (partly within gland)	Hypoglossal nerve
Superficial	Platysma muscle	Facial artery and vein	Cervical branch of VII, lymph nodes
Deep	Mylohyoid muscle, hyoglossus muscle	Lingual artery (deep to hyoglossus)	Submandibular duct

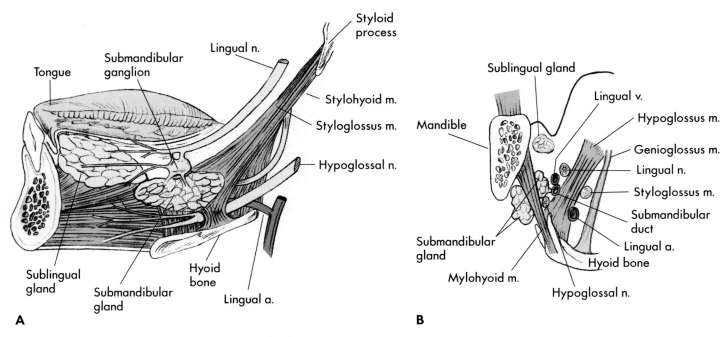

Figure 2-82   NERVE SUPPLY TO THE SUBMANDIBULAR REGION.   A, Submandibular and sublingual glands are shown in relation to the hyoglossus muscle. **B,** Coronal section shows position of several vessels and nerves in relation to the hyoglossus and mylohyoid muscles.

frenulum of the tongue. Branches of the facial and lingual arteries supply the gland with blood.

Deep to the superficial part of the gland are the mylohyoid muscle and accompanying nerves and vessels; *deep to the deep part of the gland* itself is the hyoglossus muscle, with the hypoglossal nerve, lingual vein, and lingual nerve lying just external to it on the surface of hyoglossus (Figure 2-82; listed in order, from inferior to superior). Just lateral to the submandibular gland is the medial surface of the body of the mandible. The lower three fourths of the gland is palpable through the skin and platysma muscle just inferior to the lower margin of the mandible. Across the gland passes the marginal mandibular branch of the facial nerve (see the following section).

The sublingual salivary gland (see Figure 2-80), which lies superior to the mylohyoid directly medial to the mandible, is described fully on p. 273.

Nerves in the Submandibular Triangle

The **marginal mandibular branch** of the facial nerve lies very superficial in the submandibular triangle. It travels roughly parallel to the inferior margin of the mandible. It innervates facial muscles in the area of the lower lip and chin and is especially vulnerable to traumatic injuries.

The **lingual nerve,** a branch of V3, travels on the exterior surface of hyoglossus (Figure 2-82). It is positioned superior to the hypoglossal nerve, lingual vein, and submandibular duct, all of which also travel across the external surface of the hyoglossus. More proximally, in the infratemporal fossa, the lingual nerve is joined by the **chorda tympani.** The chorda tympani branch of the facial nerve contains taste fibers for the anterior two thirds of the tongue and secretomotor axons that will synapse in the submandibular ganglion. The **submandibular ganglion** is suspended from the lingual nerve and lies above the submandibular gland and on the hyoglossus muscle. Axons originating in this ganglion then innervate the submandibular and sublingual glands. Deep to the hyoglossus are found the **glossopharyngeal nerve,** lingual artery, and stylohyoid ligament.

Nearby Vascular Structures

Lying superficial in the submandibular triangle is a plexus of veins, draining to the **facial vein.** The **lingual artery,** a major branch of the external carotid artery, is seen at the posterior margin of the hyoglossus muscle just before it passes deep to the muscle. The lingual artery then runs anterior and deep to the hyoglossus to reach the base of the tongue. Note that by contrast, the **lingual vein** runs superficial to the hyoglossus.

The submandibular triangle is generously supplied with **lymph nodes** (see Figure 2-69). Not only are these

THE SUBMANDIBULAR-SUBMENTAL REGION

THE SUBMANDIBULAR FASCIA

Fascia over the submandibular region tends to restrict edema or infectious fluids in the triangle, preventing them from tracking more inferiorly down the neck.

INFLAMMATION OF THE SUBMANDIBULAR LYMPH NODES

Infections in the floor of the mouth may cause pain and swelling in the submandibular region (a symptom known as Ludwig's angina). A similar swelling of the submandibular gland may occur in mumps as well, although the principal target of this infectious disease is the parotid gland.

CONGENITAL CYSTS IN THE LATERAL NECK

Branchial cleft cysts are common in the posterior part of the submandibular region. They represent remnants of the upper two or three original pharyngeal clefts, which normally disappear altogether.

SUBMANDIBULAR LYMPH NODES AND MALIGNANCY

Enlargement of lymph nodes in the submandibular region may be a nonspecific sign of a benign upper respiratory infection but less often will be present when there is a malignancy in the lateral part of the tongue (tumors in the *tip* of the tongue often drain to the submental region). Such findings in a patient with a history of smoking should further heighten one's suspicions.

---

nodes prone to swelling and tenderness during infections, they also are a frequent site for metastasis of tumors located deeply within the face, especially the floor of the mouth.

SUBMENTAL TRIANGLE

This triangle is bounded by the hyoid bone, anterior belly of the digastric, and the midline of the neck (alternately, some consider that we should recognize only one submental triangle—its base formed by the hyoid bone, and its two sides formed by the anterior belly of the digastric on each side [see Figure 2-61]). The submental triangle contains only fat and lymph nodes, but the muscles that make up its floor are an important part of the floor of the mouth and muscles regulating movement of the tongue. The floor of the submental triangle is formed by the medial portions of the two

mylohyoid muscles and the fibrous *raphe,* which unites them in the midline. The mylohyoid muscle joins the mental symphysis of the mandible to the hyoid bone inferiorly. The mylohyoid is quite important in (1) forming part of the floor of the mouth and (2) serving as an elevator of the hyoid bone. It also serves as a foundation, against which the tongue musculature exerts force and produces tongue movement.

The *geniohyoid* and *genioglossus muscles* lie deep to the mylohyoid muscle and form part of the floor of the mouth (geniohyoid) and the substance of the tongue (genioglossus). The geniohyoid muscles are a pair of cylindrical muscles, lying side by side in the midline. The genioglossus muscles are wider and extend from the internal surface of the mandible by a fanlike series of fibers that interdigitate with the intrinsic muscles of the tongue.

2.9

section two.nine

Ear

▶ External Ear   ▶ Inner Ear

▶ Middle Ear

The **external ear** extends from the pinna, or auricle, to the tympanic membrane, or eardrum, through the external auditory canal. The **middle ear** cavity lies on the deep side of the tympanic membrane and is connected to the mastoid air cells in the temporal bone and the pharynx through the auditory, or Eustachian, tube. The **inner ear** is an intricate series of membrane-bound spaces embedded in the petrous part of the temporal bone and abutting on the middle ear cavity. Sensory cells in the inner ear are stimulated by sound (the cochlea), position (the vestibule), and motion (the semicircular canals).

With some variations, the sensations of movement and balance are produced by a similar transduction of mechanical energy into electrical signals, transmitted through neurons from the inner ear to the brain. Elaborate structures in the vestibular apparatus permit the detection of motion of the head with respect to the ground, and interactions between the vestibular and visual systems provide information about the orientation of the head and body with respect to the horizon.

The human external ear is shaped to help collect sound waves, but in most of us there is no ability to move the external ear and direct it at the source of sound (in most other mammals, this ability is well developed). Humans do have a group of vestigial muscles surrounding the external ear, and they are innervated by proximal branches of the facial nerve, just after it emerges from the stylomastoid foramen.

EXTERNAL EAR

The external ear is known as the **pinna,** or **auricle** (Figure 2-83). The elaborate structure of the external

and middle ears is designed to transmit mechanical energy (sound waves) to the fluids of the inner ear, where changes in the membrane potential of neurons are produced. These electrical changes in the neurons of the inner ear produce a signal that is transmitted to the brainstem and thence to the higher regions of the brain, where the sensation of sound is appreciated. The external ear transmits sound to the middle ear, where the ossicles link the inner surface of the tympanic membrane to the fluid in the inner ear. The sound energy is interpreted in terms of loudness, pitch (frequency), and the direction from which it comes.

Pinna

The mammalian *pinna* (L., a feather), or external ear, has a skeleton of elastic cartilage and is covered with dense connective tissue and skin. The large posterior curved free margin of pinna is known as the **helix**

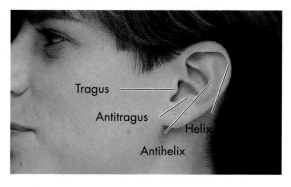

Figure 2-83 EXTERNAL EAR, OR PINNA.

(Figure 2-83). In the center of the ear is a second curved ridge of cartilage, parallel to the helix, known as the **antihelix.** Surrounding the entrance to the external auditory meatus is an anterior prominence, the **tragus,** and opposite it—at the base of the antihelix—is another prominence called the **antitragus.**

External Auditory Meatus and Canal

The **external auditory meatus** is composed of cartilage (the external third) and bone (the internal two thirds) (Figure 2-84). It is ~3.5 cm in length and in most people is in the shape of a gentle S-shaped curve. When examining the external auditory meatus, one should grasp the superior margin of the pinna and elevate it superiorly and posteriorly, resulting in a partial straightening of the canal and an improvement in view of the tympanic membrane. The coarse hairs found at the entrance to the external canal help keep foreign objects from lodging in the canal. **Ceruminous glands** lining the canal, mostly in its cartilaginous external third, produce "ear wax," which helps to prevent moisture trapped in the canal from macerating the epithelium. The epithelium is thinned to a narrow stratified layer as it continues over the external surface of the tympanic membrane (see following). *Innervation of the pinna* is provided by the greater auricular nerve of the cervical plexus, auriculotemporal branch of the trigeminal nerve, and small branches of the vagus nerve.

Tympanic Membrane (Eardrum)

The **tympanic membrane (TM)** is a bilayered disk that is concave to external view (that is, through the otoscope, viewing down the length of the external auditory canal). It is inclined at an ~50-degree angle (that is, not perpendicular to the external auditory canal), so that its inferior margin is farther from the entrance to the external meatus than is its superior margin (Figure 2-84). A small pie-shaped anterosuperior segment of the tympanic membrane is lax (and called the **pars flaccida**), while the remainder of the membrane is under considerable tension (**pars tensa**). A small inferior triangular segment of the membrane is most nearly perpendicular to the long axis of the external auditory canal and therefore reflects light directly back to the observer viewing the tympanic membrane. This area appears to be very bright when the examining light is shone on to the tympanic membrane and thus is known as the "cone of light." The **umbo** is that point in the center of the tympanic membrane, where the inferior end of the handle of the malleus is attached to the membrane on its internal surface (Figure 2-85).

The external surface of the TM is covered with a thin stratified epithelium only five to eight cells thick. The internal surface is lined by a single layer of markedly flattened cells, continuous with the lining of the middle ear cavity. In between the two is a thin layer of connective tissue fibers. *Innervation of the external surface of the TM is by branches of auriculotemporal nerve (branch of*

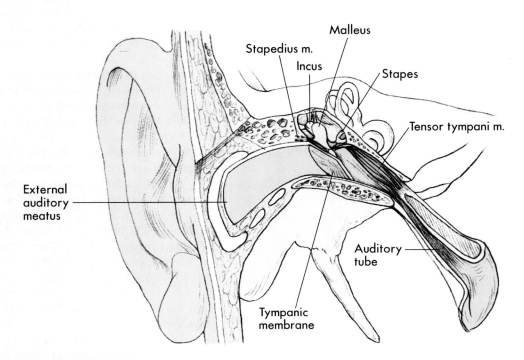

Stapedius m.
Incus
Malleus
Stapes
Tensor tympani m.
External auditory meatus
Auditory tube
Tympanic membrane

Figure 2-84   RELATIONSHIPS OF THE EXTERNAL, MIDDLE, AND INTERNAL EAR. Note that the tympanic membrane is positioned at an angle with respect to the external auditory canal not perpendicular to it.

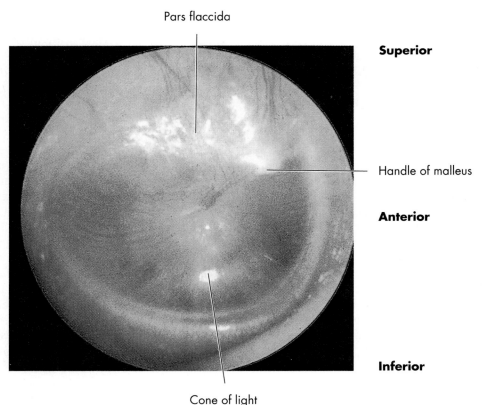

Pars flaccida

Superior

Handle of malleus

Anterior

Inferior

Cone of light

Figure 2-85 TYMPANIC MEM-BRANE. Seen through an otoscope. (From Chumbley CC, Hutchings RT: *Color atlas of human dissection,* London, 1992, Mosby.)
SEE ATLAS, FIG. 2-117

V3) and a few twigs of vagus nerve. The latter nerve (vagus) explains the tendency in some to gag or vomit with stimulation of external auditory canal. The internal surface of the TM is innervated by branches of the tympanic plexus, derived from the glossopharyngeal nerve.

Movement of the tympanic membrane in response to sound of moderate volume is measured in nanometers. The tympanic membrane oscillates as a single unit up to about 50 cycles per second (Hz), above which it begins to show regional oscillation. The human auditory system is capable of detecting sound ranging from a low-pitched sound of 25 to 30 Hz to a high-pitched sound of 15,000 to 20,000 Hz. Normal conversation and ambient sound is in the range of 500 to 200 Hz. Ability to hear the high end of the sound spectrum is lost with advancing age.

MIDDLE EAR

It is easiest to describe the middle ear cavity as a box, with six inner surfaces—the four walls, a ceiling, and a floor (Figure 2-86). This rectangle is positioned so that its long axis faces anteromedially, not in a parasagittal plane. The long axis of the middle ear cavity is also inclined downward slightly, not parallel to the ground. The major role of the middle ear cavity is to

transmit sound energy from the external canal to the inner ear. Hearing may be affected when there is inflammation and exudative fluid accumulates within the middle ear, because this tends to dampen the transmission of sound energy through the middle ear to the inner ear.

The middle ear cavity is part of the temporal bone (Figure 2-86). Specifically, it is located beneath the superior surface of the petrous part of the temporal bone, or temporal ridge (see Figure 2-10, *B*). The tympanic membrane forms its lateral wall, and the external auditory canal leads outward from the tympanic membrane to the external auditory meatus. Medial to the middle ear cavity are the **cochlea,** located anteriorly, and the **vestibule** and **semicircular canals,** located just posterior to the cochlea. Posteriorly, the middle ear cavity is continuous with the **mastoid air cells.** Anteriorly, the **auditory tube** connects the middle ear cavity with the nasopharynx. Superior is the middle cranial fossa and below is the bulb of the internal jugular vein.

Many important structures are situated close to the middle ear cavity (Figure 2-86). The **facial nerve** passes along the medial and posterior walls of the middle ear cavity, producing indentations in both. The **internal carotid artery** and **internal jugular vein** lie beneath the floor of the middle ear cavity, with the artery anterior to the vein. These vessels are close enough to the mid-

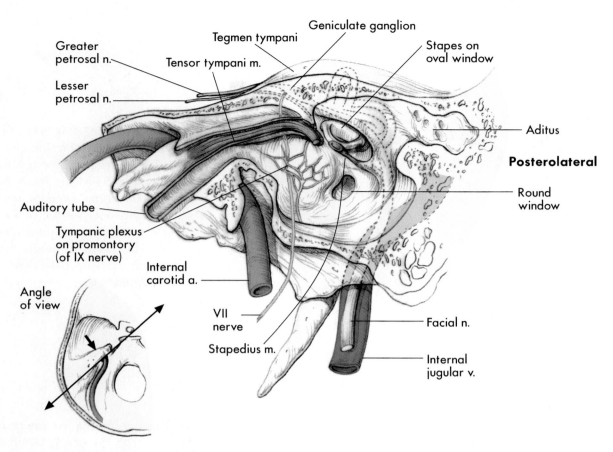

Greater petrosal n.
Tegmen tympani
Geniculate ganglion
Tensor tympani m.
Stapes on oval window
Lesser petrosal n.
Aditus
Posterolateral
Round window
Auditory tube
Tympanic plexus on promontory (of IX nerve)
Internal carotid a.
Angle of view
VII nerve
Facial n.
Stapedius m.
Internal jugular v.

Figure 2-86   MEDIAL WALL OF THE MIDDLE EAR CAVITY. See text for details.

dle ear cavity that in rare cases the turbulent flow of blood in these vessels can produce a constant annoying pulsatile buzz.

The lateral wall of the middle ear cavity consists largely of the tympanic membrane and extends upward into the epitympanic recess. The tympanic membrane is lined internally by epithelium continuous with that lining the rest of the middle ear cavity. This epithelium is innervated by the glossopharyngeal nerve through the **tympanic plexus** (Figure 2-86). The epithelium produces mucus that lubricates the interior of the middle ear cavity and ultimately drains through the auditory tube into the pharynx. Inflammation of this epithelium can cause excess mucus secretion and obstruction of this flow, causing mucus to collect in the middle ear cavity. As it accumulates, pressure builds up, causing painful sensations transmitted through the glossopharyngeal nerve.

The **chorda tympani nerve** courses across the medial surface of the tympanic membrane and is draped over the manubrium (L., handle) of the malleus. It is positioned between the malleus and the incus (Figure 2-87).

It is through an aperture in the posterior wall of the middle ear cavity, the **aditus,** that it communicates

with the mastoid air cells. The chorda tympani, later seen traveling across the medial surface of the tympanic membrane, enters the middle ear cavity through a different small lateral aperture in the posterior wall. The stapedius muscle (Figure 2-88) originates from the small **pyramidal eminence** on the medial posterior wall and extends anteriorly to attach to the neck of the stapes (one of the three ossicles). The stapedius is thought to dampen movements of the stapes and protect the tympanic membrane from injury caused by excessive excursions of the stapes. The facial nerve courses through a cylindrical channel just posterior to the thin bony surface of the posterior wall.

The **auditory tube (eustachian tube)** opens into the anterior wall of the middle ear cavity (Eustachio was a sixteenth-century Roman anatomy professor and physician to the Pope). It is a cartilaginous cylinder that travels downward and medially to open into the posterior wall of the nasopharynx. Where it opens into the nasopharynx, its opening is flared, similar to the bell of a trumpet (see Figures 2-84 and 2-120). The **tensor tympani muscle** arises from the cartilaginous part of the auditory tube (see Figure 2-87). The belly of the muscle runs in a narrow canal in the wall of the auditory tube

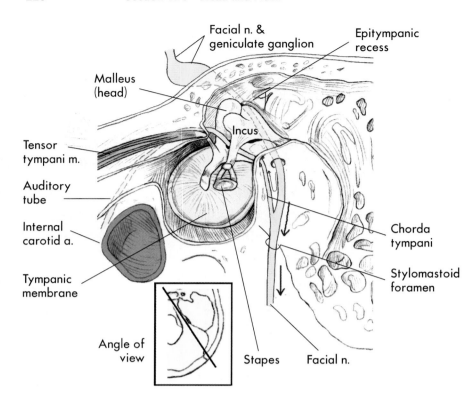

Facial n. &
geniculate ganglion

Epitympanic
recess

Malleus
(head)

Incus

Tensor
tympani m.

Auditory
tube

Internal
carotid a.

Tympanic
membrane

Chorda
tympani

Stylomastoid
foramen

Angle of
view

Stapes   Facial n.

Figure 2-87   LATERAL WALL OF THE MIDDLE EAR CAVITY. The inner surface of the tympanic membrane can be seen, with malleus, incus, stapes, and the chorda tympani coursing across the inner surface of the tympanic membrane. The main body of the facial nerve descends through the temporal bone to the right.
SEE ATLAS, FIG. 2-118

and attaches to the handle of the malleus (after looping around a small bony prominence on the anterior wall). The tensor tympani thus forms a pulleylike arrangement with the malleus. It functions to dampen tympanic movement, in turn preventing tympanic membrane rupture.

The chorda tympani, after entering the middle ear cavity posteriorly and coursing across the internal surface of the tympanic membrane and handle of the malleus, exits the middle ear cavity through a small aperture in its anterior wall. The *internal carotid artery* lies just external to the anterior wall of the middle ear cavity.

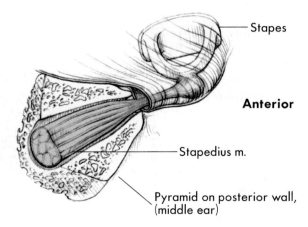

Stapes

Anterior

Stapedius m.

Pyramid on posterior wall,
(middle ear)

Figure 2-88   THE STAPEDIUS MUSCLE. The stapedius muscle emerges from the apex of a pyramidal eminence on the posterior wall of the middle ear cavity.
SEE ATLAS, FIG. 2-119

On the medial wall of the middle ear cavity is the **promontory** (see Figure 2-86), on which ramifies the *tympanic plexus* from the glossopharyngeal nerve. The promontory is an elevation on the medial wall of the middle ear cavity, adjacent to the roof, underneath which is the basal turn of the cochlea. There is also a small prominence, posterior and superior to the promontory, for the facial nerve, which passes just outside the medial wall. After it passes posteriorly, it descends and begins its course toward the stylomastoid foramen.

The medial wall of the middle ear cavity has two apertures posterior to the promontory, an **oval window** (fenestra vestibuli) above and a **round window** (fenestra cochleae) below (see Figure 2-86). The foot-plate of the **stapes** fits into the oval window, and it is here that the energy from sound waves is transferred from the ossicles to the *perilymph of the inner ear* (Figure 2-89). The inner ear consists of three membrane bound regions—the **cochlea** (for hearing), **semicircular canals** (for the detection of motion), and the **vestibule** (providing information about the positional relationship of the head to the ground and horizon). Each of these sensory structures is filled with a fluid (**endolymph**); another fluid called **perilymph** separates these sensory structures from the bony space in which each lies. Thus vibrations transmitted through the stapes to the perilymph are then transferred to the endolymph and finally produce a mechanical effect on the sensory cells in the inner ear. When these cells are activated, mechanical energy is transduced into the electrochemical ener-

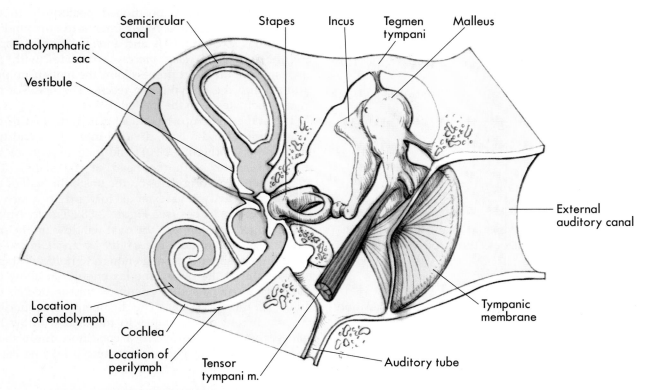

Figure 2-89 MIDDLE EAR AND INNER EAR. In schematic fashion, we see the middle ear cavity, in which the three ossicles link the tympanic membrane to the wall of the inner ear. The stapes fits over the oval window, and vibrations are here transmitted to the cochlea, where they are perceived as sound. Movements of the head cause sensory signals to be generated in the semicircular canals. SEE ATLAS, FIGS. 2-119, 2-120

gy of neuronal transmission, and the signal travels to the brain. The vibrations originally transmitted from the middle ear cavity into the perilymph later are transmitted back into the middle ear cavity when the energy passes across the membrane covering the round window. The energy is then dispersed in the middle ear cavity.

A thin, bony shelf (the tegmen tympani) forms the roof of the middle ear cavity and separates it from the middle cranial fossa (see Figure 2-89). The tegmen tympani has a small upwardly-directed evagination, the **epitympanic recess,** which accommodates the head of the malleus. In small children, the tegmen undergoes a process of sutural closure (between the squamous and petrous portions of the temporal bone). Until this closure is complete, there is an increased risk for middle ear infections to spread to the cranial cavity and produce meningitis. This is one of the factors that renders children more vulnerable to meningitis.

The floor of the middle ear cavity is elongated and narrow. Just deep to it is the bulb of the internal jugular vein, and there is a small aperture through which passes the tympanic branch of the glossopharyngeal nerve, entering the middle ear cavity to contribute to formation of the tympanic plexus. This tympanic branch provides general sensory innervation to the mucosa of the middle ear, mastoid air cells, and proximal part of the auditory tube. It also contains some parasympathetic secretomotor fibers destined for the otic ganglion.

Ossicles (Small Bones of the Middle Ear)

The ossicles form a linkage of three mobile bones, extending from the tympanic membrane to the oval window (*malleus → incus → stapes*) (Figure 2-90). They are the smallest bones of the human body. They articulate with each other by ordinary synovial joints, with surrounding ligaments. They are linked to the walls of the middle ear cavity by various ligaments and are further supported by the stapedius and tensor tympani muscles. Blood vessels, nerves, and lymphatics reach the ossicles through their ligamentous attachments to the walls of the middle ear cavity.

The ossicles amplify the force of sound waves approximately 10 times, which helps offset the impedance differential when the energy of sound waves pass from ossicles to the perilymph. The ratio of the surface area of the tympanic membrane to that of the oval window

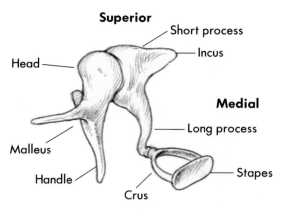

Figure 2-90   THREE OSSICLES. The malleus attaches to the inner surface of the tympanic membrane. The incus links the malleus to the stapes. The stapes is attached to the wall of the inner ear.

gives a rough idea of the degree of sound amplification produced.

The **malleus** (hammer) has a rounded *head* superiorly, a midregion in which are found the *neck, anterior* and *lateral processes,* and a *handle* inferiorly, shaped like a narrow, inverted cone (Figure 2-90). The handle is attached to the inner surface of the tympanic membrane. The head is positioned in the epitympanic recess and the tensor tympani muscle inserted in its neck. The tensor tympani muscle dampens excessive ossicular vibration. On the posteromedial surface of the head of the malleus is an *articular fossa* for the incus. The chorda tympani branch of the facial nerve travels from posterior to anterior across the medial surface of the tympanic membrane and is draped across the medial surface of the handle of the malleus just above the insertion of the tensor tympani muscle. The malleus is also held in place by anterior and superior ligaments, attached to the walls of the middle ear cavity.

The **incus** (anvil) is positioned posteriorly to the malleus and is attached by ligaments to surrounding bone. It has as central *body* and a *long* and *short process* (Figure 2-90). The *long process* articulates with the stapes, while the short process joins the malleus in protruding into the epitympanic recess. The body of the incus articulates with the malleus.

The **stapes** (stirrup) has a *foot-plate* (attached to the oval window) and a *body,* divided into a *head* and two limbs or *crura* (Figure 2-90). The long process of the incus articulates with the head of the stapes. The stapedius muscle originates on the posterior wall of the middle ear cavity and extends forward to attach to the head of the stapes (see Figure 2-88). The foot-plate of the stapes is secured in the oval window on the medial wall of the middle ear cavity by an *annular ligament.* This ligament is strong enough to hold the stapes in place but at the same time lax enough to allow the stapes to move as sound energy is transmitted to the fluids of the inner ear. The ligaments surrounding the attachment of the stapes to the oval window become calcified in *otosclerosis,* a condition diminishing ossicular movement and representing a leading cause of deafness.

Auditory Tube

This bony/cartilaginous cylinder is ~3.5 cm long and is inclined downward, forward, and medially and connects the pharynx with the anterior wall of the middle ear cavity (see Figures 2-84 and 2-86). It permits equalization of pressures between these two chambers. Its medial third (nearest the middle ear cavity) is bony; the remaining outer two thirds is cartilaginous.

The auditory tube originates in the anterior wall of the middle ear cavity and extends toward the pharynx, passing just lateral to the carotid canal. It is not a true cylinder, but rather a C-shaped tube, which broadens at

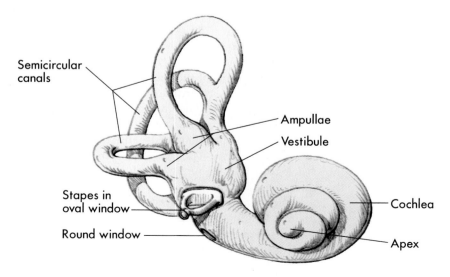

Figure 2-91   COCHLEA AND SEMICIRCULAR CANALS. This complex bony structure surrounds a membranous structure of nearly identical shape, known as the membranous labyrinth.

its pharyngeal end to form a trumpetlike opening (referred to as the **salpinx**). The medial end of the auditory tube forms the **tubal elevation** (see Figure 2-120), an inward bulging of the nasopharyngeal mucosa that surrounds the orifice of the auditory tube. The salpingopharyngeus muscle originates from the tubal elevation, and during yawning, contraction of this muscle helps open the auditory tube and equilibrate pressures between middle ear and pharynx ("popping" of your ears).

Muscles of the Middle Ear

The **tensor tympani muscle** (Figure 2-84) extends from a bony canal just superior to the auditory tube, passes through a small trochlea or pulley, and inserts on the handle of the malleus. It is innervated by nerve V (V3), and its contraction pulls inward on the tympanic membrane and makes it stiffer. This protects the tympanic membrane from tearing when very loud sound produces rapid forceful movements of the membrane.

The **stapedius muscle** (see Figure 2-88) extends from the pyramidal eminence on the posterior wall of the middle ear to the neck of the stapes. As it traverses the middle ear cavity, it lies on the posterior surface of the neck of the malleus and near the medial surface of the tympanic membrane. Innervated by nerve VII, its contraction produces stabilization of the stapes and also counteracts the inward pressure of the stapes on the oval window, which results when the tensor tympani is contracted.

Glossopharyngeal Nerve and the Middle Ear Cavity

The **glossopharyngeal nerve,** through its tympanic branch, provides general sensory innervation to the mucosa of the middle ear (see Figure 2-86). It enters the middle ear cavity through a small aperture in its floor and forms the **tympanic plexus** on the promontory of the medial wall of the middle ear. Most of the axons in the tympanic nerve are sensory and innervate the lining of the middle ear, mastoid air cells, and auditory tube. However, a small group of axons in the tympanic nerve is preganglionic parasympathetic and does *not* ramify into a plexus within the middle ear, but continues through the anterior wall of the middle ear cavity to emerge on the floor of the skull as the **lesser petrosal nerve.** This nerve travels anteromedially across the floor of the skull, enters the foramen ovale with V3, and ultimately synapses in the otic ganglion. Postganglionic axons arising in the otic ganglion, traveling with the auriculotemporal nerve, provide secretomotor innervation to the parotid gland (see Figure 2-57). This is another example of how postganglionic parasympathetic axons in the head and neck distribute with certain branches of the nerve V.

Facial Nerve and the Middle Ear Cavity

The facial nerve enters the internal auditory meatus on the medial surface of the petrous temporal bone and travels in the **facial canal,** located in the roof of the vestibule, between the cochlea and semicircular canals (see Figure 2-86). It then turns sharply in a posterior direction. Where it changes direction is located the **geniculate ganglion,** containing cell bodies of taste axons for the anterior two thirds of the tongue. These taste axons reach the tongue by eventually leaving the facial nerve as part of the *chorda tympani,* which traverses the middle ear cavity, and emerging through the petrotympanic fissure into the infratemporal fossa, where they join the *lingual nerve* to travel to the tongue.

The **geniculate ganglion** has four nerve trunks connected to it, each conveying a certain population of axons to or away from the geniculate ganglion. *First* is the body of the facial nerve itself, traveling laterally from the internal auditory meatus toward the ganglion. *Second* is the continuation of the facial nerve, which turns posteriorly away from the ganglion, traverses the temporal bone and ultimately emerges through the stylomastoid foramen. *Third* is the greater petrosal nerve, which consists of preganglionic parasympathetic axons of the facial nerve, destined to travel across the floor of the skull and ultimately to synapse in the pterygopalatine ganglion. They have no relationship to the geniculate ganglion except that they diverge from the main

---

PRINCIPLES

The ear is a most complex structure and is innervated by at least five different cranial nerves. Its complexity derives in large part from the fact that it forms from parts of the pharyngeal arches, clefts, and pouches, as well as special derivatives from both the endoderm and ectoderm of the head of the young embryo. Cranial nerves V and X supply branches that innervate the external surface of the tympanic membrane. The interior of the middle ear is innervated by nerve IX, and a major branch of nerve VII—the chorda tympani—passes through the middle ear cavity and lies on the deep surface of the tympanic membrane. The ossicles are derived from the first and second pharyngeal arches. The two small muscles attached to the ossicles, the tensor tympani and stapedius, are derived from the first and second arches, respectively, and innervated by the nerves V and VII. The auditory tube, leading from the middle ear cavity to the pharynx, is innervated by both nerves V and IX. The external auditory meatus is derived from the first pharyngeal cleft and remains innervated by the nerve of that cleft, nerve V. Nerve VIII supplies the sensory innervation to the cochlea, the true sensory portion of the ear.

THE EAR

OTITIS MEDIA

One of the most commonly diagnosed conditions in pediatrics, though less so in adult medicine, is otitis media. In otitis media, inflammation and fluid exudate are present in the middle ear cavity, producing pressure on the eardrum (and often pain) and a reduction in the movement of the ossicles.

THE AUDITORY TUBE AND OTITIS

Babies have auditory tubes which are (1) shorter than those of adults and (2) more nearly horizontal. Some believe this arrangement increases the incidence of middle ear infections in children, because pharyngeal bacteria may more easily communicate with the middle ear.

OPENINGS IN THE TYMPANIC MEMBRANE

Relief of severe otitis media is accomplished by myringotomy (L. *miringa*, a kind of membrane). This is the placement of an incision in the tympanic membrane, allowing external drainage. The incision will heal and not cause any deficit in hearing. Tears in the tympanic membrane (from infection, trauma, and so on) heal spontaneously and may not produce any effect on hearing, unless, of course, they are too large.

MASTOID INFECTIONS

Before the antibiotic era, recurrent otitis media often led to mastoiditis, necessitating surgical incision and drainage of the mastoid area.

OTITIS AND TASTE

Inflammation in the middle ear may affect the chorda tympani and alter the sense of taste.

OTITIS AND HEARING

Inadequately treated recurrent otitis media can produce impaired hearing through repeated inflammation and eventual scarring of the ossicles, limiting their ability to vibrate in response to sound.

THE STAPES AND DEAFNESS

Progressive calcification of the stapes-oval window union (otosclerosis) is a common cause of hearing loss in those of middle and older age.

INNER EAR INFECTIONS

Inflammation of the inner ear may produce a buzzing or ringing sound (**tinnitus**) when localized in the cochlea or **vertigo** (the sense of the external world moving) if centered in the semicircular canals.

MENIERE'S DISEASE

Meniere's disease is a combination of vertigo and tinnitus, thought caused by a disturbance in the normal secretion and reabsorption of fluid in the inner ear. Excessive blood levels of salicylic acid (aspirin) also characteristically produce tinnitus.

CHOLESTEATOMA

A hole in the upper part of the tympanic membrane may permit squamous epithelium from the external auditory meatus to grow into the interior of the middle ear. The keratin produced by this epithelium can form a **cholesteatoma**, a mass that can interfere with ossicular function, erode into bone, and so on.

---

body of the facial nerve near the ganglion. *Fourth* is a connecting branch to the lesser petrosal nerve, which though in contact with the geniculate ganglion is actually a branch of the glossopharyngeal nerve (see above). It represents the continuation of the tympanic nerve, containing preganglionic parasympathetic axons that "graze" the geniculate ganglion and later synapse in the otic ganglion.

As it leaves the geniculate ganglion and passes in a posterior direction, the facial nerve produces a small elevation at the junction of the roof and medial wall of the middle ear cavity. It next turns inferiorly, finally to

exit from the stylomastoid foramen on the inferior surface of the temporal bone. Before it reaches the stylomastoid foramen, however, it emits the **chorda tympani**, a small but important nerve branch that travels through the substance of the temporal bone, courses across the medial surface of the tympanic membrane, and emerges from the temporal bone through the petrotympanic fissure in the roof of the infratemporal fossa. The chorda tympani contains (1) taste axons for the anterior two thirds of the tongue, whose cell bodies are in the geniculate ganglion, and (2) preganglionic parasympathetic axons, which synapse in the submandibular ganglion and take part in secretomotor stimulation of the submandibular and sublingual salivary glands.

Blood Supply and Lymphatic Drainage of the Middle Ear Cavity

Blood supply includes branches of the maxillary, occipital, middle meningeal, ascending pharyngeal, and internal carotid arteries, which all supply the middle ear. *Venous drainage* is to the intracranial venous sinuses and the pterygoid plexus. Some remnant veins connect to the superior petrosal sinus within the cranium in children and may be a portal for production of meningitis when middle ear infections pass through unclosed sutures in the roof of the middle ear cavity in these young persons. *Lymphatic drainage* is to the parotid and retropharyngeal lymph nodes.

INNER EAR

The inner ear consists of the **membranous labyrinth** (semicircular canals and vestibule), **cochlea,** and the bony structures that surround them and mimic their shape (for example, osseous labyrinth). *Perilymph* is the clear fluid lying within the narrow space between the osseous and the membranous labyrinths and cochlea, and *endolymph* is the fluid found inside the membranous labyrinth and cochlea (Figures 2-89 and 2-91). The **semicircular** canals and **vestibule,** though not responsive to sound, respond to movement and gravitational pull by the transduction of mechanical energy (that is, waves in endolymph are transformed into neuronal membrane depolarizations and neural signals).

Vestibular Apparatus

The vestibular portion of the inner ear comprises the semicircular canals, utricle, and saccule. The **utricle** and **saccule** are two dilated sacs from which the loops of the semicircular canals originate. Endolymph flows continuously through all of these spaces. The utricle and saccule have sensory epithelia known as **maculae**. The utricle and saccule seem to respond best to static forces (for example, gravitational pull).

The **semicircular canals** are arrayed in three planes (anterior [or superior], lateral, and posterior) (Figure 2-91). Each has a dilated end (where it joins the utricle) in which is found the **crista ampullaris**, with a specialized sensory epithelium in which are found **hair cells.** The cilia that give these cells their name are activated by movements of the endolymph, and a neural signal is generated as a response. The semicircular canals seem to respond best to angular accelerations (for example, turning of head).

2.10

section two.ten

Eye and Orbit

▶ Bony Orbit

▶ Globe

▶ Eyelids and the Orbital Septum

▶ Connective Tissue and Fascia in the Orbit

▶ Muscles of the Globe and Orbit

▶ Nerve Supply of the Globe and Orbit

▶ Muscles of the Eyelids

▶ Superior Orbital Fissure and Optic Canal

▶ Lacrimal Gland and the Flow of Tears

▶ Conjunctival Membrane

▶ Vasculature of the Orbit

The eye and orbit represent an intricate and magnificently complex mechanism, the purpose of which is to protect the globe, transmit a faithful and accurate image into the globe, and position the globe so that it is directed at the appropriate part of the visual field (that is, the space at which the globe is "looking"). The **retina,** the sensory part of the eye, is itself an outgrowth of the brain. Mesenchyme on the lateral side of the developing head interacts with the developing retina to form the **lens,** the **globe,** and surrounding ligaments and fascia. The **extraocular muscles** are derived from the precervical mesodermal somites. The **walls of the orbit** are made up of contributions from several of the bones of the head. Complex fissures between these bones allow the passage of vessels and nerves in and out of the orbits. The innervation of the orbit and globe involves several of the cranial nerves—in particular, nerves II to VI.

BONY ORBIT

The orbits are often described as conical cavities with their bases at the surface of the face. Their longitudinal axis is ~23 degrees lateral to the anterior-posterior axis of the face as a whole. The globe, when we are looking at objects in the distance, face directly forward, or parallel to the anteroposterior axis of the head as a whole—that is, not parallel with the axis of the orbit.

The disparity between the visual axis of gaze and the long axis of the orbit (along which most of the extraocular muscles are aligned) accounts for much of the confusion in understanding the complex movements of the eye (Figure 2-92). The bases, or bony rims, of the orbits are circular apertures surrounding the entrance to the orbit, where the globe is located (Figure 2-93). The bony perimeter of the orbit extends farther anteriorly than the globe itself, providing the eye with protection from direct trauma anteriorly.

Walls of the Orbit

The perimeter of the orbit is composed of interlocking portions of the frontal and lacrimal bones, zygoma, and maxilla. Numerous bones interlock to form the inner walls of the orbit. The arrangement is especially complex in the medial wall, where the ethmoid, lacrimal, and palatine bones take part (Figures 2-93 and 2-94). The medial wall is characteristically thin and is referred to as the "lamina papyrecea." The roof of the orbit is also thin and is derived from the frontal bone. The lateral wall is formed by parts of the frontal zygomatic bone and greater wing of the sphenoid bone. The inferior wall is formed by the maxilla and also serves as the roof of the maxillary sinus. The orbit is bounded superiorly by the anterior fossa of the cranium, medially by the nasal cavity, inferiorly by the maxillary sinus, and laterally by the temporal fossa.

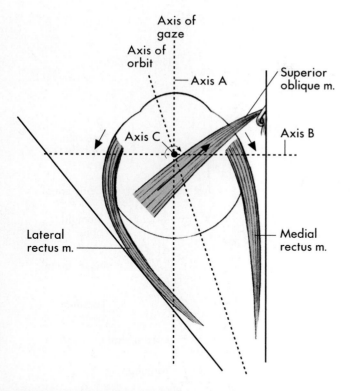

Axis of
gaze

Axis of
orbit

— Axis A

Superior
oblique m.

Axis C

Axis B

Lateral
rectus m.

Medial
rectus m.

Figure 2-92 ORBIT ANGLE OF GAZE VS. ANGLE OF ORBIT. The disparity between the long axis of orbit and the longitudinal axis of the globe accounts for much of the complexity of extraocular muscle action. *A,* Longitudinal axis of gaze; *B,* transverse axis through globe; *C,* vertical axis through globe.

The orbit is roughly in the shape of a cone, with the base facing anteriorly. The orbit narrows posteriorly to an **apex** (Figure 2-95), through which pass several important structures supplying the eye (optic and oculomotor nerves, ophthalmic artery, and so on). At the apex of the orbit are the **superior orbital fissure** and the **optic canal.** Its base faces anteriorly and forms the orbital rim. Figure 2-93 shows the composition of the orbital walls.

Three important apertures lead into the orbit from the rear (Figure 2-96). The first, the **optic canal,** transmits the optic nerve and the ophthalmic artery. The second aperture, the **superior orbital fissure,** transmits the oculomotor nerve, the trochlear nerve, branches of the V1 (ophthalmic) division of the trigeminal nerve, the abducens nerve, and the ophthalmic vein. The third aperture, the **inferior orbital fissure,** lies in the floor of the orbit. It transmits the V2 (the maxillary nerve) and certain branches of the maxillary artery. It also serves as a point of attachment for the smooth muscle of the inferior eyelid.

GLOBE

The globe is a complex structure, the role of which is to (1) *direct gaze* toward the object of interest in the visual field and (2) *transmit light* faithfully to the retina. It is equipped with mechanisms to regulate the intensity of light reaching the retina (the opening and closing of the iris) and to focus it on the retina—the process of refraction (resulting from the inherent curvature of cornea and the adjustability of the shape of the lens).

The wall of the globe consists of three layers—the external sclera (white of the eye), the intermediate choroid, and the inner retina (Figure 2-97). The **cornea** is a special clear extension of the sclera over the front of the globe, and is the most powerful refractive component in the eye. It is in the **choroid layer** that the vessels and nerves of the globe travel. The choroid layer is specialized anteriorly also to form the ciliary body and the iris. Most vessels and nerves supplying the globe enter it posteriorly and travel anteriorly toward the front of the globe in the choroid layer. The choroid, ciliary body, and iris are referred to collectively as the **uvea.** The **retina** consists of an internal sensory layer, or

CLINICAL ANATOMY OF

THE ORBIT

ORBITAL FRACTURES AND THE EYE

Fractures of the orbital walls may produce bleeding in the orbit, putting pressure on the eye and causing its protrusion (exophthalmos). When traumatic injury displaces the walls of the orbit, it is referred to as a "blowout" fracture.

ORBITAL FRACTURES AND NEARBY STRUCTURES

Whenever there is a traumatic injury to the orbit, the possibility that adjacent structures will be injured must be considered (e.g., bleeding into maxillary sinus, displacement of teeth in the upper alveolar ridge, fracture of nasal bones and subsequent airway obstruction, hemorrhage, and/or infection into cranial cavity as result of frontal bone fracture).

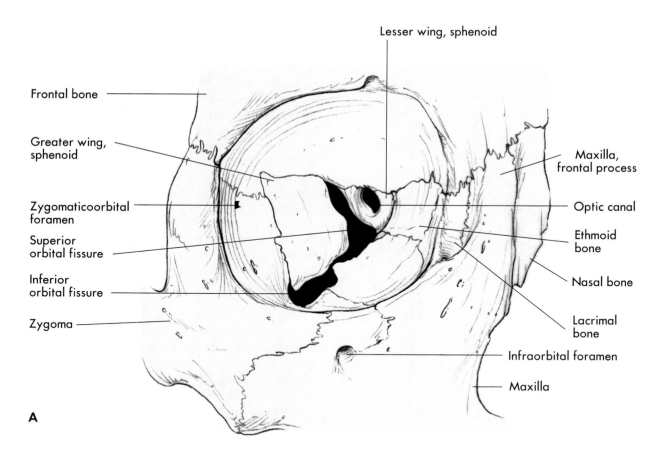

Lesser wing, sphenoid

Frontal bone

Greater wing, sphenoid

Zygomaticoorbital foramen

Superior orbital fissure

Inferior orbital fissure

Zygoma

Maxilla, frontal process

Optic canal

Ethmoid bone

Nasal bone

Lacrimal bone

Infraorbital foramen

Maxilla

A

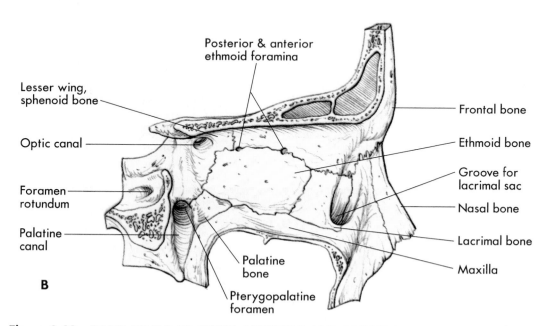

Posterior & anterior ethmoid foramina

Lesser wing, sphenoid bone

Optic canal

Foramen rotundum

Palatine canal

Frontal bone

Ethmoid bone

Groove for lacrimal sac

Nasal bone

Lacrimal bone

Maxilla

B

Palatine bone

Pterygopalatine foramen

Figure 2-93   BONY WALLS OF ORBIT, ANTERIOR AND MEDIAL VIEWS. A, Bony orbit from an anterior aspect. **B,** Medial wall of the orbit, emphasizing its relations to the anterior fossa, nasolacrimal duct, palate, and sphenoid bone.   SEE ATLAS, FIG. 2-99

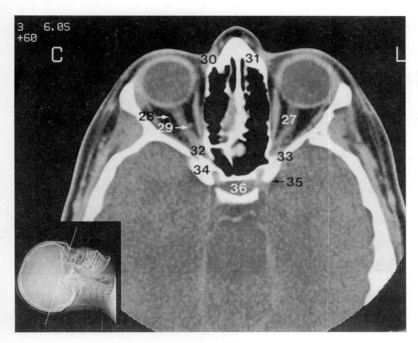

Figure 2-94 HORIZONTAL SECTION THROUGH ORBITS. CT scan through the long axis of the orbit in the horizontal plane. (From Weir J, Abrahams PH: *An imaging atlas of human anatomy,* London, 1992, Mosby.)

27 Optic nerve	**33** Superior orbital fissure
28 Long posterior ciliary artery	**34** Lesser wing of sphenoid
29 Ophthalmic artery	**35** Anterior clinoid process
30 Angular vein	**36** Pituitary gland
31 Frontal process of maxilla	
32 Optic canal	

neural retina, and a *pigment epithelium* layer located just externally to it. The retinal layer is not represented in the most anterior part of the globe, where the iris, ciliary body, and cornea are located.

Cornea

The cornea is the major refractive structure in the globe, not the lens (Figure 2-98). Visual disturbances result if the cornea has an irregular radius of curvature (*astigmatism*) or if the cornea is cloudy because of scarring or inflammation (which sometimes necessitates a transplant). Corneal lubrication (accomplished by blinking) is crucial to prevent scarring and visual loss.

Iris

Between the cornea and the lens is the iris (shaped like a flattened doughnut), the circular central aperture of which (the pupillary aperture) can widen or narrow to regulate light entry (Figure 2-99). The iris contains smooth muscle, one portion of which is arranged in a circular fashion and the other arranged radially. The former functions as a sphincter (the **sphincter pupillae,** innervated by parasympathetic nerves) and the latter as a dilator (the **dilator pupillae,** innervated by sympathetic nerves) (see Figure 2-98).

Testing of these muscles (by shining or withdrawing a light in the eye and observing changes in pupillary size—the *light reflex*) is frequently carried out as part of an evaluation of overall integrity of the brainstem. The

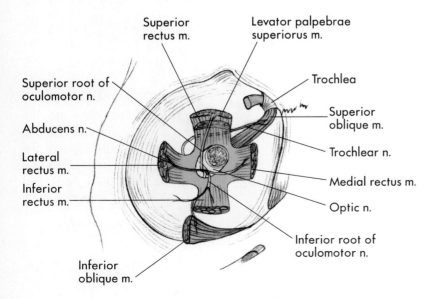

Figure 2-95 DETAIL OF APEX OF ORBIT. A fibrous ring surrounds the optic nerve as it enters the orbit and gives rise to the four rectus muscles that attach to the globe further anteriorly. Branches of cranial nerves, oculomotor (III), trochlear (IV), and abducens (VI), are also seen entering the orbit.

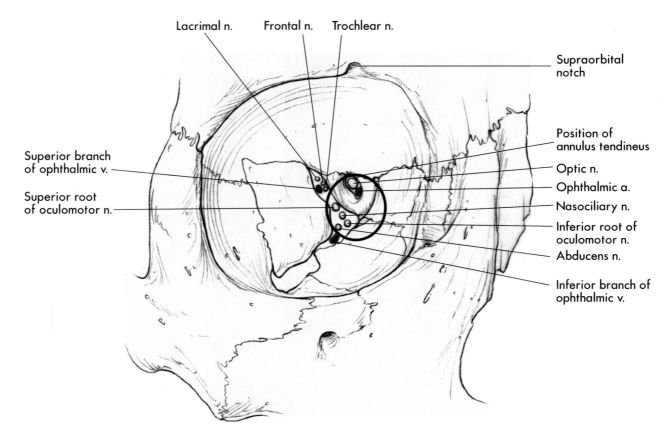

Figure 2-96 CROSS-SECTION THROUGH SUPERIOR ORBITAL FISSURE AND OPTIC CANAL. Structures entering the orbit are positioned in a highly structured way as they traverse the superior orbital fissure.

light reflex involves neural pathways and nuclei in the mesencephalon, pons, and medulla—all three major regions of the brainstem. In cases of suspected brain injury, for example, if these reflexes are impaired, we may infer that significant brainstem injury has occurred.

Lens

The lens is a thick, biconvex disk suspended from the ciliary body of the uveal layer by a series of 75 to 85 individual fibers, collectively known as the **ciliary zonule** (see Figure 2-98). The lens is flattened by the normal tension with which these fibers attach around the

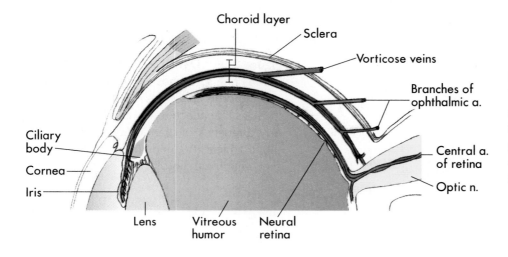

Figure 2-97 UVEAL LAYER OF THE EYE. Shown here are the several vessels and nerves that travel in the middle layer of the globe, the uvea. It is composed of the choroid, ciliary body, and iris.   SEE ATLAS, FIGS. 2-112, 2-114

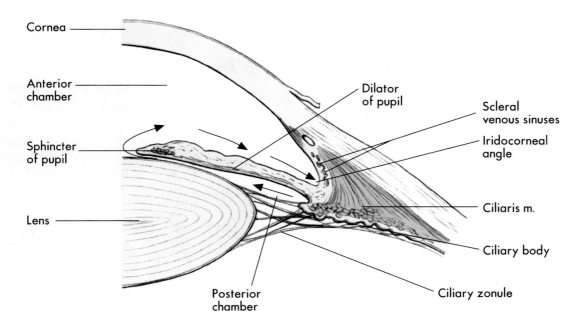

Figure 2-98 DETAIL OF CILIARY BODY AND LENS. The lens is suspended from a radially arranged series of thin fibers known as the ciliary zonule. The iris lies just anteriorly to the lens. The iris surrounds the pupil, which can be made larger or smaller by the contraction of the dilator or sphincter muscles. The anterior chamber lies between the iris and cornea. Aqueous humor originates near the ciliary body and is deposited into the posterior chamber. It drifts into the anterior chamber and then is reabsorbed into venous sinuses located in the iridocorneal angle. SEE ATLAS, FIG. 2-115

margin of the lens to the ciliary body. When the circular smooth muscle (the ciliaris) of the ciliary body contracts, the tension on the lens is relaxed. The lens then becomes more nearly spherical, making viewing of close objects possible. This process is known as *accommodation.* With age, as the lens loses its inherent elasticity, it fails to become as nearly spherical as it does in youth, and we have trouble seeing those near objects (referred to as *presbyopia;* Gr. *presbyos,* old) (Figure 2-100). With age, the lens also has a tendency to develop opacities, or *cataracts,* a common cause of blindness.

Aqueous and Vitreous Humors

The space between the cornea and the lens is filled with **aqueous humor** (Figure 2-101). Aqueous humor is produced by the ciliary body, through a filtration mechanism involving the blood vessels in the area. It is then released into the **posterior chamber** (the space between the lens and the iris). It then circulates into the **anterior chamber** (the space between the iris and the cornea), where it is reabsorbed through the venous sinuses (at the iridocorneal angle) and into the bloodstream. If its flow is interrupted or if production exceeds reabsorp-

tion, pressure builds up, leading to the condition known as *glaucoma.* The production and flow of aqueous humor resembles that of cerebrospinal fluid, because it is a filtrate of capillary blood that circulates

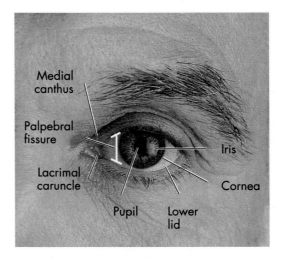

Figure 2-99 ANTERIOR VIEW OF THE EYE: THE PUNCTA AND CONJUNCTIVAL MEMBRANE.

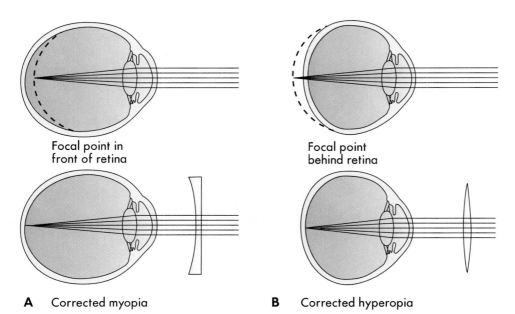

Focal point in
front of retina

A   Corrected myopia

Focal point
behind retina

B   Corrected hyperopia

Figure 2-100   REFRACTIVE ER-RORS IN VISION. A, Myopia is corrected by a concave lens. **B,** Hyperopia is corrected by a bi-convex lens. These visual problems are the result of the visual image being focused in front of (myopia) or posterior to (hyperopia) the retina.

through a set of spaces and is eventually reabsorbed back into venous blood.

Posterior to the lens is a gelatinous **vitreous humor,** posterior to which is the retina. The source of the vitreous material is not clearly known, but it is assumed to be a product of cells lining the posterior chamber. If the aqueous humor is under excess pressure (for example, from glaucoma), the pressure can be transmitted posteriorly and deprive the retina of blood supply, causing retinal ischemia and risking eventual blindness.

Visual Signal Transmission and the Retina

Light from the environment passes through the cornea and enters the interior of the eye, where both the aqueous and vitreous humors have a higher refractive index than that of the water or air. This change in refractive index bends the light rays, as does their passage through both the cornea and the lens. The cornea produces the single greatest refractive change in the entering light, but it is the lens that is adjustable, through its own intrinsic resiliency and the action of the ciliaris muscle. In mammals and birds, the design of the eye is such that it is naturally focused at infinity (defined as greater than 20-foot distance). The capability to change the shape of the lens by muscle action allows us to focus on both near and distance objects. In mammals, the ciliaris muscle is smooth muscle histologically, meaning its responses are relatively slow. In reptiles and birds, the ciliaris is striated muscle and can adapt to changes in distance much more rapidly.

Visual signal transmission begins at the **neural retina,** lining the inner surface of the posterior wall of the globe. Light stimulates receptor cells, and the depolar-

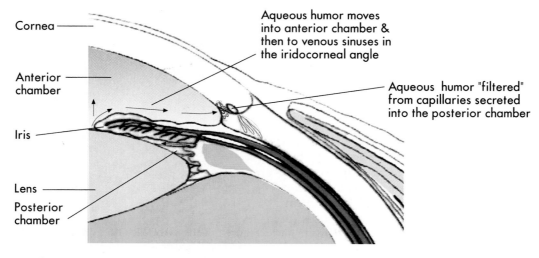

Cornea

Anterior
chamber

Iris

Lens

Posterior
chamber

Aqueous humor moves
into anterior chamber &
then to venous sinuses in
the iridocorneal angle

Aqueous humor "filtered"
from capillaries secreted
into the posterior chamber

Figure 2-101   FLOW OF AQUEOUS AND VITREOUS HUMORS.   SEE ATLAS, FIG. 2-115

ization produced activates the retinal ganglion cells. Ganglion cell axons travel across the retina and converge to form the **optic nerve,** emerging from the posterior surface of each globe, slightly to the medial side of the midline. These optic nerves then travel backward and form an **optic chiasma** (crossing) with each other at the base of the hypothalamus. The majority of the optic nerve axons then enters the thalamus (specifically the lateral geniculate nucleus [LGN]), where they synapse. Neural pathways leave the LGN and convey visual input to the cerebral cortex, particularly in the occipital region.

The retina has a relatively tenuous blood supply. Its only significant source of blood is the **central artery of the retina** (Figure 2-102), which enters the orbit through a small aperture known as the optic canal. The neural retina has direct contact with the gelatinous vitreous body. In embryonic life, there is an artery running in the anteroposterior direction through the vitreous body—the **hyaloid artery.** Occasionally, it persists into postnatal life and can obstruct vision.

EYELIDS AND THE ORBITAL SEPTUM

The gap between the free margins of the upper and lower lids (that is, the opening between the lids) is the **palpebral fissure** (see Figure 2-99). There is a medial

and lateral **canthus** (Gr. *kanthos,* corner) at the margins of the fissure. A medial canthus with a large and prominent superior fold (epicanthal fold) is characteristic in those of Asian/Native American descent. In others, the upper and lower medial folds do not overlap and are equal in size. For reasons probabily related to the smallness of the nasal bones and lower lid, people with trisomy 21, regardless of their ethnic background, have prominent medial superior epicanthal folds.

The upper and lower eyelids (**palpebrae**) are covered externally by squamous epithelium and lined internally by *conjunctiva* (a thin, moist mucous membrane). In the substance of the eyelid is a scant amount of connective tissue and fat, smooth muscle (both lids), a firm and thin quadrangular fibrous *tarsal plate* (both lids), a thin layer of striated muscle, the orbicularis oculi (both lids), and the levator palpebrae superioris (found in the upper lid only).

Along the free margins of the upper and lower lids are small apertures for the modified sebaceous (**tarsal** or **meibomian**) **glands** and modified sweat glands. There are also numerous **eyelashes,** in the free margin of both the upper and lower lids. The sebaceous secretions of the meibomian glands form a thin, oily film on the sclera and cornea and probably help to (1) lessen evaporative loss of tears and (2) prevent overflow of tears across the lower lid margin.

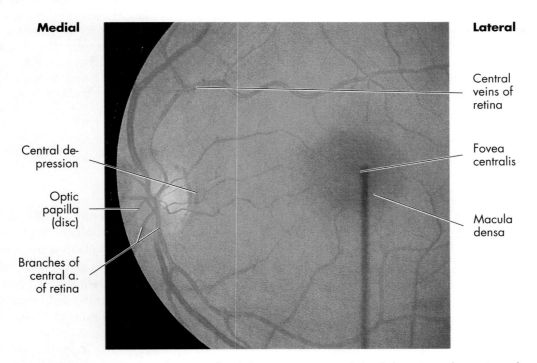

Medial   **Lateral**

Central veins of retina

Central depression

Fovea centralis

Optic papilla (disc)

Branches of central a. of retina

Macula densa

Figure 2-102 RETINA. Photograph of the appearance of the left retina when viewed through the ophthalmoscope. The macula is the area of greatest visual acuity and is unique in that no blood vessels cross it. The optic disc is the point where the optic nerve leaves the retina. (From Chumbley CC, Hutchings RT: *Color atlas of human dissection,* London, 1992, Mosby.) SEE ATLAS, FIGS. 2-113, 2-116

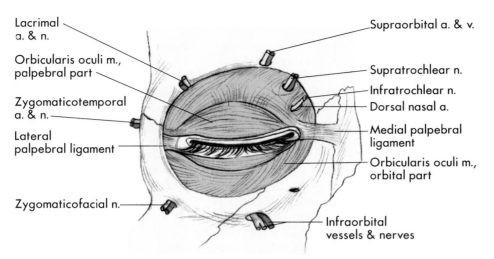

Lacrimal a. & n.

Orbicularis oculi m., palpebral part

Zygomaticotemporal a. & n.

Lateral palpebral ligament

Zygomaticofacial n.

Supraorbital a. & v.

Supratrochlear n.

Infratrochlear n.

Dorsal nasal a.

Medial palpebral ligament

Orbicularis oculi m., orbital part

Infraorbital vessels & nerves

Figure 2-103 PALPEBRAL MUS-CLES, VESSELS, AND NERVES. Here the skin has been removed from the anterior surface of the eyelids, revealing the palpebral and orbital parts of the orbicularis oculi muscle. The palpebral ligaments help hold the globe in place on its medial and lateral sides. Various terminal branches of V1, V2, ophthalmic, and maxillary arteries reach the anterior surface near the globe.
Sᴇᴇ Aᴛʟᴀs, Fɪɢs. 2-102, 2-103, 2-104

The lateral ends of the tarsal plates are attached by a **lateral palpebral ligament** to a tubercle on the zygoma, and the medial ends of the tarsal plates are joined by a strong **medial palpebral ligament** to the lacrimal bone, in the medial orbital wall (Figures 2-103 and 2-108). The proximal margins of the tarsal plates in both eyelids attach by a thin membrane to the inner margin of the orbital wall (except where the medial and lateral palpebral ligaments attach the lid to the bony orbital wall). This circumferential curtain is known as the **orbital septum.** Infections anterior to the plane of the orbital septum are said to be in the *periorbital area.* Because of the presence of the orbital septum, such periorbital infections are said to pose little danger of spreading posteriorly and causing injury to the eye. However, infections posterior to the orbital septum (or-

bital infections) do pose a risk to the eye. They require urgent attention.

CONNECTIVE TISSUE AND FASCIA IN THE ORBIT

A posterior enveloping layer of fascia (**Tenon's fascia**) covers the globe from the optic nerve root forward to near the corneal-scleral junction (Figure 2-104). This fascia splits to enclose the four rectus muscles. Extensions of these fascial envelopments from the medial and lateral rectus muscles to the lateral and medial orbital walls (respectively) form the so-called **"check" ligaments** (Figure 2-104). These are thought to limit the actions of these two muscles, though some dispute their function altogether. Tenon's fascia is especially

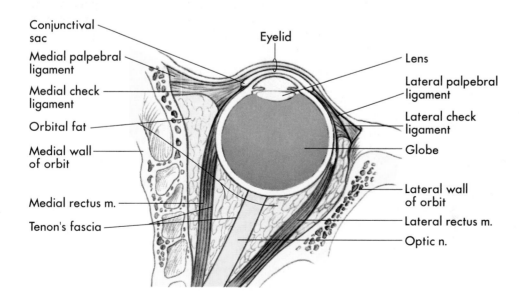

Conjunctival sac

Medial palpebral ligament

Medial check ligament

Orbital fat

Medial wall of orbit

Medial rectus m.

Tenon's fascia

Eyelid

Lens

Lateral palpebral ligament

Lateral check ligament

Globe

Lateral wall of orbit

Lateral rectus m.

Optic n.

Figure 2-104 ORBIT, HORI-ZONTAL SECTION. The orbit contains a considerable amount of fat, in which the orbital muscles, nerves, and vessels are suspended. Medial and lateral ligaments help suspend the globe from the rims of the orbit.
Sᴇᴇ ATLAS, Fɪɢ. 2-109

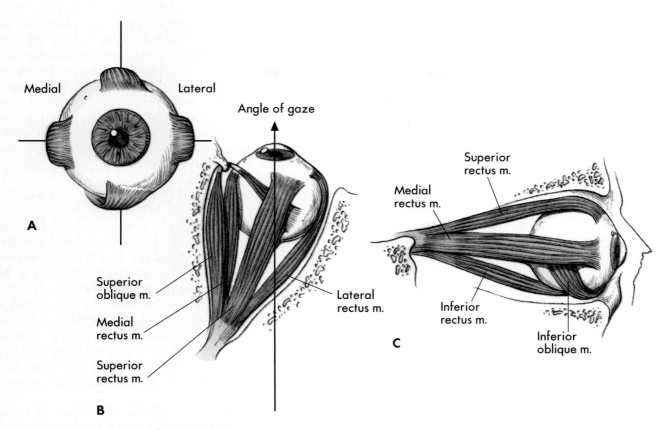

Figure 2-105 EXTRAOCULAR MUSCLES. A, Anterior view. **B,** Superior view. **C,** Lateral view. SEE ATLAS, FIGS. 2-107, 2-108, 2-109

thick underneath the globe, where it forms a sort of suspensory "sling." The orbit contains a great deal of fat, which presumably serves as a buffer, minimizing acceleration-related injuries to which the eye might be subjected when the head moves rapidly and forcefully.

MUSCLES OF THE GLOBE AND ORBIT

Both striated and smooth muscles are found in this area. Involuntary muscular action is important in several activities, such as regular lubrication of the cornea by blinking and closing the eyelids when an approaching object might strike the eye.

The *extraocular striated muscles* attaching to the eye are responsible for the positioning of the globe (Figure 2-105). They are six in number, *two oblique* and *four rectus* (L. *rectum*, straight) muscles. A seventh muscle—the *levator palpebrae superioris* (see following)—is usually described along with the extraocular muscles, though this muscle moves the upper eyelid, not the globe. The **four rectus muscles** insert on the sides of the globe anterior to its midsection. They all originate from the common tendinous ring (at the apex of the orbital

pyramid). The common flexor ring encloses the optic canal and the central part of the superior orbital fissure. The lateral and medial muscles extend toward the globe in only one plane (horizontal), but the actions of the superior and inferior recti are made complex by the disparity between the angle at which these muscles approach the globe and the visual axis of the globe itself (see Figure 2-92). The lateral rectus abducts the globe, the

Table 2-19   Muscles and Movements of the Globe

Movement	Muscle(s) Involved
Elevation	Superior rectus, inferior oblique
Depression	Inferior rectus, superior oblique
Abduction	Lateral rectus, inferior and superior oblique
Adduction	Medial rectus, inferior and superior rectus
Medial rotation ("intorsion")	Superior rectus, superior oblique
Lateral rotation ("extorsion")	Inferior rectus, inferior oblique

medial rectus adducts it, and both muscles act exclusively in the horizontal plane. The superior rectus elevates, adducts, and medially rotates the globe. The inferior rectus depresses, adducts, and laterally rotates the globe (see Table 2-19).

The **superior oblique muscle** arises on the sphenoid bone just outside the common flexor ring, on its medial side, and narrows to a tendon as it passes anteriorly through a trochlea at the superomedial portion of the orbit (the trochlea creates a pulleylike mechanism, causing the eventual direction of pull on the globe created by contraction of the superior oblique to be anteromedial, though the muscle originates posteriorly to the globe). After passing through this trochlea, the muscle inserts on the dorsal surface of the globe, deep to the insertion of the superior rectus. The superior oblique inserts on the posterolateral quadrant of the globe (viewing the globe from above). The superior oblique depresses, abducts, and medially rotates the globe.

The **inferior oblique muscle** extends from the floor of the orbit to the undersurface of the globe. It inserts on the posterolateral quadrant (when viewing the globe from below). The angle at which it pulls is parallel to that of the superior oblique. This muscle elevates, abducts, and laterally rotates the globe. The inferior oblique muscle, similar to the superior oblique, does not originate from the common tendinous ring (while the four rectus muscles do).

Just as in the case of the disparity between the axis of the orbit and the axis of gaze, the extraocular muscles approach the globe from an angle different than the axis of gaze (the anteroposterior axis of the globe itself; see Figure 2-105, B). Four of the six extraocular muscles approach the globe from the posterior apex of the orbit and therefore run parallel to the axis of the orbit itself (the remaining two extraocular muscles approach the globe from an oblique angle). This causes the muscles to pull on the globe at an angle not parallel to the axis of the globe itself, leading to the multiple actions described for each of the individual muscles.

Modern techniques of visualization are capable of resolving the individual extraocular muscles (see Figure 2-94) and allow the clinician to identify the location of tumors or other disease processes that may be putting pressure on the contents of the orbit.

NERVE SUPPLY OF THE GLOBE AND ORBIT

Innervation of the Extraocular Muscles

The **oculomotor nerve (III)** exits the brainstem ventrally, emerging between the posterior cerebral artery and the superior cerebellar artery. It travels anteriorly in the wall of the cavernous sinus (see Figure 2-26), then divides into its superior and inferi-

or roots as it passes through the superior orbital fissure. These two roots pass through the center of the common tendinous ring (see Figure 2-96), with the superior root lying somewhat superior to the inferior root. The **superior root of the oculomotor nerve** supplies the superior rectus and the levator palpebrae superioris muscles; the **inferior root** (Figure 2-106, B) supplies the rest of those muscles innervated by the oculomotor nerve (the medial and inferior rectus; inferior oblique) and in addition carries parasympathetic axons (see following).

The **trochlear nerve (IV)** has a peculiar origin on the dorsal surface of the upper brainstem (Figure 2-106, A). The nerve arches from dorsal to ventral, around the lateral surface of the brainstem, and lies imbedded in the dural margin of the tentorial notch as it travels toward the orbit. It next becomes embedded in the walls of the cavernous sinus, joining the oculomotor and abducent nerves in doing so. Similar to the oculomotor nerve, it enters the orbit through the superior orbital fissure, but above and outside the common tendinous ring. Once in the orbit, its sole purpose is to innervate the superior oblique muscle, on the superior surface of which it lies. It innervates no other muscle and carries no sensory axons.

The **abducens nerve (VI)** also innervates only one muscle, the lateral rectus, and carries no sensory axons. It first emerges from the ventral surface of the brainstem at the junction of the medulla and pons. The nerve runs anteriorly, embedded in the dura of the floor of the skull (see Figures 2-6 and 2-26), toward the cavernous sinus and the superior orbital fissure. Entering the superior orbital fissure, within the common tendinous ring, the nerve deviates to the lateral side of the orbit and becomes embedded in the substance of the lateral rectus muscle.

The oculomotor, trochlear, and abducens nerves are classified as *somatic motor*, because they innervate striated musculature of the head and/or trunk derived from somites, masses of mesoderm located embryologically along the axis of the body and in the region of the head (it is from the head somites that these muscles are derived). In addition, the oculomotor nerve carries with it some parasympathetic axons in its inferior root (see following). Most of the striated muscles in the head and neck (for example, muscles of the face, cheek, jaw, and anterior neck) are derived from mesoderm of the pharyngeal arches and are designed as *branchiomotor* for that reason. The only other muscles that are derived from somites are the intrinsic musculature of the tongue, innervated by nerve XII.

The pattern of innervation of the extraocular muscles is easily remembered according to the following "formula":

$$LR_6(SO_4)_3$$

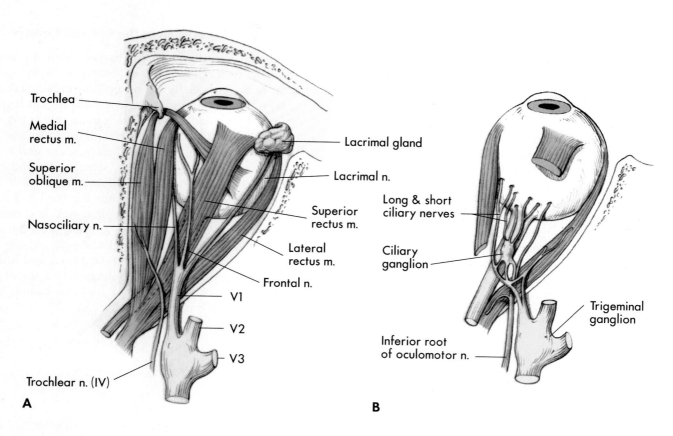

Trochlea

Medial rectus m.

Superior oblique m.

Nasociliary n.

Lacrimal gland

Lacrimal n.

Superior rectus m.

Lateral rectus m.

Frontal n.

V1

V2

V3

Trochlear n. (IV)

A

Long & short ciliary nerves

Ciliary ganglion

Inferior root of oculomotor n.

Trigeminal ganglion

B

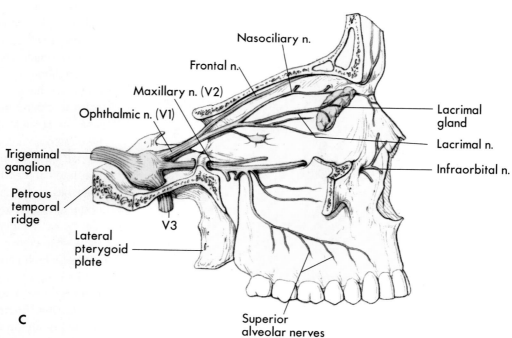

Nasociliary n.

Frontal n.

Maxillary n. (V2)

Ophthalmic n. (V1)

Trigeminal ganglion

Petrous temporal ridge

Lateral pterygoid plate

V3

Lacrimal gland

Lacrimal n.

Infraorbital n.

Superior alveolar nerves

C

Figure 2-106 NERVES OF THE ORBIT. A, Superior view. This view shows the distribution of the ophthalmic nerve and trochlear nerve in the orbit. **B,** Removal of the superior muscles shows the ciliary ganglion, positioned between the lateral rectus muscle and the optic nerve. **C,** Position of the maxillary nerve in the floor of the orbit and a view of the lateral wall of the orbit. SEE ATLAS, FIGS. 2-105, 2-106, 2-107, 2-108, 2-111

That is, the lateral rectus muscle is innervated by nerve VI, the superior oblique muscle by nerve IV, and all of the others are innervated by nerve III.

Parasympathetic Innervation of the Eye and Orbit

The **inferior root of the oculomotor nerve** conveys *preganglionic parasympathetic axons* to the ciliary ganglion, located posterior to the globe and just lateral to the optic nerve. Here, the preganglionic parasympathetic axons synapse. *Postganglionic axons* arising in the ciliary ganglion travel with the short ciliary nerves into the uvea and reach the ciliaris muscle and the pupillary constrictor. The ciliaris muscle, when it constricts, produces an increase in the spherical shape of the lens, resulting in clarity of focus on near objects (called accommodation). The pupillary constrictor causes a narrowing of the aperture of the iris.

Sympathetic Innervation of the Eye and Orbit

Postganglionic sympathetic nerves derived from the carotid plexus join various branches of the ophthalmic nerve, especially the nasociliary nerve, and accompany them to the globe and orbital region in the long and short ciliary nerves. Their main role is to regulate resistance of the vasculature in these areas and to stimulate secretion of sweat on the face, scalp, and neck (sudoriferous activity; L. *sudoris*, sweat). Sympathetic activity also produces pupillary dilation (Figure 2-107).

Preganglionic sympathetic axons for the head and neck arise in the upper thoracic spinal cord and travel upward in the sympathetic chain to synapse in the superior and middle cervical ganglia. Axons arising in these ganglia form a plexus on the external and internal carotid arteries and their branches and travel to various regions of the head and neck, including the vasculature of the brain itself.

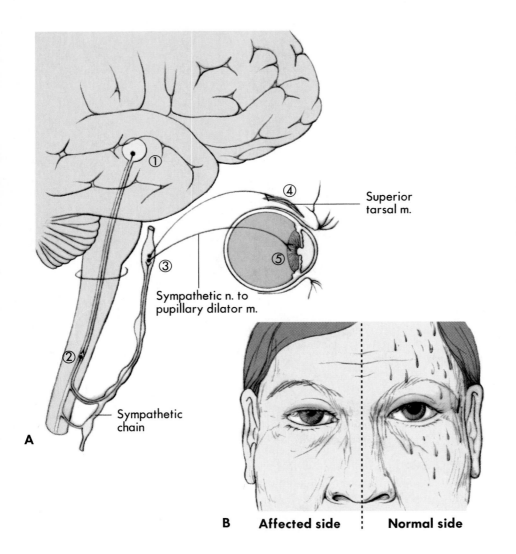

A

Superior tarsal m.

Sympathetic n. to pupillary dilator m.

Sympathetic chain

B   **Affected side** : **Normal side**

Figure 2-107 SYMPATHETIC INNERVATION IN THE ORBIT. A, Sympathetic impulses, originating in the brain (*1*), traveling down to the upper thoracic spinal cord (*2*). The preganglionic sympathetic axon originates here, travels up the sympathetic chain, and synapses in the superior cervical ganglion (*3*). From here the postganglionic axon travels, as part of a sympathetic plexus on the internal carotid artery and its branches, to the tarsal muscle of the upper eyelid (*4*) and the dilator muscle (*5*) of the pupil. **B,** The set of signs characteristic of Horner's syndrome, which can result when sympathetic input anywhere along the pathway from 1 to 4 and 5 is interrupted. The abnormalities are a constricted pupil, an absence of sweating (anhydrosis), and a drooping of the eyelid (ptosis).

Testing of the many reflexes mediated by cranial nerves affords an unparalleled opportunity for assessment of the status of the brainstem and cranial nerves I to XII. The eye in particular is the location of a variety of different responses that can be impaired when the brainstem is not functioning normally. The **corneal reflex** involves a sensory signal, generated by touching the cornea and conveyed through the ophthalmic nerve, and a blink response mediated by the facial nerve. The **pupillary reflex** (or light reaction) involves constriction of the pupil when an increased degree of light is shone upon the eye. It involves the optic nerve as a sensory nerve and the oculomotor nerve for the motor response. The **accommodation reflex** is an increase in the spherical quality of the lens, pupillary constriction, and medial deviation of both eyes (convergence). It involves the optic nerve (sensory) and the oculomotor nerve (motor). When the position of the head is rapidly changed (stimulating the vestibular system) or when an artificial stimulation is delivered to the vestibular system by placing warm or cool water in the external auditory canals ("fooling" the brain into responding as though the head were actually moving), the eyes move rhythmically from side to side. These are known as the **oculocephalic and oculovestibular reflexes,** respectively. Both involve synchronized contraction of several of the extraocular muscles.

These reflexes are commonly used in medicine to assess the status of the brainstem in the severely injured unconscious patient. The presence or absence of these reflexes also may figure in decisions about brain death in badly-injured patients.

Ophthalmic Nerve (the V1 Branch of the Trigeminal Nerve)

This nerve is entirely sensory. Though it is the smallest of the three branches of the trigeminal nerve, it innervates the globe, orbital tissues, lacrimal gland, conjunctival sac, parts of the scalp and forehead, and parts of both the inside and outside surfaces of the nose. Its cell bodies lie in the trigeminal ganglion, situated along the medial surface of the petrous temporal ridge (Figures 2-106, A and C). Axons of V1 leave the ganglion and travel anteriorly in the wall of the cavernous sinus in a position inferior to the oculomotor and trochlear nerves (see Figure 2-37). Before passing through the superior orbital fissure, it divides into the three major branches detailed below. The *lacrimal* and *frontal nerves*

pass outside the common tendinous ring (annulus tendineus), while the *nasociliary nerve* lies within it.

The first and most superficial branch, lying above the levator palpebrae superioris, is the **frontal nerve** (Figure 2-106, C). It divides early into the **supratrochlear** and **supraorbital nerves;** they supply the forehead and anterior scalp. The supratrochlear nerve passes just above the trochlea of the superior oblique muscle and then turns upward on to the forehead and scalp. The supraorbital nerve runs parallel to it and exits through the upper rim of the orbit through the supraorbital fissure. It also supplies the forehead and scalp.

The second and most medial branch of the ophthalmic nerve, the **nasociliary nerve** (Figure 2-106, C), innervates the globe and ethmoid air cells and terminates as several **internal** and **external nasal branches,** supplying the nasal mucosa, nares, and external surface of the tip of the nose. After entering the orbit, the nasociliary nerve courses forward toward the medial side of the orbital cavity, passing superiorly to the optic nerve. The two to four *long ciliary nerves* are early branches of the nasociliary nerve. They convey sensory axons to the globe (and travel in its uveal layer after penetrating the external scleral coat). In addition, the long ciliary nerves convey postganglionic sympathetic axons that innervate the dilator pupillae.

The continuation of the nasociliary nerve, now known as the **anterior ethmoidal nerve,** turns superomedially and leaves the orbital cavity through the ethmoid bone to enter the cranial cavity. It then runs forward on the cribiform plate of the ethmoid bone and then reverses its direction and once again descends through a small aperture just lateral to the crista galli into the interior of the nose. It innervates the mucosa of the upper part of the nose, and a small branch—the **external nasal nerve**—emerges on to the surface of the nose and travels downward to its tip. The anterior ethmoidal nerve is one of the few that enter the cranial cavity and then leave it again before reaching the structures or regions it innervates; the spinal root of the accessory nerve is another example.

The **lacrimal nerve,** third branch of the ophthalmic nerve, runs on the lateral side of the orbit as it conveys sensory axons to the lacrimal gland (Figure 2-106, A). It also carries postganglionic parasympathetic axons whose cell bodies are in the pterygopalatine ganglion. These travel with a branch of V2 (the zygomaticotemporal nerve), innervate the lacrimal gland, and cause lacrimation.

The **ciliary ganglion** (Figure 2-106, B) is a cluster of postganglionic parasympathetic neuron cell bodies and is an important neural element of the orbit. It is located in the center of the orbital cavity, positioned between the lateral rectus muscle and the optic nerve. These neurons receive preganglionic input from the parasympathetic component of the inferior root of the oculomotor nerve. After a synapse occurs in the ciliary ganglion, postganglionic parasympathetic axons leave the ganglion and travel toward the globe as part of the *short ciliary nerves,* of which there are normally five to eight. They are accompanied by sensory axons derived from the nasociliary nerve. These nerves penetrate the sclera near the optic nerve head. The contained parasympathetic axons then enter the uveal layer and travel anteriorly to innervate the **sphincter pupillae** (for pupillary constriction) and the **ciliaris muscle** (for changes in shape of the lens—accommodation).

The short ciliary nerves are thus composed in part of sensory branches of the nasociliary nerve, which travel forward and appear to pass through the ciliary ganglion. The sensory axons here are joined by the postganglionic parasympathetic axons that arise in the ciliary ganglion and convey them to the uveal layer of the globe and finally to the sphincter pupillae and ciliaris muscles. The short ciliary nerves also carry postganglionic sympathetic axons for the globe and its contents, particularly for the dilator pupillae muscle. The long and short ciliary nerves are compared in Table 2-20.

MUSCLES OF THE EYELIDS

The **levator palpebrae superioris** originates above the common tendinous ring and extends forward to insert into the upper eyelid. It has two layers or *lamellae,* one inserting on to the superior tarsal plate and the other to the skin of the eyelid. The muscle lies dorsally to the superior rectus and is innervated by the oculomotor nerve. Its action is to assist in elevation of the upper lid.

The inferior lamella of the levator palpebrae superioris contains smooth muscle fibers, which are also known as the **superior tarsal muscle** (of Müller). It is innervated by sympathetic nerves and helps to elevate the upper eyelid. Generalized injury to the sympathetic

nerves in various parts of the body and are difficult to detect. One of the more reliable signs, however, is the drooping of the upper eyelid, or *ptosis* (Figure 2-107, *B*), which results when the sympathetic nerve supply to the superior tarsal muscle is interrupted. In the lower eyelid is a similar layer of smooth muscle, also innervated by sympathetic nerves. Its muscle fibers attach to the inferior tarsal plate of the lower lid.

SUPERIOR ORBITAL FISSURE AND OPTIC CANAL

A variety of vascular and neural structures pass through the superior orbital fissure. The fissure is shaped like a widened letter "V" turned on its side, so that the "point" of the V faces medially. The fissure is bounded laterally by the greater wing of the sphenoid bone and medially by its lesser wing. The superior orbital fissure is continuous with the inferior orbital fissure, in the floor of the orbit (see Figure 2-96). Starting most superiorly and moving in an inferior direction, the structures in the superior orbital fissure are positioned in the following order, from most superior to most inferior:

- Lacrimal nerve
- Frontal nerve
- Superior ophthalmic vein
- Trochlear nerve
- Oculomotor nerve, superior root
- Nasociliary nerve
- Oculomotor nerve, inferior root
- Abducens nerve
- Inferior ophthalmic vein

Just medial to the "V" of the superior orbital fissure is the **optic canal,** a separate aperture in the sphenoid bone, through which pass the *optic nerve* and the *ophthalmic artery.* The *common tendinous ring (annulus tendineus)* is a circular ring of connective tissue that is positioned so that it surrounds all of the optic canal and the most medial portion of the superior orbital fissure. It serves as an origin for the four rectus muscles of the globe (medial, lateral, superior, and inferior). The supe-

Table 2-20   The Ciliary Nerves and the Globe

Long Ciliary Nerves	Short Ciliary Nerves
Arise as 4 to 8 slender branches of the nasociliary branch of V1	Arise as 8 to 12 short filaments appearing to travel from ciliary ganglion to back of globe (the nerves actually arise from the nasociliary branch of V1)
Are general sensory for most of globe, plus postganglionic sympathetic axons for innervation of dilator pupillae	Are postganglionic parasympathetic, for ciliaris and sphincter pupillae, plus some postganglionic sympathetic and sensory (proprioception for the extraocular muscles)
Pierce sclera and travel in uvea	Pierce sclera and travel in uvea

rior oblique and levator palpebrae superiorus muscles originate directly from the bone of the lesser sphenoid wing, just above the tendinous ring; the inferior oblique muscle originates more anteriorly, from the floor of the orbit.

This **common tendinous ring** (see Figure 2-96) surrounds a space through which pass all but four of the vessels and nerves supplying the orbit; only the lacrimal, frontal, and trochlear nerves and the superior and inferior ophthalmic veins lie outside. Thus, if the orbit is seen as a cone, then the tendinous ring surrounds the narrow circular aperture into the apex of the cone, through which pass the majority of the vessels and nerves supplying the orbit. The four rectus muscles originate from this same tendinous ring, while the two oblique muscles and the levator palpebrae superioris are not attached to it.

LACRIMAL GLAND AND THE FLOW OF TEARS

The **lacrimal gland** lies superolateral to the globe (Figure 2-106, *A*). It is bilobed and wraps itself around the lateral margin of the levator palpebrae superioris. The larger **orbital lobe** is superficial to the muscle and the smaller **palpebral lobe** deep to it (in a fashion similar to the submandibular gland, which has lobes both deep and superficial to the mylohyoid muscle). The

lacrimal gland "rests" in a small fossa on the inner surface of the zygoma. The lacrimal gland empties via 10 to 15 small ducts into the recess in the conjunctival sac between the upper lid and the globe (called the **superior fornix**). Ducts originating in the orbital lobe empty tears into the ducts originating into the palpebral lobe. Thus all tears eventually drain through the ducts of the palpebral lobe into the superior fornix. Tears stream from these ducts into the superior fornix and then across the cornea to collect at the medial canthus.

At the medial end of the upper and lower lid margins, there is an elevated structure known as the **lacrimal caruncle** (see Figure 2-108). At the medial end of the upper and lower lid is a pair of raised structures, the **lacrimal puncta.** A hole in the apex of each of these puncta is the entrance to the two **lacrimal ducts,** structures about 9 to 10 mm in length. After tears flow through these two canaliculi, they collect in a **lacrimal sac** (Figure 2-108). Blinking the eyelids creates suction in this sac and helps draw tears out of the palpebral fissure and across the cornea into the lacrimal sac. The lacrimal sac is nestled into the **lacrimal fossa,** located at the medial end of the orbit between the lacrimal bone and the maxilla. The lacrimal sac drains inferiorly, via the **nasolacrimal duct,** into the nose, beneath the inferior concha in the lateral wall of the nose.

Secretomotor innervation to the lacrimal gland arises in the pterygopalatine ganglion and reaches the

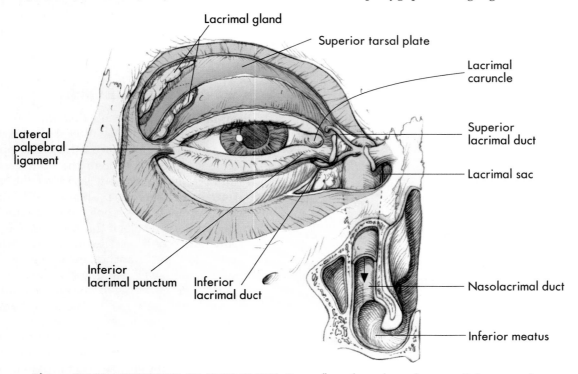

Figure 2-108 PATHWAY OF TEAR FLOW. Tears flow from lateral to medial across the front of the eye and collect in the *superior* and *inferior lacrimal ducts* into the *lacrimal sac* and thence to the *nasolacrimal duct.* SEE ATLAS, FIGS. 2-100, 2-101

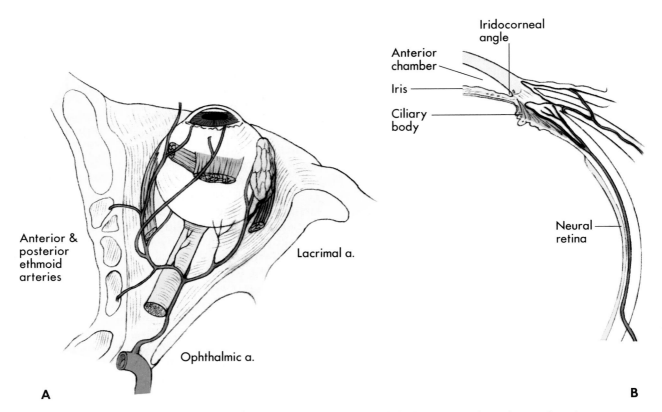

Figure 2-109   BLOOD SUPPLY TO ORBIT. A, The ophthalmic artery branches within the orbit to supply both orbital structures and the supraorbital/supratrochlear branches, which radiate over the forehead. Still other branches terminate in the nose. **B,** Termination of arterial branches in the ciliary body.   SEE ATLAS, FIGS. 2-105, 2-110

lacrimal gland by traveling with branches of V2 and finally with the lacrimal nerve of V1.

CONJUNCTIVAL MEMBRANE

The conjunctival sac is a thin transparent membrane that lines the inner surface of the eyelids (**palpebral conjunctiva**) and reflects back on to the anterior surface of the sclera (**bulbar conjunctiva**). It ends at the sclerocorneal junction (where it is continuous with the corneal epithelium), so that no conjunctival membrane is found in the direct line of vision through the cornea. On the inner surface of the eyelid, the conjunctiva is continuous with the external squamous epithelium at the lid margin. Where the upper lid palpebral conjunctiva folds back on itself to cover the sclera (a recess known as the **superior fornix**), there are numerous apertures for the ducts of the lacrimal gland. It is through these ducts that tears pass from the lacrimal gland to the anterior surface of the globe, where they moisten and provide lubrication.

VASCULATURE OF THE ORBIT

The **ophthalmic artery** is the first branch of the internal carotid artery, arising just after the latter vessel enters the cranial cavity (Figure 2-109). The ophthalmic artery enters the orbit through the optic canal, along with the optic nerve. Soon it gives off the important **central artery of the retina.** This vessel is the almost sole blood supply to the retina, and permanent retinal injury or blindness results if this tiny vessel is obstructed for any length of time. The ophthalmic artery gives off several additional branches, including the following arteries: *lacrimal, long and short ciliary, supraorbital, supratrochlear, dorsal nasal, meningeal, and anterior ethmoid* (which, like the nerve of the same name, enters and then exits the anterior cranial fossa).

The **ophthalmic veins** (superior and inferior) drain to the cavernous sinus (see Figure 2-26) and numerous anastomoses with the *angular vein* (a tributary of the facial vein) and the *pterygoid plexus* (see Figure 2-58). Considerable potential for spread of infection exists between facial and intracranial structures through the ophthalmic veins and their tributaries.

THE EYE

ABNORMALITIES OF LACRIMAL FLOW

Obstruction of the lacrimal drainage system predisposes to infection, or *dacrocystitis*. This appears as redness, tenderness, and swelling near the medial canthus. It is rather common in young children, due presumably to the small size of the lacrimal ducts.

THE CONJUNCTIVAE

Conjunctival infection and inflammation can result from a variety of sources: *Hemophilus influenzae*, *Streptococcus*, *Chlamydiae*, and *Herpes viruses*, to name a few of the most common.

ABNORMALITIES OF THE EYELIDS

Chalazion (Gr. *chalaza*, a pimple) is a lipogranuloma in one or more of the eyelid glands. **Hordoleum** (L. barleycorn) is an acute suppurative (that is, pus-producing) inflammation of the eyelid glands (in other words, a "sty"). **Entropion** (Gr. *trope*, a turning) is an outward turning of the palpebral surface of the eyelid. **Ptosis** is the drooping of one of the upper lids and can result from injury to the levator palpebrae superioris (or its innervation) or from an abnormality in the sympathetic innervation of Müller's muscle. Trauma to the eyes may produce bleeding into the dermis of the eyelids, a "black eye."

ABNORMAL GAZE

Strabismus means an abnormal deviation of one eye so that gaze is not conjugate. It may result from an imbalance of muscle tone among the extraocular muscles. **Nystagmus** is the repetitive, involuntary movement of one or both eyes. **Diplopia** is the failure to align both eyes properly, so that the brain receives two images that are out of register and therefore "double." Diplopia may result from strabismus or from other abnormalities. **Esotropia** and **exotropia** refer to abnormal inward or outward gazes, respectively.

ERRORS OF REFRACTION AND THE CORNEA

Correction of refractive errors is a common requirement. Simple situations of a mismatch between the position of the retinal and the focal points are depicted in the accompanying figure on errors of refraction, with the appropriate corrective steps shown (see Figure 2-100). Recently, radial keratotomy (the placement of incisions in the cornea) has been employed for the permanent correction of certain refractive errors. Correction for astigmatism (irregular curvature of the cornea) requires the asymmetric grinding of lenses for conventional glasses (or the construction of contact lenses) to compensate for the corneal irregularities. When irreversible injury afflicts the cornea, transplantation may be the only reasonable alternative.

PATHOLOGIES OF THE PUPIL AND IRIS

Horner's syndrome—miosis (abnormal pupillary constriction), anhydrosis (absence of sweating on affected side of face), and ptosis (drooping of upper lid)—may result from injury to any portion of the sympathetic pathway destined to supply the face (at spinal cord, sympathetic chain, and so on) (see Figure 2-107, *B*). **Miosis** is abnormal pupillary constriction; **mydriasis** is abnormal pupillary dilation.

REFLEXES INVOLVING THE EYE

The **light reflex** is the constriction of the pupil in response to light. It involves cranial nerves II and III. **Accommodation** is the constriction of the pupil as a part of an overall adjustment for near vision (which also includes convergence of the eyes and changes in the shape of the lens). The pupillary constriction involved in accommodation may remain normal while the light reflex is lost—as in advanced syphilis. The **corneal reflex** involves gently touching the cornea and producing a blink (cranial nerves V and VII).

ORBITS

Trauma involving the anterior cranial fossa may lead to periorbital bleeding—so-called "raccoon's eyes." The once frequently performed frontal lobotomy was in reality an outpatient procedure (that is, did not require overnight stay in hospital). A metal rod was inserted through the thin roof of the orbit up into the substance of the frontal lobe. The rod was then swept to and fro, transecting part of the frontal lobe. Chronic infections in the maxillary or ethmoid sinuses pose a risk to the orbit and ultimately to the cavernous sinus, because blood communicates between the orbit and cavernous sinus rather freely.

LENS

Cataracts (dense bodies) may form within the lens, in response to certain infections (for example, rubella) or simply as a part of aging. The cataracts are opaque and obstruct vision, often necessitating their removal. Some connective tissue disorders, including Marfan's syndrome, affect the strength of the fibers of the ciliary zonule. Dislocation of the lens may occur when these ciliary fibers are disturbed.

THE EYE—continued

PATHOLOGIC SIGNS AND THE RETINA

Papilledema is the abnormal swelling of the optic nerve head on the surface of the retina, interpreted as a sign of generalized increase in intracranial pressure. The retina provides our only opportunity to view blood vessels in vivo. Such systemic diseases as hypertension and diabetes mellitus often produce characteristic changes in small blood vessels, and the retinal vessels are the only ones that may be observed directly (with an ophthalmoscope).

2.11

section two.eleven

Nasal Cavity

▶ Internal Anatomy of the Nose
▶ Nasal Septum
▶ Lateral Nasal Wall
▶ Spaces in the Lateral Nasal Wall
▶ Olfactory Epithelium and Olfactory Nerve

▶ Vasculature of the Nose
▶ Innervation of the Nose
▶ Pterygopalatine Fossa

The nasal cavity is complex, because of the intricate connection of the bony and cartilaginous structures that give it shape. It is centrally located and as such is an important part of your understanding of the pterygopalatine fossa, palate, oral cavity, and orbit, all of which border on the nose. The paranasal sinuses and the lacrimal ducts drain into the nose, through apertures in its lateral wall. The considerable surface area of the inside of the nose helps it to play one of its most important roles, that of warming and humidifying inspired air. The olfactory epithelium is situated in the upper recesses of the nose and is unique because the sensory neurons that respond to odors are located in the olfactory epithelium itself, not in the CNS.

INTERNAL ANATOMY OF THE NOSE

The nose is composed of a *bony base* (nasal and frontal bones and maxillae all take part in its formation) and a mostly *cartilaginous framework*, which gives the nose its unique shape. There is a pair of anterior entrances to the nasal cavity (the **nares,** or nostrils) and a pair of posterior apertures connecting the nose with the nasopharynx (the **choanae;** Gr. *choane,* funnel). The **vestibule** is the circular enlargement enclosed by the nares. The perimeter of the vestibule on each side is made up of the major and minor **alar cartilage** and a small inferior portion of the **septal cartilage.** The floor of the nasal cavity is formed by the **hard** and **soft palates.**

The external and lateral surfaces of the nose (Figure 2-110) are formed mostly from cartilage. The two **nasal bones** form the upper bridge of the nose. The **lateral cartilages** are firmly attached to the anterior free edge of the nasal bones.

The respiratory epithelium lining the vestibules is remarkable for its coarse hairs, known as **vibrissae** (L., to vibrate). These help to filter particulate matter from the inspired air. The nasal epithelium in general has a mucociliary lining, important in removing contaminant material from inspired air and moving it toward the pharynx (where it is swallowed or spit out). The abundant vascularity of the nasal epithelium helps to warm and humidify inspired air. In the upper recess of the nasal cavity is found the **olfactory epithelium** (Figure 2-111).

The nasal cavity is "surrounded" by several *air sinuses,* the secretions of which drain into it (see Figure 2-114). The precise function of these sinuses is unknown. Their development is relatively slow, and it is not until several years after birth that a fully developed set of paranasal air sinuses is present.

NASAL SEPTUM

The nasal septum is formed by (1) the *perpendicular plate of the ethmoid bone,* (2) the *vomer* (L. *vomer,* a plowshare, or lower portion of the blade of a plow), and (3) the *septal cartilage* (Figure 2-112). The ethmoid perpendicular plate occupies the posterosuperior third of the

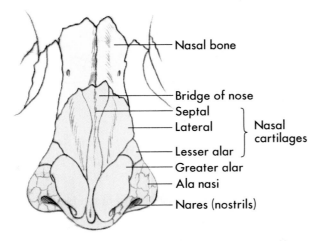

Figure 2-110   CARTILAGES AND BONES OF THE NOSE.

Labels in figure:
Nasal bone
Bridge of nose
Septal
Lateral
Lesser alar
Nasal cartilages
Greater alar
Ala nasi
Nares (nostrils)

PRINCIPLES

The nose is an organ of smell (olfaction), in which aerosolized molecules reach the olfactory epithelium, where they produce a neural response. The nose also serves to warm inspired gas. The mucosa of the nose is richly supplied with capillaries, and the flow of blood through these capillaries is increased or decreased to increase or decrease the warming of the gas being inhaled.* The moist mucus layer covering the nasal mucosa ensures that inspired gas will be almost completely humidified, lowering the risk of a drying effect on the lining of the trachea and distal airways. Inspired gas is ordinarily humidified to >90% by passing through the nose, and over 24 hours as much as 1 L of liquid is added to the inspired gas. Both the mucus layer and the coarse hairs within the nose trap foreign objects that may be inhaled with the inspired gas. The mucus layer lining the nose is renewed every 20 to 40 minutes, through secretion of mucus from the nasal epithelium, and the mucus is coated with secretory antibodies (known as IgA or immunoglobulin A) that begin the immune response to foreign organisms (such as viruses and bacteria). The interior of the nose and its connections to adjacent air sinuses lend a quality to the voice (try pinching your nose and pronouncing sounds like "c," "m," and "n."

*Interestingly, the flow of blood is maximal in one side of the nose (e.g., the right) for 3 to 5 hours, after which blood flow to the right side subsides. Simultaneously, blood flow through the opposite side of the nose (e.g., the left side) begins to increase. This alternating cycle of nasal perfusion continues indefinitely.

septum; the vomer, the posteroinferior third; and the septal cartilage, the anterior third of the septum.

The **ethmoid perpendicular plate** extends downward from the undersurface of the ethmoid bone in the midsagittal plane. The plate is seldom perfectly straight and can be permanently "remodeled" as a result of blunt trauma to the nose (fighting, auto accident, and so on). The perpendicular plate is attached inferiorly to the vomer, posteriorly to the sphenoid bone, and anteriorly to the septal cartilage.

The **vomer** is shaped like a large arrowhead, with its base facing posteriorly. It attaches to the ethmoid perpendicular plate and septal cartilage superiorly and inferiorly to the palatine bones and maxillae, because they form the hard palate. The inferior half of its posterior edge forms the posterior border of the nasal sep-

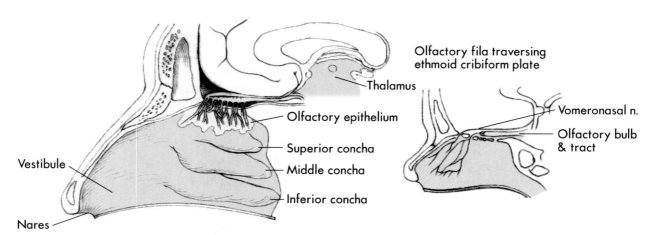

Labels in figure:
Olfactory fila traversing ethmoid cribiform plate
Thalamus
Olfactory epithelium
Superior concha
Middle concha
Inferior concha
Vestibule
Nares
Vomeronasal n.
Olfactory bulb & tract

Figure 2-111   OLFACTORY EPITHELIUM AND CRIBRIFORM PLATE.

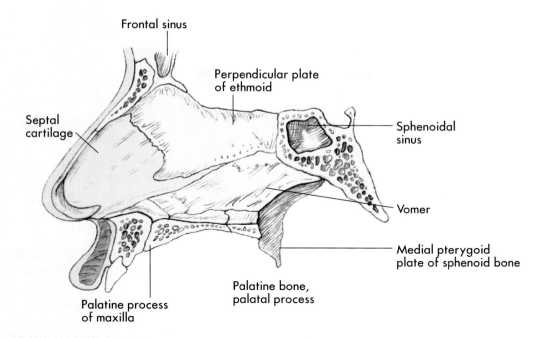

Frontal sinus

Perpendicular plate
of ethmoid

Septal
cartilage

Sphenoidal
sinus

Vomer

Medial pterygoid
plate of sphenoid bone

Palatine bone,
palatal process

Palatine process
of maxilla

Figure 2-112 COMPONENTS OF THE NASAL SEPTUM. Bones (the vomer and the perpendicular plate of the ethmoid bone) and several cartilages make up the nasal septum.

tum, and the superior half is attached to the sphenoid bone. The **septal cartilage** has a pointed posterior edge that fits in between the vomer and perpendicular plate of the ethmoid. Its anterior edge is curved and forms the lower half of the anterior margin of the nose.

The completed septum divides the nasal cavity into its left and right sides. Blood supply to the septum is rich, and the mucosa is relatively thick on the nasal septum, especially in its lower half. Arterial vessels derived from the maxillary and facial arteries supply the nasal septum (see following); recurrent nosebleeds are common, especially in the vestibule, and may bleed persistently and profusely.

The horizontal cribriform plates of the ethmoid bone form the upper recesses of each side of the nose. Perforations in these plates allow axons of the olfactory epithelium to enter the skull and convey olfactory information to the brain. The upper part of the nasal septum is formed by the thin, vertical perpendicular plate of the ethmoid bone. The lower and anterior part of the septum are completed by the independent vomer and the septal cartilage. A complex vertical wall barrier serves as part of the lateral wall of the nose and part of the medial wall of the orbit. These are the **superior** and **middle conchae** of the nasal wall, coiled ledges of bone that protrude inward into the interior of the nasal cavity. The lateral wall of the nose is completed inferiorly by the independent **inferior concha.**

The ethmoid bone, viewed anteriorly, has the appearance of three vertical components (the midline perpendicular plate/crista galli and two lateral pieces, the

superior and middle conchae) and two horizontal pieces (the cribriform plates) that join the three vertical pieces to form a single unit. The cribriform plate articulates with the frontal bones laterally, the vomer inferiorly (with the perpendicular plate), and the inferior conchae inferiorly (with the middle conchae).

LATERAL NASAL WALL

The lateral walls of the nose are of complex shape. From above downward, they are slanted outward— that is, the nose is narrower at its apex than at its base, above the hard palate. Each lateral wall has three curled inwardly-protruding shelves or conchae (Figures 2-110 and 2-113). The **inferior concha** is an independent bone, whereas the **middle and superior conchae** are parts of the ethmoid bone. The conchae are sometimes referred to as the **turbinates** (L., a whirl or coil). The conchae are lined by typical pseudostratified ciliated columnar respiratory epithelium, though in many areas the columnar cells are very short and are nearly cuboidal. The mucosa of the conchae is highly vascular. The conchae serve the purpose of increasing the surface area of the interior of the nose and increasing its ability to warm and humidify the inspired air.

SPACES IN THE LATERAL NASAL WALL

Regions on the lateral nasal walls are defined by the position of the conchae and the spaces above, between, or below them (Figure 2-114 and Table 2-21). The **sphe-**

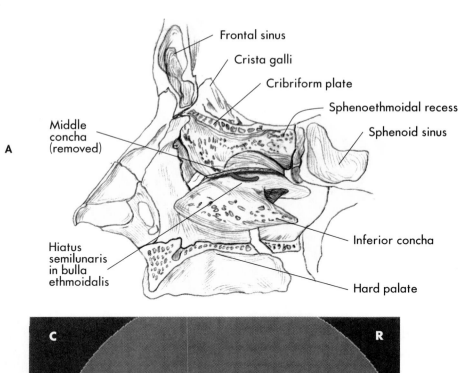

Frontal sinus
Crista galli
Cribriform plate
Sphenoethmoidal recess
Sphenoid sinus
Middle concha (removed)
Hiatus semilunaris in bulla ethmoidalis
Inferior concha
Hard palate

A

B

C   R

Inferior orbital fissure

Maxillary sinus

Perpendicular plate of ethmoid bone

Middle ethmoidal air cells

Figure 2-113 COMPONENTS OF THE LATERAL NASAL WALL. A, The superior and middle conchae (not shown) are part of the ethmoid bone, while the inferior concha is an independent bone. The middle concha has been removed to show the bulla ethmoidalis, etc. **B,** CT image through the nose. Note the coiled appearance of the turbinates. (**B** from Weir J, Abrahams PH: *An imaging atlas of human anatomy,* London, 1992, Mosby.)

SEE ATLAS, FIGS. 2-55, 2-56, 2-61

noethmoidal recess is the space superior to the superior concha; the **superior, middle, and inferior meatuses** are spaces found inferior to their respective conchae. The several **paranasal air sinuses** (frontal, maxillary, ethmoid, and sphenoid) each drains into the nose in one of these spaces, as does the nasolacrimal duct, draining tears into the nose (see Figure 2-108). If the middle concha is removed, one can see more clearly the **bulla ethmoidalis,** a raised eminence caused by the un-

derlying ethmoid air cells in the lateral wall of the nose. A curved opening, the hiatus **semilunaris,** lies just inferior to the bulla (Figure 2-113, *B*). The maxillary and anterior sinuses drain through the hiatus, while the middle ethmoid sinuses usually drain directly through the surface of the bulla.

The maxillary sinus is further notable, because its secretions must drain "uphill" to reach the **hiatus semilunaris,** a curved slitlike aperture lying just inferior to

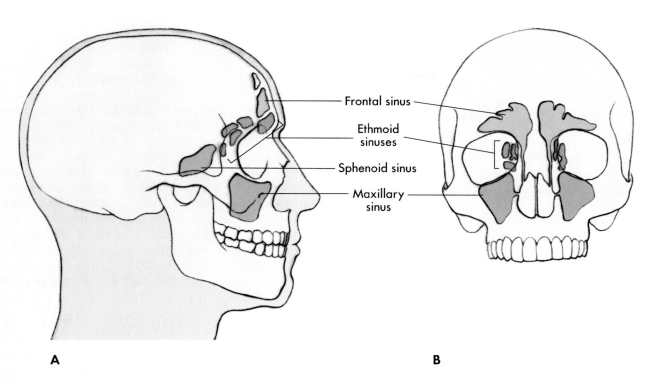

A, **B**

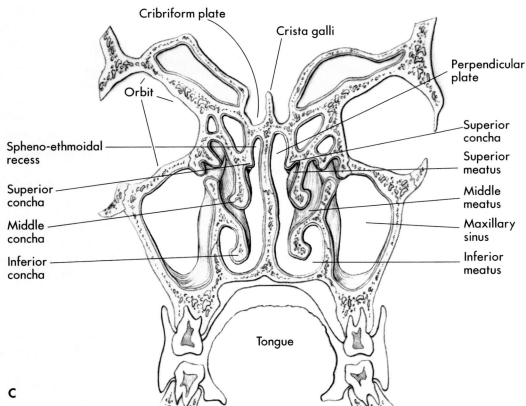

C

Figure 2-114   AIR SINUSES IN THE NOSE. A, Lateral view. **B,** Anterior view. **C,** Coronal view.   SEE ATLAS, FIGS. 2-53, 2-62, 2-63, 2-64, 2-98

Table 2-21   Sinus Drainage into the Nose

Aperture in Lateral Wall	Structure(s) Which Drain into It
Sphenoethmoidal recess	Sphenoid sinus
Superior meatus	Posterior ethmoid sinus
Middle meatus	Maxillary, frontal, and anterior/middle ethmoid sinuses
Inferior meatus	Lacrimal sac (via nasolacrimal duct)

the bulla ethmoidalis. This has implications for sufferers of chronic sinusitis, for whom it is very difficult to clear excess mucus secretions from the maxillary and other paranasal sinuses.

Near the posterior end of the superior meatus is the **sphenopalatine foramen,** through which travels the *sphenopalatine artery,* one of the end branches of the maxillary (see Figure 2-55). This vessel supplies branches to the conchae and to the base of the nasal septum.

Frontal Sinuses

The frontal sinuses are located deep to the supraorbital ridge, wholly contained within the frontal bone (Figure 2-114). They are variable in size, shape, and number. They drain into the middle meatus, by ducts that descend through the ethmoid sinuses and may even be contained within them. They do not reach full size until after puberty and are usually not present at birth.

Ethmoid Sinuses

The ethmoid sinuses comprise 10 to 20 small interconnecting chambers, positioned lateral to the lateral nasal walls (Figure 2-114). They are usually divided into anterior, middle, and posterior groups. The *anterior and middle ethmoid sinuses* drain into the middle meatus, while the *posterior ethmoid sinuses* drain into the superior meatus. In particular, the middle ethmoid air cells open through apertures on the wall of the bulla ethmoidalis. It is important to understand that the ethmoid sinuses lie between the nasal and orbital cavities and form parts of the walls of each of these important cavities (Figures 2-93 and 2-114, *C*). Very thin bony plates separate the interior of the sinuses from the structures of the orbit, such as the optic nerve and globe, and infections or inflammations in the ethmoid sinuses may pose a danger to the orbit and its contents.

Sphenoid Sinuses

There are also two sphenoid sinuses, the left and right. They are wholly contained within the sphenoid bone. The two sinuses are often confluent and may appear to be a single cavity. Their development is not complete until after puberty. Drainage is to the uppermost part of the interior of the nose, the *sphenoethmoidal recess.* Immediately superior to the sphenoid sinuses are the optic chiasma and the pituitary gland (see Figure 2-86). One can achieve surgical access to these important structures through the sphenoid sinus, by dissecting alongside the nose, entering the sphenoid sinus, and carefully removing the thin bony plate above which are found the optic nerves and pituitary gland. The **cavernous sinuses** lie on the lateral sides of each sphenoid sinus (see Figure 2-26). They contain many important structures, such as the internal carotid artery and cranial nerves III, IV, V1, V2, and VI—traveling toward the orbit.

Maxillary Sinuses

These are the largest of the air sinuses. One maxillary sinus is located on each side of the face (Figure 2-114, *A* and *B*), and they are shaped like triangles, with the middle and inferior conchae of the lateral nasal wall forming their bases. The floor of the orbit (Figure 2-114, *B*) forms the roof of the maxillary sinus. The roots of the upper teeth, embedded in the dental arch of each maxillary bone, frequently form elevations in the floor of the maxillary sinus. The maxillary sinus, as mentioned earlier, drains to the middle meatus through the hiatus semilunaris.

OLFACTORY EPITHELIUM AND OLFACTORY NERVE

The olfactory epithelium lines the upper portion of the sphenoethmoidal recess (see Figure 2-111). It is a true neuroepithelium, derived from an embryonic placode on the head surface of the embryo, rather than from the neural tube (as is the case for the great majority of the nervous system).

The neuron cell bodies for the olfactory epithelium are found in the olfactory epithelium itself; axons from these neurons traverse the cribriform plate to reach the cranial cavity. Here the majority of them synapse in the olfactory bulb, and other tracts of axons arise to travel to the base of the anterior forebrain. The neurons of the olfactory epithelium are interspersed with nonneuronal supporting cells, presumably important in maintaining the structure of the epithelium, and with mucus cells secreting lubricant mucus.

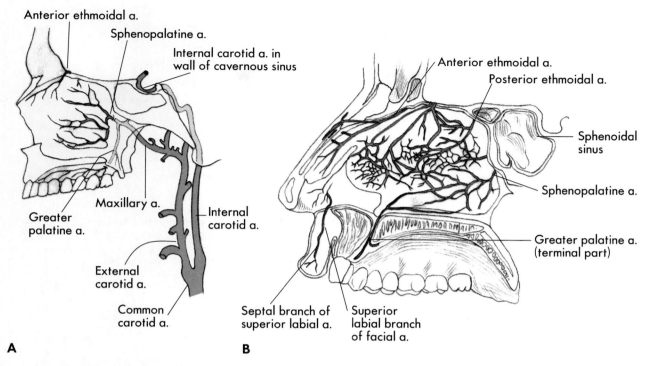

Figure 2-115   VASCULATURE TO THE NOSE: LATERAL WALL AND SEPTUM. A, Blood supply to the conchae in the lateral nasal wall. **B,** Blood supply to the nasal septum.
SEE ATLAS, FIG. 2-59

VASCULATURE OF THE NOSE

Branches derived from both the internal and external carotid arteries supply the nose. Specifically, the **ophthalmic artery** contributes the **anterior ethmoid artery** and its terminal branches, the *internal* and *external nasal arteries,* supplying the upper portions of the nose and extending as for down as the vestibule. This is one of the few examples of a structure on the exterior surface of the head and neck being supplied by a branch of the internal carotid artery. The **maxillary artery** contributes the *sphenopalatine artery,* supplying the conchae and parts of the septum (see Figures 2-55 and 2-115). It enters the nose through the sphenopalatine foramen, located just posteriorly to the superior meatus of the lateral nasal wall. The sphenopalatine artery divides into two groups of branches, the *posterior septal arteries,* to the posterior part of the nasal septum, and the *posterior lateral nasal branches,* supplying the conchae and meatuses of the lateral nasal wall, as well as the interior of the four paranasal sinuses.

The **greater palatine artery** is also a branch of the maxillary artery and descends through the greater palatine canal to supply blood to the palate. The terminal part of the greater palatine artery passes forward along the inferior surface of the palate, then turns upward to pass through the incisive foramen to supply blood to the lower part of the nasal septum and to

anastomose with terminal branches of the sphenopalatine artery. Small terminal branches of the **superior labial artery,** originally derived from the facial branch of the external carotid artery, also pass through the incisive foramen to supply the basal parts of the septum and the vestibule.

The extensive venous plexus in the submucous area vasodilates and vasoconstricts as a mechanism of heat exchange. Inflammation of this vascular plexus leads to congestion and respiratory obstruction (as in allergic rhinitis—Gr. *rhinos,* nose). Nosebleed (epistaxis) is a common clinical problem. It is frequent in an area at the base of the septum and the vestibule, supplied by branches of the superior labial artery and the sphenopalatine branch of the maxillary artery. Severe recurrent cases sometimes require external carotid ligation.

INNERVATION OF THE NOSE

Innervation of the nose is derived from numerous branches of V1 (the *ophthalmic nerve*) and V2 (the *maxillary nerve*) and from the *olfactory nerve* (for olfaction). The majority of the general sensory innervation of the nose is derived from the **maxillary nerve** (V2) (Figure 2-116). Its *nasopalatine nerve* is the major supply of the nasal septum, especially its posterior two thirds. In the

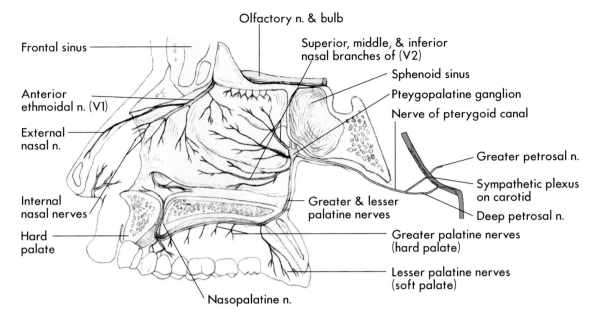

Figure 2-116   INNERVATION OF NOSE—LATERAL WALL. Branches of V1 and V2 innervate different areas of the lateral wall of the nose.   SEE ATLAS, FIG. 2-54

lateral wall, V2 innervates most of the mucosa covering the conchae, through its *anterior alveolar* and *posterior alveolar* branches. The vestibule of the nose is innervated by terminal branches of the infraorbital nerve, a more distal branch of V2.

The **ophthalmic nerve (V1)** provides innervation to the upper part of both the lateral nasal wall and the nasal septum through its *internal nasal nerve,* a branch of the anterior ethmoidal nerve. There is also a small *external nasal nerve,* supplying the upper part of the midline of the skin covering the nose.

The first cranial nerve, the **olfactory nerve,** mediates the sense of smell. The structure we recognize as the olfactory nerve is in fact a tract of the CNS that receives signals from the sensory neurons in the olfactory mucosa and conveys these signals on to the brain. The sensory neurons in the olfactory mucosa are the cells that are stimulated by odors. These cells send thin axons superiorly, through the numerous perforations of the cribriform plate, into the interior of the cranium, where they synapse on cells in the olfactory bulb. The olfactory tract, which resembles a stalk at the end of which is located the olfactory bulb, is the structure we usually identify as the "olfactory nerve."

PTERYGOPALATINE FOSSA

The pterygopalatine fossa is a complex small space, found deep within the face (Figure 2-116). It is located posterior to the maxilla, inferior to the apex of the orbit, and immediately lateral to the lateral wall of the nose. Through its many complex and small bony passages, important vessels and nerves communicate with the

oral cavity, nasal cavity, orbit, cranial cavity, infratemporal fossa, and anterior surface of the face.

The pterygopalatine fossa has the following boundaries:

Anterior: The posterior surface of the maxilla

Posterior: The base of the lateral pterygoid plate and the opening of the foramen rotundum and pterygoid canal

Inferior: The junction of the palatine perpendicular plate and the maxilla

Superior: The greater wing of the sphenoid and the inferior orbital fissure

Medial: The perpendicular plate of the palatine bone and the sphenopalatine foramen

Lateral: The pterygomaxillary fissure

The pterygopalatine fossa is more easily understood if we think of it as a space with multiple entrances and exits. In general, the vascular structures of the pterygopalatine fossa enter it through its lateral wall; the nerves of the fossa enter it posteriorly.

The major structures of the fossa are the *maxillary artery, pterygopalatine ganglion,* and *maxillary nerve.* The **maxillary artery** enters the fossa laterally, through the pterygomaxillary fissure. Before entering the pterygomaxillary fissure, the maxillary artery gives off important arterial branches for the upper and lower jaw, muscles of mastication, cranial dura mater, external ear, and tympanic membrane. The maxillary artery terminates as the *infraorbital artery,* a moderately large branch that separates from the maxillary artery just before it enters the pterygomaxillary fissure. This vessel runs across the floor of the orbit and emerges onto the face through the infraorbital foramen. The terminal part of the maxillary artery branches within the nose to supply the conchae and nasal septum (by the sphenopalatine artery), palate (by the greater and lesser palatine arteries), and nasopharynx (by the pharyngeal artery).

The sphenopalatine artery branches off of the maxillary artery within the confines of the pterygopalatine fossa, then travels medially through the sphenopalatine foramen to reach the interior of the nose (Figure 2-115). The greater palatine artery departs the maxillary artery within the fossa as well and descends through the greater palatine canal to reach the palate. The lesser palatine arteries, supplying the soft palate, are actually branches of the greater palatine arteries, supplying the hard palate. The small *pharyngeal artery* leaves the maxillary artery within the pterygopalatine fossa and enters a small passage, known as the palatovaginal canal, to emerge into the nasopharynx, which it supplies with blood.

The **pterygopalatine ganglion** is a parasympathetic ganglion, one of four found in the head and neck region. Postganglionic axons from the ganglion travel through intricate pathways to innervate the lacrimal gland and, to a lesser degree, the minor salivary glands of the soft palate. The maxillary nerve (V2) enters the upper portion of the pterygopalatine fossa through the foramen rotundum in its posterior wall. After giving off several descending branches, including the *greater palatine nerve*, it continues anteriorly and leaves the pterygopalatine fossa as the *infraorbital nerve*, accompanying the artery of the same name. Though the infraorbital nerve and artery leave the pterygopalatine fossa together, it is important to remember that they do not enter it together—the artery enters through the pterygomaxillary fissure, and the nerve enters through the foramen rotundum.

In addition to the **maxillary nerve,** the *nerve of the pterygoid canal* also enters the pterygopalatine fossa through the opening of the pterygoid canal in its posterior wall. This nerve consists of axons from (1) the *greater petrosal nerve*, composed of preganglionic parasympathetic axons derived from the facial nerve, and (2) the *deep petrosal nerve*, a collection of postganglionic sympathetic axons derived from the internal carotid plexus. Many groups of axons seem "attached" to the pterygopalatine ganglion as they pass through the pterygopalatine fossa but have no synaptic relationship to it (for example, the palatine, infraorbital, sphenopalatine, and nasal nerves—all branches of V2). Only the parasympathetic axons of the nerve of the pterygoid canal synapse in the ganglion. Axons arising from neurons in the ganglion join the continuation of the maxillary nerve as it enters the infraorbital canal. The zygomatic branch of V2 carries these postganglionic parasympathetic fibers through the lateral orbital wall. Once inside the orbit, the parasympathetic axons join the *lacrimal nerve*, a branch of V1, and accompany it to the lacrimal gland, to which the parasympathetic axons provide secretomotor innervation. The apertures in the walls of the pterygopalatine fossa and the structures traversing them are listed in Table 2-22.

CLINICAL ANATOMY OF

THE NASAL CAVITY

THE SINUSES AND MENINGITIS

Suppurative (pus-producing) infections in the sinuses, especially the ethmoid and sphenoid, pose a risk of erosion into the cranial cavity and subsequent meningitis. Barriers between these sinuses and the interior of the skull may be deficient in children, partially explaining their increased susceptibility to meningitis from organisms found in the oropharynx.

SURGERY AND THE SPHENOID BONE

Structures at the base of the brain (pituitary gland, optic nerves) may be approached surgically through the sphenoid sinus (drilling, from within the sinus, through its roof to visualize the undersurface of the brain). The sphenoid sinus is approached by dissecting between the upper lip and maxilla, and upward along the lateral side of the nose to reach the sphenoid sinus.

THE SINUSES AND TOOTHACHE

Inflammation of the maxillary sinus may produce dental symptoms, because the nerves innervating the upper jaw teeth lie in the floor of the maxillary sinus.

NOSEBLEEDS

When nosebleed (epistaxis) is persistent, packing of the nasal cavity with absorbent material promoting clot formation may be required. The anterior nares and the posterior choanae may both need packing.

OBSTRUCTIONS TO MUCUS FLOW

Any process producing obstruction to the flow of mucus from the paranasal sinuses into the nose may predispose to chronic infection in the sinuses. These may range from allergic inflammation of the nasal mucosa (especially that over the middle concha) to deviation of the nasal septum.

NASAL FRACTURES

Fracture of the nose is potentially dangerous because the bacteria-rich nasal mucus may "inoculate" the interior of the skull, through, for example, a fractured ethmoid bone. The nasal bones are among the most frequently fractured in the body.

Table 2-22   Apertures in Walls of the Pterygopalatine Fossa

Wall	Aperture	Traversed by	Comments
Lateral wall	Pterygomaxillary fissure	Maxillary artery	One of two terminal branches of external carotid artery; anesthetics can be injected into fossa through this aperture
Medial wall	Sphenopalatine foramen	Nasopalatine nerve Lateral and medial posterosuperior nasal nerves Sphenopalatine artery	Runs anteriorly along a groove on the vomer; traverses incisive foramen Innervates middle and superior conchae, upper septum, and ethmoid air cells Accompanies nasopalatine nerve
Posterior wall	Foramen rotundum Pterygoid canal Palatovaginal canal	Maxillary nerve (entering fossa) Nerve and artery of pterygoid canal Pharyngeal nerve and artery	Becomes infraorbital nerve Synapses in ganglion Supplies nasopharynx, part of auditory tube
Anterior wall	Inferior orbital fissure (actually superoanterior)	Branches of the maxillary nerve and artery, mainly the infraorbital nerve and artery	Fissure lies between maxilla and greater wing of sphenoid, innervates floor of orbit and maxilla
Inferior wall	Greater palatine canal	Greater and lesser palatine nerves and vessels	Greater palatine canal lies between palatine, maxilla, and pterygoid bones
Superior wall	Inferior orbital fissure and continuity with superior orbital fissure	Infraorbital nerve (inferior fissure) and nerves III, IV, VI, and VI (superior fissure)	Orbital fissures lie between lesser and greater sphenoid wings

2.12

Mouth and Palate

▶ Borders of the Oral Cavity

▶ Palate

▶ Teeth

▶ Cheek and its Constituent Parts

▶ Tongue

▶ Submandibular and Sublingual Glands

▶ Palatine Tonsil

The oral cavity is important in a number of vital functions, including respiration, eating, and the production of speech. Portions of the oral cavity are derived from the embryonic pharyngeal arch structures, and we find the convergence of branches from several of the cranial nerves occurring in the mouth. The three major and several minor salivary glands drain into the oral cavity, contributing to the initial stages of digestion by moistening and softening food.

BORDERS OF THE ORAL CAVITY

The roof of the oral cavity (Figure 2-117) is formed by the hard and soft palate. The tongue and the mylohyoid muscle form its floor. Laterally, the cheeks and more posteriorly the tonsillar pillars form its boundaries. Posteriorly, the oral cavity ends at the palatoglossal arches (the anterior pair of tonsillar pillars). The oral cavity may be further divided into the **vestibule** (the space between the gums and cheeks) and the **oral cavity proper** (the space interior to the gums).

PALATE

The **palate** consists of the hard and soft portions (the soft palate is about 15% of total, lying most posterior). The **hard palate** (Figure 2-118) is formed by the palatine processes of the maxillae and the horizontal

processes of the palatine bones. The *incisive foramen* is an important anterior midline palatal aperture at the junction of the primary and secondary palates (marking the border of the embryonic primary and secondary palates) (see Figure 2-122).

The substance of the **soft palate** (Figure 2-118) is muscle, connective and lymphoid tissue, and a covering squamous epithelium. The interior of the soft palate is formed by a flattened *palatine aponeurosis,* into which most of the palatal muscles are anchored. The shape of the soft palate is maintained by this aponeurosis. The posterior free margin of the palate is notable for the midline bulbous **uvula,** which extends downward and helps to seal the oropharynx from the nasopharynx during swallowing (see pp. 281–282). There are minor **salivary glands** on the inferior (oral) surface soft palate, with secretomotor innervation by branches from the pterygopalatine ganglion. There are also minor taste buds in the oral surface of the soft palate. These are diffuse clusters of glandular acini embedded in the substance of the soft palate and opening by numerous ducts onto its surface.

Muscles of the Soft Palate

The **tensor veli palatini** (Figure 2-119) muscle arises from the sphenoid spine, the scaphoid fossa at the base of the medial pterygoid plate, and the auditory tube.

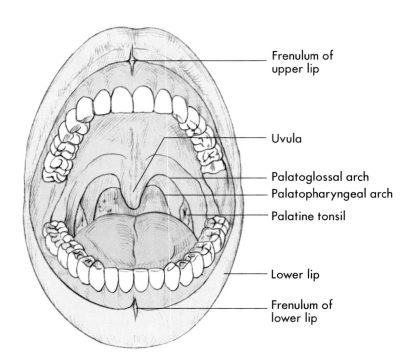

Frenulum of upper lip

Uvula

Palatoglossal arch

Palatopharyngeal arch

Palatine tonsil

Lower lip

Frenulum of lower lip

Figure 2-117   ANTERIOR VIEW OF ORAL CAVITY AND PALATAL ARCHES.

The muscle descends from the base of the skull and moves in an anterior direction, lying between the lateral and medial pterygoid plates as it does. The tensor veli palatini lies anterior to the levator veli palatini muscle as they both begin to descend toward the palate. More inferiorly, the tensor muscle moves to a position anterior and lateral to the belly of the levator muscle.

As it descends, the tensor muscle narrows to form a slender tendon that loops laterally around the hamulus of the medial pterygoid plate (Figure 2-119). The tendon now finds itself lateral to the **buccinator muscle** (which attaches to the medial pterygoid hamulus), and so it must penetrate the posterior origin of that muscle before entering the substance of the soft palate at a near-horizontal angle. The tensor muscle then terminates in the palatine aponeurosis (Figure 2-118, *A*). Because its tendon loops around the pterygoid hamulus, contraction of the tensor veli palatini *tenses the palate* in a horizontal plane and flattens the normal arch of the soft palate at rest. This is an important part of the complex act of swallowing, where the soft palate must move posteriorly and become stiffened, so that it can serve as a barrier to prevent food contents in the mouth from refluxing into the nasopharynx. Unlike most other palatal muscles, the tensor muscle is innervated by the V3 division of the trigeminal nerve.

The **levator veli palatini** muscle (Figure 2-119) arises from the base of the temporal bone and the inferior margin of the opening of the auditory tube. As it descends, the muscle lies first posterior and then medial to the tensor veli palatini and anterior to the salpin-gopharyngeus muscle. Passing posterior to the medial pterygoid hamulus, it penetrates the pharyngobasilar fascia, which fills the gap between the upper free margin of the superior pharyngeal constrictor and the base of the skull. The muscle now lies within the interior of the nasopharynx. It ends by inserting into the palatine aponeurosis of the soft palate. Because it does not loop around the medial pterygoid hamulus (as does the tensor muscle), the result of contraction of the levator muscle is *elevation of the palate.* Contraction of the levator veli palatini may also help to open the auditory tube (for example, during yawning), because of a downward pull on the rim of the auditory tube opening. This may explain the "popping of the ears" that accompanies yawning or swallowing.

The **palatopharyngeus muscle** (Figure 2-120) originates from the posterolateral aspect of the palate, very near to the point where the levator veli palatini inserts into the palate. It travels downward, passing posteriorly to the palatine tonsil, to insert on the inner wall of the pharynx and the posterior margin of the thyroid cartilage. At the level of the palatine tonsil, it forms the substance of the **posterior tonsillar pillar.** Its contraction elevates the pharynx and helps in tensing the palate, both important parts of the act of swallowing. Simultaneous contraction of the papatopharyngeus muscles causes the tonsillar pillars to move nearer to each other in the midline. Palatopharyngeus is innervated by the vagus nerve axons found in the pharyngeal plexus.

The **palatoglossus muscle** extends from the posterolateral side of the soft palate to the lateral side of the

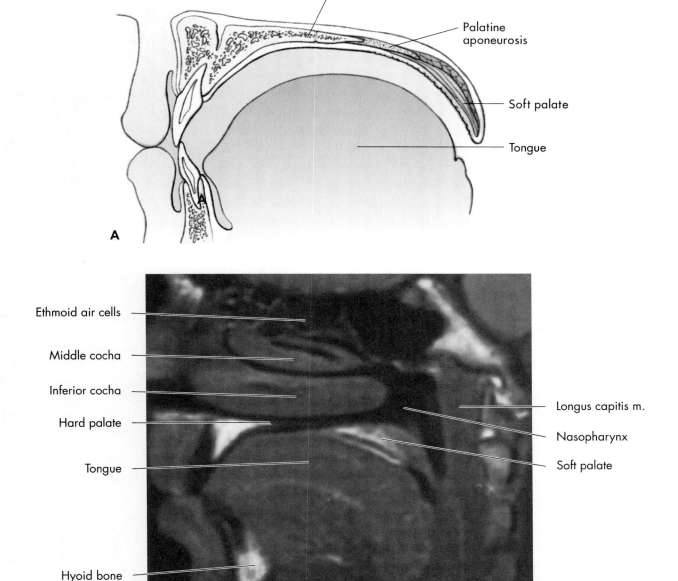

Figure 2-118 HARD AND SOFT PALATES. A, Lateral view, **B,** Sagittal MRI. (**B** from Weir J, Abrahams PH: *An imaging atlas of human anatomy,* London, 1992, Mosby.)

tongue. While descending, it forms the **anterior tonsillar pillar** (Figure 2-120), anterior to the palatine tonsil. Its contraction helps in tensing the palate and depressing it. The palatoglossus can flatten and depress the soft palate or can elevate the tongue if the palate is held rigid through the action of other muscles. It is innervated by vagal axons of the pharyngeal plexus.

The **uvula** (see Figures 2-117 and 2-119) is a bulbous midline structure that protrudes from the midline of the posterior free margin of the soft palate. It has a bilateral intrinsic muscle, the *musculis uvulae,* which is anchored in the palatine aponeurosis and extends posteriorly into the substance of the uvula. Contraction of one of these muscles alone causes deviation of the uvula to that side. Ordinarily, the two parts of the muscle act together and help in the process of tensing the palate and sealing the oropharynx from the nasopharynx.

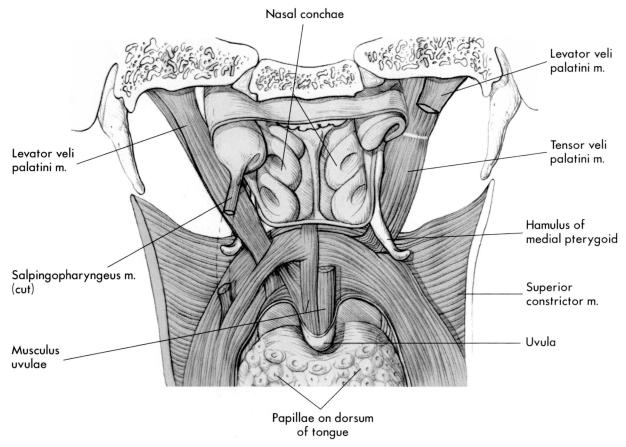

Nasal conchae

Levator veli
palatini m.

Levator veli
palatini m.

Tensor veli
palatini m.

Salpingopharyngeus m.
(cut)

Hamulus of
medial pterygoid

Superior
constrictor m.

Musculus
uvulae

Uvula

Papillae on dorsum
of tongue

Figure 2-119   LEVATOR AND TENSOR PALATINI MUSCLES, POSTERIOR VIEW.
SEE ATLAS, FIG. 2-68

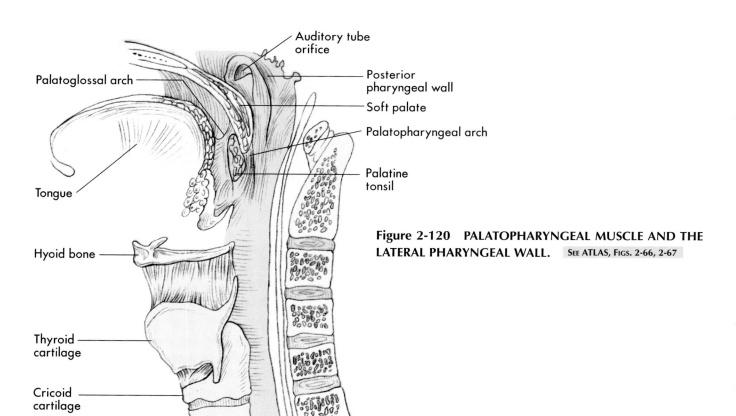

Auditory tube
orifice

Palatoglossal arch

Posterior
pharyngeal wall

Soft palate

Palatopharyngeal arch

Tongue

Palatine
tonsil

Hyoid bone

**Figure 2-120   PALATOPHARYNGEAL MUSCLE AND THE
LATERAL PHARYNGEAL WALL.**   SEE ATLAS, FIGS. 2-66, 2-67

Thyroid
cartilage

Cricoid
cartilage

Vascular Supply of the Palate

The arterial supply to the palate is by the **greater palatine artery** (Figure 2-121), a branch of the maxillary artery. This vessel descends from the pterygopalatine fossa through the greater palatine canal and, as it nears the palate, gives off several lesser palatine branches. The lesser palatine arteries turn posteriorly to supply the soft palate, while the greater palatine vessels continue anteriorly to supply the hard palate. Small branches of the ascending pharyngeal artery also supply the palate.

Venous drainage from the hard and soft palate is to the **pterygoid plexus,** located between the pterygoid muscles in the infratemporal fossa.

Nerve Supply of the Palate

Sensory innervation of the palate (Figure 2-121) is through the **greater** and **lesser palatine nerves** (to the hard and soft palate, respectively); these nerves, like the arteries of the same names, arise within the pterygopalatine fossa, as a branch of the maxillary nerve (V2). They descend through the greater palatine canal and divide into the lesser and greater branches as they approach the palate. There is also some contribution by the end branches of the **nasopalatine nerve** (also derived from V2), which travels forward near the base of the nasal septum and descends through the incisive foramen to enter the substance of the palate. It innervates the anterior half of the hard palate.

All of the intrinsic and extrinsic muscles of the palate (except one) are innervated by the motor branches of the **pharyngeal plexus**—specifically, axons that in the brainstem arise in the cranial root of the *accessory nerve* (XI) and soon after emerging from the brainstem become part of the *vagus nerve.* The exception is the tensor veli palatini, which is innervated by a small branch of the *mandibular nerve* (V3).

TEETH

In the mouth of the child, there are **20 deciduous teeth** (eight incisors, four canines, and eight molars); in the mouth of the adult, there are **32 permanent teeth** (eight incisors, four canines, eight premolars, and twelve molars) (Figures 2-122 and 2-123). Thus each half of the mandible and maxilla in the child (see Figure 2-123) has a *central and lateral incisor, one canine tooth,* and *two molars;* in the adult the comparable arrangement is a *central and lateral incisor, one canine, two premolars,* and *three molars.* The third and most posterior molar tooth in the adult emerges last (usually in the late teenage years) and is known as the *wisdom tooth.*

The term *occlusion* describes the manner in which teeth of the lower and upper jaw fit into each other during biting. On each tooth, the surfaces that come into contact with each other are the *occlusal surfaces.* The incisors have a sharp incisive surface, specialized for cutting. All of the other teeth lack a sharp edge but instead have smooth, raised prominences, known as **cusps,** on their occlusal surfaces. Canine teeth have one cusp, premolars have two (and occasionally three) cusps, and molar teeth have three to five cusps.

Each tooth has one or more elongated **roots** by which the tooth is anchored in the jaw. Typically, the incisors and canine teeth of both jaws have one root; the premolars of the mandible have one root, while those of the maxilla have two; and the molars of mandible have two roots, while those of the maxilla have three.

Most nonmammalian vertebrates have the capacity to regenerate injured or worn teeth throughout life; in mammals, however, the deterioration of the "permanent" teeth may be the direct cause of death (due to an inability to hunt and forage successfully). Most mammals produce a set of deciduous ("baby") teeth and later a permanent set. Table 2-23 describes the eruption of the deciduous and permanent teeth (also see Figure 2-123).

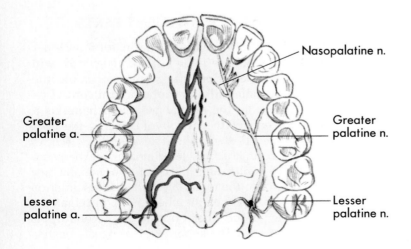

Greater palatine a.

Lesser palatine a.

Nasopalatine n.

Greater palatine n.

Lesser palatine n.

Figure 2-121 BLOOD SUPPLY AND INNERVATION OF PALATE. The greater and lesser palatine vessels and nerves descend in the palatine canal, from the pterygopalatine fossa to the undersurface of the palate (shown here), where they emerge and ramify over the inferior surface of the palate.

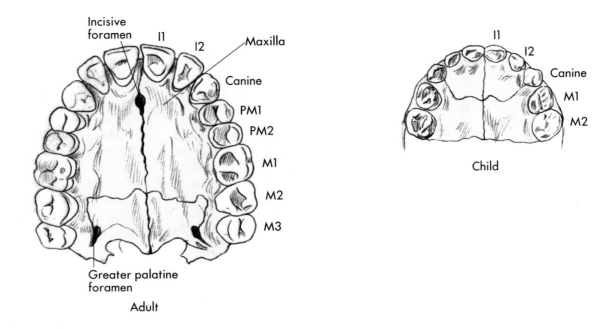

Figure 2-122   HARD PALATE AND TEETH IN THE ADULT AND CHILD. *I,* Incisor; *PM,* premolar; *M,* molar.   SEE ATLAS, FIGS. 2-39, 2-65

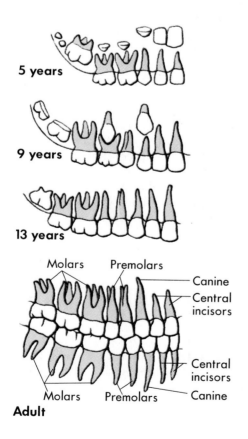

Figure 2-123   TEETH. Deciduous and permanent teeth are shown.   SEE ATLAS, FIG. 2-39

The curved portions of the maxilla and mandible, which support the teeth of each jaw, are known as the **alveolar ridges.** The space between the inner surface of the cheeks and each alveolar ridge is the **vestibule.** The space between the alveolar ridges on each side of the mouth is the oral cavity proper. Each tooth has a neurovascular core, the **pulp;** external to this, in all parts of the tooth, is the thick layer of **dentine.** Above the gingival line (that is, over the visible part of the tooth), there is an additional layer, the **enamel.**

Later in life, when teeth are lost from the mandible, the bone is extensively remodeled and in the edentulous (toothless) person, the body of the mandible is less than half the height it was earlier in life. Loss of teeth accounts for significant changes in the shape of the face in elderly persons.

CHEEK AND ITS CONSTITUENT PARTS

The cheek is composed of the buccinator muscle and surrounding connective tissue, a buccal fat pad, with epithelium on the exterior and oral mucosa on the interior. The **pterygomandibular raphe,** a firm cord of tissue extending from the medial pterygoid hamulus to the posterior end of the mylohyoid line of the mandible, forms the posterior limit of the cheek (Figure 2-124). The buccinator muscle originates on the pterygomandibular raphe and parts of the maxilla and mandible opposite the molar teeth. It extends anteriorly into the substance of the cheek. The buccinator is pierced by the parotid duct, opposite the second upper molar on each side. The superior pharyngeal constric-

Table 2-23 Eruption of the Deciduous and Adult Teeth

Type of Tooth	Deciduous Eruption	Adult Eruption
Central incisor	5-9 months	5-7 years
Lateral incisor	8-10 months	6-9 years
Canine teeth	15-20 months	8-12 years
Premolars	—	9-12 years
Molars	14-15 months (first)	5-7 years (first)
	18-24 months (second)	10-13 years (second)
		16-20 years (third, or "wisdom teeth")

tor attaches to the raphe posteriorly and extends in a posterior direction to form the upper muscular sleeve of the pharynx.

Similar to all the muscles of facial expression, the buccinator is innervated by the facial nerve, specifically by its buccal branch. In addition to its role in facial expression, it is important in chewing food (mastication), because the cheek musculature helps to position food between the alveolar ridges.

TONGUE

The tongue lies partly in the pharynx (posteriorly) and partly in the mouth (anteriorly). It participates in taste, chewing, and breakdown of ingested solids and in swallowing of both solids and liquids. It is a thick muscular structure, whose mass is made up of interlacing fascicles of striated **intrinsic musculature.** In addition, there are several additional striated muscles that attach to the tongue but originate elsewhere (the **extrinsic muscles**) (Figure 2-125).

The **base of the tongue** is a thick mass of muscle attached to the styloid process posteriorly, the hyoid bone inferiorly, and anteriorly to the inner surface of the anterior part of the mandible. It is also attached to the soft palate and pharynx by specific muscles. The more anterior mobile portion of the tongue is referred to as the oral portion. The **dorsum of the tongue** is that part facing the undersurface of the palate. The **ventral surface** (or undersurface) of the tongue faces the floor of the mouth. It is characterized by a thin midline membrane, oriented in the midsagittal plane, called the **frenulum.** It acts as a tether for the tongue and helps keep it attached to the floor of the mouth (Figure 2-126). At the base of the frenulum is a midline mass of tissue, the **sublingual papilla,** where the ducts of the two submandibular glands empty into the oral cavity.

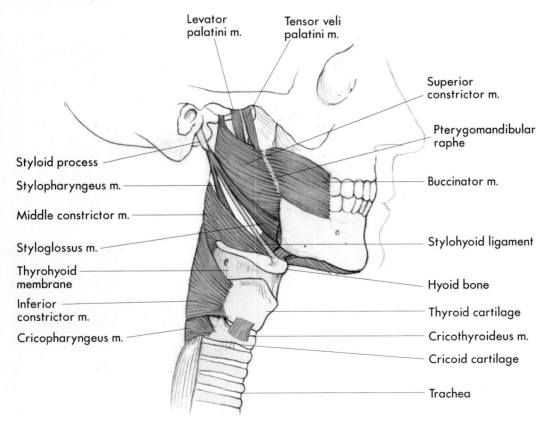

Figure 2-124 **PHARYNGEAL MUSCLES AND PTERYGOMANDIBULAR RAPHE.**

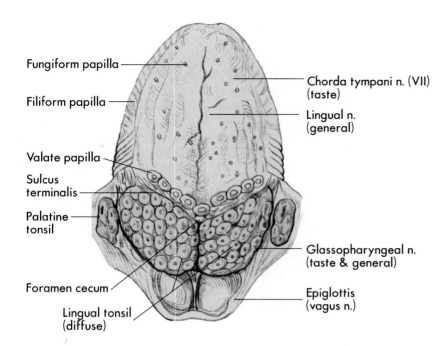

Fungiform papilla

Filiform papilla

Valate papilla

Sulcus terminalis

Palatine tonsil

Foramen cecum

Lingual tonsil (diffuse)

Chorda tympani n. (VII) (taste)

Lingual n. (general)

Glossopharyngeal n. (taste & general)

Epiglottis (vagus n.)

Figure 2-125   DORSAL VIEW OF TONGUE. The sulcus terminalis divides the posterior third from the anterior two thirds of the dorsum of the tongue. Different nerves innervate the separate regions of the tongue.
SEE ATLAS, FIG. 2-49

The undersurface of the tongue and the floor of the mouth are very vascular and therefore may be used for the administration of drugs (sublingual administration).

Dorsum of the Tongue

The surface of the tongue (Figures 2-125 and 2-126) is covered with squamous epithelium and specialized **taste buds** (classed as *filiform, fungiform,* or *circumvallate*). Circumvallate papillae are arrayed along the

sulcus **terminalis,** a V-shaped line on the dorsum of the tongue, with the **foramen cecum** at its apex. The thyroid gland begins its early development on the dorsal surface of the tongue, and the foramen cecum represents the point at which embryologic migration of the gland downward through the substance of the tongue and into the neck begins.

The dorsal surface of the tongue posterior to the sulcus terminalis (the pharyngeal portion of the tongue) has on its surface an irregular mass of lymphoid tissue known as the **lingual tonsil.** This portion of the tongue

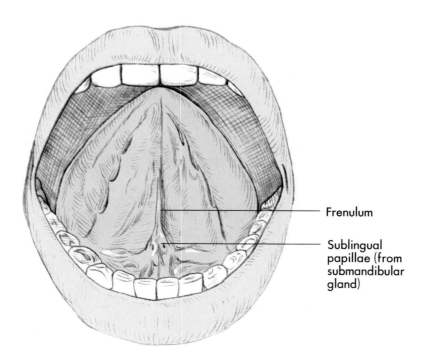

Frenulum

Sublingual papillae (from submandibular gland)

Figure 2-126   VIEW OF UNDERSURFACE OF TONGUE. A midline vertical fold of tissue, the frenulum, connects the tongue to the floor of the mouth. At its base is the sublingual papilla, where the submandibular duct opens into the oral cavity.

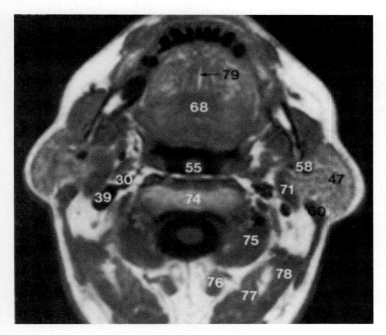

Figure 2-127 MRI OF THE OROPHARYNX. Axial image. (From Weir J, Abrahams PH: *An imaging atlas of human anatomy,* London, 1992, Mosby.)

30	Internal carotid artery	71	Posterior belly of digastric muscle
39	Internal jugular vein	74	Body of axis
47	Parotid gland	75	Inferior oblique muscle
55	Uvula	76	Rectus capitis muscle
58	Retromandibular vein	77	Semispinalis capitis muscle
60	Sternocleidomastoid muscle	78	Splenius capitis muscle
68	Intrinsic muscles of tongue	79	Lingual septum

is covered with endodermally derived third-pharyngeal arch epithelium (that is, it is the uppermost part of the embryonic gut).

The part of the tongue anterior to the sulcus terminalis (the oral portion of the tongue) is covered by epithelium derived from first pharyngeal arch epithelium. In addition to having different embryologic origins, the oral and pharyngeal portions of the dorsum of the tongue also have different sensory innervations. The glossopharyngeal nerve innervates the posterior third of the tongue, for both general and special sensation (taste). The trigeminal nerve (general sensation, through the lingual branch of V3) and facial nerve (taste) innervate the anterior two thirds of the tongue.

Musculature of the Tongue

The tongue is composed of (1) a mass of intrinsic musculature, arrayed in various directions, (2) extrinsic muscles (Table 2-24; Figure 2-127), some of which form a significant part of the tongue mass but also may alter its shape and position (genioglossus, hyoglossus), and (3) other muscles that alter the shape and position of the tongue but do not contribute significantly to its mass (styloglossus, palatoglossus). The styloglossus and palatoglossus interdigitate with hypoglossus in the substance of the tongue (Figure 2-128).

Innervation of the Tongue

The motor and sensory innervation of the tongue is complex and is shown in Table 2-25. All muscles ending in *-glossus* are innervated by the hypoglossal nerve except the palatoglossus (which is innervated by the vagus nerve). Injury to the hypoglossal nerve produces a deviation of the tongue (on voluntary protrusion) toward the side of the lesion, because of the unbalanced effect of muscle contraction on the opposite, healthy side of the tongue.

Table 2-24 Extrinsic Muscles of the Tongue

Name	Origin	Insertion	Innervation	Action
Hyoglossus	Body and greater horn of hyoid bone	Side of tongue	Hypoglossal nerve (XII)	Depresses tongue, makes dorsum convex
Genioglossus	Mental spines of mandible, near the mandibular symphysis	Body of tongue	Hypoglossal (XII)	Protrudes tongue (especially posterior fibers)
Styloglossus	Styloid process	Side of tongue	Hypoglossal (XII)	Retracts and elevates tongue
Palatoglossus	Side of soft palate	Side of tongue	Vagus (X, pharyngeal plexus)	Elevates tongue

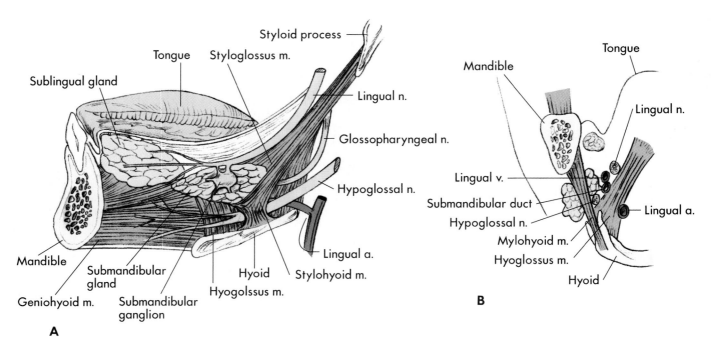

Figure 2-128   LATERAL VIEW OF THE TONGUE. A, Submandibular and sublingual glands are shown, in relation to the mylohyoid muscle. **B,** Coronal section shows the position of several vessels and nerves in relation to the hyoglossus muscle.   SEE ATLAS, FIG. 2-48

Anatomic Relationships of the Tongue

The hyoglossus muscle is a key landmark muscle for the tongue (Figure 2-128, *B*). It originates from the hyoid bone and extends upward into the substance of the tongue. Hyoglossus is a thickened quadrangular plate of muscle that is positioned in the sagittal plane. *Lateral (superficial)* to it, from inferior, are the hypoglossal nerve, deep portion of the submandibular gland, submandibular duct, submandibular ganglion, lingual vein, lingual nerve, and stylohyoid muscle (Figure 2-128). The styloglossus muscle descends to become part of the tongue by blending with the hyoglossus muscle, lying slightly lateral and posterior to it. *Medial (deep) to the hyoglossus muscle* are the lingual artery, glossopharyngeal nerve, middle constrictor muscle, and stylohyoid ligament, and more anteriorly, the genioglossus and geniohyoid muscles.

Vascular Supply of the Tongue

The **lingual artery** (Figure 2-128) is the main blood supply of the tongue, arising from the external carotid artery and coursing deep to hyoglossus. It branches extensively within the tongue. Venous drainage is by **lingual vein** (lying superficial to hyoglossus), draining to the internal jugular vein. The lingual veins may be seen easily on the underside of the tongue, running just beneath the mucosa.

Lymphatic Drainage of the Tongue

Lymphatic drainage from the posterolateral tongue is to **cervical nodes,** while the anterior tip of the tongue drains to **submental nodes** (see Figure 2-69). Submental nodes are positioned just inferior to the mental symphysis of the mandible, and any enlargements in

Table 2-25   Innervation of the Tongue

Nerve	Domain—Function
Lingual nerve (V3, general sensory)	General sensory for anterior two thirds of tongue; proprioception for intrinsic muscles
Glossopharyngeal nerve (nerve IX, general sensory and taste)	General sensory and taste for posterior third of tongue
Chorda tympani (branch of nerve VII, taste)	Taste for anterior two thirds of tongue
Hypoglossal nerve (nerve XII, motor; all but palatoglossus)	All striated muscles, intrinsic and extrinsic, except palatoglossus
Pharyngeal plexus (from nerve X, motor/palatoglossus)	Palatoglossus muscle

these nodes mandates an examination of the anterior tongue to look for possible malignancies (especially in a tobacco user).

SUBMANDIBULAR AND SUBLINGUAL GLANDS

Saliva moistens, softens, and begins the digestion of ingested carbohydrates through the action of certain enzymes. Saliva is produced by three pairs of **salivary glands** that empty into the oral cavity (Figure 2-128). The **submandibular gland** is located medial to the mandible, inferior to the mylohyoid line (line of attachment for the mylohyoid muscle on the mandible). Part of the submandibular gland is deep to the mylohyoid muscle, between it and hyoglossus, and another part is superficial to it, between the mandible and the mylohyoid muscle. The two parts are continuous with each other as they wrap around the free posterior margin of the mylohyoid muscle. It drains by a **submandibular duct** (Figure 2-128), coursing along the external surface of the hyoglossus muscle (Wharton's duct). It empties saliva in the floor of the mouth at the **sublingual papilla,** a small nodule of tissue located at the base of the

frenulum of the tongue, on its inferior surface.

The **sublingual gland** is located in a shallow depression on the medial surface of the mandible, the sublingual fossa, located just superior to the line for attachment of the mylohyoid muscle on the medial surface of the mandible (Figure 2-129). The submandibular gland lies in a similar position inferior to the mylohyoid. Lying medial to the sublingual gland are the submandibular duct and the lingual nerve. The sublingual glands drain by a series of small ducts located in the floor of the mouth, just medial to the inner surface of the mandible on each side.

Innervation of both the submandibular and sublingual glands is from the secretomotor axons originating in the *submandibular ganglion.* It lies on the lateral surface of hyoglossus, suspended from the lingual nerve, between hyoglossus and the superficial lobe of the submandibular gland. The ganglion receives its preganglionic input from the chorda tympani, originally a branch of the facial nerve. The axons of the chorda tympani are incorporated into the lingual nerve and accompany it to reach the ganglion. Both salivary glands are innervated by both adrenergic (sympathetic) and cholinergic (parasympathetic) axons. Both contribute to

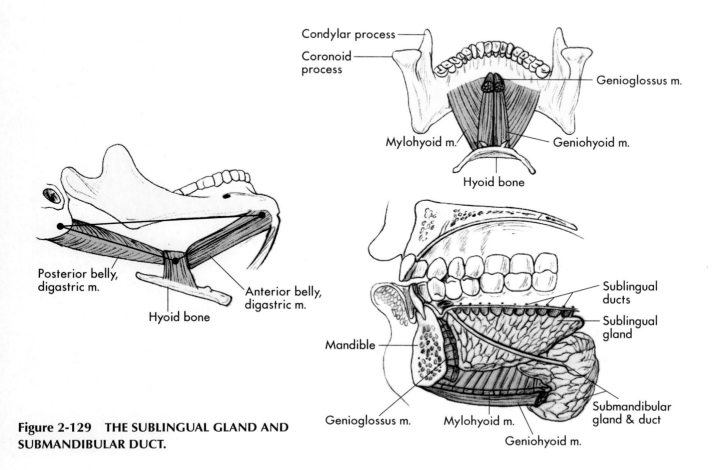

Figure 2-129   THE SUBLINGUAL GLAND AND SUBMANDIBULAR DUCT.

salivation. The adrenergic axons closely follow the distribution of arterioles within the gland, while the cholinergic axons tend to arborize around the secretory units or acini within the gland. In addition to direct neural influence (that is, parasympathetic secretomotor), vasodilation also promotes secretion of saliva (from diminished sympathetic input).

The third major salivary gland draining into the mouth is the **parotid gland.** It was described on pp. 183-186. In addition to the three major glands there are numerous **minor salivary glands** on the inferior surface of the soft palate. They are similar in structure to the mucus glands found in the mucosa throughout the digestive tract but differ in receiving postganglionic parasympathetic secretomotor innervation through the lesser palatine nerve, by axons originating in the pterygopalatine ganglion.

PALATINE TONSIL

The **palatine tonsil** (faucial tonsil) lies in a bed between two vertical muscular ridges in the lateral wall of the posterior part of the oral cavity (see Figure 2-120). These ridges are the tonsillar pillars, formed by the palatoglossus muscle (the **anterior pillar**) and the palatopharyngeus muscle (the **posterior pillar**). Each muscular pillar or arch is covered by mucosa. The floor of the bed in which the palatine tonsil is situated is part of the wall of the pharynx, specifically a part of the superior constrictor muscle. Just lateral to this muscular bed is the styloglossus muscle, as well as some large branches of the facial, lingual, and external carotid arteries. Most often the **tonsillar artery,** a branch of the facial artery, serves as the main blood supply to the palatine tonsil. A large **external palatine vein** usually lies between the deep surface of the tonsil and the superior constrictor muscle. The medial surface of the tonsil faces the interior of the oral cavity and projects a varying distance inward. It can enlarge considerably when inflammed.

The palatine and lingual tonsils, as well as the pharyngeal tonsil ("adenoid"—see p. 279) are part of a discontinuous ring of lymphoid tissue (known as Waldeyer's ring) incompletely surrounding the entrance to the pharynx. These masses of lymphoid tissue manufacture high levels of IgA, which may bind to ingested materials and prepare them for immunologic ingestion in the digestive tract.

THE MOUTH AND PALATE

MALIGNANCIES IN THE ORAL CAVITY

The oral cavity is a frequent site of malignancies resulting from environmental exposure, especially tobacco products. They occur on the lips and tongue with some frequency, especially in smokers.

SALIVARY DRAINAGE

Openings of the salivary gland ducts into the mouth may be obstructed, leading to cystic swellings (ranula). Stones may also form within the ducts of the salivary glands, sometimes necessitating surgical removal.

ECTOPIC THYROID TISSUE AND THYROGLOSSAL CYSTS

When the thyroid gland fails to migrate to the lower neck, thyroid tissue or cystic remnants may occur anywhere along its intended path of migration, or even on the dorsum of the tongue itself ("lingual thyroid").

MOBILITY OF THE TONGUE

If the frenulum of the tongue is excessively large or extends too far anterior, it may limit the mobility of the tongue and the person is said to be "tongue tied."

CLEFT LIP

Cleft lip may occur independently or accompany a cleft palate. Cleft lip occurs in 1 to 2 per 3000 live births.

CLEFT PALATE

Cleft palate is a developmental anomaly in which the midline fusion of the palatine processes of the maxillae and/or palatine bones fails; at its mildest, only the uvula is affected, while at its worst, there is a wide gap in the middle of the entire palate. In such severe cases, the base of the nasal septum may be viewed by looking upward through the oral cavity. A cleft palate permits air, liquids, or solids to pass from nose to mouth or vice versa. This leads to sucking and swallowing problems in the newborn and to difficulties in speech. Corrective devices and surgery aim to close the defect and eliminate the passage of materials between the mouth and nose.

CLEFT PALATE REPAIR

The prominent mucoperiosteum on the inferior surface of the palate may be used in surgery as a "flap" to repair congenital cleft palates.

GENIOGLOSSUS AND AIRWAY PATENCY

The genioglossus muscle protrudes the tongue, but just as importantly it is under a constant state of contraction, sufficient to prevent the tongue from collapsing posteriorly and obstructing the airway. When a patient is deeply obtuneded (due to traumatic injury or anesthesia), the genioglossus may relax completely, and when the base of the tongue moves to the posterior, the patient cannot breathe.

THE GINGIVAE

Gingivitis is an inflammation of the tissue surrounding the tooth where it "emerges" from within the bone. If untreated, it can lead to deeper inflammation (periodontitis), which can truly destroy the attachment of the teeth to the jaw.

ABNORMALITIES OF THE SOFT PALATE

Palatopharyngeal incompetency is a situation in which the soft palate does not extend far enough posterior to form a good seal with the pharynx. This problem is often associated with cleft palate. This condition is associated with problems in swallowing and speech.

TONSILLECTOMY

Enthusiasm for removal of the tonsils as a treatment for recurrent upper respiratory infections varies from decade to decade. Currently there is considerable hesitation to remove the tonsils, but in the 1950s and 1960s it was one of the most common operations performed in those in the pediatric age-group. Because of the abundant vascularity of the tonsil, the operation can be dangerous.

Pharynx

▶ Important Skeletal Structures of the Pharynx

▶ Intrinsic Pharyngeal Muscles

▶ External Muscles Forming and Acting on the Pharynx

▶ Nasopharynx

▶ Oropharynx

▶ Laryngopharynx

▶ Innervation of the Pharynx

▶ Deglutition (Swallowing)

The pharynx is a muscular tube, composed of three major intrinsic constrictor muscles, and a series of anterior cartilages and bone that form part of its perimeter. The constrictor muscles meet each other in a **posterior median raphe,** a fascial strip that extends along the dorsal midline of the pharynx. Connective tissue membranes fill in gaps between the constrictor muscles and the skeletal elements. A number of smaller muscles that serve to elevate, depress, and change the shape of the pharyngeal tube also attach to it.

The pharynx is the first part of the digestive tube to demonstrate organized *"peristaltic" contractions,* which have the effect of propelling the ingested bolus of food farther down the pharynx and into the esophagus. The pharynx is the final component in a complex and intricate process of swallowing, or *deglutition.* The pharynx communicates with the oral and nasal cavities, middle ear cavity, and the larynx. Air, food, and liquids all enter the body through the mouth and nose. It is the job of the pharynx to make sure that air and only air enters the larynx, while solid and liquid food are directed to the esophagus.

IMPORTANT SKELETAL STRUCTURES OF THE PHARYNX

Several important skeletal structures (Figure 2-130) form the framework on which the muscles and other soft tissues of the pharynx are arrayed. The **pterygomandibular raphe** extends from the medial pterygoid hamulus to the inner surface of the angle of the mandible, just above the posterior end of the mylohyoid line. This thickened fibrous cord is the main anterior attachment for the superior constrictor of the pharynx and main posterior attachment of the buccinator muscle. The sphenomandibular ligament lies just behind it.

The **hyoid bone** (Figure 2-130) is a C-shaped bone positioned in the upper neck so that its convex surface faces forward. The central third of this bone is its *body,* the *greater horns* are the curved portions of the bone extending posterosuperiorly from the body on each side, and the *lesser horns* are two small spurs of bone that protrude upward from the junction of the body and the greater horn on each side. The posterior tips of the lesser horns are suspended from the styloid process on each side of the skull by the **stylohyoid ligaments.** The hyoid bone forms the main anterior attachment for the middle constrictor muscle on each side. It is also an attachment for several other muscles of the neck. The geniohyoid, mylohyoid, and stylohyoid muscles extend superiorly from the body of the hyoid, while the sternohyoid, thyrohyoid, and omohyoid muscles attach to the body and extend inferiorly. The hyoglossus and middle constrictor muscles attach to the greater and lesser horns on each side of the hyoid bone. The **thyroid cartilage** is positioned in the anterior neck, inferior

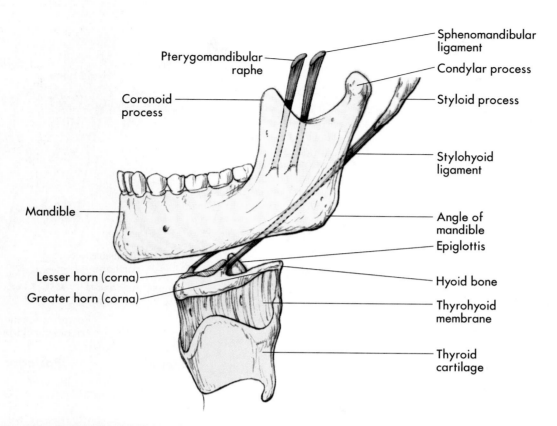

Figure 2-130 SKELETAL STRUCTURES SUPPORTING THE PHARYNX. The mandible, sphenomandibular ligament, hyoid bone, and cricoid cartilage all form anterior attachments for parts of the pharynx.

to the hyoid bone, to which it is attached by the thyrohyoid membrane (Figure 2-131). It is composed of two quadrangular plates, or *laminae,* joined in the anterior midline. Each extends posteriorly at an approximate 45-degree angle. Attached to the posterior margin of each lamina is a pair of slender vertical cylindrical processes, a larger *superior horn* or cornu, and a smaller *inferior horn.* The thyroid cartilage forms the main anterior attachment for the inferior constrictor muscle.

The **cricoid cartilage,** positioned inferior to the thyroid cartilage, is shaped like a signet ring, with a broad cartilaginous plate facing posteriorly (Figure 2-131). Because it is a closed cartilaginous ring, it is the narrowest part of the upper airway and the only one that cannot vary its size. It forms the main anteroinferior attachment for cricopharyngeus muscle (the most inferior part of the inferior constrictor muscle) and provides attachment for the cricothyroideus muscle.

INTRINSIC PHARYNGEAL MUSCLES (Table 2-26)

The **superior constrictor muscle** (Figures 2-124 and 2-132) attaches anteriorly to the pterygomandibular

raphe and to the posterior end of the mylohyoid line on the inner surface of the mandible. It sweeps posteriorly as a thin vertical plate of muscle and unites with its companion muscle from the other side in the median raphe of the pharynx. The gap between the superior constrictor and the base of the skull is occupied by the auditory tube, the levator veli palatini muscle, and the ascending branch of the facial artery; the remaining space is loosely filled with the pharyngobasilar fascia.

The **middle constrictor muscle** (Figures 2-124 and 2-132) is attached anteriorly to the hyoid bone and stylohyoid ligament. Posteriorly it surrounds the superior constrictor and attaches to its companion in the median raphe. The small gap between the superior and middle constrictors is filled with the stylopharyngeus and nerve IX; the styloglossus and the neurovascular supply of the tongue pass just external to this gap.

The **inferior constrictor muscle** (Figures 2-124 and 2-132) attaches anteriorly to the cricoid cartilage and the lateral surface of the lamina of the thyroid cartilage. The inferior constrictor also attaches to its partner in the fibrous median raphe posteriorly and lies superficial to the middle constrictor. Its lowermost fibers are

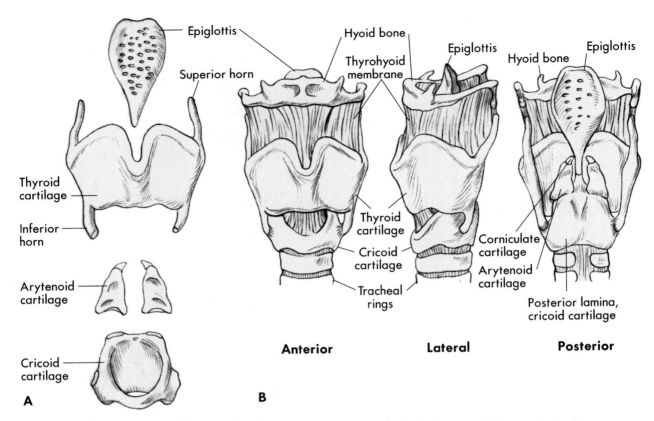

Figure 2-131   CARTILAGES OF THE LARYNX. A, "Exploded" view of the epiglottis, thyroid, arytenoid, and cricoid cartilages. **B,** Three views of the same structures assembled and attached to the underlying trachea.   SEE ATLAS, FIG. 2-80

thickened and sometimes are recognized separately as the **cricopharyngeus.** The cricopharyngeal ring is the narrowest part of the GI tract. The cricopharyngeus normally functions as a sphincter, and if it is overactive in this respect, the part of the inferior constrictor just proximal to it may become distended and form a diverticulum. By contrast, if the sphincteric activity of the cricopharyngeus is weakened, a patient may experience regurgitation of food.

The gap between the middle and inferior constrictors is large, spanned by the **thyrohyoid membrane** (Figure 2-130), which is penetrated by the internal branch of the superior laryngeal vessels and nerve.

EXTERNAL MUSCLES FORMING AND ACTING ON THE PHARYNX (Table 2-26)

The **palatopharyngeus muscle** sweeps downward from the lateral margin of soft palate to insert on internal surface of middle constrictor (Figure 2-132). It is innervated by the vagus nerve (through the pharyngeal plexus). It forms the posterior tonsillar pillar and helps to elevate pharynx. **Salpingopharyngeus** (*salpinx,*

trumpet) arises from the auditory tube and passes downward, very near to palatopharyngeus muscle, to blend into the pharyngeal musculature. It forms a raised fold in the inner mucosa of pharynx (Figure 2-132). It helps to elevate the pharynx. Contraction of salpingopharyngeus also results in opening of auditory tube orifice ("popping" of ears or swallowing after changes in atmospheric pressure). It is also innervated by the pharyngeal plexus.

The **stylopharyngeus muscle** extends from the styloid process, lies externally to the superior constrictor, and passes to the internal surface of middle constrictor to reach the posterior border of the thyroid lamina (Figure 2-132). It passes in the gap between the superior and middle constrictor muscles and blends into the musculature of the pharynx. It helps to elevate pharynx and is innervated by the glossopharyngeal nerve.

NASOPHARYNX

The pharynx is divided into three regions: the nasopharynx, oropharynx, and laryngopharynx (or hypopharynx). The **nasopharynx** (Figure 2-133) begins at

Table 2-26 Muscles of the Pharynx

Muscle	Attachments	Comments
INTRINSIC MUSCLES		
Superior constrictor	From pterygomandibular raphe and mylohyoid line of mandible to posterior median raphe and to pharyngeal tubercle on base of occipital bone	Includes a thickened band of muscle originating on the superior surface of the palate and sweeping backward to blend with the superior constrictor
Gap between superior and middle constrictors	Occupied by auditory tube, levator veli palatini, ascending palatine branch of facial artery	
Middle constrictor	From hyoid bone and stylohyoid ligament to posterior median raphe	Upper fibers overlap the superior constrictor; lower fibers are internal to inferior constrictor
Gap between middle and inferior constrictors	Occupied by stylopharyngeus muscle, glossopharyngeal nerve	
Inferior constrictor (*thyropharyngeus* part)	From thyroid lamina to the posterior median raphe	This part of the inferior constrictor sweeps upward to insert just externally to the middle constrictor; acts as the propulsive force in swallowing
Inferior constrictor (*cricopharyngeus* part)	From inferior horn of the thyroid and cricoid cartilage to the posterior median raphe of pharynx; also blends with upper fibers of esophageal musculature	This part of the inferior constrictor acts as a sphincter in swallowing, and failure of it to relax can lead to lateral diverticula in the wall of the pharynx just above it
EXTERNAL MUSCLES		
Stylopharyngeus	From styloid process to internal surface of middle constrictor	Passes between superior and middle constrictors; accompanied by nerve IX
Palatopharyngeus	From lateral surface of soft palate to internal surface of the middle constrictor	Inserts on inside of pharynx as far distal as thyroid cartilage; accompanied by salpingopharyngeus
Salpingopharyngeus	From lower margin of auditory tube prominence to inner surface of middle constrictor	Inserts on interior of pharynx near to palatopharyngeus

the posterior nasal apertures (choanae) and extends inferiorly to the level of the soft palate. Its walls are the superior constrictor and the salpingopharyngeus. The lateral wall of the nasopharynx is perforated by the aperture of the auditory tube. The opening of the auditory tube is a ring of cartilage forming a near-circular elevation in the mucosa of the pharyngeal wall (the **torus tubarius**) (see Figure 2-120). The salpingopharyngeus muscle originates from this ring of cartilage. There is often a collection of lymphoid tissue near the orifice of the auditory tube (the "tubal tonsil"). The **pharyngeal recess** ("fossa of Rosenmüller") is a depression lying between the torus tubarius and the pharyngeal wall posterior to it. There is a small single midline **pharyngeal tonsil** (adenoid) in the posterior nasopharyngeal wall. Along with the two palatine tonsils, the tubal tonsil and the midline lingual tonsil on the dorsum of the tongue, the pharyngeal tonsil contributes to the incomplete **ring of lymphoid tissue** (Waldeyer's ring) that surrounds the upper end of the digestive tract.

The superior portion of the nasopharynx is attached to the base of the skull by the *pharyngobasilar fascia*. Inflammatory swelling of the torus tubarius can occlude the orifice of the auditory tube and prevent equilibration of pressures between the middle ear and the exterior ("plugged ears"). Infection may also track upward from the nasopharynx to the middle ear and cause otitis media. Young children are more prone to frequent and recurrent infections of the middle ears; part of the cause may be that the auditory tube in children is more nearly horizontal, rather than inclined markedly downward, as in the adult. This may contribute to the migration of infectious organisms into the middle ear and to the likelihood that mucus will obstruct the auditory tube and cause fluid to accumulate within the middle ear.

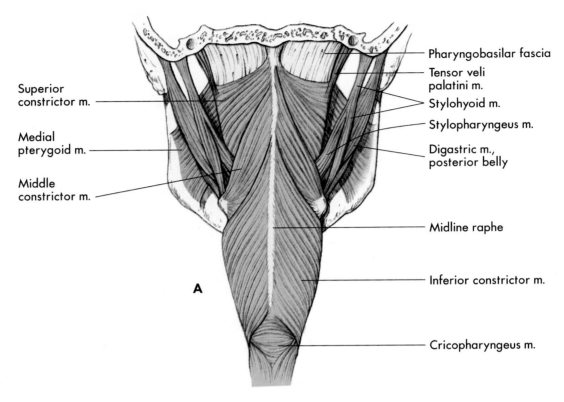

Superior constrictor m.

Medial pterygoid m.

Middle constrictor m.

Pharyngobasilar fascia

Tensor veli palatini m.

Stylohyoid m.

Stylopharyngeus m.

Digastric m., posterior belly

Midline raphe

Inferior constrictor m.

Cricopharyngeus m.

A

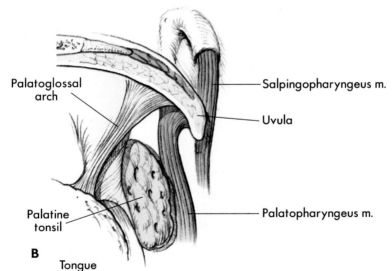

Palatoglossal arch

Salpingopharyngeus m.

Uvula

Palatine tonsil

Palatopharyngeus m.

B   Tongue

Figure 2-132 SOFT PALATE AND PALATINE TONSIL. The three pharyngeal constrictors are attached superiorly to the base of the skull by the pharyngobasilar fascia and inferiorly to the esophagus by the cricopharyngeus muscle.
SEE ATLAS, FIGS. 2-69, 2-70

OROPHARYNX

The oropharynx extends from the level of the soft palate downward to the level of the base of the tongue (Figure 2-133). Its walls are formed by the superior and middle constrictors, palatoglossus, and palatopharyngeus (comprising the tonsillar pillars), and it opens anteriorly into the oral cavity. The bed of the palatine tonsil (see Figures 2-120 and 2-133) is flanked by the anterior and posterior tonsillar pillars (the mucosa covering

palatoglossus and palatopharyngeus, respectively). The palatine tonsil bed is positioned over this gap between the superior and middle constrictors. *Stylopharyngeus* and the *glossopharyngeal nerve* pass just external to the palatine tonsillar bed. Surgery on the palatine tonsil can endanger the glossopharyngeal nerve, as well as pose a risk of hemorrhage.

The *facial artery* is the prime blood supply of the palatine tonsil, with other branches from the *lingual, as-*

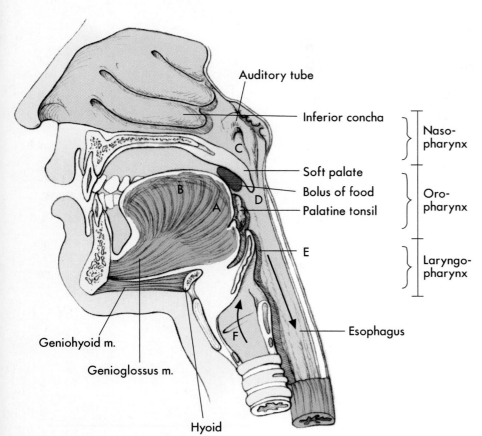

Auditory tube

Inferior concha

Naso-pharynx

Soft palate

Bolus of food

Palatine tonsil

Oro-pharynx

E

Laryngo-pharynx

Esophagus

Geniohyoid m.

Genioglossus m.

Hyoid

Figure 2-133 NASOPHARYNX, ORO-PHARYNX, LARYNGOPHARYNX, AND MECHANISM OF SWALLOWING. *A,* Posterior movement of the tongue. *B,* Upward movement of the tongue, trapping the bolus of food between it and the undersurface of the palate. *C,* Stiffening of the palate and its movement posteriorly to seal the nasal cavity from the mouth. *D,* Position and direction of movement for the bolus of food being swallowed. *E,* Posterior motion of the base of the tongue against the epiglottis and larynx to minimize the risk that the bolus of food will enter the airway. *F,* Larynx also elevated as part of this process.

<small>SEE ATLAS, FIGS. 2-78, 2-79</small>

cending pharyngeal, and *maxillary arteries.* Tonsillectomy is potentially a very bloody operation because of these vessels and a dense venous plexus.

LARYNGOPHARYNX

The laryngopharynx (or hypopharynx) extends from the base of the tongue to the origin of the esophagus (Figure 2-133). Its walls are formed by the inferior constrictor. The lowest portion of the inferior constrictor is identified as a separate muscle, the *cricopharyngeus.* It forms a sphincter at the commencement of the esophagus.

The **epiglottis** (Figure 2-134) is in the anterior wall of the laryngopharynx. It is a cartilaginous bladelike structure with a curved upper margin, often described as "omega-shaped." Between the epiglottis and the base of the tongue anteriorly is the **vallecula** or **glosso-epiglottic space** (see section on the larynx). It is a cul-de-sac that is divided into two halves by a thin membrane, the **frenulum.** The **aryepiglottic folds** are thin, raised folds of membrane that extend downward from the sides of the epiglottis posteriorly to the arytenoid cartilages of the larynx. Between the two aryepiglottic folds lies the entrance to the larynx. The areas between the aryepiglottic folds and the lateral walls of the hy-

popharynx are the **piriform recesses.** During swallowing, solid or liquid food must pass laterally or posteriorly to the aryepiglottic folds to successfully enter the upper part of the esophagus.

INNERVATION OF THE PHARYNX

The **pharyngeal plexus** is a complex network of axons to which the *vagus* and *glossopharyngeal nerves* contribute. In general, the vagal contributions are motor and the glossopharyngeal contributions sensory. The striated branchiomotor muscles composing the pharynx receive motor innervation from the pharyngeal plexus (vagal component), except stylopharyngeus, which is the one and only striated muscle to receive motor innervation from the glossopharyngeal nerve. Sensory innervation of mucosa of the nasopharynx is by V2 (pharyngeal branch of the maxillary nerve), and the pharyngeal plexus (glossopharyngeal nerve component) for the mucosa of the oropharynx and hypopharynx.

The *gag reflex* is a good illustration of how the sensory and motor innervation of the pharynx work together. It involves sensory stimulation of the pharyngeal mucosa (glossopharyngeal component) and subsequent contraction of pharyngeal musculature (vagal component).

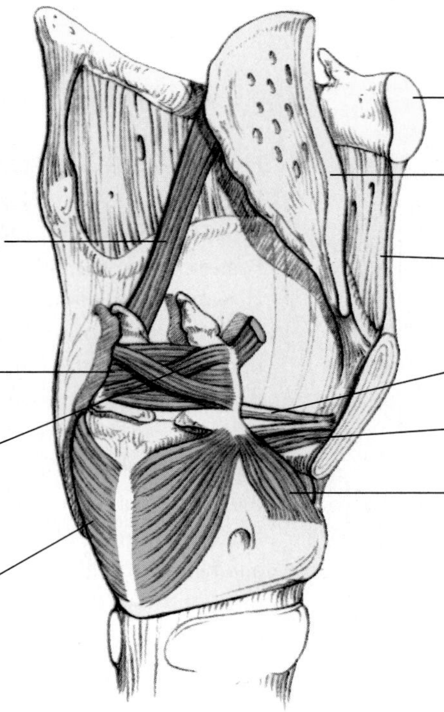

Aryepiglotticus m.

Transverse arytenoid m.

Oblique arytenoid m.

Posterior cricoarytenoid m.

Hyoid bone

Epiglottis (split in half vertically)

Thyrohyoid membrane

Vocal ligament

Vocalis m.

Lateral cricoarytenoid m.

Figure 2-134 MUSCLES OF LAR-YNX, RIGHT POSTEROLATERAL VIEW.
SEE ATLAS, FIGS. 2-82, 2-83, 2-84

The presence of a gag reflex is often used as an index of injury to the lower brainstem, where axons of these cranial nerves arise.

DEGLUTITION (SWALLOWING)

Swallowing (deglutition) is a complex act (Figure 2-133). It begins with chewing and softening of the food bolus by the masticatory muscles and moistening with saliva. The tongue then compresses the bolus against the palate and forces it posteriorly, through contraction of the intrinsic muscles of the tongue (to stiffen the tongue), the palatoglossus (to elevate the tongue against the hard palate), and the styloglossus (to retract the tongue and move the bolus of food backward along the undersurface of the palate). The soft palate is made rigid by contraction of the levator and tensor veli palatini. This seals off the nasopharynx from the oropharynx and laryngopharynx. The stylopharyngeus, salpingopharyngeus, and palatopharyngeus muscles contract and draw the pharynx superiorly, and the stylohyoid and digastric muscles elevate the hyoid bone and, by extension, the pharynx. The larynx is compressed upward against the epiglottis, and the laryngeal orifice is blocked. The food bolus then slides

PRINCIPLES ■

Innervation of the pharyngeal constrictors reflects their development from the lower pharyngeal arches. As with other structures of the head and neck, multiple cranial nerves are involved, and in many cases one nerve carries out the sensory function and another the motor. In the pharynx, the mucosal sensory function is the responsibility of the maxillary nerve (the nasopharynx) and the glossopharyngeal nerve (the oropharynx and laryngopharynx). The motor function of the pharyngeal constrictors is supplied by the vagus nerve (though the axons innervating the pharynx are in fact derived from the nerve XI and travel with the vagus nerve). Together these nerves compose the pharyngeal plexus.

posteriorly and inferiorly, passing over the posterior aspect of the closed larynx and into the hypopharynx and from there to the esophagus. Sequential contraction of the superior, middle, and inferior constrictors then forces the food bolus inferiorly into the esophagus.

THE PHARYNX

ADENOIDITIS

Inflammation of the pharyngeal tonsil, with subsequent obstruction of airflow and production of noisy breathing, is known as adenoiditis. Like inflammation of the palatine tonsils—if the obstruction is severe, there is recurrent infection, or the impairment to breathing severe enough—surgical removal may be indicated. Even more frequently, an inflamed pharyngeal tonsil can obstruct the auditory tubes.

RETROPHARYNGEAL ABSCESS

Inflammation of the posterior pharyngeal wall can cause an increase in the distance between the column of air in the pharynx and the anterior edge of the vertebral column, as visualized in a lateral x-ray of the neck. This may be the only clue to the presence of an infected area, or abscess, in a patient who demonstrates fever, pain on swallowing, and respiratory distress without any other obvious source.

PALATINE TONSILLITIS

Inflammation of the palatine tonsils is what we all refer to as "tonsillitis" and is the condition that has led to tens of thousands of surgeries to remove the inflamed tonsils. Some argue now that such surgeries are unnecessary and may be even dangerous because they remove one source of immunity for materials ingested into the GI and respiratory tracts. Proponents argue that such chronically inflamed tonsils are a site for recurrent infection that keep children out of school and keep adults from their work.

2.14 ▸ section two.fourteen
Larynx

▸ Cartilaginous Skeleton of the Larynx

▸ Glottic Region

▸ Musculature of the Larynx

▸ Innervation of the Larynx

▸ Vascular Supply of the Larynx

The larynx is a region of beautiful complexity. It is the birthplace of our speech, singing, and other forms of vocalization. Just as important, it is the means by which we protect our airways and permit nothing but inhaled air to reach the trachea and lungs. The larynx and its associated muscles are derived from the lower pharyngeal arches (specifically the fourth and sixth). The major motor innervation of the larynx is accomplished by a nerve that travels downward into the chest before returning to the larynx (the recurrent laryngeal branch of the vagus nerve). A knowledge of the anatomy of the larynx is crucial for anyone intending to practice medicine—indeed, when called on to resuscitate a critically ill patient, understanding of the structure and position of the larynx and the steps to be taken to ensure adequate respiration may well be the difference between the life and death of that patient. Numerous cartilages make up the skeleton of the larynx—the epiglottis, thyroid, and cricoid cartilages (unpaired) and the arytenoid, corniculate, and cuneiform cartilages (paired). The musculature of the larynx is striated and derived from mesoderm of pharyngeal arches four and six. Innervation of the larynx is through the superior laryngeal and recurrent laryngeal branches of the vagus nerve.

CARTILAGINOUS SKELETON OF THE LARYNX

The **thyroid cartilage** (see Figures 2-131, 2-134, and 2-135) consists of two anterior quadrangular laminae, with paired inferior and superior cornua (horns) attached along the posterior border. The superior horns attach to the hyoid bone and the inferior horns to the cricoid cartilage, both by ligaments. A strong midline thyrohyoid membrane connects the thyroid laminae superiorly to the hyoid bone. The **laryngeal prominence** ("Adam's apple") is located at the superior end of the anterior line along which the two thyroid laminae meet. It is especially large in males or in any patient being treated with androgenic hormones. The **cricoid cartilage** is shaped like a signet ring, with the broad plate (lamina) facing posteriorly. The *first tracheal ring* (see Figure 2-131) is bound to the cricoid by a strong ligament. The cricoid cartilage is the only part of the upper airway that is rigid throughout its entire circumference and therefore cannot vary its size. It is frequently the region in which objects become lodged, obstructing the airway and threatening respiration.

The paired **arytenoid cartilages** (see Figures 2-131 and 2-136) are pyramidal and sit atop the lamina of the cricoid near the midline. The base of each arytenoid cartilage has an anterior vocal process, attached to which is the **vocal ligament.** The vocal ligament extends anteriorly to attach to the inner surface of the laryngeal prominence. The base of each arytenoid cartilage also has a lateral muscular process, attached to which are the cricoarytenoid muscles (posterior and anterior). The arytenoids can rotate around their own vertical axes, in response to specific muscle actions.

The **epiglottis** (see Figure 2-131) is a flat oval-shaped cartilaginous structure, projecting upward from the an-

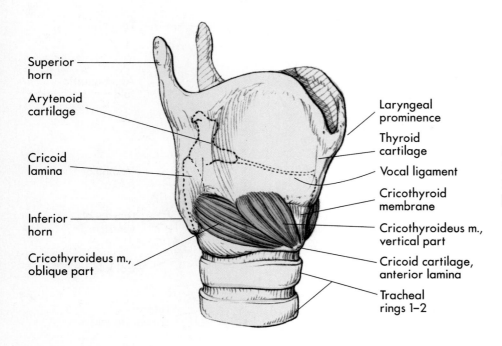

Figure 2-135 CARTILAGE OF THE LARYNX AND THE CRICOTHYROIDEUS MUSCLE.
SEE ATLAS, FIG. 2-81

terior wall of the laryngeal inlet to the level of the base of the tongue. The **aryepiglottic folds** (see Figures 2-134 and 2-137) are mucosal ridges extending superiorly from the apex of the arytenoid cartilages to each side of the epiglottis. Between the aryepiglottic folds is the **laryngeal inlet** (vestibule), leading downward into the interior of the larynx.

GLOTTIC REGION

As one views the interior of the larynx from above, the first pair of parallel mucosal folds seen is the **vestibular folds,** or **false vocal cords** (Figure 2-137).

These folds extend from posterior to anterior, in the horizontal plane. Just inferior to these, on each side, is a lateral recess, or **laryngeal ventricle,** which in other primates may extend far laterally into the neck.

Next, moving inferiorly, are found the **vocal folds,** or **true vocal cords** (Figure 2-137), another pair of parallel mucosal folds extending from posterior to anterior within the larynx, from the junction of the laminae anteriorly to the vocal processes posteriorly. The *vocal ligament* is a sturdy connective tissue band lying just deep to the mucosa of the vocal fold. The white color of the vocal cords is due to the dense collagenous fibers of the vocal ligament and the thin mucosa overlying it.

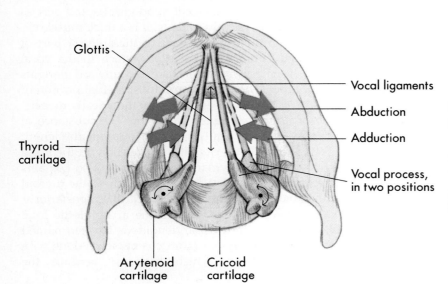

Figure 2-136 CHANGES IN GLOTTAL POSITIONS. Rotation of the arytenoid cartilages around an imaginary vertical axis results in abduction and adduction of the vocal cords, enlarging or narrowing the glottis (the space between the cords).
SEE ATLAS, FIG. 2-75

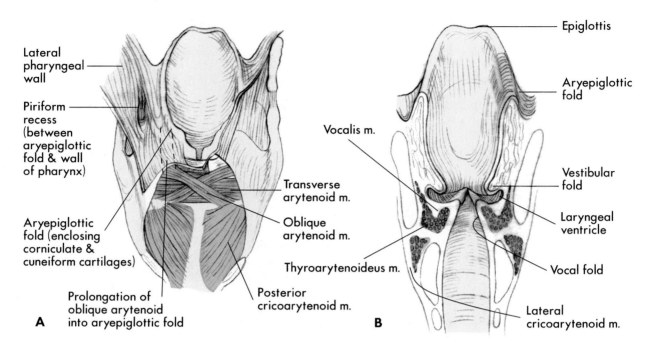

Lateral pharyngeal wall

Piriform recess (between aryepiglottic fold & wall of pharynx)

Aryepiglottic fold (enclosing corniculate & cuneiform cartilages)

Prolongation of oblique arytenoid into aryepiglottic fold

A

Transverse arytenoid m.

Oblique arytenoid m.

Thyroarytenoideus m.

Posterior cricoarytenoid m.

Epiglottis

Aryepiglottic fold

Vocalis m.

Vestibular fold

Laryngeal ventricle

Vocal fold

Lateral cricoarytenoid m.

B

Figure 2-137 POSTERIOR VIEW OF THE LARYNGEAL INLET. A, Posterior view of the larynx, including the position of the aryepiglottic fold and the piriform recess. **B,** Coronal section through midlarynx shows the vestibular folds, vocal folds, and the laryngeal ventricles. **SEE ATLAS, FIGS. 2-72, 2-74**

Deeper beneath the surface of the vocal fold is the **vocalis muscle,** a special part of the thyroarytenoideus muscle, extending from the vocal process of the arytenoid cartilage on each side anterior to attach to the inside surface of the thyroid cartilage.

The **glottis** is the thin midline space between the two vocal folds and two arytenoid cartilages (Figure 2-136). The bigger part of the glottis is that anterior space between the two vocal folds (intramembranous part); the smaller portion of the glottis is posterior and represents the space between the two arytenoid cartilages (interarytenoid part).

MUSCULATURE OF THE LARYNX

The most significant movements of the larynx occur at the cricoarytenoid and cricothyroid joints. Each arytenoid cartilage sits atop the superior edge of the cricoid cartilage and rotates around its own vertical axis. The posterior and lateral cricoarytenoid muscles (Table 2-27 and Figures 2-134 and 2-136) cause this rotary motion. These muscles both attach to the muscular process of the arytenoid. The **posterior cricoarytenoid muscles** pull the muscular processes of each arytenoid in a posterior direction, causing the vocal processes to move laterally and abduct the vocal cords. The **lateral cricoarytenoid muscles** pull the muscular processes in

an anterior direction, causing the vocal processes to move medially, adducting the vocal cords.

The thyroid cartilage also tilts anteriorly and posteriorly with respect to the cricoid cartilage. The "hinge" for this movement is at the joint between the inferior horn of the thyroid cartilage and the cricoid cartilage. The **cricothyroideus muscle** (see Figure 2-135) causes the thyroid cartilage to incline anteriorly, thus increasing the length of the vocal ligament and increasing tension on it. **Thyroartenoideus** is a complex muscle with several functionally different subdivisions and acts as an antagonist to cricothyroideus. It is a thick muscle extending from the inner surface of the anterior part of the thyroid laminae backward to attach to the vocal process of the arytenoid cartilage and upward along its lateral border. The deepest and most medial portion of the muscle is named separately as the **vocalis muscle.** Some of its muscle fibers blend into the substance of the vocal ligament. Its contraction shortens the length of the vocal fold and can alter the tension on the vocal fold as well. The thyroarytenoid muscle also contains some muscle fibers that attach anteriorly to the thyroid laminae but bypass the arytenoid cartilage posteriorly, instead sweeping upward into the aryepiglottic fold. This portion of the thyroarytenoideus is often named separately as the **thyroepiglotticus muscle.** Along with the **aryepiglotticus,** which lies just beneath the

Table 2-27   Muscles of the Larynx

Muscle	Attachments	Action(s)
Posterior cricoarytenoideus	From muscular process of arytenoid to posterior surface of cricoid lamina	Opens the glottis by laterally rotating the arytenoid cartilage
Lateral cricoarytenoideus	From muscular process of arytenoid to lateral surface of cricoid arch	Closes the glottis by medially rotating the arytenoid cartilage
Transverse arytenoideus	From posterior surface of one arytenoid cartilages to the other	Closes glottis (adducts vocal cords by bringing arytenoids together)
Oblique arytenoideus	From posterior surface of arytenoid to the opposite arytenoid cartilage	Closes glottis, pulls aryepiglottic folds toward each other
Aryepiglotticus	From the posterior surface of the arytenoid cartilage to the superior margin of the aryepiglottic fold on the opposite side of the larynx	Pulls aryepiglottic folds toward each other
Cricothyroideus	From external lateral surface of thyroid cartilage to lateral surface of cricoid cartilage (lateral surface)	Elongates and tenses the vocal cords
Thyroarytenoideus*	From inner anterior surface of thyroid cartilage to vocal process of arytenoid	Tenses and shortens vocal cords

*Vocalis is the deepest and most medial portion of thyroarytenoideus.

aryepiglottic fold and extends from the arytenoid cartilage to the epiglottis, this muscle helps regulate the size of the inlet to the larynx.

The two arytenoid cartilages can also move closer together or farther apart along a mediolateral axis. The **transverse arytenoid muscles** (Figure 2-137) connect the posterior surfaces of the arytenoid cartilages, and their contraction adducts the vocal cords by bringing the arytenoid cartilages and their vocal processes nearer to each other. The **oblique arytenoid muscles** (Figure 2-137) also originate from the posterior surface of each arytenoid cartilage, just superficial to the transverse arytenoid muscles, and sweep medially and superiorly toward the opposite arytenoid cartilage. Fibers of the oblique arytenoid muscles attach to the posterior surface of the opposite arytenoid but also continue to become part of the aryepiglotticus and the aryepiglottic fold on the opposite side. Therefore these muscles not only adduct the arytenoid cartilages, but also aid in closing off the laryngeal inlet by adducting the aryepiglottic folds.

INNERVATION OF THE LARYNX

All of the muscles of the larynx are innervated by the **vagus nerve**—the cricothyroideus by the external branch of the superior laryngeal nerve and all the remaining laryngeal muscles by the recurrent laryngeal nerve. The mucosal (sensory) innervation of the larynx above the vocal cords is by the internal branch of the

superior laryngeal nerve and below the cords by the recurrent laryngeal nerve, both of which are also branches of the vagus nerve.

The **left recurrent laryngeal nerve** (Figure 2-138)

PRINCIPLES

Speech is made up of pitch (determined by the length and tension of the vocal folds) and timbre (the "quality" of sound, determined by the shape and resonance characteristics of the laryngeal, oral, nasal, and sinus cavities and the overtones that are contained within the primary sound). The pitch created when air passes across the vocal cords is the function of both the length of the vocal cord (that is, distance from the vocal process of the arytenoid process to the inner surface of the thyroid cartilage) and the tension of the vocal cord (just as a guitar string can produce sounds of differing pitches when either its length or its tension is changed). The volume of speech is a function of the amount of air that crosses the vocal cords per unit of time and the force with which it is propelled. Whispering is accomplished by closing all but the posterior (interarytenoid) portion of the glottis (Figure 2-139). Because no vocal fold is available for vibration of air passing through this space, there can be no pitch to this form of speech although a wide range of sounds can be produced while whispering.

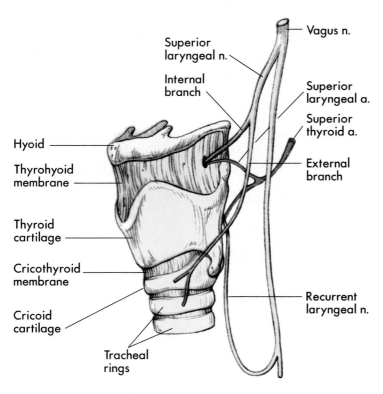

Figure 2-138   NERVE SUPPLY OF THE LARYNX. The superior laryngeal nerve has an internal and external branch, while the recurrent laryngeal nerve enters the larynx from its inferior surface.   SEE ATLAS, FIG. 2-71

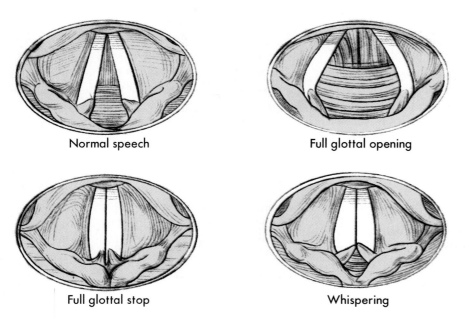

Normal speech

Full glottal opening

Full glottal stop

Whispering

Figure 2-139   DIFFERENT POSITIONS OF THE VOCAL CORDS.

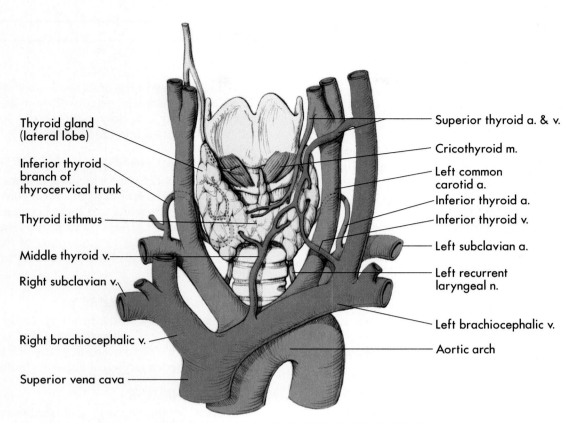

Thyroid gland (lateral lobe)

Inferior thyroid branch of thyrocervical trunk

Thyroid isthmus

Middle thyroid v.

Right subclavian v.

Right brachiocephalic v.

Superior vena cava

Superior thyroid a. & v.

Cricothyroid m.

Left common carotid a.

Inferior thyroid a.

Inferior thyroid v.

Left subclavian a.

Left recurrent laryngeal n.

Left brachiocephalic v.

Aortic arch

Figure 2-140   BLOOD SUPPLY OF THE LARYNX.

arises from the left vagus nerve in the chest and loops around the arch of the aorta to the left of the ligamentum arteriosum. The **right recurrent laryngeal nerve** loops under the right subclavian artery. Both recurrent nerves ascend into the neck by traveling in the tracheoesophageal groove (but sometimes lying more anterior or even partially embedded in the tissue of the thyroid gland). Next, they enter the interior of the larynx by passing deep to the inferior margin of the inferior constrictor muscle. The recurrent nerves innervate all of the intrinsic muscles of the larynx, save one (the cricothyroideus), and provide sensory innervation to the mucosa of the larynx inferior to the vocal folds. Each is at risk in thyroid surgery and is threatened by any space-occupying process in the neck or superior mediastinum.

The **superior laryngeal nerve** (Figure 2-138) is a branch of the vagus nerve in the upper part of the anterior neck triangle. It first travels medially, lying deep to the internal and external carotid arteries. Next, it divides into an internal and external branch. The *internal branch* penetrates the thyrohyoid membrane, accompanied by the superior laryngeal artery, and provides mucosal innervation to the epiglottis, aryepiglottic folds, and mucosa of the larynx as far inferior as the vocal

folds. It innervates no muscles. The *external branch* descends along the lateral margin of the thyroid cartilage and innervates the cricothyroid muscle. It has no sensory axons.

VASCULAR SUPPLY TO THE LARYNX

The larynx receives the majority of its blood supply from branches of the superior and inferior thyroid arteries (Figure 2-140). Specifically, the **superior laryngeal artery** is a branch of the superior thyroid artery and accompanies the internal branch of the superior laryngeal nerve in penetrating the thyrohyoid membrane. The **inferior laryngeal artery,** a branch of the inferior thyroid artery, penetrates the cricothyroid membrane to reach the infraglottic mucosa. **Laryngeal veins** drain to the thyroid veins and thence to the brachiocephalic and internal jugular veins, respectively. **Lymphatic drainage** from the supraglottic area of the larynx is to groups of nodes along the internal jugular vein and to other groups of nodes overlying the omohyoid muscle. The infraglottic region drains anteriorly into lymph nodes lying just anterior to the upper tracheal rings.

THE LARYNX

VIEWING THE LARYNX

Laryngoscopy is the visualization of laryngeal structures. It can be accomplished *directly* (by deflection of the tongue and epiglottis with a laryngoscope blade) or indirectly (through use of a mirror positioned in the posterior pharynx, while pulling the tongue forward).

TRAUMA TO THE LARYNX

Laryngeal fracture means a crushing injury of the laryngeal skeleton that threatens the patency of the airway.

CANCER OF THE LARYNX

Laryngectomy (removal of the larynx) is indicated in serious cases of malignancy, often the result of tobacco use. Whenever lymph nodes are palpable just anterior to the upper tracheal rings, suspicion of laryngeal cancer is greatly multiplied.

THE LARYNX AND THE THYROID GLAND

Note that the thyroid gland lies inferior and lateral to, not directly in front of, the thyroid cartilage. The isthmus lies in front of the first one to three tracheal rings.

ESTABLISHING AN AIRWAY

Tracheostomy (or tracheotomy) is a procedure designed to secure a reliable opening to the trachea when trauma, infection, or other illness has blocked it or where the patency of the oral/nasal areas is not reliable. An opening is made, usually through the upper tracheal rings, and a hollow rigid plastic or metal curved tube is inserted into the trachea.

MATURATIONAL CHANGES IN THE LARYNX

The larynx undergoes considerable change at puberty in the male. The length of the vocal cord nearly doubles, and the supporting cartilages become thicker and stronger. Similar changes occur in the female but to a lesser degree. Similar to other parts of the body, cartilaginous components of the larynx tend to calcify with age.

SURGICAL RISK TO THE LARYNX

Thyroidectomy may result in injury to the recurrent laryngeal nerves. Surgery on the common carotid, usually for arteriosclerosis, places the internal branch of the superior laryngeal nerve at similar risk.

VALSALVA MANEUVER

Contraction of the thoracic and abdominal wall muscles, accompanied by forced closure of the glottis, leads to a marked increase in intrapleural and intraabdominal pressure (Valsalva maneuver). This is a necessary part of several human functions, including urination, defecation, and childbirth. Closure of the glottis is crucial because otherwise the pressure within the chest and abdomen would be dissipated as air escaped through the trachea.

2.15

Systems Review and Surface Anatomy of the Head and Neck

▶ Musculoskeletal Anatomy of the Head and Neck

▶ Vascular Supply of the Head and Neck

▶ Lymphatic Drainage of the Head and Neck

▶ Innervation of the Head and Neck

▶ Surface Anatomy and Physical Examination of the Head and Neck

MUSCULOSKELETAL ANATOMY OF THE HEAD AND NECK

The **skeleton of the head and neck** consists of the cranial vault, the bones of the orbit, nose and jaws, and the skeletal elements of the neck. The frontal, parietal, temporal, and occipital bones form the rounded dome of the skull, while the ethmoid, frontal, sphenoid, temporal, and occipital bones form the base of the skull. The floor of the skull contains numerous **apertures** through which pass important vessels and nerves entering and leaving the skull. All of these apertures are either in or along the adjacent borders of four bones—the ethmoid, sphenoid, temporal, and occipital. In the head and neck, the only mobile bones are the **mandible** (see Figure 2-50), **ossicles** of the middle ear (see Figure 2-90), and the **hyoid bone** of the neck.

The bones of the face are unique in possessing **air sinuses** (see Figure 2-114), all of which drain into the in-terior of the nose. The purpose of these sinuses is unclear, but they do have the effect of changing the quality of the voice, and in other species (for example, birds) may be valuable in making the head lighter.

The bones of the cranial vault are joined to each other along **suture lines**—the sites of fibrous joints earlier in life, when the bones of the cranial vault are more widely separated (see Figures 2-1, *A*; 2-2; and 2-3). The only major synovial joint in the face is the **temporomandibular joint** (Figure 2-51), by which the mandible is suspended beneath the temporal bone. The mandible is also attached to the base of the skull by the sphenomandibular and stylomandibular ligaments, the pterygomandibular raphe, and several of the muscles of mastication (see Figure 2-53). The joints between the ossicles are synovial also, but the remaining bones of the face and skull are virtually immobile.

Individual bony anatomy in the head and neck can be complex. The **orbit** (see Figure 2-93) is made up of parts of the frontal, zygomatic, maxillary, lacrimal, palatine, sphenoid, and ethmoid bones. The **nose** consists of parts of the ethmoid, maxillary, and inferior concha bones, as well as nasal cartilages (see Figure 2-110).

Groups of **superficial striated muscles** are found in the scalp and face. Those embedded in the superficial fascia of the face are known as the muscles of facial expression. Movements of the mandible (see Figure 2-50), so important in chewing of food, are controlled by the **muscles of mastication** (see Figure 2-53). The **floor of the mouth** and the **tongue** also consist of striated muscle. The orbit contains a variety of striated muscles (the **extraocular muscles**), whose collective task it is to position the globe. The neck contains many striated muscles. Both the anterior and posterior surfaces of the cervical vertebral column are covered with **longitudinal muscles.** They are important in maintaining head position and in moving the head and neck. The **scalene muscles** (see Figure 2-62) of the neck are positioned anterolaterally and connect the cervical vertebrae with the upper two ribs. In the anterior midline of the neck is a group of vertical striated muscles known as the **"strap" muscles** (see Figure 2-77). The large **sternocleidomastoid** and **trapezius muscles** (see Figure 2-61) connect the skull to the vertebral column and shoulder girdle.

The **pharynx** (see Figures 2-124 and 2-130) is a muscular cylinder extending from the base of the skull to the midpoint of the neck. Muscles from the base of the skull and the soft palate attach to the outer surface of the pharynx and help control it. The **larynx** (see Figure 2-134) also has a specialized group of striated muscles, devoted to protecting the entrance to the airway and taking part in vocalization and respiration.

Smooth muscle associated with blood vessels and hair arrector muscles are found throughout the head and neck, but independent groupings of smooth muscle are found only in certain areas. The eye contains three important smooth muscle groups—the constrictors and dilators of the **pupil** (see Figure 2-99); the **ciliaris** muscles (see Figure 2-98), which help to control the shape of the lens (influencing focus of the eye); and the smooth muscles found in each of the **eyelids** (see Figure 2-107), especially the upper eyelid.

VASCULAR SUPPLY OF THE HEAD AND NECK

The arterial blood flow to the head and neck derives largely from four vessels—the two **carotid arteries** and the two **vertebral arteries** (themselves derived from the subclavian artery—see Figure 2-64). The common carotid arteries originate in the upper part of the thorax

and ascend into the neck, where at about C6 they divide into the **internal** and **external carotid arteries** (see Figure 2-66). The internal carotid artery supplies structures inside the cranial cavity and most of the orbit and globe. The external carotid supplies the face and scalp. The vertebral arteries supply the spinal cord, brainstem, cerebellum, and other structures of the posterior fossa. They then anastomose with the internal carotid arteries in the crucially important **circulus arteriosus** (see Figure 2-24), a vascular anastomotic arcade surrounding the sella turcica. In general, the brainstem, cerebellum, parts of the temporal lobe, and the occipital lobe receive most of their blood from branches of the vertebral artery; the frontal, parietal, and some of the temporal lobe, plus deep structures in the anterior part of the brain, are supplied by branches of the internal carotid artery.

In the neck, branches of the **subclavian artery** supply the thyroid gland and nearby areas. The posterior scalp and neck are supplied mainly by branches of the **external carotid artery** (see Figure 2-25), but other branches derived from the costocervical trunk and the inferior thyroid artery (each originally branches of the subclavian artery) also supply the neck.

Venous drainage of the head and neck is complex. Inside the cranial cavity, most venous blood collects into **cerebral venous sinuses,** which ultimately converge and help form the **internal jugular vein** (see Figure 2-23). A smaller amount of venous blood enters the **cavernous sinus** and drains anterior toward the orbit and posterior to the petrosal sinuses. The cavernous sinus (see Figure 2-26) is a spongelike vascular structure applied to the base of each side of the sella turcica. It has special significance because it is intimately associated with cranial nerves III, IV, and VI and V1 and V2, as well as the internal carotid artery. The veins of the surface of the face converge on the internal jugular vein and drain to the base of the neck. Veins of the anterior scalp drain forward, across the forehead and into the **ophthalmic veins** or the **superficial temporal veins.** The posterior part of the scalp drains to the **external jugular veins** in the anterolateral part of the neck.

LYMPHATIC DRAINAGE OF THE HEAD AND NECK

The brain itself has no lymphatic drainage—the cerebrospinal fluid appears to fill that role for the brain. Structures outside the cranial cavity do have ordinary lymphatic drainage, which converges on the deep and superficial lymph nodes located along the carotid artery in the anterolateral part of the neck. The anterior midline parts of the upper neck, including the tip of the tongue, drain to the **submental nodes** located just inferiorly to the chin (see Figure 2-69).

INNERVATION OF THE HEAD AND NECK

The majority of the structures in the head and neck are innervated by **cranial nerves**. The cranial nerves may be grouped according to several different criteria. **Nerves I and II** are not true cranial nerves, but tracts of the central nervous system (see Figures 2-102 and 2-111). They are concerned with smell and sight, respectively. **Nerves III, IV, and VI** (see Figure 2-106) and **XII** (see Figure 2-74) innervate the extraocular muscles and the tongue, respectively. Nerve III also contains some autonomic axons that participate in the regulation of pupillary size and regulation of the shape of the lens. **Nerve V** (see Figure 2-41) is the major sensory nerve of the anterolateral part of the face and the anterior half of the scalp. It also provides motor innervation to the muscles of mastication and several other muscles related to the middle ear and the palate. **Nerve VII** (see Figures 2-44 and 2-86) is responsible for part of taste, innervation of the striated muscles of facial expression, and autonomic innervation of the lacrimal, submandibular, and sublingual glands. **Nerve VIII** (see Figure 2-29) is a pure sensory nerve, innervating the cochlea and organs of balance and equilibrium. **Nerve IX** (see Figure 2-71) is responsible for part of taste; innervation of a single striated muscle related to the pharynx; sensory innervation of the pharynx, posterior tongue, and middle ear; and autonomic innervation of the parotid gland. **Nerve X** (see Figures 2-70 and 2-72) innervates much of the striated muscle of the pharynx and larynx, provides some sensory innervation to the epiglottis and larynx, and provides autonomic innervation to many of the thoracic and abdominal viscera. **Nerve XI** (see Figure 2-70) is a pure motor nerve. Its spinal root innervates the sternocleidomastoid and trapezius muscles, and its cranial root joins the vagus nerve.

Certain regions of the head and neck are not innervated by branches of cranial nerves. Sensory innervation of the posterior scalp is the responsibility of **dorsal primary rami** from the upper cervical segments (see Figure 2-40). Innervation of certain striated muscles in the anterior neck and the lateral scalp posterior to the ear is the responsibility of the **motor fibers of the cervical plexus** (derived from C1 to C4). Sensory innervation of the anterior part of the neck is the responsibility of cutaneous branches of C3 to C4, part of what is known as the cervical plexus (see Figure 2-63). Thus the cranial nerves and the upper cervical spinal nerves form a continuum, especially in the upper regions of the neck.

Autonomic innervation of head and neck structures varies from structure to structure. **Sympathetic innervation** reaches the head and neck by forming a plexus on the various branches of the internal and external carotid arteries and their branches. In addition to the usual sympathetic functions of vasoconstriction, stimulation of hair arrector muscles, and production of sweating, sympathetic axons play a special role in dilating the pupil and elevating the upper eyelid. **Parasympathetic innervation** of head and neck structures (Figure 2-141) is confined to cranial nerves III, VII, and IX (cranial nerve X contains parasympathetic axons, but they affect thoracic and abdominal visceral, not head and neck structures. **Parasympathetic axons of nerve III** synapse in the ciliary ganglion of the orbit and ultimately cause pupillary constriction and an increase in the roundness of the lens. **Parasympathetic axons of nerve VII** synapse in the pterygopalatine and submandibular ganglia and ultimately cause tears to flow from the lacrimal gland and salivation in the submandibular and sublingual glands. **Parasympathetic axons of nerve IX** synapse in the otic ganglion and ultimately cause salivation in the parotid gland. **Parasympathetic axons of nerve X** synapse on collections of nerve cells in the walls of thoracic and abdominal viscera and produce a wide variety of effects (see sections on thorax and abdomen).

The upper ends of the respiratory and digestive systems (often called the **aerodigestive system**) are found in the head and neck region. Both the nasal and oral cavities can lead into either the trachea or the esophagus. The passage of materials (air, liquids, solids) into one of these two cylinders is directed by muscular contraction in the palate, pharynx, and larynx.

SURFACE ANATOMY AND PHYSICAL EXAMINATION OF THE HEAD AND NECK

The **dermatomal pattern** familiar in other parts of the body is preserved in the head and neck as well (see Figure 2-40). The **V1, V2,** and **V3** branches of the **trigeminal nerve** innervate the anterolateral part of the face, anterior to the ear—V1 innervating the region above the eye, V2 innervating the area between the eye and the midcheek, and V3 innervating the region inferior to this, including the skin over the mandible. Spinal segments C2 and C3 are represented on the superior and inferior portions of the posterior scalp, respectively. A wide strip of skin extending from the area posterior to the ear downward into the anterolateral neck is the province of the lower two segments of the cervical plexus, segments C3 and C4. These areas of skin may be tested as part of the neurologic examination to determine specific injury to cranial nerves or spinal segments. Such diseases as herpes zoster (shingles) produce skin eruptions in a dermatomal pattern.

Certain bony landmarks may be palpated in the head and neck (see Figures 2-1, *A*; 2-2; 2-3; and 2-142). The supraorbital ridges, over which the eyebrows grow, are parts of the frontal bone. At the medial end of each supraorbital ridge are small notches through which pass the supraorbital and supratrochlear branches of

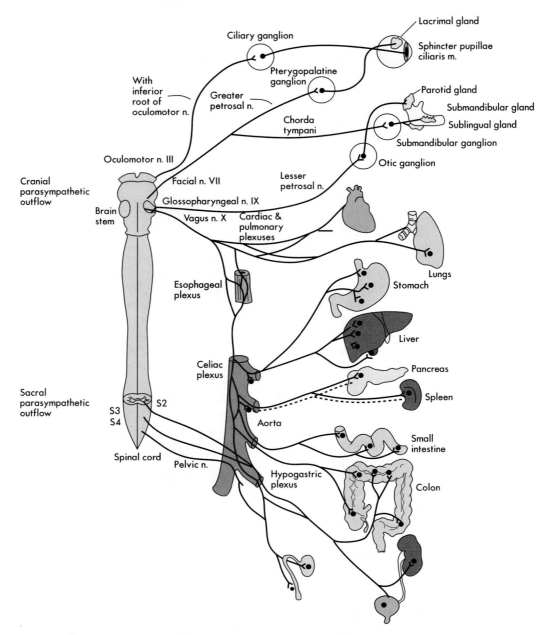

Figure 2-141   PARASYMPATHETIC INNERVATION TO HEAD AND BODY.

the ophthalmic nerve. Because these nerves extend upward across the forehead and on to the superior surface of the scalp, injection of local anesthetic around these nerves as they pass the supraorbital ridge can produce anesthesia in the scalp, a very useful adjunct, for example, to suturing wounds in the skin of the forehead. The superior, lateral, and inferior margins of the **orbit** are formed principally by parts of the frontal, zygomatic, and maxillary bones. Trauma to the face may fracture part of the margin of the orbit, which may be detected by gentle palpation. The **zygomatic arch** is formed by parts of the maxillary and temporal bones and the zygoma itself and also is vulnerable to fracture in traumatic facial injury.

The **maxilla** (Figure 2-142) forms the substance of the upper jaw, and teeth should be palpated gently to determine whether they are firmly seated in the maxilla and/or whether there is infection present in the socket of each tooth, located deeper within the bone. Approximately 2 cm inferior to the midpoint of the lower margin of the orbit is the **infraorbital foramen,** through which emerges the cutaneous branch of the maxillary nerve, the **infraorbital nerve** (see Figure 2-45), plus accompanying vessels. This foramen is in a vertical line with the supraorbital and supratrochlear notches above. The **nasal bones** (see Figure 2-110) form the upper third of the midline of the nose and are among the most frequently fractured bones in the body.

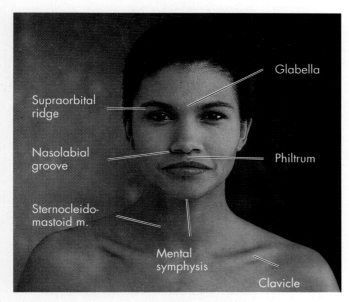

Glabella

Supraorbital
ridge

Nasolabial
groove

Philtrum

Sternocleido-
mastoid m.

Mental
symphysis

Clavicle

Figure 2-142 BONY LANDMARKS OF THE HEAD AND NECK.

They too are examined by palpation. Examination of the **mandible** (see Figure 2-50) should involve palpation of the **temporomandibular joint** (see Figures 2-51 and 2-52). Asking the patient to clench his/her teeth should cause a slight forward movement of the mandible, but an exaggerated forward movement suggests dislocation of the joint. As with the maxilla, the seating of teeth in the mandible should be assessed by pressing gently on each tooth. About 2 cm from the midline, on its anterior surface, each mandible has a **mental foramen,** through which passes the **mental nerve** (see Figure 2-45), the cutaneous branch of the inferior alveolar nerve (branch of the mandibular nerve). This foramen is in a vertical line with the infraorbital and supraorbital/supratrochlear foramina above, and together these foramina represent the points of exit for the **cutaneous branches of V1, V2, and V3** (see Figure 2-45).

Palpation of the scalp and skull should be performed to determine any points of tenderness or skeletal deformity. In the adult, only a limited number of skull landmarks may be palpated, but in the infant the **anterior and posterior fontanelles** (see Figure 2-4) should be assessed to determine whether they are closing in an appropriate fashion or whether the skull is showing any signs of deformation. In the infant the widened **sagittal suture** (see Figure 2-3) is also easily palpable.

In the anterior neck, the **hyoid bone** (at vertebrae level C3 to C4) (see Figures 2-130 and 2-131) is easily palpable, as is the **laryngeal prominence of the thyroid cartilage** (at vertebral level C4) (see Figure 2-131). Further inferior, the anterior lamina of the **cricoid cartilage** may be palpated (at vertebral level C5 to C6) (see Figure 2-131).

The **facial muscles (of expression)** are organized around the orifices of the head and neck and act to open or close these orifices (see Figures 2-42 and 2-43). The examiner should test each of these. Squinting the eyes is a good test of the **orbicularis oculi muscle,** innervated by the upper branches of the facial nerve. Elevation of the eyebrows is a test of the **occipitofrontalis muscle.** The levator labii superioris alaquae nasi muscle is capable of flaring the nostrils. The **oral cavity** has the largest number of muscles regulating its shape and degree of opening and is capable of modifying speech and of a large variety of expressions, which are also important to human communication. Asking a patient to smile, purse the lips, grimace, and so on can effectively test the function of this complex group of muscles. A group of muscles also surround the external ear, but few human subjects can exert voluntary control of these muscles.

Among the muscles of mastication, the **temporalis and masseter** can be examined by palpation (see Figure 2-53). Asking the patient to forcefully press his/her teeth together, as in biting down hard on something, the fan-shaped belly of temporalis may be palpated in the temporal fossa, above the zygoma. Similarly, the masseter can be palpated, extending from the zygoma downward toward the angle of the mandible. By placing one's finger over the upper end of the condylar process of the mandible, the slight anterior movement of the mandible during clenching of the jaw may be detected. Excess anterior movement suggests dislocation or laxity in the **temporomandibular joint** (see Figure 2-51). By palpating along the anterior edge of the masseter muscle, one can usually locate the **parotid duct** (see Figure 2-48, *A*) as it passes the anterior margin of the muscle and descends into the buccal fat pad toward the cheek.

A closer examination of the eye reveals the **sclera, iris,** and **pupil** (see Figure 2-99). The latter two should be circular and symmetric in appearance. The pigmentation in the iris is often not uniform, however. The gap between the upper and lower eyelids is the **palpebral fissure** (see Figure 2-108), which is limited by the **medial** and lateral **canthus** at each side. At the medial canthus are the two lacrimal punctae, through which tears drain into the lacrimal canaliculi and ultimately the lacrimal sac. The **conjunctival membrane** covers the anterior portion of the sclera and then reflects onto the deep surface of each eyelid. It may be inflamed and show increased vascularity.

Eye movements should be assessed by asking a patient to follow an object as the examiner moves it through the full extent of the patient's visual field. Eye movements should be synchronized or *conjugate*—that is, left and right eye move together. Isolated injury to nerves and muscles often can be detected as a deficit in conjugate movements—for example, when a patient is asked to follow an object being moved to the far left side of the visual field, if the right eye adducts maximally but the left eye does not abduct fully, it is presumptive evidence of an injury to nerve VI on the left. *Constriction* and *dilation* of the pupil should also be conjugate. Recall that the pupil may constrict in response to a light shone in the patient's eyes or as a part of the *accommodation reflex,* when viewed objects are moved closer and closer to the patient's eyes. Certain conditions affect pupillary constriction in response to light but not as a part of the accommodation reflex.

Inspection of the **oral cavity** (see Figure 2-117) should include assessment of the dorsal surface of the tongue, where certain infectious diseases and dietary deficiencies may produce changes in the appearance of the mucosa. The parotid ducts open into the oral cavity through a small papilla located opposite the second upper molar on each side of the mouth. The patient should be asked to protrude his tongue; injury to cranial nerve XII produces a *deviation of the tongue* toward the injured side. Mobility and strength of the tongue can also be tested by asking the patient to press his/her tongue into his/her cheek. Asking the patient to press his/her tongue up against his/her palate reveals the underside of the tongue, where the two **lingual veins** are usually prominent and visible. In the midline is the **frenulum** (see Figure 2-126), a thin membrane that attaches the tongue to the floor of the mouth. At the base of the frenulum are the paired **sublingual papillae,** where the **submandibular ducts** open into the mouth. The **soft palate** should be symmetric, and the pendulous **uvula** should be in a midline position (see Figure 2-117). Deviation of the uvula can indicate injury to cranial nerve X. The gag reflex can be tested by gently touching the posterior wall of the pharynx with a soft cotton swab or tongue depressor.

The **sternocleidomastoid** is the major landmark in the neck, separating the anterior and posterior triangles. The **submandibular gland** may be palpated externally or even more effectively by placing one finger inside the mouth, along the medial surface of the mandible, and the other finger over the surface of the submandibular triangle. The pulse of the **facial artery** (see Figure 2-45) crossing the inferior border of the mandible is palpable in the middle third of the inferior margin of the mandible. The pulse of the **common carotid artery** may be located by first palpating the trachea, in the midline, and gently sliding the fingers laterally until the pulse is felt. Using the arterial pulse as a guide, the **internal jugular vein** (see Figure 2-47) may be located 1 to 2 cm lateral to the arterial pulse. The internal jugular vein is commonly used for placement of venous catheters. The **external jugular vein,** crossing the sternocleidomastoid superomedially, may also be cannulated

In the posterior triangle, located posteriorly to the sternocleidomastoid muscle, the **cervical plexus** (see Figure 2-63) emerges along the posterior margin of the muscle at its midpoint. The branches of the plexus pass anteriorly, superiorly, posteriorly, and inferiorly from this point. The **spinal accessory nerve** (cranial nerve XI) also emerges from the midpoint of the posterior border of sternocleidomastoid and passes posteroinferiorly to pass deeply to the anterior surface of the trapezius muscle (see Figure 2-73). The **phrenic nerve** lies on the anterior surface of scalenus anterior, in the inferomedial corner of the posterior triangle. The trunks and divisions of the **brachial plexus** also move inferolaterally to pass beneath the midpoint of the clavicle into the axilla (see Figure 2-62).

The **thyroid gland** is positioned in the anterior neck—not over the thyroid cartilage—but consists of lateral lobes that extend upward as high as the midpoint of the thyroid cartilage, and a midline isthmus centered over the second to third ring of the trachea, giving the gland the appearance of an inverted "U" (see Figure 2-78). Palpation of the thyroid gland is carried out by locating the thyroid cartilage and passing the fingers inferolaterally, examining for abnormal masses or overall thyroid size.

2.16

Head and Neck

■ CASE 1

DISTURBED SKULL GROWTH

A 6-month-old male child was noted to have a head that seemed to "bulge" to each side, and the condition seemed to have worsened over 3 to 4 months. The parents felt that the skull was not enlarging in the antero-posterior direction. The grandmother thought that the child's skull felt "funny" and that the separation between the right and left side of the skull seemed to be widening. A visit to the pediatrician resulted in a referral to the neurologist, who examined the patient and ordered an x-ray and CT scans, which led to an elucidation of the source for this problem.

Questions

1. What normal developmental processes are at work in the development of the skull over the first 14 to 18 months of life?
2. What might account for the enlargement of the skull in one dimension but not another?
3. What are the surgical options for this baby's condition, and what are the anatomic principles involved?

■ CASE 2

SUDDEN CHANGE IN MENTAL STATUS

An 11-month-old female child was brought to her pediatrician by her parents because they noted that she seemed lethargic and had lost some of her appetite. In addition, she had begun to vomit in the last 24 hours even though her intake had been limited to an occasional sip of fluid and only a small amount of solid food. She had no fever nor other sign of infectious ill-ness. She responded to stimulation and recognized her parents when they spoke, but her attention seemed to drift when not being talked to directly. Her neck was not stiff on physical examination, but she did seem to the pediatrician to be drowsy. Her head circumference was well above the 95th percentile for age, and her anterior fontanelle was bulging. Further examination of her scalp revealed that her sagittal suture seemed widened. Examination of her eyes showed papilledema (forward bulging of the optic discs anterior to the level of the retina). While being examined further, she became agitated and cried and experienced a generalized convulsion, with shaking of both upper and lower limbs and rolling of her eyes backward.

There was no recent history of head trauma or exposure to any medications or toxins. Review of her past history was significant for no prior hospitalizations, nothing but normal childhood illnesses, and completely normal physical and intellectual development up to this point.

She was taken immediately to the local hospital, where a series of tests revealed the diagnosis.

Questions

1. What anatomic alterations might produce a bulging fontanelle, splitting of the sagittal suture, and papilledema?
2. The following tests were included in the workup of this child: lumbar puncture and CT scan of the head. Based on the symptoms revealed here, in which order should these two tests be performed and why?
3. Assume that this baby's lateral ventricles and third ventricle are greatly enlarged but not the fourth ventricle. In what single anatomic location might a tumor be found that would produce these findings?

■ CASE 3

A HEADACHE, WITH SEVERE COMPLICATIONS

A 17-year-old football player had a vigorous contact practice and felt good at the conclusion of the afternoon. At home that evening, however, he did not feel good and vomited his dinner. He began to complain of a headache and declined an offer to go to a movie that night. He went to bed early and fell asleep quickly. When his parents returned from the movie at around 11:00 PM, they looked in on him and saw that he was sleeping very soundly. His mother was worried, however, and at about 2:00 AM she arose again and went to her son's room to check on him. She was unable to arouse him and found him to be breathing slowly and irregularly. She called 911, and the boy was taken to the local emergency room. An emergency CT scan revealed the diagnosis.

Questions

1. Given the recent history, what is the most likely explanation for this young man's serious problems?
2. Why did his condition take several hours to develop fully?
3. What is the anatomic basis for the bleeding process most likely to be involved in his illness?

■ CASE 4

UNUSUAL APPEARANCE IN A NEWBORN BABY

A 3-week-old baby was brought to the hospital for evaluation. His parents thought that his ears seemed placed too low on the side of his head, that the shape of his external ear was unusual, and that a small aperture in the upper neck was slowly dripping a clear fluid. His mouth did not seem to open fully, and the mother stated that the child seemed to have an excessive overbite.

Questions

1. What developmental process might explain the findings in the ear, the lower jaw, and the neck?
2. What other structures, not evident on external examination, might also be abnormal?

■ CASE 5

FACIAL WEAKNESS

A 39-year-old female noted that she occasionally drooled from the left side of her mouth. She could not raise the corner of her mouth on that same side when trying to smile, and her husband told her that her facial expression seemed to be "flat" on that side. On exami-

nation, the physician noted some small areas of dryness and scaling on the left cornea and palpated a small nontender mass just anterior to the left ear.

Questions

1. What single lesion can explain abnormalities in the mouth, cheek, and eye?
2. How might the mass palpated be related to the symptoms seen here?
3. What are the treatment options for this patient?

■ CASE 6

HEAD INJURY AND RAPID LOSS OF CONSCIOUSNESS

A 9-year-old girl was out riding her bicycle when she was struck by a car speeding through an intersection. She had no broken bones but did have numerous bruises, scrapes, and a bleeding area of injury just above her ear on the left side. She did not lose consciousness at the scene of the accident, and her parents decided they would just take her home rather than go to the emergency room. However, the ambulance personnel persuaded them to take her to the emergency room for an examination. On the way to the emergency room, in the ambulance, she began to vomit, appeared more drowsy, and lost consciousness. When she arrived at the hospital, she was responsive only to deep pain and a few minutes after arrival began to have a seizure. While waiting for the CT scanner to be set up, someone ordered an anteroposterior and lateral skull film, and the diagnosis was revealed.

Questions

1. What kinds of postinjury complications might lead to the early appearance of full consciousness in this patient, followed by a rapid deterioration?
2. Which of the listed injuries is most likely to have contributed to the progression of symptoms, and by which process or processes is the injury likely to have taken place?
3. What surgical-anatomic principles are involved in an understanding of this condition?

■ CASE 7

PROBLEMS COMBING HAIR

A 27-year-old woman had a dark nevus (discolored spot on the skin) removed from the skin of her neck. The nevus was located in the skin along the posterior border of the sternocleidomastoid muscle on the right side. The surgeon found that the nevus was tightly adherent to the underlying fascial tissue, and, because of concern that the nevus might be a malignant melanoma, an extensive tissue dissection was performed. Study of the tissue in the pathology laboratory suggested that all of the tumor had been removed successfully. The woman was of course pleased with this result but noted that after she went home from the hospital, she had trouble combing her hair. She could not grasp the hairbrush well and particularly was weak in lifting the brush to the top of her head. Because she experienced this weakness with her right but not with her left hand, she called her surgeon and asked whether she had any idea why this should be happening.

Questions

1. What muscle or muscles would be involved in the motions with which this patient was having difficulty?
2. Considering the recent history of surgery, what structure(s) might have been injured to produce this outcome?

■ CASE 8

AN UNEXPECTED POSTOPERATIVE COMPLICATION

A 57-year-old man underwent surgery for removal of several malignant nodules on his thyroid gland. The surgery involved opening the pretracheal fascia, removing the many nodules, and examining the rest of the thyroid gland for any remaining disease. The fascia was closed and the operation completed. The patient was returned to his room and seemed to be recovering well until about 4 hours afterward, when his breathing became very raspy and he started to turn blue. He was in obvious respiratory distress, and the resident on call for the night decided that an emergency reopening of the surgical wound was required. After the decompression, a tracheotomy was required. The patient was much more stable, appeared well oxygenated, and was out of danger.

Questions

1. What was the reason for the development of acute respiratory distress in the postoperative period?
2. What anatomic landmarks guide the physician in the performance of a tracheotomy?

■ CASE 9

DANGER IN "SIMPLE" EAR INFECTIONS

The mother of a 3-year-old child brought her son to the pediatrician to express some concerns about his be-

havior. He had been progressing normally from the standpoint of walking, manipulating objects, and so on, but seemed to be having trouble with language. He had started to babble at the usual time (a few months of age) but seemed to have trouble forming words and putting phrases together. He was also easily distracted and did not always pay attention when people spoke to him. The pediatrician performed an office physical examination and found no abnormalities. In taking the history, it developed that the family had moved around a good bit, and there had never been consistent medical care. The boy had been healthy, except for frequent and nagging ear infections. The mother had always treated these with antibiotics from the public health clinic, but she estimated he had experienced 10 to 12 infections per year and in many cases was never truly free of symptoms. The pediatrician ordered a series of special tests, and the diagnosis became clear.

Questions

1. What is meant by the common "ear infection" of childhood? Are there other types of infections in the ear as well?
2. What is the risk in frequent and repeated ear infections, and how could it be assessed?
3. What can be done to treat this problem? What options are available to correct such hearing loss once it has occurred?

■ CASE 10

EYE MOVEMENT ABNORMALITIES AND SUDDEN DETERIORATION AFTER SURGERY

A patient underwent neurosurgery for removal of a large cyst and was returned to her room after surgery in seemingly good condition. However, over the next several hours, she became less alert, and her physician was summoned. On physical examination the most remarkable finding was her inability to carry out a full range of eye movements. In particular, she could not medially deviate her right eye, though it did abduct normally. At rest, her right eye seemed increasingly to point downward and laterally. Her right eye also seemed to have some difficulty looking upward. Finally, several of the attending nurses felt that the right pupil was becoming increasingly constricted in comparison with the left eye.

Questions

1. What structure or structures probably have been injured to produce the set of findings seen here? What accounts for the inability to adduct her eye? For the

resting position of inferolateral gaze? Why are her pupils now not equal in size?

2. What overall clinical condition is probably occuring in this case?

■ CASE 11

DIFFERENCES IN APPEARANCE OF THE EYES

A 54-year-old man visited the company doctor because he felt tired and had lost his usual energy level. Further, his vision "just didn't seem right," and his wife had noted that his left eye "looked funny" and seemed to be partly closed. A review of his health history showed that he was in good general health, though he had been a heavy smoker for more than 20 years. His cough had increased in recent months. His physical examination revealed a thin, well-muscled man. Examination of his head and neck was remarkable for a left pupil 3 mm in diameter and a right pupil 5 mm in diameter at rest. Both pupils constricted with light stimulation. His left eyelid seemed to droop a bit, and he could not fully elevate it when asked to do so. Extraocular muscle function was normal, with a full range of eye movements.

Questions

1. What can we infer about the location of any likely pathology on the basis of the "one-sidedness" of the abnormalities?
2. What single innervation of the eye might explain the combination of symptoms seen here?
3. What does the health history have to do with the diagnosis?

■ CASE 12

SUDDEN ONSET OF EYE PAIN AND BLURRED VISION

A 9-year-old boy from Central America had recently emigrated to the United States and was seen in an emergency clinic for sudden pain in his right eye and some blurriness and loss of vision. He had received little health care in his native land, and examination of the patient showed a swollen painful right eye, bulging forward of the eye, and discoloration of the adjacent skin. Examination of his mouth showed several dead-looking teeth, including two molars in his upper jaw on the right that were mobile to gentle pressure. Pus appeared to exude from around the bases of these same teeth when gentle pressure was applied with a tongue depressor blade. The oral mucosa was tender to touch, with several open weeping lesions and a foul odor to his breath.

Questions

1. What anatomic concept can explain the appearance of symptoms involving the teeth and the eyes?
2. What nerve or nerves might mediate painful sensations arising from the abnormalities described in this case?
3. Precisely where is pressure applied to the globe in this lesion?

■ CASE 13

A TRIP TO THE DENTIST

A 3-year-old male child was scheduled for a trip to the dentist. He was complaining of a sharp pain in a tooth in his lower jaw in the back of his mouth on the left side. The father asked the dentist whether it would be possible to provide pain relief for his son, if the tooth had to be drilled and a cavity filled. The dentist said that if the tooth were in the lower jaw, it would likely be easier to anesthetize it than if it were in the upper jaw. She further said that if the tooth were toward the back of the mouth, it would be easier to anesthetize than if it were one of the central incisors. The father looked skeptical and asked the dentist why this should be so.

Questions

1. What anatomic factors influence the dentist's capability to provide anesthesia for the teeth of the upper and lower jaws?
2. In the lower jaw, why should anterior teeth be harder to anesthetize than posterior teeth?

■ CASE 14

A "SIMPLE" CASE OF TONSILITIS

A 7-year-old boy was suffering from recurrent sore throats, often missing school to a considerable degree and being treated with antibiotics repeatedly. His physician suggested a tonsillectomy, and the parents agreed. The surgery was planned for the next week, and the boy reported to the hospital early one morning and went to the operating room. The removal of his tonsils seemed to be going well, but suddenly there was massive bleeding and the surgeons had to resuscitate the patient with numerous transfusions. He survived the operation, but the physicians had to explain to the family how such a serious complication could have occurred.

Questions

1. What are the "tonsils" anatomically, and where are they located?

2. Which blood vessels lie near to the tonsils and are at risk in a surgery of this kind?

CASE 15

BABY MAKES A FUNNY NOISE WHEN BREATHING

A 6-week-old baby was taken to the doctor's office because of noisy breathing. The parents reported that the breathing noise was present almost all of the time, though the mother stated that it did get somewhat better when she held the baby up on her shoulder. It was worst when the baby was placed on his back (the supine position). The noise was described as a raspy, grating sound and occurred only when the baby was breathing in. It clearly emanated from the upper airway (larynx and/or trachea) because the noise was faint and distant when the stethoscope was placed to the baby's chest. There was no recent history of cough, runny nose, fever, or illness in the household. The baby never turned blue. The baby displayed some signs of extra respiratory effort, especially when the noise was loudest. The doctor referred the baby to a pulmonary specialist, who performed a procedure that confirmed the diagnosis of laryngomalacia. The parents were reassured that the condition would get better with time and that no surgery would be required.

Questions

1. What can account for noisy breathing in the upper airway?
2. What are the signs of abnormal respiratory effort?
3. What sort of procedure was performed, and what is laryngomalacia? Why did the symptoms occur only during inspiration, and why did putting the baby on the mother's shoulder help?

ANSWERS AND EXPLANATIONS

CASE 1

1. The individual bones of the cranial vault—the frontal, parietal, temporal, and occipital bones—are not fused to each other along their adjacent margins at birth and undergo a gradual process of closure over the first 14 to 18 months of life. They fuse along adjacent borders, the most prominent of which are along the sagittal midline of the skull, where the parietal bones face each other, and along a transverse line where the anterior borders of the two parietal bones face the posterior border of the frontal bone. These lines of apposition are known respectively as the sagittal and coronal sutures.
2. When one of the skull's sutures closes well in advance of the others, the skull may no longer enlarge in the dimension perpendicular to the suture. Thus premature closure of the sagittal suture prevents further side-to-side growth, and the skull elongates from anterior to posterior. In this situation, the child's skull has enlarged in the left-to-right dimension; this indicates that the coronal suture has fused prematurely, and the continued growth of the brain has separated and widened the sagittal suture. A widened gap in this suture would be indicative of premature coronal sutural closure.
3. When a decision is made to reopen prematurely closed sutures, the skull is widely exposed and the fused suture is reopened. If necessary, long strips of bone are removed to make the skull a more nearly normal size.

CASE 2

1. The bulging fontanelle, split sutures, and papilledema all suggest a process producing increased pressure inside the cranium. The possibilities include an enlargement of the brain itself (as in cerebral edema), an increase in the size of the ventricles (as in hydrocephalus), and the presence of a space-occupying lesion inside the cranium (for example, a hemorrhage or tumor).
2. When there are mental status changes accompanied by physical signs of increased pressure within the cranium, physicians are interested in knowing whether the process is infectious (as in meningitis), or is a space-occupying lesion (such as a tumor or a hemorrhage). A lumbar puncture samples cerebrospinal fluid and allows detection of microorganisms that might be causing meningitis. A CT scan or other imaging study allows visualization of a hemorrhage, tumor, or ventricular enlargement. When pressure inside the cranium is increased, the performance of a lumbar puncture poses the risk of acute herniation of the lower brainstem through the foramen magnum, due to the sudden decompression experienced when a needle is placed in the lumbar subarachnoid space. Therefore, in most cases, an imaging study should *precede* the lumbar puncture. If signs of increased intracranial pressure are found, steps can be taken to reduce that pressure before the lumbar puncture is attempted.
3. The most likely location of a lesion producing these

findings is in the fourth ventricle or in the narrow passage connecting the third and fourth ventricles (known as the cerebral aqueduct). The most common sources of this sort of lesion are (1) congenital stenosis (blockage or narrowing) of the cerebral aqueduct and (2) a tumor in the posterior fossa of the skull, putting pressure on the fourth ventricle and/or cerebral aqueduct.

■ CASE 3

1. The history of contact football practice raises the likelihood of trauma to the head, most likely resulting in intracranial bleeding.
2. When head trauma leads to a slowly developing loss of consciousness, it is likely to be the result of venous bleeding, most commonly resulting from a subdural hematoma.
3. A subdural hematoma means that one of the cranial venous sinuses has been damaged, but the resultant bleeding accumulates between the dura mater and the arachnoid mater. The venous bleeding is slower than arterial bleeding and produces the dangerous situation described here—a patient who may seem only mildly or moderately ill at first and subsequently goes to bed, only to have the bleeding continue, the space-occupying hemorrhage increase in size, and the patient lapse into unconsciousness and be threatened with death as time passes.

■ CASE 4

1. The lower jaw, parts of the external ear, and the neck are derived from the first pharyngeal arch. The external ear develops from a series of tissue masses surrounding what will be the entrance into the external auditory canal. The mandible is derived from cartilage, which in turn forms from mesoderm of the first arch. The skin of the anterolateral neck forms in part from the skin surrounding the pharyngeal clefts. The normal process of closure of this skin of the neck involves the obliteration of the pharyngeal clefts. When one persists, it forms a pharyngeal arch cyst, which in rare instances is open to the exterior through a small pore and may communicate internally with the oropharynx.
2. Because the malleus and incus are derived in part from the first pharyngeal arch, it might be expected to be abnormal. This could cause hearing deficits. The maxilla is also a derivative of the first arch and might be malformed. The auditory (Eustachian) tube is similarly vulnerable to abnormal growth.

■ CASE 5

1. The numerous symptoms and signs in this patient are best explained by a lesion involving the facial nerve. It has five branches—the temporal, zygomatic, buccal, mandibular, and cervical. The temporal branches innervate some muscles of the eyelid; the buccal and mandibular branches, the skin around the mouth. When the eyelid does not periodically lubricate the eye, the cornea may become dried and damaged.
2. The facial nerve traverses the parotid gland after it emerges from the stylomastoid foramen and "fans out" to divide into its five branches described above. Therefore a tumor in the parotid gland may compress and damage any or all of these nerves.
3. The facial nerve and its branches will be permanently injured if the tumor is allowed to remain in place and grow. Surgical removal is usually recommended and does pose a considerable risk to the branches that run through the parotid gland.

■ CASE 6

1. The progression of symptoms suggests that immediately after the accident, the pathologic processes that were set in motion were not as severe as they subsequently became. This would most strongly imply bleeding because it is a process that takes several minutes to hours to produce its full pathologic effect. Moreover, the relatively rapid sequence of change suggests arterial, rather than venous, bleeding. The loss of consciousness and vomiting are clear signs of increases in intracranial pressure, resulting in this case from the accumulation of blood inside the skull. The arterial pressure of the severed vessel means that larger amounts of blood will hemorrhage than would occur if the hemorrhage were venous. In fact, the bleeding may continue to a point at which the flow of blood into the cranial cavity (in the carotid and vertebral arteries) is threatened, which will lead to generalized injury to the brain, beyond areas directly affected by the pressure of the local arterial hemorrhage.
2. The bruises and scrapes alone are unlikely to have produced the severe injuries described here. The obvious suspect is the injury above the left ear, where we presume that a fracture of the underlying skull (in the temporal region) has caused a tear in the middle meningeal artery. This artery runs in a groove on the inner surface of the skull in the temporal region, and because this area of the skull is especially prone to fracture, the vessel is similarly put at risk. This injury is known as an epidural

hematoma (epidural, "above" or outside the dura mater) blood accumulates between the skull and the dura mater. When an artery is severed, it bleeds forcefully and the progression of symptoms is likely to be more rapid (see Case 4 for a contrast in the progression of symptoms).

3. The middle meningeal artery is vulnerable to this injury because it crosses the inner surface of the squamous part of the temporal bone. This bone is thin in this area and exposed, so that it frequently receives traumatic blows in processes like vehicular accidents. This sort of hemorrhage poses a serious and immediate threat to the brain, and the appropriate treatment is a surgical opening of the lateral side of the skull and removal of the large accumulation of blood and blood clot that will collect there in a matter of only a few hours. The bleeding in the artery must also be stopped. Failure to recognize this possibility can have tragic results, either in the death of the patient or permanent severe injury to the brain. This bleeding is known as epidural, but recall that inside the skull, the dura consists of two layers—one that follows the contours of the outer surface of the brain, and the second that is identical to the endosteum of the inner surface of the cranial bones themselves (endosteal dura). In these hemorrhages, the bleeding dissects into the potential space between the outer surface of the endosteal dura and the inner surface of the skull bone itself.

■ CASE 7

1. The elevation of the brush up over the top of the head involves the abductors of the shoulder and those muscles which can elevate the shoulder girdle. Included would be the deltoid muscle, the trapezius muscle, and several muscles that rotate the scapula (involved in elevation of the upper limb).

2. The most likely candidate for injury is the accessory nerve (cranial nerve XI). It emerges from the midpoint of the posterior border of the sternocleidomastoid muscle and is embedded in the thick cervical fascia that extends off of the posterior border of the sternocleidomastoid. It is most likely that the surgeon accidentally transected the nerve, rendering the sternocleidomastoid and trapezius muscles severely weakened. Often a surgeon may face just such a difficult choice—to dissect aggressively, hoping to remove all of a tumor and knowing full well that an important structure may be injured in the process.

■ CASE 8

1. The thyroid gland, subject of the surgery in this case, is enclosed in a layer of cervical fascia known as the pretracheal fascia. It also encloses the trachea. In surgery of the thyroid gland, considerable postoperative bleeding may occur, and if the fascial layer is sutured closed, there is a risk that bleeding within the pretracheal fascia will develop and obstruct the trachea. Patients undergoing these surgeries must be monitored closely to prevent such an occurrence.

2. A tracheotomy is the creation of an opening in the trachea, through which a hollow cylinder can be passed to ensure the movement of air in and out of the tracheobronchial tree. It is indicated in any circumstance that leads to obstruction of the trachea and subsequent difficulties moving air into and out of the lungs. While many sites may be chosen, the two most common are (1) the central midline portion of the trachea inferior to the cricoid cartilage at the second or third tracheal ring and (2) the midline cricothyroid membrane, filling the space between the cricoid and thyroid cartilages. In region #1 the person performing the procedure must take care not to lacerate the isthmus of the thyroid gland, as it passes in front of the upper tracheal rings. Performing a tracheotomy in region #2 entails some risk of damaging the larynx. Current recommendations for performance of tracheotomy indicate a preference for region #1, inferior to the cricoid cartilage.

■ CASE 9

1. An inflammation of the middle ear cavity is known as otitis media and is the most common infection of childhood. The vast majority are caused by bacteria or viruses. The infection produces inflammatory fluid in the middle ear, which dampens the vibrations of the ossicles, diminishing hearing. When the pressure in the middle ear cavity builds up, it causes tension and stretching of the tympanic membrane, causing pain. The inflammatory fluid can also interrupt the function of the chorda tympani, leading to a loss of taste sensation. Otitis externa is an inflammation of the external auditory canal, usually caused by fungi or bacteria. It is very painful, especially if the external ear is tugged on (which will not cause pain in otitis media). An inner ear inflammation (involving the cochlea and/or the semicircular canals) is most often viral and causes disturbances in hearing and equilibrium, without causing any pain.

2. Frequent and persistent middle ear infections cause scarring to the tympanic membrane and increase the chance that it may even be perforated. With such re-

peated infections, the ossicles and the foot-plate of the stapes as it attaches to the oval window suffer permanent loss of mobility, and hearing acuity is lost. The astute physician will be concerned about repeated otitis media and assess the child's hearing as soon as it is practical to do so.

3. Recurrent otitis media can be treated initially with very aggressive antibiotic therapy. If this fails, then small tubes are often inserted through the tympanic membrane to drain pus from the middle ear into the external auditory canal (in an attempt to minimize damage to the ossicles and oval window). The small holes created in the tympanic membrane will heal and do not cause hearing loss themselves. Loss of hearing has an adverse effect on language development because language is an imitative skill. Deaf babies coo and make nonspecific sounds identical to those of the hearing baby but only with the ability to hear and imitate can the complexities of language develop normally.

■ CASE 10

1. The right oculomotor nerve (III) appears to be dysfunctional because the eye cannot medially deviate, an action that is most imputed to the medial rectus, innervated by nerve III. The superior rectus muscle is responsible for moving the eye upward and inward, and when it cannot contract normally, the eye at rest drifts downward and outward. Superior rectus is innervated by nerve III. Last, the ability to point the eye upward is limited, and the inferior oblique is probably involved. It too is innervated by nerve III. The ability to move the eye laterally is preserved, because the lateral rectus muscle is innervated by nerve VI, not III.

2. In this patient's case, with a major neurosurgical procedure just completed and with the relatively rapid onset of symptoms, one should assume that there has been postoperative hemorrhage inside the skull or some other source of suddenly increased intracranial pressure.

■ CASE 11

1. Abnormalities in the function of complex structures like the eye are likely to be bilateral and symmetric if they are the result of system-wide abnormalities (for example, a toxin, poison, or infection) and likely to be unilateral and asymmetric if they are the result of focal lesions (such as tumors and hemorrhages).

2. The simplest explanation for the constricted left pupil (miosis), drooping eyelid (ptosis) on the left, and the "funny" look of the left eye is an injury to

the sympathetic innervation of that eye. The "funny" look is taken to be a retraction or skining of the eye back into the orbital cavity, known as enophthalmos. Not reported here but also a part of this symptom complex in others is anhydrosis, or a lack of sweating, on the affected side. All of these symptoms result from an interruption of sympathetic innervation on the left. This constellation of problems is known as Horner's syndrome.

3. Having established that an interruption of sympathetic function to the left eye explains this patient's history and examination, we need to look along the pathway for sympathetic innervation to the eye and realize that an injury anywhere along that path could cause the symptoms. Thus an injury to the preganglionic sympathetic axons near the spinal cord would be a candidate, as would injury to the cervical sympathetic chain or a lesion to the sympathetic axons on branches of the carotid artery. Finally, an injury near the eye might produce these symptoms, though it would be likely to affect other visual functions as well.

This patient's history of smoking and a progressive cough, coupled with a loss of energy, are worrisome for lung cancer. Lung cancers located near the apex of the lung can put pressure on the sympathetic chain as it passes through the thoracic outlet, which was found to be the location of the tumor in this patient. This case is a good illustration of how symptoms and signs in one system of the body (the eye) may point to a disease process in an entirely different part of the body (the lungs).

■ CASE 12

1. The posterior teeth of the upper jaw and the orbital cavity are separated by a thin sheet of bone, most of it part of the maxilla. When oral infections become chronic and involve the maxillary sinus, the destructive effect of the infection can erode through this thin sheet of bone and invade the overlying orbit. Such infections can initially cause considerable pain in the jaw and teeth, but if the nerves are destroyed by the infection, the patient may feel less—rather than more—pain as the infection progresses.

2. The nerves involved are the middle and posterior superior alveolar branches of the maxillary nerve, or V2.

3. The danger in these lesions is that they are posterior to the orbital septum and thus pose a direct threat to the globe and the patient's vision. Remember that those infections which are anterior to the orbital septum are classed as periorbital cellulitis and may be painful but do not threaten one's vision.

CASE 13

1. The teeth of the lower jaw are innervated by the inferior alveolar nerve, a branch of the mandibular nerve, or V3. The inferior alveolar nerve enters the interior of the mandible at the mandibular foramen, which is palpable on the medial surface of the mandible. The dentist can bathe the nerve in anesthetic at this point and produce near-complete anesthesia for the teeth of the lower jaw on one side.

   The upper jaw's teeth are innervated by a series of branches that descend from the posterior, middle, and anterior superior alveolar nerves, all derived from the maxillary nerve. There is no easily accessible place where the dentist might bathe the entire maxillary nerve in anesthetic; therefore the nerves to each teeth must be bathed by injecting anesthetic into the gum, always more tedious and usually less effective in providing complete anesthesia.

2. In both jaws, the midline teeth receive some innervation from the nerves innervating the other side of the jaw. Thus, even in the lower jaw, the central incisor will not be fully anesthetized if the inferior alveolar nerve on one side only is anesthetized. The opposite inferior alveolar nerve may be anesthetized or local anesthetic infiltrated around the central incisor to fully deaden the tooth.

CASE 14

1. The tonsils are masses of lymphoid tissue located in the posterior part of the oral cavity. The palatine tonsils, most commonly the subject of a tonsillectomy, are located in a recess between two vertical folds of mucosa, the palatoglossal and palatopharyngeal folds (or anterior and posterior tonsillar pillars). The palatine tonsils lie just medially to a portion of the superior pharyngeal constrictor muscle, and arteries supplying the palatine tonsil penetrate this muscular wall to enter the tonsil. The pharyngeal tonsil, or adenoid, is located on the upper part of the posterior pharyngeal wall. Finally, there is a mass of lymphoid tissue on the posterior surface of the tongue, the lingual tonsil. Together, these lymphoid masses form an incomplete ring of tissues that "guards" the entrance to the pharynx. All of them secrete antibody (IgA) on to their surfaces, which helps to neutralize ingested or inhaled antigens.

2. The tonsils receive blood from the tonsillar branch of the facial artery (which penetrates the wall of the tonsillar bed and enters the lateral surface of the tonsil). Also supplying arterial blood are branches of the ascending pharyngeal, lingual, and ascending palatine arteries. The external palatine vein descends on to the tonsil from the soft palate and is the vessel most likely to cause bleeding during surgery.

CASE 15

1. Abnormal noises during breathing usually result from the vibration as air moves past a surface in the wall of the airway (indeed, "normal" respiratory sounds—for-example, speech—result from vibration of air as it passes over the vocal cords) or from excessive narrowing of some part of the airway, also producing extra sounds as the air moves past the point of narrowing.

2. When a patient must expend extra effort to move air past an area of narrowing or obstruction, the clinical signs are tachypnea (breathing rapidly), retractions (heaving of the chest so that the ribs show through the chest wall skin or visible contraction of accessory respiratory muscles like sternocleidomastoid), and flaring of the nostrils.

3. The procedure was a bronchoscopy, which involves direct visualization of the larynx through a narrow tube inserted through the nose or mouth. Laryngomalacia is a condition of immaturity of the cartilage in such structures as the epiglottis, arytenoid cartilages, and aryepiglottic folds. Because the cartilage in these structures is immature, they tend to collapse in front of the glottis during inspiration, producing an obstruction to the easy flow of air into the lungs. The problems occurred during inspiration because that is the time at which pressures within the distal trachea and lungs are momentarily subatmospheric, which encourages the walls of the larynx and trachea to collapse. Placing the baby in a vertical position might help because in that position the epiglottis (attached to the tongue) tends to fall forward, widening the opening into the airway and lessening the likelihood of obstruction. Similarly, placing the baby on his back allows the epiglottis to fall posteriorly, narrowing the opening into the larynx and making the abnormal sounds worse.

SECTION THREE

Upper Limb

▶ **3.1** Shoulder

▶ **3.2** Axilla

▶ **3.3** Brachial Plexus

▶ **3.4** Arm

▶ **3.5** Forearm

▶ **3.6** Wrist

▶ **3.7** Hand

▶ **3.8** Systems Review and Surface Anatomy of the Upper Limb

▶ **3.9** Case Studies: Upper Limb

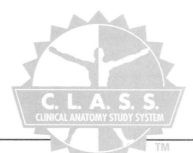

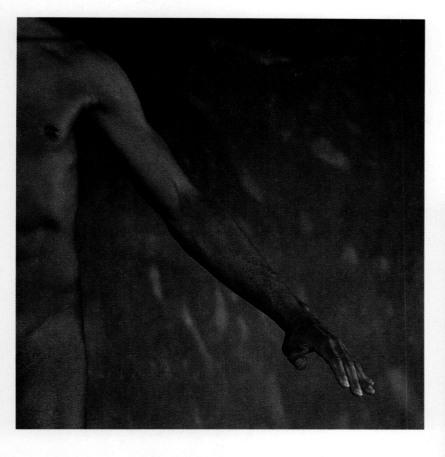
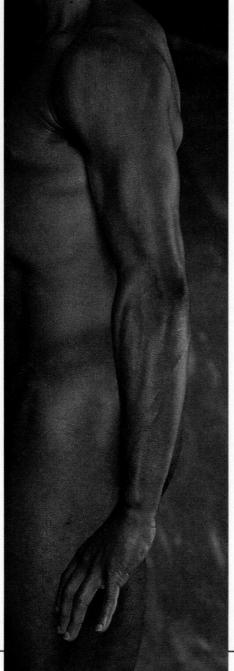

3.1

Shoulder

▶ Introduction to the Upper Limb

▶ Shoulder (Pectoral) Girdle

▶ Humerus

▶ Joints of the Shoulder Girdle

▶ Shoulder Muscles and Shoulder Movement

▶ Arterial Blood Supply to the Shoulder

▶ Venous Drainage of the Shoulder

▶ Nerve Supply to the Shoulder

INTRODUCTION TO THE UPPER LIMB

The upper limb is a highly mobile and flexible appendage with which we carry out the majority of physical interactions with our environment. Anatomically, it consists of the **hand,** whose digits represent the maximum in dexterity and manipulation of objects; the **forearm,** between wrist and elbow joints, a bony platform to which are attached many of the most important muscles for movement of the digits; the **arm,** lying between the elbow and shoulder joints, in which are located several strong muscles acting on the forearm; and the **shoulder** and **shoulder girdle,** a complex of several bones, ligaments, and muscles that serve as a bridge between the upper limb and the trunk. The bones of the shoulder girdle are the **clavicle** and **scapula;** in the **arm,** the **humerus** is the single bone; in the **forearm** are found the **ulna** and **radius;** in the **wrist,** there is a set of eight bones known as the **carpal bones;** and the **hand** is made up of **metacarpal bones** and **phalanges** (Figure 3-1).

Of the large joints in the upper limb, the hingelike **elbow joint** is relatively simple, with a limited range of movement. By contrast, the **shoulder joint, radioulnar joints, wrist joint,** and some of the **individual joints** of the five digits have higher degrees of flexibility and permit greater dexterity. Not surprisingly, among the joints of the five digits, the **carpometacarpal** joint of the thumb allows the greatest range of movement.

The upper limb works as a large **lever,** with joints, at the end of which is a sophisticated grasping tool, the hand. The hand is able to grasp objects of various sizes and shapes, and the forearm's ability to carry out pronation (palm down) and supination (palm up) allows objects to be examined very thoroughly or brought to the mouth for ingestion. The rich variety of capabilities that the upper limb and hand possess enable the immense range of interactions with the environment that are so characteristic of human existence.

Structures of the upper limb cannot be understood without reference to the neck and thorax, two regions with which the upper limb is intimately connected. For example, the major nerves and vessels of the upper limb are derived from parent nerves and vessels in the neck and thorax. The major arteries and veins for the upper limb are derived from vessels passing through the thoracic inlet (Figure 3-2), a bony aperture at the apex of the upper thoracic cage. Its bony perimeter is formed by the *first ribs, manubrium* of the sternum, and body of the *T1 vertebra.* Because the thoracic inlet is a relatively small rigid cylinder, *structures passing through it can be compressed and injured if there is any disruption of their relationship to each other*—by bleeding, growth of a

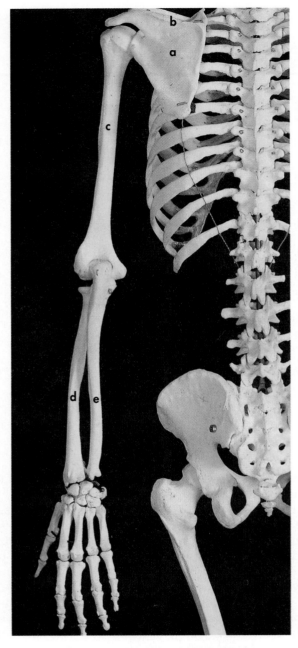

Figure 3-1 BONES OF THE UPPER LIMB. Posterior view. *a*, Scapula; *b*, clavicle; *c*, humerus, *d*, radius; *e*, ulna. (From Chumbley CC, Hutchings RT: *Color atlas of human dissection*, ed 2, London, 1992, Mosby.)

SEE ATLAS, FIG. 3-1

A patient's degree of skeletal maturation has a great influence on the type of fracture that may result from trauma, and the concern physicians have about the sequelae (i.e., aftereffects) of such injuries. First, the relative softness of the bones of newborns and toddlers increases the likelihood of trauma producing a *"greenstick fracture"* rather than an ordinary fracture completely separating the two bone fragments. A greenstick fracture is so named because the injured bone shaft, at the point of injury, becomes soft and pliable but does not separate. In this it resembles what happens to a newly grown branch of a tree when you try to "snap" it in two. Similarly, the halves of the injured bone do not separate because the walls of the bone separate incompletely, and the soft tissues surrounding the shaft of the bone remain attached as well.

Another crucial consideration in the evaluation of fractures in children is the possible involvement of the epiphyseal (growth) plates (see p. 10) of the bone in the fracture. If the line of a fracture crosses one of these areas of bone growth, the posthealing alignment of the bone on opposite sides of the plate is disturbed, and the subsequent growth and development of the bone will be asymmetric.

nerable to injury from pathologic processes in the neck as well as in the upper limb itself.

SHOULDER (PECTORAL) GIRDLE

The shoulder girdle consists of the two bones that attach the upper limb to the thoracic wall—the **scapula** and **clavicle**. The **glenoid fossa** of the scapula forms the articulation of the shoulder girdle with the head of the humerus. The medial end of the clavicle has a strong and complex articulation with the sternum at the **sternoclavicular joint,** forming the only true skeletal linkage of the trunk to the upper limb. The pelvis is the comparable "bony girdle" for the lower limb. *The pectoral and pelvic girdles provide strength, support, and contribute to mobility.* Each half of the pelvis derives from three separate bones that are fused in adult life (see Section 6, Pelvis and Perineum). Because these component bones are fused, the pelvis provides great strength but lacks mobility. In the upper limb, the weaker but more flexible articulations between bones of the pectoral girdle and the humerus provide greater mobility than in the pelvis (Figures 3-3 and 3-4).

Scapula

The **scapula** (Figure 3-5) is an inverted thin triangle of bone positioned on the posterolateral surface of the

tumor, or compression against the bones surrounding the inlet.

Virtually all of the nerves supplying the upper limb originate from the **brachial plexus,** a complex of nerves arising principally from spinal cord segments C5 to T1. This complex group of nerves traverses the posterior triangle of the neck and passes beneath the clavicle to reach the upper limb. Thus the brachial plexus is vul-

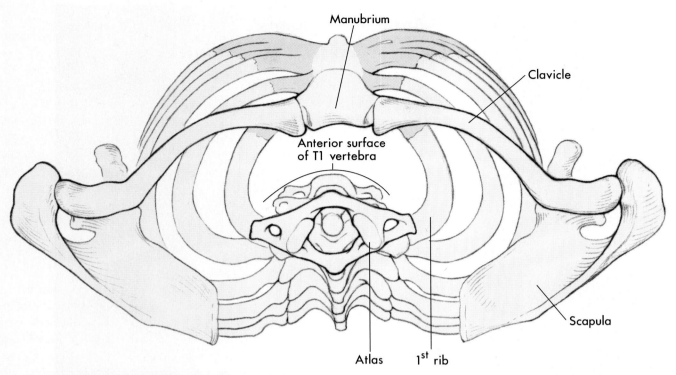

Figure 3-2 THORACIC INLET. This space is bounded by the T1 vertebra, the first ribs, and the manubrium of the sternum. Through it pass all the structures connecting the neck and thorax, as well as several that link thorax to upper limb.

PRINCIPLES ▪

The shoulder and pelvic girdles both attach the limb to the vertebral column, and facilitate movement. The functional differences between the forelimbs and hindlimbs of man are reflected in the specialization of different elements of the limb girdle:

UPPER LIMB GIRDLE

1. Made up of the scapula and clavicle (on each side)
2. No direct articulation with vertebral column
3. Emphasizes mobility over strength
4. Anterior components strongly attached to sternum by costal cartilages
5. Joint with limb (glenoid fossa) is shallow, maximizing movement

LOWER LIMB GIRDLE

1. Made up of the pubis, ischium, and ilium (on each side), which fuse to form a single bone (hip bone)
2. Articulates directly with vertebral column (i.e., sacro-iliac joint)
3. Emphasizes strength over mobility
4. Anterior components articulate directly and strongly (i.e., pubic symphysis)
5. Joint with limb (acetabulum) is deep, allowing less movement

upper chest wall. The base of the triangle is the **superior border.** The scapula has two other borders, the **vertebral** or **medial border,** facing the vertebral column and roughly parallel to it, and the **lateral border,** facing the lateral body wall. As the lateral and vertebral borders descend they converge and meet to form a 45 degree angle at the *inferior angle* of the scapula. The *superior angle* is found at the intersection of the superior and vertebral borders. The flattened surface of the scapula facing the chest wall is the *costal surface*, while the surface facing outward is the *dorsal surface*. On the upper part of the lateral border, where it meets the superior border, is the glenoid fossa (see Figures 3-3 and 3-4).

The **glenoid fossa** is an ovoid, slightly concave depression, facing anterolaterally, which forms a shallow ball-and-socket joint between scapula and head of the humerus (the **glenohumeral joint;** Figure 3-6). The dimensions of the glenoid fossa are about $3\frac{1}{2} \times 2$ cm, with its long axis running superoinferior. The glenoid fossa is very shallow, but in life a fibrocartilaginous **glenoid labrum** (Figure 3-7) attaches around its perimeter, deepening the glenoid fossa and helping to protect against disarticulations of the head of the humerus.

Arising close to the superior aspect of the glenoid fossa and from the lateral end of the superior border of the scapula is a strong and broad pedicle of bone, the **coracoid process** (see Figures 3-2, 3-4, and 3-5), extending in an anterior and slightly superior direction away

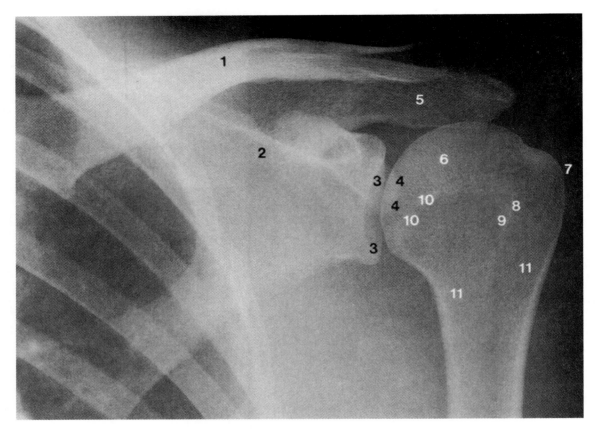

Figure 3-3   SHOULDER JOINT. Anteroposterior (AP) x-ray. (From Weir J, Abrahams PH: *An imaging atlas of human anatomy,* London, 1992, Mosby.)   SEE ATLAS, FIG. 3-65

1 Clavicle	**7** Greater tubercle of humerus
2 Scapula	**8** Intertubercular groove
3 Glenoid fossa	**9** Lesser tubercle of humerus
4 Humeral head, articular surface	**10** Anatomic neck
5 Acromion	**11** Surgical neck
6 Head of humerus	

from the glenoid fossa. The rounded end of the coracoid process, lying about 3 cm anterior to the glenoid fossa, is a point of attachment for the pectoralis minor, short head of biceps, and coracobrachialis muscles. Also attaching here are the coracohumeral, coracoacromial, and coracoclavicular ligaments. Just medial to the base of the coracoid process, on the superior scapular border, is a shallow depression, the **suprascapular notch** (see Figure 3-5). Through this notch passes the suprascapular nerve. A small **transverse scapular ligament** connects the two sides of the notch, and the suprascapular artery and vein pass just above this ligament (see Figure 3-10).

The **supraglenoid tubercle** is a small bony prominence at the "12 o'clock" position near the perimeter of the glenoid fossa. To it attaches the tendon of the long head of the biceps brachii muscle. At the opposite "6 o'clock" position around the perimeter of the glenoid fossa is another small bony prominence, the **infragle-**

noid tubercle. To it attaches the long head of the triceps brachii muscle.

The **scapular spine** (see Figures 3-5 and 3-10) is a raised ridge of bone running across the dorsal surface of the scapula. As it travels from medial to lateral across this surface, the ridge is inflected superiorly at a 25 to 30 degree angle. The scapular spine begins on the medial scapular border, about 2 to 3 cm inferior to the superior angle of the scapula. As it extends from medial to lateral it remains attached by a thin bony strut to the dorsal scapular surface. The most lateral 2 to 3 cm of the scapular spine, however, lack this underlying bony strut, although the spine itself continues laterally uninterrupted. The spine terminates about 3 cm lateral and posterior to the glenoid fossa as the **acromion,** a thick flattened bony process, which articulates with the lateral end of the clavicle. The deltoid and trapezius (see Figure 3-16) muscles attach to the scapular spine and acromion.

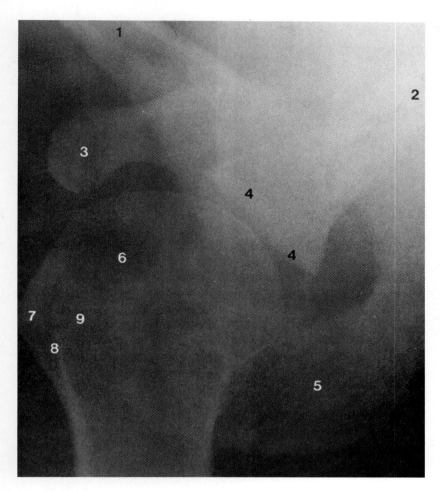

Figure 3-4 GLENOHUMERAL JOINT. X-ray looking down on the left shoulder from above. (From Weir J, Abrahams PH: *An imaging atlas of human anatomy,* London, 1992, Mosby.)

1	Clavicle	6	Head of humerus
2	Spine of scapula	7	Lesser tubercle
3	Coracoid process	8	Intertubercular
4	Glenoid fossa		groove
5	Acromion	9	Greater tubercle

That part of the dorsal scapular surface lying superior to the scapular spine is the **supraspinous fossa.** The dorsal scapular surface inferior to the scapular spine is the **infraspinous fossa.** Vessels and nerves in the supraspinous fossa can reach the infraspinous fossa by traveling around the lateral edge of the bony pedicle supporting the acromion. The small gap between the lateral end of the spine and the underlying posterior surface of the scapula is known as the **scapular notch** (also called the **supraglenoid notch**).

Movements of the scapula are complex. It can "slide" anteriorly and posteriorly along the surface of the chest wall, movements known respectively as *protraction* and *retraction*. It can be *elevated* or *depressed,* as in the repeated shrugging of the shoulders. Additionally, to a limited degree, the scapula can *rotate* in its own horizontal plane so that the glenoid fossa faces almost directly upward. This rotation is important in movements such as abduction of the upper limb (Table 3-1).

Clavicle

The **clavicle** (see Figure 3-2) is a bony strut, in the shape of a very gentle S, extending from the *acromion* of the scapula laterally to the *manubrium* of the sternum medially (its articulation with the sternum is the only synovial joint uniting the upper limb and trunk) (see Figure 3-13). The clavicle suspends the upper limb at a considerable distance from the trunk, permitting a greater range of upper limb movements. The medial two thirds of the clavicle is nearly cylindrical in cross-section and is convex anteriorly. On the medial end of the clavicle are regions for attachment of the *pectoralis major* and *sternocleidomastoid* muscles and for the *costoclavicular ligament* (which binds the clavicle to the first rib). The *subclavius* muscle is attached to the inferior surface of the medial one third of the clavicle. The lateral one third of the clavicle is flattened in cross-section and is concave anteriorly. It has surfaces for the attachment of *deltoid* and *trapezius muscles* superiorly and special surfaces for the *coracoclavicular ligaments* inferiorly.

The **acromioclavicular joint** (Figure 3-8; see also Figure 3-12) links the **acromion** (the lateral end of the scapular spine) to the lateral end of the **clavicle.** There is an ovoid flattened surface on the lateral end of the clavicle, intended to articulate with a similar flattened fossa on the anteromedial edge of the acromion. Both joint surfaces are covered with fibrocartilage. The small synovial cavity of this joint occasionally contains an ar-

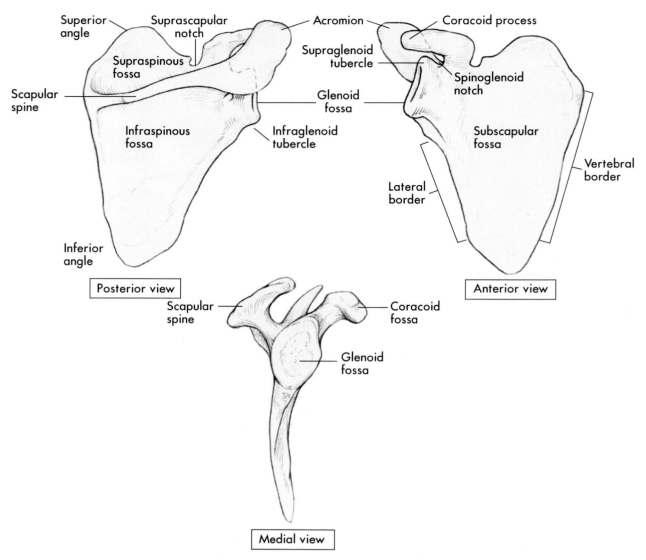

Figure 3-5   SCAPULA. Three views.   See ATLAS, Fig. 3-95

ticular disk. A capsule encircles the entire joint, and a strong acromioclavicular ligament covers its superior surface. The **coracoclavicular ligaments** (see Figure 3-10) also reinforce the glenohumeral articulation although they are not in direct contact with it. The coracoclavicular ligament has two distinct components, the *conoid* and *trapezoid* ligaments. The conoid ligament extends from the superior surface of the coracoid process near its base to the conoid tubercle, located on the inferior surface of the clavicle ~2 to 3 cm medial to its lateral end. Extending laterally from the conoid tubercle on the inferior surface of the clavicle is a *trapezoid line,* to which the *trapezoid ligament* attaches. The trapezoid ligament attaches inferiorly to the coracoid process.

HUMERUS

The humerus (Figure 3-9) is the sole bone of the arm. In its midportion, the humerus has a relatively simple cylindrical shape. At both its proximal and distal ends are specializations for the attachment of muscles and articulation with other bones.

At its proximal end, the anterior surface of the humerus has three important specialized features. From roughly medial to lateral, they are the rounded head of the humerus, the lesser tubercle, and the greater tubercle. The **head of the humerus** is a smooth rounded hemisphere facing superomedially. It articulates with the glenoid fossa of the scapula. The head of the humerus is much larger than the fossa, and the two fit together like a large grapefruit placed in a shallow bowl, not as a true ball-and-socket. This joint is described more completely on p. 318.

The **anatomic neck of the humerus** lies just inferior to the head (see Figure 3-9). Lateral and slightly inferior to the humeral head is the **lesser tubercle.** The lesser tubercle is a raised hillock, about 1 cm high, situated above the midshaft at the proximal end of the humerus.

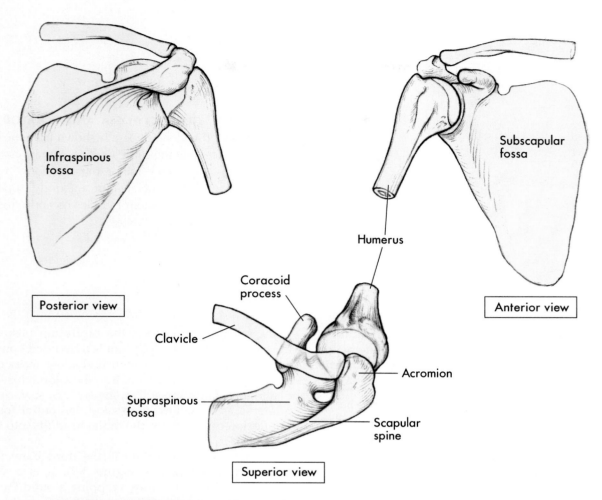

Infraspinous fossa

Posterior view

Subscapular fossa

Anterior view

Humerus

Coracoid process

Clavicle

Supraspinous fossa

Acromion

Scapular spine

Superior view

Figure 3-6   GLENOHUMERAL JOINT. Three views. The shallowness of the glenoid fossa predisposes to easy dislocation of the humeral head. This tendency is compensated by the lateral ends of the clavicle and acromion, which partially overlie the joint, and the rotator cuff muscles (not shown here; see Figure 3-7).   SEE ATLAS, FIGS. 3-92, 3-93, 3-94

Lateral to the lesser tubercle and separated from it by the **intertubercular (bicipital) groove** is the **greater tubercle.** The greater tubercle is slightly larger than the lesser and lies on the anterolateral surface of the humerus, extending around to its posterior surface. The *transverse humeral ligament* spans the gap between the lesser and greater tubercles and converts the intertubercular groove into a canal. The tendon of the long head of the biceps passes through this canal. Just inferior to the tubercles is the **surgical neck of the humerus** (see Figure 3-9), much more frequently a site of humeral fracture than is the anatomic neck (at the junction of the head and shaft of the humerus). The surgical neck of the humerus is in reality the uppermost portion of its shaft.

The **shaft of the humerus** extends from the surgical neck inferiorly to the **supracondylar ridges** of the humerus (see Figure 3-9). It is roughly cylindrical although it becomes more triangular distally. The medial edge of the humerus is smooth, with no distinguishing features. The lateral edge features a midshaft rough-

ened prominence, the **deltoid tuberosity,** where the *deltoid muscle* attaches. The *brachialis* and *coracobrachialis muscles* attach to the anteromedial surface of the humeral shaft (see Figure 3-9). On its posterior surface there is a slightly raised diagonal ridge, running from the medial side of the surgical neck downward and laterally to a region just proximal to the deltoid tuberosity. To this ridge attaches the *lateral head of the triceps muscle.* Inferior to this is the **musculospiral (or radial) groove** for the *radial nerve.* Much of the remainder of the posterior surface of the humerus is occupied by attachment of the *medial head of the triceps muscle.*

At its distal end, the cylindrical shaft of the humerus is broadened into a flattened triangle in the frontal plane, whose lateral and medial sides are the **lateral** and **medial supracondylar ridges,** respectively (see Figure 3-9). At the distal end of the anterior surface of the humerus are four bony prominences. Most lateral is the **lateral epicondyle,** positioned at the inferior end of the lateral supracondylar ridge. Many *extensor muscles of the forearm* are attached to the lateral epicondyle. The

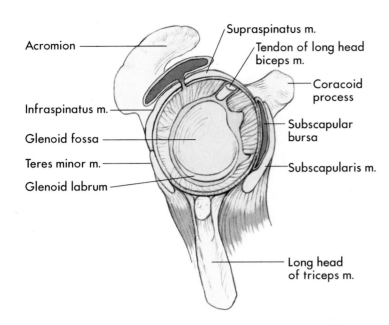

Acromion

Supraspinatus m.

Tendon of long head biceps m.

Coracoid process

Infraspinatus m.

Glenoid fossa

Teres minor m.

Glenoid labrum

Subscapular bursa

Subscapularis m.

Long head of triceps m.

Figure 3-7   GLENOID FOSSA AND ROTATOR CUFF MUSCLES. The glenoid fossa is shown from the lateral aspect. Note how the subscapularis, supraspinatus, infraspinatus, and teres minor muscles form a collar around the glenohumeral joint anteriorly, superiorly, and posteriorly. These four muscles comprise the **rotator cuff.**   SEE ATLAS, FIGS. 3-96, 3-97

lateral epicondyle does not take part in formation of the elbow joint, however. Just medial to the lateral epicondyle, on the anterior surface of the distal humerus,

is the second prominence, the **capitulum** (also called the **capitellum**). The capitulum is a rounded bony eminence, which articulates with a shallow fossa on the head of the radius, as part of the elbow joint. Just proximal to the capitulum, still on the anterior surface of the humerus, is a shallow depression, the **radial fossa.** In full flexion of the elbow, the radial head fits into the radial fossa.

Medial to the capitulum is the third bony prominence, the **trochlea** (see Figure 3-9). It is a smooth curved spool-like structure wrapping around the distal end of the humerus onto its posterior surface. Just above the trochlea is a shallow depression on the anterior surface of the humerus, the **coronoid fossa.** The coronoid process of the ulna fits into the coronoid fossa during full elbow flexion. On the medial side of the dis-

PRINCIPLES ■

Especially in the case of long bones such as the humerus, maturation is a slow and gradual process that extends well into the third decade of life for certain bones (see Introduction). From the clinical standpoint, the continued maturation of bones means that diseases or traumatic injuries of bones may injure these growth regions (*epiphyseal plates*) and distort continued growth and development of the bone. Growth centers located in the midshaft of a long bone are known as the primary ossification centers; those located near the ends of the long bone are secondary ossification centers. Certain prominent features of individual bones (e.g., coracoid process of the scapula, the greater tuberosity of the humerus, the greater trochanter of the femur) have their own ossification centers. At each ossification center, preexisting cartilage is replaced by bone. Throughout life, bone is constantly regenerated and replaced from a collection of germinative cells that lie along the surface of existing bone tissue.

The most common process that injures growth regions of bones is trauma. If a fracture line extends across one of these growth regions, then the clinician must make every effort to realign the fractured fragments. An infection of bone (osteomyelitis) also poses special threats if the inflammation involves the epiphyseal plate. Bones depend on a rich blood supply, and any interruption of the numerous vessels that enter the interior of bones through nutrient foramina can also threaten bone.

Table 3-1   Movements of the Shoulder Girdle

Movement	Involved Muscles	Illustration of Movement
Protraction	Serratus anterior Pectoralis minor	As in doing a "push-up" or a "bench press"
Retraction	Trapezius Rhomboid major Rhomboid minor	As in pulling the oars in a rowboat
Elevation	Trapezius Levator scapulae	As in lifting a weight over the head
Depression	Pectoralis minor Serratus anterior Latissimus dorsi	As in doing a "pull-up"
Rotation	All of muscles above, contracted in a sequential fashion	As in circumduction at the shoulder joint

---

THE SHOULDER

SEPARATED SHOULDER

A separated shoulder is an injury to the **acromioclavicular joint,** often the result of forceful trauma to the "point" of the shoulder, as when the shoulder strikes the ground. The remedy for a separated shoulder is simply rest, sling immobilization, and avoidance of further trauma. As with all injuries to ligaments, the healed tear is usually not as strong as the ligament was before the injury.

DISLOCATED SHOULDER (GLENOHUMERAL JOINT)

A dislocated shoulder is a disturbance of the articulation of the **humeral head** with the **glenoid fossa.** Because the glenohumeral joint is reinforced superiorly, posteriorly, and anteriorly by the **rotator cuff,** the most frequent dislocation of the glenohumeral joint occurs in the anteroinferior direction. Greater than 95% of shoulder dislocations cause the humeral head to slide inferiorly or to slide anteriorly, to lie deep to the coracoid process and the origin of pectoralis

minor. The shoulder is the most frequently dislocated joint in the body.

FRACTURES OF THE CLAVICLE

The clavicle is often fractured as a result of a forceful blow to the "point" of the shoulder. It may also result from a fall on outstretched hands, the force of the fall being transmitted from hand to radius to humerus and then to shoulder girdle. Because the **sternoclavicular joint** is the only true skeletal articulation of the upper limb with the trunk, numerous disruptions of this joint might be expected when forceful trauma occurs. However, the sternoclavicular joint is so strong that it is the **clavicle** that is fractured much more often. Fractures of the clavicle usually occur in midshaft, medial to the attachment of the coracoclavicular ligament. The medial clavicular segment of the clavicle is displaced upward due to the pull of the sternocleidomastoid, and the lateral segment pulled downward by gravity, with inability of the trapezius to elevate it.

---

tal humerus is the fourth prominence, the **medial epicondyle,** appearing to be a continuation of the medial supracondylar ridge. More prominent than the lateral epicondyle, the medial epicondyle serves as an important attachment for many of the *flexor muscles of the forearm.* It does not take part in the elbow joint. The *ulnar*

nerve descends just posterior to the medial epicondyle and passes behind it in the **medial epicondylar groove,** against which the nerve may be compressed (the "funny bone").

On the posterior surface of the distal end of the humerus is the posterior surface of the trochlea and the

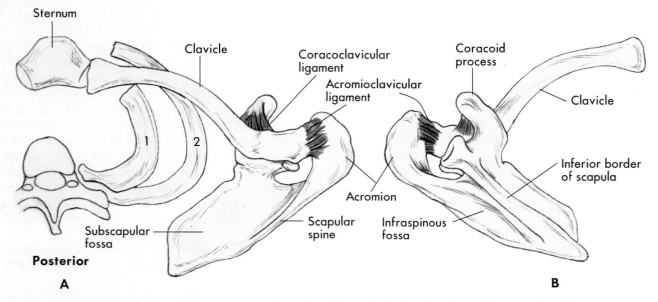

Figure 3-8 SHOULDER GIRDLE. Superior (**A**) and inferior (**B**) views. The superior view illustrates the attachments of the lateral end of the clavicle, especially to the acromion and coracoid process. SEE ATLAS, FIG. 3-8

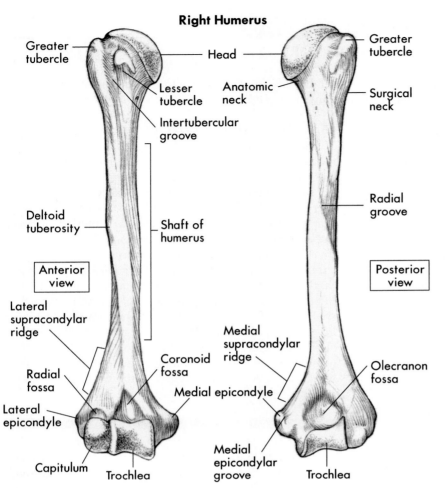

Right Humerus

Greater tubercle

Head

Greater tubercle

Lesser tubercle

Anatomic neck

Surgical neck

Intertubercular groove

Deltoid tuberosity

Shaft of humerus

Radial groove

Anterior view

Posterior view

Lateral supracondylar ridge

Medial supracondylar ridge

Radial fossa

Coronoid fossa

Olecranon fossa

Lateral epicondyle

Medial epicondyle

Capitulum

Trochlea

Medial epicondylar groove

Trochlea

Figure 3-9 HUMERUS. Anterior and posterior views. SEE ATLAS, FIGS. 3-73, 3-74

olecranon fossa. This fossa lies just proximal to the trochlea and into it fits the olecranon process of the ulna during full extension.

JOINTS OF THE SHOULDER GIRDLE

The articulation of the shoulder girdle and upper limb is not sturdy, a fact that maximizes upper limb mobility but makes the upper limb to trunk attachment less stable than the comparable attachment in the lower limb. As if to compensate for this, the upper limb and its girdle are extensively tethered to the trunk by muscles. There are three major joints through which the upper limb and the upper limb girdle are attached to the trunk, the **glenohumeral joint,** the **acromioclavicular joint,** and the **sternoclavicular joint.** Of these, the acromioclavicular and glenohumeral joints in reality unite the upper limb and bones of the shoulder girdle, while *the sternoclavicular joint is the only true articulation of the upper limb girdle with the trunk.*

Glenohumeral Joint

The glenohumeral joint is the articulation of the *head of the humerus* with the *glenoid fossa* of the scapula

(Figure 3-11). It is a joint of the ball-and-socket variety, but the socket is very shallow, allowing a maximum of mobility. The glenoid fossa is pear-shaped rather than circular and is deepened by the **glenoid labrum,** a fibrocartilaginous rim attached around the margin of the glenoid fossa (see Figure 3-7). The part of the head of the humerus and the surface of the glenoid fossa that it faces are both covered with hyaline cartilage. A synovial membrane lines the rest of the joint space, except for these articular surfaces. A strong **joint capsule** lies external to the synovial membrane and encloses the entire joint. The capsule is attached to the scapula just external to the rim of the glenoid labrum. It attaches laterally to the anatomic neck of the humerus, except on the medial surface of the humerus, where it attaches 1 to 2 cm inferior to the plane of the anatomic neck. The joint capsule is loose and allows considerable range of motion.

There are 2 to 3 small apertures in the joint capsule. The first is for the *tendon of the long head of the biceps brachii muscle,* which originates from the supraglenoid tubercle on the margin of the glenoid fossa. This tendon actually traverses the joint cavity, and although it appears to be inside the joint, it is actually surrounded by synovial membrane and is not in true contact with

CLINICAL ANATOMY OF

THE HUMERUS

THE BIRTH PROCESS AND SHOULDER TRAUMA

The passage of a baby's head through the birth canal is not always a smooth and effortless process, and one frequent source of difficulty is the delivery of the shoulder once the head has emerged. The obstetrician must sometimes apply force to the baby to facilitate the delivery, and it is possible for the shaft of the humerus to be fractured as part of this process. The baby's clavicle may also be fractured in this same fashion.

MIDSHAFT FRACTURE OF THE HUMERUS

The radial nerve runs a spiral course around the posterior surface of the humerus as it descends toward the elbow, and, when the humerus is fractured in midshaft, it may injure the radial nerve as well. Such an injury would be expected to produce a weakness in the extensor muscles of the forearm and a *"wrist drop"* or inability to maintain the wrist in a position midway between true flexion and extension.

There would also be sensory loss on the dorsum of the forearm and the dorsal side of the lateral 3 1/2 digits of the hand.

FRACTURES AND THE HEAD OF THE HUMERUS

In patients under 20 years of age but especially in children of preschool and early school age, a fracture of the humerus may displace the head of the humerus along its epiphyseal line. In severe cases the humeral head slides anteriorly, and the examiner can palpate the edge of the humeral shaft posteriorly along the proximal end of the humerus. The surgical neck of the humerus is also crossed anteriorly by the radial nerve, and it may be torn or stretched if there is a fracture at the surgical neck. The axillary nerve may also be damaged by fractures of the neck of the humerus, leading to weakness in the deltoid muscle and a loss of sensation on the lateral surface of the skin over the shoulder.

---

the joint space and the synovial fluid within it. This tendon arches across the superior surface of the head of the humerus, reinforcing the joint to some degree. Joining the short head of the biceps, it attaches distally to the radial tuberosity of the radius. There are usually one or two other small apertures in the joint capsule

through which pass thin extensions of the synovial membrane. This allows the interior of the joint to be continuous with **bursae** (flattened sacs lined with synovial membrane) beneath the subscapularis tendon and between the tubercles of the humerus, surrounding the tendon of the long head of the biceps. The largest bursa

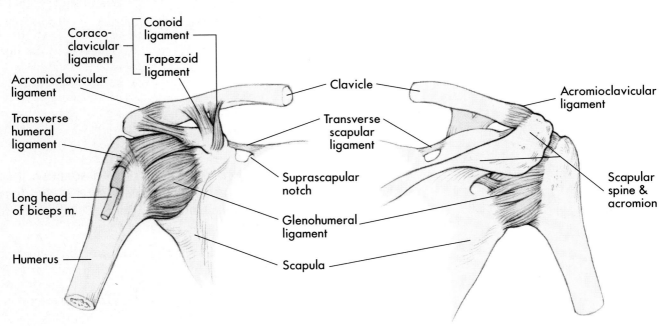

Figure 3-10 LIGAMENTS OF THE SHOULDER. Anterior and posterior views.

SEE ATLAS, FIG. 3-90

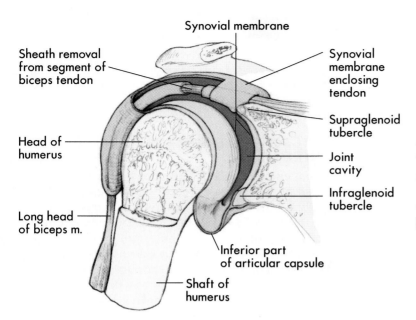

Synovial membrane

Sheath removal
from segment of
biceps tendon

Head of
humerus

Long head
of biceps m.

Synovial
membrane
enclosing
tendon

Supraglenoid
tubercle

Joint
cavity

Infraglenoid
tubercle

Inferior part
of articular capsule

Shaft of
humerus

**Figure 3-11   INTERIOR OF THE GLENOHUMER-
AL JOINT.** Note that the long head of the biceps
tendon travels across the synovial space of the
glenohumeral joint but is covered by synovial
membrane as it does and is not in direct contact
with the synovial fluid of the glenohumeral joint.
SEE ATLAS, FIG. 3-91

of the shoulder region, the **subacromial bursa,** is sometimes not continuous with the glenohumeral joint space
(see Figure 3-7).

The capsule of the glenohumeral joint is reinforced
posteriorly, superiorly, and anteriorly by a group of
tendons that blend with the joint capsule and strength-
en it. The **rotator cuff** (see Figures 3-7 and 3-15), as this
group of tendons is known (see pp. 324-325 for a fuller
description of the individual muscles), comprises the
tendons of the teres minor and infraspinatus muscles posteriorly, the *tendon of the supraspinatus muscle* superiorly,
and the *tendon of the subscapularis muscle* anteriorly. The
tendons of the long head of the triceps and biceps
brachii muscles provide some reinforcement on the inferior and superior aspect of the joint capsule, respec-

tively, although neither is attached directly to the joint
capsule (see Table 3-3). The long head of the triceps
muscle is separated from the joint capsule by the axillary nerve and posterior humeral circumflex vessels. As
a consequence, the inferior aspect of the joint capsule is
weakest. *Most shoulder dislocations are inferior,* occurring
through this area of capsular ligamentous weakness.

Acromioclavicular Joint

The **acromioclavicular joint** permits small degrees
of angular movement in all directions (i.e., a change in
the angle between the acromion and the lateral end of
the clavicle) (see Figure 3-8). Up to 30 degrees of such
movement can be achieved at the acromioclavicular

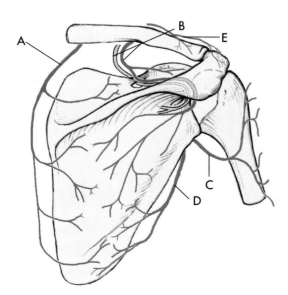

Figure 3-12   JOINTS OF THE CLAVICLE AND SCAPULA. Posterior
view of the scapula. *A,* Dorsal scapular artery. *B,* Suprascapular
artery. *C,* Posterior humeral circumflex artery. *D,* circumflex scapular artery. *E,* Branches of thoracoacromial artery.

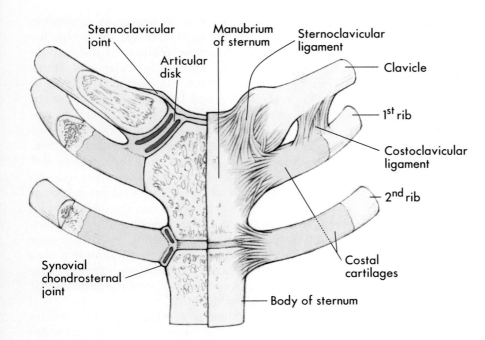

Figure 3-13 JOINTS OF THE STERNUM. The sternoclavicular joint is a double synovial joint, with an articular disk dividing the synovial cavity into two distinct compartments.

See Atlas, Fig. 3-87

joint. This angular motion is essential for rotation of the scapula in its own horizontal plane, which in turn is necessary for maximal shoulder joint abduction and adduction. Similarly, protraction and retraction of the scapula would not be possible without movement at the acromioclavicular joint, permitting the scapula and humerus to move as a unit with respect to the clavicle.

Sternoclavicular Joint

The **sternoclavicular joint** is exceedingly strong and is the only true articulation of the upper limb and its girdle to the trunk (Figure 3-13). Despite its strength, it must be significantly mobile, so as to allow maximum range of motion for the upper limb girdle and the limb itself. Movement can occur in several planes, and up to 25 to 30 degrees of motion is possible. During full abduction of the shoulder, the clavicle must rotate superiorly through 30 to 40 degrees of arc, along its long axis. This motion takes place at the sternoclavicular joint. The joint itself involves the *medial end of the clavicle,* part of the *costal cartilage of the first rib,* and the lateral surface of the *manubrium* (see Figure 3-13). The interior of the joint is divided into two separate compartments by the thick **articular disk** (see Figure 3-13). A tough **capsule** surrounds the joint, and there are *anterior* and *posterior sternoclavicular ligaments* just exterior to it.

A *costoclavicular ligament* unites the inferior surface of the medial end of the clavicle with the superior sur-

---

CLINICAL ANATOMY OF

THE SHOULDER JOINT

BURSITIS AROUND THE SHOULDER JOINT

Like many other important joints, many of the major muscles surrounding the shoulder joint are "cushioned" by a bursal sac, which minimizes friction and subsequent irritation associated with movement. The most important bursae at the shoulder joint are the **deltoid bursa** and the **subacromial bursa** (see Figure 3-7). They are subject to inflammation (bursitis).

ROTATOR CUFF INJURIES

The **rotator cuff** is a mantle of the tendons of four muscles (subscapularis, supraspinatus, infraspinatus, and teres minor), which enclose the glenohumeral joint on its posterior, superior, and anterior aspects. It is in fact the strongest element engaged in reinforcing the shoulder joint. The muscles of the rotator cuff, especially the supraspinatus, are frequently torn during forceful exercise (throwing a ball, lifting a heavy weight, or direct trauma). Degenerative inflammatory changes in the tendons of the rotator cuff muscles may also predispose them to rupture.

face of the medial end of the first rib and its cartilage. Abduction of the shoulder requires elevation of the lateral end of the clavicle. As this occurs, the costoclavicular ligament is progressively tensed and ultimately prevents further elevation of the clavicle, helping to limit abduction of the shoulder.

SHOULDER MUSCLES AND SHOULDER MOVEMENT

A variety of muscles passes across the shoulder joint, linking the arm, scapula, clavicle, neck, and thoracic wall in various arrangements. Shoulder movement is defined as the set of movements that occur between the head of the humerus and the scapula. However, many shoulder movements may not be completed unless there is coordinated movement at other joints, particularly the acromioclavicular and sternoclavicular joints. Abduction of the shoulder is a good example of a complex movement.

Shoulder abduction is the movement of the upper limb away from the center of the trunk at the gleno-humeral joint. The first 20 to 30 degrees of abduction take place solely at the glenohumeral joint, but, for greater degrees of abduction, rotation of the scapula and movement at the acromioclavicular and sternoclavicular joints must also occur. Beyond 30 degrees of abduction, each incremental 15 degrees of shoulder abduction involves 10 degrees of glenohumeral movement and 5 degrees of scapular rotation. This combined movement is known as the **scapulohumeral rhythm.** Beyond 90 degrees of abduction, both the humerus and the clavicle rotate laterally around their long axes, to permit full abduction to occur. The maximal degree of effective abduction is achieved when the vertebral column is laterally flexed to the opposite side. This complex of movements allows a person to reach high over his or her head. The return of the upper limb to a neutral position, by a process of adduction, involves a reversal of the complex sequence of joint movements that produced maximal abduction.

Glenohumeral movement (Figure 3-14) occurs through a wide variety of planes and is not easily described in conventional terms of flexion-extension,

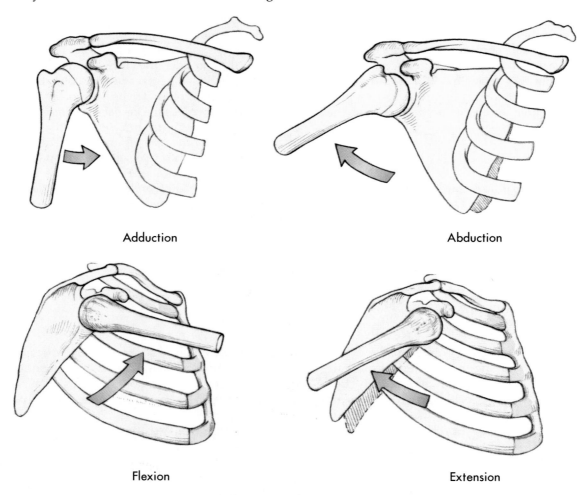

Adduction

Abduction

Flexion

Extension

Figure 3-14   GLENOHUMERAL MOTIONS. Adduction and abduction occur in the mediolateral axis; flexion and extension in the anteroposterior axis.

Table 3-2   Movements of the Glenohumeral Joint

Movement	Muscles Involved	Illustration of Movement
Flexion	Pectoralis major Deltoid (anterior fibers) Coracobrachialis	Moving the arm in the anteroposterior plane from posterior to anterior
Extension	Deltoid (posterior fibers) Teres major	Moving the arm in the anteroposterior plane from anterior to posterior
Abduction	Deltoid (central fibers) Supraspinatus	Holding the arm out to the side of the body, held parallel to the ground in the mediolateral plane
Adduction	Pectoralis major Latissimus dorsi Infraspinatus, teres major, subscapularis (Gravity also plays a role)	Moving in the mediolateral plane, starting from the position of abduction, so that the arm is held snugly against the side of the trunk

Rotation of the humerus	Medial: pectoralis major, latissimus
	    dorsi, deltoid, teres major
	Lateral: infraspinatus, subscapularis,
	    deltoid, teres minor
		Holding the upper limbs straight overhead, as in signalling a "touchdown" in football, requires lateral humeral rotation

Circumduction	Produced by a sequential combination of
	    flexion → abduction → extension →
	    adduction
		Combined serial flexion, abduction, extension, adduction

adduction-abduction, etc. The glenoid fossa faces anterolaterally at a 45 degree angle. An imaginary axis that passes through the head of the humerus perpendicular to the plane of the fossa defines the axis for flexion and extension. Thus *flexion* of the upper limb causes it to move both anteriorly and in part across the front of the chest, parallel to the plane of the glenoid fossa. *Extension* is a movement in the opposite direction. In practice, any movement of the humerus in an anterior (ventral) direction is usually referred to as *flexion*, even when the movement is not in a plane exactly parallel to the glenoid fossa. *Abduction* is movement of

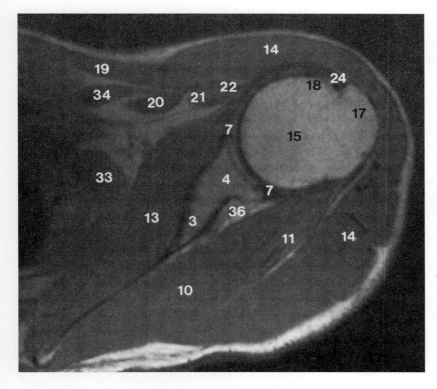

Figure 3-15 MRI SCAN OF SHOULDER, TRANSVERSE PLANE. The MRI technique allows differentiation of muscle and other soft tissue structures. (From Weir J, Abrahams PH: *An imaging atlas of human anatomy,* London, 1992, Mosby.)

3 Body of scapula	**20** Pectoralis minor muscle
4 Glenoid fossa	**21** Coracobrachialis muscle
7 Glenoid labrum	
10 Infraspinatus muscle	**22** Short head of biceps brachii muscle
11 Teres minor	
13 Subscapularis muscle	**24** Tendon of long head of biceps brachii muscle
14 Deltoid muscle	
15 Head of humerus	**33** Serratus anterior muscle
17 Greater tubercle	
18 Lesser tubercle	**34** Subclavius muscle
19 Pectoralis major muscle	**36** Suprascapular artery

Table 3-3   Muscles of the Rotator Cuff

Name	Origin	Insertion	Innervation	Action(s)
Teres minor	From lower portion of infraspinous fossa, along lower lateral border	Posterior surface of greater tubercle of humerus, and on humeral shaft just inferior (passes posterior to humerus)	Axillary nerve (C5 to C6)	Laterally rotates humerus; weak adductor of humerus; stabilizes glenohumeral joint, especially during abduction; may be partly fused with infraspinatus
Infraspinatus	Medial two thirds of infraspinous fossa	By a tendon to posterior surface of greater tubercle of humerus	Suprascapular nerve (C5 to C6)	Laterally rotates humerus; may be partly fused with teres minor; stabilizes glenohumeral joint
Supraspinatus	Medial two thirds of supraspinous fossa	By a tendon, to the greater tubercle of humerus; lies superior to glenohumeral joint	Suprascapular nerve (C5 to C6)	Important abductor of shoulder, with deltoid; reinforces joint capsule superiorly
Subscapularis	From medial three fourths of subscapular fossa, on anterior surface of scapula	To lesser tubercle of humerus and shoulder joint capsule	Upper and lower subscapular nerves (C5 to C7)	Medial rotation and weak adduction of humerus; stabilizes glenohumeral joint

the upper limb away from the trunk in the horizontal (coronal) plane. *Adduction* is movement of the arm toward the trunk in the same plane.

The humerus can also *rotate* around its long axis, especially when the humerus is at rest along the side of the body. As the humerus is flexed, extended, or abducted, the maximum degree of humeral rotation is diminished. *Circumduction* is a continuous sequence of flexion-extension and abduction-adduction movements, as in swinging one end of a jump rope around

in circles. A more detailed description of movements at the glenohumeral joint is found in Table 3-2.

Rotator Cuff Muscles

In some cases muscles may stabilize joints as efficiently as ligaments and capsules. The **rotator cuff muscles** form a continuous "collar" of reinforcement

---

PRINCIPLES

Muscles must pass across joints to produce movement at that joint. In some areas of the body, however, the muscles are also significant for the stability they provide to the joint. Not surprisingly, this occurs most often in joints of minimal strength and maximum flexibility. At the *shoulder,* a particularly effective group of muscles and their tendons (known as the rotator cuff) is in place. These muscles are very important to the movements of the upper limb, and, if the muscles are injured (torn or stretched), the entire joint becomes unstable.

The *hip* joint is crossed posteriorly by a number of small muscles and their tendons, but the muscles are so small that they provide little joint reinforcement. The *knee* is another example of a joint in which the muscles and tendons crossing over the joint provide a great deal of the stability.

CLINICAL ANATOMY OF

THE SHOULDER MUSCLES

WINGING OF THE SCAPULA

One of the most important motions of the scapula is its ability to "slide" anteriorly and posteriorly along the posterolateral surface of the chest wall (protraction and retraction), as part of the complex of movements that give the upper limb such a high degree of mobilty. The serratus anterior muscle extends from the deep surface of the scapula to the upper eight or nine ribs, and, when this muscle does not function, the scapula is not held tightly against the chest wall and protrudes outward or *"wings"* when protraction is attempted. The most common cause of such an abnormality is injury to the *long thoracic nerve* (which innervates the serratus anterior), usually as the result of surgical dissection in the axilla as part of a mastectomy (breast removal).

Table 3-4   Additional Shoulder Muscles

Name	Origin	Insertion	Innervation	Action(s)
Serratus anterior	Anterolateral surface, ribs one to eight or nine	Medial border of scapula	Long thoracic nerve (C5 to C7)	Protracts and medially rotates scapula
Pectoralis major	Medial one third of clavicle, costal cartilages one to eight, external oblique fascia	Intertubercular groove	Medial and lateral pectoral nerves (C5 to T1)	Flexes, adducts, and medially rotates humerus
Pectoralis minor	Ribs three, four, and five near their costal cartilages	Coracoid process	Medial pectoral nerve (C6 to C8)	Protracts and depresses scapula; elevates ribs
Teres major	Dorsal surface of inferior angle of scapula	Lesser tubercle and intertubercular groove of humerus (passes anterior to humerus)	Lower subscapular nerve (C6 to C7)	Adducts, extends, and medially rotates humerus
Trapezius	Occiput, vertebral spines, and ligaments of cervical and thoracic vertebrae	Lateral one third clavicle, acromion, most of the scapular spine	Accessory nerve (motor) and branches of C3 to C4 (sensory)	Can exert force on head, spine, or scapula; elevates shoulder, rotates scapula medially (inferior fibers), or laterally (superior fibers)
Latissimus dorsi	Lumbar aponeurosis, lumbar spines, and posterior iliac crest	Intertubercular groove of humerus; its tendon blends variably with teres major	Thoracodorsal nerve (C6 to C8)	Extends, adducts, and medially rotates the humerus; aids in lateral scapular rotation
Deltoid	Lateral one third of clavicle; acromion; most of scapular spine	By a strong tendon (aponeurosis) to the deltoid tuberosity of humerus	Axillary nerve (C5 to C6)	Abducts humerus; flexes humerus (anterior fibers); extends humerus (posterior fibers)
Sternocleidomastoid	Medial end of clavicle (clavicular head) and manubrium (sternal head), with small triangular gap between	The mastoid process of skull and lateral one third of the superior nuchal line	Accessory nerve (motor), and branches of C3 to C5 (sensory, ?motor)	Rotates head to opposite side; tilts head to same side; major neck landmark
Rhomboid major	Spines of vertebrae T2 to T5	Vertebral border of scapula, lower two thirds	Dorsal scapular nerve (C4 to C5)	Retracts scapula; aids in scapular elevation and lateral rotation
Rhomboid minor	Spines of vertebrae C8 and T1	Vertebral border of scapula opposite root of spine	Dorsal scapular nerve (C4 to C5)	Retracts scapula; aids in scapular elevation and lateral rotation
Levator scapulae	Transverse processes, vertebrae C1 to C4	Superior angle, scapula, and upper one fourth of vertebral border of scapula	Branches of C3 to C4; occasionally from branch of dorsal scapular nerve (C4 to C5)	Elevation of scapula; laterally rotates scapula so that acromion is depressed

around the anterior, superior, and posterior surfaces of the glenohumeral joint (Figure 3-15). Each muscle has important actions on the humerus, but their role in stabilizing the joint prompts consideration of them separate from the other shoulder muscles (Table 3-3).

Other Shoulder Muscles

Several other muscles act on the shoulder girdle and influence upper limb movement but are not strictly speaking muscles acting directly on the glenohumeral joint. These shoulder muscles are described in Table 3-4 and Figure 3-16.

This diverse group of additional muscles may flex, extend, medially rotate, laterally rotate, adduct, or abduct the upper limb. Some act on the glenohumeral joint (teres muscles, latissimus dorsi, deltoid) while others act on the scapula (rhomboids, levator scapula). Still others attach to the clavicle (sternocleidomastoid, part of deltoid) and influence upper limb movement by moving or stabilizing this part of the shoulder girdle (see Figure 3-16).

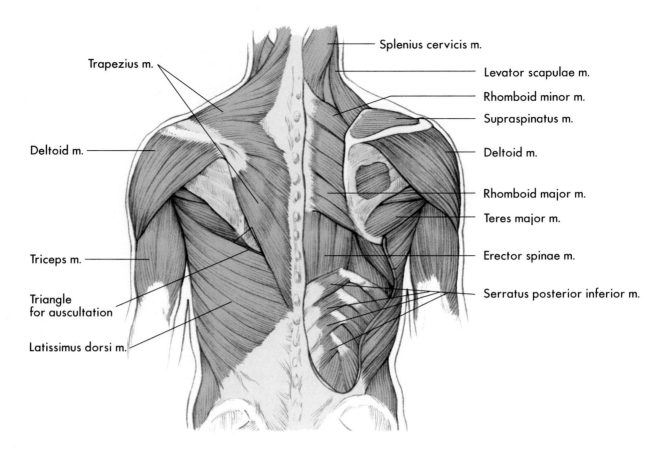

Figure 3-16   BACK MUSCULATURE. On the left side of the specimen are more superficial muscles; on the right are deeper muscles.   SEE ATLAS, FIGS. 3-61, 3-62, 3-63, 3-64

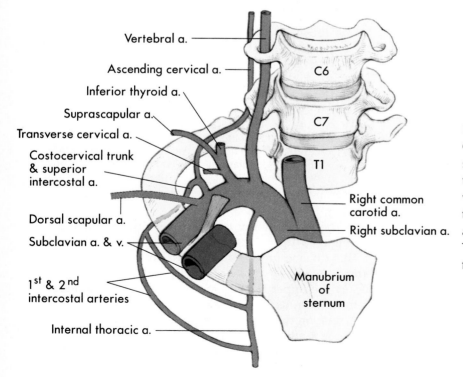

Figure 3-17   BRANCHES OF THE SUB-CLAVIAN ARTERY. Shown here is the subclavian artery on the right. The position of the scalenus anterior muscle divides the artery into its first, second, and third parts (proximal to, posterior to, and distal to the muscle, respectively). The vessel ends at the distal end of the first rib.

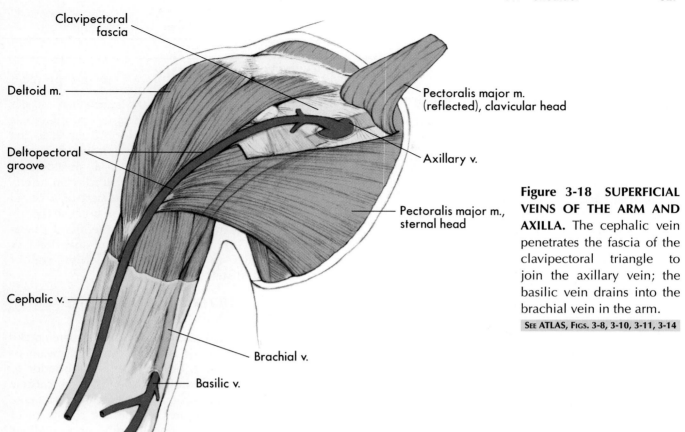

Clavipectoral fascia

Deltoid m.

Deltopectoral groove

Cephalic v.

Pectoralis major m. (reflected), clavicular head

Axillary v.

Pectoralis major m., sternal head

Brachial v.

Basilic v.

Figure 3-18 SUPERFICIAL VEINS OF THE ARM AND AXILLA. The cephalic vein penetrates the fascia of the clavipectoral triangle to join the axillary vein; the basilic vein drains into the brachial vein in the arm.

Sᴇᴇ ATLAS, Fɪɢs. 3-8, 3-10, 3-11, 3-14

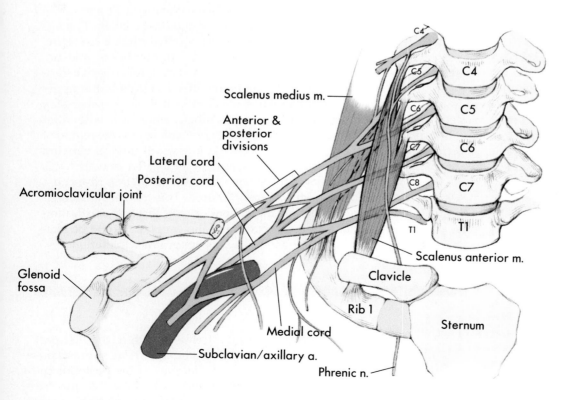

Scalenus medius m.

Anterior & posterior divisions

Lateral cord

Posterior cord

Acromioclavicular joint

Glenoid fossa

Medial cord

Subclavian/axillary a.

Phrenic n.

C4

C5

C6

C7

C8

T1

C4

C5

C6

C7

T1

Scalenus anterior m.

Clavicle

Rib 1

Sternum

Figure 3-19 BRACHIAL PLEXUS. Relationships to nearby structures.

Sᴇᴇ ATLAS, Fɪɢs. 3-16, 3-17

THE NEUROVASCULAR SUPPLY OF THE SHOULDER

EXTENT OF COLLATERAL BLOOD FLOW

Anastomotic flow in the shoulder region is quite well developed. The suprascapular and dorsal scapular arteries supply blood to the scapula and anastomose extensively with branches of the subscapular artery that also supply the scapula. The internal thoracic artery and its anterior intercostal branches anastomose with the posterior intercostal branches of the aorta (and the costocervical trunk, for the upper two intercostal spaces). This collateral circulation is so good that in a **Blalock-Taussig shunt** (a common operation performed to provide relief for a variety of congenital heart diseases), the subclavian artery is disconnected completely from the distal circulation to the upper limb and anastomosed surgically with the pulmonary artery. Despite this drastic rearrangement, the upper limb remains well perfused through these and other channels for collateral blood flow.

IMPORTANCE OF THE NEUROVASCULAR "PEDICLE" OF A MUSCLE

Knowledge of the blood supply to certain muscles has made it possible for reconstructive surgeons to move entire muscles to different parts of the body to replace muscles that have been surgically removed or injured through disease or trauma. For example, the removal of the pectoralis major and minor is often necessary as part of the total mastectomy for breast cancer. In these surgeries, it is possible to take the latissimus dorsi muscle, with its intact **neurovascular "pedicle"** entering the muscle on its inferior surface, and move the latissimus muscle around to the anterior chest wall to replace the surgically removed pectoral muscles. This gives the patient a more natural look to the chest wall after the breast and underlying muscles have been surgically removed.

CERVICAL RIBS AND SUBCLAVIAN CIRCULATION

The subclavian vessels normally must pass over the first rib, which in the best of circumstances is a tight fit. If a cervical rib (a rib related to the seventh cervical vertebra) is present, the subclavian vessels must also pass over the superior surface of this rib as well, and the likelihood of some obstruction to the flow of blood through the subclavian vessel is even greater. This may also result in a **poststenotic aneurysm** in the third part of the subclavian artery. Aneurysms commonly form in that part of a vessel just distal to the site of an obstruction because the velocity of blood flow is increased as the blood passes through the point of narrowing, and this "jet" of blood is thought to put special stress on the wall of the vessel just distal to the obstruction.

CARDIAC CATHETERIZATION AND THE SHOULDER VEINS

Cardiologists and cardiovascular surgeons make use of the subclavian or axillary veins as a means of access when threading catheters into the interior of the heart. This procedure is known as a **cardiac catheterization,** and is commonly employed to make measurements of pressures within the chambers of the heart and carefully define anatomic abnormalities before surgery is planned.

STELLATE GANGLION BLOCK

The stellate ganglion is the combined T1 and inferior cervical ganglia of the sympathetic chain. Patients suffering from vascular obstructive disease involving the upper limb (producing pain, numbness, and tingling in the upper limb) may derive relief from a variety of steps that dilate the blood vessels in the upper limb and therefore increase blood flow. One such step is the **stellate ganglion block,** where a needle is inserted through the posterior triangle into the region of the transverse process of the seventh cervical vertebra (since the stellate ganglion is located between this transverse process and the neck of the first rib), and a local anesthetic agent infused. This may provide long-term relief for the patient or may serve as verification that a surgical removal of the ganglion would be likely to improve the patient's upper limb circulation.

ARTERIAL BLOOD SUPPLY TO THE SHOULDER

An important arterial anastomotic network exists around the shoulder. Several branches of the **subclavian artery** (Figure 3-17) contribute to the blood supply of the shoulder. The **suprascapular artery** is a branch of the thyrocervical trunk, itself a branch of the first part of the subclavian artery (Figure 3-17). The suprascapular artery arises in the medial part of the posterior triangle of the neck, then courses laterally across this triangle, passing anterior to the scalenus anterior muscle and the roots of the brachial plexus. It then passes just above the transverse ligament of the scapula (see p. 312) to enter the *supraspinous fossa*. From here some branches pass around the lateral side of the scapular notch to reach the *infraspinous fossa*. The suprascapular artery provides blood supply to structures in both of these fossae.

The **superficial cervical artery** also arises from the thyrocervical trunk, near to the origin of the suprascapular artery, and passes laterally across the posterior triangle of the neck. It follows the posterior belly of the omohyoid muscle as it turns posteriorly, toward the scapula. It supplies the trapezius and levator scapulae muscles, but, unlike the suprascapular artery, it neither passes close to the scapular notch nor does it supply muscles of the supra- and infraspinous fossae. The **dorsal scapular artery*** arises from the third part of the subclavian artery. This vessel turns backward and travels among the proximal components of the brachial plexus, as it courses toward the superior angle of the scapula. On reaching the scapula it descends deep to the rhomboid muscles, near their attachments to the vertebral border of the scapula.

The suprascapular and dorsal scapular arteries take part in the **scapular anastomosis,** which receives additional major blood supply from the subscapular artery and from some posterior branches of the upper thoracic intercostal vessels. *This anastomosis protects the upper limb from the harmful effects of insufficient blood supply (ischemia)* when obstruction of blood flow in the subclavian or axillary arteries distal to the thyrocervical trunk occurs.

VENOUS DRAINAGE OF THE SHOULDER

The shoulder region, like most parts of the body, has a set of *deep veins*, usually accompanying the major arterial trunks, and a set of *superficial veins*, draining the skin and subcutaneous tissues. The superficial veins ultimately drain into the deep veins (Figure 3-18). The

---

*Occasionally the superficial cervical and dorsal scapular arteries are not present. In their place there is a unique common parent vessel, a branch of the thyrocervical trunk known as the **transverse cervical artery**. In these cases, the **superficial branch** of the transverse cervical is equivalent to the missing superficial cervical, and the **deep branch** of the transverse cervical artery is equivalent to the missing dorsal scapular artery.

brachial and axillary veins and their tributaries represent the *deep veins* of the shoulder.

There are two prominent *superficial veins* of the upper limb, the **cephalic vein** and the **basilic vein.** They are more fully described on p. 347. At the level of the shoulder, the basilic vein has already penetrated the deep fascia to join the brachial vein. The cephalic vein travels in a shallow **deltopectoral groove** between the adjacent sides of the deltoid and pectoralis major muscles (see Figure 3-18). Just distal to the clavicle, in a small depression known as the **deltopectoral triangle,** the cephalic vein penetrates the clavipectoral fascia and joins either the axillary or subclavian vein.

NERVE SUPPLY TO THE SHOULDER

The **brachial plexus** is the major structure for innervation of the shoulder area (Figure 3-19). It is described fully on pp. 336-341, as are the individual branches supplying shoulder muscles (see Tables 3-3, 3-4, and 3-5). A few of the shoulder muscles are not supplied by brachial plexus branches, however. For example, the *levator scapulae muscle* is innervated by small branches of **cervical nerves C3 to C4.** The *trapezius muscle,* important in elevation of the shoulder and stabilization during other movements, is innervated by the spinal root of cranial nerve 11 (the accessory nerve). Most believe that its motor innervation arises in the **accessory nerve** while its sensory innervation (proprioception, etc.) derives from small branches of **cervical nerves C3 and C4.**

The cutaneous innervation of the shoulder area is also derived from branches of the cervical plexus, intercostal nerves, and branches of the brachial plexus. The **supraclavicular nerves,** derived from segments C3 to C4 of the cervical plexus, innervate the *skin on the upper aspect of the shoulder,* extending as far laterally as the skin over the acromion and inferiorly as far as the second intercostal space. On the *lateral aspect of the shoulder,* extending inferiorly from acromion to mid-humerus, the skin is innervated by a cutaneous branch of the **axillary nerve (C5 to C6)** (see Figure 3-26). The *upper medial aspect of the arm,* extending upward into the axilla, is innervated by a branch of T2, the **intercostobrachial nerve.** *Distally the arm* is innervated by various cutaneous branches of the **brachial plexus,** detailed on pp. 338-340.

3.2

section three . two

Axilla

- ▶ Walls of the Axilla
- ▶ Spaces in the Axilla
- ▶ Axillary Artery

- ▶ Axillary Vein
- ▶ Lymphatic Drainage of the Axilla
- ▶ Fasciae in the Axilla

*T*he axilla is a space, surrounded by four walls, in the shape of a pyramid (Figure 3-20), with its tip cut off (i.e., a "truncated" pyramid). At its apex (which is triangular, however), the axilla is continuous with the posterior triangle of the neck (see pp. 198-205). The base of the axilla is at the level of the lower margins of the pectoralis major and latissimus dorsi/teres major muscles, which form parts of the anterior and posterior walls of the axilla, respectively. The axilla is a conduit for the passage of structures between the upper limb and root of the neck, including many important structures of the head, neck, and thorax. The *brachial plexus* and the *subclavian vessels* enter the axilla through a relatively narrow space between the first rib, scapula, and clavicle. Extreme shoulder extension or depression can cause compression of these vessels and nerves between the clavicle and the first rib (the *costoclavicular syndrome*).

WALLS OF THE AXILLA

The **anterior wall** of the axilla is composed of the *pectoralis major* and *pectoralis minor muscles*, plus the lower margin of the *subclavius muscle* and the *clavipectoral fascia*. The **posterior wall** is made up of the *latissimus dorsi, teres major, and subscapularis muscles*. The **medial wall** is formed by the *serratus anterior muscle*, covering the upper eight to nine ribs (Figure 3-21). The **lateral wall** of the axilla is formed by the *coracobrachialis muscle* and the shaft of the *humerus*. The **apex** of the axilla is surrounded by the *clavicle, scapula,* and *first rib* (forming its triangular walls). SEE ATLAS, FIG. 3-15

The lower margin of the pectoralis major forms the sharp **anterior axillary fold.** The lower margins of the latissimus dorsi and teres major form the rounded **pos-**terior axillary fold. The **axillary fascia** extends across the space between these two folds, forming a concave **axillary floor.**

SPACES IN THE AXILLA

The axillary muscles are arrayed in a manner that creates several consistent spaces or passages in the walls of the axilla. These spaces are defined by the structures forming their borders and are important for the structures that pass through them. Understanding these spaces and the structures passing through them is very helpful in comprehending the anatomy of the axilla.

The **quadrangular** (or **quadrilateral**) **space** (Figure 3-22) is in the posterior wall of the axilla and is bounded laterally by the *humerus*, medially by the *long head of the triceps muscle*, inferiorly by the *teres major muscle*, and superiorly by the *subscapularis* (when viewed from anterior) and *teres minor* (when viewed from posterior) *muscles*. Through the quadrangular space pass the axillary nerve and the posterior humeral circumflex vessels.

The **triangular space** is best seen when viewed from the posterior aspect (see Figure 3-22). Its lateral border is formed by the *long head of the triceps,* while the *teres major* and *teres minor muscles* form its lower and upper borders. Its "apex" is that point, medially, where the borders of the teres major and minor muscles meet. Through this space passes the subscapular artery or its large circumflex scapular branch.

The **triangular interval** is bounded laterally by the *humerus* and medially by the *long head of the triceps muscle.* Its base is formed by the inferior margin of the *teres*

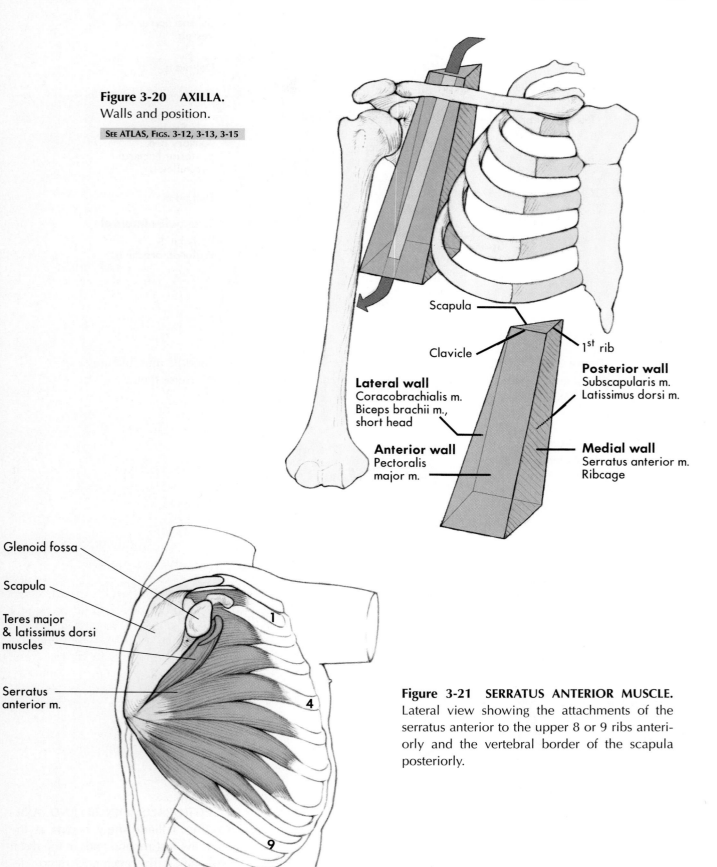

Figure 3-20 AXILLA.
Walls and position.

SEE ATLAS, FIGS. 3-12, 3-13, 3-15

Scapula

Clavicle

1st rib

Lateral wall
Coracobrachialis m.
Biceps brachii m.,
short head

Posterior wall
Subscapularis m.
Latissimus dorsi m.

Anterior wall
Pectoralis
major m.

Medial wall
Serratus anterior m.
Ribcage

Glenoid fossa

Scapula

Teres major
& latissimus dorsi
muscles

Serratus
anterior m.

1

4

9

Figure 3-21 SERRATUS ANTERIOR MUSCLE.
Lateral view showing the attachments of the
serratus anterior to the upper 8 or 9 ribs anteriorly and the vertebral border of the scapula
posteriorly.

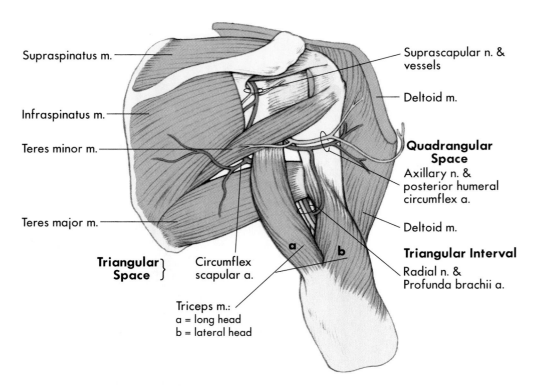

Supraspinatus m.

Infraspinatus m.

Teres minor m.

Teres major m.

Suprascapular n. & vessels

Deltoid m.

Quadrangular Space
Axillary n. & posterior humeral circumflex a.

Deltoid m.

Triangular Interval
Radial n. & Profunda brachii a.

Triangular Space }

Circumflex scapular a.

Triceps m.:
a = long head
b = lateral head

Figure 3-22 AXILLARY SPACES. This posterior view of the scapula and its musculature illustrates the three important muscular spaces and the structures that traverse them.
SEE ATLAS, FIGS. 3-69, 3-70

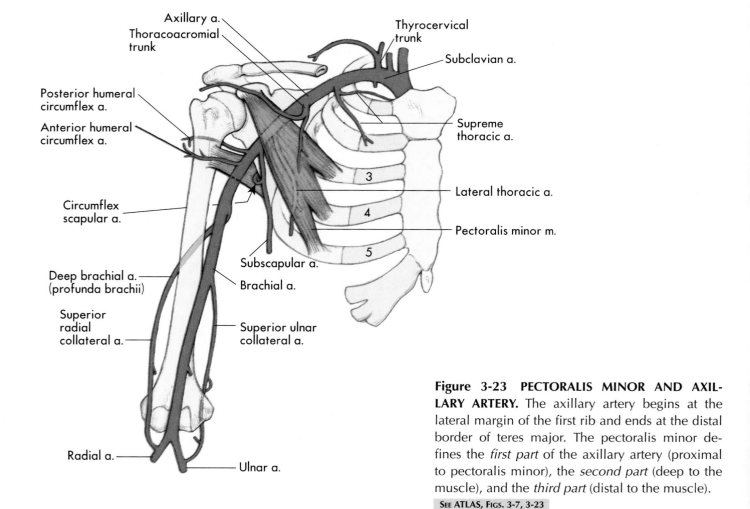

Axillary a.
Thoracoacromial trunk

Thyrocervical trunk

Subclavian a.

Posterior humeral circumflex a.

Anterior humeral circumflex a.

Supreme thoracic a.

Circumflex scapular a.

Lateral thoracic a.

Pectoralis minor m.

Deep brachial a. (profunda brachii)

Subscapular a.

Brachial a.

Superior radial collateral a.

Superior ulnar collateral a.

Radial a.

Ulnar a.

Figure 3-23 PECTORALIS MINOR AND AXILLARY ARTERY. The axillary artery begins at the lateral margin of the first rib and ends at the distal border of teres major. The pectoralis minor defines the *first part* of the axillary artery (proximal to pectoralis minor), the *second part* (deep to the muscle), and the *third part* (distal to the muscle).
SEE ATLAS, FIGS. 3-7, 3-23

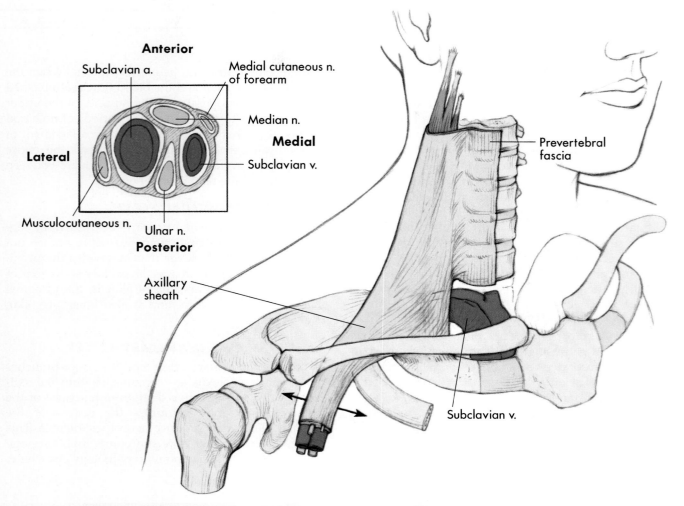

Figure 3-24 CERVICAL FASCIA AND THE AXILLARY SHEATH. *Inset* in the upper left shows the relationships of structures within the axillary sheath, cut in cross-section where marked by the arrows.

major muscle. It is traversed by the radial nerve and the profunda brachii artery, as they spiral posteriorly around the shaft of the humerus.

AXILLARY ARTERY

The axillary artery is the central structure of the axilla. For example, the cords of the brachial plexus (see pp. 336-341) are named according to their relationship to the axillary artery. The subclavian artery becomes the **axillary artery** at the *lateral border of the first rib* and extends as far as the *inferior border of the teres major muscle,* where the axillary artery becomes the **brachial artery** (Figure 3-23). The pectoralis minor muscle crosses anterior to the axillary artery and, in so doing, defines the three parts of the artery. The *first part of the axillary artery* extends from the lateral border of the first rib to the medial border of pectoralis minor; it lies anterior to the first intercostal space and is posterior to the clavicular fibers of the pectoralis major. The *second part of the axillary*

artery is deep to pectoralis minor. The posterior cord of the brachial plexus lies deep (posterior) to the artery. At this point the coracobrachialis muscle lies superolateral to it. The *third part of the axillary artery* lies between the distal border of pectoralis minor and the inferior border of the teres major muscle. Anterior to it is the pectoralis major; posterior to it are the teres major and latissimus dorsi muscles.

The first part of the axillary artery has one branch, the second part two, and the third part three. The **superior thoracic** (or **supreme thoracic**) **artery** is the sole branch of the *first part of the axillary artery.* It divides into several branches, which supply the pectoralis major and minor muscles and anastomose with the first posterior intercostal artery.

The *second part of the axillary artery* gives rise to two vessels, the **thoracoacromial trunk** and the **lateral thoracic** artery. The thoracoacromial trunk passes around the medial border of the pectoralis minor muscle, then divides into four branches—**deltoid, acromial, clavicu-**

THE AXILLA

LYMPH NODES AND THE AXILLA

Axillary lymph node dissection is an important part of many cancer operations, particularly those involving removal of the breast since breast cancers frequently spread to the axillary lymph nodes. A **complete axillary dissection** involves exposure and risk to many important structures. Most such operations intentionally sacrifice the following: pectoralis major and minor, nerves to pectoral muscles, axillary tail of the breast, thoracoacromial vessels to axilla, many tributaries to axillary vein, many smaller branches of axillary artery. Surgeons make every effort to preserve and protect the following: brachial plexus, axillary vein and artery, thoracodorsal nerve (to latissimus dorsi), and long thoracic nerve (to serratus anterior).

AXILLARY NERVE BLOCK (FIGURE 3-24)

Anesthetic blocks of the brachial plexus may be accomplished by infusing local anesthetic into the **axillary sheath,** an extension of the prevertebral fascia of the neck, which encloses the major branches of the brachial plexus and the axillary artery. Such an anesthetic block, combined with an occlusive tourniquet technique to completely block blood flow to the upper limb, allows the surgeon to operate on the upper limb without having to place the patient under general anesthesia. The upper limb can tolerate 1 to 2 hours

without blood flow and be entirely normal when the tourniquet is relaxed and the blood flow reestablished at the end of the operation. This capacity of the upper limb tissues to tolerate prolonged periods of no blood flow is also what makes possible the reattachment of traumatically severed fingers (or indeed the entire upper limb), even when considerable delay between the injury and the reattachment occurs.

INTERCOSTOBRACHIAL NERVE

The intercostobrachial nerve is derived from segment T2 and is the first cutaneous nerve branch not part of the brachial plexus that innervates the proximal arm and axilla. It crosses the axillary space to provide innervation to an area of skin in the proximal medial skin of the arm, and it also innervates skin over the axilla.

ANEURYSM OF THE AXILLARY ARTERY

Because the axillary artery and the major branches of the brachial plexus are contained within the axillary sheath, a progressive dilation (**aneurysm**) of the axillary artery may compress the nerves of the brachial plexus and produce neurologic deficits. This is a good example of how symptoms involving one system of the body may point to pathology elsewhere.

lar, and **pectoral.** These vessels also anastomose with other vessels of the anterior chest wall. The lateral thoracic artery emerges on the lateral border of the pectoralis minor and travels downward on the surface of serratus anterior to supply it and the pectoral muscles with blood.

The *third part of the axillary artery* gives rise to three branches—the subscapular artery, posterior humeral circumflex, and anterior humeral circumflex. The **subscapular artery** is so named because it arises at the lower border of the subscapularis muscle and lies on the surface of serratus anterior, descending along the anterior border of the subscapularis toward the inferior angle of the scapula. About 4 cm from its origin the subscapular artery gives rise to the **circumflex scapular artery,** an important component of the scapular anastomosis (see p. 329). This vessel hooks around the lateral scapular border, deep to teres minor, and enters the **infraspinous fossa** deep to the infraspinatus. Here it anastomoses with branches of the suprascapular and dorsal scapular arteries.

The **posterior humeral circumflex artery** is larger than its anterior companion. It accompanies the axillary nerve through the quadrangular space and travels partway around the surgical neck of the humerus. Here it lies deep to the deltoid and gives off several branches to that muscle and adjacent structures. The **anterior humeral circumflex artery** crosses the anterior surface of the surgical neck of the humerus, gives off small branches to the head of the humerus, and anastomoses with the posterior humeral circumflex artery.

AXILLARY VEIN

The axillary vein is the proximal continuation of the brachial veins and, in turn, continues medial to the lateral border of the first rib as the **subclavian vein.** The **cephalic vein** penetrates the **clavipectoral fascia** and joins the **axillary vein** (the **basilic vein** drains into the brachial vein at a point more distal in the arm). The axillary vein lies medial to the axillary artery, and it is flanked by the medial cutaneous nerves of the arm and forearm. Normal variations in the arrangements of these veins are common and often the brachial vein is double, flanking the brachial artery as venae comitantes. **Venae comitantes** is the name applied to the veins, often double or triple, which accompany major arteries.

LYMPHATIC DRAINAGE OF THE AXILLA

The **axillary lymph nodes** are important targets of lymphatic drainage from the breast (see Figure 1-7). These nodes must always be examined carefully in patients with breast cancer, since axillary nodes are a frequent site for metastasis (spread of the tumor cells). Axillary lymph nodes also receive drainage from the anterior and posterior chest wall (from clavicle to umbilicus) and the upper limb. Lymph leaves the axilla and drains into the **subclavian lymph duct,** which empties into the subclavian vein on each side.

FASCIAE IN THE AXILLA

The **axillary fascia** covers the space between the anterior (pectoralis major) and posterior axillary folds (latissimus dorsi) and splits to enclose the pectoralis minor. The **clavipectoral fascia** spans the gap between the upper margin of the pectoralis major and the clavicle and splits to encircle the subclavius muscle. The **axillary sheath** is an extension of the prevertebral fascia of the neck down into the axilla, where it encloses the first part of the axillary artery and the proximal portions of the brachial plexus (Figure 3-24). The **axillary tail of the breast,** enclosed in its own fascial jacket, also extends to a variable extent into the axilla, wrapping around the inferolateral margin of the pectoralis major muscle as it does.

Brachial Plexus

▶ Components of the Brachial Plexus

▶ Brachial Plexus in the Neck

▶ Brachial Plexus in the Axilla

*T*he brachial plexus is the most important neural plexus in the body. It is not necessarily the most complex, but the overwhelming importance of the innervation of the upper limb, especially the hand, gives the brachial plexus its unique significance. The brachial plexus is formed from the entire anterior primary rami of **C5 to C8** and most of the anterior primary ramus of **T1.** In addition, the plexus usually receives some axons from both the **C4** and **T2** segments. Moving from medial to lateral, it consists of *roots, trunks, divisions, cords,* and *nerves,* arranged in a characteristic pattern that defines the brachial plexus. The axons of the brachial plexus contain sensory and motor axons from C5 to T1 and carry sympathetic axons arising in the **inferior** (or stellate—inferior plus first thoracic ganglion) and **middle cervical sympathetic ganglia.**

COMPONENTS OF THE BRACHIAL PLEXUS

The brachial plexus begins in the neck. The **roots of C5, C6, C7, C8, and T1** emerge between the scalenus anterior and scalenus medius muscles and combine with each other near the lateral border of scalenus medius as they begin to move laterally across the floor of the posterior triangle of the neck. The *C5* and *C6 roots* combine to form the **upper** or **superior trunk;** the *C7 root* continues laterally, without combining with any other root, but nonetheless, lateral to the scalene muscles, changes its name to the **middle trunk,** and the *roots of C8 and T1* combine to form the **lower** or **inferior trunk.** As these trunks continue in a lateral direction, they are positioned just deep to the inferior belly of the omohyoid and the suprascapular artery; by contrast,

the dorsal scapular artery lies just deep to the roots of the brachial plexus. The trunks then pass beneath the clavicle to enter the axilla. As they do, each trunk divides into an **anterior** and **posterior division** (Figure 3-25; see also Figure 3-19).

Just proximal to the medial edge of the pectoralis minor muscle, the *posterior divisions of all three trunks* combine to form the **posterior cord,** lying posterior to the second part of the axillary artery. This large struc-

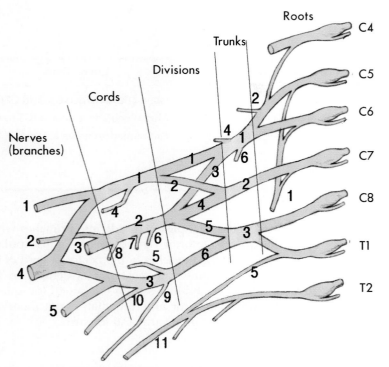

Roots

Trunks

Divisions

Cords

Nerves
(branches)

C4
C5
C6
C7
C8
T1
T2

Roots	Cords
1 Long thoracic nerve	1 Lateral cord
2 Dorsal scapular nerve	2 Posterior cord
	3 Medial cord
Trunks	4 Lateral pectoral nerve
1 Upper trunk	5 Medial pectoral nerve
2 Middle trunk	6 Upper subscapular nerve
3 Lower trunk	7 Thoracodorsal nerve
4 Suprascapular nerve	8 Lower subscapular nerve
5 First intercostal nerve	9 Medial cutaneous nerve of arm
6 Nerve to subclavius	10 Medial cutaneous nerve of forearm
Divisions	11 Intercostobrachial nerve
1 Anterior division, upper trunk	**Nerves (branches)**
2 Anterior division, middle trunk	1 Musculocutaneous nerve
3 Posterior division, upper trunk	2 Axillary nerve
4 Posterior division, middle trunk	3 Radial nerve
5 Posterior division, lower trunk	4 Median nerve
6 Anterior division, lower trunk	5 Ulnar nerve

Figure 3-25 STRUCTURE OF THE BRACHIAL PLEXUS. Semischematic view of the brachial plexus, with its roots, trunks, divisions, cords, and branches.

SEE ATLAS, FIGS. 3-9, 3-19, 3-20

ture then continues laterally, lying on the anterior surface of the subscapularis muscle. While traveling beneath the pectoralis minor muscle, the posterior cord gives off one of its most important branches, the **axillary nerve,** which traverses the quadrangular space to exit the axilla (see Figures 3-22 and 3-26).

The *anterior divisions of the upper and middle trunks* unite deep to the pectoralis minor muscle to form the **lateral** or **anterolateral cord,** lying lateral to the second part of the axillary artery. Just distal to the lateral border of pectoralis minor, the **musculocutaneous nerve** branches away from the lateral cord. The remainder of the lateral cord continues laterally to form a major part of the **median nerve** (see Figures 3-19 and 3-25).

The *anterior division of the lower cord* continues laterally across the axilla and forms the **medial** or **anteromedial cord,** also related to the axillary artery, on its medial side. The main derivatives of the medial cord are the **ulnar nerve** and a portion of the **median nerve.** As it reaches the lateral border of the subscapularis muscle, the brachial plexus has formed all of its major branches and beyond this point ceases to exist as a plexus.

In relation to the *second part of the axillary artery* (i.e., deep to pectoralis minor), the lateral, medial, and posterior cords of the brachial plexus lie lateral, medial, and posterior, respectively (see Figure 3-19). The posterior cord of the plexus is actually superolateral to the *first part of the axillary artery,* however, because the artery turns inferiorly toward the chest. Also, at

the level of the *third part of the axillary artery,* the cords begin to branch and lose their relationship to the artery.

BRACHIAL PLEXUS IN THE NECK

Above the clavicle, the brachial plexus gives rise to relatively few branches. The **dorsal scapular nerve** arises from the *C5 root,* pierces the scalenus medius and comes to lie posterior to levator scapulae; it continues over to the back, descending on the anterior (i.e., deep) surface of the rhomboid muscles, just medial to the vertebral scapular border. It innervates the rhomboid muscles. The **long thoracic nerve** arises from branches of *roots C5 to C7* and moves posterior to pass deep to the first part of the axillary artery and the lateral continuation of the brachial plexus itself. It then descends on the external surface of the serratus anterior muscle, which it innervates. The long thoracic nerve is somewhat unique in lying superficial to the muscle it innervates. Individual small branches of the roots supply the scalene muscles and other deep neck muscles. These are not considered part of the brachial plexus since they have no anatomic connection with it.

The trunks are relatively short sections of the brachial plexus (see Figure 3-25) and give rise to only two individual nerves. The **suprascapular nerve** (*C4 to C6*) arises from the upper trunk, just before it divides into its anterior and posterior divisions. It passes posterior, deep to trapezius, and passes through the *suprascapular notch* to reach the *supraspinous fossa.* It inner-

Table 3-5   Branches of Cords of the Brachial Plexus

Posterior Cord	Medial Cord	Lateral Cord
Upper subscapular nerve (C5 to C6)	Medial pectoral nerve (C8 to T1)	Lateral pectoral nerve (C5 to C7)
Thoracodorsal nerve (C6 to C8)	Medial antebrachial cutaneous nerve (C8 to T1)	Musculocutaneous nerve (C5 to C7)
Lower subscapular nerve (C5 to C6)	Medial brachial cutaneous nerve (C8 to T1)	Part of median nerve (C5 to C7)
Axillary nerve (C5 to C6)	Part of median nerve (C5 to C7)	
Radial nerve (C5 to T1)	Ulnar nerve (C8 to T1)	

vates the *supraspinatus,* then loops laterally around the root of the scapular spine to reach the *infraspinous fossa.* Here it innervates the *infraspinatus* muscle and supplies small twigs to the scapula and glenohumeral joint. The **nerve to subclavius (C5 to C6)** is a small filament arising from the medial end of the upper trunk. It descends deep to the subclavian artery and enters the substance of the subclavius muscle.

As the three trunks course laterally, they pass deep to the clavicle and divide into their anterior and posterior divisions. At this point the brachial plexus leaves the neck.

BRACHIAL PLEXUS IN THE AXILLA

Distal to the clavicle, the brachial plexus continues through the axilla. Its divisions combine into the **lateral, medial,** and **posterior cords,** which in turn give rise to the definitive branches of the brachial plexus. These branches are shown in tabular form in Table 3-5. The cords of the brachial plexus divide into branches while they lie on the anterior surface of the subscapularis muscle. In general, branches of the posterior cord of the brachial plexus innervate posterior structures in the arm and forearm. Branches from the lateral (or anterolateral) and medial (or anteromedial) cords innervate anterior structures in the arm and forearm.

Posterior Cord

The posterior cord (Figure 3-26) branches into an **upper subscapular nerve** (*C5 to C6*), supplying subscapularis alone, and a **lower subscapular nerve (**C5 to C6*)*, supplying both subscapularis and teres major (which lies along the inferolateral border of the subscapularis). Between the two subscapular nerves arises the important **thoracodorsal nerve** (*C6 to C8*). It travels downward along the chest wall, in company with the subscapular artery and its thoracodorsal branch, to innervate the latissimus dorsi muscle. The **axillary nerve**

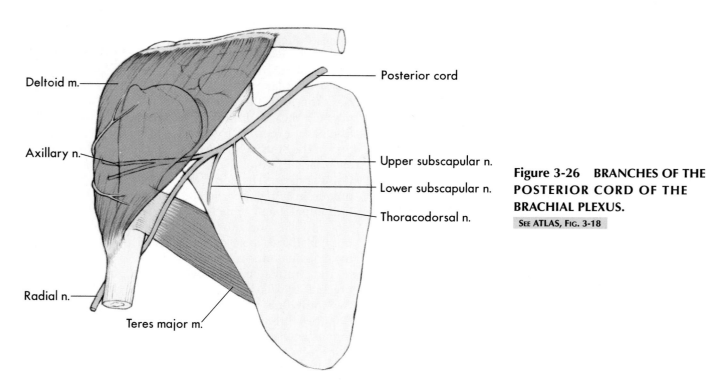

Deltoid m.

Axillary n.

Radial n.

Teres major m.

Posterior cord

Upper subscapular n.

Lower subscapular n.

Thoracodorsal n.

Figure 3-26   BRANCHES OF THE POSTERIOR CORD OF THE BRACHIAL PLEXUS.
Sᴇᴇ Aᴛʟᴀs, Fɪɢ. 3-18

THE BRACHIAL PLEXUS

VARIATIONS IN BRACHIAL PLEXUS STRUCTURE

The contributions of segmental nerves and T2 to the brachial plexus vary; when C4 provides a significant input, the plexus is said to be **prefixed.** When C4 contributes few axons but T2 contributes many, the plexus is **postfixed.** The posterior cord and its branches innervate the postaxial or extensor muscles; the lateral and medial cords innervate the preaxial or flexor muscles.

INJURY TO THE UPPER ROOTS OF THE PLEXUS

Erb-Duchenne palsy is a tearing or traction injury involving the upper roots of the brachial plexus (C5, C6). It results from stretching forces applied to the shoulder that pull the head away from the shoulder (i.e., exaggerated lateral flexion of the shoulder). This can occur as a result of a forceful fall onto the shoulder or, during childbirth, when the obstetrician applies force to the baby's head while the shoulder has not yet been delivered. The result of this injury is dysfunction in those muscles innervated by segments C5 and C6. The usual clinical picture is an upper limb with an adducted shoulder, medially rotated arm, extended elbow, and flexed wrist.

INJURY TO THE LOWER ROOTS OF THE PLEXUS

Klumpke's paralysis is the result of injury to the lower roots of the brachial plexus (C8, T1). This affects mainly the intrinsic muscles of the hand, and the clinical picture is that of a "claw hand" (Figure 3-27). This syndrome results from any injury which forcefully abducts the shoulder joint. Again, it can occur during a difficult childbirth, especially when the delivery is breech (lower limbs and buttocks delivered first), and the obstetrician pulls forcefully on the trunk while the upper limb remains inside the birth canal.

(*C5 to C6*) separates from the posterior cord and deviates further posteriorly (see Figure 3-26), where it traverses the quadrangular space (along with the posterior humeral circumflex artery). The axillary nerve innervates the deltoid and teres minor muscles and a considerable area of skin over the shoulder, just below the plane of the acromion.

The **radial nerve** (*C5 to C8; T1*) is the largest single derivative of the posterior cord. It travels laterally across the anterior surface of subscapularis and crosses anterior to the lateral ends of latissimus dorsi and teres major. It then passes between the humerus and the long head of the triceps (in the triangular interval), to reach the *posterior compartment* of the arm. Here it travels with the profunda brachii artery in a shallow groove on the humerus, deep to the lateral head of the triceps. As it wraps around to the lateral side of the humerus, it passes through the lateral intermuscular septum to reenter the *anterior compartment* of the arm. At the lateral epicondyle of the humerus, it emits branches for nearby posterior compartment muscles (e.g., triceps, extensor carpi radialis longus) and divides into its terminal superficial and deep branches (see p. 365). The radial nerve innervates the triceps muscle in the arm and all of the posterior musculature of the forearm (including brachioradialis, which is functionally an elbow flexor muscle). It also has posterior cutaneous branches for part of the arm, all of the forearm, and for the skin on the lateral side of the dorsum of the hand. It occasionally sends branches to the brachialis muscle.

Medial Cord

The medial cord of the brachial plexus (see Figure 3-25) provides branches that innervate structures in the chest wall, arm, forearm, and hand. The **medial pectoral nerve** (*C8 to T1*) arises from the proximal medial cord and travels between the axillary artery and vein to penetrate the undersurface of the pectoralis minor (and innervate it). Some of its branches loop around the inferolateral border of pectoralis minor and go on to innervate the pectoralis major muscle as well (the medial pectoral nerve, which actually lies lateral to the **lateral pectoral nerve,** so named not by its position but because of its origin from the lateral cord—see following). Further laterally, the medial cord gives rise to a **medial cutaneous nerve of the arm** (*C8 to T1*) and shortly thereafter a **medial cutaneous nerve of the forearm** (*C8 to T1*). The medial cord continues onward to provide two final branches—the **ulnar nerve** (*C8 to T1*) and the medial cord's contribution (C6 to C8) to the **median nerve** (*C5 to C8; T1*). The ulnar nerve descends in the upper arm just medial to the brachial artery but midway down the arm penetrates the medial intermus-

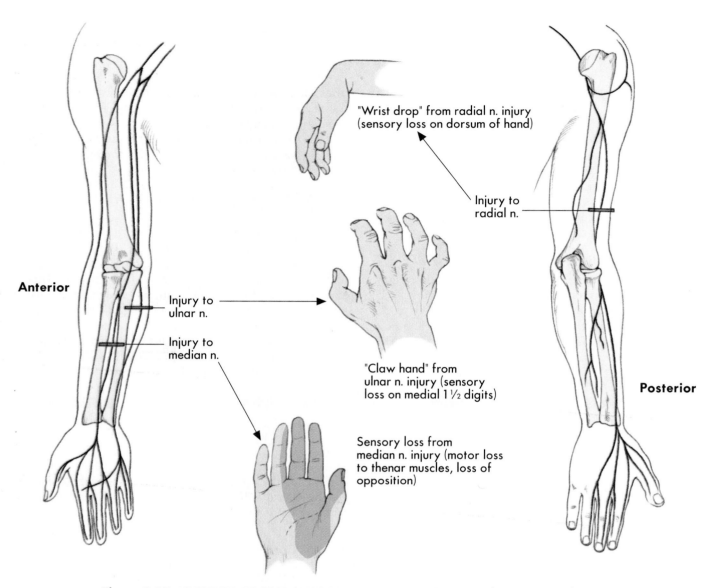

Anterior

Injury to
ulnar n.

Injury to
median n.

"Wrist drop" from radial n. injury
(sensory loss on dorsum of hand)

Injury to
radial n.

Posterior

"Claw hand" from
ulnar n. injury (sensory
loss on medial 1 ½ digits)

Sensory loss from
median n. injury (motor loss
to thenar muscles, loss of
opposition)

Figure 3-27   INJURIES TO THE MAJOR UPPER LIMB NERVES. Both sensory and motor
loss are described for each injury.   **SEE ATLAS, FIG. 3-72**

cular septum and enters the *posterior compartment of the
arm.* It then descends further and passes between the
medial epicondyle and the olecranon of the ulna,
where it is vulnerable to compression (the "funny
bone"). It passes behind the elbow joint in the **medial
epicondylar groove** and then reenters the forearm *anterior compartment* by passing between the two heads of
the flexor carpi ulnaris muscle. The ulnar nerve innervates the flexor carpi ulnaris and the medial two or
three elements of the flexor digitorum profundus. In
the hand, the ulnar nerve innervates all of the intrinsic
muscles (excepting the thenar muscles and the lateral
two lumbricals). It provides cutaneous innervation to
both the anterior and posterior surfaces of the medial
side of the hand and the little finger as well as the medial half of the ring finger. The ulnar nerve also sup-

plies the majority of innervation to the wrist and hand
joints and to the blood vessels of the hand. The median
nerve is discussed following.

Lateral Cord

The lateral cord gives rise to two derivative branches
and contributes to the median nerve. The **lateral pectoral nerve (***C5 to C7***)** emerges where the anterior divisions of the upper and middle trunks unite to form the
lateral cord. The lateral pectoral nerve then passes anterior to the axillary artery and pierces the clavipectoral
fascia to emerge along the superomedial border of the
pectoralis minor (which it usually does not innervate).
It does go on to innervate the pectoralis major muscle.
Confusingly, it actually lies medial to the medial pec-

PRINCIPLES ■

Just as defined regions of the skin are innervated by given spinal nerve segments—regions defined as dermatomes—it is possible to list groups of muscles innervated by each spinal nerve segment, a grouping defined as a **myotome**. In fact, what is represented by a myotome is the muscle(s) derived from the mesoderm developing in each individual body segment. Most muscles of the limbs can be said to derive their innervation predominantly, but not exclusively, from one or two spinal cord segments. Below are some of the upper limb muscles innervated by such segments:

C3 to C4: Trapezius, levator scapulae

C5: Rhomboids, deltoid, biceps, supraspinatus, infraspinatus, teres minor

C6: Serratus anterior, latissimus dorsi, teres major, brachialis, brachioradialis, supinator, biceps, pectoralis major

C7: Pectoralis minor, triceps, pronator teres, serratus anterior, latissimus dorsi, flexor and extensor carpi radialis, extensor carpi radialis longus/brevis, extensor digitorum

C8: Pectoralis minor, triceps, flexor digitorum superficialis and profundus, pronator quadratus, most forearm extensor muscles, thenar muscles, flexor carpi ulnaris

T1: Most intrinsic hand muscles except thenar muscles (i.e., hypothenar muscles, lumbricals, interossei)

Knowledge of myotomal patterns of innervation helps explain functional losses when there is injury to a spinal cord segment.

toral nerve as they both reach the anterior chest wall. The second branch, the **musculocutaneous nerve** (C5 to C7), arises just distal to the lateral border of pectoralis minor muscle; it courses in a lateral direction, pierces the coracobrachialis muscle (which it inner-

vates), and continues laterally and distally between the biceps and brachialis muscles (both of which it innervates). It reaches the lateral side of the arm and, near the elbow, forms the **lateral cutaneous nerve of the forearm**. This nerve runs distally along the border of the radius as far as the wrist. It innervates the skin of the lateral forearm, especially on the anterior side.

The **lateral cord** (see Figure 3-25) ends by contributing to the **median nerve** (*C5 to C8; T1*). The median nerve is formed when the roots from the lateral and medial cords unite on the anterior surface of the third part of the axillary artery. In the upper half of the arm the median nerve is lateral to the brachial artery; at about midarm it crosses in front of the artery and thereafter lies medial to the artery, as far as the elbow joint. It crosses the elbow joint lying just anterior to the tendon of the brachialis muscle and enters the forearm by passing between the two heads of the pronator teres muscle (which it innervates). In the forearm, the median nerve descends on the deep surface of the flexor digitorum superficialis, between it and the flexor digitorum profundus muscle. About 4 cm above the wrist it emerges on the lateral border of the flexor digitorum superficialis to lie progressively more superficial as it approaches the wrist. The median nerve is the most superficial of the structures passing deep to the flexor retinaculum (the palmaris longus muscle is more superficial at the wrist, but it is superficial to the flexor retinaculum and does not traverse the carpal tunnel).

In the arm, the median nerve has no branches other than small twigs to the brachial artery. Sometimes a small branch to the pronator teres arises proximal to the elbow. In the forearm, there are branches to all the anterior muscles (except the flexor carpi ulnaris and the two medial components of the flexor digitorum profundus). In the hand, the thenar muscles and the lateral two lumbrical muscles are supplied by the median nerve. The median nerve provides innervation of the anterior palmar surface of the wrist. On the anterior side of the hand it innervates the thumb, index, middle and lateral half of the ring fingers; the innervation extends over to the distal phalanx on the dorsal surface of these same digits.

3.4 ◀ Arm

▸ Humerus

▸ Muscles of the Arm

▸ Brachial Vessels

*T*he arm extends from the shoulder joint to the elbow joint (Figure 3-28). It has a single bony element, the **humerus** (described on p. 314), and its musculature is segregated by fascial barriers into **anterior** and **posterior compartments.** The musculature of the arm is largely devoted to movement at the elbow joint, with some contribution to shoulder movement and stability. The arm also helps make the forearm stable and helps position the forearm and hand for effective function of the digits. The **brachial artery** is a continuation of the axillary artery in the arm and gives rise to the important **deep brachial artery** (also known as the **profunda**

brachii). Just distal to the elbow the brachial artery divides into the **radial** and **ulnar arteries,** the major arterial supply of the forearm and hand. Several large branches of the **brachial plexus** descend through the arm as well (see p. 337, and following).

The **cubital fossa** is a shallow triangular depression on the anterior surface of the elbow joint. The "apex" of this imaginary triangle points distally. The base of the triangular cubital fossa is at the distal end of the humerus, and the two sides are formed by the pronator teres and the brachioradialis muscles (see Figure 3-29). It is an important region of the proximal forearm, and

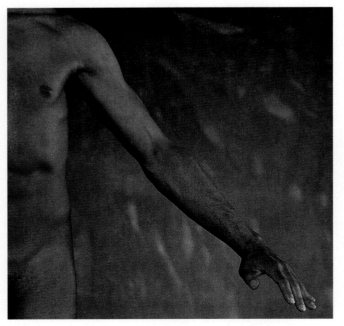

Figure 3-28 BOUNDARIES OF THE ARM. The arm extends from the shoulder joint proximally to the elbow joint distally. Its axis is the humerus, and muscles originating in the arm mediate flexion and extension of the elbow joint.

Both the forelimbs and hindlimbs in humans show evidence of **compartment formation**—the presence of fascial sheets or septa, which divide the limb segment into spaces occupied by functionally similar groups of muscles, vessels, and nerves. For example, in the arm the anterior compartment contains muscles that are flexors, and all are innervated by the same nerve (the musculocutaneous). The posterior compartment of the arm is occupied by the triceps muscle, innervated by the radial nerve.

The septa extend from the central bone in the limb outward to the deep fascia. This compartmental arrangement can prove to be a threat to the patient, however. For example, in traumatic injury to the limbs, there may be progressive bleeding confined to one of these compartments. As bleeding continues, pressure within the compartment builds up and the muscles, nerves, and vessels are threatened by the high pressure within that space (**compartment syndrome**). The corrective procedure applied is a **fasciotomy**—the placing of an incision in the enclosing fascia, to relieve the pressure in the compartmental space.

many of the important vessels and nerves of this area are described with reference to the cubital fossa.

HUMERUS

A description of the bony anatomy of the humerus is found on pp. 314-318. The **medial intermuscular septum** originates from the medial side of the humerus, along an imaginary line connecting the intertubercular groove and the medial epicondyle. This septum extends medially to blend with the subcutaneous tissues. A similar **lateral intermuscular septum** extends away from the lateral side of the humerus. These septa, and the humerus to which they are anchored, constitute a *barrier between the posterior and anterior compartments of the arm*. These compartments are seen most clearly along the distal half of the humerus. The barrier is not complete, however; for example, the ulnar nerve penetrates the medial septum in the lower arm, passing from the anterior to the posterior compartment. The radial nerve passes from the posterior to the anterior compartment by penetrating the lateral septum at midarm level.

With a few exceptions, the *proximal half* of the humerus is a site for the *insertion of muscles*, most of

Table 3-6　Muscles of the Arm

Name	Origin	Insertion	Innervation	Action(s)
Deltoid	Lateral one third of clavicle; acromion; most of scapular spine	By a strong tendon to the deltoid tuberosity of humerus	Axillary nerve (C5 to C6)	Abducts shoulder; flexes shoulder (anterior fibers); extends shoulder (posterior fibers)
Coracobrachialis	From coracoid process of the scapula	At midpoint of medial humeral border	Musculocutaneous nerve (C5 to C6)	Flexes and, to a degree, adducts shoulder
Brachialis	Anterior surface of distal one half of humerus	Tuberosity and coronoid process of ulna	Musculocutaneous nerve (C5 to C7)	Flexes elbow
Biceps brachii	Short head: coracoid process Long head: supraglenoid tubercle	Tuberosity of radius By bicipital aponeurosis to fascia over pronator teres	Musculocutaneous nerve (C5 to C6)	Supination; flexion of the elbow; weak shoulder flexor; long head helps stabilize shoulder
Triceps brachii	Long head: infraglenoid tubercle Medial head: broad strip on posterior humerus Lateral head: raised ridge on upper posterior one third of humerus	To olecranon process of ulna	Radial nerve (C6 to C8)	Extension of elbow joint (forearm)

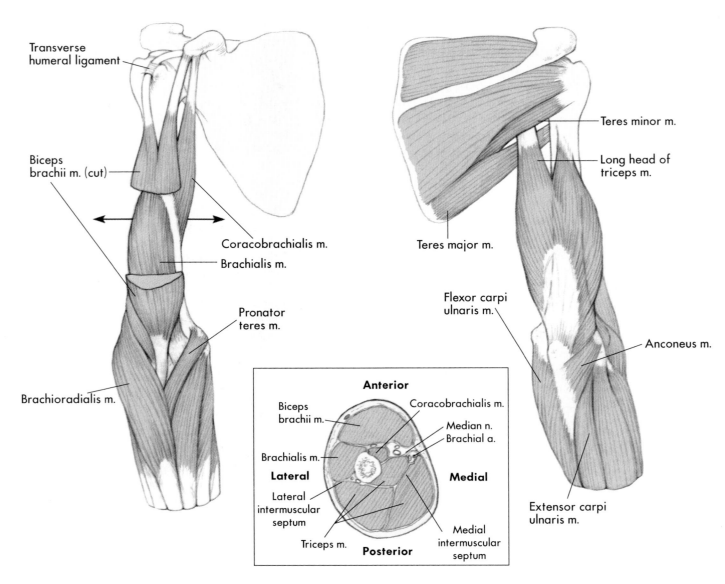

Transverse
humeral ligament

Biceps
brachii m. (cut)

Coracobrachialis m.

Brachialis m.

Pronator
teres m.

Brachioradialis m.

Teres minor m.

Long head of
triceps m.

Teres major m.

Flexor carpi
ulnaris m.

Anconeus m.

Extensor carpi
ulnaris m.

Anterior

Biceps
brachii m.

Coracobrachialis m.

Median n.
Brachial a.

Brachialis m.

Lateral

Medial

Lateral
intermuscular
septum

Triceps m.

Posterior

Medial
intermuscular
septum

Figure 3-29   ANTERIOR AND POSTERIOR MUSCLES OF THE ARM. *Inset* is a cross-
section through the arm, showing the fascial compartments.
SEE ATLAS, FIGS. 3-21, 3-22, 3-27, 3-29

which originate from the scapula or the trunk. The *distal half* of the humerus, with a few exceptions, is primarily a site of *origin for muscles* extending more distally into the forearm (Figure 3-29).

MUSCLES OF THE ARM

The arm is divided by fascial septa into an anterior and posterior compartment. The **lateral** and **medial intermuscular septa** (see Figure 3-29) attach to the humerus and radiate medially and laterally to the skin, dividing the arm. The *median nerve* and *brachial vessels* lie in a fascial space between the two compartments, on the medial side of the arm. The *ulnar nerve* travels through the arm anterior to the medial-side fascia, be-

tween the brachialis and triceps. It then passes through the fascia to enter the posterior compartment and passes into the forearm posterior to the medical epicondyle. The *radial nerve* curves posteriorly around the humerus, from medial to lateral, and at the elbow passes anterior to the lateral humeral epicondyle. The *musculocutaneous nerve* lies in the anterior compartment between the brachialis and biceps muscles.

Anterior Compartment

The principal muscles in the anterior compartment (Table 3-6) are the biceps brachii, coracobrachialis, and brachialis. **Biceps brachii** originates from the coracoid process and the supraglenoid tubercle of the scapula. It

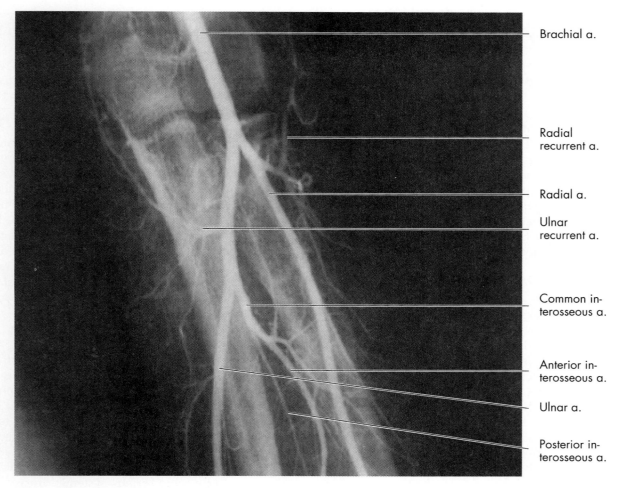

Brachial a.

Radial recurrent a.

Radial a.

Ulnar recurrent a.

Common interosseous a.

Anterior interosseous a.

Ulnar a.

Posterior interosseous a.

Figure 3-30 **BRACHIAL ARTERY ARTERIOGRAM.** An arteriogram is produced by injecting dye into a vessel as an x-ray is taken. Shown here is the bifurcation of the brachial artery into its radial and ulnar branches. (From Weir J, Abrahams PH: *An imaging atlas of human anatomy,* London, 1992, Mosby.) SEE ATLAS, FIG. 3-36

passes over both the shoulder and elbow joints and inserts on the radial tuberosity in the upper forearm. It is a major flexor of the elbow and an important supinator as well (see pp. 353-354). **Coracobrachialis** originates from the coracoid process and inserts along the middle half of the humerus on its medial side. It is a weak shoulder flexor and medial rotator of the arm. **Brachialis** originates on the distal half of the anterior humerus. It inserts on the anterior surface of the coronoid process of the proximal ulna. It is a powerful elbow flexor.

Several additional muscles pass through the anterior compartment. The **supraspinatus** tendon inserts most laterally, on the highest facet of the greater tubercle. The **pectoralis major** inserts on the humerus by an elongated aponeurosis along the lateral border of the intertubercular groove on the proximal third of the humerus. Just medial to this is the insertion of **latissimus dorsi,** on the floor of the intertubercular groove,

although the site of attachment is not broad as is that for pectoralis major. Medial to the insertion of latissimus dorsi is the insertion of **teres major** on the medial border of the intertubercular groove. Teres major originates on the posterior side of the scapula and forms part of the posterior axillary wall as it passes in a lateral direction. The tendon of **subscapularis** inserts squarely onto the lesser tubercle of the humerus. The **deltoid** originates from the lateral clavicle and scapular spine and terminates as a tendon with a broad insertion on the **deltoid tuberosity,** a roughened prominence about halfway down along the lateral margin of the humerus. Opposite the deltoid tuberosity, on the medial side of the shaft at midhumerus, is the site for insertion of the **coracobrachialis muscle.**

The distal half of the anterior surface of the humeral shaft is almost completely covered by the origin of the **brachialis muscle.** The **brachioradialis muscle** originates from the proximal half of the lateral supracondy-

THE ARM

DISTAL FRACTURES OF THE HUMERUS

Fractures near the distal end of the humerus, near the supracondylar ridges, produce a distal humeral fragment that can be displaced anteriorly or posteriorly with respect to the rest of the humerus. Especially when the displacement is posterior, the action of the brachialis and triceps muscles tends to pull the distal fragment superiorly, so that it rides over the edge of the proximal humeral segment. Any of the nerves (ulnar, radial, median) or branches of the brachial artery may be pinched between these moving fragments or stretched over them.

A COMMON MEANS OF MEASURING BLOOD PRESSURE

Blood pressure commonly is measured by encircling a body part, usually the arm, with an inflatable cuff and inflating it to the point that arterial flow downward into the arm is occluded. Then the pressure in the cuff is slowly released, while listening or feeling for a pulse in a vessel distal to the cuff (the brachial, radial, or ulnar artery). The brachial artery is palpated against the medial surface of the distal humerus, the radial artery just medial to the radial styloid process, and the ulnar artery just lateral to the pisiform bone and the tendon of flexor carpi ulnaris at the wrist. The first point at which the pulse can be felt or heard again (as the pressure in the cuff is released) is the systolic pressure. As the pressure is released even further, the point at which the pulse can no longer be heard with the stethoscope is the diastolic pressure.

A COMMON SITE FOR SAMPLING BLOOD

Sampling of blood is commonly performed by taking blood from one of the veins in the anterior forearm, usually the **median antecubital vein** or the **basilic vein** (see Figure 3-45). A tourniquet is placed over the arm *above* the intended site of blood sampling (i.e., proximal to the intended site). This forces blood to accumulate in and distend the veins distal to the tourniquet (including the vessels listed previously). Once the vessel has been successfully entered and the blood flow established, the tourniquet should be loosened, so that when the needle is removed the vein will not bleed excessively.

PATHOLOGIC FRACTURES

When a patient appears before you with a definite fracture, and a thorough history does not explain how the fracture might have occurred, you should consider the possibility of a pathologic fracture. These fractures suggest some weakness in the bone itself, so that ordinary forces are sufficient to cause a fracture. Bone cancers often present this way, when what seems to be a common fracture of a long bone proves to be the signal of a more serious systemic disease. Prolonged use of medications that lower bone density can also produce pathologic fractures.

---

lar ridge, while **extensor carpi radialis longus** originates from the distal half of the lateral supracondylar ridge. Still further distally, on the lateral epicondyle itself, is the origin for several more of the forearm extensor muscles (**"common extensor origin"**). To the medial epicondyle attaches the humeral head of the **pronator teres.** The medial epicondyle is the **common flexor origin** for many of the anterior forearm muscles. A more complete description of the forearm flexor and extensor muscles is found on pp. 356-363.

Posterior Compartment

In the posterior compartment, the major muscle group is the **triceps brachii** (see Figure 3-29). The triceps consists of three heads. The *lateral head* originates from a narrow raised diagonal ridge above the musculospiral groove on the upper third of the posterior humeral shaft. The *medial head* originates from a broad area extending from just distal to this diagonal groove to a point just proximal to the two humeral epicondyles. The *long head* originates from the infraglenoid tubercle. The posterior compartment also receives the **infraspinatus** and **teres minor** muscles, both of which insert on the greater tubercle.

BRACHIAL VESSELS

Distal to the inferolateral border of teres major, the axillary artery becomes the **brachial artery.** In the proximal part of the arm it lies medial to the humerus, anterior to brachialis, but in the distal humerus it lies anteriorly, between the two epicondyles. The median nerve lies lateral to the brachial artery high in the arm, but at midhumerus the nerve crosses anterior to the brachial artery, and distal to this the median nerve is medial to the brachial artery. Throughout its course the artery lies near the humerus, and its pulse can be palpated by pressing it gently against the underlying bone. The most important branch of the brachial artery is the **deep brachial artery** or **profunda brachii.** It arises from the proximal brachial artery, passes posterior between the long and medial heads of the triceps in the triangular interval, and joins the radial nerve in the **spiral groove** of the humerus, deep to the lateral head of triceps. From its medial side, the brachial artery also gives off the **superior** and **inferior ulnar collateral arteries** (see Figure 3-23), which anastomose with branches of the radial and ulnar arteries at the elbow.

As it crosses the cubital fossa at the elbow, the brachial artery remains superficial, covered only by the bicipital aponeurosis and the median cubital vein. The **cubital fossa** is a triangular depression with its base at the distal end of the humerus and the two sides formed by the pronator teres and the brachioradialis. In the upper forearm, the brachial artery deviates toward the "apex" of the cubital fossa, and finally 3 to 4 cm below the elbow it terminates by dividing into the **radial** and **ulnar arteries** (Figure 3-30).

The brachial artery is accompanied by a **brachial vein** or **vena comitantes,** deep in the arm, but the larger veins of the arm are actually those found in the superficial tissues, the cephalic vein and the basilic vein. The **cephalic vein** travels in the superficial tissues along the lateral margin of the arm and penetrates the clavipectoral fascia to drain into the axillary vein just distal to the clavicle (see Figures 3-18 and 3-45). The **basilic vein** travels in the superficial tissues on the medial side of the arm. Less than halfway up the arm it penetrates the superficial fascia and assumes a position medial to the brachial artery. The smaller brachial vein actually joins the basilic vein to become the **axillary vein,** superior to the teres major muscle (Figure 3-18).

3.5

Forearm

▶ Radius

▶ Ulna

▶ Elbow Joint

▶ Radioulnar Joints

▶ Movements at the Radioulnar Joints

▶ Interosseous Membrane

▶ Muscles of the Forearm

▶ Blood Supply to the Forearm

▶ Venous Drainage of the Forearm

▶ Nerve Supply in the Forearm

*T*he forearm extends from the elbow to the wrist and is framed on two bones, the **radius** and the **ulna.** Most of the muscles in the forearm are intended to manipulate the wrist and digits. The wrist is positioned by these muscles for integrated function of the digits by extrinsic muscles of the forearm and intrinsic muscles of the hand. The location of the bellies of these muscles in the forearm, not in the hand itself, prevents the mass of these muscles from limiting the flexibility and mobility of the fingers. The forearm is capable of motion at three major joints: the **elbow joint,** the **radioulnar joints,** and the **wrist joint.**

RADIUS

The radius is an elongated cylindrical bone, lying on the lateral side of the forearm (see Figure 3-36). The proximal end of the bone forms a thick circular disk, the **radial head.** The head of the radius articulates with the **capitulum,** the more lateral of the two prominences on the distal end of the humerus, and the medial side of the radial head nestles into a shallow depression on the ulna, the **radial notch.** Just distal to the head of the radius is the constricted **radial neck** and about 2 cm distal to the head is the **radial tuberosity,** a rounded eminence on the anteromedial aspect of the radial shaft. The tendon of biceps brachii attaches here. The shaft of the radius is triangular in cross-section and broadens distally. On the medial side of the distal end of the radius is a short, shallow groove, the **ulnar**

notch, which takes part in the distal radioulnar joint, and serves as a site of attachment for the **triangular fibrocartilage** that separates the distal ulna from the carpal bones. On the lateral side of the distal radius is the **radial styloid process,** a bony prominence that projects further distally than the rest of the radius. The distal end of the radius presents a flattened ovoid surface to the carpal bones, with two of which (the scaphoid and lunate) the radius articulates.

ULNA

The ulna lies in a medial position in the forearm. It has a large, expanded upper end, which is most important in the articulation with the humerus at the elbow joint (see following). The most prominent feature of the ulna is a large curved C-shaped process, concave anteriorly, known as the **trochlear notch.** The curved projection of bone forming the superior part of the trochlear notch is the **olecranon.** In full elbow extension, the olecranon fits into the **olecranon fossa** on the posterior surface of the humerus, and the trochlea of the humerus fits into the **trochlear notch** of the ulna. The lower lip of the trochlear notch is formed by a bony prominence, the **coronoid process.** Just lateral to it is a small concave depression, the **radial notch,** into which the head of the radius fits when the forearm bones are articulated. The **shaft of the ulna** is triangular in cross section and slightly narrowed just below the radial notch to accommodate movements of the radial tuberosity during pronation and supination. On the posteromedial aspect of the distal ulna is a small peglike prolongation, the **styloid process,** to which the ulnar collateral ligament of the wrist attaches. The distal end of the ulna is broadened and rounded (although less so than the radius) and articulates with the distal end of the radius. The ulna does not articulate directly with any of the carpal bones because it is separated from them by the **triangular fibrocartilage,** extending from the ulnar styloid process to the distal lip of the **ulnar notch** of the radius. The medial surface of the ulna lies just beneath the skin and is easily palpable, from the olecranon to the styloid process.

The adjacent sides of the ulna and radius are joined along most of their length by a strong **interosseous membrane** (see pp. 355-356 for a more complete description).

ELBOW JOINT

The elbow is a compound joint (Figure 3-31), comprising the (1) articulation of the **trochlea** of the humerus with the **trochlear notch** of the ulna and (2) the articulation of the **capitulum** of the humerus with the superior surface of the **radial head** (Figure 3-32).*

These two articulations are enclosed in a single synovial membrane, reinforced outwardly by an *articular capsule* and by *radial collateral* and *ulnar collateral ligaments.* The elbow joint functions as a hinge, with its transverse axis lying slightly inferior to the line connecting the two epicondyles of the humerus. There is little or no rotary movement in the elbow joint. *Extension* of the elbow (i.e., "straightening" the elbow) is limited by the olecranon of the ulna as it contacts the olecranon fossa of the humerus; *flexion* of the elbow (as in doing a "curl" in weightlifting) is limited only by the apposition of the muscle masses of the arm and forearm, and the bones themselves.

A **synovial membrane** lines the joint cavity, and just external to it there is a moderately thick **joint capsule.** Between the synovial membrane and the capsule there are several consistent **fat pads,** especially over the olecranon fossa posteriorly and the coronoid fossa anteriorly. The joint is further strengthened by ligaments (Figure 3-33). The **medial (ulnar) collateral ligament** extends from the medial epicondyle of the humerus to the coronoid process and olecranon of the ulna. The **lat-**

*Some include the proximal radioulnar joint as part of the elbow.

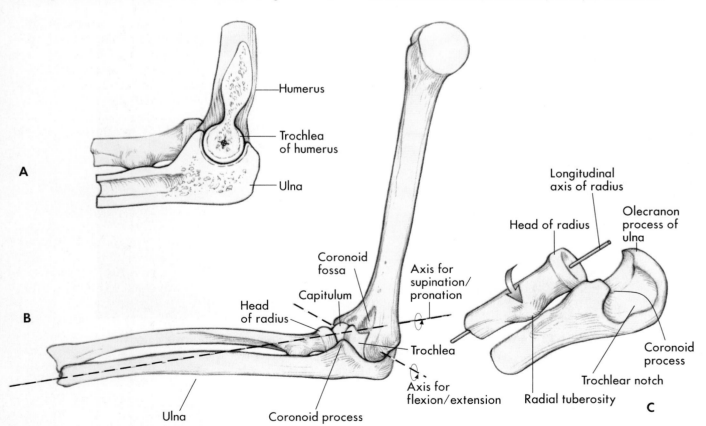

Figure 3-31 MOVEMENTS AT THE ELBOW. A, Longitudinal section. **B,** Medial view. **C,** Detailed anteromedial view of proximal ulna and radius.

SEE ATLAS, FIGS. 3-98, 3-99, 3-100, 3-101

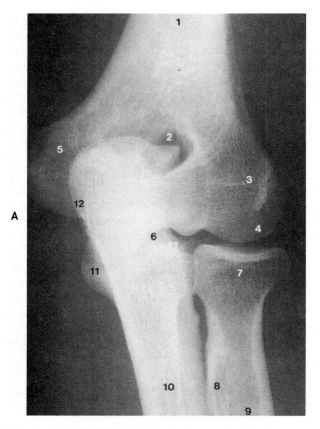

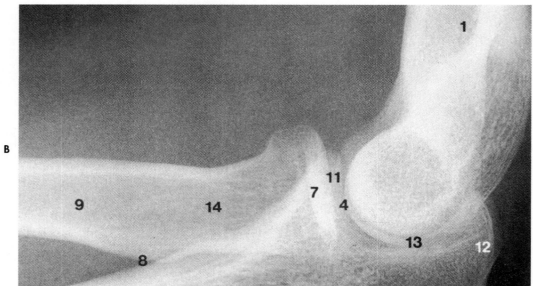

Figure 3-32   RADIOGRAPHS OF THE ELBOW JOINT. Shown here are two x-ray views of the elbow, an anteroposterior view (**A**) and a lateral view (**B**). (From Weir J, Abrahams PH: *An imaging atlas of human anatomy,* London, 1992, Mosby.)

1 Humerus	**5** Medial epicondyle	**10** Ulna
2 Olecranon fossa	**6** Trochlea	**11** Coronoid process of ulna
3 Lateral epicondyle of	**7** Head of radius	**12** Olecranon
humerus	**8** Tuberosity of radius	**13** Trochlear notch
4 Capitulum	**9** Radius	**14** Neck of radius

THE FOREARM

TRANSMISSION OF FORCE IN THE FOREARM

The radius represents more direct continuity with the hand, distally, while the ulna represents a continuation of the humerus proximally and has less to do with direct transmission of force from the hand. When a patient has fallen on the ground and braced the fall with the hands, a strong force is transmitted upward into the radius. As a result of this arrangement, forceful falls onto the outstretched hands are much more likely to cause fracture of the radius than of the ulna. Via the **interosseous membrane,** force applied to the hand is transmitted to the ulna and thence to the arm and shoulder.

FRACTURES OF THE RADIUS

The sequelae of a radial fracture depend to a large degree on the location of the fracture. If it is *distal to the insertion of the pronator teres,* then the pronator muscle tends to "pronate" the now-loosened proximal fragment, moving it medially and rotating it although biceps and supinator oppose this). The distal fragment of the radius is usually pulled toward the ulna by the pronator quadratus.

When the fracture is *proximal to the insertion of the pronator teres* but distal to the insertion of the biceps and supinator, the proximal fragment is forcefully supinated by the unopposed action of the biceps and supinator. The distal fragment is forcefully pronated due to the unopposed action of the two pronator muscles.

FRACTURES OF THE ULNA

The ulna is vulnerable to fracture because its posteromedial border is so close to the surface of the forearm (although its posteromedial position tends to reduce the number of direct blows to this part of the upper limb).

FRACTURE OF BOTH THE RADIUS AND ULNA

Usually as a result of a fall on outstretched arms, a person may simultaneously fracture both the styloid process of the ulna and the distal radius. The result of this fracture is that the radius and ulna lie side-by-side, instead of the usual arrangement where the radius extends further distally than does the ulna. This type of injury is known as a **Colles' fracture.**

COMPRESSION OF THE MAJOR FOREARM NERVES

Nerve compressions in the forearm can occur wherever a nerve passes through a confined space. Most often this results from **muscular hypertrophy** (the result of repeated muscle efforts on the job or as a result of weightlifting). At the elbow, the median nerve passes between the two heads of pronator teres and again is vulnerable to compression as it passes between the ulnar and radial heads of the flexor digitorum superficialis, the ulnar nerve between the two heads of the flexor carpi ulnaris, and the radial nerve through the supinator.

COMPARTMENT SYNDROMES IN THE FOREARM

When there is bleeding within one of the compartments of the forearm (the anterior/flexor or the posterior/extensor), structures within that compartment may be impaired by the rising pressure. Thus, if there is a forceful blow to the anterior surface of the forearm producing a tear in the radial artery and if the fascial septae, which define the flexor compartment are still intact, then the hemorrhaging into the flexor compartment ultimately will compress the median and/or ulnar nerves.

---

eral **(radial) collateral ligament** extends from the lateral epicondyle to the annular ligament on the head of the radius. The capsule of the elbow joint blends with the upper margin of the **annular ligament** (see Figure 3-33), a structure involved with reinforcement of the proximal radioulnar joint (see next section). There is typically a large **olecranon bursa** (an isolated synovium-lined flattened sac of clear fluid) between the olecranon process and the skin, which dissipates the pressure produced when one leans on the elbows.

In full extension of the elbow, the forearm and arm are not exactly aligned. It is normal for the forearm to deviate laterally some 12 to 15 degrees from the long axis of the arm as the elbow moves from a flexed to a fully extended position (the **"carrying angle"** of the forearm). This disparity is the result of the fact that (1) the trochlea of the humerus does not form a precise "fit" into the olecranon fossa of the ulna and (2) the medial edge of the trochlea extends further distally than does the lateral edge of the trochlea, meaning that the

THE ELBOW

DISLOCATION OF THE ELBOW

Dislocation of the elbow joint occurs when the proximal end of the ulna (the olecranon) becomes disarticulated from the trochlea of the humerus. The olecranon then may slide along the posterior surface of the humerus, and the coronoid process of the ulna may "lock" itself into the olecranon fossa on the posterior surface of the humerus. When this occurs, it is difficult to reduce the dislocation (that is, return the bones to their proper relationship), and open reduction (surgery) may be necessary.

"TENNIS ELBOW" OR LATERAL EPICONDYLITIS

"Tennis elbow" is a painful irritation of the lateral epicondyle of the humerus at the site of the common extensor muscle attachment. This condition is called "tennis elbow" because it may be precipitated by repeated supination/extension of the forearm, as in hitting the backhand shot in tennis. It is not restricted to athletics, however; a repeated motion such as tightening wood screws with the right arm will produce the same condition.

OLECRANON BURSITIS AT THE ELBOW

When pressure is applied to the back of the elbow joint, as in leaning forward on the elbows for a prolonged period, the bursal sac between the olecranon process and the skin can become irritated, filled with fluid, and give a distinctly swollen appearance to the back of the elbow. Less often, with repeated flexion-extension of the elbow joint (as when doing weightlifting "curls" repeatedly), a deeper olecra-non bursa, between the posterior humerus and the ulna, may also become inflamed, swollen, and painful.

DISLOCATION OF THE RADIAL HEAD

When a strong pull is applied to the forearm while it is held in the extended and supinated position, the head of the radius is likely to slide past or rupture the annular ligament, which surrounds it in its articulation with the capitulum of the humerus. It is usually dislocated from its normal position in the proximal radioulnar joint as well. This dislocation is the commonest upper limb dislocation in children but occurs less often in adults. This is probably due to the fact that in the child the head of the radius is not fully ossified and, therefore, more deformable and able to slip under the annular ligament and out of the articular fossa on the side of the ulna.

AVULSION FRACTURES AT THE ELBOW

The medial epicondyle of the humerus is the common origin for the superficial flexor muscles of the forearm, while the lateral epicondyle is a similar common origin for the superficial extensor muscles of the forearm. In both places the force of muscle contraction can be so great that small chips of bone are actually pulled away from the epicondyle—an **avulsion fracture.** They appear as small irregularly shaped fragments adjacent to the condyle itself. The other most common fractures around the elbow are (1) a fracture of the capitulum and (2) a fracture of the radial head at the level of its epiphyseal plate.

---

ulna comes to rest at an angle lateral to the long axis of the humerus. The carrying angle is characteristically increased in Turner syndrome, an "XO" chromosome disorder.

RADIOULNAR JOINTS

Separate from the elbow joint, the radius and ulna articulate with each other at two distinct joints, the **proximal** and **distal radioulnar joints.** At these joints, and not at the elbow or wrist joints, supination and pronation take place. These movements are unique to the forearm. At rest, in *supination,* the radius and ulna are parallel to each other, and the palm of the hand faces anteriorly. *Pronation* occurs when the radial side of the forearm (i.e., the lateral side), moves anteriorly and medially, in effect "rolling" in front of the ulna, causing the palm of the hand to face posteriorly or downward (see Figure 3-35). When pronation is complete, the distal end of the radius has moved from a position lateral to the distal ulna (where it is at rest, in supination) to a position medial to the distal ulna.

The **proximal radioulnar joint** (Figure 3-34) is the articulation of the medial side of the radial head into an ovoid depression, the **radial notch,** on the lateral side of the coronoid process of the ulna. The radial notch shares part of its border with the trochlear notch. The **annular ligament,** a semicircular ligament surrounding the head of the radius, stabilizes the articulation of the radial head with the radial notch of the ulna. Movement in the proximal radioulnar joint is part of pronation-supination and is described following (pp. 353-354).

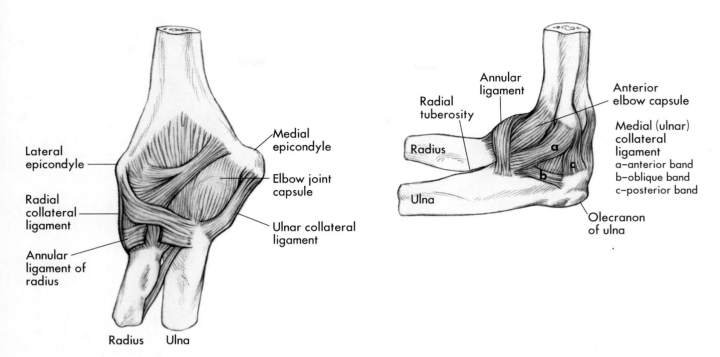

Figure 3-33 LIGAMENTS OF THE ELBOW JOINT. Anteroposterior and lateral views.
See Atlas, Fig. 3-102

The **distal radioulnar joint** (see Figure 3-34) is formed by the distal head of the ulna and the ulnar notch on the medial side of the distal end of the radius. The interior of the joint is lined by a synovial membrane, and a typical *joint capsule* surrounds it. Movement at the distal radioulnar joint is part of pronation-supination and is described following (p. 354). The distal limit of the distal radioulnar joint is formed by a thick fibrocartilaginous **triangular fibrocartilage** (also known as the **triangular articular disk**). This disk attaches medially to the lateral side of the ulnar **styloid process** and laterally to the rim of the **ulnar notch** on the radius, just adjacent to the border of the larger radiocarpal joint surface (see following). No true "ulnocarpal" joint exists because this disk separates the carpal bones from the distal end of the ulna.

MOVEMENTS AT THE RADIOULNAR JOINTS

Pronation and supination are complex movements (Figure 3-35) occurring simultaneously around an axis best described as an imaginary line between the head of the radius proximally and the medial end of the triangular articular disk distally. In the proximal radioulnar joint, the head of the radius can rotate within the perimeter created by the annular ligament. At the distal radioulnar joint, the ulna remains nearly stationary, as the distal radius and the articular disk move through an arc anterior to the distal end of the ulna. This means that as pronation/supination take place, the thumb side of the wrist and hand are permitted to move through a wider arc than is the fifth finger side of the hand. This makes possible the greatest degree of mobility for the thumb. In addition to pronation/supination, a negligible degree of forward and backward sliding of the ulna and radius can occur at both the distal and proximal radioulnar joints.

The main value of pronation/supination is to provide a wide range of motion for the palm of the hand—that is, to maximize the range of directions in which the palm of the hand may face. Supination would seem to be the more significant movement of the two, since actions like bringing food to the mouth and picking up objects to bringing them closer to the eyes for examination are primarily movements of supination. Pronation and supination alone (that is, involving only the proximal and distal radioulnar joints) can result in a change in position of the palm of the hand through an arc of about 180 degrees. Movements of other joints in the upper limb can add to the degree of supination and pronation possible. For example, if the elbow is extended, the humerus is allowed to rotate around its long axis, and the shoulder girdle is pulled anteriorly, the total arc through which the palm of the hand may move increases to greater than 350 degrees. You can verify this by holding your straightened upper limb out in front of you, palm up, and rotating your entire upper limb medially. At the extreme of this medial rotation, the palm nearly achieves its original position (facing upward), using not only the mobility of the radioulnar joint but also that of the shoulder joint and even the shoulder girdle.

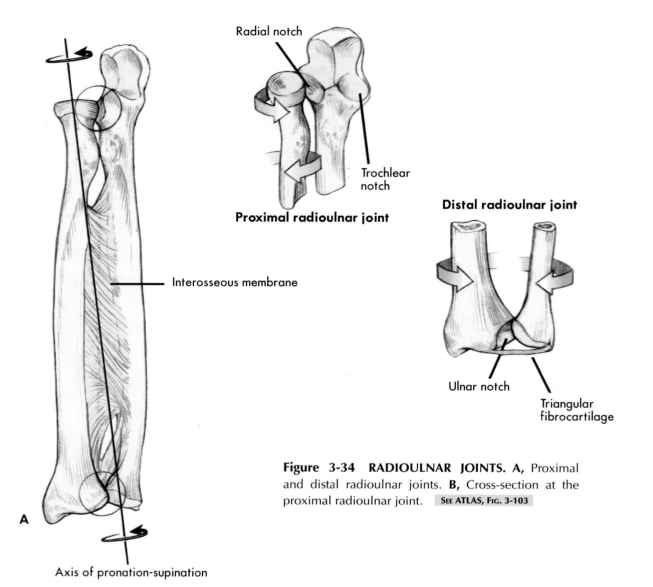

Radial notch

Trochlear notch

Proximal radioulnar joint

Distal radioulnar joint

Interosseous membrane

Ulnar notch

Triangular fibrocartilage

Figure 3-34 RADIOULNAR JOINTS. A, Proximal and distal radioulnar joints. **B,** Cross-section at the proximal radioulnar joint. SEE ATLAS, FIG. 3-103

Axis of pronation-supination

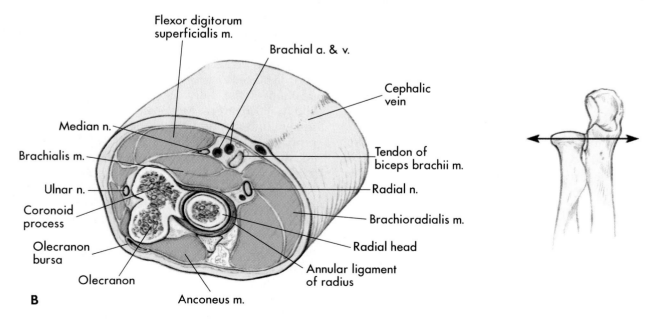

Flexor digitorum superficialis m.

Brachial a. & v.

Cephalic vein

Median n.

Brachialis m.

Tendon of biceps brachii m.

Ulnar n.

Radial n.

Coronoid process

Brachioradialis m.

Olecranon bursa

Radial head

Olecranon

Annular ligament of radius

Anconeus m.

B

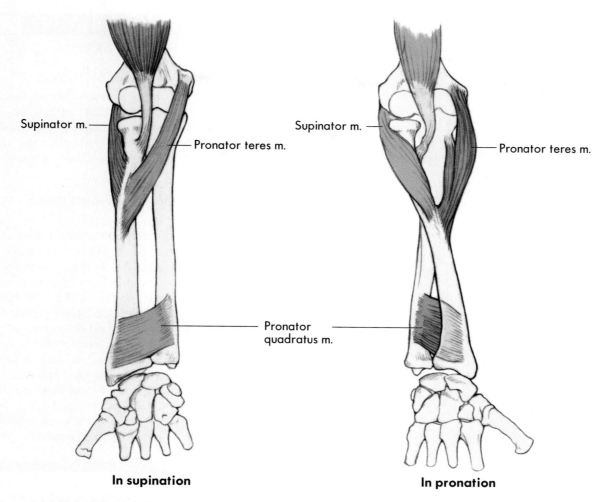

Supinator m.

Pronator teres m.

Supinator m.

Pronator teres m.

Pronator
quadratus m.

In supination

In pronation

Figure 3-35   MUSCLES MEDIATING PRONATION AND SUPINATION. When the elbow is extended, the supinator is the prime supinating muscle, but, with the elbow flexed, the biceps brachii becomes the most important supinating muscle. Note how pronator teres and supinator appear to be antagonists, as judged by their relative position and insertion on the radius.   SEE ATLAS, FIG. 3-33

INTEROSSEOUS MEMBRANE

Along a considerable distance, the adjacent sides of the radius and ulna are linked to each other by a flat, tough **interosseous membrane,** attached along most of the adjacent borders of the radius and ulna (Figure 3-36). The upper margin of the interosseous membrane lies about 2 cm below the radial tuberosity. Beyond this upper margin, the membrane extends all the way distally to the ends of the two bones and is intact except for a small ovoid aperture at the distal end. The gap above the proximal end of the interosseous membrane allows the passage of the **posterior interosseous vessels** (branches of the common interosseous artery and vein, see p. 363 and Figure 3-30). The small distal aperture in the interosseous membrane permits passage of terminal parts of the **anterior interosseous vessels** to the posterior compartment of the forearm.

While providing considerable strength and stability between radius and ulna, the interosseous membrane nonetheless permits supination and pronation to occur. The collagenous fibers of the membrane are oriented in an inferomedial direction, descending as they travel from radius to ulna. Forces against the hand (e.g., falling on outstretched forearms and hands) are transmitted primarily to the radius and then are transferred to the ulna through the interosseous membrane. The interosseous membrane also increases the surfaces for attachment of muscles in both the anterior and posterior compartments of the forearm.

MUSCLES OF THE FOREARM

Muscles found in the forearm have a variety of attachments. They are found in two large groupings, the

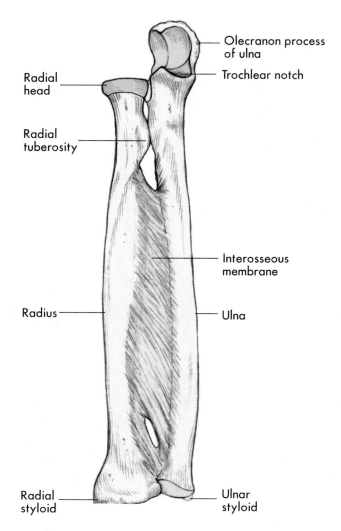

Figure 3-36   INTEROSSEOUS MEMBRANE.

THE FOREARM

AN EFFUSION IN THE ELBOW JOINT

When the elbow joint becomes inflamed, fluid accumulates in the joint cavity. This can be seen on x-rays of the elbow because the excess synovial fluid causes an elevation of the fat pads near the elbow joint, especially that over the olecranon fossa posteriorly.

SUPINATION/PRONATION AND DAILY ACTIVITIES

Right-handed carpenters may have a distinct advantage! The muscles for supination are more numerous and more powerful than those for pronation and placing screws into lumber (which involves supination) will be much easier for the right-hander than for a left-handed colleague. Motor-driven tools have probably eliminated this bit of vocational prejudice! Note also that turning a screwdriver is a good deal more difficult if the elbow is fully extended than if it is partly flexed, because the supinator force of the biceps muscle is greatly diminished in full extension. Thus reaching into a confined space (with full elbow extension) to turn a screw is more difficult than when the elbow can be held in partial flexion.

anterior and posterior forearm muscles. Several of the muscles actually originate from a part of the humerus and insert distally on the bones of the wrist or the hand (Figure 3-37). In such cases, these "forearm muscles" in fact do not attach to any of the bones in the forearm at all. Other muscles originate from the radius, ulna, and/or the interosseous membrane and insert distally on the forearm bones or the bones of the hand or wrist.

Anterior Forearm Muscles

In the superficial layer, all of the anterior muscles originate (Table 3-7), at least in part, from the medial epicondyle of the humerus (Figure 3-38). The most lateral of the muscles is the **pronator teres.** This muscle pulls the radius medially with respect to the ulna and is the major pronator muscle. It actually originates as two heads, one from the common flexor origin on the radial epicondyle of the humerus and the second from the medial side of the ulna about 2 cm below the lip of

the coronoid process. The two heads unite and course laterally across the forearm to insert along the anterior border of the middle third of the radius. The pronator teres forms the medial border of the cubital fossa of the elbow. The *median nerve,* which innervates the pronator teres, passes through a small proximal gap between the two heads of the muscle and enters the forearm. The median nerve may be compressed in this gap (see Figure 3-47).

The **flexor carpi radialis** lies just medial to pronator teres. It originates from the medial epicondyle of the humerus, narrows to a tendon about halfway down the forearm, and passes through the lateral wall of the **flexor retinaculum** in a small tunnel separate from the carpal tunnel (a bony ligamentous passage at the wrist through which all other extrinsic flexors of the digits and the median nerve pass, see pp. 370-372). Flexor carpi radialis inserts distally on the bases of the second and third metacarpal bones. Lying medial to flexor carpi radialis is **palmaris longus,** a long slender tendon and small muscle, which originates from the medial epicondyle. Descending in the forearm, palmaris longus passes anterior to the flexor retinaculum (i.e., it does not traverse the carpal tunnel) to insert distally in the **palmar fascia,** a strong plate of connective tissue

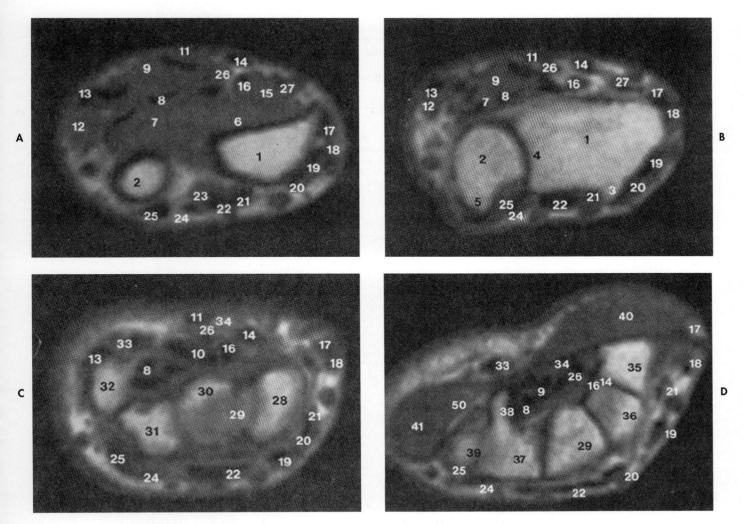

Figure 3-37 MRI STUDIES OF THE FOREARM. Shown here are four MRI transverse sections, moving from proximal to distal, through the forearm and wrist. **A,** Mid-forearm. **B,** Distal radioulnar joint. **C,** Proximal carpal row. **D,** Distal carpal row. (From Weir J, Abrahams PH: *An imaging atlas of human anatomy,* London, 1992, Mosby.)

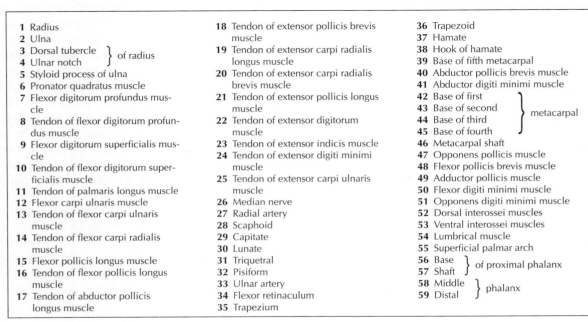

1 Radius
2 Ulna
3 Dorsal tubercle ⎫ of radius
4 Ulnar notch ⎭
5 Styloid process of ulna
6 Pronator quadratus muscle
7 Flexor digitorum profundus muscle
8 Tendon of flexor digitorum profundus muscle
9 Flexor digitorum superficialis muscle
10 Tendon of flexor digitorum superficialis muscle
11 Tendon of palmaris longus muscle
12 Flexor carpi ulnaris muscle
13 Tendon of flexor carpi ulnaris muscle
14 Tendon of flexor carpi radialis muscle
15 Flexor pollicis longus muscle
16 Tendon of flexor pollicis longus muscle
17 Tendon of abductor pollicis longus muscle

18 Tendon of extensor pollicis brevis muscle
19 Tendon of extensor carpi radialis longus muscle
20 Tendon of extensor carpi radialis brevis muscle
21 Tendon of extensor pollicis longus muscle
22 Tendon of extensor digitorum muscle
23 Tendon of extensor indicis muscle
24 Tendon of extensor digiti minimi muscle
25 Tendon of extensor carpi ulnaris muscle
26 Median nerve
27 Radial artery
28 Scaphoid
29 Capitate
30 Lunate
31 Triquetral
32 Pisiform
33 Ulnar artery
34 Flexor retinaculum
35 Trapezium

36 Trapezoid
37 Hamate
38 Hook of hamate
39 Base of fifth metacarpal
40 Abductor pollicis brevis muscle
41 Abductor digiti minimi muscle
42 Base of first ⎫
43 Base of second ⎬ metacarpal
44 Base of third ⎪
45 Base of fourth ⎭
46 Metacarpal shaft
47 Opponens pollicis muscle
48 Flexor pollicis brevis muscle
49 Adductor pollicis muscle
50 Flexor digiti minimi muscle
51 Opponens digiti minimi muscle
52 Dorsal interossei muscles
53 Ventral interossei muscles
54 Lumbrical muscle
55 Superficial palmar arch
56 Base ⎫ of proximal phalanx
57 Shaft ⎭
58 Middle ⎫ phalanx
59 Distal ⎭

Table 3-7   Individual Forearm Flexor Muscles

Muscle	Origin(s)	Insertion(s)	Nerve	Action(s)
SUPERFICIAL LAYER				
Pronator teres	Medial epicondyle of humerus and small ulnar head	Middle third of radius	Median (C6 and C7)	Pronation of forearm
Flexor carpi radialis	Medial epicondyle	Base of the second and third metacarpal	Median (C6 and C7)	Flexion of wrist, abduction of wrist
Palmaris longus	Medial epicondyle	Palmar fascia	Median (C7 and C8)	Flexion of wrist, tension on palmar fascia, and supplemental thumb abduction
Flexor carpi ulnaris	Medial epicondyle and ulna (two heads)	Pisiform, hamate, and to base of metacarpal fifth	Ulnar (C7 and C8)	Flexion wrist, adduction of wrist (ulnar deviation)
MIDDLE LAYER				
Flexor digitorum superficialis	Medial epicondyle, ulna, and oblique line of radius	Middle phalanx of digits two to five	Median (C7, C8, T1)	Flexes middle phalanx of digits two to five (rest of hand/wrist)
DEEP LAYER				
Flexor digitorum profundus	Ulna and interosseous membrane	Distal phalanx of digits two to five	Median (digits two to three) and ulnar (digits four to five); (C8, T1)	Flexes distal phalanx of digits two to five (hand and other phalanges also)
Flexor pollicis longus	Upper radius and interosseous membrane	Distal phalanx of thumb	Median (C8 to T1)	Flexes distal phalanx of thumb (also other phalanges and wrist)
Pronator quadratus	Distal ulna	Distal radius	Median (C8 to T1)	Pronates the forearm

covering the palm. Palmaris longus is absent on one or both sides in as many as 15% of individuals. **Flexor carpi ulnaris** is the most medial of the superficial muscles. It originates from two heads, one from the humerial medial epicondyle and the other from the humeral upper half of the posterior subcutaneous border of the ulna, distal to the olecranon process. Its distal half is mostly tendinous, and it inserts on the pisiform bone of the wrist and, by ligaments, to the hamate and fifth metacarpal bones as well.

In the middle plane, **flexor digitorum superficialis** is just medial to the palmaris longus and lies in a slightly deeper plane than the superficial flexor muscles (Figure 3-39). This muscle has multiple origins, from the medial epicondyle, from the ulna just inferior to the coronoid process, and laterally from a narrow strip on the radius inferior to the radial tuberosity. The median nerve passes between these medial and lateral origins to adopt a position deep to the flexor digitorum superficialis. Near the wrist the median nerve emerges along the lateral border of the muscle and becomes more superficial. The four tendons of the muscle are destined for the middle phalanges of digits two to five. Distally, as they pass through the carpal tunnel, the tendons for digits three

and four are superficial to those for digits two and five.

The deep plane of forearm flexor muscles consists of flexor digitorum profundus, flexor pollicis longus, and pronator quadratus (Figure 3-40). None of the deep muscles has an origin on the medial epicondyle of the humerus. Instead, they originate from various parts of the ulna, radius, and from the interosseous membrane that tethers the two bones. **Flexor digitorum profundus** arises from the upper two thirds of the anterior surface of the ulna and the middle half of the interosseous membrane adjacent to the ulna. The upper border of its origin on the ulna is in the shape of a U, which partially surrounds the insertion of the *brachialis muscle* on to the ulna. It travels down the forearm deep to the flexor digitorum superficialis, and, throughout most of the forearm, the median nerve is sandwiched between the superficial and deep flexor muscles. The four tendons of flexor digitorum profundus traverse the carpal tunnel deep to the tendons of flexor digitorum superficialis. In the hand, the four lumbrical muscles arise from the four tendons of the flexor digitorum profundus. The four tendons of flexor digitorum profundus insert onto the distal phalanges of digits two to five (see Figure 3-40).

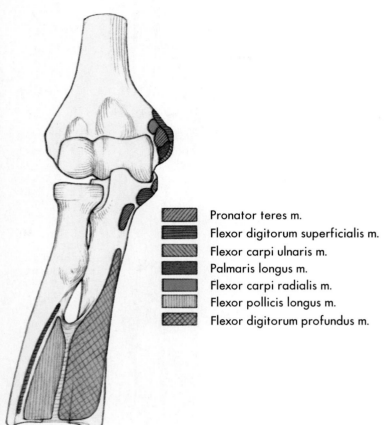

Pronator teres m.
Flexor digitorum superficialis m.
Flexor carpi ulnaris m.
Palmaris longus m.
Flexor carpi radialis m.
Flexor pollicis longus m.
Flexor digitorum profundus m.

Figure 3-38 PROXIMAL ATTACHMENTS OF THE ANTERIOR FOREARM MUSCLES, ANTERIOR VIEW. Shown here are the origins of the superficial and deep flexor muscles of the forearm.

The **flexor pollicis longus** muscle originates on the anterior radius from the radial tuberosity as far distally as the level of the pronator quadratus muscle (see following) and on the interosseous membrane adjacent to it. It narrows to a tendon in midhumerus and travels distally through the carpal tunnel in a lateral position. The tendon then travels deep to the opponens pollicis, lies in a groove between the two sesamoid bones anterior to the thumb M-P joint, and reaches the distal phalanx of the thumb, on which it inserts. The attachments of the long flexor tendons to the digits, in structures known as the fibrous flexor sheaths, are described on p. 389.

Pronator quadratus originates from a narrow oblique strip on the anterior surface of the ulna, about 5 to 7 cm from the distal end of the bone. The muscle is situated on the floor of the deep compartment of the forearm. It crosses transversely to insert on a broad rectangular plane covering the distal 5 to 6 cm of the radius.

Posterior Forearm Muscles

Of the 12 muscles in the posterior compartment of the forearm (Table 3-8), three are exceptional because they insert proximally, not at the level of the hand or wrist, as do the remaining nine muscles. The first of these three muscles, **anconeus,** originates from the pos-

terior surface of the lateral epicondyle and inserts on the upper fourth of the posterior surface of the ulna. It is active in extension. The **supinator** muscle arises from two overlapping heads, a superficial tendinous and a deep muscular one. The superficial head arises from the lateral epicondyle and the radial collateral ligament of the elbow. The deep head arises from the annular ligament of the radius and a small crest on the ulna. The supinator attaches to the lateral surface of the upper radius. The two heads are separated by the *posterior interosseous nerve* (the deep branch of the radial nerve). The supinator is of course involved in supination, although biceps brachii is the prime muscle for supination when the elbow is flexed.

Brachioradialis is the third exceptional muscle in the posterior forearm. It originates from the upper lateral supracondylar ridge of the humerus. The radial nerve passes between it and the brachialis muscle. The brachioradialis then courses downward, forming the lateral border of the forearm, and inserts on the lateral surface of the radius just proximal to the styloid process. It is an exceptional muscle because, although it is innervated by the radial nerve and lies in the posterior compartment, it is a *flexor* of the elbow joint.

The remaining nine posterior muscles of the forearm act as extensors of the wrist and/or digits. Each of these extensor muscles may be placed into one of two categories—the superficial and deep. Most of the **su-**

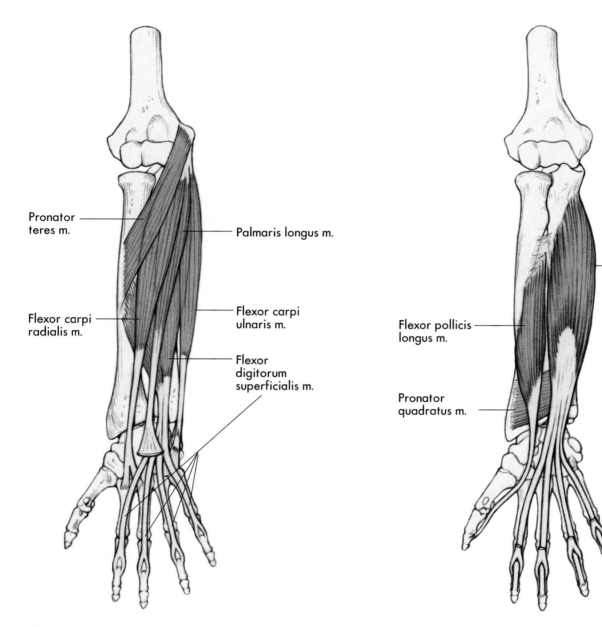

Figure 3-39   SUPERFICIAL FOREARM FLEXOR MUSCLES.
Anterior view.   SEE ATLAS, FIG. 3-30

Pronator teres m.

Palmaris longus m.

Flexor carpi radialis m.

Flexor carpi ulnaris m.

Flexor digitorum superficialis m.

Figure   3-40   DEEP   FOREARM   FLEXOR   MUSCLES.
Anterior view.   SEE ATLAS, FIGS. 3-32, 3-35

Flexor digitorum profundus m.

Flexor pollicis longus m.

Pronator quadratus m.

perficial muscles (Figure 3-41) originate from a **common extensor origin** (also referred to as the common extensor tendon) on the lateral epicondyle of the humerus, while most of the **deep muscles** (Figure 3-42) originate from specific regions on the ulna, radius, and interosseous membrane and not from the lateral epicondyle. As with the flexor muscles, the long extensor tendons pass deep to a rectangular retinaculum at the wrist. This **extensor retinaculum** attaches laterally to the distal radius and medially to the pisiform and hamate bones. It is divided into six separate compartments, each containing certain tendons, by fascial septae that extend downward and are anchored to the ulna or radius. This helps prevent the long exten-

sor tendons from "bowstringing" when the wrist is extended.

Brachioradialis (see Figure 3-41), described on p. 359, is positioned along the posterolateral border of the radius and is sometimes classified as a superficial extensor muscle. Moving medially, the next superficial posterior muscle is **extensor carpi radialis longus.** It arises on the lateral supracondylar ridge of the humerus, and, in the distal third of the forearm, it becomes a tendon. Descending the forearm, the tendon passes deep to the "outcropping" muscles of the thumb—abductor pollicis longus and extensor pollicis brevis—and then passes deep to the extensor retinaculum with the extensor carpi radialis brevis. It extends

Table 3-8   Individual Posterior Compartment Muscles

Muscle	Origin(s)	Insertion(s)	Nerve	Action(s)
SUPERFICIAL LAYER				
Extensor carpi radialis longus	Lateral supracondylar ridge	Base of second metacarpal	Radial (C6, C7)	Extends wrist
Extensor carpi radialis brevis	Lateral epicondyle of humerus	Bases of second and third metacarpals	Radial (C7 to C8)	Extends the wrist
Extensor digitorum	Lateral epicondyle of humerus	Extensor sheath, distal two phalanges of fingers two to five	Radial (C7 to C8)	Extends phalanges and wrist
Extensor digiti minimi	Lateral epicondyle of humerus	Extensor sheath	Deep radial (C7 to C8)	Extends digit five
Extensor carpi ulnaris	Lateral epicondyle and ulna	Base of fifth metacarpal	Deep radial (C7 to C8)	Extends/adducts wrist
Brachioradialis	Lateral supracondylar ridge	Just proximal to radial styloid process	Radial (C5, C6)	Flexes elbow (note "flexor" action of a posterior muscle)
DEEP LAYER				
Extensor indicis	Lower third of ulna and interosseous membrane	Extensor digitorum tendon	Deep radial (C7 to C8)	Extends, adducts second finger
Extensor pollicis longus	Middle third of ulna and interosseous membrane	Base of distal phalanx of thumb	Deep radial (C7 to C8)	Extends thumb
Extensor pollicis brevis	Radius and adjacent interosseous membrane	Base of proximal phalanx of thumb	Deep radial (C7 to C8)	Extends thumb
Abductor pollicis longus	Upper ulna and radius and interosseous membrane	Base of first metacarpal and trapezium	Deep radial (C7 to C8)	Abducts thumb and wrist
Anconeus	Lateral epicondyle of humerus	Olecranon and posterior ulna	Radial (C7 to C8)	Extends elbow
Supinator	Lateral epicondyle and small head from ulna	Radius (oblique line)	Deep radial (C6)	Supinates

further beyond the wrist to insert on the base of the second metacarpal bone. The tendon of extensor carpi radialis longus lies just lateral to the tubercle on the dorsum of the distal radius (Lister's tubercle). **Extensor carpi radialis brevis** originates on the lateral epicondyle of the humerus and travels down the forearm just medial to the extensor carpi radialis longus. In the forearm, it follows the same course as extensor carpi radialis longus and within the same compartment passes deep to the extensor retinaculum. Its tendon then inserts on the bases of the second and, to a lesser extent, the third metacarpal bones. **Extensor digitorum** originates from the lateral epicondyle and becomes a broad flat muscle coursing down the middle of the posterior forearm. It passes deep to the extensor retinaculum with the extensor indicis and divides into four tendons, destined for the **extensor sheaths** (see p. 390 for complete description) of digits two to five. Each tendon is linked to adjacent tendons by intertendinous connections, which tether the tendons to each other to limit lateral mobility. These attachments also limit independent actions of the tendons. **Extensor digiti minimi** originates on the lateral epicondyle and the common extensor origin and travels down the forearm just medial to extensor digitorum (to which it is often attached by a small muscular slip). It passes deep to the extensor retinaculum and usually splits into two tendons that end by attaching to the extensor sheath of the fifth digit. Lying most medial in the superficial group is **extensor carpi ulnaris,** arising from the lateral epicondyle and the posterior subcutaneous ulnar border. Distally, it passes beneath the extensor retinaculum between the head of the ulna and its styloid process and inserts on the base of the fifth metacarpal bone.

The deep group (see Figure 3-42) of posterior forearm muscles arises from areas on the proximal ulna, ra-

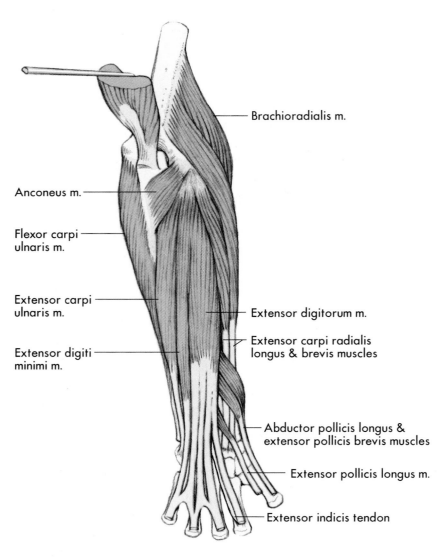

Brachioradialis m.

Anconeus m.

Flexor carpi
ulnaris m.

Extensor carpi
ulnaris m.

Extensor digiti
minimi m.

Extensor digitorum m.

Extensor carpi radialis
longus & brevis muscles

Abductor pollicis longus &
extensor pollicis brevis muscles

Extensor pollicis longus m.

Extensor indicis tendon

**Figure 3-41   SUPERFICIAL FOREARM EX-
TENSOR MUSCLES.** Posterior view.
SEE ATLAS, FIGS. 3-76, 3-77, 3-78

dius, and interosseous membrane. Many of the muscles are devoted to thumb movements, whereas none of the superficial extensors inserts on the thumb. **Supinator,** which arises from the lateral epicondyle, is described on p. 359. Most medial in the deep group is the **extensor indicis.** It arises from the posterior surface of the lower ulna and the adjacent interosseous membrane. Distally, as it attaches to the extensor sheath of the index finger, it blends with the index finger tendon of extensor digitorum. Just lateral to extensor indicis lies **extensor pollicis longus,** arising from the middle third of the posterior ulnar surface and the adjacent interosseous membrane. It travels under the extensor retinaculum just medial to a tubercle on the dorsal surface of the distal end of the radius (Lister's tubercle) and crosses superficial to the tendons of extensor carpi radialis longus and brevis on the posterior surface of the wrist. It then inserts on the base of the distal phalanx of the thumb. Extensor pollicis longus forms the medial border of the anatomic "snuff-box." The **anatomic "snuff-box"** is a triangular depression on the

dorsum of the hand at the base of the thumb. The lateral border of the snuff-box is formed by the tendons of extensor pollicis brevis and abductor pollicis longus (see following). Pulsations of the radial artery may be palpated in the floor of the snuff box.

Extensor pollicis brevis arises on the posterior surface of the radius and adjacent interosseous membrane, just lateral to extensor indicis. It descends along the lateral margin of the forearm, travels deep to the extensor retinaculum, and inserts on the base of the proximal phalanx of the thumb. The most lateral of the deep forearm extensors is **abductor pollicis longus.** Its origin is from the middle portion of the interosseous membrane, with small areas of the adjacent radius and ulna. It descends along the lateral margin of the forearm, passes beneath the extensor retinaculum with extensor pollicis brevis, and inserts on the base of the first metacarpal and the trapezium.

As the tendons of the long posterior forearm muscles pass across the dorsum of the wrist, they are grouped into specific compartments, each surrounded

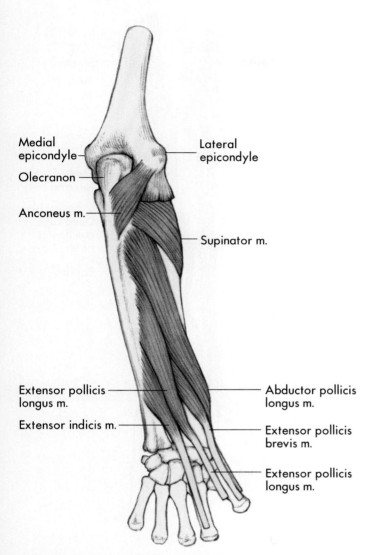

Medial epicondyle

Olecranon

Anconeus m.

Lateral epicondyle

Supinator m.

Extensor pollicis longus m.

Extensor indicis m.

Abductor pollicis longus m.

Extensor pollicis brevis m.

Extensor pollicis longus m.

Figure 3-42 DEEP FOREARM EXTENSOR MUSCLES. Posterior view. SEE ATLAS, FIGS. 3-79, 3-80

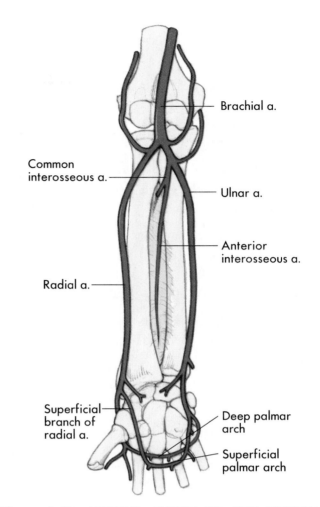

Brachial a.

Common interosseous a.

Ulnar a.

Anterior interosseous a.

Radial a.

Superficial branch of radial a.

Deep palmar arch

Superficial palmar arch

Figure 3-43 ARTERIAL SUPPLY TO THE FOREARM. Anterior view.

by fascia derived from the extensor retinaculum. These are described on p. 375 in Table 3-10.

BLOOD SUPPLY TO THE FOREARM

Arterial supply to the forearm depends entirely on branches of the brachial artery. After crossing the cubital fossa, the brachial artery divides into two branches, the radial and ulnar arteries, about 2 cm below the elbow (Figure 3-43).

The **radial artery** courses to the lateral side of the forearm and aligns itself with the radius. It lies deep to the brachioradialis muscle and emerges along its medial border in the distal half of the forearm to lie between brachioradialis and flexor carpi radialis tendons. Just proximal to the wrist, it lies on the radius where it is palpable. Near the wrist, the artery gives off a **superficial branch** which travels anterior to the surface of the flexor retinaculum to supply the thenar muscles (Figure

3-44) and then participates in the **superficial palmar arch.** Approaching the wrist, the **deep branch of the radial artery** deviates laterally and passes deep to the radial collateral ligament of the wrist. It then moves laterally along the surface of the scaphoid bone and lies in the floor of the anatomic "snuff box" (see p. 362). It then passes between the two heads of the first dorsal interosseous muscle to become the major contributor to the **deep palmar vascular arch.** The radial artery is most often the major blood supply to the thumb.

The **ulnar artery** also originates 1 to 2 cm below the elbow and moves medially deep to pronator teres and the other superficial forearm flexors. The ulnar artery is the larger of the two branches of the brachial artery. About 2 to 3 cm distal to its origin the ulnar artery gives off the **common interosseous artery,** which shortly divides into the **anterior and posterior interosseous arteries.** The latter artery arches over the upper margin of the interosseous membrane to reach the posterior compartment of the forearm. The anterior interosseous artery moves distally in the anterior forearm compartment, accompanied by the deep branch of the median nerve. The posterior interosseous artery also descends,

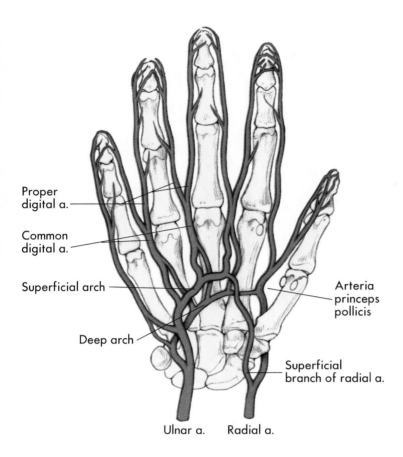

Proper
digital a.

Common
digital a.

Superficial arch

Deep arch

Arteria
princeps
pollicis

Superficial
branch of radial a.

Ulnar a.   Radial a.

Figure 3-44   ARTERIAL SUPPLY TO THE HAND. Anterior view.   See ATLAS, Figs. 3-57, 3-58, 3-59

but in the posterior forearm compartment, accompanied by the deep branch of the radial nerve.

As it descends toward the wrist, the ulnar artery lies deep to the flexor carpi ulnaris and is joined on its medial side by the ulnar nerve. Near the wrist, the ulnar artery and nerve pass superficial to the medial end of the flexor retinaculum (often partially embedded in it) and then pass just lateral to the pisiform bone. The main portion of the ulnar artery then continues distally into the hand and is the major source of the **superficial palmar arch** (see Figure 3-44). Along with the deep branch of the ulnar nerve, a **deep branch of the ulnar artery** then passes between abductor digiti minimi and flexor digiti minimi, between the heads of opponens digiti minimi, and contributes to the formation of the **deep palmar arch,** passing deep to the long flexor tendons (see Figure 3-44). Both of the vascular arches in the hand contribute to the formation of digital arteries, supplying the individual fingers (see pp. 391-392).

VENOUS DRAINAGE OF THE FOREARM

In the forearm, as in the arm, there is a set of **deep veins** accompanying the deep forearm arteries. These deep veins often occur as double or even triple groups of vessels, collectively representing the "vein," or **venae**

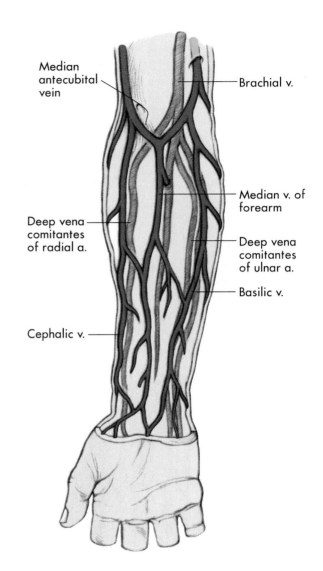

Median
antecubital
vein

Brachial v.

Median v. of
forearm

Deep vena
comitantes
of radial a.

Deep vena
comitantes
of ulnar a.

Basilic v.

Cephalic v.

Figure 3-45   SUPERFICIAL AND DEEP VEINS OF THE FOREARM. Anterior view.   See ATLAS, Figs. 3-8, 3-25

comitantes. There is also a set of **superficial veins,** lying in the superficial fascia, and not accompanying arteries (Figure 3-45). These two systems of veins anastomose at several points. The deep veins are the **ulnar** and **radial** and are named for the arteries they accompany.

The major superficial veins are the cephalic, basilic, and the median vein of the forearm. The **cephalic vein** originates on the dorsolateral aspect of the wrist and travels up the lateral margin of the forearm. The **basilic vein** arises near the base of the little finger and ascends along the medial border of the forearm. Between the two is the **median vein of the forearm,** which arises from a collection of small vessels in the palm of the hand. It ascends in the middle of the forearm and, just below the cubital fossa, courses to the medial side and joins the basilic vein. A **median antecubital vein,** lying just distal to the elbow, connects the cephalic vein with the basilic vein. The median cubital vein usually cross-

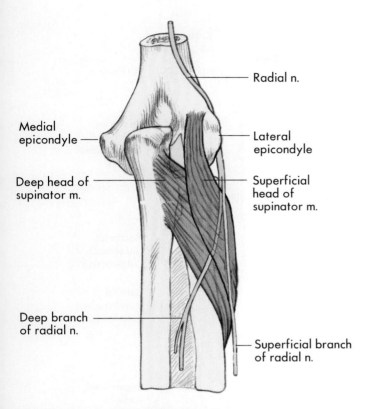

Figure 3-46   RADIAL NERVE AT THE ELBOW.
SEE ATLAS, FIGS. 3-82, 3-83

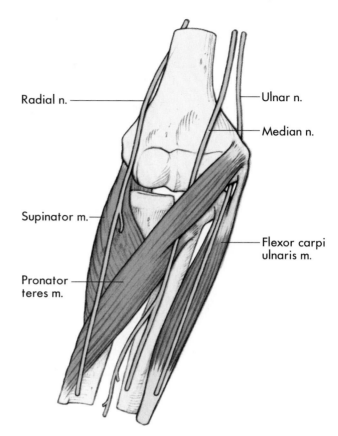

Figure 3-47   POTENTIAL SITES FOR COMPRESSION OF NERVES IN THE PROXIMAL FOREARM. Anterior view, right elbow.

PRINCIPLES ■

In many areas of the body, peripheral nerves pass through muscles, ligaments, bony spaces, or other narrow passages. When the narrowness of these passages is exacerbated, the result can be an impediment to the function of the nerve. In the forearm, all three major nerves (median, ulnar, and radial) pass through or between certain muscles of the forearm. When a patient exercises vigorously or repeatedly, the result may be pressure on the nerve and impairment of the nerve's function, affecting the distal forearm and hand. A similar process can occur in the anterior abdominal wall, where tight clothing can put pressure on the lateral femoral cutaneous nerve as it passes deep to the lateral end of the inguinal ligament, or in the middle ear cavity, where inflammation and irritation can impair the sense of taste mediated through the chorda tympani, a small nerve that traverses the middle ear cavity.

Cases such as these underscore the importance of taking a thorough patient history. In the first example, numbness, tingling, and muscle weakness experienced in the hand and distal forearm might be well described but unexplained until the careful physician learned that the patient had been doing some particularly stressful weight training over the past few days.

es the cubital fossa just superficial to the bicipital aponeurosis. It is often used for blood sampling.

NERVE SUPPLY IN THE FOREARM

The three major deep nerves of the forearm are the radial, median, and ulnar. The **radial nerve** lies anterior to the lateral epicondyle in the arm in its anterior compartment. It passes into the forearm beneath the brachioradialis muscle. As it does, it provides several direct branches to nearby muscles (anconeus, brachioradialis, extensor carpi radialis longus and brevis). It then divides into a superficial and deep branch. The **deep branch** passes between the two heads of supinator and emerges in the posterior compartment of the forearm, where it is known as the **posterior interosseous nerve** (Figures 3-46 and 3-47). This nerve supplies nearly all the muscles of the posterior forearm but has few cutaneous branches. It does not provide muscular or cutaneous innervation beyond the wrist. It dwindles in size as it descends the forearm, ending as a tiny thread over the dorsum of the wrist. The **superficial branch** of the radial nerve passes over the surface of the supinator muscle and descends through the forearm deep to the brachioradialis, lying lateral to the radial artery. It has

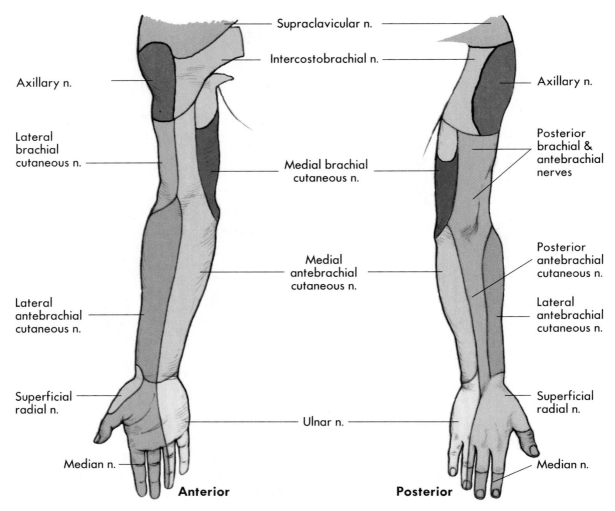

Supraclavicular n.

Intercostobrachial n.

Axillary n.

Axillary n.

Lateral brachial cutaneous n.

Posterior brachial & antebrachial nerves

Medial brachial cutaneous n.

Medial antebrachial cutaneous n.

Posterior antebrachial cutaneous n.

Lateral antebrachial cutaneous n.

Lateral antebrachial cutaneous n.

Superficial radial n.

Superficial radial n.

Ulnar n.

Median n.

Median n.

Anterior

Posterior

Figure 3-48   CUTANEOUS INNERVATION OF THE UPPER LIMB.
See Atlas, Figs. 3-5, 3-6, 3-85

no muscular and only a few cutaneous branches in the forearm but ends by providing cutaneous innervation of the dorsum of the wrist, hand, and the lateral 3½ digits (see Figure 3-48) (i.e., the thumb, index, and middle fingers, and the lateral side of the ring finger).

The **median nerve** (see Figure 3-46) enters the forearm by passing between the two heads of pronator teres and descends in the anterior compartment of the forearm, traveling between the flexor digitorum superficialis and flexor digitorum profundus muscles. In the forearm, the median nerve supplies branches to all of the anterior forearm flexors except flexor carpi ulnaris and the medial two slips of the flexor digitorum profundus. It provides a small cutaneous branch for the thenar eminence (see following). Near the wrist the median nerve becomes more superficial, emerging along the lateral border of the flexor digitorum superficialis muscle, where it is very vulnerable just proximal to the wrist. The median nerve is the most superficial structure in the carpal tunnel, deep to the flexor retinaculum. It generally lies between the tendons of the flexor

digitorum superficialis and the flexor carpi radialis. Just distal to the flexor retinaculum is a short, curved **recurrent branch,** arising on the lateral side of the nerve and arching over the medial border of flexor pollicis brevis. The recurrent branch supplies the superficial head of this muscle as well as the opponens pollicis and abductor pollicis brevis. Beyond this, the median nerve divides into three **common digital branches.** These nerves are responsible for cutaneous innervation of the lateral 3½ digits (the thumb, index, long, and lateral ½ of ring finger). Each common digital nerve divides into two **proper digital nerves,** each of which supplies the skin and subcutaneous tissues on one side of each digit. For example, a common digital nerve divides into two proper digital nerves, innervating the adjacent sides of the second and third digits.

At the elbow, the **ulnar nerve** lies in a groove on the posterior surface of the medial epicondyle of the humerus and travels between the two heads of the flexor carpi ulnaris to enter the forearm (see Figure 3-46). It descends through the forearm between the flexor carpi

THE NEUROVASCULAR SUPPLY TO THE FOREARM

VENOUS ACCESS IN THE FOREARM

The superficial veins in the anterior forearm are commonly used for collection of blood samples. Most frequently used is the median cubital (or antecubital) vein, which runs a diagonal course across the cubital fossa, linking the cephalic vein to the basilic vein. Ascending from the wrist toward the cubital fossa are three major superficial veins: (1) the **cephalic vein** on the lateral margin, (2) the **basilic vein** on the medial margin, and (3) the **median vein of the forearm** ascending up the midline of the anterior forearm.

In a small number of individuals, the ulnar artery passes anterior to the bicipital aponeurosis and descends in the forearm anterior to the flexor carpi ulnaris muscle. If this is so, then this artery may be mistaken for a vein (though its pulsations should indicate otherwise). The danger here is that a medication that results in vasoconstriction might be injected into this artery and jeopardize the blood flow to structures distal to the site of injection.

AN ALTERNATE SITE FOR ARTERIAL CANNULATION

The radial artery at the wrist is the most frequently employed site for arterial blood sampling. If the radial artery is not available, an attempt can be made to cannulate the brachial artery, lying on the medial side of the brachialis muscle in the distal arm and deep to the bicipital aponeurosis in the proximal forearm. There are two potential risks to using the brachial artery. First, since the radial and ulnar arteries both arise from the brachial artery, a failed attempt to cannulate the brachial artery could potentially obstruct flow of blood distally into the forearm and hand. Second, if there is substantial bleeding from the brachial artery after attempts to cannulate it, this blood can accumulate in the small space just deep to the bicipital aponeurosis, compressing the median nerve.

BRACHIORADIALIS REFLEX

In addition to the more familiar testing of reflexes at the elbow, the function of the C5 to C6 nerve roots can be assessed by eliciting the brachioradialis reflex. This is performed by holding the palm in a vertical position, holding the forearm parallel to the ground, and tapping gently on the distal radius with a rubber hammer. The brachioradialis muscle overlies the radius at this point, and the force of the hammer will cause a reflex contraction in the brachioradialis muscle (assuming the appropriate nerve segments—C5 and C6—are intact).

HIGH AND LOW LESIONS TO THE MEDIAN NERVE

If the median nerve is injured high in the forearm, the patient will experience sensory loss to the thenar region, muscle weakness on the lateral side of the hand, and substantial muscular weakness in the muscles on the anterior side of the forearm. A median nerve lesion low in the forearm will *not* involve the long flexor muscles since the fibers innervating those muscles will have left the median nerve more proximally in the forearm.

---

ulnaris and the flexor digitorum profundus. It lies just medial to the ulnar artery throughout most of the forearm. In the forearm, it provides branches for the flexor carpi ulnaris and the medial two or three slips of the flexor digitorum profundus. At the wrist, it passes superficial to the flexor retinaculum in a canal with the ulnar artery and enters the hand along the lateral border of the hypothenar muscles, deep to the palmaris brevis muscle (a small superficial muscle in the medial palm). Shortly after passing lateral to the pisiform bone, the ulnar nerve and the ulnar artery divide into deep and superficial branches. The **deep branch** of the nerve and artery pass lateral to the pisohamate ligament and lateral to the hook of the hamate bone, where they are palpable. The nerve then descends between the two heads of opponens digiti minimi muscle to reach the deep muscles of the palm. It innervates all of the intrinsic muscles of the hand, except the thenar muscles and the lateral two lumbrical muscles. The **superficial branch** of the ulnar nerve is described following.

The *cutaneous innervation of the forearm* is shared by branches of the radial, musculocutaneous, median, and ulnar nerves as well as direct branches of the brachial plexus (Figure 3-48). The radial nerve contributes the **posterior cutaneous nerve of the forearm,** arising above the elbow and coursing down the posterior aspect of the forearm. It provides cutaneous innervation of the distal third of the arm and most of the dorsal forearm. The **superficial branch of the radial nerve** descends through the forearm deep to the brachioradialis and then emerges proximal to the wrist to innervate the rest of the dorsal forearm skin and the skin on the lateral half of the dorsum of the hand extending as far as the middle phalanx of the thumb, index, long, and lateral half of ring fingers (see following). The **musculocutaneous nerve** lies in a lateral groove between brachialis and biceps in the distal arm. It then passes into the forearm and just below the elbow pierces the deep fascia to become the **lateral cutaneous nerve of the forearm.** It innervates the lateral half of the anterior surface of the forearm and a narrower strip on the lateral side of the posterior forearm. The medial half of both the anterior and posterior surface of the forearm is innervated by the **medial cutaneous nerve of the forearm,** a branch of the medial cord of the brachial plexus. It arises in the arm and travels along with the basilic vein.

The *anterior surface of the hand* is innervated by three nerves. The **superficial radial nerve** innervates a small crescent on the lateral edge of the thenar eminence plus the dorsolateral surface of the hand and the dorsal surface of the thumb, index, long, and lateral half of ring fingers as far distal as the distal interphalangeal joint. About 5 cm above the wrist is a **palmar cutaneous branch of the median nerve,** which deviates laterally and ramifies over the thenar eminence. In contrast, the main *median nerve* provides cutaneous innervation to the ventral surface of the thumb, index, long, and lateral half of ring fingers and the skin over the distal phalanx on the dorsal surface of those same digits. The skin over the hypothenar eminence, the ventral surface of the medial half of the hand, and the ventral surface of the little finger and medial half of the ring finger is innervated by the *ulnar nerve.* The dorsal skin on the medial part of the hand is innervated by the **dorsal branch of the ulnar nerve,** a branch that arises in midforearm and descends to the level of the hand.

Wrist

▶ Bones of the Wrist

▶ Radiocarpal Joint

▶ Flexor Retinaculum

▶ Extensor Retinaculum

▶ Anatomic "Snuff Box"

▶ Blood Vessels and Nerves of the Wrist

BONES OF THE WRIST

There are eight wrist or **carpal bones** (Figures 3-49 and 3-50), arranged in two roughly parallel rows, each row extending from lateral to medial (Table 3-9). Each of the carpal bones articulates with adjacent carpal bones by small *synovial joints,* and small individual *ligaments* unite adjacent bones (Figure 3-51). The **triquetrum, lunate,** and **scaphoid** are linked, on their anterior surfaces, to the distal end of the radius by the **palmar radiocarpal ligament.** The **scaphoid** and **lunate** bones lie most directly opposite the distal radius. The bones of the distal row form a relatively strong and rigid arch, with the **capitate** as the keystone. The second and third metacarpals and the carpal bones lying posterior to them form a relatively immobile or "fixed" unit of the hand, while the carpals, metacarpals, and digits to each side of this fixed unit are much more mobile. The wrist transmits force between the hand and forearm. The line of force (Figure 3-52) passes through the **capitate** bone of the distal carpal row, the **scaphoid** and **lunate** bones of the proximal carpal row, and onward proximally to the distal end of the radius. These carpal bones are the most likely to be fractured or dislocated in traumatic injury to the hand and wrist.

The **pisiform** is positioned atop the **triquetrum** and projects anterior to the plane of the other seven carpal bones. Some consider the pisiform to be a **sesamoid bone** (bones in various parts of the body, embedded in tendons and usually located in places where tendons are subjected to pressure and stress—e.g., the patella and sesamoid bones in the short flexor muscles of the foot and here at the wrist) in the tendon of flexor carpi ulnaris. The pisiform and the **hamulus** (or hook), an anterior extension of the **hamate bone,** form two processes projecting anterior to the plane of the wrist on the medial side. On the lateral side of the wrist, the tubercle of the trapezium and tubercle of the scaphoid bone project anterior to the plane of the wrist, the former lying distal to the latter. The **pisiform** and **hamulus** thus serve as the medial attachments for the flexor retinaculum, while the tubercles of **trapezium** and **scaphoid** serve as lateral attachments (see section on the flexor retinaculum, pp. 370-371).

With the wrist bones articulated to form an inverted arch and the flexor retinaculum in place, a **carpal tunnel** (see Figures 3-52 and 3-54) is created. The anterior surfaces of the carpals and their covering palmar radiocarpal ligament form the *posterior wall* or *floor* of the carpal tunnel, the pisiform and hamulus form the *medial wall,* and the tubercles of trapezium and scaphoid form the *lateral wall.* The *anterior wall* is formed by the flexor retinaculum. The long flexor tendons for the thumb and fingers and the median nerve traverse this narrow carpal tunnel and are vulnerable to injury by compression ("carpal tunnel syndrome"—see following discussion).

The medial and lateral aspects of the wrist joint (Figure 3-53, see also Figure 3-51) are reinforced by (1) a **lateral collateral ligament** (extending between the scaphoid bone and radial styloid process) and (2) a **medial collateral ligament** (connecting the triqetrum/pisiform and ulnar styloid process). What appear to be two individual ligaments of the pisiform bone, linking it to two distal structures—the **pisohamate ligament** and the **pisometacarpal ligament**—are in reality pro-

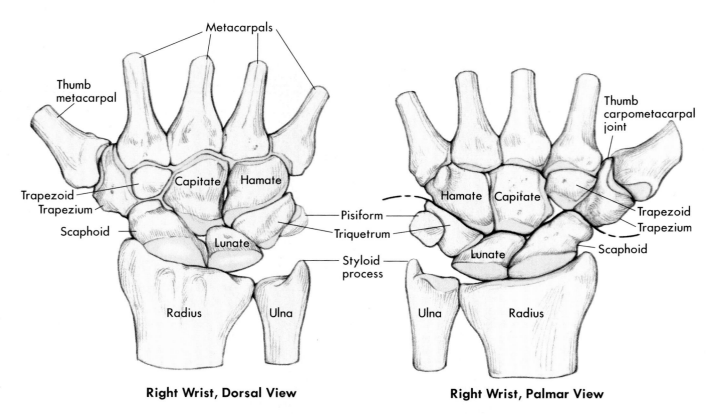

Right Wrist, Dorsal View   **Right Wrist, Palmar View**

Figure 3-49   CARPAL BONES. Dorsal and palmar views.   SEE ATLAS, FIGS. 3-40, 3-105

longations of the **flexor carpi ulnaris tendon,** with the pisiform acting as a sesamoid bone within the tendon. The **pisohamate ligament** is an important landmark for the deep branch of the ulnar nerve.

The wrist, acting as a unit, can flex and extend, important elements of the overall mobility of the hand. The tendon of *flexor carpi radialis* passes over the wrist anteriorly and inserts on the bases of metacarpals two and three, and *flexor carpi ulnaris* inserts on the fifth metacarpal, pisiform, and hamate bones. These two muscles aid in wrist flexion. Similarly, the *extensor carpi radialis longus* and *brevis* and the *extensor carpi ulnaris* pass over the dorsum of the wrist and insert on the bases of the same metacarpals two, three, and five. They are important in wrist extension.

The hand and wrist can also deviate medially or laterally, in the plane of the hand itself. These movements are referred to as *ulnar deviation (adduction)* and *radial deviation (abduction).* Ulnar deviation is produced by the flexor and extensor carpi ulnaris, acting together; radial deviation results from combined contraction of the extensor carpi radialis longus and brevis muscles and the flexor carpi radialis, significantly aided by abductor pollicis longus and extensor pollicis brevis. A greater range of ulnar deviation is possible (up to 45 degrees) because on the radial side the styloid process extends more distally and blocks radial deviation past 10 to 15 degrees.

RADIOCARPAL JOINT

Of the two long bones in the forearm, only the radius has true articulation with the carpal bones. The **radiocarpal joint** (see Figure 3-53) involves (1) the distal surface of the *radius,* facing (2) the *scaphoid* and *lunate* bones, and (3) the *triangular fibrocartilage* connecting the medial side of the distal radius with the ulnar styloid process, facing (4) the *triquetrum.* The articular disk prevents any direct articulation of the ulna and the carpal bones. The distal surface of the articular disk is parallel to the surface of the distal end of the radius, and the two create a composite smooth concave joint surface. The proximal surfaces of the scaphoid, lunate, and triquetrum are roughly parallel, and together create a congruent convex surface.

The radiocarpal and intercarpal joints act together to allow a wide range of flexion, extension, ulnar deviation, and radial deviation. A combination of these movements is known as **circumduction,** produced by moving the wrist through a repetitive sequence of flexion, radial deviation, extension, ulnar deviation, etc.

FLEXOR RETINACULUM

The **flexor retinaculum** (Figure 3-54) is a strong fibrous ligament extending across the anterior surface of the wrist, connecting the *tubercles of the scaphoid and trapezium* laterally with the *pisiform and hamulus of the*

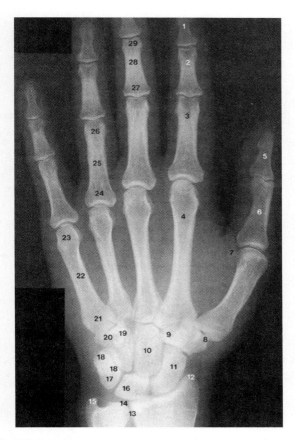

Figure 3-50 X-RAY OF THE HAND, ADULT. Anteroposterior view. (From Weir J, Abrahams PH: *An imaging atlas of human anatomy,* London, 1992, Mosby.)   SEE ATLAS, FIG. 3-37

1 Distal ⎫ phalanx of	**11** Scaphoid	**21** Base ⎫
2 Middle ⎬ index finger	**12** Styloid process ⎫ of radius	**22** Shaft ⎬ of fifth metacarpal
3 Proximal ⎭	**13** Ulnar notch ⎭	**23** Head ⎭
4 Second metacarpal	**14** Head ⎫ of ulna	**24** Base ⎫ of proximal phalanx
5 Distal ⎫ phalanx	**15** Styloid process ⎭	**25** Shaft ⎬ of ring finger
6 Proximal ⎭ of thumb	**16** Lunate	**26** Head ⎭
7 Sesamoid bone	**17** Triquetrum	**27** Base ⎫ of middle phalanx
8 Trapezium	**18** Pisiform	**28** Shaft ⎬ of middle finger
9 Trapezoid	**19** Hook of hamate	**29** Head ⎭
10 Capilate	**20** Hamate	

hamate bones medially. It is a prolongation of the deep fascia of the forearm. The flexor retinaculum, the bones to which it is anchored, and the palmar radiocarpal ligament surround the **carpal tunnel.** The tendons of flexor digitorum superficialis, flexor digitorum profundus, flexor pollicis longus, and the median nerve pass through the carpal tunnel. The tendon of flexor carpi radialis is also deep to the flexor retinaculum but is contained within its own canal laterally where the retinaculum splits to enclose the groove on the trapezium.

The long flexor of the thumb, flexor pollicis longus, is encased in its own synovial sheath as it traverses the

Table 3-9   Bones of the Wrist

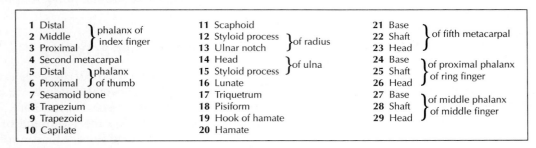

	Lateral Side	←—————————————————————————————————→		Medial Side
Proximal row	Scaphoid	Lunate	Triquetrum	Pisiform
Distal row	Trapezium	Trapezoid	Capitate	Hamate

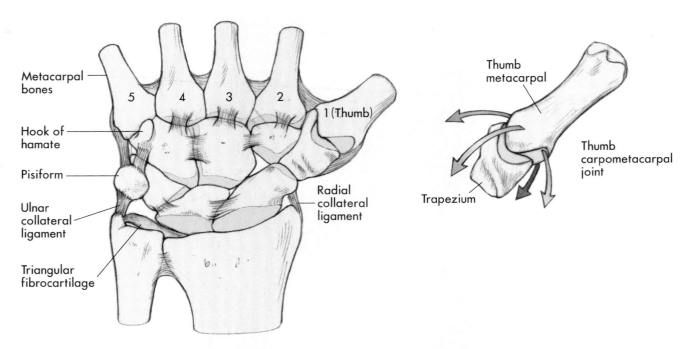

Figure 3-51   WRIST LIGAMENTS AND THE CARPOMETACARPAL JOINT OF THE THUMB. Anterior view.   SEE ATLAS, FIG. 3-111

carpal tunnel, and the sheath is continuous along the anterior surface of the thumb. The deep and superficial tendons for the fingers are enclosed in a **common sheath** at the wrist but only that for the fifth digit is continuous on to the anterior surface of the finger. The sheaths for digits two to four end at the base of the hand, and new synovial sheaths for these fingers commence at the level of the metacarpophalangeal joints.

The tendons of *palmaris longus* and *flexor carpi ulnaris* approach and blend with the flexor retinaculum from its proximal side; the *thenar* and *hypothenar muscles* attach to its distal margin. The ulnar nerve, ulnar vessels, and palmar cutaneous branches of the median nerve lie just superficial to the flexor retinaculum and are often blended into it.

EXTENSOR RETINACULUM

On the dorsum of the wrist is a thickened oblique band of the deep fascia, the **extensor retinaculum,** extending from the radius inferiorly and laterally to the pisiform and hamate medially (Figure 3-55). In reality it is a side-by-side series of longitudinal fibrous tunnels through which pass the various extensor tendons and their synovial sheaths to the wrist and hand, in a regular arrangement, shown in Table 3-10.

The extensor retinaculum prevents "bowstringing" of the extensor tendons during wrist extension, much like the metal loops on a fishing rod. Its obliquity means it remains taut while the movements of the hand and radius occur about the ulna in pronation and supination.

ANATOMIC "SNUFF BOX"

On the posterolateral side of the wrist is a triangular region bounded by several tendons, known as the **anatomic "snuff box"** (see Figure 3-55). The *base* of the triangle is formed by the distal end of the radius; the *medial side* is the tendon of extensor pollicis longus and the *lateral side* the tendons of extensor pollicis brevis and abductor pollicis longus. The *apex* of the triangle is over the thumb metacarpal. The tendons of extensor carpi radialis longus and brevis lie in the floor of the snuff box, as does the scaphoid bone and the radial artery.   SEE ATLAS, FIG. 3-81

BLOOD VESSELS AND NERVES OF THE WRIST

The **ulnar** and **radial arteries** both supply small branches to the wrist (see Figures 3-43 to 3-45). The **anterior interosseous artery,** itself a branch of the ulnar artery, also supplies branches to the wrist. Innervation is supplied by small filaments arising from both the **anterior** or **posterior interosseous nerves** (derived from the median and radial nerves, respectively).

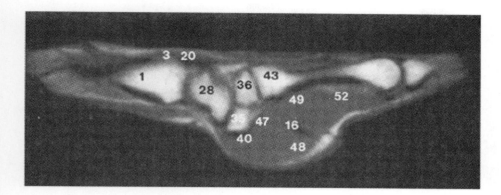

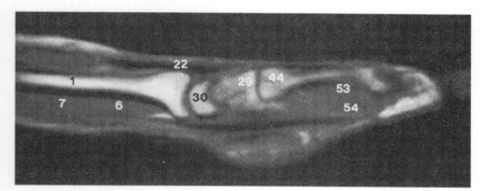

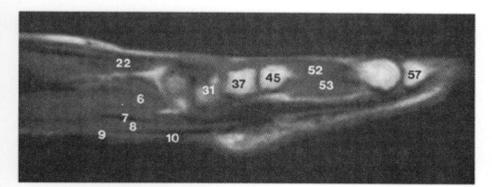

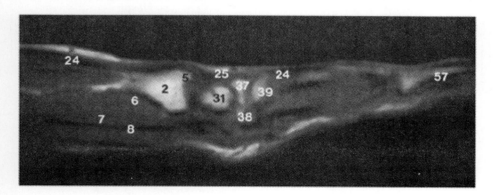

Figure 3-52 MRI THROUGH THE WRIST. Sagittal sections. (From Weir J, Abrahams PH: *An imaging atlas of human anatomy,* London, 1992, Mosby.)

1 Radius
2 Ulna
3 Dorsal tubercle of radius
5 Styloid process of ulna
6 Pronator quadratus muscle
7 Flexor digitorum profundus muscle
8 Tendon of flexor digitorum profundus muscle
9 Flexor digitorum superficialis muscle
10 Tendon of flexor digitorum superficialis muscle
16 Tendon of flexor pollicis longus muscle
20 Tendon of extensor carpi radialis brevis muscle
22 Tendon of extensor digitorum muscle
24 Tendon of extensor digiti minimi muscle
25 Tendon of extensor carpi ulnaris muscle
28 Scaphoid
29 Capitate
30 Lunate
31 Triquetral
35 Trapezium
36 Trapezoid
37 Hamate
38 Hook of hamate
39 Base of fifth metacarpal
40 Abductor pollicis brevis muscle
43 Base of second ⎫
44 Base of third ⎬ metacarpal
45 Base of fourth ⎭
47 Opponens pollicis muscle
48 Flexor pollicis brevis muscle
49 Adductor pollicis muscle
52 Dorsal interossei muscles
53 Ventral interossei muscles
54 Lumbrical muscle
57 Shaft of proximal phalanx

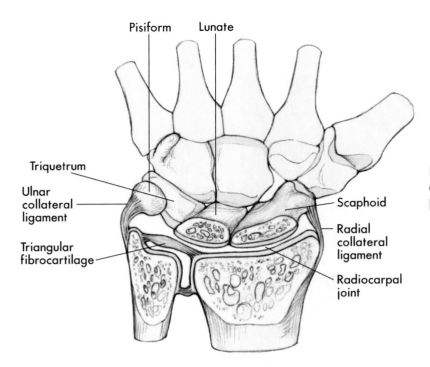

Pisiform   Lunate

Triquetrum

Ulnar
collateral
ligament

Triangular
fibrocartilage

Scaphoid

Radial
collateral
ligament

Radiocarpal
joint

**Figure 3-53 INTERIOR OF THE RADIO-
CARPAL JOINT.** Anterior view, right wrist.

See Atlas, Figs. 3-104, 3-106, 3-107

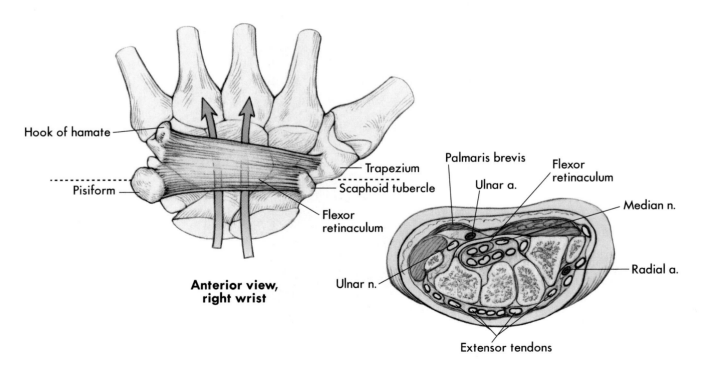

Hook of hamate

Pisiform

Trapezium

Scaphoid tubercle

Flexor
retinaculum

**Anterior view,
right wrist**

Palmaris brevis

Ulnar a.

Flexor
retinaculum

Median n.

Radial a.

Ulnar n.

Extensor tendons

Figure 3-54   FLEXOR RETINACULUM AND WRIST IN CROSS-SECTION.
See Atlas, Figs. 3-43, 3-109, 3-110

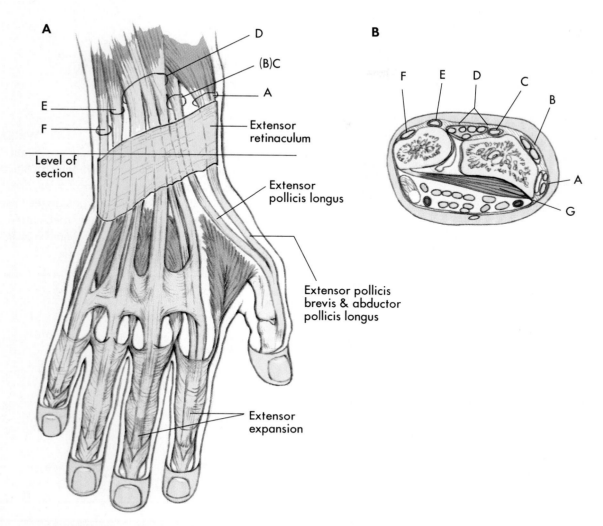

Figure 3-55 **DORSUM OF THE HAND AND WRIST AND CROSS-SECTION THROUGH DISTAL ULNA AND RADIUS. A,** Dorsal view. **B,** Cross-section. Cross-section through the distal forearm shows the following synovial compartments: *A,* abductor pollicis longus and extensor pollicis brevis; *B,* extensor carpi radialis longus and extensor carpi radialis brevis; *C,* extensor pollicis longus; *D,* extensor digitorum and extensor indicis; *E,* extensor digiti minimi; *F,* extensor carpi ulnaris; *G,* pronator quadratus muscle. See ATLAS, FIGS. 3-75, 3-86, 3-109

Table 3-10 Wrist Extensor Synovial Compartments

←Lateral Side	Opposite Radius				Between Radius and Ulna	Opposite Ulna	Medial→ Side
	First (A) (Two sheaths)	Second (B) (Two sheaths)	Third (C) (One sheath)	Fourth (D) (Two sheaths)	Fifth (E) (One sheath)	Sixth (F) (One sheath)	
	Abductor pollicis longus Extensor pollicis brevis	Extensor carpi radialis longus and brevis	Extensor pollicis longus	Extensor digitorum Extensor indicis	Extensor digiti minimi	Extensor carpi ulnaris	

*Letters A to F indicate the position of the six tendon compartments located on the dorsum of the wrist, shown in Figure 3-55, *B.*

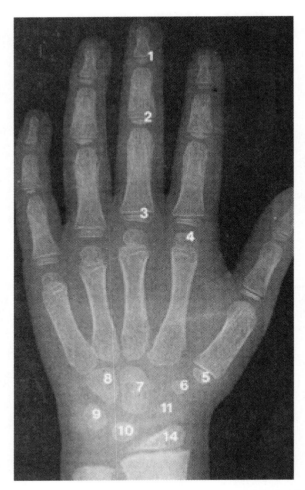

Figure 3-56 X-RAY OF THE HAND AND WRIST, 3-YEAR-OLD CHILD. Note the incomplete ossification of the carpal bones. Also, note the proximal position of the epiphyseal plate in the thumb metacarpal. Embryologically, this bone resembles the phalanges (also with proximal epiphyses) not the other metacarpals. (From Weir J, Abrahams PH: *An imaging atlas of human anatomy,* London, 1992, Mosby.)   SEE ATLAS, FIG. 3-37

Epiphyseal plates	Ossification centers
1 Distal phalanx	**6** Trapezium
2 Middle phalanx	**7** Capitate
3 Proximal phalanx	**8** Hamate
4 Head of metacarpal	**9** Pisiform
5 Base of thumb metacarpal	**10** Lunate
	14 Scaphoid

CLINICAL ANATOMY OF

THE WRIST

CARPAL TUNNEL SYNDROME

Structures within the carpal tunnel are vulnerable to compression and subsequent injury. The synovial sheaths within the carpal tunnel may become swollen and inflamed (tenosynovitis), from fluid retention, excessive exercise, or infection. Changes in hormonal status, as in pregnancy or menopause, increase the incidence of carpal tunnel syndrome in females. The median nerve is most superficial in the carpal tunnel and is first affected by such processes. Compression of the median nerve leads to sensory changes over the lateral side of the hand and muscle weakness in the thenar eminence (known as "**carpal tunnel syndrome**").

FRACTURE OF THE SCAPHOID BONE

Fracture of the scaphoid bone occurs as a consequence of a fall on outstretched arms; the scaphoid is the most commonly fractured carpal bone. In some in-dividuals the scaphoid bone receives its blood supply exclusively along its distal margin (while in most, blood is supplied to the bone from both the proximal and distal margins) and, if a fracture is severe enough, the proximal portion of the bone may fail to receive adequate blood flow to heal properly. The proximal fragment of bone will then become necrotic and may become a locus of infection and/or inflammation to the wrist. Surgical removal of the dead fragment of bone is sometimes necessary.

DISLOCATION OF THE LUNATE BONE

When the lunate bone is loosened from its surrounding companion carpal bones, it most often moves anteriorly and protrudes through the "floor" of the carpal tunnel. This further increases the pressure inside the carpal tunnel and may lead to carpal tunnel syndrome (see previously).

CLINICAL ANATOMY OF
THE WRIST (continued)

FUSION OF WRIST BONES OR "ARTHRODESIS"

In patients whose carpal bones are chronically inflamed, producing pain and lack of motion, it is sometimes necessary to surgically fuse the carpal bones to each other. This is known as an **arthrodesis.** Chronic recurrent inflammation may spontaneously fuse the carpal bones even without surgical assistance.

CYCLIST'S HAND

Long-distance cycling, in which the rider holds the hands in an extended position against the handle grips, produces pressure on the hook of the hamate and injures the ulnar nerve. This can lead to sensory loss on the medial side of the hand and weakness in the intrinsic hand muscles.

"GANGLIA" AT THE WRIST

In many people bulbous swellings on the dorsal surface of the wrist appear periodically. These ganglia are not painful but may be "inconvenient" because a patient will bump them against something and cause some discomfort. They are misnamed because they are not neural tissue at all but cystic extensions of the synovial sheaths enclosing the long extensor tendons of the wrist. They may be evacuated with a fine needle, or they sometimes recede spontaneously. They are not a forerunner of malignant disease or any other serious complication.

ARTERIAL PULSES AT THE WRIST AND THE ALLEN TEST

Pulses are commonly palpated at the wrist in three places: (1) the radial artery, which passes toward the hand lying just medial to the radial styloid process; (2) the ulnar artery, which passes just lateral (in the anatomic position) to the pisiform bone; and (3) the deep radial artery, which crosses the floor of the "anatomic snuff box." The radial artery is often chosen for blood sampling and/or placement of an indwelling catheter to permit additional blood sampling and to measure blood pressure continuously.

Before performing such a puncture or cannulation, it is important to check that the circulation delivered to the hand through the ulnar artery will suffice to keep the hand well perfused even if the radial artery should be totally obstructed as a result of the procedure. This is checked by the *Allen test.* The examiner should wrap his or her hand around the dorsum of the patient's wrist, positioning his or her thumb over the radial artery and the long finger over the ulnar artery (or vice versa) and compress both vessels. The patient is then asked to make a fist repeatedly, removing most of the venous blood from the hand. The hand should now appear pale. Next the examiner should release the pressure over the radial artery and verify that radial artery flow alone can perfuse the hand (by observing the skin flush). Next the process is repeated, this time releasing the ulnar artery and verifying that it too can support the entire vascular circulation to the hand. In this manner, the examiner is assured that cannulating the radial artery will be safe because the ulnar artery can support adequate blood flow to the hand.

LACERATION OF THE WRISTS

Accidental or purposeful lacerations of the wrist often fail to produce fatal exsanguination but do cause injury to the median nerve since it is so close to the surface at the wrist, between the palmaris longus and flexor carpi radialis tendons.

BONE MATURATION AND THE WRIST

The carpal bones undergo a well-understood sequence of ossification, a sequence which may be employed to estimate the age of a child of unknown age (e.g., in a forensic case or in studies of bony remains in physical anthropology). Figure 3-56 illustrates an x-ray of the wrist of a 3-year-old child. Compare it with Figure 3-50, a similar x-ray of the wrist of an adult. In the child's wrist, note the epiphyseal centers in both the metacarpals and the phalanges.

section three.seven

Hand

▶ Metacarpal Bones

▶ Carpometacarpal (CM) Joints Two to Five

▶ Carpometacarpal (CM) Joint of the Thumb

▶ Metacarpophalangeal (MP) Joints

▶ Phalanges

▶ Fascial Structures in the Hand

▶ Thenar Muscles

▶ Hypothenar Muscles

▶ Interosseous and Lumbrical Muscles

▶ Muscle Insertions on Individual Digits

▶ Fibrous Flexor Sheaths

▶ Extensor Expansions

▶ Blood Vessels of the Hand

▶ Nerves in the Hand

▶ Movements and Functions of the Hand

*T*he human hand represents a highly sophisticated blend of biology and engineering—something which we, despite great strides in robotics and bioengineering, have not yet been able to duplicate. The fingers of the hand are exquisitely sensitive instruments, densely supplied with sensory receptors and nerves. A complex array of muscles, tendons, and specialized ligamentous structures produces a capacity for very fine control of the movement and position of the digits. Our ability with our hands to manipulate objects in the environment has long been recognized as one of the hallmarks of the human species.

METACARPAL BONES

The skeleton of each of the five digits or "rays" of the hand consists of a **metacarpal bone** and two or three **phalanges** (Figures 3-57 and 3-58). The metacarpal bones articulate with the distal surfaces of the carpal bones (the **carpometacarpal joints**—see following) and extend distally to form the base for each digit. Each metacarpal has a proximal concave **base,** a **shaft,** and a rounded **head** distally. The base of each metacarpal bone is slightly broadened to articulate with the carpal bones and with each other on the lateral or medial surfaces of their adjacent sides.

The metacarpal **shafts** are slightly bowed toward the posterior, which helps create space for the intrinsic hand muscles in the hollow of the palm. It is the **heads** of the metacarpals that form what we commonly recognize as "knuckles." The head of the first metacarpal has two additional shallow depressions on its anterior surface, to accommodate the two sesamoid bones embedded in the palmar joint capsule and the heads of the flexor pollicis brevis (see pp. 383-384). Distally, each metacarpal head articulates with the proximal phalanx of its digit, forming a **metacarpophalangeal joint** (see following).

The **thumb metacarpal** stands apart from the other four and possesses several unique qualities. The metacarpal bones for the digits are nearly parallel to each other, but the thumb metacarpal projects laterally at a 70 to 80 degree angle. In addition, in comparison to metacarpals two to five, the shaft of the first metacarpal is rotated approximately 90 degrees around its own long axis. As a result, the *lateral-facing surface of the first metacarpal is equivalent to the posterior-facing surface of the second to fifth metacarpals.* This difference in orientation helps give humans the ability to grasp objects between thumb and other digits (see fuller discussion following) and is also the basis of the unique terminology applied to thumb movements.

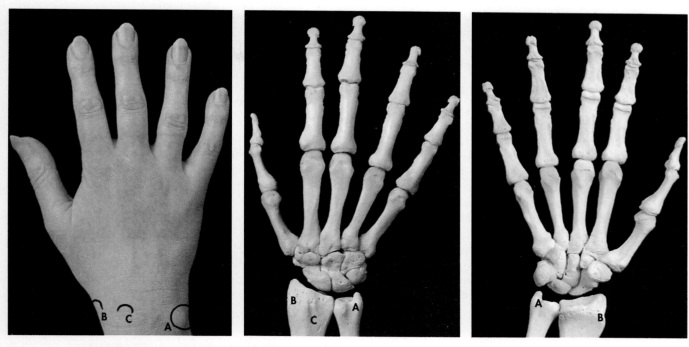

Figure 3-57 HAND, SKELETAL STRUCTURE AND INTACT HAND. A, Skin intact, dorsal view. **B,** Skeleton of hand, dorsal view. **C,** Skeleton of hand, palmar view. *A,* Ulnar styloid; *B,* radial styloid; *C,* Lister's tubercle. (From Chumbley CC, Hutchings RT: *Color atlas of human dissection,* ed 2, London, 1992, Mosby.)   **SEE ATLAS, FIG. 3-57**

CARPOMETACARPAL (CM) JOINTS TWO TO FIVE

The CM joints for the index and long fingers have little mobility. The ring and little finger CM joints move in the anterorposterior plane about 15 to 30 degrees. For the second through the fifth digits, the majority of motion occurs at the metacarpophalangeal joints (MP joints) not the CM joints. The **second metacarpal** artic-

ulates principally with the trapezoid bone and, to a lesser degree, with the trapezium and capitate bones, the **third metacarpal** articulates with the capitate bone alone, the **fourth metacarpal** articulates with both the capitate and hamate bones, and the **fifth metacarpal** articulates with the hamate bone alone.

Each CM joint has a **synovial cavity** and a surrounding fibrous **joint capsule.** Often the synovial cavities of

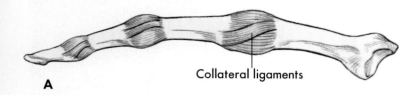

Collateral ligaments

A

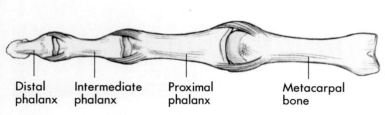

Distal phalanx | Intermediate phalanx | Proximal phalanx | Metacarpal bone

B

Figure 3-58 METACARPOPHALANGEAL AND IN-TERPHALANGEAL JOINTS, WITH LIGAMENTS. A, Lateral view. **B,** Dorsal (posterior) view.

SEE ATLAS, FIG. 3-38

adjacent CM joints are continuous. CM joints are reinforced by overlying **dorsal** and **palmar ligaments,** plus **medial** and **lateral collateral ligaments.**

The capitate is joined, by special short ligaments, to the bases of the second and third metacarpal bones. Partially as a consequence of these ligaments, the index and long finger metacarpals have reduced mobility. They represent the stable "backbone" of the hand around which the other fingers and thumb move more freely. In addition, the adjacent sides of the bases of metacarpals two to five have small facets where they articulate with each other. There are no such facets on the lateral side of the second metacarpal base and the medial side of the fifth metacarpal base. There are none at all on the thumb metacarpal base, underscoring its independence and resultant wide range of motion (see following). The metacarpophalangeal joint ligaments of digits 2 to 5, on their palmar surfaces, are joined by **deep transverse metacarpal ligaments.** These also con-

nect fibrous plates of the metacarpophalangeal (MP) joints of the digits and are notably strong between the fourth and fifth digits. Consequently, independent movement of these two metacarpals is limited.

CARPOMETACARPAL (CM) JOINT OF THE THUMB

The CM joint of the thumb (see Figure 3-57) is more complex than the other CM joints and permits a very wide range of motion. Indeed, for the thumb it is the CM joint that provides the greatest degree of mobility, whereas for the other four digits there is greater mobility at the metacarpophalangeal (MP) joints than at the CM joint.

The thumb CM joint involves the articulation of the (1) base of the *first metacarpal bone* and (2) an articular surface on the distal and somewhat lateral side of the *trapezium.* A **lateral ligament** reinforces the joint, run-

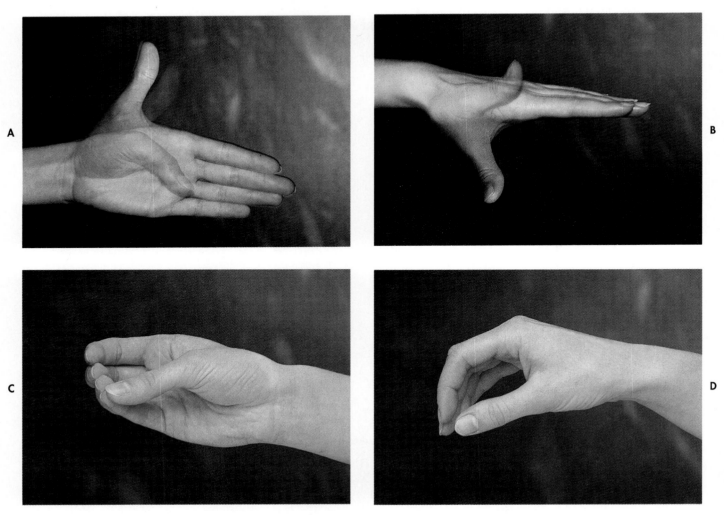

Figure 3-59   EXAMPLES OF THUMB MOVEMENTS. A, Flexion-extension. **B,** Abduction-adduction. **C,** Opposition. **D,** Hand in neutral position.

ning from the lateral side of the trapezium to the base of the first metacarpal. As with the other CM joints, there are **palmar** and **dorsal ligaments** as well.

Both joint surfaces are oval saddlelike depressions, arranged so that their long axes are perpendicular to each other. The joint is often called a **"double saddle" joint** (see Figure 3-51). The geometry of the joint surfaces is not perfectly symmetric, however, as is illustrated by the mandatory medial rotation of the thumb during its full flexion. Indeed, this medial rotation of the thumb along its long axis is essential for opposition of the thumb (see following).

Movements of the thumb are different than for the fingers (Figure 3-59). *Flexion* is the act of sweeping the thumb across the palm toward the little finger, in the plane of the palm and perpendicular to the plane of the thumbnail. *Extension* is the reverse of this motion. *Abduction* occurs by moving the thumb away from the hand through an arc perpendicular to the palm; *adduction* is that movement bringing the thumb into contact with the palm of the hand, moving along the same axis. *Circumduction* is the sequence of flexion, abduction (also known as radial deviation), extension, adduction (also known as ulnar deviation) (or in reverse order).

METACARPOPHALANGEAL (MP) JOINTS

In the metacarpophalangeal joints (MP), the rounded heads of the metacarpals fit into the shallow concave proximal surfaces of the phalanges. Although each of the five MP joints has a different range of mobility, *flexion, extension, abduction, adduction,* and *circumduction* are possible. Flexion of the MP joint and simultaneous extension of the interphalangeal (IP) joints produces straightened fingers, flexed at the knuckle. This position is crucial for many five movements of which the hand is capable, including threading a needle, manipulating a knife, etc.

Each MP joint has **medial** and **lateral collateral ligaments** (see Figure 3-58). Unlike similar ligaments for the IP joints, the collateral ligaments of the MP joints are taut in flexion and relaxed in extension (Figure 3-58). It is this quality that makes adduction-abduction movement at the MP joint nearly impossible if the MP joint is flexed. A much greater range of adduction/abduction is possible when the MP joints are extended. A strong **palmar ligament** or plate passes over and reinforces the anterior surface of each MP joint (see Figure 3-66). Between metacarpals two and three, three and four, and four and five, a strong **deep transverse metacarpal ligament** unites the palmar ligaments to each other. *The MP joint of the thumb is not tethered to the others in this fashion,* permitting the thumb to move in and out of the plane of the palm. In actuality, however, the MP joint of the index finger has even a greater range of mobility than the MP joint of the thumb (but

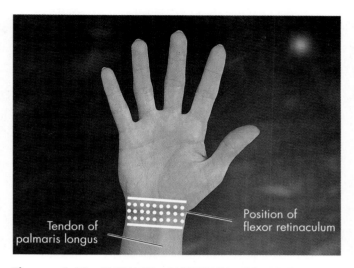

Figure 3-60 SURFACE ANATOMY OF THE PALM. Flexor retinaculum indicated.

remember that the CM joint of the thumb gives it an overall range of mobility that exceeds that for any other digit).

PHALANGES

There are three phalanges in each finger, termed the **proximal, middle,** and **distal** (see Figures 3-56 and 3-57). For the thumb there are only two phalanges, termed the **proximal** and **distal** (however, a study of comparative anatomy shows that the "true" proximal phalanx of the thumb is the thumb metacarpal bone, and parts of the trapezium are the "true" metacarpal for the thumb). The phalanges also have an expanded base, a shaft, and a rounded head. Each base has a shallow concave surface facing proximally, to articulate with the head of the metacarpal or phalanx proximal to it. At the distal end of each digit, the "tip" of each distal phalanx is not rounded but instead is in the form of a thickened rough-surfaced tuft. Numerous tendons and ligaments attach to both the dorsal and palmar surfaces of the phalanges. The specific attachments of the long flexor tendons allow for independent and separate movement of individual phalanges in one digit (see the following section on hand movement).

The **interphalangeal joints (IP joints)** consist of a small head, from the proximal phalanx, and a base from the distal phalanx. Each has a **synovial cavity** and **capsule** and is reinforced by a **palmar ligament or plate** and two **collateral ligaments**—on the medial and lateral sides of the joint. The collateral ligaments remain taut both in extension and in flexion. There is no ligament on the dorsum of the joint, but the **extensor expansion** (see p. 390), present on the dorsum of each digit, serves this purpose. IP joint movement is hingelike, permitting 100 to 150 degrees of flexion but little extension past the neutral point—that is, when all phalanges are in longitudinal alignment—because of the tough fibrocartilaginous palmar plate or capsule.

FASCIAL STRUCTURES IN THE HAND

On the dorsum of the hand, both the deep and superficial fascial layers are very thin, loose, and attached to the synovial sheaths passing through the extensor retinaculum. The laxity of this layer means that when there is swelling or hemorrhage in the hand, on either the palmar or dorsal side, it is usually the dorsum of the hand where swelling becomes visible.

By contrast, the **palmar fascia** (or **aponeurosis**), on the anterior surface of the hand, is thick and sturdy. It is triangular in shape with its base distally, at the level of the metacarpal heads. Its apex is at the level of the flexor retinaculum, to which it attaches. The palmaris longus muscle inserts into the palmar fascia at its proximal convergence, and the palmaris brevis muscle lies medial to the palmar fascia, extending medially to the ulnar side of the hand (see Figure 3-54)

SEE ATLAS, FIG. 3-42

In the palmar fascia, collagenous fibers run in longi-

tudinal, transverse, and vertical planes. The **longitudinal fibers** run from proximal to distal, and at the level of the metacarpal heads divide into separate slips that extend subcutaneously into the digits. The slip to the thumb is smaller than that for the fingers. The **transverse fibers** are found distally in the palm, deep to the longitudinal fibers. They help prevent lateral-medial stretching of the palmar fascia. Most distally, at the level of the MP joints, these transverse fibers form the **superficial transverse metacarpal ligament.** This structure helps the fibrous flexor sheaths of the four fingers to prevent "bowstringing" of the long flexor tendons.

The **vertical fibers** in the palmar fascia attach it to the overlying skin of the palm, helping to stabilize the palmar skin when handling objects. **Deep vertical fibers** descend and attach to the fibrous flexor sheaths and the deep transverse metacarpal ligaments. On the lateral side, the **lateral palmar septum** extends deep and attaches the palmar aponeurosis to the first metacarpal bone; on the medial side, the **medial palmar septum** extends deep and attaches the palmar aponeurosis to the fifth metacarpal bone. An **intermediate palmar septum** passes from the palmar aponeu-

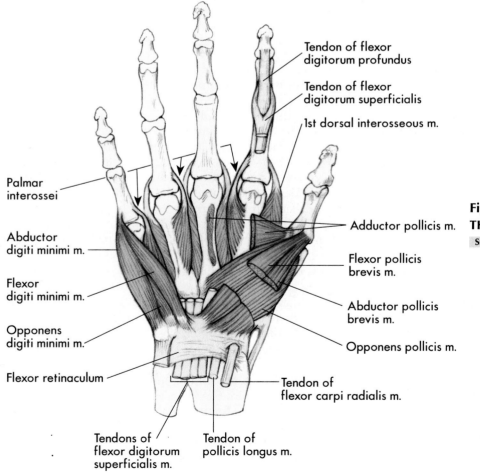

Palmar
interossei

Abductor
digiti minimi m.

Flexor
digiti minimi m.

Opponens
digiti minimi m.

Flexor retinaculum

Tendons of
flexor digitorum
superficialis m.

Tendon of
pollicis longus m.

Tendon of flexor
digitorum profundus

Tendon of flexor
digitorum superficialis

1st dorsal interosseous m.

Adductor pollicis m.

Flexor pollicis
brevis m.

Abductor pollicis
brevis m.

Opponens pollicis m.

Tendon of
flexor carpi radialis m.

Figure 3-61 DEEPER MUSCLES OF THE PALM.   Anterior view.

SEE ATLAS, FIGS. 3-49, 3-50

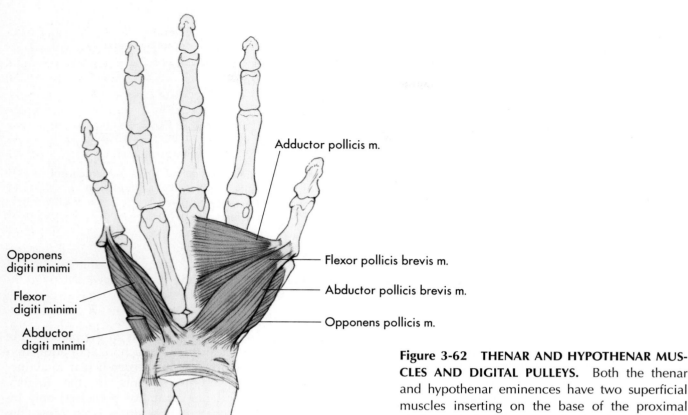

Adductor pollicis m.

Opponens
digiti minimi

Flexor
digiti minimi

Abductor
digiti minimi

Flexor pollicis brevis m.

Abductor pollicis brevis m.

Opponens pollicis m.

**Figure 3-62   THENAR AND HYPOTHENAR MUS-
CLES AND DIGITAL PULLEYS.** Both the thenar
and hypothenar eminences have two superficial
muscles inserting on the base of the proximal
phalanax and a deeper single muscle terminating
on the metacarpal shaft.   **SEE ATLAS, FIGS. 3-48, 3-51**

rosis deep and attaches to fascia covering the second
lumbrical and the long flexor tendons of the long
finger.

The region medial to the intermediate septum is
sometimes called the **midpalmar space** or **central palmar space** and the region lateral to it the **thenar space**
(Figure 3-60), although in fact both are really potential
spaces, containing the long flexor tendons and the lumbricals, surrounded by loose fascia.

The floor of the palm is formed by a series of strong
ligaments lying just anterior to the carpal bones, the
most prominent being the **palmar radiocarpal ligament.** Further distal, the **deep transverse metacarpal
ligament** binds the heads of the metacarpals to each
other. Just anterior to this ligament pass the long flexor
tendons and anterior to these is the **superficial transverse metacarpal ligament.**

THENAR MUSCLES

The raised area between the midpalm and the base
of the thumb is the **thenar eminence,** formed by the
underlying thenar muscles—**abductor pollicis brevis,
flexor pollicis brevis,** and **opponens pollicis** (Figure 3-
61). These muscles, along with the **adductor pollicis,**
lying deep to these three (and technically part of the
group of intrinsic hand muscles not the thenar muscle

group), are responsible for positioning of the thumb for
opposition. The thumb is capable of a rich and unique
variety of motions and has a unique terminology to describe them.

In the thenar eminence, the abductor pollicis brevis
and superficial head of the flexor pollicis brevis are
most superficial, and the opponens pollicis lies deep.
Abductor pollicis brevis and **flexor pollicis brevis**
share an insertion on the proximal phalanx of the
thumb, while **opponens pollicis** inserts on the
metacarpal of the thumb. All three muscles originate
from various parts of the flexor retinaculum and the
lateral bones in the distal carpal row. The **flexor pollicis
brevis** has two heads. The **superficial head** originates
from the trapezium and flexor retinaculum and passes
lateral to the flexor pollicis longus tendon to insert on
the proximal phalanx. The **deep head** originates from
the capitate and trapezoid, passes deep to the flexor
pollicis longus tendon, and joins the superficial head to
insert on the proximal phalanx. Part of the deep head
of flexor pollicis brevis is now considered to be the **first
palmar interosseous muscle.** Details of their attachments, innervation, and actions are described in Table
3-11 and Figure 3-62. **Adductor pollicis** is a triangular
muscle, whose base (origin) extends along the shaft of
the third metacarpal bone and also includes the bases
of the second and third metacarpals, small areas of the

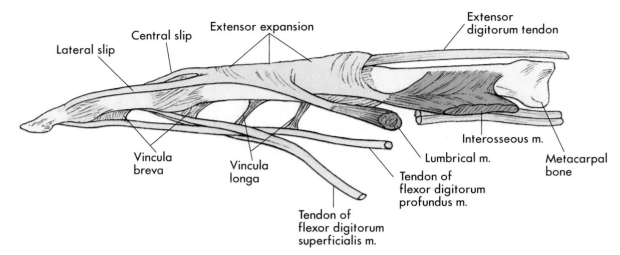

Figure 3-63   EXTENSOR SHEATHS AND THE LONG FLEXOR TENDONS.   Lateral view.
SEE ATLAS, FIGS. 3-47, 3-56

trapezoid and the capitate bones, and the flexor retinaculum. It narrows into a slender tendon that inserts on the base of the thumb proximal phalanx.

Movements of the thumb (see Figure 3-59) are described in terms different from those applied to the other digits because (1) the thumb is positioned differently than the fingers and (2) the thumb is capable of unique movements not possible in the other digits (Table 3-12). In the anatomic position, the thumbnail faces in a lateral direction, while the nails of the fingers face to the posterior. If, for example, one defines abduc-

tion and adduction as movements in the plane of the nail, then it is clear that abduction and adduction movements of the thumb are perpendicular to abduction and adduction movements of the fingers. Opposition is a unique capability, possessed only by the thumb. The goal of opposition is to cause the "pulp" surface (i.e., the rounded eminence directly opposite the nail) of the distal phalanx to face the pulp surfaces of the other digits. This capability is essential to realizing the full range of capabilities for grasping and manipulating objects with the hand.

Table 3-11   Thenar Muscles

Muscles	Origin(s)	Insertion(s)	Nerves	Action(s)
Abductor pollicis brevis	Trapezium, trapezoid, flexor retinaculum	Base of proximal phalanx, thumb, and extensor sheath	Median nerve (C6, C7)	Abducts thumb, extends thumb IP joint
Opponens pollicis	Trapezium, flexor retinaculum	Medial side of thumb metacarpal	Median nerve (C6, C7), radial nerve?	Opposition
Flexor pollicis brevis	Superficial head: trapezium and flexor retinaculum; Deep head: trapezoid and capitate bones; (previously the first palmar interosseous, originating on the thumb metacarpal, was considered part of the deep head of flexor pollicis brevis)	Both heads converge on to base of proximal phalanx of thumb; has small sesamoid bone in distal tendon, just before insertion	Median nerve (C7-8, T1)	Flexes thumb at MP joint; aids in opposition
Adductor pollicis	Transverse head: distal one-half of third metacarpal Oblique head: capitate; trapezoid, base of metacarpal two and three; flexor retinaculum	Base of proximal phalanx, thumb; distal tendon has small sesamoid bone	Ulnar nerve (C8, T1)	Adducts and flexes MP joint

Note: all thenar muscles insert on the proximal thumb phalanx except opponens pollicis.

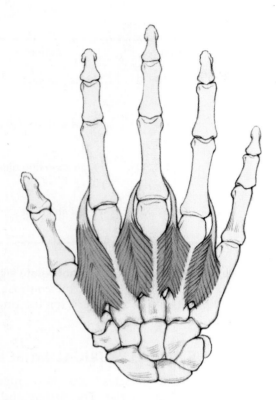

Dorsal interossei muscles
(dual origins)

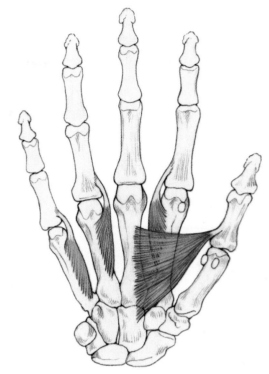

Palmar interossei
& adductor pollicis muscles
(single origin)

Figure 3-64   INTEROSSESOUS MUSCLES AND ADDUCTOR POLLICIS.
SEE ATLAS, FIGS. 3-52, 3-53

The hands of several other primates are specialized for grasping, as these animals "swing" through the trees from branch to branch. This form of locomotion is known as "brachiation" and requires the hand to be flattened, with very strong finger flexor musculature to ensure a good grip on the branch. In these animals the thenar eminence is negligible, the palm is flat, and the thumb cannot be opposed effectively. Neither abduction nor opposition is well developed in these animals.

Table 3-12   Movements of the Thumb

Movement	Description
Flexion	The "sweeping" motion in which the thumb moves from lateral to medial in the plane of the palm of the hand. Involves movement at carpometacarpal (CM) and metacarpophalangeal (MP) joints. Carried out by flexor pollicis brevis and longus.
Extension	Movement of the thumb from medial to lateral in the plane of the palm of the hand. Involves both CM and MP joints. Carried out by extensor pollicis brevis and longus and to a lesser degree by abductor pollicis longus.
Abduction	Movement of the thumb away from the palm of the hand, in a plane perpendicular to the palm. In full abduction, the thumb metacarpal rotates medially. Occurs mainly at CM joint. Carried out by abductor pollicis brevis and longus.
Adduction	Movement of the thumb toward the palm of the hand in a plane perpendicular to the palm, the reverse of abduction. Occurs at CM joint. Carried out by adductor pollicis.
Circumduction	A consecutive combination of flexion, extension, adduction and abduction, in which the thumb moves through a 360 degree arc, with the thumb CM joint as the reference point for this movement.
Opposition	Opposition or a combination of flexion and medial rotation of the thumb (often as part of thumb abduction). This causes the "pulp" surface of the thumb's distal phalanx to face the similar pulp surface of any of the other digits. This capability is central to the unique capabilities of the hand. Carried out by the thumb abductors and opponens pollicis, principally at the thumb carpometacarpal joint.

Table 3-13   Hypothenar Muscles

Muscles	Origin(s)	Insertion(s)	Nerve(s)	Action(s)
Palmaris brevis	Transverse carpal ligament/palmar aponeurosis	Skin on medial border of hand	Ulnar nerve (C8, T1)	Tenses palmar skin
Abductor digiti minimi	Pisiform, pisohamate ligament	Base of proximal phalanx fifth digit	Ulnar nerve (C8, T1)	Abducts, flexes fifth digit
Opponens digiti minimi	Hook of hamate, flexor retinaculum	Lateral margin metacarpal five	Ulnar nerve (C8, T1)	Opposition fifth digit
Flexor digiti minimi brevis	Hook of hamate, flexor retinaculum	Base of proximal phalanx fifth digit	Ulnar nerve (C8, T1)	Flexes fifth digit

HYPOTHENAR MUSCLES

On the medial side of the hand, between the mid-palm and the base of the fifth digit is a raised area known as the **hypothenar eminence.** Beneath it lie three muscles—the **abductor digiti minimi, flexor digiti minimi,** and the **opponens digiti minimi** (Table 3-13 and Figure 3-62; see also Figure 3-61). Although it does not act on the fifth digit, the **palmaris brevis** muscle is usually included in this group. It is a superficial muscle, attaching to the palmar fascia on the medial side of the hand. It forms the roof of a tunnel for passage of the ulnar nerve and vessels from wrist to palm. The other three muscles (abductor digiti minimi, flexor digiti minimi, and opponens digiti minimi) originate from medial carpal bones and flexor retinaculum. The opponens muscle is deep to the other two. The pattern of insertion is mirror image of the thenar muscles—the opponens muscle inserts on the metacarpal, and the other two muscles insert on the proximal phalanx. The fifth digit is capable of a wider range of motion than any of the other fingers, but it does not approach the capabilities of the thumb because of reduced mobility of the fifth finger metacarpal. The CM joint of the fifth finger is less mobile, and the fifth finger cannot rotate significantly around its long axis (which, by contrast, the thumb can). This rotation is necessary for the opposition of the thumb and the four digits.

INTEROSSEOUS AND LUMBRICAL MUSCLES

The **"intrinsic hand muscles"** are those muscles confined to the hand and wrist. The thenar and hypothenar muscles are discussed previously (pp. 383-

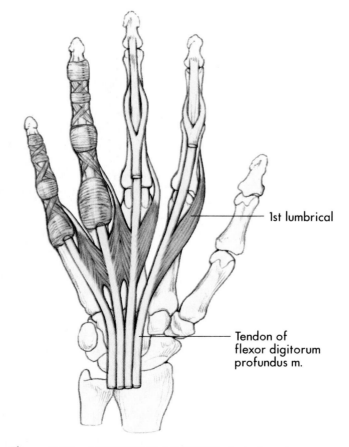

1st lumbrical

Tendon of flexor digitorum profundus m.

Figure 3-66   LUMBRICAL MUSCLES. Anterior view. See Atlas, Figs. 3-44, 3-46

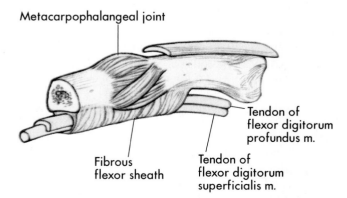

Metacarpophalangeal joint

Tendon of flexor digitorum profundus m.

Fibrous flexor sheath

Tendon of flexor digitorum superficialis m.

Figure 3-65   FLEXOR TENDONS AND THE DIGITS. Lateral oblique view.   See Atlas, Figs. 3-45, 3-113

386). The lumbricals and interossei are sometimes referred to as the "deep hand muscles" (adductor pollicis was described with the thenar muscles, on p. 383).

The **lumbrical muscles** (see Figure 3-66) are four elongated cylindrical muscles of the distal half of the palm. **Lumbricals one and two** originate from and lie on the lateral side of each of the two lateral tendons of flexor digitorum profundus (i.e., those for the second and third digits). **Lumbricals three and four** originate from the adjacent sides of flexor digitorum profundus tensons two and three and three and four, respectively. The bellies of these muscles lie parallel to the long flexor tendons and pass lateral to their MP joints and insert on to the dorsolateral surface of the extensor sheath for the same digit (see Figure 3-63; see also p. 390). They are unique in that they link a flexor tendon directly to an extensor tendon and are not attached directly to bone. Because they pass from the anterior surface of the palm across the palmar side of the MP joint to the dorsal surface of the digits, they can flex the MP joints; their insertion on the extensor sheath causes extension of the IP joints. Their innervation is from the *median nerve* (lumbricals one and two) and *ulnar nerve* (lumbricals three and four)—the same nerves innervating the muscles and tendons from which they arise.

The **interosseous muscles** are arranged in two groups, the **dorsal** and **palmar** (although they may also be described as **proximal** and **distal,** respectively, based on the position at which they each insert into the extensor sheath) (Figure 3-64). The **dorsal interossei muscles,** each with two heads of origin, lie in the spaces between adjacent metacarpal bones, while the **palmar interossei,** each with a single head of origin, lie on the palmar surfaces of the metacarpals. The interossei are the most deeply placed muscles in the hand; for example, the first palmar interosseous muscle lies deep to the oblique head of adductor pollicis. The attachments, innervations, and actions of the interossei and lumbricals are described more fully in Table 3-14.

The interossei and lumbricals are important in fine movements of the digits but, in addition, make possible the reshaping of the hand into a "cup." In mammals who lack this ability, the movements of the digits, though varied, are confined to the horizontal plane of the palm. This means that in such creatures the hand is little more than a static platform for the fingers. In man, where three of the metacarpals are able to move independently, a wide range of movements is possible for the thumb and fingers. The deep hand muscles and their innervation (predominantly ulnar nerve) are thus key elements in one of our most vital human capabilities.

MUSCLE INSERTIONS ON INDIVIDUAL DIGITS

Each of the five digits, on its flexor side, receives several tendons (Table 3-15). The arrangement and relationships of these tendons is intricate and permits

Table 3-14 Lumbrical and Interosseous Muscles

Muscle(s)	Origin(s)	Insertion(s)	Nerve(s)	Action(s)
Lumbricals	Tendons of flexor digitorum profundus	Extensor expansion	Median nerve (#one, two) Ulnar nerve (#three, four)	Flex MP joint, extend IP joints
Dorsal interossei (four)	From adjoining sides of metacarpals one to two, two to three, three to four, four to five.	Extensor expansions of digits two, three, and four; base of proximal phalanx of digits two, three, four Note that first dorsal interosseous inserts on the index finger, the second and third interossei converge on the third digit, and the fourth interosseous inserts on the ring finger	Ulnar nerve (C8, T1)	Abduct digits, flex MP and extend IP joints "DAB" (i.e., Dorsals ABduct)
Palmar interossei (four)*	First: from base of metacarpal one Second: from medial side of metacarpal two Third to fourth: lateral side of metacarpals four and five.	First: base of thumb proximal phalanx and extensor expansion Second to fourth: extensor expansion of digits; base of proximal phalanx of index, ring, and little finger expansion	Ulnar nerve (C8, T1)	Adduct digits, flex MP, and extend IP joints "PAD" (i.e., Palmars ADduct)

*In the past, the first palmar interosseous muscle was considered part of the flexor pollicis brevis. The *true deep head* of the flexor pollicis brevis originates from the *carpal bones* not from the first metacarpal bone.

Table 3-15   Muscle Insertions on to the Digits

Digit	Inserts on Metacarpal	Inserts on Proximal Phalanx	Inserts on Middle Phalanx	Inserts on Distal Phalanx	Inserts on Extensor Expansion
Thumb	Abductor pollicis longus Opponens pollicis	Extensor pollicis brevis Abductor pollicis brevis Flexor pollicis brevis (deep and superficial heads) Adductor pollicis (oblique and transverse heads)	(Thumb has no middle phalanx)	Flexor pollicis longus Extensor mechanism Extensor pollicis longus (some fibers of extensor pollicis brevis may join as well)	First palmar interosseous* Abductor pollicis brevis (primary insertion is on thumb proximal phalanx)
Index finger	Flexor carpi radialis Extensor carpi radialis longus Extensor carpi radialis brevis	Second* dorsal interosseous Second palmar interosseous	Flexor digitorum superficialis Central slip, extensor expansion	Flexor digitorum profundus Lateral slips, extensor expansion	Extensor digitorum Extensor indicis First dorsal interosseous Second palmar interosseous* First lumbrical
Long finger	Flexor carpi radialis Extensor carpi radialis brevis	Second and third dorsal interossei	Flexor digitorum superficials Central slip, extensor expansion	Flexor digitorum profundus Lateral slips, extensor expansion	Extensor digitorum Second and third dorsal interossei Second lumbrical
Ring finger	No muscle inserts on the fourth metacarpal bone; however, both the palmar and dorsal interosseous muscles originate from it	Fourth dorsal interosseous Fourth palmar interosseous	Flexor digitorum superficialis Central slip, extensor expansion	Flexor digitorum profundus Lateral slips, extensor expansion	Extensor digitorum Fourth dorsal interosseous Third palmar interosseous* Third lumbrical
Little finger	Flexor carpi ulnaris Extensor carpi ulnaris Opponens digiti minimi	Abductor digiti minimi Flexor digiti minimi brevis Fourth palmar interosseous	Flexor digitorum superficialis Central slip, extensor expansion	Flexor digitorum profundus Lateral slips, extensor expansion	Extensor digiti minimi Extensor digitorum Fourth palmar interosseous* Fourth lumbrical

*In the past, the first palmar interosseous muscle was considered part of the flexor pollicis brevis. The *true deep head* of the flexor pollicis brevis originates from the *carpal bones,* not from the first metacarpal bone. According to the previous system, there are only three palmar interossei, corresponding to palmar interossei 2 to 4 as described here.

many tendons to exert an independent action on the digit. The **thumb** receives one *long flexor tendon* (flexor pollicis longus), the three *thenar muscles* (abductor pollicis brevis, flexor pollicis brevis, and opponens pollicis), the *adductor pollicis,* and *first palmar interosseous muscles.* The **fifth finger** receives tendons of two *long flexors* (flexors digitorum superficialis and profundus), the three *hypothenar muscles* (abductor digiti minimi, flexor digiti minimi brevis, and opponens digiti minimi), and the *fourth palmar interosseous muscle.* The **index, long, and ring fingers** receive *two long flexor tendons* (flexor digitorum superficialis and profundus), all of the four *dorsal interosseous tendons,* and two of the *palmar interosseous tendons.* The long flexor tendons attach to the digit after traversing a specialized structure, the **fibrous flexor sheath,** while the thenar, hypothenar, and intrinsic hand muscles attach independently to various bones of the hand.

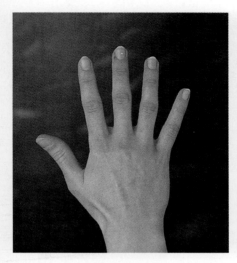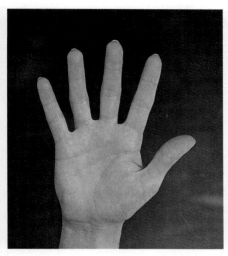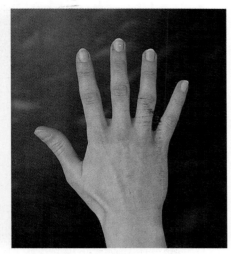

Figure 3-67 **CUTANEOUS DISTRIBUTION OF THE MEDIAN AND RADIAL NERVES IN THE HAND.**

FIBROUS FLEXOR SHEATHS

As the long flexor tendons and their synovial sheaths reach the level of the MP joints, each enters a cylindrical "canal" and travels more distally along the anterior surface of the digit (Figures 3-65 and 3-66). These canals are known as the **fibrous flexor sheaths.** The sheaths are anchored along both sides of the phalanges, and a fibrous band arches anteriorly, creating a closed cylinder over each phalanx through which the long tendons pass. The fibrous sheath is thickened on its anterior surface into five discrete **annular bands** or pulleys (see Figure 3-66). The first two are positioned over the level of the MP joint and proximal part of the proximal phalanx. The third pulley is at the level of the proximal IP joint, the fourth on the middle phalanx, and a small fifth pulley near the distal IP joint. Between

these annular pulleys are three crossed thin pulleys called **cruciate pulleys.** The rest of the fibrous flexor sheath is very thin, consisting largely of synovial membrane. This complex arrangement of pulleys allows the digits to flex fully without the individual pulleys interfering with each other's movements.

As **tendons of flexor digitorum superficialis** approach the middle phalanx, they split into two slips, which straddle the profundus tendon and attach to either side of the middle phalanx. This split permits the **tendon of flexor digitorum profundus** to pass between the two slips of the superficialis tendon and advance distally, where it will attach to the distal phalanx of the digit. The flexor synovial sheath of the fifth digit is continuous with the synovial space of the palm. Those of digits 2 to 5 are interrupted, while that of the thumb is separate altogether.

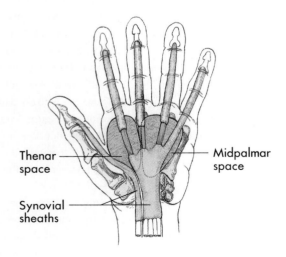

Thenar space

Midpalmar space

Synovial sheaths

Figure 3-68 SYNOVIAL SHEATHS AND FASCIAL COMPARTMENTS IN THE PALM.

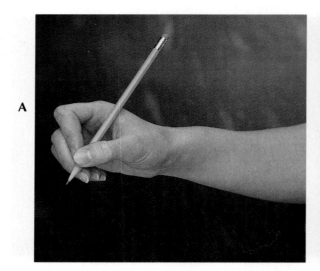 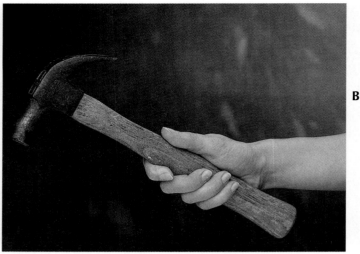

Figure 3-69 PRECISION AND POWER GRIPS. A, In the precision grip, the wrist and fingers are fixed by the larger muscles, and the intrinsic hand muscles make small incremental movements of the fingers. **B,** The power grip involves the long flexor tendons and the palmar muscles, and the object is to create a rigid grip on the object being held.

EXTENSOR EXPANSIONS (Sheaths or Hoods)

The extensor tendons for the index, middle, ring, and little fingers all insert on an **extensor expansion** (see Figure 3-63), an elongated triangular aponeurotic structure that extends from the level of the MP joint along the dorsal surface of the three phalanges of the digits. At the level of the MP joint, the base of the extensor expansion for each digit is tethered to the **deep transverse metacarpal ligament** (which links the palmar surfaces of the finger MP joints).

For the fingers, the **extensor digitorum tendon** is the central structure in the extensor mechanism. The extensor digitorum tendon passes over the dorsal surface of the MP joint and extends outward along the dorsal midline of the proximal phalanx. As it approaches the proximal IP joint the extensor digitorum tendon trifurcates. A **central slip of the tendon** crosses the proximal IP joint and inserts into the base of the middle phalanx. The two **lateral slips** pass along the lateral margin of the proximal IP joint and continue distally. These two slips cross the distal IP joint, are joined by the intrinsic muscle lateral bands, and insert into the base of the distal phalanx. Thus the expansion is loosely attached to the digits but still has considerable mobility. When the digits are flexed, the expansion slides distally, and, when the digits are extended, the expansion slides proximally.

The **dorsal** and **palmar interosseous muscles** insert on the extensor expansions, the dorsal group inserting more proximally than the palmar. For the *index, long,* and *ring fingers,* there are interosseous insertions on *both* sides of the expansion; for the *little finger,* the ab-

ductor digiti minimi inserts on the medial side of the expansion. The four **lumbrical muscles** insert on the lateral sides of the extensor expansions just distal to the interosseous insertions. Both the interossei and lumbricals make possible the simultaneous *flexion of the MP joints and extension of the IP joints,* a posture so important to the capabilities of the hand for fine manipu-

---

PRINCIPLES

TENDONS AND ABDOMINAL VISCERA

The long flexor tendons in the hand are encircled by a thin layer of synovium (the *"visceral mesotendon"*), a double layer of which reflects off of the tendons and then turns to form a lining of the interior of the flexor sheath through which the tendon passes (the *"parietal mesotendon"*). The small "pedicle" that connects the visceral and parietal mesotendons is discontinuous, so that the tendon appears to be "suspended" from the lining of the flexor sheath by a series of tiny strands of connective tissue. These are known as the **vincula** (L. *vincere,* to bond or join) (see Figure 3-63). Vascular and neural structures reach the tendon by sending small branches to the tendon through the vincula. The arrangement is exactly analogous to the mesenteries of the intestine and the pleural membranes in the chest. This arrangement greatly facilitates the easy movement of the tendon within the fibrous flexor sheath, just as the abdominal peritoneum and thoracic pleura facilitate movement of viscera within those body spaces.

THE OPPOSABLE HUMAN THUMB

Opposition is a combination of thumb flexion and abduction and involves the rotation of the thumb along its own long axis (during thumb flexion-extension) that prepares the "pulp" of the thumb (i.e., the surface opposite the nail) to meet the pulp surface of the other digits. More than any other movement, opposition greatly expands the opportunity to use the upper limb for grasping and manipulation of objects in the environment. The key evolutionary adaptations making opposition possible are (1) the increasing angle between the index finger and the thumb, and (2) the great flexibility of the carpometacarpal joint of the thumb.

Creating a cup-shaped recess in the palm of the hand requires movement of the other four digits as well. The hypothenar muscles allow the little finger to rotate around its long axis as well, to prepare for opposition with the thumb. The central digits are able to flex at the metacarpophalangeal joints while maintaining extension of the interphalangeal joints through the unique interactions of the long flexors, long extensors, and the interosseous/lumbrical muscles. The latter muscles permit flexion at the metacarpophalangeal joints while the long extensors maintain extension at the interphalangeal joints. This allows an object to be "cradled" in the palm before the fingers are closed over it (i.e., the interphalangeal joints are flexed) to secure it in place.

lation of small objects. The lumbrical muscles are unique in having a movable origin (the deep flexor tendons) and the ability to maintain a constant state of tension through a wider range of motion than can the interossei.

The extrinsic extensor tendons end and become part of the substance of the **extensor expansions** (or extensor hoods, extensor sheaths) **for digits two to five.** The extensor sheath is a triangular expansion of connective tissue positioned over the dorsum of each digit, with its base at the level of the metacarpophalangeal joint. The *lumbrical muscles,* the *interosseous muscles,* and the *long tendons of extensor digitorum, extensor indicis, extensor digiti minimi, and part of abductor digiti minimi* all attach to the extensor expansions rather than inserting directly on the bones of the digits. This extensor expansion is loosely attached proximally, by thin filaments, to the **deep transverse metacarpal ligament,** and covers the dorsal and lateral surfaces of the metacarpophalangeal joints. The tendons of **extensor digitorum, extensor indicis,** and **extensor digiti minimi** all attach to the proximal margin of the extensor expansion on their

respective digits. The **lumbrical muscles** and **interossei** attach to the expansion at its posterolateral angle (the **dorsal interossei** have an additional slip by which they attach directly to the proximal phalanx as well).

The extensor mechanism causes contraction of the long extensor muscles, the interossei, and the lumbricals to affect the entire digit and eliminates the necessity for each of these muscles to have separate tendinous insertions on the three phalanges of each digit. This economy of structure adds to the mobility of each digit. This mechanism also prevents any hyperextension of individual interphalangeal joints—but the joint anatomy does not permit any significant degree of extension anyway, and such movement would not add to the important capabilities of the hand.

BLOOD VESSELS OF THE HAND

The hand is supplied with blood through **deep** and **superficial palmar arches** (see Figure 3-44). The radial and ulnar arteries contribute to both arches, but in most cases the radial artery is the prime source to the deep arch and the ulnar artery the prime supply to the superficial arch. The superficial arch lies just deep to the palmar aponeurosis, while the deep arch is positioned more proximally deep to the long flexor tendons.

The **superficial branch of the radial artery** branches from the parent vessel just above the wrist. It runs across the base of the thenar muscles and joins the superficial palmar arch. The **deep branch of the radial artery** continues across the floor of the anatomic snuff box (see pp. 372-373), then passes between the two heads of the first dorsal interosseous muscle to reach the deep space of the palm. Variably it gives off a large *princeps pollicis branch* and then continues medially as the **deep palmar arch.** Three **common digital arteries** arise from the arch, and each travels distally toward the webspaces between the digits. Here they anastomose with similar branches from the superficial arch. At the base of the digits, each common digital artery divides into a pair of **proper digital arteries,** which travel distally along the adjacent sides of each pair of digits. In addition, the deep arch emits single branches for the lateral side of the second digit and the medial side of the fifth digit.

The **ulnar artery** lies lateral to the ulnar nerve at the wrist, where both pass across the surface of the flexor retinaculum deep to palmaris brevis. The artery then passes just lateral to the pisiform bone, between it and the hamate bone. The **deep branch of the ulnar artery** separates and descends between the flexor digiti minimi and the abductor digiti minimi to anastomose with the larger deep branch of the radial artery, to complete the deep palmar arch. It is accompanied by the **deep branch of the ulnar nerve.** The **superficial branch of**

THE HAND

DUPUYTREN'S CONTRACTURE

Dupuytren's contracture is a tightening of the palmar fascia, resulting in a forced partial flexion of the metacarpophalangeal and proximal interphalangeal joints, commonly involving the ring (fourth) finger. The skin of the palm displays a raised vertical ridge extending from the heel of the hand to the base of the ring finger. Surgical removal of the contracted connective tissue is often necessary to loosen the contracted finger.

MEDIAN NERVE INJURY AT THE WRIST

A low median nerve injury, such as the one that occurs via compression in carpal tunnel syndrome, affects the tone and strength of the thenar muscles and the sensory innervation of the lateral three and one-half digits. The long forearm flexor muscles are not involved because the branches of the median nerve innervating them depart from the parent nerve before it reaches the wrist.

HIGH AND LOW LESIONS IN THE ULNAR NERVE

An injury to the ulnar nerve low in the forearm or at the wrist denervates most of the intrinsic hand muscles and leads to a *claw hand*. This results because the long deep flexor tendons on the medial side of the hand, also innervated by the ulnar nerve, remain intact and exert an unopposed flexor pull on the ring and little fingers. If the ulnar nerve injury is high enough in the forearm, however, it injures the branches to the two medial tendons of the flexor digitorum profundus as well as the more distal branches to the intrinsic hand muscles, and less claw hand deformity results.

TROPHIC RELATIONSHIPS BETWEEN NERVES AND MUSCLES

Muscle wasting in carpal tunnel syndrome is a good illustration of the **trophic relationship** that exists between striated muscle and the nerves that innervate them. When the nerve input to such a muscle is interrupted, the muscle wastes away, loses its strength, and in time becomes much reduced in size. Even when the nerve-muscle relationship remains intact, if physiologic transmission of impulses is blocked, the muscle similarly wastes away. Smooth muscle is innervated by autonomic nerves, but no such trophic relationship exists in the case of smooth muscle.

INFECTIONS IN THE HAND

The palmar fascia is such a thick and strong sheet of tissue that even when infections or other sources of irritation are localized on the palmar side of the hand, the swelling appears on the dorsum of the hand, where the fascial covering is very much thinner and less strong.

COMMON CONGENITAL DEFORMITIES IN THE HAND

Since the development of the hand is so intricate, and involves a highly synchronized series of events, it is no surprise that a variety of developmental errors occurs. The upper limb develops along a proximal to distal gradient. Earlier developmental errors tend to affect the shoulder and arm, and later developing errors involve the forearm and hand. The bones of the arm, forearm, wrist, and hand may be duplicated or absent in part. The symmetry of the hand may be altered, or certain segments of the upper limb may be small in comparison to other parts of the limb. One of the most common errors is **syndactyly,** when digits are fused along their adjacent sides.

the **ulnar artery** arises lateral to the hook of the hamate bone, travels distally on the surface of the flexor digiti minimi, and forms the superficial palmar arch at the midpoint of the metacarpals, distal to the level at which the deep arch lies. From the arch originate three **common digital arteries** (for webspaces between the digits), accompanied by like branches of the ulnar and median nerves. Similar to branches of the radial artery, these common digital arteries divide into **proper digital arteries** for the adjacent sides of the digits. There is also a single proper digital artery for the medial surface of the fifth digit.

NERVES IN THE HAND

The cutaneous innervation of the hand is provided by superficial branches of the **ulnar, median,** and **radial nerves,** as shown in Figures 3-67 and 3-68. All of the intrinsic muscles in the hand are innervated by branches of the median or ulnar nerves. Interruption of muscular innervation may be inferred by the functional losses characteristic of injuries to the individual nerves. Thus interruption of the *median nerve* (see Figure 3-27) affects the *thenar muscles* most dramatically and leads to loss of sensation on the *lateral side* of the anterior surface of the hand. Low injury to the *ulnar nerve* causes sensory loss on the *medial side* of the hand, on both anterior and posterior surfaces, and loss of function of the *hypothenar muscles* and most of the *intrinsic muscles* of the hand (lumbricals, interossei). The latter loss produces a characteristic "claw deformity" appearance of the hand.

MOVEMENTS AND FUNCTIONS OF THE HAND

The **central fixed unit of the hand,** consisting of the distal row of carpal bones and the second and third metacarpals, is a relatively immobile point around which the thumb, fourth, and fifth fingers move. The carpometacarpal joints of the index and middle fingers are relatively less mobile than those for the thumb, ring, and little fingers; the middle, ring, and little fingers flex as a unit and serve to stabilize objects for manipulation by the index finger and thumb.

The myriad muscles attaching to the hand give it the ability to participate in a wide variety of positions and movements. The hand may be used to grab hold of an object and grip it firmly while muscles of the forearm, arm, and shoulder contract to move the object in space. In this motion, little or no fine control is produced. Examples of this movement are (1) pulling downward on the cord of a window shade and (2) pushing or pulling on the oars while rowing. This function is known as the **power grip** (Figure 3-69, *B*). A second type of "nonprecision" grip is used when carrying a briefcase or lifting a bucket by its handle. This grip is similar to the "brachiation" described earlier (see p. 385) because the emphasis is on strength of the digits. Precise hand movements are not produced through these mechanisms.

In comparison, the **precision grip** (Figure 3-69, *A*) relies heavily on the thenar, hypothenar, lumbrical, and interosseous muscles. These intrinsic hand muscles assume prime importance and control the digital movements, while the long flexor and extensor tendons help stabilize the hand. The tip of the thumb is brought into opposition with the distal ends of the other digits, and a maximum of fine control is made possible. The concavity of the hand is created by the carpal bones, which are fixed in position and create a concave shape, and the intrinsic muscles of the hand, which can cooperate to create a "cup-shape" further distal in the palm of the hand. The **opposition** between the thumb and the other digits is in large measure made possible by the unique movements of the thumb. The various muscles that act on it do not function strictly in flexion-extension or abduction-adduction but rather act like a set of guy-wires, which can pull on the thumb from a variety of angles. Crucial to opposition is the ability of the thumb to rotate around its long axis, so that the "pad" of the thumb can face the other digits. The metacarpals of the ring and little fingers are also capable of a limited degree of rotation.

The metacarpal bone of the thumb, from an evolutionary viewpoint, resembles the proximal phalanx of the other digits, and the trapezium is the bone comparable to the metacarpal bone of the other digits. This is supported by the fact that (1) for the thumb, the extensor expansion runs along the dorsal surface of the metacarpal and the two phalanges (whereas it runs along the dorsum of the three phalanges for the other digits), and (2) the epiphyseal plate of the thumb metacarpal is proximal, like that of the proximal phalanges for the other digits, and does not resemble the pattern of maturation for the metacarpals of digits two to five (see Figures 3-50 and 3-56).

Systems Review and Surface Anatomy of the Upper Limb

▶ Musculoskeletal Anatomy of the Upper Limb

▶ Vascular Supply of the Upper Limb

▶ Lymphatic Drainage of the Upper Limb

▶ Innervation of the Upper Limb

▶ Surface Anatomy and Physical Examination of the Upper Limb

MUSCULOSKELETAL ANATOMY OF THE UPPER LIMB

The **shoulder girdle** (see Figure 3-1) comprises the **clavicle** and **scapula.** The shoulder girdle attaches the upper limb to the trunk and increases the mobility of the upper limb by suspending it at some distance from the surface of the chest wall. The scapula is capable of *retraction* and *protraction* (backward-forward sliding along the curved surface of the chest wall), *elevation* and *depression,* or *rotation* in its own horizontal plane (Table 3-16). This rotation is integral to full abduction of the upper limb. The clavicle has little intrinsic movement, but it serves as the only true articulation of the entire upper limb complex with the trunk (the **sternoclavicular joint**). Most of what holds the upper limb to the body wall is represented by muscles. Separate groups of muscles attach the upper limb to the shoulder girdle (e.g., the **deltoid** and **rotator cuff muscles**), the shoulder girdle to the chest wall (e.g., **serratus anterior,** the **rhomboid muscles**), and the upper limb directly to the chest wall (e.g., **pectoralis major, latissimus dorsi**).

The **glenohumeral** joint can flex, extend, adduct, abduct, and circumduct. It achieves a maximum of mobility and flexibility but does so at the expense of strength and stability.

The **humerus** is characterized by a proximal rounded head, directed superomedially, and a straight and relatively simple shaft with a marked groove on its upper anterior head, the **intertubercular groove.** Its distal end flares into a pair of triangular ridges, the **lateral** and **medial epicondyles.** The distal surface of the humerus is made up of two rounded swellings, the **capitulum** and the **trochlea.** The former articulates with the head of the radius and the latter with the olecranon process of the ulna.

The two forearm bones are the medially placed **ulna** and the laterally placed **radius.** The ulna forms the major articulation with the humerus; the radius is represented by only the articulation of the radial head with the capitulum of the humerus. Distally, however, it is the radius that articulates with the carpal (wrist) bones, while the ulna has no direct articulation with them. The **interosseous membrane** links the ulna and radius and transfers forces between them.

The **wrist** consists of eight bones arranged in two rough curved parallel rows of four bones each. The proximal row includes the **scaphoid, lunate, triquetrum,** and **pisiform,** while the distal row includes the **trapezium, trapezoid, capitate,** and **hamate.** Each is linked by a series of small synovial joints and reinforcing ligaments to its neighboring bones. It is the scaphoid and lunate bones that form most of the articu-

Table 3-16   Movements at Upper Limb Joints

Joint	Flexion	Extension	Adduction	Abduction	Other
Shoulder (glenohumeral joint)	Pectoralis major Deltoid (anterior) Coracobrachialis	Deltoid (posterior) Teres major Latissimus dorsi	Pectoralis major Latissimus dorsi Teres major/minor Coracobrachialis	Supraspinatus Deltoid	Medial rotation: pectoralis major, subscapularis, teres major Lateral roation: teres minor, infraspiratus Circumduction: serial flexion, abduction, extension, adduction
Elbow	Biceps brachii Brachialis Brachioradialis	Triceps brachii Anconeus	—	—	Pronation*: pronator quadratus, pronator teres Supination*: biceps brachii, supinator
Wrist (radiocarpal joint)	Flexor carpi ulnaris Flexor carpi radialis	Extensor carpi radialis longus and brevis Extensor carpi ulnaris	Flexor carpi ulnaris Extensor carpi ulnaris	Flexor carpi radialis Extensor carpi radialis longus and brevis	Circumduction: serial flexion, abduction, extension, adduction, etc.
Carpo-metacarpal	Thumb: flexor pollicis longus, flexor pollicis brevis Little finger: flexor digiti minimi Digits 2-5: long flexor tendons	Thumb: extensor pollicis longus and brevis; abductor pollicis longus Fingers: long extensor tendons	Thumb: adductor pollicis	Thumb: abductor pollicis longus and brevis Digit 5: abductor digit minimi	Opposition (thumb): opponens pollicis, abductor pollicis brevis and longus Opposition (digit 5): opponens digiti minimi
Metacarpo-phalangeal	Thumb: flexor pollicis longus, flexor pollicis brevis, abductor pollicis brevis, adductor pollicis Digits 2-5: interossei, lumbricals, flexor digitorum profundus and superficialis Digit 5: flexor digiti minimi	All long extensor tendons for digits 2-5	Thumb: adductor pollicis Digits 1, 2, 4, 5: palmar interossei	Thumb: abductor pollicis longus and brevis, flexor pollicis brevis Digits 2-4: dorsal interossei	—
Inter-phalangeal	Flexor digitorum profundus and superficialis	Interossei Lumbricals All long extensors inserting on extensor expansions	—	—	—

*Pronation and supination occur at the *radioulnar* joints.

lation with the distal end of the radius (the **radiocarpal joint**). The distal row of carpal bones articulates with the bases of the five metacarpal bones. The trapezium articulates only with the thumb metacarpal at a special saddle-shaped joint.

The numerous muscles acting on each of the joints of the upper limb have been described elsewhere in the text. Here are indicated the spinal cord segments that innervate the groups of muscles acting on certain joints. Even when many seemingly disparate muscles cooperate to act on a joint, it is understandable that this particular set of muscles works as a group because they share a common innervation (Table 3-17).

VASCULAR SUPPLY OF THE UPPER LIMB

The upper limb is supplied with arterial blood through the subclavian artery and its numerous branches. Several important branches of the **subclavian artery,** including the suprascapular, transverse cervical, and dorsal scapular, supply structures of the scapula and its attached muscles. The continuation of the subclavian

Table 3-17   Segmental Innervation of Muscles Acting on Joints

Movement(s)	Segments	Representative Muscles
Shoulder abduction	C5	Deltoid, supraspinatus
Shoulder adduction	C6 to C8	Teres muscles, pectoralis major
Elbow flexion	C7 to C8	Biceps, brachialis
Elbow extension	C6	Triceps
Supination	C6	Biceps, supinator
Pronation	C7 to C8	Pronator teres, pronator quadratus
Wrist flexion	C6 to C8	Flexor carpi radialis/ulnaris
Wrist extension	C6 to C7	Extensor carpi radialis/ulnaris
Digital flexion (long muscles)	C7 to C8	Flexor digitorum superficialis and profundus
Digital extension (long muscles)	C7 to C8	Extensor digitorum, extensor indicis, extensor digiti minimi
Digital abduction	C8 to T1	Dorsal interossei, lumbricals 1 and 2
Digital adduction	C8 to T1	Palmar interossei, lumbricals 3 and 4

artery, the **axillary artery,** also contributes several branches to the same region. An important **anastomosis** exists around the **scapula,** including the **subscapular artery** (from the axillary), the **suprascapular** and **dorsal scapular** (from the subclavian), the **thoracoacromial** and **humeral circumflex arteries** (from the axillary), and various other smaller branches of the axillary artery.

The **brachial artery** supplies the arm and gives off the **deep brachial artery,** which accompanies the radial nerve in a spiral course around the posterior surface of the humerus. At its termination, the brachial artery gives off the **superior ulnar** and **radial collateral** branches, which descend and take part in the important anastomosis around the elbow.

In the upper forearm the brachial artery divides into the radial and ulnar arteries. The **radial artery** descends in the anterior forearm, lying just deep to the medial edge of the brachioradialis muscle. Near the wrist it gives off a **superficial branch,** which courses across the flexor retinaculum to enter the thenar muscles, finally to contribute to the superficial palmar arterial arch at the level of the midshaft of the metacarpal bones. The **deep branch** (the continuation of the radial artery) descends in a posterior direction and crosses the scaphoid and trapezium on the floor of the "anatomic snuff box," passes between the two heads of the first dorsal interosseous muscle, and terminates in the deep palmar arterial arch at the level of the metacarpal bases in a plane just anterior to the interosseous muscles.

The **ulnar artery** descends in the forearm deep to the flexor carpi ulnaris and, on reaching the wrist, divides into a larger superficial and a smaller deep branch. The **deep branch** passes lateral to the hamate bone and descends into the palm to join the deep palmar arch. The larger **superficial branch** forms the majority of the **superficial palmar arch.**

LYMPHATIC DRAINAGE OF THE UPPER LIMB

Most of the lymphatic drainage of the upper limb converges on lymph nodes and vessels in the **axilla.** There are several distinct groups of axillary lymph nodes, including the **pectoral, subscapular, lateral,** and **apical.** These communicate with lymphatic channels on the breast, anterior chest wall, and regions near the clavicle. Lymph from all these regions eventually converges on a **right lymphatic duct** and the **thoracic duct** on the left, both of which enter the venous circulation near the junction of the subclavian and internal jugular veins on their respective sides (see Thorax, Section One, for more details).

INNERVATION OF THE UPPER LIMB

The entire upper limb is innervated by branches of the **brachial plexus,** with the exception of a few twigs that innervate the skin of the medial arm (where the innervation arises from T2). The brachial plexus arises from the roots of spinal segments C5 to C8 and T1, with inconsistent contributions from C4 and T2. The five major roots of the plexus rearrange themselves into superior, middle, and inferior **trunks.** Each trunk gives off an anterior and a posterior **division,** which in turn reassemble into the lateral, medial, and posterior **cords** (the cords are named for their relationship to the second part of the axillary artery). The primary spinal roots responsible for movements at the joints of the upper limb are listed in Table 3-17.

Table 3-18 lists all of the muscles derived from the posterior or anterior (**postaxial** or **preaxial**) side of the developing limb. The pattern of branching within the brachial plexus is complex but not chaotic; in fact, the posterior divisions of each of the trunks contain axons that innervate striated muscles derived from the posterior or dorsal mesoderm of the developing limb.

Table 3-18 Mesodermal Origin and Innervation of Upper Limb Muscles

Muscles Derived from Posterior Mesoderm (Postaxial) and Innervated by Branches of Posterior Cord		Muscles Derived from Anterior Mesoderm (Preaxial) and Innervated by Branches of Lateral or Medial Cord	
Muscle	Nerve	Muscle	Nerve
Deltoid	Axillary		
Supraspinatus	Suprascapular	Pectoralis major	Lateral and medial pectoral
Infraspinatus	"	Pectoralis minor	Lateral pectoral
Subscapularis	Upper subscapular	Coracobrachialis	Musculocutaneous
Latissimus dorsi	Thoracodorsal	Biceps brachii	"
Teres major	Lower subscapular	Pronator teres	Median
Teres minor	Axillary	Flexor carpi radialis	"
Triceps	Radial	Palmaris longus	"
Anconeus	"	Flexor digitorum superficialis	"
Extensor carpi radialis longus	"	Flexor digitorum profundus	Median and ulnar
Extensor carpi radialis brevis	"	Flexor carpi ulnaris	Ulnar
Extensor digitorum	"	Flexor pollicis longus	Median
Extensor digiti minimi	"	All thenar muscles	Median
Extensor carpi ulnaris	"	Adductor pollicis	Ulnar
Brachioradialis	"	All hypothenar muscles	Ulnar
Supinator	"	All interossei	Ulnar
		Lateral two lumbricals	Median
		Medial two lumbricals	Ulnar
		Palmaris brevis	Ulnar

In the upper limb, this is the **posterior cord,** which branches into a variety of nerves, the largest of which are the **axillary nerve** and the **radial nerve.** In like fashion, the anterior divisions of the brachial plexus combine and form the **lateral** and **medial cords.** The major branches of these cords are the **musculocutaneous, median,** and **ulnar nerves.**

The **cutaneous innervation** of the upper limb creates the **dermatomes** of the upper limb. The C5 root is represented on the lateral border of the shoulder and upper arm, the C6 root is represented on the lateral border of the forearm and the thumb side of the hand, C7 is represented in midpalm, C8 on the ulnar side of the hand and up the medial side of the forearm, and T1 on the upper medial forearm and part of the medial side of the arm. T2 innervates the remainder of the medial arm up to the axilla.

SURFACE ANATOMY AND PHYSICAL EXAMINATION OF THE UPPER LIMB

Surface anatomy and physical examination of the upper limb include assessment of the shoulder region, the arm, forearm, wrist, and hand. The **vertebral border** and **inferior angle of the scapula** are easily palpable in almost all patients (Figure 3-70). On the anterior surface of the shoulder region, the **acromion** should first be located at the lateral end of the **scapular spine.**

Moving the hand medially on to the **clavicle** allows palpation of the **acromioclavicular joint,** reinforced heavily by ligaments. The joint should be firm and nearly immobile.

The **coracoid process** of the scapula is palpable just inferior to the lateral third of the clavicle. Feeling further medially along the **clavicle,** note the *sigmoid-shaped curve* at the midpoint of the clavicle and the medial third, which protrudes further forward than the lateral third. Just deep to this S-shaped curve in the midclavicle lies the **subclavian vein,** and palpation of this clavicular curve is a significant landmark to placement of a catheter into the vein, located by passing a needle just deep to the clavicle and passing it medially, in the direction of the acromion on the opposite shoulder. A catheter placed in the subclavian vein may be threaded into the heart. This vein is frequently cannulated as part of the care of the seriously ill patient, where frequent blood samples and measurement of pressures within the heart are useful in patient management. At the medial end of the clavicle is the **sternoclavicular joint.** The mobility of this joint can be appreciated by placing an examining finger on the anterior surface of the joint while the upper limb is rotated through a wide range of motion.

The medial end of the **clavicle** can be palpated, moving in its shallow socket on the lateral side of the **manubrium** of the **sternum.** Passing on to the surface

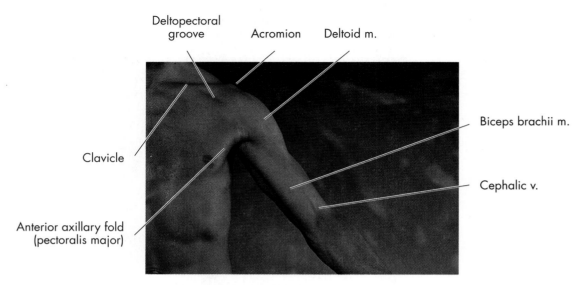

Deltopectoral groove   Acromion   Deltoid m.

Biceps brachii m.

Cephalic v.

Clavicle

Anterior axillary fold
(pectoralis major)

Figure 3-70   SURFACE ANATOMY OF THE UPPER LIMB.   Anterior view.

of the manubrium, slide the fingers inferiorly and ap-preciate the horizontal raised bony ridge known as the **sternal angle.** Just lateral to the sternal angle is the ar-ticulation of the **second rib** with the sternum.

Sliding the examining hand inferiorly across the an-terior chest wall allows identification of the thick **pec-toralis major** muscle. It originates from the medial third of the clavicle, the upper eight costal cartilages and sternum, and the external oblique fascia. The mus-cle passes laterally and, as it does, narrows into a thick-ened cylinder, which attaches to the **medial border of the intertubercular groove** of the upper end of the **humerus.** The free inferior margin of the pectoralis major is felt as the **anterior axillary fold,** defining the anterior border of the axillary space. By inspection, it is often possible to identify a shallow groove lying along the upper border of the pectoralis major and inferior border of the deltoid muscle. This is the **deltopectoral groove,** and it is filled in life with the **cephalic vein,** a major superficial vein of the arm and forearm, which here penetrates the deep fascial layer and drains into the **axillary vein.**

Moving to the posterior surface of the shoulder (Figure 3-71), palpate the **scapular spine** to the point where it blends with the medial border of the scapula. Inferior to the scapular spine is the **infraspinous fossa,** filled in life with the infraspinatus and teres muscles. Inferior to the inferior angle of scapula, the substance of the body wall is formed by the latissimus dorsi mus-cle, which sweeps upward and laterally from the small of the back to insert on the proximal humerus. The in-ferior margin of the latissimus dorsi forms the posterior axillary fold, the posterior limit of the axilla. Near the

inferior angle of the scapula is the so-called **triangle of auscultation,** a small gap in the otherwise thick muscu-lature of the posterior wall. This small gap is bounded by the latissimus dorsi and trapezius muscles along with the edge of the scapula and is the best place in which to examine the posterior segments of the lungs with the stethoscope since it is a small gap in the other-wise thick musculature overlying the back. Above the scapular spine is the **supraspinous fossa,** filled in life with the supraspinatus muscle. The upper contour of the shoulder, extending from the acromion to the base of the neck, is formed by the trapezius muscle. Extending laterally from the acromion, forming the rounded contour on the top of the shoulder, is the del-toid muscle.

The hand can be placed on the scapular spine and the person being examined can be asked to move his or her upper limb through a wide range of motions—flex-ion, extension, adduction, etc.—to note the unique movements of the scapula itself. The scapula can slide anteriorly or posteriorly around the chest wall (*protrac-tion* and *retraction*), be *elevated* or *depressed,* and can *ro-tate* around its own horizontal plane.

Moving on to the arm (see Figure 3-71), it is some-times possible to palpate the greater tubercle at the proximal humerus but only when the deltoid muscle is rather thin. The **deltoid tuberosity** is usually palpable on the anterolateral aspect of the shaft of the humerus near its midpoint. Inferiorly, one can palpate the **lateral** and **medial supracondylar ridges** and the **lateral** and **medial epicondyles.** On the posterior side of the arm, one can palpate the shaft of the humerus and appreci-ate its articulation with the prominent olecranon

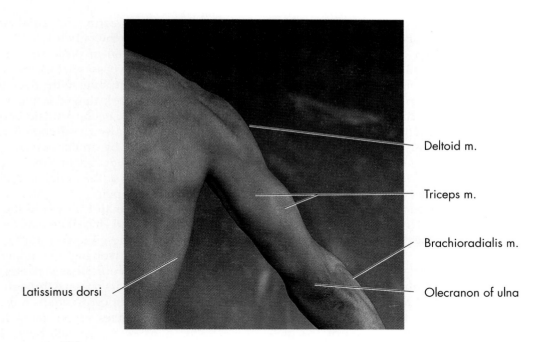

Figure 3-71 **SURFACE ANATOMY OF THE UPPER LIMB.**   Posterior view.

process of the ulna, forming the major component of the elbow joint. Anteriorly, in the crook of the elbow, is the **cubital fossa** (see Figure 3-29), a depression that deepens as the elbow joint is flexed. The cubital fossa is bounded laterally by the brachioradialis muscle and medially by the pronator teres. The biceps muscle forms a flattened distal sheetlike extension, the **bicipital aponeurosis** (also called **lacertus fibrosus**), downward on to the fascia covering the pronator teres on the medial side of the upper forearm. The **brachial artery** and **median nerve** lie just deep to this fibrous sheet.

By applying a tourniquet to the upper arm the many **superficial veins** of the forearm and elbow region can be distended. These vessels are frequent sites for both blood sampling and the infusion of drugs and fluids. The pattern of superficial venous anatomy is quite variable, but most individuals have a laterally placed **cephalic vein** running the length of the arm and forearm, a medial **basilic vein** occupying the superficial tissues in the forearm and lower arm but ascending into the deep compartment in midarm, a **median cubital vein** traveling diagonally across the cubital fossa of the elbow, and a **median vein of the forearm** lying in between the cephalic and basilic veins and roughly parallel to them (see Figure 3-45).

The hand can be placed on the proximal radius (see Figure 3-71) and the patient asked to **pronate** and **supinate** several times. The **radius** can be felt rotating around its own long axis as it moves medially, across the ulna in pronation, and returns to a more lateral position in supination. The whole subcutaneous shaft of the ulna is easily palpable on the posteromedial side of

the forearm, while the radius is less easily palpable along the lateral margin of the forearm. Distally, the **radial styloid process** is clearly palpable as a small rounded eminence just proximal to the wrist on its lateral border. The **ulnar styloid process** is easily palpable and visible as a smaller rounded eminence protruding posteromedially just proximal to the wrist, with the head of the ulna on the posterior aspect, especially prominent on pronation.

At the wrist, on its anterior surface, the **pisiform bone** and hook process of the **hamate bone** are palpable on the medial side. They represent the two medial bony attachments of the **flexor retinaculum** (see Figure 3-54). Less easy to palpate are the **scaphoid tubercle** and **trapezium,** the two lateral attachments of the flexor retinaculum. Moving further distally, the thumb metacarpal is easily palpable, while the metacarpals of the fingers are palpable dorsally. The metacarpophalangeal and interphalangeal joints of each digit are easily palpable as well.

The upper limb offers several opportunities to assess the function of the **deep tendon reflexes.** With the patient's upper limb resting on a table with the elbow flexed, the examiner's thumb can be placed on the **biceps tendon,** and the thumb tapped with a reflex hammer. The patient's biceps muscle should twitch in response to the stimulus. This tests the integrity of spinal *cord segments C5 to C6* in the musculocutaneous nerve. Next, the patient's relaxed elbow should be lifted off the table with the olecranon pointing skyward. Tapping on the distal tendon on the **triceps muscle** as it blends into the olecranon process of the ulna should elicit a twitch contraction of the belly of the triceps. This tests the integrity of the radial nerve and the spinal *cord segments C7 and C8,* which innervate this muscle. The **brachioradialis muscle** can be tested in a similar fashion by resting the upper limb in a flexed elbow position with the hand held in a vertical plane. Tapping on the radius a few centimeters inferior to the elbow produces a stretch in the muscle and results in a reflexive contraction of the brachioradialis muscle. This tests the integrity of spinal *cord segments C5 to C6 to C7* in the radial nerve.

Refer to Figure 3-48 and review the **cutaneous innervation of the upper limb.** Deficits in sensory testing can suggest damage to particular nerves or to spinal cord segments, depending on the pattern of sensory abnormality observed.

Pulses are palpable at several points in the upper limb. The overall integrity of the circulation to the upper limb may be assessed first by noting the color of the digits and the **capillary refill time** in them. This is determined simply by pressing on the skin of one of the digits, temporarily blanching that area of skin, and noting the time required for the color to return to the skin when the pressure is released. A normal circulatory system produces capillary refill in 1 to 2 seconds. Significantly longer filling times suggest that the patient's heart is not beating strongly, or that the patient's vascular system (i.e., the total capacity of the blood vessels and heart) is not adequately filled with blood (as a result of severe vomiting, diarrhea, or hemorrhage).

Beginning proximally, one may palpate a strong pulse along the medial side of the upper arm (the **brachial artery**). The second opportunity for location of the **brachial pulse** is as it courses along the medial side of the distal humerus and passes beneath the bicipital aponeurosis into the forearm. The **radial artery** may be palpated just medial to the radial styloid process in the distal forearm and again in the base of the anatomic snuff box as the artery passes across the scaphoid and trapezium bones to contribute to the deep palmar arch. The **ulnar artery** may be palpated in the distal forearm just lateral to the hook of the hamate bone. Here the artery divides into its deep and superficial branches, accompanied as it does by similar branches of the ulnar nerve. The deep and superficial palmar arterial arches, derived from branches of the radial and ulnar arteries, are not palpable at any point.

The location of the **major nerves** in the upper limb should be borne in mind since they may be injured as a result of trauma or exposed to risk during a variety of invasive procedures involving the upper limb. The **ulnar nerve** is very superficial as it passes posterior to the medial epicondyle. Its passage through the forearm is protected by the flexor carpi ulnaris muscle, but near the wrist it again becomes superficial as it passes just lateral to the hook of the hamate bone. The **median nerve** lies just deep to the bicipital aponeurosis in the cubital fossa and may be injured with repeated needle sticks in an attempt to cannulate the median cubital vein. The nerve is deep to the flexor digitorum superficialis throughout most of the forearm, but near the wrist it lies very near to the surface, just medial to the tendon of flexor carpi radialis, just before passing beneath the flexor retinaculum. The **recurrent motor branch** of the median nerve, responsible for innervation of the thenar muscles, is just below the skin about midway along the medial surface of the thenar eminence. It is quite vulnerable to injury in lacerations of the palm.

3.9

Upper Limb

CASE 1

A 17-YEAR-OLD HIGH SCHOOL FOOTBALL PLAYER GETS HURT

A 17-year-old male football athlete was engaged in a "blocking drill," where he was asked to "drive" his shoulder repeatedly into a thin pad attached to a metal frame. He experienced considerable pain on one impact and heard a "cracking" noise at that same time. He was taken to the locker room, and, on removal of his shirt and pads, it was noted that his right upper limb seemed to be "hanging" low, and there was a conspicuous bump on the top of his shoulder. Attempts to abduct the shoulder, whether carried out by the patient or by his examiners, caused extreme pain. On examination, the shoulder was exquisitely tender (painful) near the bump and less so on nearby areas of skin.

Questions

1. What is the nature of the injury, and what anatomic structures are involved?
2. What accounts for the protuberant "bump" on the crown of the shoulder?
3. What sort of treatment is recommended for injuries of this sort?

CASE 2

FACILITATING THE REPAIR OF EXTENSIVE WRIST AND HAND INJURIES

A 24-year-old farmer inadvertently had his left hand and wrist run over by a tractor and the blade attached to its front end. He suffered numerous superficial lacerations on both the anterior and posterior sides, and it was clear that certain deeper blood vessels and tendons had been lacerated as well. His surgeon realized that a prolonged period of repair of these tendons and vessels and the cleaning and closure of more superficial lacerations would be required. The anesthesiologist recommended that a single injection of anesthetic agent might be used to make these repairs possible with no discomfort to the patient.

Questions

1. In what single region might an anesthetic be injected to produce anesthesia throughout the forearm, wrist, and hand?
2. What anatomic landmarks guide the placement of this anesthetic agent?

CASE 3

INABILITY TO MOVE ONE ARM IN A NEWBORN INFANT

A large female newborn infant (nine and one-half pounds) was delivered vaginally with some difficulty. In particular, after the baby's head had emerged from the birth canal, the shoulders seemed to be "stuck." The obstetrician gently turned the baby's head so that it was facing to the left and then pulled downward on the head and neck in an effort to get the upward-facing (anterior or right) shoulder of the baby to emerge next. After a few moments this was accomplished, and thereafter the left shoulder emerged relatively easily, as did the trunk and remainder of the body. The baby cried immediately, was active and vigorous, and was pronounced in good health. Later that day, however, it was noticed that the baby seemed not to move her right upper limb very well, while she freely moved her left upper limb and both lower limbs. Moreover, the right upper limb seemed to be held close alongside the body, with the elbow extended and the forearm pronated.

Questions

1. What accounts for the combination of upper limb abnormalities observed in this baby?
2. What mechanism likely produced the injuries seen here?
3. What is the likely outcome in cases such as these?

■ *CASE 4*

A 27-YEAR-OLD MALE INVOLVED IN A SERIOUS AUTOMOBILE ACCIDENT

A 27-year-old male was a belted passenger in an auto crossing an intersection when the car was hit on the rider's side by a speeding car running through a red light. The impact occurred directly on the young male passenger's right arm. He was removed from the auto by ambulance personnel and transported to a local hospital. His head and neck were uninjured, apart from superficial abrasions and a "whiplash." His right upper limb, however, had a spreading hematoma on the lateral surface of the arm, and an x-ray confirmed a clean midshaft fracture of the humerus. It was noted on the x-ray that the proximal fragment of the humerus was tightly applied to the wall of the axilla and that the upper end of the distal humeral fragment seemed to have slipped superior and lateral to the proximal humeral fragment. Over the course of the next several hours, the patient experienced a progressive weakness in extension of his right elbow, and he noted that his wrist began to drop (wrist in a flexed position). The patient was unable to extend his wrist. He could still flex his elbow on command, though weakly in comparison to normal. He could still supinate and pronate his forearm. He still could curl his fingers into a partial fist although he could not close his fist tightly. Sensation was intact on the anterior surfaces of his arm and hand but inconsistent on the dorsal surface of the forearm and hand.

Questions

1. Why is the proximal humeral fragment adducted? Why did the distal fragment slide superior and lateral to the proximal fragment?
2. What accounts for the weakness in elbow flexion?
3. Why are supination and pronation intact?
4. Why was he unable to extend his wrist, and why was wrist flexion limited? Why was finger flexion limited?

■ *CASE 5*

EXCESSIVE EXERCISE AT THE ELBOW JOINT

A 46-year-old right-handed college professor decided that he would show his 15-year-old son, a new member of the high school tennis team, that he could still provide him with some high-level competition on the tennis courts. The professor had not played tennis regularly for years but felt he could rely on his always-strong serve to impress his son. The two volleyed for a long period and then played two vigorous sets of tennis. The son diplomatically allowed his father to pre-vail in the first set, and then darkness mercifully fell so the match was discontinued. The next morning the father found it very painful to attempt to grasp something with his right hand, his elbow joint was visibly swollen, and he was forced to withdraw from the planned completion of the tennis match with his son. After taking some antiinflammatory medication, the pain abated and he was able to hold things in his hand. He tried to do some work in his shop later in the afternoon and found that use of a screwdriver produced excruciating pain in his elbow once again.

Questions

1. What is "tennis elbow"?
2. Which particular stroke in tennis is most likely to produce it?
3. What anatomic facts explain why the attempt to use a screwdriver exacerbated the pain?

■ *CASE 6*

A 77-YEAR-OLD FEMALE SLIPS ON THE ICE

A 77-year-old female was walking outside her home during winter and slipped on a hidden patch of ice. She used outstretched arms to break her fall and heard a cracking sound. After the fall, she observed that the dorsal surface of her left wrist seemed to protrude posteriorly in an unnatural fashion. She went to the doctor's office, and she noted further that her right and left upper limbs were no longer of the same length. An x-ray of her wrist was taken, and it showed bony damage to both radius and ulna. She was intrigued when her doctor told her that if such an injury occurred in a 7-year-old child, it would actually be more worrisome and potentially more serious.

Questions

1. What part of the radius is fractured in this sort of injury?
2. How does the injured limb come to be shorter than the normal limb?
3. Why is such an injury more serious in a young child than in an older adult?

■ *CASE 7*

A MOTORCYCLE FALL WITH A DELAYED COMPLICATION

A 19-year-old motorcycle enthusiast was riding on a slick pavement street after a light rain. Attempting to negotiate a turn at high speed, the motorcycle spun out and the rider was thrown, landing on the pavement on his outstretched hands. He had gloves on, and suffered no abrasions. He checked himself over, seemed to be in one piece, and retrieved his motorcycle and went on his way. Later that evening, while watching TV, his left wrist began to throb, and the pain increased steadily. He could move all his fingers, and decided to "tough it out" and see how things were in the morning, realizing that he had no health insurance. He took aspirin and some Percodan (a strong opiate painkiller) left over from some dental work he had undergone some months before, and controlled the pain. This went on for several days, and the pain then seemed to improve and he forgot about the injury in the ensuing weeks.

About 3 months later, however, he began to notice renewed pain in the wrist, and it began to be more difficult to carry out a full range of motion. He was also having some intermittent fevers. By this time he had acquired a job offering health insurance, and he went to the doctor. Examination of the wrist revealed pain to passive motion in several directions and point tenderness over the "anatomic snuff box." The patient also showed some redness over the wrist, and blood tests showed signs of inflammation (an elevated white count).

Questions

1. What was the differential diagnosis for the original injury?
2. How did the patient endure the early symptoms and seemingly recover?

3. What was the particular injury suffered by this patient?
4. What accounts for the late-onset symptoms?

■ CASE 8

THE EFFECTS OF PREGNANCY ON WRIST MOBILITY

A 24-year-old female office worker became pregnant, and as her pregnancy progressed she noticed that her fingers seemed stiffer and it was hard for her to type on her word processor. She found that she could only type for 5 or 10 minutes at a time, and her wrist would begin to ache and further typing would be impossible. Subsequently she began to notice that her index and ring fingers seemed numb and on closer examination that her thumb was also partially numb as well. She was surprised that her doctor prescribed diuretics or "water pills," and she was further advised that wearing a splint on her wrist while sleeping would also be useful.

Questions

1. Why should pregnancy have an effect on this woman's ability to type?
2. Why are the fingers on the lateral side of her hand affected most?
3. What is the rationale behind prescription of the diuretics and use of the splint?

ANSWERS AND EXPLANATIONS

■ CASE 1

1. This young athlete has suffered a forceful blow to the crown of the shoulder and has torn the **acromio-clavicular** and **coracoclavicular ligaments,** producing a **shoulder separation.** This is really a misnomer, because the shoulder joint (i.e., glenohumeral joint) is not involved. Instead, the lateral end of the clavicle and the acromion (distal part of the scapular spine) have been separated.
2. In this injury, when both the acromioclavicular and coracoclavicular ligaments are torn, then the scapula/humerus "sags" below the level of the lateral end of the clavicle, which produces the observed "bump" on the top of the shoulder in this patient. If only the acromioclavicular ligament is torn, then the clavicle and the scapula still move as a unit, since

the coracoclavicular ligament is intact, and the bump on the shoulder would not be visible.
3. Injuries of this sort heal themselves if the upper limb is immobilized (usually by holding it high against the anterolateral chest wall), and the patient is instructed to avoid any further impact on the shoulder, usually for a matter of several weeks.

■ CASE 2

1. Effective anesthesia of the upper limb is very useful for repair of traumatic injuries, such as those indicated here, and can also be employed for invasive surgery on the upper limb, if anesthetic plus a tight occlusive tourniquet are used to minimize the risk of bleeding. The most effective place to insert local

anesthetic is in the upper axilla before the major branches of the brachial plexus have separated. Here the branches of the plexus are encased in the axillary sheath, a downward extension of the cervical fascia. The goal of the technique is to localize the axillary sheath, introduce a small needle into its interior, and gently inject several milliliters of anesthetic solution. The fluid drifts upward and downward within the axillary sheath, further increasing the efficiency of the anesthetic.

2. An **axillary block** is achieved by abducting the shoulder and exposing the upper axilla. The axillary pulse is localized, and a small needle inserted through the anesthetized skin in the direction of the pulse. When the needle reaches the axillary sheath a "pop" is usually felt by the person advancing the needle. Some prefer to intentionally penetrate the artery with the needle, then withdraw it until the tip of the needle is safely outside the arterial lumen (injection of anesthetic directly into the arterial blood may cause dangerous cardiac dysrhythmias). With the tip of the needle within the sheath but not in the artery, the anesthetic is then injected slowly and allowed to bathe the nerve roots. Depending on the anesthetic agent chosen, the effect can persist for several hours.

■ CASE 3

1. When the obstetrician pulled forcefully on the head of the baby, in a downward direction, it caused a severe lateral flexion of the head to the right. Very forceful falls on the ground can produce a similar momentary lateral flexion. This risks the upper roots of the brachial plexus and has produced in this baby **Erb-Duchenne palsy.** Nerve roots C5 to C7 are usually involved. Axons in these roots innervate the shoulder abductors, the elbow flexors, and the wrist extensors. Weakness in these muscle groups produces the combination of positional abnormalities described in this baby.

2. As mentioned, the forceful downward traction of the head with the right shoulder still engaged in the birth canal produced an effective severe lateral flexion of the right shoulder.

3. In the large majority of cases such as these the nerve roots have been stretched but not actually torn. If such is the case, then time (several weeks or months) will be sufficient for the nerves to repair themselves. If significant restoration of neurologic function does not occur over the first few weeks, however, then the prospects for permanent neurologic loss increase significantly.

■ CASE 4

1. This patient underwent a **transverse fracture through the shaft of the humerus.** The location of the fracture determines how the bone fragments will be positioned afterward. In this case, the fracture is across the humeral shaft superior to the level of the deltoid insertion on the deltoid tubercle. Because of this, the rotator cuff tendons pull the proximal fragment medially and the deltoid tendon exerts an upward pull on the distal fragment, pulling it along the lateral surface of the proximal fragment.

2. Elbow flexion is partially mediated by the **brachioradialis,** innervated by the **radial nerve** (even though this is typically the nerve of extension in the upper limb). The fracture of the humerus had injured the radial nerve as it travels in a **musculospiral groove** on the posterior surface of the humerus in the vicinity of the fracture.

3. Supination is still functional because the biceps brachii is a very efficient supinator, particularly if the elbow is partly flexed. Pronation is intact because the muscles that mediate it, pronator quadratus and pronator teres, are not innervated by the radial nerve.

4. Damage to the radial nerve means that all of the forearm extensor muscles are weakened, and therefore wrist extension is not possible. When the wrist is partly flexed, there is passive stretch on the long extensor tendons. This prevents the long flexor tendons from achieving full finger flexion since the long extensor tendons cannot stretch, and they are made taut near the midpoint of flexion.

■ CASE 5

1. "Tennis elbow" is **lateral epicondylitis.** Literally, this phrase means that tissues at or near the lateral epicondyle of the humerus are inflamed. The long superficial extensor muscles of the forearm originate from the lateral epicondyle. The actual mechanism of injury is still open to debate, but it is likely that small "microtears" are produced, pulling the extensor muscle tendons away from the bone.

2. The supinator is one of the important muscles originating in part from the lateral epicondyle. Of the various tennis strokes, the backhand is the one that produces a forceful supination (the racket is rotated laterally as the elbow fully extends).

3. For a right-handed person, "screwing" a screw inward is also the motion of supination and is painful for someone whose lateral epicondylar area is already inflamed. For a left-handed person, turning a

screw clockwise in an effort to penetrate wood requires pronation, not supination.

▮ *CASE 6*

1. This is a **Colles' fracture** or fracture of the distal radius just proximal to the styloid process. In about 40% of the cases there is injury to the ulnar styloid process as well.
2. When this part of the radius is fractured, the radius "buckles" in a dorsal direction. A lateral view of the wrist will yield an image of a "dinner fork deformity" where the wrist bulges dorsally because of the fracture.
3. This fracture is one of many that results from a fall on outstretched hands. In the elderly, where bones are usually somewhat demineralized, the fracture may occur with a fall of less force than would be required to produce a similar fracture in the young. If this occurs in a school-age child, there is additional fear that the fracture line will cross the distal epiphyseal plate of the radius, and the healing process will result in malalignment of the plate and disturbance to the continued growth of the radius. In the worst cases, the radius will develop in a deformed fashion.

▮ *CASE 7*

1. This patient has suffered one of the various fracture injuries to the distal forearm, wrist, and/or hand. Among the most frequently injured structures in accidents of this type are (1) fracture of the distal radius, (2) fracture of the lunate, scaphoid, or capitate bones, or (3) damage to the metacarpal row or the phalanges.
2. By self-administration of analgesics, the patient may have masked painful symptoms sufficiently that he did not seek medical evaluation in the immediate few days after the accident occurred. The initial fracture which occurred produced an inflammatory response, which is the body's way of removing injured tissue and repairing damage. Part of this inflammatory response is the production of pain, which is intended to cause the patient to behave appropriately to protect the injured limb. Unfortunately, this patient overrode these natural "warning systems" by use of the pain medication.

3. The pain over the anatomic snuff box is diagnostic for **fracture of the scaphoid bone** since it may be palpated in the base of this region. The scaphoid is the most frequently fractured wrist bone, and injury to it produces injury to several of the adjacent intercarpal joints.
4. The scaphoid bone receives its blood supply from a small series of vessels that enter the bone along its distal margin. When the scaphoid is fractured, there is a very real possibility that the proximal fragment of bone will not be able to reestablish blood supply and will undergo irreversible death. This is known as **avascular necrosis** of the scaphoid bone and accounts for the later onset of renewed painful symptoms. Often this avascular fragment will have to be removed surgically since its continued presence in the wrist will be seen by the body as a "foreign object," stimulating a continuing inflammatory response. If allowed to worsen, this reaction may injure the intercarpal joints and lead to permanent immobility ("freezing") of these joints.

▮ *CASE 8*

1. Pregnancy leads to a considerable accumulation of fluid in the body due to the high levels of estrogenic hormones in the woman's system and the venous obstruction resulting from the enlarging uterus within the abdominal cavity. At the wrist, the edema has affected the synovial sheaths of the long flexor tendons in the **carpal tunnel,** through which the long tendons of the forearm and the median nerve pass. This is one mechanism underlying **carpal tunnel syndrome.**
2. The pressure exerted on the **median nerve,** where it passes beneath the flexor retinaculum, produces sensory loss in the hand, on the anterior surface of the thumb, index and middle finger and the medial half of the ring finger. More chronic compression of this nerve can lead to **muscle wasting** in the thenar eminence, a symptom of long-standing carpal tunnel syndrome. This muscle wasting results from the chronic lack of intact innervation of these muscles, a situation which invariably leads to the shrinking and scarring of striated muscles.
3. The diuretics encourage the kidneys to increase fluid output from the body as a whole, and this will have a helpful effect on the swelling in the carpal tunnel. The splint helps place the wrist in a neutral position, which encourages reduction of the swelling.

Back and Spinal Cord

▶ **4.1** Back and Vertebral Column

▶ **4.2** Spinal Cord

▶ **4.3** Systems Review and Surface Anatomy of the Back and Spinal Cord

▶ **4.4** Case Studies: Back and Spinal Cord

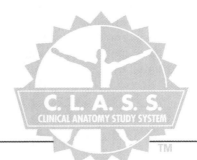

C. L. A. S. S.
CLINICAL ANATOMY STUDY SYSTEM

™

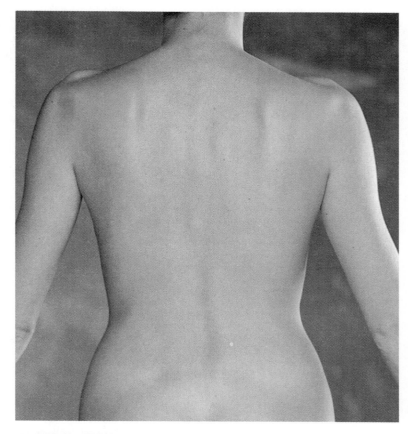

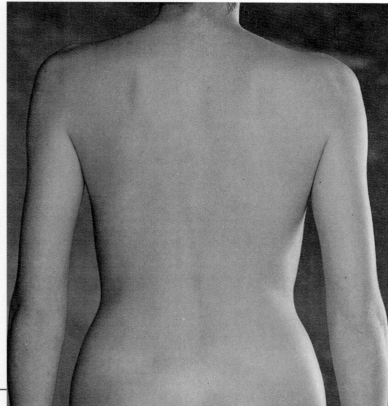

Back and Vertebral Column

▶ Normal Vertebral Column

▶ "Typical" Vertebra

▶ Cervical Vertebrae

▶ Thoracic Vertebrae

▶ Lumbar Vertebrae

▶ Sacrum

▶ Vertebral Ligaments and Articulations

▶ Musculature of the Back and Vertebral Column

▶ Blood Supply of the Back and Vertebral Column

▶ Innervation of the Back and Vertebral Column

The **back** consists of the spinal cord, its encircling meninges, the vertebral column, and the muscles and ligaments that surround it. The **vertebral column** is the *axis* around which the limbs perform movements and is, of course, an important *support* for both the head and the thoraco-abdominal viscera (Figure 4-1). The vertebral column also serves the very important function of cushioning and protecting the **spinal cord.** Many muscles that move the upper limb course across the back to attach to the vertebral column. The back's own **muscles** and **ligaments** are involved in virtually every movement of the head, limbs, and trunk, because the axis of the body must be stabilized to maintain desired posture during such movements. Ailments of the back account for a large share of visits to doctors' offices and are the single greatest cause of lost working time in industry.

NORMAL VERTEBRAL COLUMN

The vertebral column consists of **33 vertebrae—7 cervical, 12 thoracic, 5 lumbar, 5 sacral** (fused into a single bone, the **sacrum**), and **2 to 4 coccygeal** (fused to form the **coccyx**) (see Figure 4-1). The individual vertebral bodies are linked by the flexible fibrocartilaginous **intervertebral disks.** Longitudinal **ligaments** span the gaps between the vertebral bodies and help keep the vertebrae and disks in alignment.

The vertebral column has four normal **curvatures** in the sagittal plane (see Figure 4-1), all named for the region of the vertebral column in which they occur—a **cervical** curvature (convex anterior), a **thoracic** curvature (convex posterior), a **lumbar** curvature (convex anterior), and the fixed curve of the sacrum (convex posterior). These curvatures are barely present in the newborn infant but become more prominent as the child begins to walk and increasingly relies on the vertebral column to support the weight of his or her head and body. There is a normal **lumbosacral angle** at the union of the L5 vertebra and the sacrum, with the sacrum inflected in a posterior direction (see Figure 4-1; see also Figure 4-13).

Any **abnormal curvature** (or an exaggeration of a normal curvature) that is *convex ventrally* is known as a **lordosis;** an abnormal curvature *convex dorsally* is a **kyphosis.** Any significant *lateral curvature* of the spine is abnormal and is known as **scoliosis.**

"TYPICAL" VERTEBRA

A typical vertebra consists of a **body** and a **neural arch** (composed of a **pedicle** and a **lamina**). The **spinal**

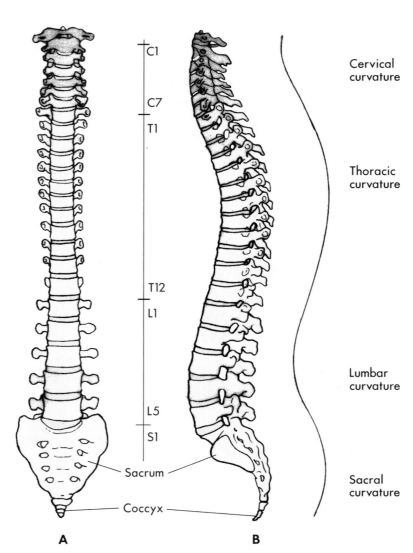

A

B

Figure 4-1   TWO VIEWS OF THE VERTEBRAL COLUMN. A, Articulated vertebral column viewed from the anterior aspect. **B,** Left lateral view of the vertebral column. In the lateral view, note the four normal curvatures of the vertebral column.   SEE ATLAS, FIG. 4-2

Cervical curvature

Thoracic curvature

Lumbar curvature

Sacral curvature

cord lies in a protected space, the **vertebral foramen,** protected anteriorly by the vertebral body and posterolaterally by the neural arch (Figure 4-2). The neural arch usually supports a dorsal midline **spinous process** (although the spinous process is absent in some vertebrae). Many muscles producing extension and rotation of the vertebral column attach to the spinous processes.

The superior and inferior edges of the pedicles are curved rather than straight (forming the **superior** and **inferior vertebral notches**), so that, when adjacent vertebrae are articulated with each other, there is a gap between the inferior vertebral notch of the vertebra above and the superior vertebral notch of the vertebra below—the **intervertebral foramen** (Figure 4-3). Nerve roots enter and leave the spinal cord by passing through these intervertebral foramina.

At the junction of the pedicle and the lamina, on each lateral side of the vertebra, arises the **transverse process** (see Figure 4-2). Many muscles producing lateral flexion and rotation of the vertebral column attach to the transverse processes.

Thoracic vertebrae have well-developed **costal processes,** which develop into fully formed **ribs** (see Figure 4-21). The other vertebrae have only small remnants of these costal processes, normally incorporated into the transverse processes. In cervical vertebrae, however, there is a unique aperture apparently within the transverse process, the **foramen transversarium** (transverse foramen), which is in reality a gap between the costal process and the true transverse process. The **costal process** is a mesodermal condensation lying anterior to the transverse process. In the thoracic region, it forms the heads of the ribs; in the cervical region it forms part of the perimeter surrounding the transverse foramen. The vertebral artery and vein travel through the foramina transversaria of vertebrae C1 to C6, usually bypassing the C7 vertebra, even though C7 does have a foramen in its transverse process. When occa-

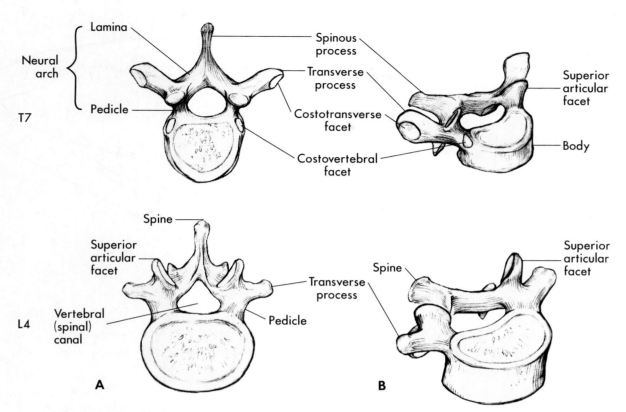

Figure 4-2   REPRESENTATIVE VERTEBRAE. Two views of T7 and L4 vertebrae. **A,** Superoinferior views. **B,** Right anterior oblique views.   SEE ATLAS, FIGS. 4-3, 4-16

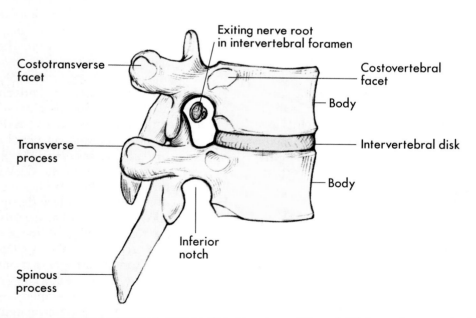

Figure 4-3   INTERVERTEBRAL FORAMEN. Vertebrae T5 and T6 have been articulated and the resultant intervertebral foramen is shown with a segmental nerve in place. The intervertebral foramen also permits blood vessels (not shown here) to enter and leave the interior of the vertebral canal.

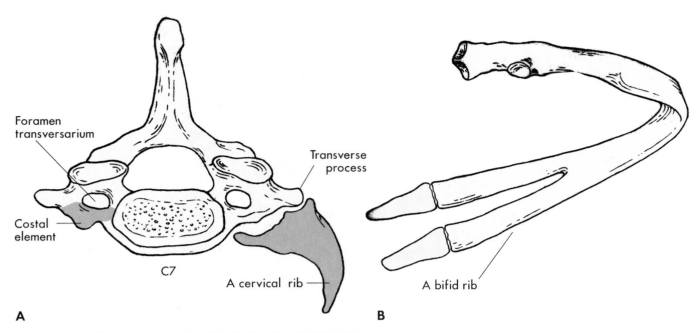

Foramen
transversarium

Transverse
process

Costal
element

C7

A cervical rib

A bifid rib

A

B

Figure 4-4   VARIATIONS IN RIB STRUCTURE. A, A cervical rib, which represents an exaggerated growth of the costal element that normally forms part of the perimeter of the transverse foramen. **B,** A bifid rib with two costal cartilages.

sional **lumbar** or **cervical ribs** form (usually in C7 or L1), they represent an anomalous exaggerated growth of the costal process of these vertebrae into a full rib (Figure 4-4).

Each vertebra has a **superior** and **inferior articular facet,** with which it articulates with the vertebra above and below it (see Figures 4-2 and 4-14). Articular facets of adjacent vertebrae are congruent with each other. A synovial joint exists between them, allowing for a small degree of movement at the joint. Collectively, the movement of large numbers of these joints permits considerable overall movement of the spine. Table 4-1 shows the variations in structure exhibited by vertebrae found in different regions of the vertebral column.

CERVICAL VERTEBRAE
Atlas and Axis (C1 and C2)

The **atlas** in reality consists of a pair of strong **lateral masses,** which are linked anteriorly by the anterior arch and posteriorly by the posterior arch (Figure 4-5). On each side, lateral to the lateral mass, the atlas has a large ovoid **articular facet,** which faces upward to articulate with the congruent occipital condyle on each side of the base of the occipital bone. Just lateral to the articular facets are the **transverse foramina** (or **foramina transversaria**), through which pass the vertebral

artery and vein. After they emerge superior to the foramen transversarium of the atlas, the vertebral arteries travel posterior to the lateral mass of the atlas and enter the skull through the foramen magnum. On each side, the **transverse process** of the atlas lies still further lateral to the foramen transversarium. The **vertebral veins** do not originate inside the skull or traverse the foramen magnum to reach the neck. Instead, the vertebral veins are made up of vessels originating from the cervical **internal vertebral venous plexus** that drain inferiorly to the brachiocephalic veins (see Figure 4-30).

The atlas is unique among vertebrae in having no body, its place being taken by the **dens** or **odontoid process** (see Figure 4-5) of the C2 vertebra (the axis). The **anterior arch of the atlas** has a small **anterior tubercle** in the midline. Posteriorly, in place of a true spinous process, the atlas has a midline **posterior tubercle** where the two halves of the posterior arch meet. The **posterior arch of the atlas** is attached to the posterior rim of the foramen magnum by the **atlanto-occipital membrane** (see Figure 4-15).

The **axis** (C2 vertebra) is similar to other typical cervical vertebrae in having **transverse foramina,** a posterior **bifid spine,** and a typical cylindrical **body** located anteriorly (see Figure 4-5). It is unique, however, because its **dens** or **odontoid process** protrudes upward from the body into the space left by the "missing" body of C1 (Figure 4-6).

Table 4-1 Structural Features of Individual Vertebrae

Vertebrae	Spinous Process	Transverse Process	Articular Process	Vertebral Body	Comments
C1 (atlas)	Absent	Long/stout; has a transverse foramen	Has unique superior facet (occipital); inferior facet for axis	Lacks a body; has anterior and posterior arches	Vertebral canal large and triangular
C2 (axis)	Bifid; laminae serve as attachment for ligamentum flavum	Short; has transverse foramen facing superolateral	Facets face in horizontal plane	Has a dens (odontoid process) extending upward into C1	Posterior longitudinal ligament starts here Anterior longitudinal ligament begins at skull
C3 to C7	Bifid (except C7)	Small and short	Facets face in horizontal plane	Small and transversely broad	Vertebral canal is heart-shaped
Thoracic vertebrae	Single, downswept from T1 to T12, spines get progressively longer	Large; T1 to T9 have articular facets for rib heads	Facets face in frontal plane (i.e., anterior to posterior)	Bodies cylindrical, and heart-shaped; costal facets on body	Vertebral canal is round and relatively small
Lumbar vertebrae	Short, stout, almost horizontal	Thin, relatively long	Facets face in sagittal plane (i.e., left to right)	Relatively large, wide, and kidney-shaped	Vertebral canal is triangular

Other Cervical Vertebrae (C3 to C7)

The remaining cervical vertebrae (**C3 to C7**) resemble each other (Figure 4-7) except that, while the **spinous processes** of C3 to C6 are **bifid,** that of the seventh cervical vertebra is usually not (see Figure 4-5). Also C7 may lack transverse foramina altogether. In C3 to C6, the transverse foramina are occupied by the **vertebral artery** and **vein,** but in C7, even though transverse foramina are usually present, the vessels usually do not pass through them (see Figure 4-29). C7 is sometimes called the "vertebra prominens" because its spine protrudes posteriorly quite markedly (although, in fact, the T1 spine often seems to protrude further when the spines of the vertebral column are being palpated during physical examination). The superior and inferior articular facets of cervical vertebrae face each other in a generally horizontal plane. The **costal element** in C7 is one of the most common from which **accessory ribs** may form (e.g., a "cervical rib"). Such accessory or cervical ribs often are more than just interesting variants; when they are present, the large vessels and nerves destined for the upper limb cross superior to the cervical rib or its cartilaginous anlage (these vessels and

nerves ordinarily pass over the *first thoracic rib* to enter the axilla). This abnormal positioning heightens the risk of compression of the nerves and vessels (see Figure 4-4).

Figure 4-8 shows a magnetic resonance image (MRI) of the cervical spine, revealing the relationships of the vertebrae and important soft tissues in this region.

THORACIC VERTEBRAE

There are 12 thoracic vertebrae (Figure 4-9). They are characterized by **downswept spines,** prominent **transverse processes,** heart-shaped **bodies,** and are unique in articulating with the normal 12 pairs of **ribs.** Ribs 1 to 10 articulate both with the vertebral body and its transverse process. Ribs 11 and 12 articulate only with the vertebral body and are not joined to the transverse processes on these vertebrae. Review the section on the chest wall (Section One, Thorax) for details of these articulations. The **superior** and **inferior intervertebral articular facets** of thoracic vertebrae face forward and backward in the **frontal** plane (Figure 4-10; see also Figure 4-14).

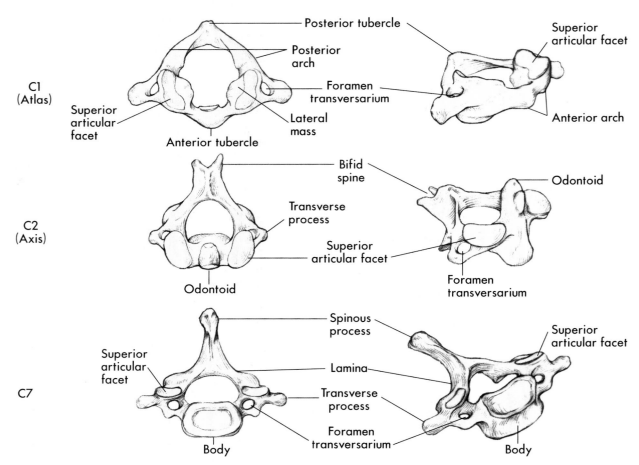

Figure 4-5   CERVICAL VERTEBRAE C1, C2, AND C7. Vertebra C1 is unique for the broad articular facets with which it articulates with the occipital condyles of the base of the skull (see also Figure 4-16) and the absence of a body, the space for which is occupied by the dens (odontoid process) of C2. C2 possesses the bifid spines typical of cervical vertebrae. All of the vertebrae shown possess the foramen transversarium unique to cervical vertebrae.   **SEE ATLAS, FIGS. 4-6, 4-7, 4-8, 4-13**

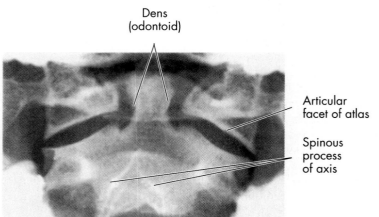

Figure 4-6   C1 AND C2, ANTERIOR VIEW. Close-up x-ray shows the odontoid process (dens) of C2 extending upward into the center of the atlas. A mobile odontoid process places the spinal cord in jeopardy, usually when the transverse ligament of the atlas is damaged. (From Weir J, Abrahams PH: *An imaging atlas of human anatomy,* London, 1992, Mosby.)   **SEE ATLAS, FIG. 4-9**

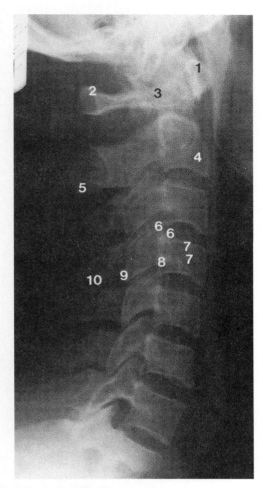

Figure 4-7 LATERAL CERVICAL SPINE FILM. In the lateral x-ray of the cervical spine (C-spine), the physician is interested in the alignment of the vertebral bodies as an indication that no trauma to the neck has occurred. Accident victims are often kept in support collars or otherwise restrained from moving their necks fully until such C-spine films have been taken and declared normal ("cleared"). (From Weir J, Abrahams PH: *An imaging atlas of human anatomy,* London, 1992, Mosby.) SEE ATLAS, FIG. 4-10

1 Anterior arch of atlas	**6** Superior articular facet, C4
2 Posterior arch of atlas	**7** Body of C4
3 Dens of axis (odontoid process)	**8** Posterior limit of body
	9 Inferior articular facet, C4
4 Body of axis	**10** Spinous process, C4
5 Spinous process of axis	

LUMBAR VERTEBRAE

Lumbar vertebrae are specialized for weight bearing and strength. They have strong, thick **bodies** (Figures 4-11 and 4-12; see also Figure 4-2) and stout **spines** and **transverse processes** to which attach several large paravertebral muscles. The transverse processes are also an attachment for some of the muscles and fasciae of the

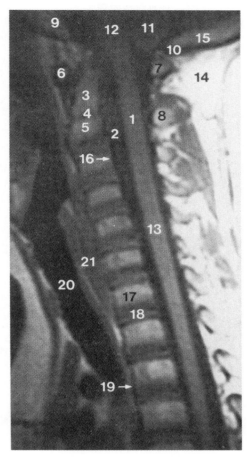

Figure 4-8 CERVICAL SPINE MRI. MRI allows visualization of many different tissues that cannot be distinguished on conventional x-ray or CT scan. (From Weir J, Abrahams PH: *An imaging atlas of human anatomy,* London, 1992, Mosby.) SEE ATLAS, FIGS. 4-10, 4-12

1 Spinal cord
2 Cerebrospinal fluid in subarachnoid space
3 Odontoid process (dens)
4 Synchondrosis
5 Body of axis, C2
6 Anterior } Arch of atlas, C1
7 Posterior }
8 Spinous process of axis
9 Clivus
10 Posterior margin of foramen magnum
11 Cerebellar tonsil
12 Brainstem
13 Cervical expansion
14 Suboccipital fat
15 Occipital bone
16 Posterior longitudinal ligament
17 Body, C7
18 Nucleus pulposus of intervertebral disk (between C7 and T1)
19 Anterior longitudinal ligament and cortical bone
20 Trachea
21 Esophagus

anterolateral abdominal wall (internal oblique, transversus abdominus). The **superior** and **inferior intervertebral articular facets** are characteristically positioned in the sagittal plane (see Figure 4-2).

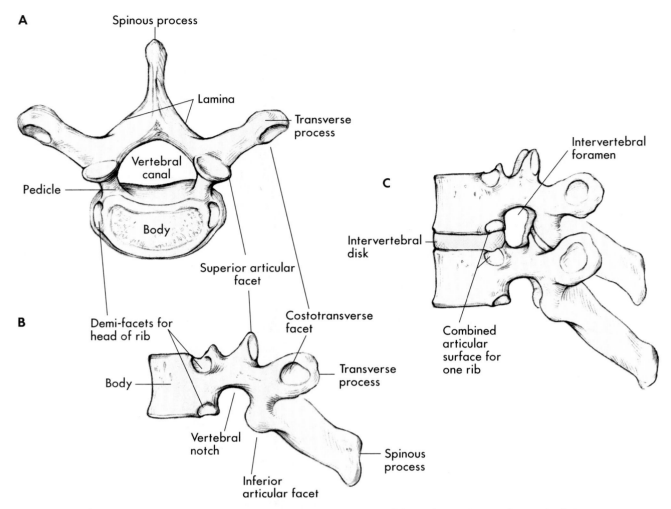

A
Spinous process

Lamina

Transverse
process

Vertebral
canal

Pedicle

Body

C

Intervertebral
foramen

Intervertebral
disk

Superior articular
facet

B

Demi-facets for
head of rib

Body

Costotransverse
facet

Transverse
process

Combined
articular
surface for
one rib

Vertebral
notch

Spinous
process

Inferior
articular facet

Figure 4-9   THORACIC VERTEBRAE. Superior (**A**) and lateral (**B**) views of a typical thoracic vertebra. **C,** Two articulated thoracic vertebrae. Note how the superior and inferior vertebral notches combine to form an intervertebral foramen.   See ATLAS, Fig. 4-15

SACRUM

The **sacrum** represents the fusion of five separate sacral vertebrae (Figure 4-13). The sacrum displays a marked anterior concavity. **Anterior** and **posterior sacral foramina** are the equivalent of the intervertebral foramina of the separate vertebrae in cervical, thoracic, and lumbar regions. **Anterior primary rami** of sacral spinal nerves (those branches of the segmental spinal nerve that innervate the anterolateral areas of the body—see p. 436 for further discussion) exit through the **anterior sacral foramina** and **posterior primary rami** (branches of spinal nerves that innervate posterior regions of the body) through the **posterior sacral foramina.** The laminae of S5, and sometimes S4, fail to meet in the midline, creating a gap known as the **sacral hiatus.** This hiatus leads into the vertebral canal.

A normal part of sacral structure is a prominent anterior convexity, the **sacral promontory,** which is the

part of the sacrum closest to the pubic symphysis. On each side of the sacrum there is a large **lateral process,** whose rough articular surface articulates with the ilium, to form the **sacroiliac joint** (see Figure 4-13). This joint is reinforced by very strong ligaments and transmits the weight of the trunk to the lower limbs. The lateral processes (also known as the *ala*) are formed by fusion of the transverse and costal elements of the upper sacral vertebrae.

The **sacral canal** is the equivalent of the vertebral canal in the other parts of the vertebral column. The sacral canal is in the shape of a flattened triangle, and at its inferior end there is a free dorsal opening, the **sacral hiatus** (see Figure 4-13). Within the sacral canal is a wide bundle of nerve roots descending from higher levels of the spinal cord, the **cauda equina** (see Figure 4-13; see also Figure 4-38).

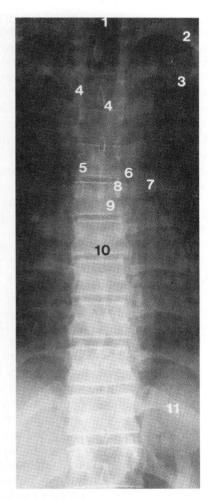

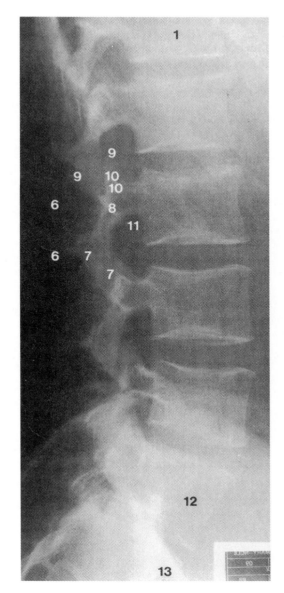

Figure 4-10 THORACIC SPINE X-RAY, ANTERIOR VIEW. Thoracic vertebrae and the rib heads that articulate with them are revealed in this x-ray. (From Weir J, Abrahams PH: *An imaging atlas of human anatomy,* London, 1992, Mosby.)

Figure 4-11 LUMBAR SPINE, LATERAL VIEW. Lateral x-ray of the lumbar spine is often used to confirm proper vertebral alignment. (From Weir J, Abrahams PH: *An imaging atlas of human anatomy,* London, 1992, Mosby.) **SEE ATLAS, FIG. 4-16**

1 C7 vertebra	**7** Transverse process, T6
2 First rib	**8** Pedicle, T6
3 Clavicle	**9** Body, T6
4 Trachea, walls	**10** Spinous process, T6
5 Right main bronchus	**11** Tenth rib
6 Left main bronchus	

1 Body, T12	**10** Mamillary process
6 Spinous process, L2	**11** Inferior vertebral notch
7 Inferior articular facet, L2	**12** Lumbar vertebra, L5
8 Transverse process, L2	**13** Sacral promontory
9 Superior articular facet, L2	

VERTEBRAL LIGAMENTS AND ARTICULATIONS

The articulations of the vertebral column are of great importance. Figure 4-14 shows how the vertebrae articulate and reveals how these articulations give the ver-

tebral column flexibility. The vertebral column *supports much weight,* serves as an *axis for movements* of the limbs, trunk, head, and neck, and *protects the spinal cord from trauma.* The specific structures listed in Table 4-2, all involved in vertebral attachment, are the most important means by which the bodies of vertebrae in the

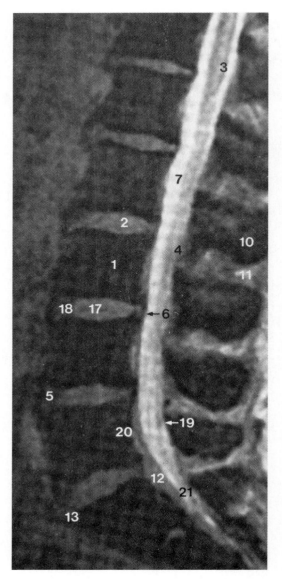

Figure 4-12   LUMBAR SPINE, LATERAL MRI IMAGE. The MRI study has largely replaced the myelogram as a means of diagnosing herniated disks and nerve compression. The MRI is noninvasive, painless, and free of radiation. A myelogram involves placement of a needle in the subarachnoid space, injection of dye, and several x-rays. (From Weir J, Abrahams PH: *An imaging atlas of human anatomy*, London, 1992, Mosby.)

1	Body, L3
2	Nucleus pulposus, L2-L3 disk
3	Conus medullaris
4	Cauda equina
5	Anterior longitudinal ligament
6	Posterior longitudinal ligament and annulus fibrosus
7	Cerebrospinal fluid
10	Spinous process
11	Interspinous ligament and bursa
12	Epidural space (fat filled)
13	Sacral promontory
17	Internuclear cleft, L3-L4 disk
18	Annulus fibrosus, L3-L4 disk
19	Nerve root
20	Basivertebral veins
21	Caudal lumbar thecal sac

vertebral column are secured to each other. More detailed description of these ligaments follows.

Attachments of the Vertebral Column to the Skull

The **dens** lies just posterior to the anterior tubercle of the atlas and is held in this position by the strong **transverse ligament of the atlas.** This ligament lies just posterior to the dens and prevents it from moving backward, where it might crush the upper cervical spinal cord (see Figure 4-5). The transverse ligament extends from one lateral mass of the atlas across to the other. It has both an upward and downward extension, attaching to the anterior edge of the foramen magnum and the body of the axis, respectively. These extensions give the transverse ligament of the atlas the look of a cross, and for this reason this group of ligaments is often called the **cruciform ligament** (Figure 4-15).

The apex of the dens is attached to the anterior lip of the foramen magnum by the **apical ligament of the dens** (see Figure 4-15). The **alar ligaments** extend superolaterally from the apex of the dens to the medial sides of the occipital condyles (Figure 4-16). More posteriorly, the **tectorial membrane** extends vertically from the base of the dens across its posterior surface to the anterior lip of the foramen magnum. It is an upward continuation of the posterior longitudinal ligament.

Two other specialized ligaments originate from C1 and C2: (1) the **atlanto-axial membrane,** extending from the anterior arch of C1 to C2, and (2) the **atlanto-occipital membrane,** extending from the anterior and posterior arches of the atlas to the anterior and posterior margins of the foramen magnum (see Figure 4-15).

All of these ligaments help to secure the upper cervical vertebral column firmly to the base of the skull. The **dens** serves as a *pivot* for **side-to-side movements** of the head (as in shaking the head "no"); so in reality this movement is best described as the movement of the combined skull/C1 unit with respect to C2 (at the **atlanto-axial joint**). **Flexion** and **extension** of the head (as in nodding the head "yes"), by contrast, involve movement of the skull with respect to the C1 vertebra (at the **atlanto-occipital joint**).

Attachments of the Vertebrae to Each Other

The **anterior** and **posterior longitudinal ligaments** run as two flattened vertical bands of fibrous tissue on the anterior and posterior surfaces of the adjacent vertebral bodies, respectively (Figures 4-17 and 4-18). The **anterior longitudinal ligament** extends all the way from the sacrum to the inferior surface of the occipital bone. The **posterior longitudinal ligament** extends from the sacrum to the body of C2. Above C2, the **tec-**

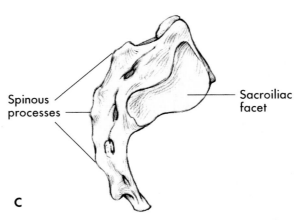

Figure 4-13 THREE VIEWS OF THE SACRUM. Note the anterior (**A**) and posterior (**B**) sacral foramina, which transmit the anterior and posterior divisions, respectively, of the sacral spinal nerves. Note also the large articular surface for the important sacroiliac joint, seen in the lateral view (**C**). SEE ATLAS, FIG. 4-20

torial membrane represents a continuation of the posterior longitudinal ligament.

The **intervertebral disks** are *fibrocartilaginous flattened structures* interposed between adjacent vertebral bodies (see Figure 4-12). Each disk consists of a gelatinous inner region, the **nucleus pulposus,** surrounded by a solid ring of stiffer material, the **annulus fibrosus** (Figure 4-19; see also Figure 4-18). Because they each are somewhat flexible, the disks give the vertebral column considerable mobility in all planes.

The disks are tightly bound to the hyaline cartilage lining the facing surfaces of adjacent vertebrae. All around their perimeter they are attached to the curved rim of the vertebral bodies above and below by an **annular ligament.** They are also held in place anteriorly and posteriorly by the longitudinal ligaments (see previously), lying just external to the annular ligaments.

PRINCIPLES

The nucleus pulposus at the center of each intervertebral disk is a vestige of the notochord. The **notochord** is a cylindrical midline mass of tissue, which forms early in the development of the embryo. It lies between the endodermal and ectodermal layers and plays an important role in the **induction** of surrounding tissues to form important adult structures such as the vertebral column. (Induction is the process by which one collection of tissue exerts an influence on the development of another.) The cylindrical notochord causes the somitic mesoderm near it to condense into masses that begin the process of forming the vertebral bodies and neural arches. The notochord itself disappears almost completely in the adult human.

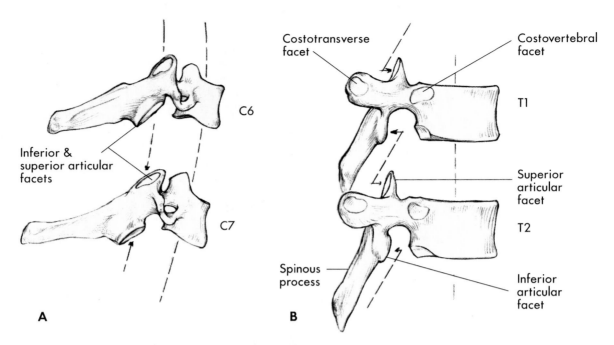

Figure 4-14   VERTEBRAL ARTICULATIONS. In these two examples, pairs of articulated cervical and thoracic vertebrae are separated to show their points of attachment. In cervical vertebrae (**A**), the superior and inferior articular facets are nearly in the horizontal plane, while for thoracic vertebrae (**B**) they are in the frontal plane. (In lumbar vertebrae [not shown] the articular facets are in the sagittal plane.) In **A**, the *dashed lines* indicate the position of the anterior and posterior borders of the spinal cord. In **B**, the *vertical dashed line* indicates the articulation of adjacent vertebral bodies. The *jagged dashed lines* indicate how articular facets align with each other.

The disks are thickest in the regions of most mobility, the cervical and lumbar areas, and thinner in the thoracic area. They become progressively flattened with age and allow correspondingly less mobility. A weakened annulus fibrosus may allow the gelatinous nucleus pulposus to herniate posterolaterally, compressing nearby spinal nerves (Figure 4-20).

The **ligamentum flavum** attaches the *laminae* of adjacent vertebrae (thus there are two ligamenta flava, on right and left, between each pair of vertebrae) (see Figure 4-18). This ligament is thickest in the lumbar area. It is yellowish in color, owing to a high percentage of elastic fibers in its makeup. The **supraspinous** and **interspinous ligaments** join the *spines* together. A spe-

Table 4-2   Ligaments of the Vertebral Column

Ligament	Attachments
Transverse ligament of atlas	Extends from one lateral mass of the atlas to the other; secures dens in anterior position
Apical/alar ligaments of dens	Connect apex of dens to foramen magnum, occipital condyles on base of skull
Anterior longitudinal ligament	Runs along anterior surface of vertebral bodies
Posterior longitudinal ligament	Runs continuously along posterior surface of vertebral bodies; continues cephalically as tectorial membrane
Intervertebral disks	Provide "cushion" between vertebral bodies; important as shock absorbers; prone to herniation and pressure on nerve roots
Ligamentum flavum	Connects neural laminae to each other
Supraspinous ligaments	Connects tips of vertebral spinous processes
Interspinous ligaments	Connects shafts of spinous processes

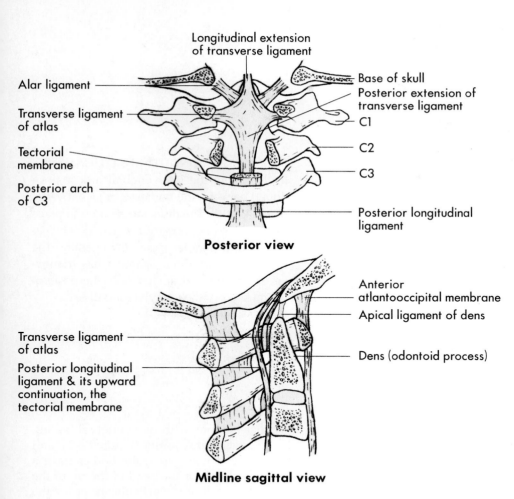

Longitudinal extension
of transverse ligament

Alar ligament

Transverse ligament
of atlas

Tectorial
membrane

Posterior arch
of C3

Base of skull
Posterior extension of
transverse ligament

C1

C2

C3

Posterior longitudinal
ligament

Posterior view

Transverse ligament
of atlas

Posterior longitudinal
ligament & its upward
continuation, the
tectorial membrane

Anterior
atlantooccipital membrane

Apical ligament of dens

Dens (odontoid process)

Midline sagittal view

Figure 4-15 LIGAMENTS CON-NECTING THE SKULL AND VER-TEBRAL COLUMN. Both C1 and C2 vertebrae are separately attached to the base of the skull to ensure maximum stability. The transverse ligament of the atlas prevents the dens from moving posteriorly and crushing the spinal cord as it passes through the lumen of the C1 vertebra. With its upward and downward extensions, the transverse ligament forms the **cruciform ligament**. SEE ATLAS, FIG. 4-11

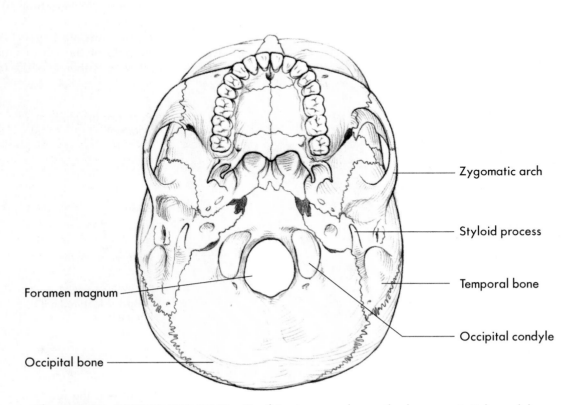

Zygomatic arch

Styloid process

Temporal bone

Occipital condyle

Foramen magnum

Occipital bone

Figure 4-16 BASE OF THE SKULL. On this view are shown the large occipital condyles, the surfaces at which the skull articulates with the C1 vertebra, the atlas.

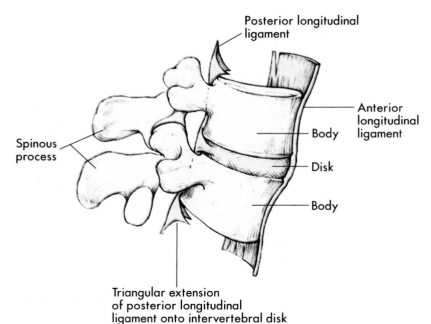

Posterior longitudinal ligament

Spinous process

Anterior longitudinal ligament

Body

Disk

Body

Triangular extension of posterior longitudinal ligament onto intervertebral disk

Figure 4-17   LONGITUDINAL LIGAMENTS. In this figure the intervertebral disk is positioned between the bodies of adjacent vertebrae L4 to L5. The disks are secured in place by anterior and posterior longitudinal ligaments, and annular ligaments laterally. The posterior longitudinal ligament has triangular extensions that anchor onto the posterolateral sides of the intervertebral disks. See Atlas, Figs. 4-17, 4-24, 4-25

cialized thick part of the supraspinous ligament is the **ligamentum nuchae,** a thick ligament in the cervical region that is crucial for quadripeds in supporting the head in a "forward-looking" position. The **intertransverse ligaments** attach adjacent transverse processes.

Articulations of Ribs and Vertebrae

The **heads** of the first, tenth, eleventh, and twelfth ribs articulate with one **vertebral body** only; the other rib heads have articulations with two vertebral bodies. These are the **costovertebral joints** (Figures 4-21 and 4-22). For thoracic vertebrae 1 to 9, the bodies have a large upper articular facet for the head of the rib of the same number and a small lower articular facet for the head of the rib one number lower. Vertebrae 10 to 12 articulate with one rib head only.

On their **transverse processes,** vertebrae T1 through T10 articulate with **tubercle** of the rib to which each corresponds numerically (e.g., tubercle of the fourth rib

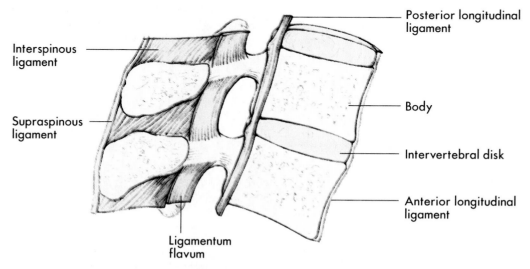

Interspinous ligament

Supraspinous ligament

Posterior longitudinal ligament

Body

Intervertebral disk

Anterior longitudinal ligament

Ligamentum flavum

Figure 4-18   MIDSAGITTAL SECTION THROUGH A VERTEBRA. In this view, the vertebra is sectioned in the midline, permitting a view of the ligamentum flavum and the interspinous and supraspinous ligaments.   See Atlas, Figs. 4-24, 4-25

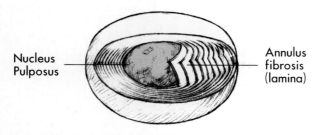

Figure 4-19 INTERVERTEBRAL DISK. The intervertebral disk consists of a laminated outer annulus fibrosus and an inner gel-like nucleus pulposus. SEE ATLAS, FIG. 4-22

articulates with the transverse process of T4). These are the **costotransverse joints** (see Figures 4-21 and 4-22). Ribs 11 and 12 articulate only with the *bodies* of T11 and T12, respectively, not with their transverse processes.

MUSCULATURE OF THE BACK AND VERTEBRAL COLUMN

For any individual pair of vertebrae, the amount of motion is small. In the aggregate, however, quite appreciable movement of the vertebral column as a whole is allowed, when muscles at many segments contract in unison. The muscles of the vertebral column are frequently in a increased state of contraction in order to stiffen the vertebral column because it serves as a "base" against which movements of the head or limbs occur. This is an example of an **isometric contraction,** in which muscle tone increases, but no movement actually occurs. Isometric contraction may also occur if a person voluntarily contracts a muscle and its antagonistic muscles simultaneously, preventing any movement from occurring. See p. 427 for a fuller description of movements of the vertebral column.

PRINCIPLES

Muscles that develop in the dorsal midline of the body, usually extending no further laterally than the tip of the transverse process, are designated **epaxial muscles.** In the adult these are the **erector spinae,** the **transversospinal muscles** of the vertebral column, as well as certain individual muscles that attach to the posterior surface of the skull. Epaxial muscles are innervated by the posterior primary rami of spinal nerves. Epaxial muscles, especially those in the cervical region, are of great importance in four-footed animals (i.e., **quadripedal**) since extension of the neck is crucial in providing the animal a forward gaze. **Hypaxial muscles** are all those muscles that lie lateral to the transverse process of the vertebrae. They comprise the lateral and anterior body wall muscles and include the muscles of the limbs as well. Hypaxial muscles are innervated by anterior primary rami of spinal nerves. Hypaxial muscles, especially those of the upper limbs, are of great significance in animals that stand on two feet (i.e., **bipedal**) since the upper limbs are the means of exploring and manipulating the environment.

Extrinsic Muscles of the Vertebral Column

The vertebral muscles are divided into two large groups—(1) the **extrinsic muscles,** which are important in the attachment of limbs and limb girdles to the vertebrae and contribute to motions of the trunk, and (2) the **intrinsic muscles,** which stabilize and carry out motions of the vertebral column itself. The extrinsic muscle group includes muscles such as **latissimus dorsi,** the **rhomboid muscles,** and **levator scapula** (Figure 4-23). The remainder of this chapter reviews the **intrinsic**

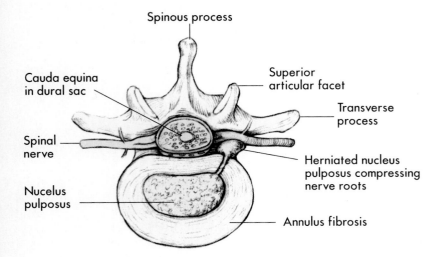

Figure 4-20 HERNIATION OF AN INTERVERTEBRAL DISK. The posterolateral margin of the annulus fibrosus has become weakened, and the inner nucleus pulposus has herniated through this weakness. It commonly puts pressure on the nerves exiting the vertebral canal at this level, leading to the symptoms of a "slipped disk." These occur most frequently in the cervical and lumbar regions. SEE ATLAS, FIG. 4-26

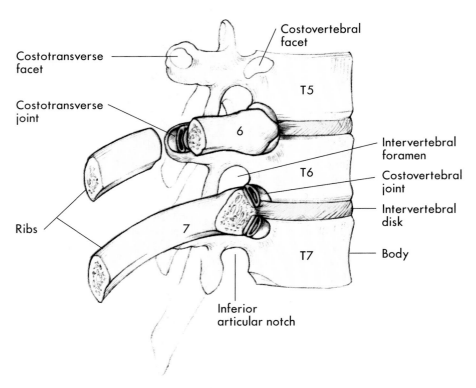

Figure 4-21   COSTOVERTEBRAL AND COSTOTRANSVERSE JOINTS, LATERAL VIEW.
Both these joints are synovial joints, and the costovertebral joint is complex because the articular surface involves small areas on each of two vertebral bodies, the intervening intervertebral disk, and the head of the rib as well.

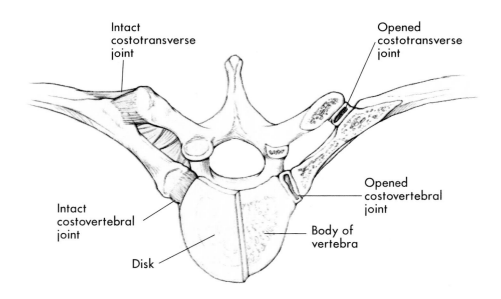

Figure 4-22   COSTOVERTEBRAL AND COSTOTRANSVERSE JOINTS, SUPERIOR VIEW.
This figure should be compared with Figure 4-21. On the left are the intact joints, enclosed by ligaments, and on the right are the joints that have been opened to reveal the interior synovial cavity.

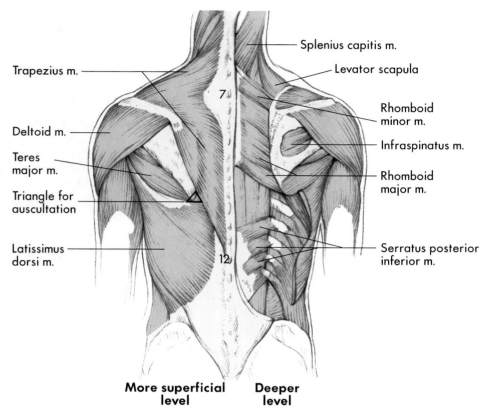

Trapezius m.

Deltoid m.

Teres major m.

Triangle for auscultation

Latissimus dorsi m.

Splenius capitis m.

Levator scapula

Rhomboid minor m.

Infraspinatus m.

Rhomboid major m.

Serratus posterior inferior m.

7

12

More superficial level   **Deeper level**

Figure 4-23   SUPERFICIAL BACK MUSCLES. On the left are shown the most superficial back muscles, including latissimus dorsi, trapezius, deltoid, and the teres muscles. On the right, slightly deeper, are the levator scapula, rhomboid muscles, serratus posterior inferior, and the oblique muscles of the abdominal wall. Note the small triangle on the left side, representing a small gap among the large muscles at which breath sounds may be heard best.   SEE ATLAS, FIGS. 4-4, 4-27, 4-28, 4-29, 4-33

muscles; descriptions of the extrinsic muscles are found in other sections (e.g., muscles of the shoulder, the gluteal region, etc.)

Intrinsic Muscles of the Vertebral Column

The intrinsic **longitudinal** vertebral muscles, placed more superficially, are collectively called the **erector spinae.** The erector spinae muscles originate caudally from the lower *lumbar vertebrae*, the *sacrum,* and *iliac crest.* The muscle fibers ascend varying distances and attach to medial portions of ribs and vertebrae above (Figure 4-24). The fibers can extend over two to three intervertebral spaces or more. The fibers of erector spinae tend to run vertically and interconnect similar regions of vertebrae or ribs (i.e., spines to spines, transverse processes to transverse processes, etc.). The individual **longitudinal muscle groups** within erector spinae are **iliocostalis, longissimus,** and **spinalis,** ar-

rayed from lateral to medial. The *iliocostalis* muscles connect the ilium and lumbar fascia with ribs. The *longissimus* muscles connect the transverse processes and the proximal ribs of adjacent segments to each other. The *spinalis* group of muscles connects the spines of various vertebrae to each other. In the upper thoracic and cervical region there are elongated muscles originating from the spinous process (the **splenius** muscles) and others from the transverse processes (the **semispinalis** muscles) (see Figure 4-24). These ascend and attach to the posterior aspect of the skull, helping to extend the neck and turn the head. The splenius muscles are unique in that they deviate laterally as they ascend. The semispinalis capitis is part of the transversospinal muscle group (see following discussion).

Second is a more deeply placed set of muscles known collectively as the **transversospinal group.** Its defining characteristic is that its fibers travel **superomedially** as they ascend, crossing one to six interverte-

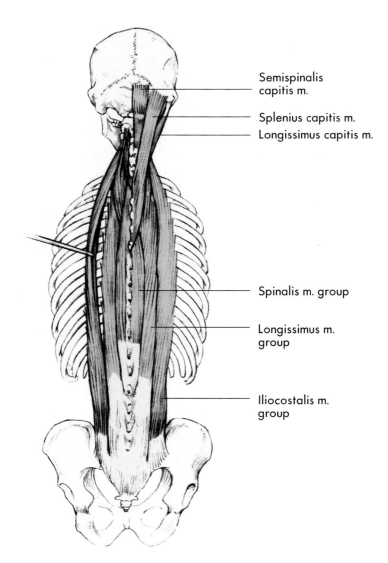

Semispinalis
capitis m.

Splenius capitis m.
Longissimus capitis m.

Spinalis m. group

Longissimus m.
group

Iliocostalis m.
group

Figure 4-24   ERECTOR SPINAE MUSCLES. The large longitudinal set of muscles of the back, located between the midline and the angles of the ribs, is known as the erector spinae. It consists of several subdivisions, based on the position the muscles occupy (see text).   SEE ATLAS, FIGS. 4-4, 4-31

bral spaces, and connect a transverse process with the spinous process of a vertebra above (Figure 4-25). This group of muscles can rotate the vertebrae with respect to each other. Named muscles within this group, moving from superficial to deep, are **semispinalis, multifidus,** and the **long** and **short rotator** muscles. Semispinalis spans three to six intervertebral spaces and is most prominent in the thoracic and cervical regions. Multifidus (most prominent in the thoracic region) spans two to four intervertebral spaces and the rotators (present throughout) one to two. In reality what is present is a continuum of muscles spanning as many as six interspaces and as few as one.

Muscles Controlling Head Movement

The **suboccipital muscles** are a special group of muscles linking the **atlas,** the **axis,** and the **base of the skull** (Figure 4-26). The muscles are special versions of muscles found in the rest of the vertebral column. Muscles extending from the spinous processes of C1 and C2 upward to the base of the skull are known as the **rectus capitis posterior** muscles (major and minor). They mediate **extension** of the skull on the vertebral column. The wide transverse processes of C1 have two attached muscles: a smaller **obliquus capitis superior,** extending upward to the base of the skull, and an

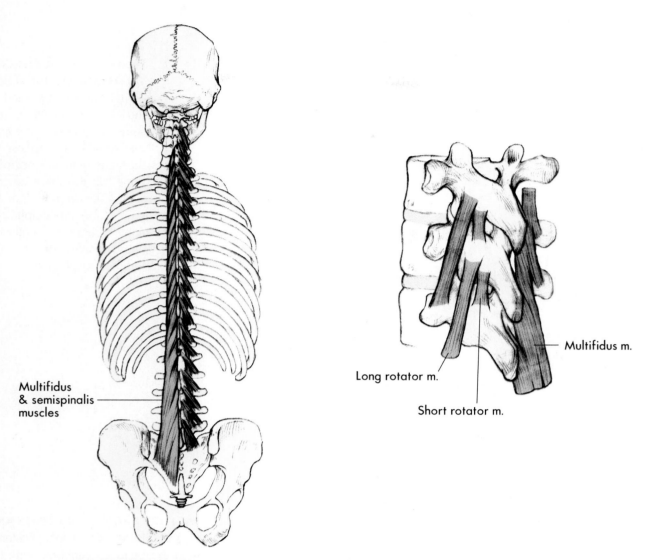

Multifidus & semispinalis muscles

Long rotator m.

Short rotator m.

Multifidus m.

Figure 4-25   TRANSVERSOSPINAL MUSCLES. Deep to erector spinae is the transverso-spinal group of muscles. In general these muscles connect the transverse processes to the spines and so run superomedially at an oblique angle. They are named separately (semi-spinalis, multifidus, long rotators, and short rotators) on the basis of the number of inter-vertebral spaces they span (see text). **SEE ATLAS, FIGS. 4-4, 4-34, 4-35**

obliquus capitis inferior, sloping medially and inferi-orly to attach to the spine of C2. Obliquus capitis supe-rior is a weak *extensor* of the neck; obliquus capitis infe-rior is a strong *rotator* of the atlas around the dens or odontoid process. Rotation of the head on the spine is produced by coordinated contraction of the splenius capitis and sternocleidomastoid muscles.

The vertebral column can **flex** (bend anteriorly), **ex-tend** (bend posteriorly), **lateral flex** to either side, and **rotate** around its own vertical axis to a limited degree. **Psoas major** mediates flexion, along with many other anterior muscles of the trunk. The **erector spinae** medi-ates extension, and the **transversospinal** group of mus-cles mediate rotation.

BLOOD SUPPLY OF THE BACK AND VERTEBRAL COLUMN

Within the vertebral canal, there is on each side a **longitudinal arterial vessel,** which is positioned on the medial side of the base of each pedicle, and travels the length of the vertebral column from cervical to sacral regions. These vessels are supplied by each of the **radicular arteries** (Figure 4-27), which enter the vertebral canal by traversing the intervertebral fora-men. The radicular arteries are derived from a variety of sources (in the midthorax and abdominal regions from the descending aorta; in the cervical area from

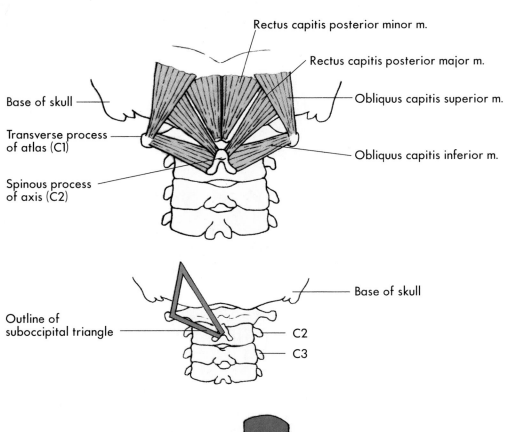

Rectus capitis posterior minor m.

Rectus capitis posterior major m.

Base of skull

Transverse process of atlas (C1)

Spinous process of axis (C2)

Obliquus capitis superior m.

Obliquus capitis inferior m.

Outline of suboccipital triangle

Base of skull

C2

C3

Figure 4-26 SUBOCCIPITAL TRIANGLE. The suboccipital triangle is formed by muscles connecting the spinous process of the axis, the transverse process of the atlas, and the occipital bone of the base of the skull. The vertebral artery crosses the suboccipital triangle obliquely to enter the cranial cavity through the foramen magnum.

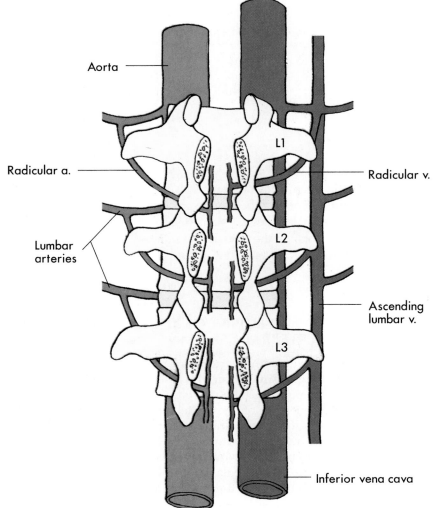

Aorta

Radicular a.

Lumbar arteries

L1

L2

L3

Radicular v.

Ascending lumbar v.

Inferior vena cava

Figure 4-27 RADICULAR VESSELS AND THE VERTEBRAL COLUMN. Posterior view of the L1 to L3 vertebrae with the neural arches removed to allow a view into the vertebral canal. On the left is the descending aorta, with its segmental lumbar arteries, each of which emits a radicular artery that enters the vertebral canal by traversing the intervertebral foramen. On the right is the inferior vena cava and ascending lumbar vein, receiving blood from the spinal cord and vertebral canal via the radicular veins from each vertebral level.

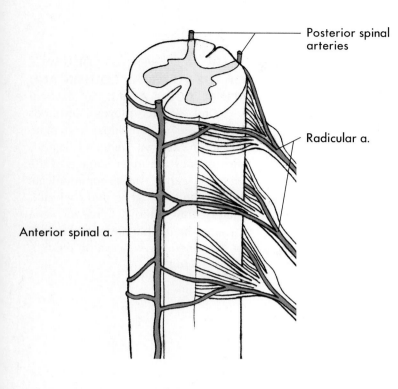

Figure 4-28 FORMATION OF THE ANTERIOR SPINAL ARTERY. Radicular arteries supply the anterior and posterior spinal arteries by entering the vertebral canal through the intervertebral foramina.

branches of the occipital and vertebral arteries) (Figures 4-28 and 4-29). Within the vertebral canal, branches from these longitudinal vessels supply the bodies, pedicles, and laminae of each vertebra. These vessels supply the spinal cord as well (see pp. 439-441).

There is a venous plexus just external to the dura mater of the vertebral canal (the **internal vertebral venous plexus;** see p. 441). In addition, a second profuse plexus of veins lies on the external surface of each vertebra (the **external vertebral venous plexus** (Figure 4-30). This plexus is found anterior to the vertebral bod-

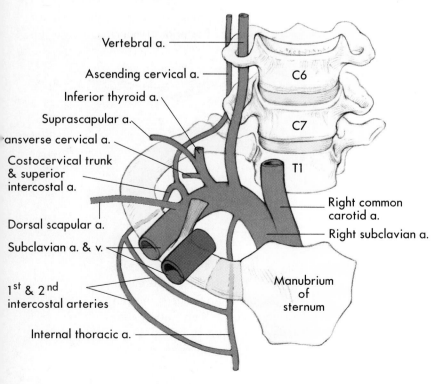

Figure 4-29 VERTEBRAL ARTERY AND CERVICAL VERTEBRAE. The branches of the proximal portion of the subclavian artery are shown. The vertebral artery traverses the foramina transversaria in six of the seven cervical vertebrae. The costocervical trunk divides into an ascending cervical branch and a superior intercostal artery, which then divides into the upper two intercostal arteries. The internal thoracic artery provides anterior intercostal arteries, which anastomose with the posterior intercostal arteries.

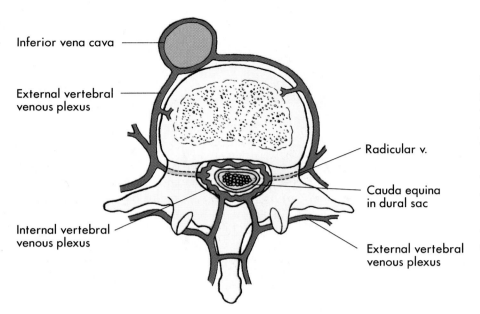

Inferior vena cava

External vertebral venous plexus

Internal vertebral venous plexus

Radicular v.

Cauda equina in dural sac

External vertebral venous plexus

Figure 4-30 VENOUS DRAINAGE OF THE VERTEBRAL COLUMN AND SPINAL CORD AT L3. An external vertebral venous plexus surrounds the surface of individual vertebrae, while an internal vertebral venous plexus lines the inner surface of the vertebral canal. These communicate freely with each other, and each ultimately drains into the inferior vena cava (in the lumbar and sacral areas), or the superior vena cava (in the thoracic region).

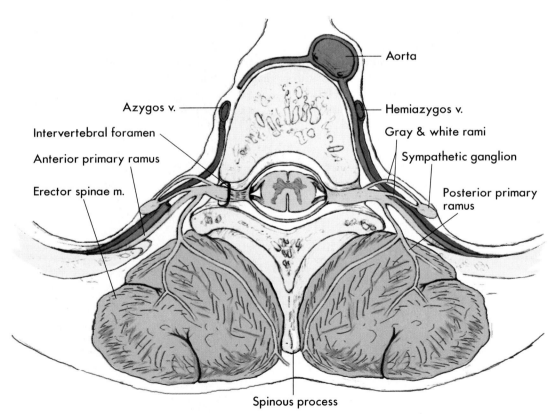

Aorta

Azygos v.

Intervertebral foramen

Anterior primary ramus

Erector spinae m.

Hemiazygos v.

Gray & white rami

Sympathetic ganglion

Posterior primary ramus

Spinous process

Figure 4-31   SPINAL CORD AND THE INTERCOSTAL SPACE. The spinal cord is shown within the vertebral canal, and the spinal nerve, encased in dura mater, escapes to either side through the intervertebral foramen. Note the division of each spinal nerve into an anterior and posterior primary ramus. Also shown are the sympathetic chains, aorta with its paired posterior intercostal arteries, and the azygos/hemiazygos veins draining the intercostal spaces. The nearby intercostal arteries and azygos/hemiazygos veins provide branches that bring blood into the vertebral canal. **SEE ATLAS, FIGS. 4-1, 4-5, 4-30**

ies, alongside the transverse processes, and around the base of the spinous processes. Both the internal and external venous plexuses anastomose freely with segmental veins of the body wall at all levels of the posterior thoracic and posterior abdominal walls. These rich anastomoses are a valuable mechanism for collateral blood flow but unfortunately also make it possible for malignant cells to spread from one region of the body to another.

INNERVATION OF THE BACK AND VERTEBRAL COLUMN

The intrinsic musculature of the back is innervated by the **posterior primary rami** of segmental spinal nerves (Figure 4-31). These nerves also innervate the skin and subcutaneous tissues overlying the intrinsic muscles of the back, the vertebral column, and the meninges. Posterior primary rami contain the full variety of somatic motor, autonomic, and sensory axons found in the anterior primary rami. Few of the posterior primary rami have specific names, and most are identified by the spinal cord segments they represent.

CLINICAL ANATOMY OF

THE VERTEBRAL COLUMN

LUMBAR PUNCTURE/SPINAL TAP

This procedure is performed to remove cerebrospinal fluid (CSF) for diagnostic purposes, to measure pressure within the subarachnoid space, or to administer drugs directly into the CSF (indicated for spinal anesthesia or in treatment of certain malignancies). The lumbar puncture (LP) is performed by passing a long, thin needle (3 to 4 inches long for an adult) between adjacent lumbar spines (usually L4 to L5 or L5 to S1) and entering the subarachnoid space. This area of the vertebral column is used because the spinal cord itself ends at the L1 to L2 vertebral level and the inserted needle cannot injure the spinal cord. The lumbar puncture (LP) is a procedure highly dependent on a knowledge of anatomy (Figure 4-32).

CONGENITAL ABNORMALITIES OF THE VERTEBRAL COLUMN

Spina bifida is a spectrum of congenital abnormalities in which the neural arch fails to close. If serious enough, the spinal nerves or even the spinal cord itself may protrude backward out of a defect in the posterior midline of the vertebral column, most commonly in the lumbar region.

Occasionally the vertebrae do not separate from each other successfully or develop only partially. The result is development of only a part of the vertebra (called a **hemivertebra**) or an abnormal fusion of parts of adjacent vertebrae. In either case the result is a progressive malalignment of the vertebral column, due to the asymmetry and the imbalance of muscle forces acting on the vertebral column.

Certain chromosomal conditions (e.g., trisomy 21) are characterized by **laxity** in intervertebral ligaments, creating the risk of spinal cord injury even with apparently "normal" ranges of movement. This is especially true at the atlanto-occipital joint.

INJURIES TO THE VERTEBRAL COLUMN

A *"whiplash" injury* of the cervical spine is a forceful extension, then flexion of the cervical spine. It often involves no permanent displacement of vertebral structures, but muscles and ligaments are injured usually followed by inflammation and muscle spasm. It occurs during rapid decelerations (such as a car hitting a tree), where the driver's head and neck snap forward, then backward forcefully. It is treated by immobilization and rest.

Traumatic forces applied along the vertebral column (as when jumping from a height and landing on the feet) commonly result in **crush** or **compression fractures** of vertebral bodies or the breaking of small fragments away from the body of a vertebra. Painful symptoms are caused by inflammation, nerve compression, and muscle spasm.

Trauma to the upper back and neck poses a special risk to **alignment** of the cervical vertebrae. When vertebral articulations are disrupted, the vertebrae may move with respect to each other, and the spinal cord may be compressed or even severed. This process can occur at any vertebral level but is particularly catastrophic in the **cervical region** because the entire spinal cord below may be affected. Movements of injured patients, therefore, must be minimized until x-rays confirm proper alignment of the cervical spine.

Spondylolysis is a *separation* of parts of a vertebra (spinous process, laminae, and inferior articular facet) from the remaining anterior portion of that vertebra (body, transverse processes, pedicles, and superior articular facet). The defect occurs in the *interarticular*

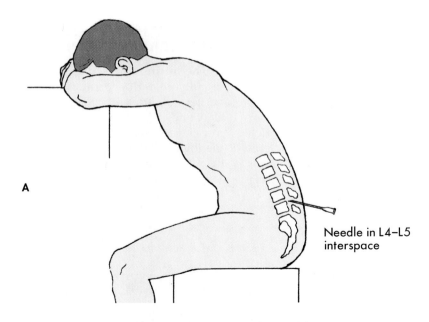

A

Needle in L4–L5
interspace

Lumbar puncture, upright position

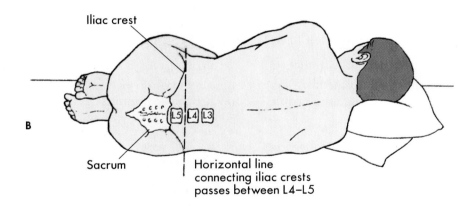

Iliac crest

B

L5 L4 L3

Sacrum

Horizontal line
connecting iliac crests
passes between L4–L5

Lumbar puncture, lateral position

Figure 4-32   LUMBAR PUNCTURE. The lumbar puncture may be performed with the patient sitting upright (**A**) or lying on his or her side (**B**). The upright position is used most often in adults. The lateral position is used most often in children. A line connecting the iliac crests passes through the L4 to L5 interspace, which, along with L5 to S1, is the most commonly chosen interspace for a lumbar puncture. See text for details of the procedure.

THE VERTEBRAL COLUMN (continued)

area. In spondylolysis, there is no true separation of these fragments and no misalignment of the vertebral column.

If the anterior fragment moves anteriorly, taking with it all of the vertebral column superior to it, **spondylolisthesis** exists. Spondylolisthesis threatens the nerve roots of the cauda equina or may cause a narrowing of the pelvic outlet in important situations such as childbirth.

Age and/or trauma lead to weakening of the **annulus fibrosis** of intervertebral disks, causing the **nucleus pulposus** to "herniate" or protrude abnormally into the intervertebral foramina, producing nerve compression. Symptoms can include sensory loss, muscle weakness, and pain (see Figure 4-20).

CONTROL OF HEAD POSITION

Muscles on both the posterior and anterior side of the cervical vertebral column ascend and attach to various points on the base of the skull. On the posterior side muscles, such as **semispinalis**, exemplify this function (see Figure 4-24), while anteriorly muscles, such as **longus capitis,** play this role (see Figure 4-43).

These complex muscles help to support the head and turn it from side to side.

JOINTS OF THE UPPER VERTEBRAL COLUMN

The **transverse ligament of the atlas** (Figure 4-15) normally secures the dens, preventing it from crushing the spinal cord; the act of hanging often fractures this ligament, allowing the cord to be crushed, leading to death.

BLOOD SUPPLY OF THE VERTEBRAL COLUMN

Surgery involving the posterior abdominal wall can represent a threat to radicular arteries in this area, particularly the large **arteria radicularis magna** usually found in the lower thoracic or upper lumbar region. If this vessel is damaged, the spinal cord inferior to this level may be damaged and paralysis may ensue.

The vertebral venous plexus (see Figure 4-30) is a valveless network of vessels that unfortunately can permit malignant cells from one part of the body to travel to another part of the body and spread the disease (*metastasize*).

4.2

section four.two

Spinal Cord

- Structure of the Spinal Cord
- Spinal Nerves and the Spinal Cord
- Spinal Cord and the Meninges
- Spinal Cord and Vertebral Canal

- Blood Supply to the Spinal Cord and Vertebrae
- Sympathetic Nervous System and the Spinal Cord
- "Typical" Spinal Nerve

STRUCTURE OF THE SPINAL CORD

The **spinal cord** is a tapered solid cylinder of neural tissue, continuous superiorly with the brainstem at the level of the foramen magnum of the skull and ending inferiorly at vertebral level L1 to L2 in the adult. The tapered inferior end of the spinal cord is known as the **conus medullaris.** In early stages of development, the spinal cord is a true cylinder, with a hollow interior (the **central canal**). In the adult human, this space is usually obliterated completely, represented only by a small tuft of cells in the center of the spinal cord. The spinal cord contains tens of thousands of **neuron cell bodies,** an **even greater number of axons,** and a variety of **nonneuronal cells and processes,** including **glial cells** and **connective tissue** elements. These nonneuronal cells usually outnumber the neurons approximately 10:1. One of the important roles of glial cells is to create the **myelin** that surrounds individual axons and improves the speed and precision of nerve impulse conduction. The spinal cord is enclosed by three meningeal jackets (see Figure 4-36)—the **pia mater, arachnoid mater,** and **dura mater.** These are described following.

When viewed in cross section, the central **gray matter** of the spinal cord is arranged into a roughly **H-shaped** body (called gray because of its color in the fresh state) (Figure 4-33). This H-shaped body of gray matter contains nearly all of the **neuron cell bodies** of the spinal cord, along with an interlacing network of

axons and glial cell processes. The two posterior vertical elements of the H are the **dorsal** or **posterior horns,** regions of the gray matter where neuron cell bodies concerned with *sensory function* are located. The two anterior vertical elements of the H are the **ventral** or **anterior horns** and contain most of the neuron cell bodies concerned with *motor activity.* In the thoracic and upper lumbar regions of the spinal cord, there is a small **intermediate** or **lateral** horn positioned between the dorsal and ventral horns, along the lateral margin of the gray matter (see Figures 4-33 and 4-35). The intermediate horns contain **sympathetic preganglionic** neuron cell bodies. The lateral horn is absent in other parts of the spinal cord (i.e., cervical, lumbar below L3, sacral, and coccygeal).

Surrounding the gray matter is a mantle of spinal cord **white matter** (so named because its high myelin content makes it appear white in the fresh state; see Figure 4-33). The white matter of the spinal cord consists of many large and important bundles of axons (often called "columns") ascending toward the brain and descending from the brain to the spinal cord. Still other groups of axons ramify within nearby regions of the spinal cord.

In the anterior midline of the cord, there is a vertical fissure, the **anterior median fissure,** and a comparable **posterior median fissure** on the dorsum of the cord. Blood vessels descend into each of these fissures, gaining more ready access to the deepest structures within the spinal cord (see Figure 4-33).

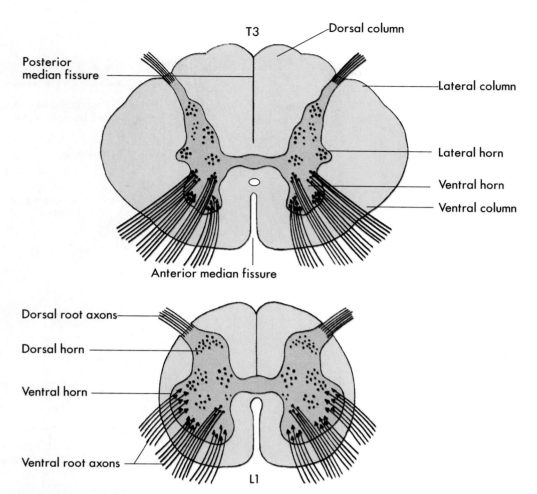

Figure 4-33   INNER STRUCTURE OF THE SPINAL CORD. Clusters of neurons in the ventral horn of the spinal cord can be demonstrated to innervate individual groups of muscles or even single individual muscles. The same is true for the dorsal horn, where sensory axons enter the spinal cord in an organized fashion representing discrete regions of the body.

SPINAL NERVES AND THE SPINAL CORD

Many spinal cord neurons produce axons traveling away from the spinal cord and out into the tissues of the body, where they provide motor innervation to various structures or tissues (also called *efferent* axons). These motor axons—the **ventral roots**—form a continuum of small nerve roots exiting along each ventrolateral surface of the spinal cord (see Figures 4-35 and 4-36). All ventral root axons have their cell bodies in the anterior or lateral horns of the spinal cord. Ventral root axons innervate muscles, glands, or other neurons, located in various regions of the periphery of the body. The ventral roots are surrounded and supported by so-called **nonneuronal tissues—meningeal coverings, Schwann cells, connective tissue elements,** and **small blood vessels** (Figure 4-34).

Emerging along the *dorsolateral margin* of each side of the spinal cord is a set of nerve fibers that comprise the **dorsal roots** (Figure 4-35). The dorsal roots consist exclusively of **sensory axons,** bringing neural signals from the periphery into the spinal cord (also called *afferent* axons). Near where the dorsal and ventral roots unite to form the spinal nerve is found the **dorsal root ganglion (DRG),** an ovoid swelling on the dorsal root. The **neuron cell bodies** of all dorsal root axons are found in the DRG, not in the spinal cord. Sensory neurons emit only two processes (see Figure 4-34). First is a short **central process,** traveling from the DRG along the dorsal root and into the spinal cord. Some central processes synapse on neurons in the spinal cord, while others ascend in the spinal cord all the way up into the brainstem, where they then synapse. Second is the

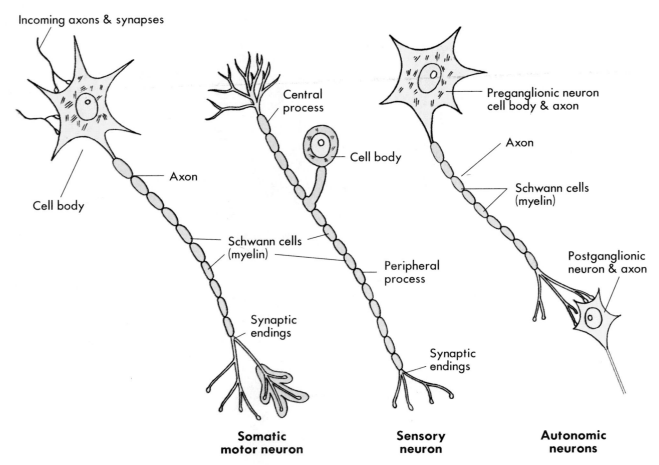

Figure 4-34   VARIETIES OF NEURONS. Three of the most commonly encountered neurons in the peripheral nervous system. On the left is the typical **somatic motor neuron,** the axon of which directly innervates striated muscle. In the center is a typical **sensory neuron,** with a central and peripheral process. On the right are **two autonomic neurons,** with a ganglionic synapse connecting the two. (See text for details.)

longer **peripheral process** of the DRG neuron. The peripheral process travels outward from the DRG in the dorsal root and into the spinal nerve (see following) later to ramify within the tissue the axon innervates. Like the ventral roots, dorsal roots contain many **non-neuronal tissues.** In sensory neurons, the neural impulse originates in the periphery, is conducted along the peripheral process, travels past the cell body in the DRG, and travels medially along the central process to enter the spinal cord.

Within the **intervertebral foramina,** the ventral and dorsal roots of each segment unite to form a true **spinal nerve** (see Figure 4-35). Spinal nerves represent all of the axons leaving and entering the spinal cord at that level. The spinal nerve quickly divides into two unequal derivative branches—the **posterior primary ramus,** supplying tissues adjacent to the posterior midline of the trunk, and the **anterior primary ramus,** supplying tissues in the lateral and anterior parts of the body wall and all of the limbs.

In the cervical and upper thoracic regions, the intervertebral foramina are almost directly adjacent to the corresponding segment of the spinal cord, but, in the lower thoracic, lumbar, sacral, and coccygeal segments, the intervertebral foramina are often many centimeters below the section of the spinal cord with which they are connected. Since the formation of the true spinal nerve always occurs within the intervertebral foramen, dorsal and ventral roots in these segments descend for many centimeters (forming the **cauda equina**) before they join to form the spinal nerve (see Figure 4-38).

SPINAL CORD AND THE MENINGES

There are **three meningeal layers** surrounding the spinal cord (Figure 4-36). The innermost and thinnest layer is the **pia mater.** It is closely applied to the surface of the spinal cord, and a thin **sleeve** of pia extends outward for a short distance encircling each dorsal and

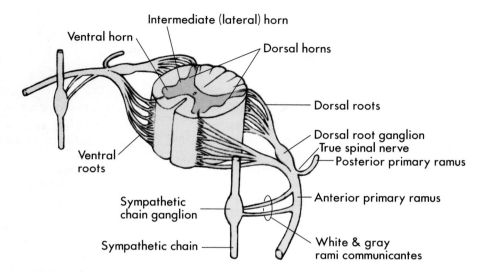

Figure 4-35   SPINAL CORD AND SYMPATHETIC CHAINS. Each spinal segment consists of paired dorsal and ventral rootlets, each of which collects into a single bundle known as the dorsal and ventral root of each side. The dorsal root ganglion is located just proximal to the junction of the dorsal and ventral roots. The sympathetic ganglia are connected to the spinal nerve by rami communicantes. In the thoracic region, there are both white and gray rami, while above T1 and below L2 there are only gray rami communicantes.   SEE ATLAS, FIG. 4-38

ventral root as it leaves the lateral surface of the cord. In the cervical and thoracic regions, there is a flattened midline extension of pia on each side of the spinal cord in the frontal plane. This extension or shelf, known as the **denticulate ligament,** extends laterally to attach to the inner surface of the dura, lining the vertebral canal (see Figure 4-36, *A*). While the shelflike denticulate ligament has a continuous medial origin from the pia covering the spinal cord, its lateral attachments are interrupted, forming a series of toothlike connections to the dura. Its name (*denticulate*) is derived from these interrupted lateral attachments. The denticulate ligament helps stabilize the spinal cord within the vertebral canal. The important **accessory nerve** (cranial nerve XI), arising from the upper five to six cervical spinal cord segments, ascends along the dorsal surface of the denticulate ligament. This **spinal root of the accessory nerve** eventually traverses the foramen magnum and is reunited with the cranial root of the accessory nerve (cranial nerve XI), forming the complete cranial nerve XI.

There is another set of strands of pia mater, the incomplete **subarachnoid septum,** extending from the dorsal midline of the cord in the sagittal plane and attaching posteriorly to the dura. It is most reliably present in the cervical region but may be missing elsewhere (see Figure 4-36, *A*). There is a similar set of pial filaments in the ventral midline.

The **arachnoid mater** is the intermediate of the three meningeal layers (see Figure 4-36, *B*). It is also delicate although stronger than the pia. It is called *arachnoid* because of the lacy irregular strands of tissue (like a spider web) that extend from the inner surface of the arachnoid membrane, crossing the subarachnoid space to attach to the pia. The arachnoid is notable for enclosing the **arteries** whose branches supply the brain and spinal cord (Figure 4-37). Paradoxically, the arachnoid itself is very poorly vascularized. Also important is the fact that the arachnoid encloses the layer of **cerebrospinal fluid (CSF)** surrounding the brain and spinal cord. The CSF occupies a wide fluid-filled gap between the pia and arachnoid mater. This is known as the **subarachnoid space.** Although not numerous in the area of the spinal cord, along the superior surface of the brain the arachnoid forms small tufts that protrude through the outer dural covering and lie within the lumina of large dural venous sinuses. These structures (the **arachnoid granulations**) allows CSF to diffuse back into the bloodstream, preventing a build-up of CSF pressure within the brain. The arachnoid mater, like the dura mater, extends inferiorly to the level of the S2 vertebra.

The thickest and strongest of the meningeal layers is the **dura mater.** It has two layers in the cranial cavity (where it is known as **cranial dura**) but only one surrounding the spinal cord. While the outer layer of the cranial dura is tightly adherent to the inner periosteal layer of the skull, the single layer of dura found surrounding the spinal cord is separated from the inner surfaces of the bones comprising the vertebral column

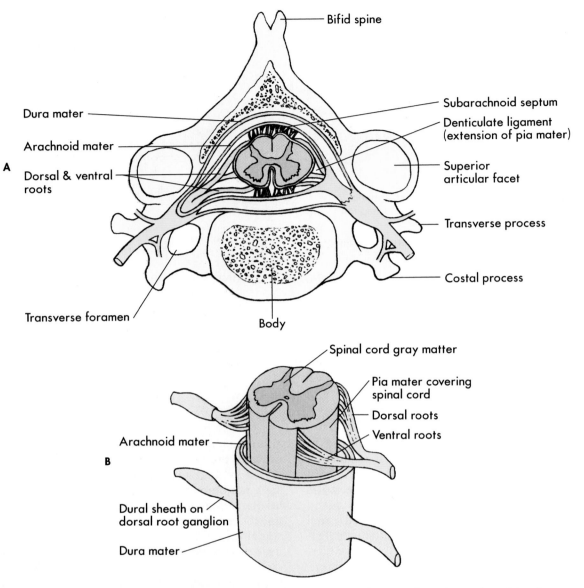

Figure 4-36   CERVICAL SPINAL CORD (IN SITU).   A, The spinal cord is tethered by the denticulate ligaments and the subarachnoid septum. Extensions of pia, arachnoid, and dura mater enclose the spinal nerves as they exit through the intervertebral foramina. The dura becomes continuous with the epineurium, the connective tissue sheath enclosing peripheral nerves. **B,** The spinal cord is covered by three layers of meningeal tissue—the pia mater, arachnoid mater, and the dura mater.   SEE ATLAS, FIG. 4-5, 4-32, 4-37

by a wide space, the **epidural space,** in which lie fat and elements of the internal vertebral venous plexus (see Figure 4-30). The dura is closely adherent to the arachnoid membrane, which lies just interior to the dura. At the base of the skull, the dura of the vertebral canal is attached to the perimeter of the foramen magnum. Within the vertebral canal, the dura and arachnoid membranes form a wide cylinder enclosing the spinal cord and surrounding the subarachnoid space in

which CSF lies. The dural and arachnoid membranes extend inferiorly to vertebral level S2 to S4, where the dura narrows considerably. Below this level, the dura closely surrounds the **filum terminale** (a downward extension of pia mater), which terminates lower still near the second coccygeal vertebra (Co2).

Extensions of the dura form sleeves around the dorsal and ventral roots as they move away from the spinal cord toward the intervertebral foramina at each

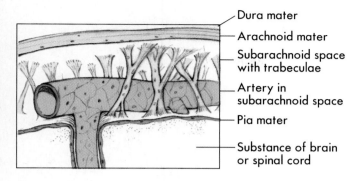

- Dura mater
- Arachnoid mater
- Subarachnoid space with trabeculae
- Artery in subarachnoid space
- Pia mater
- Substance of brain or spinal cord

Figure 4-37   SUBARACHNOID SPACE. The major arteries supplying the spinal cord lie in the subarachnoid space and emit branches that descend into the substance of the spinal cord. The pia mater covers the spinal cord itself.

level (see Figure 4-36, *B*). The dura encloses the dorsal root ganglion on the dorsal root, but, distal to this point, the dural sheath blends with a thick connective tissue sheath (the *epineurium*), which encloses the nerves as they travel further out into the periphery.

Elements of the spinal cord and its meninges continue inferiorly inside the vertebral canal of the sacrum. Below the **conus medullaris** (inferior end of the spinal cord, usually at vertebral level L2), the pia mater is continued as the **filum terminale,** anchored inferiorly to the second coccygeal vertebra (see Figure 4-38). For the upper two thirds of its course, the filum is very loosely surrounded by the CSF and sheaths of arachnoid and dura mater. In the upper two thirds of the filum, therefore, the **subarachnoid space** (between the filum and the arachnoid/dura) is particularly wide, which is fortuitous because this is the region where the needle enters the subarachnoid space during a **lumbar puncture** (see Figure 4-32; see also section on clinical anatomy of the spinal cord). In its lower third (opposite S3 and below), the arachnoid/dura lies closer to the filum, and the subarachnoid space is absent.

SPINAL CORD AND VERTEBRAL CANAL

The **spinal cord** lies protected within the **vertebral** or **spinal canal.** Between each pair of vertebrae there is a gap on the left and right side of the vertebral column, the **intervertebral foramina** (see Figure 4-9). Through these, the left- and right-sided spinal nerves for that segment escape the vertebral canal and begin their journey to the areas of the body wall or limbs that they innervate. The vertebral canal is found throughout the length of the vertebral column, but the spinal cord itself extends only from the first cervical (C1) level to the level of the first or second lumbar vertebra (L1 to L2). This results from the **differential growth** of the vertebral column and spinal cord, especially in the later stages of prenatal development. Below L2, the vertebral canal contains the many nerve roots that comprise the **cauda equina** (so named because it resembles the many hairs in a horse's tail). The cauda equina (Figure 4-38) is made up of all those descending nerve roots that are destined to exit the vertebral canal below vertebral

level L2, although they originated from the spinal cord at levels superior to vertebral level L2. This arrangement is created because the vertebral column and the spinal cord, although each consists of cervical, thoracic, lumbar, sacral, and coccygeal segments, are "out of register" with each other. In the cervical region, corresponding levels of the spinal cord and vertebral column lie nearly adjacent to each other, and a nerve root such as C3 exits the vertebral canal through the C2 to C3 intervertebral foramen, lying almost directly lateral to the C3 segment of the spinal cord. Further down the spinal cord, however, intervertebral foramina are found more and more inferior to the corresponding spinal cord level. This creates a situation where a nerve root, having emerged from the spinal cord, must descend within the vertebral canal for a considerable distance before exiting the vertebral canal through its corresponding intervertebral foramen. The newborn human child demonstrates only a mild degree of this disparity between spinal cord and vertebral column. With growth and increased body length, the disparity between levels of the vertebral column and spinal cord becomes greater (Figure 4-39).

The numbering of spinal nerves and vertebral segments is sometimes confusing. In the cervical region, where there are *seven cervical vertebrae,* there are in fact *eight cervical nerves.* The C1 cervical nerve exits the vertebral canal above the C1 vertebra (i.e., between it and the skull), the C2 nerve above the C2 vertebra (or between vertebrae C1 and C2), and so on. However, the nerve exiting below the C7 vertebra (and above the T1 vertebra) is designated C8. Below this point, spinal nerves share a name with the vertebra *below which* they exit the vertebral canal (e.g., the T5 nerve exits between T5 and T6, the L3 nerve between L3 and L4, etc.)

BLOOD SUPPLY TO THE SPINAL CORD AND VERTEBRAE
Arterial Supply

The spinal cord is supplied with blood by a series of paired arterial branches, entering the vertebral canal by traversing the intervertebral foramina on each side. At

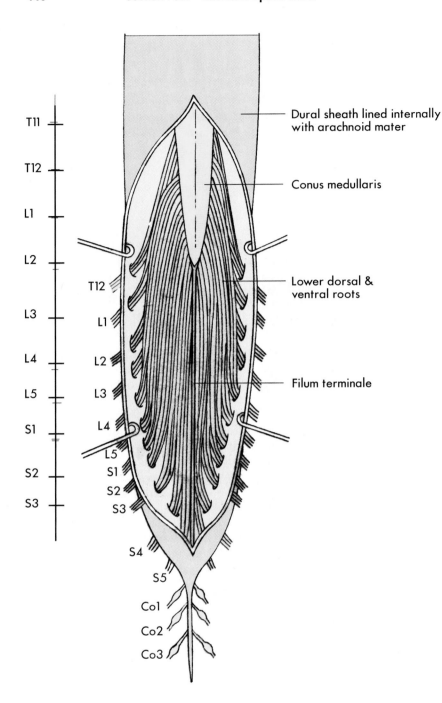

T11

T12

L1

L2

L3

L4

L5

S1

S2

S3

Dural sheath lined internally with arachnoid mater

Conus medullaris

T12
L1
L2
L3
L4
L5
S1
S2
S3

Lower dorsal & ventral roots

Filum terminale

S4
S5
Co1
Co2
Co3

Figure 4-38   CAUDA EQUINA. At the inferior end of the spinal cord, segmental nerve roots must descend considerably before they exit the vertebral canal and travel out into the periphery. The spinal cord ends at L2, and the dural sac surrounding the cord ends at S2 to S4, but the pia mater extends further inferiorly as the filum terminale, which ultimately attaches to the coccygeal vertebrae. The conus medullaris is the inferior-most end of the spinal cord proper.   See Atlas, Fig. 4-36

each level these **radicular arteries** give direct blood supply to the dorsal roots, ventral roots, and the adjacent areas of the spinal cord and, in addition, contribute to the **anterior** and **posterior spinal arteries,** longitudinal vessels that travel up and down most of the length of the spinal cord (Figure 4-40). Branches of the **vertebral, deep cervical, intercostal,** and **lumbar arteries** contribute branches to the spinal cord and to the anterior and posterior spinal arteries in this way. The single **anterior spinal artery** is positioned directly anterior to the cord in the anterior median fissure. The two **posterior spinal arteries** are positioned on each

side of the dorsal root at its entry into the spinal cord (see Figure 4-40). The anterior spinal artery is responsible for the blood supply to the anterior two thirds of the spinal cord, while the posterior spinal arteries supply the rest. These anterior and posterior spinal arteries also provide blood supply to the surrounding vertebral column. A particularly large radicular artery in the lower thoracic or upper lumbar region is often responsible for blood supply to most of the spinal cord at that level and below. Injury to this largest radicular artery can result in permanent injury to the spinal cord.

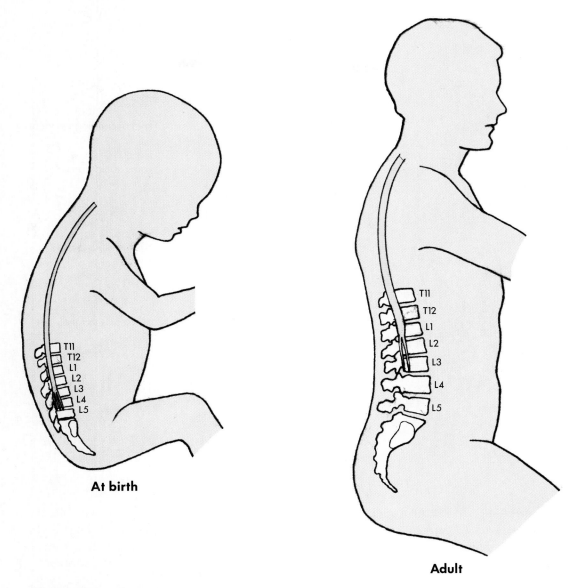

At birth

Adult

Figure 4-39 SPINAL CORD IN THE INFANT AND THE ADULT. In the newborn, the spinal cord ends at the L3 to L4 vertebral level, but in the adult it terminates at the L1 to L2 vertebral level.

Venous Drainage

Radicular veins drain each section of the spinal cord, traveling through the intervertebral foramina to contribute to the formation of the **anterior spinal vein** and multiple **posterior spinal veins.** These drain freely into the external and internal vertebral venous plexuses (see Figure 4-30). For a more detailed discussion of venous drainage, see p. 429.

SYMPATHETIC NERVOUS SYSTEM AND THE SPINAL CORD

The **sympathetic chains,** and the axons that link them to the spinal cord and to exiting spinal nerves, represent part of the **sympathetic division** of the **auto-**nomic nervous system. The sympathetic division is also known as the **thoracolumbar outflow** because only cord segments T1 to L2 contribute preganglionic axons to the sympathetic chain. Sympathetic innervation has widespread effects on most areas of the body (excluding only the brain itself). In general, sympathetic activity produces an increase in various aspects of body metabolism and increases in the "vital signs" of body function—*heart rate, respiratory rate, blood pressure,* and *temperature.* These effects are produced by neural influence on the organs and tissues involved—for example, sympathetic innervation of the heart increases its rate of beating, and contraction of the smooth muscle in the walls of blood vessels (vasoconstriction) produces a de-

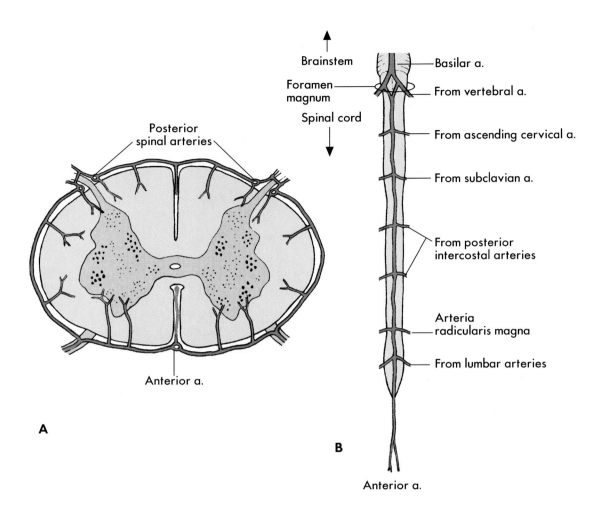

Figure 4-40   ARTERIAL SUPPLY OF THE SPINAL CORD. A, Spinal cord receives blood from a series of perpendicular branches that arise on the outer surface of the cord and penetrate inward. The principal parent vessels from which these branches arise are the single anterior spinal artery and the paired posterior spinal arteries. **B,** Numerous sources of blood supply the anterior spinal artery along its course.

crease in the collective volume in the vascular system and increases blood pressure.

Somatic Nerves and Autonomic Nerves

Spinal nerves that innervate striated muscle (**somatic nerves**) have their cell bodies in the spinal cord and have axons that leave the spinal cord in the ventral roots to innervate the striated muscle directly. The regulation of striated muscle contraction is thus carried out by a **single neuron,** whose cell body is in the spinal cord and whose axon directly enters the substance of the target striated muscle (see Figure 4-34). By contrast, sympathetic innervation of smooth muscle or glands involves not one but **two neurons** in the transmission of the neural signal from the spinal cord to the target

tissue (smooth muscle, cardiac muscle, or gland). The first of the two neurons (and its axon) is called the **preganglionic element** (because the synapse between these two neurons often but not always occurs in a ganglion). The neuron on which the preganglionic axon synapses (and its axon) is known as the **postganglionic element.***

In the case of sympathetic nerves, the preganglionic cell body lies in the **intermediate** or **lateral horn** of

---

*The terms **preganglionic** and **postganglionic** are established in medical terminology because in most cases the preganglionic axon synapses on the postganglionic cell body *in a ganglion.* In certain cases involving both sympathetic and parasympathetic axons, this synapse does not occur within a ganglion, but the terms are employed nonetheless.

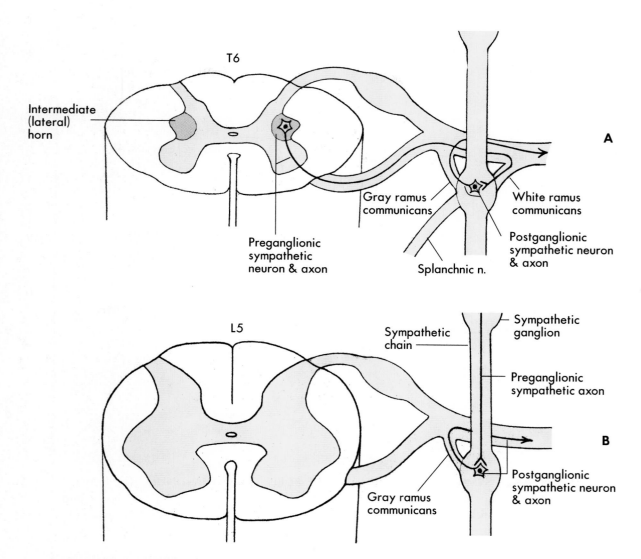

Figure 4-41 SYMPATHETIC NERVES AT DIFFERENT VERTEBRAL LEVELS. A, At vertebral levels T1 to L2, preganglionic sympathetic neuron cell bodies are located in the intermediate horn, and their axons travel in the ventral root to reach the sympathetic chain. The axons then traverse the white ramus communicans to enter the sympathetic ganglion and, as shown here, synapse in a neuron in that ganglion (other options would be to enter the splanchnic nerve or to ascend or descend in the sympathetic chain). When they synapse in the sympathetic ganglion, the postganglionic axon then traverses the gray ramus communicans to reenter the spinal nerve. **B,** At a level where no lateral horn exists, the sympathetic ganglion receives preganglionic input through the sympathetic chain. The postganglionic axons traverse the gray ramus to enter the spinal nerve for that level.

the spinal cord (found only at levels T1 to L2). **Preganglionic sympathetic axons** arising from these neurons leave the spinal cord as part of the ventral roots of those spinal segments. As they approach the vicinity of the sympathetic chain, these preganglionic sympathetic axons depart from the spinal nerve and enter the sympathetic chain (traveling through **white rami communicantes** as they do) (Figure 4-41).

Sympathetic Chains

An elongated chain of **sympathetic ganglia** lies along the left and right sides of the vertebral column, extending all the way from the upper cervical region downward to the level of the lower part of the sacral region, where they unite to form the **ganglion impar** (see Figure 4-44). Bundles of axons connect the individual ganglia, creating the **sympathetic chain** (see Figure 4-35).

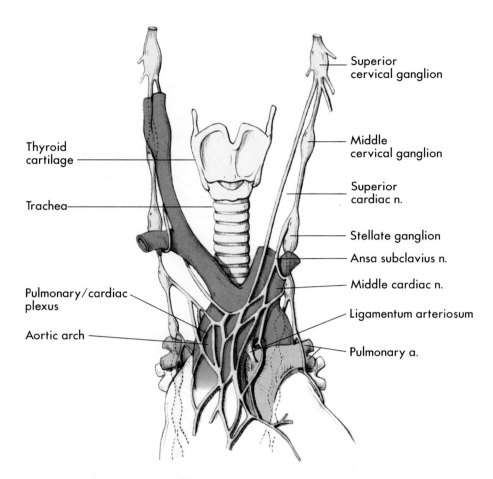

Figure 4-42   SYMPATHETIC NERVES IN THE SUPERIOR MEDIASTINUM. The cervical sympathetic ganglia supply postganglionic branches (the cardiac nerves), which descend through the neck and enter the mediastinum. Here they enter plexuses that innervate the heart and lungs.

A **sympathetic ganglion** is a cluster of several hundred **multipolar neuron** cell bodies, along with hundreds of smaller **interneurons** whose dendrites and axons are confined within the ganglion. Each ganglion in the chain (excepting those at the cervical and caudal ends of the chain) is joined to the ganglion above and the ganglion below by a continuous bundle of axons known as the **sympathetic chain.** The sympathetic chain is made up of many axons, ascending or descending from one level to another. Early in development, there is one sympathetic ganglion for each spinal level, but in adulthood some of the ganglia fuse. As a result, the total number of sympathetic ganglia along each side of the vertebral column is somewhat less than the total number of spinal cord segments. This is most evident in the cervical region, where there are three ganglia in the adult (the **superior, middle,** and **inferior**) representing the eight cervical segments of the spinal cord (Figure 4-42). The **superior cervical ganglion** represents the fusion of the original cervical ganglia one to four, the **middle cervical ganglion** ganglia

five and six, and the **inferior cervical ganglion** ganglia seven and eight (Figure 4-43). To complicate matters further, the inferior cervical ganglion is usually fused with the first thoracic ganglion, to form the **stellate ganglion.** In the thoracic and lumbar regions, there is usually a 1:1 relationship between spinal cord segments and sympathetic chain ganglia. In the sacral region, the original five ganglia are often partially fused so that only three or four ganglia are present in the adult (Figure 4-44).

Connections of the Sympathetic Chains and Spinal Nerves

At all levels there is a **gray ramus communicans** linking the segmental spinal nerve at that level to the sympathetic chain. These rami contain **postganglionic** sympathetic axons leaving the sympathetic ganglion and entering the spinal nerve. For those sympathetic ganglia opposite spinal cord levels T1 to L2, however, there are also one or two **white rami communicans**

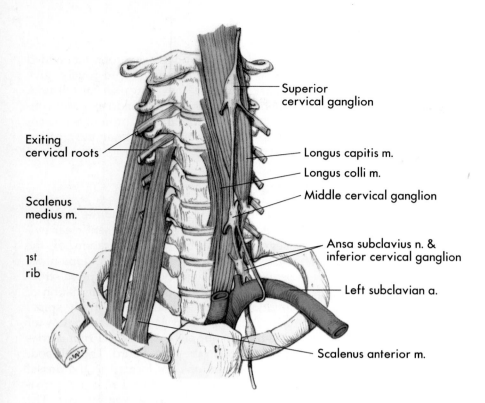

Superior
cervical ganglion

Longus capitis m.

Longus colli m.

Middle cervical ganglion

Ansa subclavius n. &
inferior cervical ganglion

Left subclavian a.

Scalenus anterior m.

Exiting
cervical roots

Scalenus
medius m.

1st
rib

Figure 4-43 ANTERIOR CERVICAL MUSCLES AND THE SYMPATHETIC CHAIN. The anterior cervical muscles (e.g., **longus colli, longus capitis**) lie on the anterior surfaces of the bodies and transverse processes of the seven cervical vertebrae. They mediate flexion (i.e., forward bending) of the head on the trunk and are innervated by individual twigs of the cervical spinal nerves. Also shown is the sympathetic chain in the neck, where the ganglia are collected into a superior, middle, and inferior cervical ganglion. The small axonal loop encircling the subclavian artery is known as the **ansa subclavius**. Also shown are the cervical roots emerging through the intervertebral foramina.

connecting the spinal nerve to the sympathetic ganglion. Axons in these rami are **myelinated** (hence the descriptive term "white"). These are **preganglionic sympathetic axons,** whose cell bodies are in the **lateral horn** of the spinal cord gray matter in cord segments T1 to L2. Since there is no lateral horn in spinal cord segments above T1 or below L2, it follows that there are no white rami communicans with sympathetic ganglia above T1 or below L2.

Having reached the sympathetic chain ganglion, the white ramus axon follows one of three paths: *first,* it may synapse on one of the neurons in that sympathetic ganglion. *Second,* the axon may travel upward or downward through the sympathetic chain and then synapse upon a neuron in another sympathetic ganglion. *Third,* the axon may pass through the sympathetic ganglion (without synapsing) and exit along the medial border of the ganglion to help form the **greater, lesser,** or **least splanchnic nerves,** which travel to the abdomen and synapse on specialized sympathetic ganglia located along the abdominal aorta (known as **prevertebral ganglia**). These splanchnic nerves issue only from sympathetic ganglia opposite spinal segments T6 to T12 and are not found in other areas of the sympathetic chain. Every sympathetic ganglion issues postganglionic splanchnic axons along its medial border—axons that innervate structures in the posterior midline of the body. The **cardiac nerves** arise from the superior and middle cervical ganglia and innervate the heart and lungs. Apart from these, no splanchnic nerve has an individual name.

All of the sympathetic ganglia in the chain are connected to nearby spinal nerves by one or more **gray rami communicans.** These rami contain mostly unmyelinated axons (hence the descriptive term "gray"), whose cell bodies are in the sympathetic ganglia. These are **postganglionic sympathetic axons** which, after rejoining the spinal nerves, travel along with those nerves and innervate **smooth muscle** (as in the wall of blood vessels), **arrector pili** muscles of hair follicles, and **sweat glands.** Gray rami are found at *every level* of the spinal cord, and they represent the path by which postganglionic sympathetic axons are distributed in *all spinal nerves* (in contrast to preganglionic sympathetic axons, which are found only in ventral roots from segments T1 to L2).

Parasympathetic Nerves and the Spinal Cord

Parasympathetic neurons of the spinal cord are found only in **sacral segments two, three,** and **four** and their derivative nerves. Other parasympathetic axons arise in cranial nerves three, seven, nine, and ten. The parasympathetic system is also known as the **craniosacral outflow.** The spinal parasympathetic axons originate from the gray matter of the cord in a region comparable to the *lateral horn* from which sympathetic axons originate in the thoracic and upper lumbar spinal cord. Parasympathetic axons travel outward in sacral spinal roots two, three, and four and a few centimeters from the spinal cord separate and travel medially across the pelvic floor as the **pelvic nerve** (also

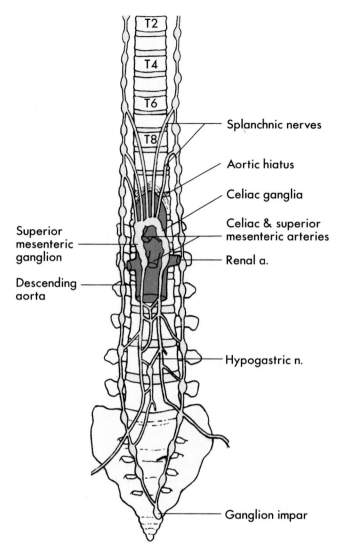

Splanchnic nerves

Aortic hiatus

Celiac ganglia

Celiac & superior
mesenteric arteries

Renal a.

Superior
mesenteric
ganglion

Descending
aorta

Hypogastric n.

Ganglion impar

**Figure 4-44   SYMPATHETIC CHAINS AND SPLANCHNIC
NERVES.** The sympathetic chains emit medial branches
from the T6 to T12 levels (the splanchnic nerves). These
synapse in ganglia positioned at the origin of branches of
the abdominal aorta, especially the celiac ganglion. The
sympathetic chains continue inferiorly in the abdomen
and eventually meet in the midline, anterior to the coccyx (the ganglion impar).

known as **pelvic splanchnic nerves** or **nervi erigentes**).
Some of these preganglionic parasympathetic axons
contribute to a neural plexus on the urinary bladder
neck, while others ascend in the posterior abdominal
wall and innervate the *descending colon.* Axons innervating the *sigmoid colon* travel within the two leaflets of
the sigmoid mesocolon. On reaching the descending
colon, sigmoid colon, urinary bladder, and other pelvic
floor viscera, these axons synapse on clusters of neurons embedded in the walls of these organs. The axons
of the pelvic nerve represent the *preganglionic element* in

this autonomic pathway, and the neurons embedded
in the walls of the organs listed previously give
off axons that represent the *postganglionic element.*
Parasympathetic innervation of the bladder causes contraction of bladder wall musculature, promotes muscular activity in the colon, and participates in the creation
of erections in the genitalia.

"TYPICAL" SPINAL NERVE

The paired dorsal and ventral roots and the region of
the spinal cord to which they join represent clear evidence of **segmentation** in the organization of the
human body. Especially in the thorax and abdomen, we
can see most clearly the evidence of a repetitive structure in adjoining parts of the body. The foundation of
this segmentation is the **spinal nerve.** Each spinal
nerve contains the motor and sensory innervation for
the part of the body it supplies. The **dorsal root** carries
sensory axons inward to the spinal cord. The cell bodies of these sensory neurons are located in the **dorsal
root ganglia,** positioned on the dorsal root just proximal to the point where it joins the ventral root. The
ventral roots carry motor axons away from the spinal
cord toward the structures in the periphery. **Somatic
motor nerves** have their cell bodies in the ventral horn
of the spinal cord, at all levels, and travel outward in
the ventral roots, eventually to innervate striated muscles in various parts of the body. A special subclass of
motor axons, the **preganglionic sympathetic axons,** is
found only in the ventral roots of cord segments T1 to
L2. These preganglionic axons leave the ventral root
and enter the sympathetic chain ganglion at the same
segment, to be distributed as described in the preceding section.

The vertebral column provides a clear illustration of the
segmental organization of the body. The segments are
roughly disk-shaped, and the vertebra for each segment
provides a posterior attachment for many of the muscles that encircle the trunk. Each segment, which is
manifested as an intercostal space on the surface of the
thorax and a similar horizontal band on the wall of the
abdomen, is innervated by a segmental spinal nerve
and receives blood supply from a single intercostal
artery and vein (although each individual nerve, artery,
and vein have collateral branches that also supply the
adjacent spaces on each side). In the limbs and the
head and neck, the segmental nature of the body is distorted and difficult to appreciate, though evidence of
segmentation still remains. Appreciation of the segmentation of the body clarifies, at least in part, the many
complexities of human structure.

THE SPINAL CORD

SPINAL CORD COMPRESSION

When disk herniation occurs in a posterior direction, the spinal cord itself may be compressed and permanently injured. This condition is a true emergency and requires rapid diagnosis and corrective surgery if permanent injury is to be avoided.

DISEASES OF SPINAL MOTOR NEURONS

Certain infectious diseases (e.g., **poliomyelitis**) or inborn conditions (**Werdnig-Hoffman disease, amyotrophic lateral sclerosis or ALS**) have a predilection for the ventral horn motor neuron, whose axons innervate striated muscles. These conditions produce progressive and irreversible loss of function of these muscles. When they involve the muscles crucial for breathing (the diaphragm, abdominal and thoracic wall muscles, etc.), then the conditions become truly life-threatening.

DERMATOMES

The region of skin innervated by the nerves arising in a single segment of the spinal cord is defined as the **dermatome** of that segment. In the thoracic and upper abdominal wall the dermatomes are clearly defined, and the dermatomes in these areas look like thick disks stacked one atop the other.

REFERRED PAIN

Referred pain is defined as a sensation of pain in one area of the body that is produced by a pathologic process in a different area of the body. Common examples are the arm or shoulder pain experienced as the result of injury to the heart, or shoulder pain associated with pathologic processes involving the diaphragm. The explanation for these phenomena is not clear. It appears that incoming sensory signals from the area of true pathologic disturbance (e.g., the heart, during the interruption of coronary blood flow that occurs during a "heart attack") reach the spinal cord and produce excitation in adjacent neurons in that part of the spinal cord (in this case, neurons that innervate areas of the arm or shoulder). The brain interprets the excitation of the neurons innervating the arm or shoulder as evidence of a real pathologic condition in the arm or shoulder. As further evidence that the brain can be "fooled," consider the phenomenon observed in cases of **"phantom limb pain,"** where amputees continue to experience feelings in a limb that has been removed because stimulation of the nerves that formerly supplied the amputated part is interpreted by the brain as sensation occuring in that removed limb.

REMOVAL OF CEREBROSPINAL FLUID (THE "LUMBAR PUNCTURE" OR "SPINAL TAP")

The **cauda equina** is made up of all those descending nerve roots that are destined to exit the vertebral column below vertebral level L2, although they originated from the spinal cord at levels superior to vertebral level L2 (see Figure 4-38). This arrangement creates the opportunity for physicians to remove samples of cerebrospinal fluid by inserting needles into the vertebral canal below L2, safe in the knowledge that the needle will not jeopardize the spinal cord itself. Nerve roots rarely might be damaged by the needle, but these can regenerate—unlike the spinal cord itself, which would be permanently injured by a needle puncture. For this reason, lumbar punctures (see Figure 4-32) are nearly always performed below vertebral level L2.

EPIDURAL AND SPINAL ANESTHESIA

Using a knowledge of the spinal nerve roots, meninges, and the vertebral column, it is possible to anesthetize large regions of the body without having to place the patient under general anesthesia. This is desirable in surgeries involving the abdomen, pelvis, or lower limbs, and is used frequently in childbirth. **Epidural anesthesia** is produced by infusing local anesthetic agents into the space between the dura and the bony interior of the vertebral canal. **Spinal anesthesia** is produced by injecting local anesthetics into the subarachnoid space. In each case, the goal is to bathe nerve roots in the anesthetic medication, blocking signal transmission. This produces anesthesia for those areas of the body supplied by the nerve roots involved. It is especially useful in childbirth, where the mother can remain awake during the birth but have excellent pain relief at the same time. Other pain-killing medications (e.g., morphine) can also be administered in this fashion.

4.3

Systems Review and Surface Anatomy of the Back and Spinal Cord

▶ Musculoskeletal Anatomy of the Back and Spinal Cord

▶ Vascular Supply of the Back and Spinal Cord

▶ Lymphatic Drainage of the Back and Spinal Cord

▶ Innervation of the Back and Spinal Cord

▶ Surface Anatomy and Physical Examination of the Back and Spinal Cord

MUSCULOSKELETAL ANATOMY OF THE BACK AND SPINAL CORD

Individual vertebrae can be understood if they are seen as variations on a basic structural plan—an anterior **body,** a pair of **pedicles** supporting a neural **lamina** or arch, and **transverse** and **spinous processes.** In the center is the spinal or **vertebral canal,** in which is situated the spinal cord. Each pair of vertebrae fit together in such a way that a lateral gap, the **intervertebral foramen,** is formed; through this foramen passes the **spinal nerve** for that segment. Equally important are the arteries and veins that traverse the intervertebral foramen to convey blood between the vertebral canal and the areas external to the vertebral column.

Movements of the vertebral column include **flexion** (bending forward, as in reaching down to touch the toes), **extension** (the opposite of flexion), **lateral flexion** (bending of the vertebral column to the left or right in the coronal plane), and a composite **twisting** motion that revolves around the long axis of the vertebral column itself. The complex **erector spinae** muscles, arrayed in the vertical axis posterior to the vertebral col-

umn, are responsible for extension. Flexion of the lumbar vertebral column is produced by groups of muscles that attach the vertebral column anteriorly to the pelvis or lower limb (e.g., iliopsoas). Lateral flexion is caused by contraction of abdominal wall muscles on one side at a time. Flexion of the spine as a whole is accomplished by contraction of all the muscles lying anterior to the vertebrae. This includes the scalene muscles and sternocleidomastoid in the neck, for example. Twisting motions of the vertebral column result from contraction of the **transversospinal** group of muscles, positioned deep to the erector spinae.

VASCULAR SUPPLY OF THE BACK AND SPINAL CORD

The vertebral column and spinal cord are both supplied with **arterial blood** by the series of **radicular arteries** that enter the vertebral canal through the intervertebral foramen at each spinal level. The radicular arteries are derived from various large arteries, including the **vertebral, deep cervical, posterior intercostal,** and **lumbar arteries. Venous drainage** from the spinal cord and vertebral column collects into an **internal** and **external vertebral venous plexus**. Venous blood from these plexuses mingles with blood in the cranial venous sinuses, the vertebral veins, the deep cervical veins, the posterior intercostal, and the lumbar veins.

LYMPHATIC DRAINAGE OF THE BACK AND SPINAL CORD

The spinal cord lacks lymphatic drainage, and the vertebral column has only scant lymphatic drainage directed at the tributaries emptying into the lumbar lymphatic chains and the thoracic duct.

INNERVATION OF THE BACK AND SPINAL CORD

The vertebrae receive innervation similar to other bones throughout the body, the periosteum being the most richly innervated and the most sensitive to pain. Numerous small branches of individual spinal nerves perform this function. At each vertebral level there are also **recurrent meningeal** branches that depart from the spinal nerve and reenter the vertebral canal through the intervertebral foramen. These recurrent meningeal nerves innervate the dura mater, arachnoid mater, pia mater, and tissues associated with the blood vessels inside the vertebral canal.

The erector spinae and transversospinal group of muscles comprise the "paraspinous" muscles and are notable for being innervated by the **posterior primary rami** of spinal nerves, whereas the remainder of structures on the lateral and anterior parts of the body wall and all of the limbs are innervated by branches of the **anterior primary rami** of spinal nerves. These anterior primary rami are the branches that we commonly refer to as the "nerves" of the body wall and trunk (e.g., the phrenic nerve, the intercostal nerves, etc.).

SURFACE ANATOMY AND PHYSICAL EXAMINATION OF THE BACK AND SPINAL CORD

The **spinous processes** of the vertebral column may be palpated in the posterior midline of the back, even in an obese person, since fat does not accumulate along the midline (Figure 4-45). The first clearly palpable vertebral spine is that of the C7 vertebra—known as the "vertebra prominens." In some individuals it may be possible to palpate the necks and angles of the **ribs,** as they extend laterally away from the vertebral column. Anteriorly, it is possible to palpate the skin over the **costochondral** and **chondrosternal joints.** In patients with inflamed joints (arthritis), palpation in these areas may produce pain.

In examining a newborn, the examiner should always confirm that the vertebral column is intact from cervical to sacral regions by palpating the adjacent spines and determining that there is no discontinuity. Occult cases of **spina bifida** (a congenital failure of certain vertebrae to create a complete neural arch) may be detected in this fashion.

When performing a **lumbar puncture** or spinal tap, the clinician should approach posteriorly, aiming the needle at the L4 to L5 or L5 to S1 interspace. To locate this vertebral level accurately, he or she should palpate the iliac crests of the pelvis. An imaginary horizontal line connecting the two iliac crests passes through the

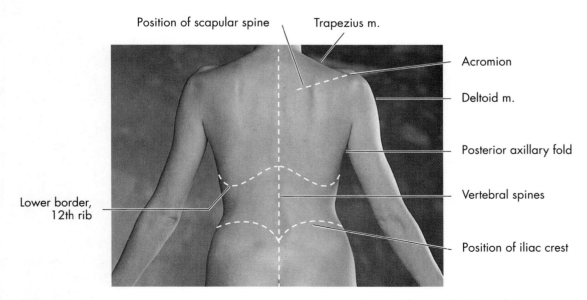

Position of scapular spine · Trapezius m. · Acromion · Deltoid m. · Posterior axillary fold · Vertebral spines · Position of iliac crest · Lower border, 12th rib

Figure 4-45 SURFACE ANATOMY OF THE BACK. Inspection and examination of the posterior trunk should always include confirmation of the straightness of the spine, the position of the scapular spine and iliac crests, and the position of the twelfth rib.

L4 vertebra. With this as a reference, the spinal needle may be inserted in the correct intervertebral space.

By asking the patient to stand with straightened lower limbs and flex the hips as far as possible (i.e., trying to touch the toes with the knees locked), an examiner may observe the alignment of the vertebrae or palpate along the vertebral column to confirm that the vertebrae are vertically aligned. A common abnormality of vertebral alignment is **scoliosis** or abnormal lateral flexion of the spine. This simple and noninvasive test is an accurate way to assess patients for scoliosis.

The **segmental nature** of the body's organization is revealed best in the trunk, beginning with the intercostal nerves and vessels, which emerge between pairs of vertebrae and course anterolaterally around the body wall. Clinical conditions that affect segmental nerves (such as herpes zoster or shingles) may manifest themselves by causing skin eruptions in a pattern reminiscent of a dermatome. A clinician who is aware of these segmental patterns is more likely to recognize the disease for what it is.

A patient should be able to carry out a wide range of movements involving his or her vertebral column—flexion (bending forward), extension (bending backward), lateral flexion (to the left or right side), and rotation. The examiner must be careful not to confuse movement taking place at the atlantooccipital joint (between C1 and the skull) or in the pelvis with true movements of the vertebral column. In the cervical region a patient can normally touch his or her chin to the chest, point the chin laterally at nearly a 45 degree angle, and flex the neck and head to the side so that the face is nearly parallel to the ground. Motion in the thoracic spine is limited by the ribs, and in the lumbar region the articular facets limit lateral flexion.

Back and Spinal Cord

■ *CASE 1*

ABNORMAL SENSATIONS IN THE UPPER LIMBS

A middle-aged male began to experience tingling sensations and some pain in both shoulders, right worse than left, and reported that his right upper limb felt "weaker." The pain was often worse in the morning, on awakening, and could usually be worsened by jogging. Reflexes in the upper limbs were normal, and there was no obvious muscle wasting. His health was otherwise good. There was no history of trauma, other than what might result from a mild exercise program. A lateral MRI scan was ordered.

Questions

1. What is the abnormality?
2. What are some of the surgical approaches available to treat this problem?

■ *CASE 2*

VERTEBRAL COLUMN

A 45-year-old male who works on a receiving dock at a department store was in the process of moving some crates and felt a strong painful shock in his lower back, radiating to the posterior leg on the right side. He took the rest of the day off, rested, applied heat to his back, and returned to work 2 days later. Thereafter he continued to work for several weeks, seemingly without impairment. However, he slowly began to note several disturbing symptoms. His right leg seemed to be weak, he had constant moderate pain in his lower back, and he noted an enlarging area of numbness along the lateral side of his right leg. On visiting his doctor, he was found to have absent reflexes in his right ankle and signs of muscle wasting in the right calf. He also was unable to fully flex and extend his lumbar spine because of pain.

Questions

1. What accounts for the absent ankle reflex and muscle wasting of the right calf? What about the affected skin areas?
2. Where is the exact location (i.e., vertebral level) of the herniated disk?
3. In what direction must the disk herniation have been in order to produce these symptoms?

■ *CASE 3*

LOWER BACK PAIN

A male in his 50s reported to his physician that he had been suffering from low back pain, occasionally radiating into the lower limbs, for about 2 years. He had been reluctant to come to the doctor for fear surgery would be ordered. Of late, however, the pain had become more frequent and more intense. There were no abnormalities in sensation in the back or lower limbs, and all reflexes were intact. Lifting objects did exacerbate the pain, however. A set of x-rays of the lumbar spine were ordered.

Questions

1. What is the abnormality?
2. Why are the ordinary signs of low back disease not present here (weakness, loss of sensation, absence of reflexes)?
3. What is the origin of this condition?

■ *CASE 4*

VERTEBRAL COLUMN AND LUMBAR PUNCTURE

A 6-month-old female who was previously in good health became sleepy and did not nurse well, something very different from her normal behavior. Over the course of the next several hours she became more and more lethargic, and late in the evening her parents took her to the emergency room. The doctors there felt she was seriously ill and informed the parents that their daughter needed a lumbar puncture.

Questions

1. Where, within the vertebral canal, is cerebrospinal fluid located?

2. At what vertebral level should a lumbar puncture be performed and why?
3. What is the goal in performing a lumbar puncture—that is, where should the tip of the needle be placed?
4. What anatomic structures are encountered in passing the needle through the skin to reach the subarachnoid space?

ANSWERS AND EXPLANATIONS

■ CASE 1

1. This scan reveals a **herniated disk** in the midcervical spine, probably involving the disk between cervical vertebrae five and six. The herniated disk puts pressure on the nearby nerves. The most directly adjacent are the roots of C5, which would make the symptoms consistent with the anatomic diagnosis.
2. Surgery in this area is often approached from anterior, rather than from posterior as would be the case in thoracic or lumbar vertebral surgery. This places many crucial structures (trachea, vagus nerves, recurrent nerves, etc.) at risk during this sort of surgery.

■ CASE 2

1. The innervation of the posterior calf muscles is carried out by segments **L4 to L5 to S1,** as part of the tibial division of the sciatic nerve. The tibialis posterior, gastrocnemius, and soleus muscles are involved in ankle flexion. Prolonged injury to these nerve roots leads to wasting of the muscles innervated since the muscles depend on intact innervation to maintain their size and bulk. The same spinal cord segments provide cutaneous innervation to the lateral side of the leg and foot.
2. In the lower lumbar and sacral spine, nerve roots exit the intervertebral foramen very high up in the foramen. Consequently, herniated disks often compress not the nerve that exits at the same level but the nerve passing inferior to exit at the level below. In this case, a **herniated disk** at the L4 to L5 interspace affects not the L4 nerve but the L5 nerve (and perhaps S1 as well). A herniated disk at the L5 to S1 interspace affects not the L5 nerve but the S1 nerve. The herniated disks in this patient are most likely at both the L4 to L5 and the L5 to S1 interspace.
3. The **anatomic relationships** in the region of the intervertebral foramen are very significant in the

pathology of herniated disks. The central **annulus fibrosus** of the disk must herniate posterolaterally if it is to put pressure on the exiting nerve roots. If the disk herniates directly posteriorly, it presses on the spinal cord itself (or the cauda equina at lower segments). Fortunately this is rare.

■ CASE 3

1. This patient's x-rays showed that the body of L5 seemed to lie anterior to the plane of the vertebral bodies immediately above. The spinous process, however, was not projected forward. This is a condition known as **spondylolisthesis,** where the vertebral bodies (usually of lower lumbar segments) move anterior with respect to the rest of the vertebral column and to the sacrum, lying just inferior.
2. The ordinary signs of nerve compression are often mild or not present because the lesion does not necessarily produce pressure on exiting nerve roots.
3. Most agree that this condition results from a failure of the vertebral body to fuse to the pedicles that support the neural arch of the affected vertebra. This is a failure of the normal embryologic processes by which separate ossification centers of what will eventually be one bone fail to fuse properly.

■ CASE 4

1. Cerebrospinal fluid lies deep to the arachnoid membrane, in the subarachnoid space, and bathes the spinal cord and the spinal nerves in the vertebral canal. The subarachnoid space extends superiorly into the cranial cavity as well, and CSF surrounds the brain in a similar fashion.
2. A lumbar puncture must be performed safely below the level where the spinal cord itself has ended, usually at ~L3 vertebral level in an infant (see Figure 4-32). Below this level, the vertebral canal contains

the many nerve roots destined to exit the vertebral canal at lower levels—the **cauda equina** (see Figure 4-38). When the spinal needle is inserted into the subarachnoid space at this level, it may brush against some of the roots of the cauda equina. This usually does no harm, but even if the needle were to impale one of the nerve roots, that nerve could regenerate since it is a peripheral nerve. Were the spinal tap performed at a higher level and the spinal cord itself injured, it has no such capacity to regenerate.

3. The tip of the needle must be positioned in the subarachnoid space. Fluid will slowly flow outward through the needle since the CSF normally is under a small degree of pressure within the subarachnoid space.

4. The spinal needle is placed through the skin at the **L4 to L5 or L5 to S1 vertebral level,** because this will ensure that the spinal needle will not jeopardize the spinal cord itself (see answer #2; Figure 4-32). The skin over the chosen interspace is infiltrated with local anesthetic and sterilized. The spinal needle first enters the skin, passes through the superficial fascia, and then encounters the **supraspinous ligament,** which is felt by the person passing the needle as an increase in resistance. It descends through the **interspinous ligament,** and at the level of the neural lamina passes through the **ligamentum flavum** (see Figure 4-18). Just deep to the ligamentum flavum lies the **internal vertebral venous plexus,** and next the **dura mater.** Although the **arachnoid membrane** is separate from the dura, it normally is closely applied to the inner surface of the dura. The clinician usually feels a "pop" when the needle enters the subarachnoid space. This "pop" probably results from the needle emerging on the inner surface of the combined ligamentum flavum–dura mater–arachnoid mater. Once in the subarachnoid space, the CSF begins to flow.

SECTION FIVE

Abdomen

▶ **5.1** Abdominal Wall

▶ **5.2** Inguinal Canal and Descent of the Testes

▶ **5.3** Peritoneal Membranes and Development of the Gut

▶ **5.4** Liver, Gallbladder, Spleen, and Pancreas

▶ **5.5** Esophagus, Stomach, and Lesser Sac

▶ **5.6** Small Intestine

▶ **5.7** Colon and Anorectal Region

▶ **5.8** Kidneys and Suprarenal Glands

▶ **5.9** Posterior Wall and Diaphragm

▶ **5.10** Systems Review and Surface Anatomy of the Abdomen

▶ **5.11** Case Studies: Abdomen

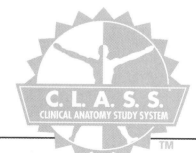

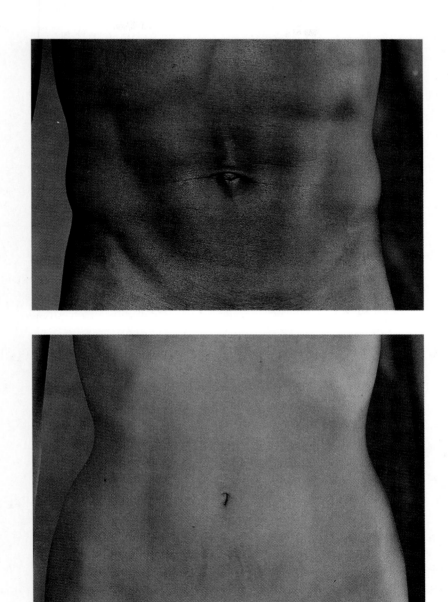

5.1 ◀ Abdominal Wall

▶ Layers of the Abdominal Wall

▶ Neurovascular Supply of the Abdominal Wall

*T*he abdominal wall is an inferior continuation of the thoracic wall and resembles it closely (with the major difference, of course, that no ribs are present). It has a similar set of three fundamental muscle layers (Figure 5-1; see also Figure 5-3). Like the thoracic wall, the abdominal wall plays a pivotal role in the maintenance of posture and the movements of the limbs. It is centrally involved in respiration, urination/defecation, and childbirth. At the inferolateral margin of the abdominal wall is a unique region known as the *inguinal canal* (see Figure 5-8). Especially in the male, it is an important site of pathology, as it marks the area in which the migration of the testis toward the scrotum occurs.

The abdominal wall is a muscular sheath that attaches superiorly to the *xiphoid cartilage* and *costal margin* (Figure 5-2), laterally and posteriorly to the *lumbar fascia,* inferiorly to the *inguinal ligament,* and in the midline to the *linea alba* (thickened fascial cord in the anterior midline of abdominal wall) (see Figure 5-5).

The abdominal wall encloses the contents of the abdominal cavity but also is an active muscular participant in urination, defecation, parturition (childbirth), vocalization, and multiple movements of the trunk.

LAYERS OF THE ABDOMINAL WALL

The skin of the abdominal wall features a dermis with dermal fibers arrayed preferentially along *cleavage lines (of Langer).* When the skin is incised, healing will produce a smaller scar if the incision has been made parallel to the lines and a larger scar if the incision was transverse to these lines.

The **superficial fascia** has two layers: a *superficial layer* (Camper's fascia) that is mostly fat and a *deep layer* (Scarpa's fascia) that is predominantly fibrous (Figures 5-3 and 5-4). This latter layer is strong enough to hold sutures and may be closed independently when suturing an abdominal incision. Scarpa's fascia is continuous laterally with the thoracolumbar fascia, and inferiorly with the deep fascia of the thigh. The **thoracolumbar** [or just "lumbar"] **fascia** is an important expanse of tissue lying in the wide area between the iliac crest and the transverse processes of the lumbar vertebrae. Many large muscles of the abdominal wall are attached to this fascia. The **deep fascia** is the investing fascia of the abdominal wall muscles.

The **external oblique muscle** is the most superficial of the three muscle layers. Its fibers run in general from superolateral to inferomedial (see Figures 5-1, 5-3, and 5-4). Superiorly, it attaches to the anterior tips of ribs 5 to 12, and inferiorly it attaches to the iliac crest. The external oblique has a free posterior border extending from rib 12 to the iliac crest; the other muscles of the anterolateral abdominal wall do not have such a free posterior edge. The external oblique is muscular laterally and posteriorly but becomes aponeurotic about halfway between the anterior superior spine (ASIS) and the pubis and extends from there medially to the linea alba as an aponeurosis. Anteromedially, the external oblique attaches to the xiphoid cartilage, downward along the linea alba, and inferiorly to the pubic tubercle. The lower border of muscle is coiled internally on itself to form a thick cord, the *inguinal ligament,* extending from the pelvis to the pubic tubercle (see Figure 5-8).

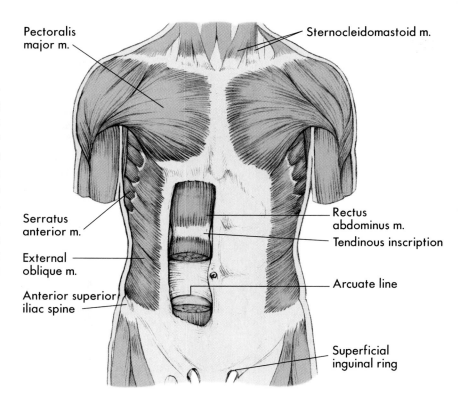

Figure 5-1 THE ANTERIOR ABDOMINAL WALL. Pectoralis major is the most external muscle of the chest wall, with external oblique and serratus anterior contributing part of the lower half of the chest wall. The most external muscle layer of abdominal wall is formed by the musculature and aponeurosis of the external oblique and the paired rectus abdominus muscles extending from the xiphoid process superiorly to the pubic tubercle inferiorly. On the right side, the rectus sheath is incised to show the tendinous inscriptions on the surface of the muscle and the arcuate line.

SEE ATLAS, FIG. 5-10, 5-14

Pectoralis major m.

Sternocleidomastoid m.

Serratus anterior m.

External oblique m.

Anterior superior iliac spine

Rectus abdominus m.

Tendinous inscription

Arcuate line

Superficial inguinal ring

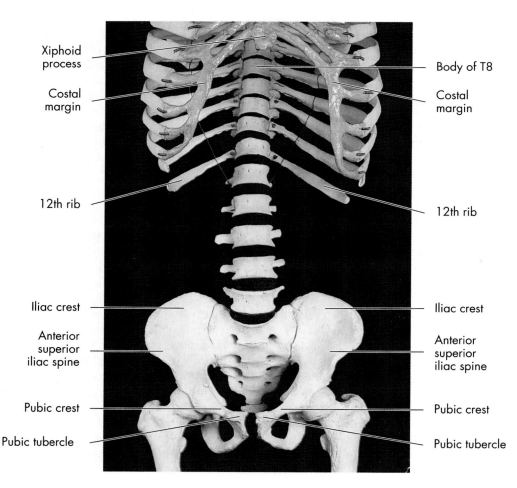

Xiphoid process

Costal margin

12th rib

Iliac crest

Anterior superior iliac spine

Pubic crest

Pubic tubercle

Body of T8

Costal margin

12th rib

Iliac crest

Anterior superior iliac spine

Pubic crest

Pubic tubercle

Figure 5-2 SKELETON OF THE ABDOMINAL WALL. The costal margin, lumbar vertebrae, and upper surface of the pelvis are the attachments for the muscles forming the abdominal wall. (From Chumbley CC, Hutchings RTV: *Color atlas of human dissection*, ed 2, London, 1992, Mosby.)

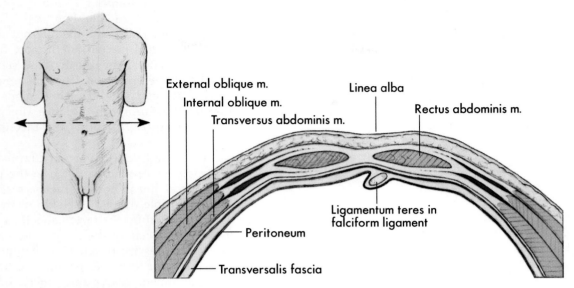

Figure 5-3 LAYERS OF THE ABDOMINAL WALL. *Inset* shows level of cross-section. Falciform ligament is visible in this section because it is just above the level of the umbilicus. Above the umbilicus, the falciform ligament extends from the interior of the abdominal wall upward to the liver.

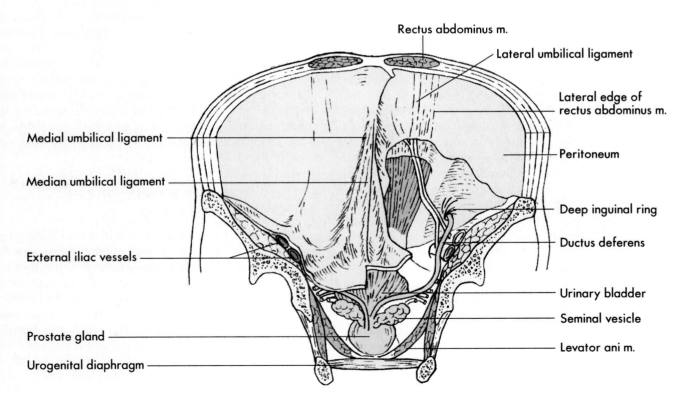

Figure 5-4 ANTERIOR ABDOMINAL WALL. This is a view of the anterior abdominal wall as seen from inside the abdominal cavity. The peritoneum has been removed partially on the right. SEE ATLAS, FIG. 5-37

It is instructive to look on the thoracic and abdominal anterior walls as a unit because they share many structural similarities. In each there is a basic structure of *three concentric muscle layers,* the external intercostal/external oblique, internal intercostal/internal oblique, and the innermost intercostal/transversus abdominus. The *vessels and nerves* coursing through the thoracic and abdominal walls lie in a plane between the deepest and the intermediate layers of muscle. In both the thorax and abdomen there is an *internal lining of smooth membrane* (the parietal pleura/parietal peritoneum) and just external to it a layer of *loose connective tissue* (the transversalis fascia of the abdominal wall; the loose connective tissue in the thoracic wall has no special name). The abdominal wall lacks *skeletal elements,* but they are present in the thoracic wall (ribs, costal cartilages, sternum). The abdomen has an external *vertical muscle* in the midline (the rectus abdominus), although a similar muscle is usually absent in the human thorax (see footnote below). The horizontal *segmentation* of the human trunk is evident in both abdomen and thorax, especially in the latter (with its ribs, intercostal vessels, and so on). Both the abdominal and thoracic walls play important roles in positioning of the trunk, contraction to support movements of the limbs, and contraction as a part of breathing, urination, defecation, and childbirth.

The **internal oblique muscle** is in the intermediate position of the muscles in the abdominal wall. Its muscle fibers appear to fan out as they extend from posterior around the abdominal wall toward the linea alba (Figure 5-5). Superiorly they run from inferolateral to superomedial, although in the region of the inguinal ligament its muscle fibers parallel those of the external oblique. The internal oblique originates from the lumbar fascia, the iliac crest, and the lateral one third of the inguinal ligament. Like the external oblique, the internal oblique is muscular posteriorly and laterally but becomes aponeurotic about 4 cm lateral to the linea alba, to which it eventually attaches. Its lower margin joins with fibers from the transversus abdominus muscle to form the important **falx inguinalis**, a fibromuscular arch that passes from the lateral part of the inguinal ligament medially to insert on the pecten pubis (a narrow ridge of bone extending laterally from the pubic tubercle a short distance along the superior pubic ramus). The falx provides strength and reinforcement where the weight of the abdominal contents puts greatest pressure on the anterior abdominal wall. Its role in the formation of the inguinal canal is described in Chapter 5.2.

The **transversus abdominus** is the deepest of the three muscles in the anterolateral abdominal wall and is often fused significantly with the internal oblique. It extends from the costal margin, the lumbar fascia, the iliac crest, and the lateral one fourth of the inguinal ligament forward to the linea alba. Its fibers are predominantly horizontal and like its companions become aponeurotic as they approach the linea alba. With the internal oblique muscle, it forms the **falx inguinalis** (see previous discussion).

The **rectus abdominus** is a vertical straplike muscle extending from the xiphoid cartilage to the pubic tubercle. Its vertical linear border, the *linea semilunaris* (Figure 5-6), is visible through the skin of the slender subject. It is encircled by the **rectus sheath**, a complex derivation of the fasciae of the three other abdominal wall muscles. The fasciae of all three abdominal wall muscles pass anterior to the rectus muscle in the lower third of the abdomen. Above this, in the upper two thirds of the abdomen, the fasciae are arranged as follows: external oblique fascia is anterior, internal oblique fascia splits to lie both anterior and posterior, and transversus fascia lies posterior. The area where this transition occurs is the *arcuate line.* It is a landmark for the location of the *inferior epigastric vessels* as they begin to ascend on the posterior surface of the rectus abdominus by passing between the posterior rectus sheath and the muscle itself (see later discussion).*

Deep to the muscles is the **transversalis fascia.** It is a loose connective tissue layer containing a small amount of fat. Structures we describe as being "in" the walls lining the abdominal and pelvic cavities are embedded in this layer of tissue. Lining the inner surface of the transversalis fascia is the **peritoneum.** The *parietal division of the peritoneum* lines the walls surrounding the abdominal and pelvic cavities, and the *visceral division of the peritoneum* reflects inward to partially surround some of the abdominal and pelvic viscera.

NEUROVASCULAR SUPPLY OF THE ABDOMINAL WALL

The posterior part of the abdominal wall is supplied with blood by the 3 to 4 segmental **lumbar vessels,** comparable to the intercostal arteries of the thoracic wall. The lateral and anterior parts of the abdominal wall are supplied with blood by the lower 5 to 6 **intercostal vessels.** These emerge from the intercostal spaces and course anteromedially across the anterior body wall to the midline. Their pattern is suggestive of

---

*There is occasionally present a vertically oriented midline muscle in the chest, *sternalis,* which is the homolog of the rectus abdominus in the abdomen. It is regularly present in carnivores and some other mammals.

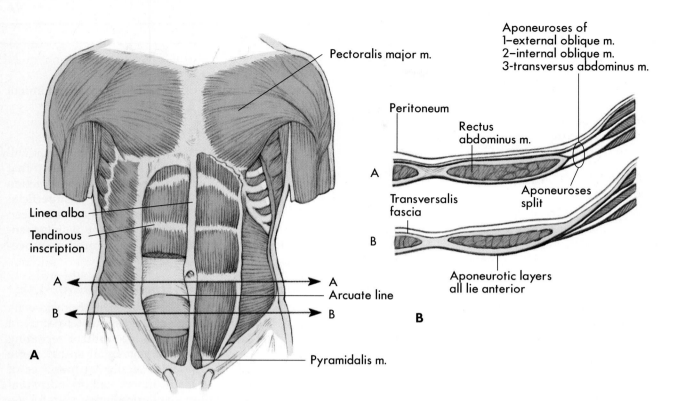

Pectoralis major m.

Aponeuroses of
1–external oblique m.
2–internal oblique m.
3–transversus abdominus m.

Peritoneum

Rectus
abdominus m.

A

Transversalis
fascia

B

Aponeuroses
split

Aponeurotic layers
all lie anterior

B

Linea alba

Tendinous
inscription

A

A

Arcuate line

B

B

A

Pyramidalis m.

Figure 5-5 THE RECTUS ABDOMINUS MUSCLE. A, The anterior abdominal wall is made up on each side of three layers of flattened muscle and a pair of elongated vertical muscles, each known as **rectus abdominus.** The rectus muscle has two or three transverse whitish bands, the tendinous inscriptions, between the level of the umbilicus and the xiphoid. In cross-section A-A, just inferior to the umbilicus, the external oblique aponeurosis lies anterior to the rectus; the aponeurosis of the internal oblique splits to pass both in front of and behind the rectus and the aponeurosis of the transversus abdominus passes posterior to the rectus. In cross-section B-B, all three of these aponeurotic layers lie anterior to the rectus; only the transversalis fascia and peritoneum lie posterior. **B,** A portion of the rectus muscle has been removed to reveal the arrangement of aponeuroses derived from the more lateral abdominal muscles. The gently curved aponeurotic edge, the **arcuate line,** represents the point at which all of the aponeurotic layers first lie anterior to the rectus. Viewed from the interior, the arcuate line marks the point at which the inferior epigastric vessels enter and lie in the transversalis fascia posterior to the rectus. The small **pyramidalis muscle** lies anterior to the lower end of the rectus abdominus muscle. Sᴇᴇ Aᴛʟᴀs, Fɪɢs. 5-11, 5-12, 5-14, 5-15, 5-16

the repeating segmental arrangement of the body wall, and there are anastomoses between these vessels just as there are anastomoses between the intercostal vessels in the thoracic wall.

The rectus muscle and its fascial coverings receive vascular supply through the **superior epigastric artery** (a branch of internal thoracic artery) from above and the **inferior epigastric artery** (branch of external iliac artery) from below. These vessels run along the deep surface of the rectus muscle and anastomose within its substance (see Figure 5-4).

Other arteries supplying the abdominal wall include the **superficial epigastric** (from the external iliac artery), **deep iliac circumflex** (from the external iliac artery), and **musculophrenic** (from the internal thoracic artery). Venous drainage parallels the arterial supply. The superficial epigastric veins may be hypertrophied in cases of portal hypertension, creating tortuous vessels visible through the anterior abdominal wall.

Intercostal nerves T7 to T12 and the **upper one or two lumbar nerves** innervate the abdominal wall and its musculature (see Figure 5-59).

THE ABDOMINAL WALL

INCISIONS IN THE ABDOMINAL WALL

Incisions are planned to expose the desired area of the abdomen with the smallest possible opening, and with reference to the Langer lines, to promote healing with the smallest possible scar.

IMPORTANCE OF ABDOMINAL MUSCULATURE

The abdominal musculature is important in a variety of functions, including respiration, defecation, urination, and parturition (childbirth). All of these share the characteristic of utilizing the abdominal muscles to increase intraabdominal pressure. This is transmitted to adjacent tissues (e.g., the pelvic viscera, the thoracic cavity). In addition, the abdominal muscles are very important in positioning of the trunk, and the maintenance of equilibrium when arms or legs are moved. They are also key in gait, where truncal position must be controlled.

THE URACHUS

The **urachus** is a cordlike remnant of the narrow connection between the primitive gut and the allantois. Normally the urachus degenerates, but it may persist and present as an infected cystic structure attached to the interior of the infraumbilical abdominal wall in the midline.

THE CREMASTER REFLEX

Gentle stroking of the skin near the umbilicus will elicit a contraction of abdominal wall muscles on that side and a "pulling" of the umbilicus to the direction of the stimulus. This is an example of a **superficial muscular reflex**. By contrast, the more familiar deep tendon reflex is best exemplified by the patellar tendon reflex (i.e., tapping on the knee to produce movement at the knee).

SEGMENTATION AND THE ABDOMINAL WALL

The abdominal wall, along with the thoracic wall, exhibits the best evidence of the segmental nature of the human body. These areas are built of repeating units, each innervated by a segmental spinal nerve and supplied with blood by segmental branches of the aorta. The skin domains innervated by individual spinal nerves are known as **dermatomes**. Careful examination of a patient may reveal segmental (dermatomal) areas of anesthesia and provide evidence that there may be an injury to that particular nerve or to the part of the spinal cord from which it arose.

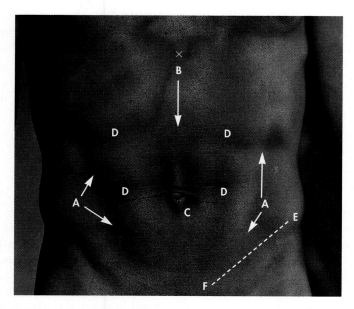

Figure 5-6   THE LINEA ALBA AND LINEA SEMILUNARIS. The positions of these lines are projected onto the anterior abdominal wall. *A*, Linea semilunaris; *B*, linea alba; *C*, umbilicus; *D*, tendinous inscriptions; *E*, anterior superior iliac spine; *F*, pubic symphysis. *Dashed line*, position of inguinal ligament.

PRINCIPLES

Hernias tend to form where a layer of tissue separates one region from another (e.g., thorax from abdomen, abdomen from outside). They are the more likely to form if there is pressure inside one space or cavity of the body. Hernias are most likely to form where there is already a weakness in a tissue layer separating two chambers or spaces. For example, *congenital diaphragmatic hernias* (Figure 5-7) form where there is a congenital gap in the diaphragm (usually along the posterior margin of the diaphragm on the left) or where a structure passes through the diaphragm, creating a weakness (e.g., the gastroesophageal junction, where *hiatus hernias* form). *Inguinal hernias* are the most common because there is the combination of a natural weakness in the lower abdominal wall and the force of gravity that focuses the weight of the abdominal contents on this part of the anterior abdominal wall.

Herniation of intestinal contents into the inguinal canal and beyond into the scrotum is a common occurrence in males. The comparable process in females, which would result in herniation of abdominal contents through the inguinal canal and into the labium majus, is rare. This is the case presumably because the size of the male spermatic cord creates a natural weakness in the lower abdominal wall of the male, but in the female only the small round ligament passes through the inguinal canal. More common in females is herniation of abdominal contents through the space between the inguinal ligament and the upper surface of the superior pubic ramus, resulting in a *femoral hernia*. These hernias usually pass through the femoral canal, a space lying just medial to the femoral vein.

Anterior abdominal hernias also can occur through the umbilical area (*umbilical hernias*) and also in a gap between the two rectus abdominus muscles (*rectus diastasis hernias*), usually superior to the umbilicus.

A large potential gap in the posterior abdominal wall is filled by the psoas major and quadratus lumborum muscles, which fill the space between the twelfth rib and the iliac crest of the pelvis on each side. Posterior abdominal wall hernias (*lumbar hernias*) do occur occasionally in a small triangle bounded by the lateral edge of the latissimus dorsi, the free posterior edge of the external oblique muscle, and the upper edge of the iliac crest (see Figure 4-23).

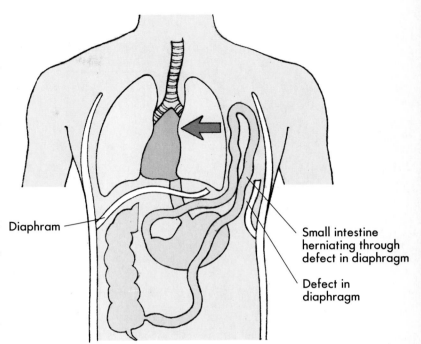

Figure 5-7 DIAPHRAGMATIC HERNIA. Here much of the small intestine has herniated through a defect in the left side of the diaphragm into the chest, pushing the lungs and mediastinum to the right. Such patients usually have severe respiratory distress, and often succumb because their lungs are severely hypoplastic (underdeveloped).

5.2

section five.two

Inguinal Canal and Descent of the Testes

▶ Walls of the Inguinal Canal

▶ Arrangement of Layers in the Inguinal Canal

▶ Relations of Inferior Epigastric Vessels

▶ The Spermatic Cord

▶ The Scrotum

▶ Descent of the Ovary

*T*he **inguinal canal** is the site of inguinal herniation, one of the most common problems of men. This canal is the site through which the testis and spermatic cord migrate, during development, to reach the scrotum. As such, it is a natural "weak spot" in the abdominal wall. Our upright posture adds to the pressure exerted on this region of natural weakness. The surgical repair of an inguinal hernia is a very "anatomic" operation because it is designed to recreate a nearly normal anatomic situation by repositioning layers of muscle and fascia where weakening has occurred. The **spermatic cord,** which descends through the inguinal canal, consists of the *ductus deferens* and several concentric layers of *muscle* and *fascia* with accompanying vessels and nerves.

WALLS OF THE INGUINAL CANAL

The inguinal canal forms a complex passage through which descends the testis (in the male) (Figure 5-8) or round ligament (in the female) (Figure 5-9), accompanied by layers of muscle and fascia (Table 5-1). In the female these layers are very thin and hardly distinguishable; thus our discussion will focus on the male.

The testis in the male and the round ligament in the female appear to penetrate the abdominal wall as they descend into the scrotum or labia. In reality, however, various layers of the abdominal wall are "pushed"

ahead of them, so that concentric layers of muscle or fascia surround the testis or round ligament as it descends into the scrotum. An exception to this is the peritoneum itself, a narrow "neck" that descends into the scrotum *alongside* the testis, rather than being "pushed" ahead of the testis (see later discussion).

ARRANGEMENT OF LAYERS IN THE INGUINAL CANAL

The arrangement of muscle layers in the inguinal canal is complex. The **external oblique** has a fascial extension known as the *external spermatic fascia* traveling downward into the scrotum with the testis. The external oblique also forms the *external* or *superficial ring* at the medial end of the inguinal canal. This is better described as a triangular thickened edge of fascia that is concave medially and is positioned inferomedially just superior to the inguinal ligament, and immediately lateral to the pubic tubercle (see Figure 5-8). Radiating away from the "apex" of the triangle are the two sides of the superficial ring, separately named as the *lateral* and *medial crus* (see Figure 5-8). The palpable external ring does not represent a true aperture in the external oblique but rather a thickened margin from which the much thinner external spermatic fascia originates and descends into the scrotum.

464

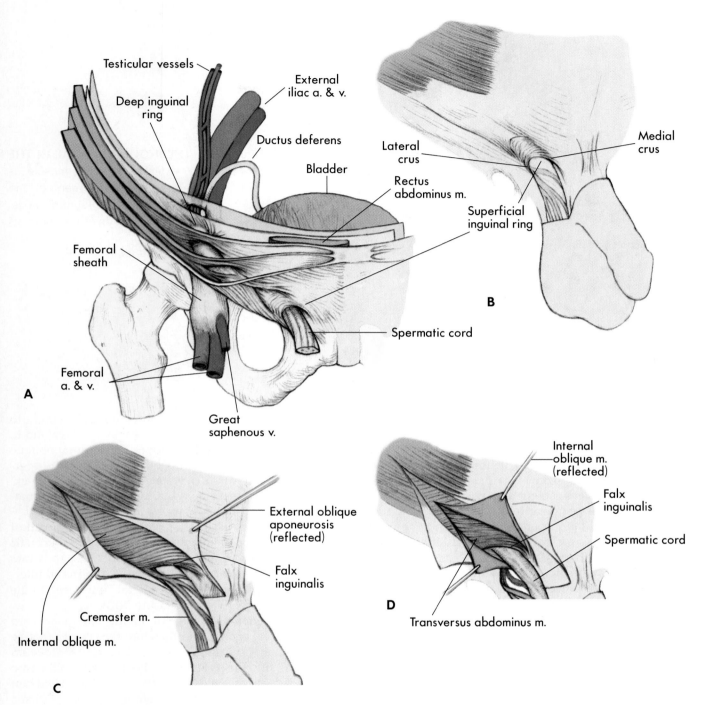

Figure 5-8 THE INGUINAL CANAL IN THE MALE. A, The inguinal region is fully dissected, with the various layers separated for clarity. The external iliac vessels are shown passing beneath the inguinal ligament, where they become the femoral vessels. **B,** Shown are the superficial inguinal ring and the external oblique muscle/aponeurosis. The tissue of the external spermatic fascia has been removed, which more sharply defines the superficial ring and reveals the fibers of the spermatic cord. **C,** The fibers of the external oblique have been split and pulled apart, to reveal the fibers of the internal oblique muscle. The falx inguinalis is the lower margin of the internal oblique, along with underlying fibers of the transversus abdominus, and the cremaster muscle is shown as a continuation of the internal oblique down into the spermatic cord. **D,** The dissection is completed by splitting the fibers of the internal oblique and spreading them to show the underlying fibers of the transversus abdominis muscle. SEE ATLAS, FIG. 5-20

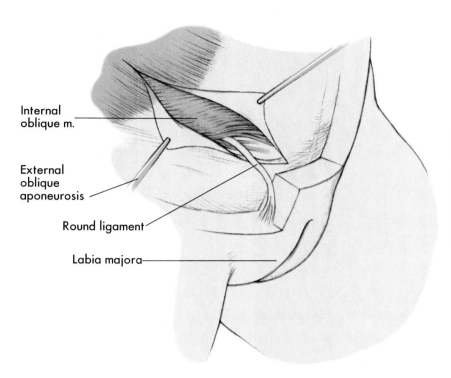

Internal
oblique m.

External
oblique
aponeurosis

Round ligament

Labia majora

Figure 5-9   THE INGUINAL CANAL IN THE FEMALE. The external oblique muscle is split to reveal the round ligament of the uterus as it terminates in the labium majus. This structure is the homolog of the spermatic cord in the male.
SEE ATLAS, FIGS. 5-26, 5-27, 5-28

The coiled inferior margin of the external oblique muscle is the **inguinal ligament** (of Poupart); it extends from the anterior superior spine to the pubic tubercle (see Figure 5-8). The **lacunar ligament** (of Gimbernat) is a crescent-shaped ligament originating at the medial end of the inguinal ligament and extending laterally to attach along the pectineal line on the superior pubic ramus. Between the inguinal ligament and the upper surface of the pubis is the space for the iliopsoas muscle and the femoral canal.

In the inguinal region, the **internal oblique muscle** is anterior to the spermatic cord laterally. As we follow the lower edge of the internal oblique, moving from lateral to medial, the free lower edge of the muscle arches over the spermatic cord and at the medial end of the inguinal canal lies posterior to the spermatic cord. The lower margin of the internal oblique, along with the similar lower margin of the **transversus abdominus** muscle, constitutes what is known as the **falx in-**

guinalis. The falx appears to provide reinforcement to the abdominal wall in this potentially weak area and to help prevent intestinal herniation. The internal oblique layer of muscle also extends downward into the spermatic cord as the thin *cremaster muscle*. There is *no* extension of the transversus abdominus into the spermatic cord, either as a muscular or a fascial layer.

The **transversalis fascia** forms the posterior wall of the inguinal canal, remaining posterior to the spermatic cord as it passes from lateral to medial. It extends into the cord as the *internal spermatic fascia*. It forms an internal or *deep inguinal ring* at the lateral "entrance" to the inguinal canal (see Figures 5-5 and 5-13).

The **peritoneum** is internal to the spermatic cord throughout its course, and therefore the cord cannot be visualized as "pushing" an extension of peritoneum ahead of it into the scrotum (see Figure 5-13). In the case of the peritoneum, a narrow extension of the peritoneum (the *processus vaginalis*) travels alongside the spermatic

Table 5-1   Walls of the Inguinal Canal

Anterior Wall	Superior Wall (roof)	Posterior Wall	Inferior Wall (floor)
External oblique (throughout)	Falx inguinalis (as it arches over the spermatic cord, moving from lateral to medial)	Transversalis fascia (laterally)	Inguinal ligament (throughout)
Internal oblique and transversus abdominus (falx inguinalis) (laterally)		Internal oblique and transversus abdominus (falx inguinalis) (medially)	

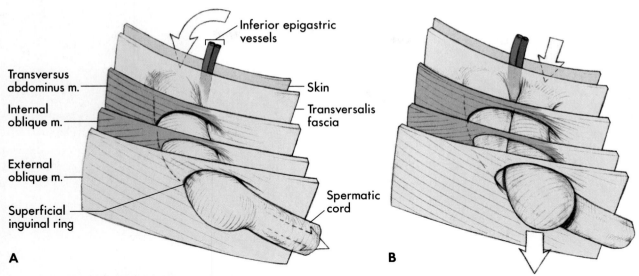

Figure 5-10 INGUINAL HERNIAS. A, Indirect inguinal hernia. An indirect hernia replicates the pathway by which the developing testis descends through the abdominal wall into the scrotum. The peritoneal membrane, sometimes including a part of the intestine, descends along this same path. The *top curved arrow* shows the deep inguinal ring, where the herniating loop of intestine would enter the inguinal canal. The *bottom arrow* shows the path by which the herniated segment of intestine would enter the scrotum, having passed through the superficial inguinal ring. **B,** Direct inguinal hernia. In a direct inguinal hernia, the herniating segment of intestine passes *medial* to the inferior epigastric vessels, not lateral as in the case of the indirect hernia. The direct hernia does not enter the deep inguinal ring and does not dissect within the layers of the spermatic cord. Note that the "swelling" caused by the herniation is at nearly the same point as the herniation of the indirect type. This means that the examiner may detect a hernia in the root of the scrotum, and even follow it, by palpation, toward the superficial inguinal ring, but not be able to tell if it is a direct or an indirect hernia. In theory, at least, the direct hernia does not dissect within the spermatic cord but passes lateral or medial to it.

cord down into the scrotum. It later becomes isolated from the peritoneal cavity and persists as a "bubble" of peritoneum in the scrotum, alongside the testis.

RELATIONS OF INFERIOR EPIGASTRIC VESSELS

The **inferior epigastric vessels** arise from the external iliac vessels, just before they pass beneath the inguinal ligament (see Figure 5-4) to enter the thigh as the femoral vessels. The inferior epigastric vessels course superiorly and medially, departing from the external iliac vessels at a point just medial to the deep inguinal ring. The **spermatic cord,** moving toward the external inguinal ring, appears to pass in front of the inferior epigastric vessels as it moves from lateral to medial. Surgeons dissecting in this area, as part of an inguinal hernia repair surgery, use these vessels as a convenient landmark for distinguishing indirect from direct inguinal hernias.

An inguinal hernia results when there is a weakness in the abdominal wall, in the region of the inguinal ligament, so that the layers of the abdominal wall and sometimes portions of the intestinal tract may protrude forward. Often such hernias track downward into the root of the scrotum. *Indirect* or *congenital hernias* (Figure 5-10, *A*) retrace the descent of the testis (and therefore pass lateral to the inferior epigastric vessels on their way to the scrotum), while *direct* or *acquired hernias* (Figure 5-10, *B*) pass medial to the inferior epigastric vessels.

THE SPERMATIC CORD

The **spermatic cord** is a composite of several structures and layers of tissue, arranged in concentric fashion. Central is the **ductus (vas) deferens**, conveying semen from the testis to the urethra. The ductus is accompanied by fascial layers, muscles, vessels, nerves, and an extension of the peritoneum. The arrangement

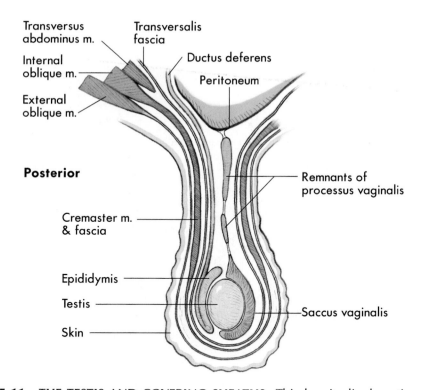

Transversus
abdominus m.

Transversalis
fascia

Internal
oblique m.

Ductus deferens

Peritoneum

External
oblique m.

Posterior

Remnants of
processus vaginalis

Cremaster m.
& fascia

Epididymis

Testis

Saccus vaginalis

Skin

Figure 5-11   THE TESTIS AND COVERING SHEATHS. This longitudinal section through the scrotum shows the testis, the adjoining layers of peritoneum, and the downward extensions of tissue derived from the layers of the abdominal wall. The posterior part of the drawing shows the abdominal wall, and how its various layers extend downward into the scrotum. Anteriorly, the layers of the scrotal wall attach to the pubis. Just interior to the skin and superficial fascia is the external oblique muscle and its continuation, the external spermatic fascia. Internal to these are the internal oblique muscle and the cremaster muscle and fascia in the scrotum. Next is the transversus abdominus muscle, which has no continuation into the scrotum. Internal to these is the transversalis fascia, and its continuation, the internal spermatic fascia. Next are the ductus deferens and the testis itself, which in effect are at the center of the concentric layers of tissue that make up the spermatic cord. There is a slim neck of peritoneum (the processus vaginalis), extending downward into the scrotum. Directly adjacent to the testis, the processus vaginalis dilates to form an ovoid expansion, the saccus vaginalis. In time the testis "sinks" into the saccus vaginalis, and simultaneously the saccus vaginalis is isolated from the peritoneal cavity because the processus vaginalis becomes obliterated.   SEE ATLAS, FIGS. 5-31, 5-32

of these various structures can be understood only with reference to embryology: The testis (or the round ligament in the female) migrates from a position in the upper posterior abdominal wall (originally near the kidney) to the scrotum (or labium in the female), and in so doing creates the **inguinal canal.**

Contents of the Spermatic Cord

The spermatic cord can be visualized as a series of concentric layers of tissue and/or structures (Figure 5-11). Those layers are, moving from *central to peripheral:*

- Ductus deferens (vas deferens)
- Testicular arteries (branch of aorta)
- Artery to the ductus deferens (branch of inferior vesical artery)
- Internal spermatic fascia (branch of transversalis fascia)
- Artery to the cremaster (branch of inferior epigastric artery)
- Pampiniform venous plexus (to gonadal veins, left renal vein, IVC)
- Ilioinguinal nerve (from T12 to L1)
- Genital branch of genitofemoral nerve (from L1 to L2)
- Autonomic nerves, lymphatics

- Cremaster muscle (extension of internal oblique)
- External spermatic fascia (from external oblique)
- Superficial fascia
- Skin

In theory, there can be a fascial remnant of the processus vaginalis lying just external to the ductus deferens, but in most males this is obliterated and no longer identifiable.

Nerves in the Spermatic Cord

The **ilioinguinal nerve** (T12 to L1) innervates the skin and subcutaneous tissues of the medial thigh, base of penis, and scrotum/labia (see Figure 5-59). The **genital branch** of the *genitofemoral nerve* (L1 to L2) innervates the cremaster muscle and mediates the motor limb of the *cremaster reflex* (where stroking of the medial thigh leads to retraction of testis toward inguinal canal). It is believed that this ability to regulate the position of the testis is important in temperature regulation and spermatogenesis. Successful sperm formation depends on the testis being 2° to 3° cooler than the core body temperature.

Vasculature of the Spermatic Cord

The **pampiniform plexus** drains blood from the testis and cord into the testicular veins. It is important in the regulation of temperature in the testis, a key variable in sperm production. The *right testicular vein* drains superiorly into the IVC, while the *left testicular vein* drains into the left renal vein, often at a right angle (Figure 5-12). This makes varicoceles more common on the left (see following).

The **testicular arteries** arise in the upper abdomen, from the abdominal aorta, reminding us of the embryologic origin of the testis (see Figure 6-16 for diagram of testicular arteries and Figure 6-20 for drawing of ovarian arteries). The testicular arteries arise from the anterolateral surface of the aorta, at a level just inferior to that of the renal arteries (usually L1 or L2). One also should remember that lymphatic drainage generally follows arterial supply, so lymph nodes in the groin or perineum will *not* enlarge in response to testicular inflammation or malignancy (instead, paraaortic nodes in the posterior abdominal wall become enlarged).

THE SCROTUM

The **scrotum** contains the testes. It is covered with skin, has virtually no subcutaneous fat, and has a thin fascial layer known as the *dartos tunic* (a continuation and fusion of both layers of abdominal wall superficial fascia) (see Figure 5-11). In this dartos layer, there is also some smooth muscle that can wrinkle the skin of the scrotum.

The layers of the spermatic cord were described previously. While descending into the scrotum, the testis "pushes" ahead of it several layers of the abdominal wall, so in theory, most of these layers could be identified surrounding the testis as well. In reality, they are usually fused to the testis and cannot be distinguished.

·CLINICAL ANATOMY OF

THE INGUINAL REGION

VENOUS DRAINAGE AND VARICOCELES

The right angle at which the left testicular vein drains into the left renal vein is thought to predispose the left testicular vein to venous obstruction and the occurrence of varicoceles (tortuous dilated pampiniform plexus; see Figure 5-12) more frequently on the left than the right. Varicoceles can cause infertility (presumably because of temperature disregulation on the affected side).

CANCER OF THE TESTIS

Testicular cancer is often clinically "silent," in part because any lymphatic spread that might occur is to the paraaortic nodes (because of the embryologic origin of the testis), not to the groin or scrotum, where the enlarged nodes might be seen or palpated.

INGUINAL HERNIAS

Inguinal hernias can be palpated in the male patient by placing the fingertip over the superficial inguinal ring and asking the patient to cough. This increase in intraabdominal pressure makes the hernia "bulge" against the fingertips. Inguinal hernias are much more common in adult males than in adult females, but this strong gender difference is not the case in the inguinal hernias common in *small premature infants*. In these children, often only 1 or 2 pounds in weight, the many weeks they spend on the mechanical ventilator produces constant high intraabdominal pressures and puts stress on the inguinal region, causing an equal risk of inguinal herniation in these small premature infants, both male and female.

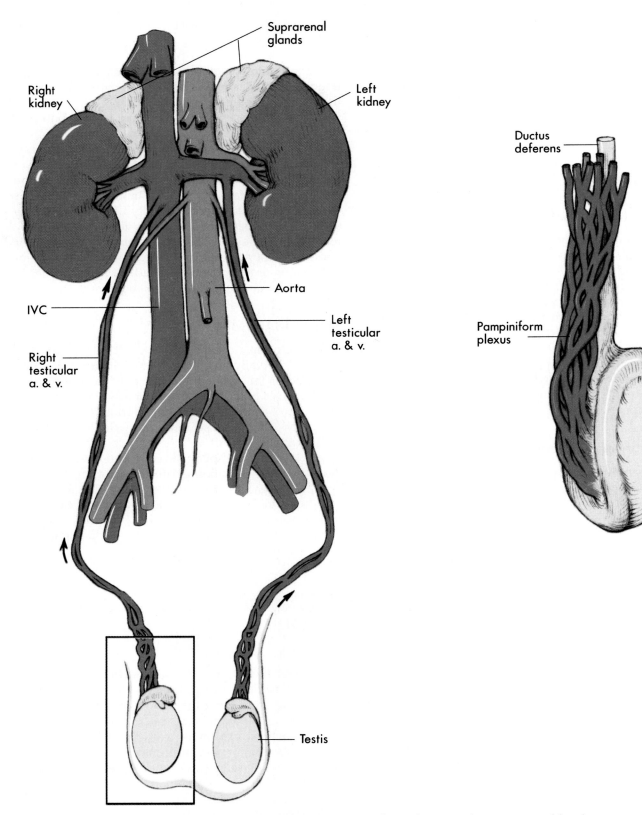

Figure 5-12 BLOOD SUPPLY TO THE TESTIS. The right testis drains venous blood upward to the inferior vena cava (IVC), and the right testicular artery arises from the aorta. The left testicular vein usually drains to the left renal vein, and the left testicular artery arises from the aorta. Recall that lymphatic drainage follows the arterial vessels and drains to lymph nodes in the retroperitoneal tissue near the kidneys. The enlargement at right shows the right testis, viewed posterolaterally. This view allows us to see the *pampiniform plexus*, the complex tangle of small veins that drain the testis and converge on the testicular veins, traveling upward to the IVC. These veins may become tortuous and dilated and impede the venous return on that side (a *varicocele*). Such a condition can raise the temperature in the testis and jeopardize fertility. <small>SEE ATLAS, FIGS. 5-35, 5-105, 5-106</small>

The Processus Vaginalis

As the testis migrates to the scrotum, a slender evagination of the peritoneal membrane (the **processus vaginalis**) migrates into the scrotum along with the testis. In the normal course of development, the processus vaginalis is later separated from the rest of the peritoneal cavity (see Figure 5-11). There then remains a "bubble" of peritoneal membrane in the base of the scrotum, lying directly anterior to the testis. The testis "sinks" into this peritoneal remnant, resulting in the coverage of the testis on all but its posterior surface. This peritoneal investment of the testis is known as the **tunica vaginalis.**

Occasionally the connection between the peritoneal cavity and the tunica vaginalis can remain after birth (*persistent processus vaginalis*). In this situation, the likelihood of inguinal herniation (of the congenital variety—see previous discussion and Figure 5-10) is increased.

The Testis and Ductus Deferens

Each testis is approximately 4 by 3 by 2.5 cm. The testis is covered externally by the thin *tunica vaginalis*, except posteriorly, where the tunica is deficient as it folds back on itself (see Figures 5-11 and 5-13). On this posterior uncovered portion of the testicular surface is positioned the **epididymis** (Figure 5-13). This uncovered part of the testis is analogous to the hilum of the lung (where vessels, nerves, and lymphatics gain access to the lung).

Just as was the case with the pleural and peritoneal membranes, the portion of the tunica vaginalis adherent to the testis is the *visceral portion,* and that not adherent to the testis is the *parietal portion.* The outer fibrous covering of each testis is a thick *tunica albuginea,* lying just internal to the tunica vaginalis.

Passing from the Testis to the Ductus Deferens

Each testis (see Figure 5-13) is divided internally into several hundred lobules, each containing tightly coiled *seminiferous tubules.* Sperm are formed here. The seminiferous tubules converge on a *rete testis,* a network of ducts, which in turn drain into a set of *ductuli efferenti,* which empty into the *head of the epididymis.*

The **epididymis** is a highly coiled collection of

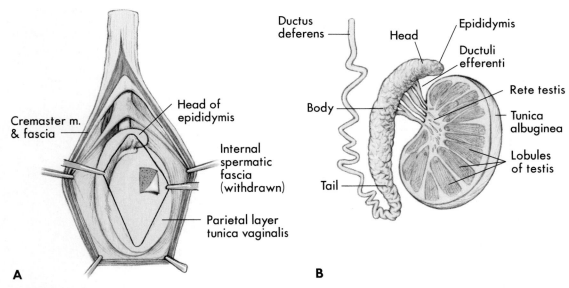

Figure 5-13 THE TESTIS AND EPIDIDYMIS. A, Parasagittal section through the testis, showing its fibrous septae, dividing the testis into lobules. The lobules contain densely coiled seminiferous tubules, in which the sperm develop. The lobules converge on a region near the surface on the side of the hilus of the testis (that is, along the concave edge). Sperm are collected into other sets of tubules and finally emerge from the hilus of the testis as the ductuli efferenti. These ductuli enter the head of the epididymis. Within the epididymis, sperm descend through its body and tail, where they emerge in the thick-walled ductus deferens (vas deferens). **B,** The layers of fascia and muscle surrounding the testis have been incised and pulled aside to reveal the interior to the saccus vaginalis. The curved epididymis is visible on the posterior pole of the testis. A small "window" of the visceral layer of the tunica vaginalis has been reflected upward to show the parenchyma of the testis, lying just underneath.

tubules through which sperm must pass to mature and be functional. The epididymis has a head, body, and tail. The **ductus deferens** (or **vas deferens**) is a duct exiting the epididymis and is central in the spermatic cord. It is highly muscular, innervated by sympathetic nerves, and contracts forcefully as a part of ejaculation.

DESCENT OF THE OVARY

The ovary normally descends only partway along the posterior abdominal wall. Very rarely, it may descend into the inguinal region (into the "canal of Nuck," normally occupied only by the processus vaginalis and the round ligament in the female).

Peritoneal Membranes and Development of the Gut

▶ The Parietal and Visceral Mesenteries

▶ The Dorsal and Ventral Mesenteries

▶ Growth and Rotation of the Gut

▶ Vascular Supply of the Mesenteries

▶ The Parietal Peritoneum

▶ The Greater Omentum

▶ The Lesser Omentum

▶ Peritoneal and Retroperitoneal Structures

*O*ne of the most intricate aspects of human anatomy is the rotation of the gut and the subsequent positioning of membranes that suspend parts of the intestinal tract within the abdominal cavity. The intra-abdominal gut, which begins as a simple tube extending from the diaphragm to the anus, undergoes a complex process of growth, folding, and rotation that results in the adult pattern of gut position in the abdominal cavity. The gut actually herniates outside the body at the sixth embryologic week and returns at the tenth week, rotating as it does. Because of the intricacy of this process, there are many developmental "errors," such as obstructions, abnormal rotation and fixation, and duplications of segments of the gut. The gut consists of foregut, midgut, and hindgut (see Table 5-3).

Also important is the concept that structures such as the gallbladder, liver, and pancreas may be viewed as *exocrine glands* for the GI tract because they secrete enzymes and other substances into the gut to take part in the digestive process. These organs form as branched outgrowths of the GI tract, forming the duct systems that drain materials from these organs into the gut (e.g., bile, pancreatic enzymes). They develop into mature glands as mesoderm condenses around the original outgrowths of the endodermal lining of the gut. The liver and pancreas also synthesize a number of substances that are secreted into the bloodstream, meaning that these organs also function as *endocrine glands.*

THE PARIETAL AND VISCERAL MESENTERIES

The peritoneal membrane is subdivided into the **parietal portion** (lining the walls of the abdominal cavity) and the **visceral portion** (covering the intraperitoneal abdominal viscera) (see Figure 5-14, *D*). **Mesenteries** are double-layered leaflets of peritoneum that connect the parietal to the visceral peritoneum, forming a kind of "sling" in which the organ is suspended.

Just as in the pleural cavity, no organ in the abdominal cavity is *completely* surrounded by mesentery. There must be (and always is) at least a small area on the surface of the organ where mesentery is not tightly affixed (i.e., the **hilum** of the organ; [*hilum*, L., a small thing]. In these areas, the two layers of mesentery (Figure 5-14)

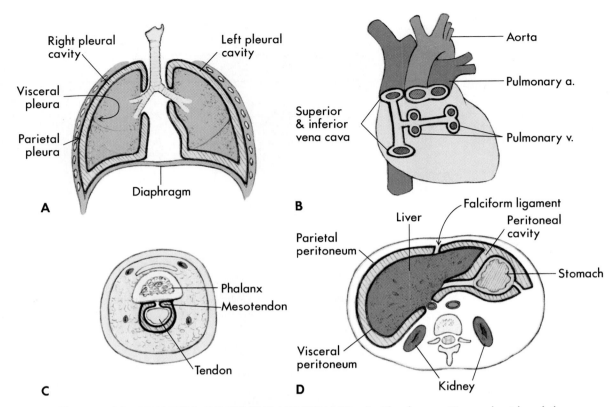

Figure 5-14   EXAMPLES OF SEROUS MEMBRANES. A, The lungs. On each side of the chest a lung is suspended within a *pleural cavity.* **B,** Posterior view of the heart. The aorta and pulmonary artery are encircled in a common pericardial collar. The six venous vessels bringing blood to the heart (four pulmonary veins and the superior and inferior vena cavae) are encircled in a second pericardial collar. Nerves and lymphatics supplying the heart do so by traveling in one or both of these two *stalks* for the heart. **C,** The digits. The tendon is encircled in a serous membrane, except for a hilum, where the membrane doubles back on itself and forms a serous cavity in which the tendon may move with a minimum of friction. Vessels, nerves, and lymphatics reach the tendon at the hilus. When growth is complete, the longitudinal membrane at the hilum of the tendon becomes interrupted, so that instead of a continuous sheath of double membrane, there is a series of small stalks known as *vinculae,* through which the vessels, nerves, and lymphatics travel. **D,** The peritoneal membrane in the abdomen. Here organs are encircled by peritoneum except where a double layer of peritoneum (*mesentery*) connects them to the posterior abdominal wall. In the foregut, a similar double layer of peritoneum connects them to the anterior abdominal wall (exemplified here by the falciform ligament).

are reflected off the surface of the organ and are continuous with the parietal peritoneum lining the body cavity (forming the aforementioned mesenteric "sling" for the organ). Neural, vascular, and lymphatic supply to such organs travels within the leaflets of this sling to reach the organ itself. Such organs or structures are said to be **intraperitoneal** (or are said to be "peritonealized"). Organs tightly affixed to the body wall and covered with peritoneum on their inwardly facing surface only are said to be **retroperitoneal**. These two terms are fundamental to understanding the anatomy of the abdominal cavity. Furthermore, some organs

(e.g., kidney) are retroperitoneal throughout development and are thus *primarily retroperitoneal*. Others (e.g., pancreas) are initially intraperitoneal but later in development become *secondarily retroperitoneal* by "sinking" into the posterior abdominal wall, acquiring as they do an anterior peritoneal covering (see Figure 5-16).

THE DORSAL AND VENTRAL MESENTERIES

Much of the peritoneal membrane in the adult is the derivative of the embryonic dorsal and ventral mesen-

Particular segments of the mesentery are named for the part of the gut to which they are related (e.g., *mesogastrium,* stomach; *mesoduodenum,* mesocolon. The mesentery of the jejunum and ileum is unique and is known as *The Mesentery* (capital M). Between the two thin layers of mesentery travel the nerves, lymphatics, and blood vessels that supply the intestines. Organs supported and surrounded by mesenteries are able to change size and position and to move around within the abdominal cavity with a minimum of friction. This ability is necessary for the intestinal tract, which is alternately filled with and then empty of food, and which moves about considerably during the peristaltic contractions important to digestion.

teries (Figure 5-15). Early in development, the **dorsal mesentery** is comprised of a pair of parallel membranes that reflect anteriorly from the right and left sides of the posterior abdominal wall and travel forward as two thin membranous sheets in the sagittal plane. As they approach the intestine, they pass to the left and right sides of it (see Figure 5-15). In the foregut, these two leaflets of dorsal mesentery split to surround the gut, then approach each other and continue toward the anterior abdominal wall as the ventral mesentery. Remember that the **ventral mesentery** exists only in the foregut region. In the midgut and hindgut (i.e., *distal to the second part of the duodenum*), where no ventral mesentery exists, the two leaflets of the dorsal mesentery simply encircle the intestine and form a *true sling.*

The two leaflets of the *dorsal mesentery* reflect onto the interior of the left and right sides of the *posterior ab-dominal wall,* and the two leaflets of the *ventral mesentery* reflect onto the interior of the left and right sides of the *anterior abdominal wall.* Each is continuous with the parietal peritoneum lining the lateral body wall (see Figure 5-14). Thus, where there is *both* a ventral and dorsal mesentery (i.e., in the region of the foregut), the visceral peritoneum covering the gut is continuous with them both, and the dorsal and ventral mesenteries in turn are continuous with the parietal peritoneum lining the body wall. Distal to the foregut, the visceral peritoneum forms a sling around the gut, and the two leaflets of the dorsal mesentery (forming the "sling") are continuous with the parietal peritoneum lining the entire abdominal cavity.

Organs Developing Within Peritoneal Leaflets

Important structures (e.g., spleen, pancreas) develop from mesodermal condensations within the two leaflets of either the dorsal or the ventral mesentery. With the subsequent rotation of the gut, the position of these organs becomes very difficult to understand and is best clarified through study of embryology. Table 5-2 describes the mesenteries more exactly, in relation to the part of the gut they support. For example, the term "dorsal mesoduodenum" means the dorsal mesentery adjacent to the developing duodenum.

GROWTH AND ROTATION OF THE GUT

The abdominal gut begins as a *simple cylinder* (except where it opens ventrally to be continuous with the yolk sac) extending from the esophageal hiatus in the diaphragm to the anus (see Figure 5-15). Over the first 8 weeks of development, there is differential growth and rotation of the intestine. As an example, we might

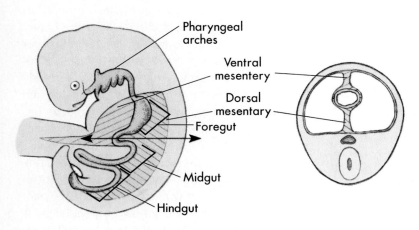

Figure 5-15 DEVELOPMENT OF THE MESENTERIES. On the left is a lateral view of a human embryo at approximately 5 to 6 weeks of development. The double-headed arrow shows the level at which the cross-section on the right side was made. The gut is supported by the bilayered dorsal mesentery along its entire length, and by a continuous ventral mesentery only as far inferior as the second part of the duodenum. Thus above the level of the second part of the duodenum (at the level of section), the two sides of the abdominal cavity are separate, but at a more inferior level the two sides are in direct communication.

Table 5-2   Structures Developing Within the Mesenteries

Structure	Description
IN DORSAL MESENTERY	
Pancreas	Develops in the dorsal mesoduodenum (dorsal pancreatic bud) and a smaller part in the ventral mesoduodenum (ventral pancreatic bud)
Spleen	Develops in the dorsal mesogastrium
IN VENTRAL MESENTERY	
Liver	Develops in the ventral mesogastrium (membranes related to the lesser curvature of the stomach)
Gallbladder	Develops in the ventral mesogastrium as an outgrowth of the liver bud

imagine the simple gut tube undergoing more rapid growth on its left side than its right. As this proceeds, the tube will begin to form a curve that is concave on the side of less growth. In this manner, several regions of the gut become curved and enlarged. Simultaneously, in places the gut tube begins to rotate around its own vertical axis, so that in the stomach, for example, the primitive anterior surface of the gut is rotated to the right (Figure 5-16). Third, the gut elongates considerably and begins to fold back on itself. The pattern of this folding is far from random and produces a predictable pattern of coiling and rotation, especially in the small intestine.

Fixation and Suspension

At 6 weeks of gestation, the midgut is herniated outside the body (see Figure 5-15) in the umbilical stalk. As it returns to the abdominal cavity, by the tenth week, the rotation of the gut takes place. The process of **gut herniation and rotation** is divided into three stages. *First,* the entire small intestine and much of the large intestine leave the abdominal cavity and herniate outside the body wall. The intestinal loops are suspended in their mesenteric slings, and the *superior mesenteric artery (SMA)* becomes a longitudinal axis around which the intestinal loops soon will rotate (Figure 5-17). The SMA leads from the umbilicus outward to a point in the distal ileum, the segment of intestine that migrates *furthest* away from the umbilicus. With the SMA serving as an axis, the intestinal loops begin to rotate counterclockwise, with the cecum (proximal large intestine) serving as the "leading" segment of the rotation.

Second, from weeks 9 to 12, the intestinal loops return into the abdominal cavity, and cecal rotation is advanced to the point that the cecum is positioned in the right upper quadrant (that is, through about 180 degrees). *Third,* from about 13 weeks onward, the cecum migrates to the right lower quadrant, the ascending colon is created, and the small intestinal mesentery is fixed against the posterior wall. The rotation of these gut loops normally occurs in a counterclockwise direction, around the axis of the superior mesenteric artery. When complete, the cecum will rotate through 270 degrees, and the large intestine will create an inverted V-shaped "frame" in which the small intestinal loops will

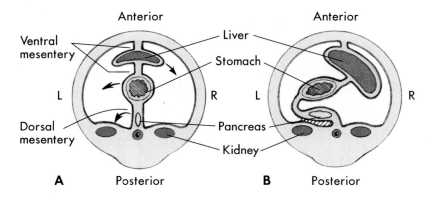

A   Anterior / Posterior   **B**   Anterior / Posterior

Figure 5-16   ROTATION OF THE STOMACH. A, Pancreas, stomach, and liver are shown in the midline, enclosed by the two leaflets of the ventral and dorsal mesenteries. At this point, the pancreas is not incorporated into the posterior wall. **B,** The stomach has rotated around its own long axis, and the dorsal mesentery has "swung" to the left as well. The liver enlarges and moves to the right. As a result of this rotary movement, the formerly sagittal ventral mesentery of the stomach (connecting the liver and stomach) has now become the horizontal lesser omentum. In addition, the pancreas "sinks" back into the posterior wall, obliterating as it does the space between the dorsal mesentery and the body wall. The pancreas is then no longer suspended by a mesentery into the abdominal cavity.

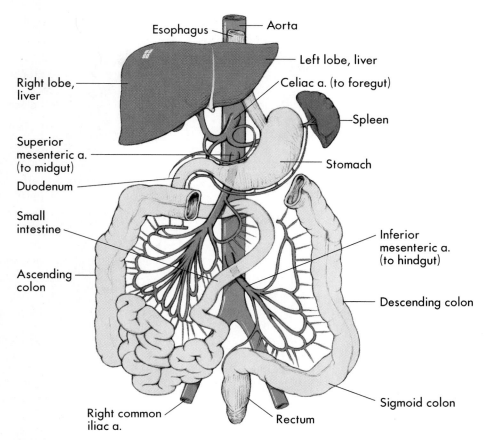

Figure 5-17   THE GASTROINTESTINAL TRACT. This drawing shows the gastrointestinal tract and the three major arteries that supply it. Derivatives of the primitive foregut are supplied by the celiac artery and its branches. The midgut, extending from the duodenum to the midtransverse colon, is supplied by branches of the superior mesenteric artery. The hindgut, extending from the midtransverse colon to the lower rectum, is supplied by branches of the inferior mesenteric artery.   SEE ATLAS, FIGS. 5-7, 5-59

be contained (see Figures 5-18, 5-43). Many variations in the pattern of rotation occur, however, some benign, but some causing pathology.

In addition, at this time, the ascending and descending colons are fixed against the posterior wall and become *secondarily retroperitoneal* (Figure 5-18). The duodenum becomes fixed to the posterior wall (secondarily retroperitoneal), while the rest of the small intestine (jejunum and ileum) stays *intraperitoneal* (i.e., suspended within a peritoneal sling).

Rotation of the Stomach: The Greater and Lesser Sacs

As the liver, gallbladder, pancreas, and spleen are growing and distorting the mesenteries in which they lie, the stomach is rotating around its superoinferior axis (see Figure 5-16) so that the *dorsal mesentery is swung toward the left*. Eventually the stomach rotates through 90 degrees, and a space between the posterior surface of the stomach and the posterior abdominal wall is created. This is the **lesser sac,** or the **omental bursa.** The remainder of the intraabdominal cavity is known as the **greater sac.** The growth of the liver subdivides the ventral mesentery into two subregions, the falciform ligament (from liver to anterior wall) and the lesser omentum (from stomach to liver, see p. 481).

Before the growth and rotation of the stomach and the adherence of the duodenum to the posterior abdominal wall, the inferior margin of the ventral mesentery is in the sagittal plane. *After the rotation of the stomach and the movement of the duodenum to a retroperitoneal position,* however, the free margin of the ventral mesentery is in the coronal plane and has moved to the right. It is represented as the right-side free margin of the **lesser omentum.** Passing around the right side of the lesser omentum gains entrance to the lesser sac (Figure 5-19). This passage is limited superiorly by the liver and inferiorly because the duodenum is embedded in the posterior abdominal wall. Therefore the entrance to the lesser sac has become a relatively narrow passage known as the *epiploic foramen* (of Winslow; see Figures 5-19 and 5-37).

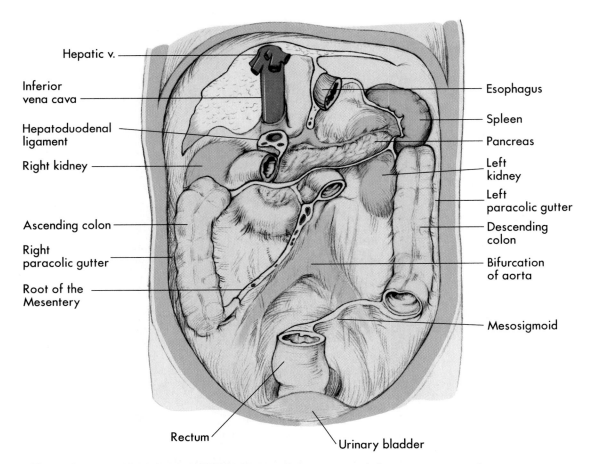

Hepatic v.

Inferior vena cava

Hepatoduodenal ligament

Right kidney

Ascending colon

Right paracolic gutter

Root of the Mesentery

Esophagus

Spleen

Pancreas

Left kidney

Left paracolic gutter

Descending colon

Bifurcation of aorta

Mesosigmoid

Rectum

Urinary bladder

Figure 5-18   RETROPERITONEAL STRUCTURES. Many of the intraperitoneal organs in the abdominal cavity have been removed, and what remains are the several retroperitoneal organs and their peritoneal coverings. The inferior vena cava is shown, with the hepatic veins draining into it just before it passes through the diaphragm. The stump of the esophagus lies to its left, sectioned where it is continuous with the stomach. The two peritoneal layers surrounding the esophageal stump course to the left and right and describe a broad horizontal diamond-shaped area. This area is that part of the diaphragm that abuts directly on the liver without any intervening peritoneum (known as the bare area of the liver). Further still to the left is the spleen. The duodenum is transected shortly distal to the pylorus, and the peritoneally enclosed hepatoduodenal ligament lies just above it. The root of the transverse mesocolon runs transversely across the mid-abdomen, and just inferior to it is the distal end of the duodenum, as it continues into the jejunum. The root of the mesentery extends at a 45-degree angle from the mid-abdomen toward the right lower quadrant. In the left lower quadrant, we see the root of the sigmoid mesocolon.   SEE ATLAS, FIGS. 5-41, 5-42, 5-43, 5-52, 5-77, 5-81

Fixation vs. Suspension

After the tenth week of gestation, when the intestines return to the abdominal cavity, certain parts of the gut become *fixed* to the posterior abdominal wall, and others remain *suspended* in a peritoneal sling within the abdominal cavity (the former are *retroperitoneal*, the latter, *intraperitoneal*).

Normally, the duodenum is fixed to the posterior wall, and the cecum also is attached. Between these two points, the intestine is suspended in a peritoneal sling.

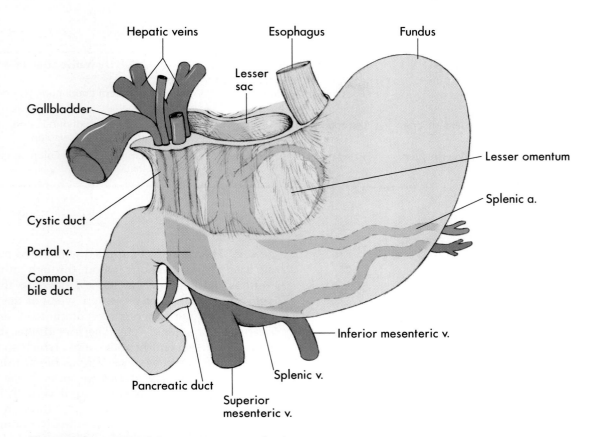

Figure 5-19 THE LESSER OMENTUM. The lesser omentum joins the lesser curvature of the stomach to the undersurface of the liver. Note that the splenic, inferior mesenteric, and superior mesenteric veins converge to form the portal vein.

SEE ATLAS, FIGS. 5-9, 5-48, 5-52, 5-53, 5-90, 5-91

Giant "Glands" of the GI Tract

Both the pancreas and the liver/gallbladder are essentially "glands" of the gastrointestinal tract because they drain by ducts into the second part of the duodenum at the *ampulla of Vater* (see Figures 5-19 and 5-24). The ducts of these structures travel within the free right-side margin of the lesser omentum, derived from the ventral mesentery.

Regions of the Developing Gut

In embryologic terms, we speak of the **foregut, midgut,** and **hindgut.** Although the intestinal tube becomes exceedingly complex as it grows and rotates, it is still possible (and useful) to recognize these three areas (Table 5-3).

VASCULAR SUPPLY OF THE MESENTERIES

All intraperitoneal parts of the intestinal tract depend entirely on **vascular supply** traveling between the two leaflets of the mesenteries in which these segments

of the intestine are suspended. The **arteries** supplying these sections of the intestinal tract are derived from the *celiac, superior mesenteric,* and *inferior mesenteric arteries.* If the intestinal tract were removed from the abdomen and laid out in a straight line, we could see how these arteries supply adjacent and continuous domains for which they are responsible for blood supply and that there is considerable opportunity for *collateral circulation,* if any particular arterial branch should be occluded. The demands for blood supply to the intestinal tract are unique because inadequate blood supply to even a small area reduces overall gut activity. Even if an *ischemic* (i.e., lacking necessary blood supply) area is small, the intestinal tract cannot function properly because enzyme *secretion,* mucus secretion, and peristalsis are necessary in every part of the gut to assure proper function. This is not the situation in other vital organs, such as brain, heart, liver, and kidney, where damage to one area will not necessarily prevent the other healthy parts of the organ from functioning normally.

The inferior and superior mesenteric arteries have companion veins of the same name, but there is *no* celi-

Table 5-3   Derivatives of the Developing Gut

Region of Gut	Blood Supply	Function	Adult Derivative Structures
Foregut	Celiac artery	Digestion-absorption	Stomach, first part of duodenum, part of second part duodenum
Midgut	Superior mesenteric artery	Absorption	Remaining second part of duodenum, and distally to midpoint of transverse colon
Hindgut	Inferior mesenteric artery	Excretion; H_2O reabsorption	Gut distal to mid-transverse colon, as far as anorectal junction

PRINCIPLES ■

Apart from the digestive tube itself, several of the major organs in the abdomen (liver, gallbladder, and pancreas) deposit a secretion into the lumen of the gut. In this sense they resemble the salivary glands of the upper digestive tract. The **liver** manufactures *bile,* which is stored and concentrated in the gallbladder. Bile helps to emulsify fats and make them more digestible. It also serves as a means of ridding the body of used blood proteins (hemoglobin). Bile lends color to the stool, and when there is obstruction to bile flow, the stools appear abnormally pale or even chalk-white. The **gallbladder** is a reservoir for bile, concentrating it while it is stored there. When food enters the duodenum, a hormonal signal travels from the duodenum through the bloodstream to stimulate the transport of bile from the gallbladder into the duodenum. In addition to its role in manufacturing bile, the **liver** secretes a tremendous variety of substances into the bloodstream (e.g., proteins, enzymes, clotting factors).

The **pancreas** synthesizes a number of powerful *digestive enzymes,* which are also released into the duodenum on the signal of circulating hormones that are released into the bloodstream in response to eating. Special layers of mucus within the pancreas itself help to prevent these powerful enzymes from digesting the pancreas itself (*autodigestion*). Obstruction to the normal flow of pancreatic secretions can make this autodigestion possible because the enzymes are prevented from flowing out of the pancreas into the duodenum. In addition to this exocrine function, the pancreas also has a crucial endocrine function, secreting *insulin* and other glucose-regulating hormones into the bloodstream.

ac vein. The structures supplied with blood by the celiac artery drain venous blood through other veins. **Venous drainage** of the *stomach* flows to the splenic vein and the superior mesenteric vein, of the proximal *duodenum* to the superior mesenteric vein, and of the *spleen* to the splenic vein. The *liver* drains its venous blood to the several hepatic veins, which soon empty into the inferior vena cava. Venous blood from the *entire small intestine, half of the large intestine, and the spleen* combine to form the hepatic **portal vein.** This venous blood is unique because it will pass through a second capillary bed, in the liver, before finally draining to the heart. Venous blood from the *distal half of the large intestine* drains to the inferior mesenteric vein, which itself contributes to the portal vein by joining the superior mesenteric vein (see Figure 5-19).

Lymphatic drainage of the intestine is doubly important because small globules of fat, absorbed directly from ingested foods, are transported through the lymphatic channels of the mesentery to be deposited in the portal bloodstream. From here they go to the liver to be digested.

THE PARIETAL PERITONEUM

Mesenchyme that condenses and forms a thin layer lining the interior of the abdominal cavity becomes the **parietal peritoneum.** It is continuous with the **visceral peritoneum,** which covers the intraabdominal organs. The processus vaginalis is an outward evagination of the peritoneum into the scrotum (see Figure 5-11).

The parietal peritoneum is innervated by somatic nerves of the body wall (e.g., intercostal nerves), making it exquisitely sensitive to pain and other stimuli. The visceral peritoneum is innervated by autonomic nerves and has a much higher threshold of response to pain and other stimuli.

THE GREATER OMENTUM

The **greater omentum** is an outward evagination of a section of the *dorsal mesentery* lying along the

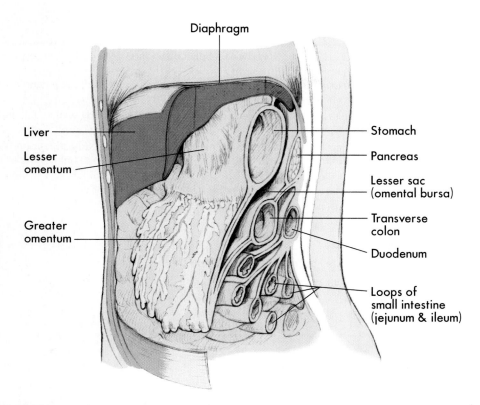

Figure 5-20 THE GREATER OMENTUM. This oblique cutaway view of the abdomen shows the many reflections of the mesentery (in which the small bowel is suspended) and the greater omentum, an evagination of the dorsal mesentery that creates a broad drape hanging downward in front of the transverse colon and small intestine. The drawing also shows a parasagittal section through the lesser sac, showing how the retroperitoneal pancreas is in its posterior wall and the stomach in its anterior wall.

SEE ATLAS, FIGS. 5-39, 5-40, 5-45

greater curvature of the stomach (Figure 5-20). This evagination becomes massive in size and drapes downward in front of the loops of the small intestine. As an outward evagination of the dorsal mesentery, which then extends downward in the abdomen, the greater omentum represents a total of *four layers of peritoneum*—because the two-layered mesentery is folded back on itself.

The four layers of the greater omentum usually fuse into a single fat-laden membrane. The **gastroepiploic arteries** lie within the leaflets of the greater omentum, about 3 to 5 cm inferior to the greater curvature of the stomach. The space (or potential space) within the leaflets of the greater omentum is continuous with the lesser sac (although this connection is obliterated as layers fuse).

THE LESSER OMENTUM

This derivative of the *ventral mesentery* conects the lesser curvature of the stomach with the posteroinferior

surface of the liver. It has a right-side free margin in which are found the common bile duct, portal vein, and hepatic artery (see Figure 5-19). It is a two-layered membrane, derived from the right and left sides of the ventral mesentery. The ventral mesentery is represented between the anterior surface of the liver and the anterior body wall by the **falciform ligament.**

PERITONEAL AND RETROPERITONEAL STRUCTURES

In addition to recognizing which structures are retroperitoneal and which are intraperitoneal (Table 5-4), one should recognize and distinguish those that are *primarily retroperitoneal* (are now and always were retroperitoneal) and those that are *secondarily retroperitoneal* (during development they were intraperitoneal but as part of normal development have become retroperitoneal). No structures change from retroperitoneal to intraperitoneal status during development.

Table 5-4   The Peritoneum, Structure by Structure

Structure	Peritoneal Specialization(s)
Stomach	Suspended within the dorsal mesentery; the greater omentum extends off the greater curvature of the stomach, and the lesser omentum off the lesser curvature
Liver	Suspended within leaflets of ventral mesentery; attached to anterior body wall by falciform ligament and to stomach by lesser omentum
Pancreas	Originally within leaflets of dorsal and ventral mesentery, in adult is nearly all retroperitoneal (by "falling" backward to blend into the posterior abdominal wall); small portion of tail is intraperitoneal, within lienorenal ligament
Duodenum	Becomes secondarily retroperitoneal as it "falls" back against posterior wall
Jejunum and ileum	Suspended within the abdominal cavity (intraperitoneal or "peritonealized")
Cecum	Nearly all is secondarily retroperitoneal
Ascending colon	Secondarily retroperitoneal
Transverse colon	Peritonealized, suspended by transverse mesocolon
Descending colon	Secondarily retroperitoneal
Sigmoid colon	Intraperitoneal
Rectum	Retroperitoneal

CLINICAL ANATOMY OF

ABDOMINAL DEVELOPMENT

SPECIAL REGIONS WITHIN THE PERITONEAL CAVITY

The complex attachments of the mesenteries and the peritoneum create some channels and "gutters" along which fluids (e.g., pus, blood) will flow most easily, if they are present in the abdominal cavity. The most easily understood of these are the (1) paracolic gutters, in the depressions between the ascending and descending colon and the abdominal wall; and (2) the supracolic space, between the diaphragm and the transverse mesocolon. In cases of peritonitis, an understanding of these may help predict where the infectious exudates or other fluids will accumulate.

PARACENTESIS

Paracentesis is the process of withdrawing fluid from the abdominal cavity. It is most often performed in the midline below the level of the umbilicus or just superior to the inguinal ligaments in the inferolateral quadrants of the abdomen.

MALROTATION OF THE GUT

There is a large variety of congenital malrotations of the gut, the most common of which is a failure of the cecum to rotate through the normal full 270 degrees of counterclockwise rotation. Malrotations are significant because they predispose to the formation of abnormal adhesions and/or obstructions of the gut.

HERNIATIONS

The gut may fail to return from its normal herniation through the umbilicus during the sixth to the tenth week, producing an *oomphalocoele,* or congenital persistence of the gut outside the abdominal cavity. A similar condition is *gastroschisis,* which may appear identical to oomphalocoele but really represents a later reherniation of the intestines through a defect in the abdominal wall resulting from abnormal muscle growth (not a persistence of herniation through the umbilicus, which defines an oomphalocoele).

Intraperitoneal Structures

The **stomach** is suspended along its lesser curvature by the hepatogastric ligament (derived from ventral mesentery and part of the lesser omentum) and along its greater curvature by the dorsal mesogastrium (from dorsal mesentery).

The **liver** is suspended within leaflets of ventral mesentery; it is attached to anterior body wall by the falciform ligament and to stomach by the lesser omentum.

The **jejunum and ileum** are suspended within the abdominal cavity ("peritonealized") by the Mesentery (note the capital M specifies that this is the mesentery of the jejunum and ileum) (see Figure 5-18). The **transverse colon** is peritonealized and is suspended by the transverse **mesocolon**. The **sigmoid colon** is peritonealized.

Retroperitoneal Structures

The **pancreas** is originally within leaflets of dorsal and ventral mesentery but in the adult has become nearly all retroperitoneal (by "falling" backward to blend into the posterior abdominal wall) (see Figure 5-16). A small portion of the pancreatic tail is within lienorenal ligament and should be isolated and protected during *splenectomy* (where part of the procedure involves ligating the vessels in the lienorenal ligament). The **cecum** and **ascending** and **descending colon** are secondarily retroperitoneal, in the same fashion (except for a small part of the cecum that is intraperitoneal).

section five.four
Liver, Gallbladder, Spleen, and Pancreas

▶ The Liver

▶ The Gallbladder and Biliary Tree

▶ The Spleen

▶ The Pancreas

*T*he **liver, gallbladder,** and **pancreas** develop within the leaflets of the dorsal or ventral mesentery. Each organ drains into the duodenum, their secretions playing an important role in digestion. The **spleen,** by contrast, creates no secretions but instead conveys partially metabolized products of hemoglobin breakdown to the liver via the portal circulation. The liver and pancreas are both **exocrine** (secreting substances into an open cavity—in this case the gut) and **endocrine** organs (producing substances to be excreted into the bloodstream). The gallbladder stores and concentrates bile (formed in the liver).

THE LIVER

The liver is largely protected by the ribcage although it is wholly within the abdominal cavity (Figure 5-21). It is covered over much of its surface by peritoneal membranes (see later discussion). Just deep to these peritoneal coverings is a thin capsule of connective tissue (Glisson's capsule). The average liver weighs 3 to 4 lb in the male, and 2.5 to 3 lb in the female.

The anterior edge of the liver, especially on the right, is normally palpable at the costal margin or slightly inferior to it. The liver is a compound gland lying within the leaflets of the ventral mesentery. It is connected to the digestive tract by its duct, the *bile duct.* Bile is its exocrine secretion. **Bile** contains (1) bile pigments, the breakdown products of hemoglobin catabolism, and (2) bile salts (formed from cholesterol and helping to emulsify ingested fats). The average adult produces 700 to 1000 ml of bile per day. In addition, bile is the vehicle

in which several drugs and toxins are excreted from the body.

The cells of the liver also carry out a complex and varied set of metabolic functions, including carbohydrate, protein, and lipid degradation and synthesis, production of clotting factors, and detoxification of various compounds.

Lobes of the Liver

The lobes of the liver are traditionally defined by the obvious surface features, especially on the inferior surface. The **right lobe,** lying to the right of a line connecting the inferior vena cava and the gallbladder, is the largest anatomic lobe of the liver. The **left lobe** lies to the left of the line created by the ligamentum venosum and ligamentum teres. Two much smaller lobes are defined by anatomic criteria: The **quadrate lobe** lies between the gallbladder and ligamentum teres, and the **caudate lobe** lies between the inferior vena cava and ligamentum venosum, posterior to the quadrate lobe. Both the quadrate and caudate lobes are visible only on the inferior surface of the liver (see Figure 5-21).

Surgeons operating on the liver, especially in operations involving removal of a part of the liver, soon discovered that the blood and bile flow do not segregate according to these anatomic criteria. For example, the blood flow to the left lobe of the liver is not confined to the left lobe alone, so that there may be bleeding problems if one attempts to remove the left lobe by making a surgical incision along the line connecting the ligamentum venosum and ligamentum teres.

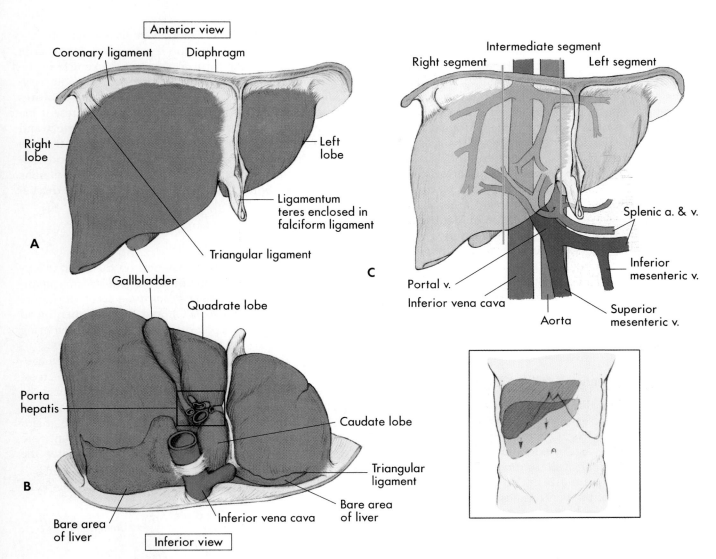

Anterior view

Coronary ligament   Diaphragm

Right
lobe

Left
lobe

Ligamentum
teres enclosed in
falciform ligament

A

Gallbladder   Triangular ligament

Quadrate lobe

Porta
hepatis

Caudate lobe

Triangular
ligament

B

Bare area
of liver   Inferior vena cava

Bare area
of liver

Inferior view

Intermediate segment

Right segment   Left segment

Splenic a. & v.

Inferior
mesenteric v.

C

Portal v.

Inferior vena cava

Aorta

Superior
mesenteric v.

Figure 5-21   THE LIVER. *Inset* shows the position of the liver at *full inspiration* (*dotted lines*) and at *full expiration* (*solid lines*). **A,** Anterior view of the liver showing the falciform ligament extending anteriorly to the inner surface of the anterior chest wall. The ligament's lower free edge contains the round ligament of the liver (ligamentum teres). The peritoneum covering the liver reflects onto the inferior surface of the diaphragm, and where it does it is known as the coronary ligament. Its right-side free edge is the right triangular ligament. **B,** Inferior view of the liver showing the space in which the substance of the liver is in direct contact with the diaphragm. This is known as the bare area, and its perimeter is outlined by a dark line. **C,** View of the liver showing the relationship of the three major vessels and how their branching defines the right, intermediate, and left segments. These subdivisions are very important for surgeons operating on the liver.

SEE ATLAS, FIG. 5-68

More recent studies show that the left lobe, quadrate lobe, and nearly all of the caudate lobe share a *common blood supply* (from the left hepatic artery and left major branch of the portal vein) and biliary drainage. The right hepatic artery and right-side branch of the portal vein supply the entire right lobe and a small posterior area of the caudate lobe, and biliary drainage in these areas also follows the arterial pattern. The *hepatic veins,* however, do *not* follow these patterns and may present intraoperative bleeding problems in liver surgery, even if knowledge of the arterial and biliary patterns is respected. There is wide disagreement among surgeons about the importance of this system of identifying liver lobes on the basis of incoming blood supply. Several investigators have defined from 6 to 15 "lobes" of the liver, reminiscent of the basis for identifying bronchopulmonary segments of the lung. In the liver, each of these segments is defined by an incoming branch of the hepatic artery, portal vein, and biliary duct. Except for the hepatic veins, there is little communication between these segments.

Peritoneal Reflections and the Liver

Recalling that the liver develops within the leaflets of the ventral mesentery, we can see that the *falciform, triangular,* and *coronary ligaments* represent that portion of the ventral mesentery extending from the liver to the anterior abdominal wall or undersurface of the diaphragm (see Figure 5-21). The *lesser omentum* represents that part of the ventral mesentery connecting the liver and the stomach.

The **triangular ligaments** connect the upper surface of the liver with the inferior surface of the diaphragm. On the left, the two leaflets of the triangular ligament are close together, and no important structures are found between the two leaflets. On the right, the two leaflets are widely separated medially and are fused to form a true double-layered membrane only most laterally. More medially, the two layers of membrane are separated and surround the *bare area* (containing the IVC and hepatic veins). Each leaflet of the triangular ligament is called a **coronary ligament.** The bare area represents that part of the liver in direct contact with the diaphragm (i.e., no intervening layer of peritoneum).

The **falciform ligament** is a continuation of the ventral mesentery that "emerges" from the ventral surface of the liver from a fissure between the left lobe and the quadrate lobe (see Figure 5-21). It has a scythe-shaped free inferior margin, extending from the liver to the umbilicus. Within this lower margin is the thickened *round ligament of the liver,* a remnant of the left umbilical vein in the fetus and newborn.

The **lesser omentum** is a double layer of peritoneum connecting the undersurface of the liver and the lesser curvature of the stomach (see Figure 5-19). The lesser omentum contains many blood vessels and lymphatics. Notable among them are the *hepatic artery, portal vein,* and *bile duct.* These form a palpable thickening in the right-side free margin of the lesser omentum—the *hepatoduodenal ligament.* These three important structures travel as a unit throughout the liver and represent the important functions of the liver—the hepatic artery and portal vein delivering blood to the liver, and the bile ducts draining bile away from it. The liver's blood supply is unique in that about 70% of it is portal venous blood, and about 30% is arterial blood (see later discussion).

The Porta Hepatis

The **porta hepatis** is that region on the inferior surface of the liver where one finds the *gallbladder, ligamentum teres* (round ligament), *ligamentum venosum* (Figure 5-22), *inferior vena cava* (IVC), and the aforementioned structures of the hepatoduodenal ligament entering and leaving the liver (Figure 5-23).

The porta hepatis lies between the quadrate and caudate lobes of the liver. It may be visualized as the crosspiece in an H, where the IVC and gallbladder form the right-side vertical piece and the falciform ligament and ligamentum venosum the left-side piece. The major components of the hepatoduodenal ligament are arranged in a predictable fashion as they enter the

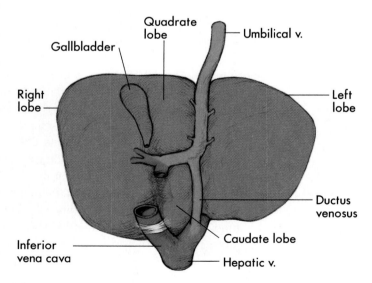

Figure 5-22   BLOOD FLOW AND THE FETAL LIVER. The ductus venosus is a fetal vessel that shunts umbilical venous blood, returning from the placenta, past the liver and directly into the inferior vena cava. After the child is born, the ductus venosus closes, and its proximal remnant persists as a slender fibrous cord, the ligamentum venosum, while the final segment of the umbilical vein becomes the ligamentum teres of the liver.

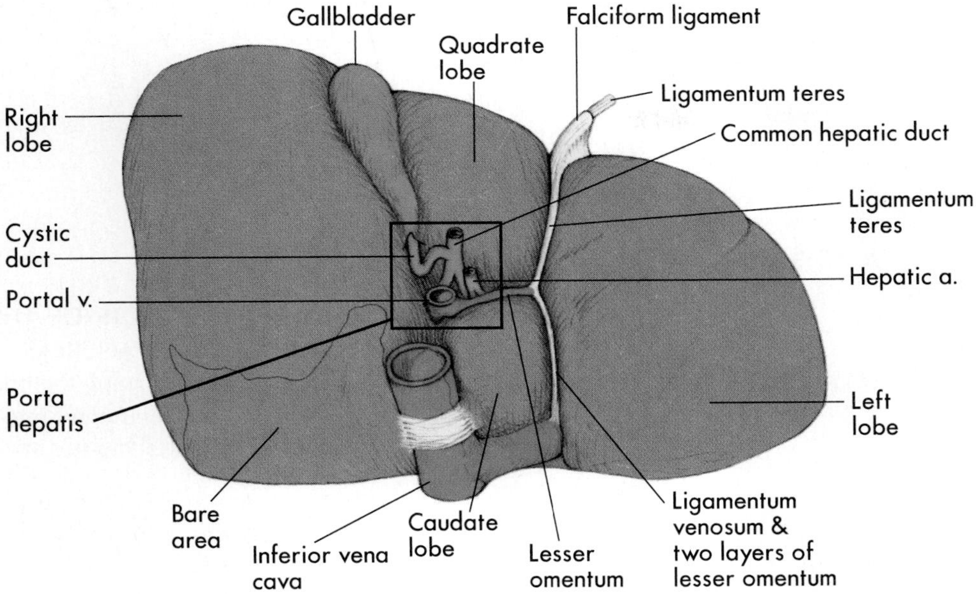

Figure 5-23 THE LIVER AND PORTA HEPATIS. The undersurface of the liver. The area within the box is the porta hepatis or "door to the liver." The gallbladder and ligamentum teres form the upper two vertical limbs; the ligamentum venosum and inferior vena cava form the lower two vertical limbs; and the porta hepatis forms the cross-bar of the H.
SEE ATLAS, FIGS. 5-71, 5-73

porta hepatis—the *portal vein* lies posterior, the *hepatic artery* anterior and to the left, and the *common bile duct* anterior and to the right. The porta hepatis is analogous to the hilum of the lung (i.e., a "root," or place where neurovascular structures enter and leave the organ).

The Hepatic and Common Bile Ducts

The *right* and *left hepatic ducts* unite just inferior to the porta hepatis to form the **common hepatic duct** (Figure 5-24). The *left hepatic duct* drains the left lobe, all of the quadrate, and most of the caudate lobe (in conventional gross anatomic terms), and the *right hepatic duct* drains the right lobe and a small part of the caudate lobe. The union of the left and right hepatic ducts produces the **hepatic duct.** A short distance from the porta hepatis, the *cystic duct* and the *hepatic duct* unite to form the **common bile duct.**

The **common bile duct (CBD)** is about 10 cm in length. It lies to the right and anterior in the hepatoduodenal ligament, the thickened free right margin of the lesser omentum (see Figure 5-19). As it travels toward the duodenum, it lies posterior to the first part of the duodenum, just to the right of the gastroduodenal artery, and anterior to the head of the pancreas.

As the CBD approaches the duodenum, it is joined by the pancreatic duct and the **hepatopancreatic ampulla of Vater** (L. *ampulla,* narrow-necked globular

flask) is formed. Together, these two ducts enter the wall of the duodenum on its posterior side and form a visible prominence on its lumen (the *greater papilla*) (see Figure 5-24). A circular smooth muscle *sphincter (of Oddi)* forms the wall of the ampulla and contracts and relaxes to regulate bile flow. It is believed that hormonal influences are much more important than neural inputs in the regulation of this sphincter tone.

PRINCIPLES

The portal vein, hepatic artery, and bile duct compose a trio of structures that travel together through the liver (the *portal triad*). These three structures are seen in the hepatoduodenal ligament, in the right-hand free margin of the lesser omentum. The internal architecture of the liver is organized around these three structures as well. Liver cells are arrayed in longitudinal cords, converging on a tributary of the hepatic vein in the center. Around the periphery are several portal triads. The hepatic artery and portal vein branch release blood into spaces that run between the liver cords, ultimately converging on the central hepatic vein. Bile manufactured by the liver cells, flows outward between these cords of liver cells and is collected in the bile ducts that compose the third element of the portal triad. Bile ducts in turn drain into larger ducts that leave the liver as the right and left hepatic ducts.

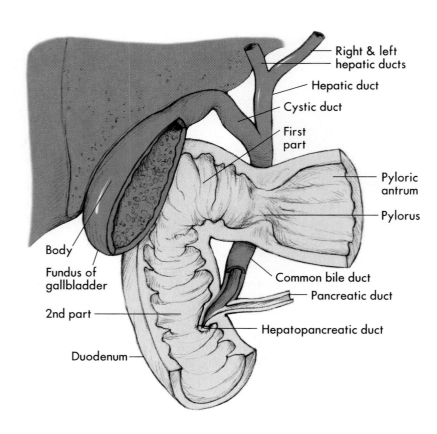

Right & left
hepatic ducts

Hepatic duct

Cystic duct

First
part

Pyloric
antrum

Pylorus

Body

Fundus of
gallbladder

Common bile duct

Pancreatic duct

2nd part

Hepatopancreatic duct

Duodenum

Figure 5-24   DUCTS OF THE LIVER, GALL-BLADDER, AND PANCREAS. Close-up of the pyloric region showing the bile ducts, pancreatic ducts, and their entry into the duodenum.
SEE ATLAS, FIGS. 5-60, 5-61, 5-66, 5-67

PRINCIPLES ■

A *portal venous system* is one in which blood collected from one set of capillary beds passes through a second set of capillary beds before it reaches the vena cava and drains to the heart. In the abdominal cavity, blood drained from the capillary beds of the intestine, where so much digestion of food products has occurred, is drained not to the heart but to the cells of the liver, through a set of vessels that collect this blood from the intestine and then branch to form the second set of capillary vessels. This unusual vessel is the *hepatic portal vein.* It forms from the union of the superior mesenteric and splenic veins and travels in the posterior part of the hepatoduodenal ligament to reach the liver. Although it is a vein by histologic criteria, it is unusual in breaking up into a successively smaller and smaller set of branches, which in fact are capillaries. Blood released from the portal vein is allowed to bathe the cells within the liver, where nutrients are metabolized. This blood is then collected into the tributaries of the hepatic veins, which do empty into the inferior vena cava, just inferior to the right atrium. An important portal system is also found in the *pituitary gland,* where the purpose of the double system of capillaries is to deliver a specific group of trophic hormones from the hypothalamus to the pituitary gland.

Blood Supply of the Liver

The liver is unique in receiving both arterial and venous blood (portal), in a ratio of about 3:7. The portal venous blood is rich in nutrients absorbed in the gut. Blood from these two sources passes through capillary beds in the liver and is drained by the hepatic veins into the inferior vena cava.

Arterial blood supply to the liver is derived from the celiac trunk, which normally arises from the aorta at T12-L1 and divides into the *splenic, left gastric,* and *common hepatic arteries* (see Figures 5-17 and 5-27). The *proper hepatic artery* is derived from the common hepatic artery and lies in the left side of the hepatoduodenal ligament. It in turn divides into the right and left hepatic arteries. The *right hepatic artery* supplies the right lobe and part of the caudate lobe, and the *left hepatic artery* supplies the rest of the liver. Over 50% of individuals will have some variation from the textbook pattern of blood supply from the celiac trunk.

The **hepatic portal vein** usually arises from the union of the *splenic* and *superior mesenteric veins,* taking place posterior to the pancreas (although there is much variation here also). It drains into capillary beds in the liver. From these arise the tributaries of the *hepatic veins,* which drain into the IVC.

The *portal vein* is positioned posterior in the hepatoduodenal ligament (see Figure 5-21). It delivers to the liver venous blood that has already traversed the capillary beds of the GI tract and spleen. Portal blood sup-

CLINICAL ANATOMY OF

THE LIVER

RESISTANCE TO BLOOD FLOW THROUGH THE LIVER

Portal hypertension results when there is an obstruction to the easy flow of blood through the portal vein into the liver. There are many possible causes, including intrinsic liver disease (e.g., cirrhosis) and vascular obstruction. Signs of portal hypertension include hemorrhoids and gastroesophageal bleeding. Both of these result from the obstruction of portal venous blood flow through the liver and the increased flow of blood through alternate paths to reach the vena cava (e.g., the rectal veins and the esophageal veins). When these alternate paths receive more blood than they normally would, the veins dilate, distend, and become more prone to hemorrhage. This is especially likely to happen in the esophagus, where the ingestion of hot or cold substances or even coughing may precipitate life-threatening bleeding.

BYPASSING THE LIVER'S NORMAL BLOOD FLOW

Portocaval shunts are vascular surgical procedures in which the portal vein is anastomosed to the inferior vena cava, renal vein, or other suitable vein eventually draining to the vena cava (hence the "caval" in portocaval). Such procedures are indicated for those with serious portal venous obstruction, often caused by liver disease.

JAUNDICE

When the amount of hemoglobin breakdown products exceeds the ability of the liver to metabolize and excrete it or when the hepatic and bile ducts are obstructed, the hemoglobin products accumulate in the blood and from there into the tissues. This produces jaundice (Middle English, *jaundys*, yellow), often accompanied by itching. Jaundice is often interpreted as a sign of serious liver dysfunction.

INFLAMMATION OF THE LIVER

Several viruses and bacteria can produce direct liver infection (hepatitis). Abscesses in the liver can erode through Glisson's capsule and even cross the diaphragm and cause pleuritis (pleural inflammation) or empyema (pus in the pleural space).

LIVER TRANSPLANTATION

Liver transplantation is used increasingly for cases of irreversible acquired liver disease (e.g., mushroom poisoning) or congenital abnormality (e.g., lack of extrahepatic biliary system in biliary atresia). The vascular anatomy of the liver determines the strategy of the surgical approach to liver transplantation.

THE LIVER AND HEART FAILURE

When the heart performs inefficiently as a pump, blood literally "backs up" in the inferior vena cava and the hepatic veins. Pressure within the lumen of the hepatic veins increases, and fluid passes from the intravascular space out into the substance of the liver. This causes the liver to enlarge, which may be ascertained by palpating its anterior edge well down in the abdomen (instead of just below the costal margin, where the liver edge normally is located). Thus an enlarged liver is a common sign of cardiac dysfunction.

"FUNCTIONAL RESERVE" IN THE LIVER

The liver is essential to life, but metabolic and synthetic demands of the body can be met even when as much as 70% of it is removed or nonfunctional. This property also explains why eventually fatal diseases (such as cirrhosis) may progress to a point of near-total liver destruction before producing symptoms or signs in the patient.

THE LIVER AND METASTATIC CANCER

Because the liver takes part in the hepatic portal system, blood that has just traversed the gut is delivered directly to the capillary beds of the liver. Thus the liver is a very frequent locus for metastasis (Gr., a shifting or a departure) of cancer originating in the GI tract.

---

plies many substances to the liver for metabolic processing. The passage of blood from one capillary bed through a second capillary bed before its return by systemic veins to the heart is the defining feature of a *portal system*. In clinical medicine, the hepatic portal system is the most significant of the portal systems in the body.

THE GALLBLADDER AND BILIARY TREE

The **biliary tree** is a multiply branched network of passages that originate in the liver parenchyma and converge ultimately on the bile duct, draining bile from the liver to the duodenum (see Figure 5-24). Those biliary passages within the liver are said to be *intrahepatic;*

those outside the liver are *extrahepatic*. Intrahepatic and extrahepatic biliary obstruction are different physiologically and require different diagnostic/therapeutic approaches.

The **gallbladder** serves as a storage and concentrating reservoir for bile produced within the liver. Through its cystic duct, the gallbladder can (1) receive bile from the hepatic ducts or (2) deliver bile back into the hepatic duct and on into the duodenum (see Figure 5-24). Bile is released into the duodenum when appropriate hormones are released from the duodenum in response to ingestion of food. Bile also is released upon accumulation of too much bile in the gallbladder (generally about 100 ml or more).

The gallbladder is a saclike organ divided into a *fundus*, a *body*, and a *neck*. The *infundibulum* connects the body and the neck. The position of the gallbladder varies with its fullness. Its fundus may extend well down into the pelvis in some individuals. The gallblad-

der, in its bed on the inferior surface of the liver, forms one of the landmarks defining the porta hepatis. It lies in a groove on the right side of the liver, separating the right lobe from the quadrate lobe.

The Cystic Duct

The **cystic duct** is 4 to 5 cm long and connects the gallbladder to the common hepatic duct (see Figure 5-24). The junction of the cystic and hepatic ducts usually occurs near the porta hepatis but may occur more inferiorly, nearer to the duodenum. The mucosa of the cystic duct is thrown into a series of crescentic folds, which form a *spiral valve* (of Heister), believed to open and close in response to hormonal stimuli connected with digestion (i.e., the ingestion of food into the duodenum stimulates the release of hormones, which relax the spiral valve of Heister).

CLINICAL ANATOMY OF

THE GALLBLADDER

ROLE OF THE GALLBLADDER

The gallbladder is not a vital organ and may be removed surgically, with only mild changes in dietary practices necessary for good postoperative functioning (e.g., avoidance of high-fat, large meals).

GALLSTONES

Stones may form in the gallbladder and obstruct the normal flow of bile, leading to enlargement of the gallblader and inflammation. These stones may be made of bilirubin metabolites, cholesterol, or various calcium salts. They frequently obstruct the gallbladder, leading to bile retention and the risk of rupture into the peritoneal cavity. This can lead to peritonitis.

DILATION OF THE GALLBLADDER

Hartmann's pouch is the abnormal dilation of the usually narrow portion of the gallbladder connecting the body to the neck (infundibulum). It may obstruct nearby structures.

GALLBLADDER INFLAMMATION

Cholecystitis is inflammation of the gallbladder; cholecystostomy is placement of an external drain from the gallbladder to the gut or the exterior of the body to prevent recurrent build-up of bile; cholecystectomy is removal of the gallbladder. Remember the variants in the association of the cystic artery and right hepatic duct. A surgeon must be careful, while

ligating the cystic artery as part of a cholecystectomy, not to ligate the hepatic duct as well.

CHOLECYSTECTOMY

If most of the gallbladder must be removed, it is possible to connect the remaining "stump" to the duodenum, ensuring some bile flow to the intestine (although the flow will be continuous, not coordinated with the ingestion of food).

DIAGNOSTIC IMAGING OF THE GALLBLADDER

Ultrasound imaging has become the method of choice for examining the gallbladder. A CT scan of the abdomen also will provide valuable information noninvasively. If a patient swallows a liquid containing radiopaque materials that are extracted from the bloodstream by the liver and concentrated in the bile, an x-ray taken some time later will show the position of the gallbladder because the gallbladder will be filled with the radiopaque material. More directly, a catheter tip may be inserted into the greater papilla and dye can be injected, which will highlight the biliary tree on subsequent x-ray. Placement of this catheter tip may be performed directly, as during surgery, or through use of an endoscope (a flexible hollow tube passed down the esophagus and into the duodenum, with the patient moderately sedated).

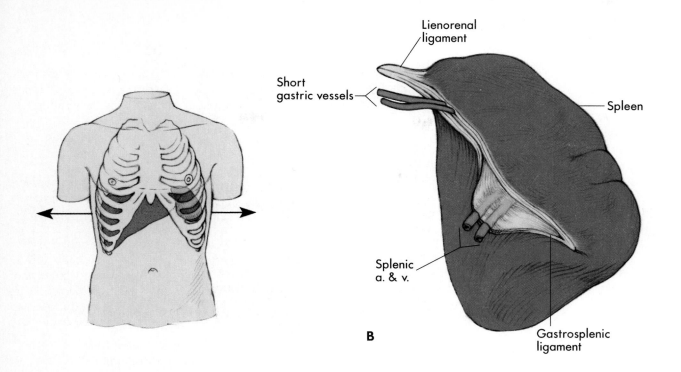

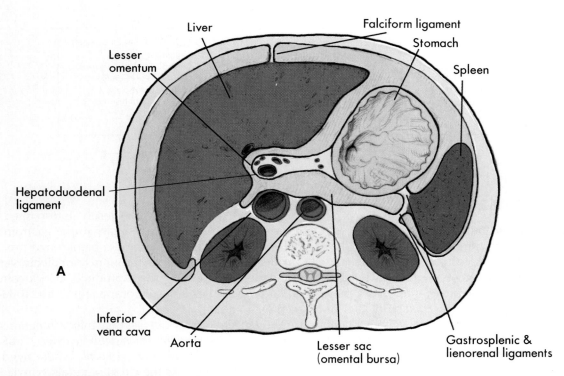

Figure 5-25   THE SPLEEN. A, Cross-section is displayed as though we were looking upward, from the feet, toward a body lying on its back (supine). The lesser omentum is seen here as a bilayered membrane extending medially from the lesser curvature of the stomach. Its right-side free margin, called the hepatoduodenal ligament, contains the portal vein, hepatic arteries, and bile ducts. Just to the right of the hepatoduodenal ligament is the entrance to the lesser sac or omental bursa. From the left side of the stomach a double layer of peritoneum extends backward to attach to the posterior wall in the vicinity of the left kidney. The spleen develops within these two leaflets and grows so large that it dwarfs the enclosing peritoneal covering. The gastrosplenic and lienorenal ligaments make it impossible to pass out of the lesser sac around the left side of the stomach. **B,** The lienorenal and gastrosplenic ligaments, containing the branches of the splenic artery and short gastric arteries, respectively.   Sᴇᴇ **ATLAS, Fɪɢs. 5-3, 5-46, 5-55, 5-56**

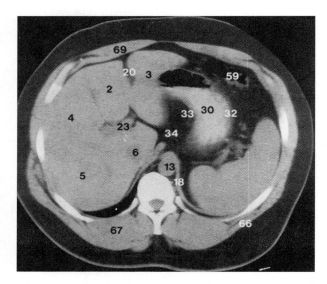

Figure 5-26   ABDOMINAL CT SCAN, L1 LEVEL. The crura of the diaphragm label this section as the L1 level of the abdominal wall. Note the individual muscles discernible within the abdominal wall. (From Weir J, Abrahams PH: *An imaging atlas of human anatomy,* London, 1992, Mosby)   SEE ATLAS, FIG. 5-3

2 Medial segment of left lobe ⎫ **3** Lateral segment of left lobe ⎪ **4** Anterior segment of right ⎬ Liver 　 lobe ⎪ **5** Posterior segment of right ⎭ 　 lobe **6** Inferior vena cava **13** Aorta	**18** Left crus of diaphragm **20** Fissure for ligamentum veno- 　 sum **23** Portal vein **30** Body of stomach **32** Greater curvature of stom- 　 ach	**33** Lesser curvature of stomach **34** Left gastric artery **59** Left colic (splenic) flexure **66** Latissimus dorsi muscle **67** Erector spinae muscle **69** Rectus abdominis muscle

Blood Supply to the Gallbladder

The blood supply to the gallbladder is by the **cystic artery,** normally a branch of the right hepatic artery (in about 70% of cases). In the majority of individuals, the cystic artery passes posterior to the common hepatic and cystic ducts. In others, however, the vessel may arise from the common hepatic artery (about 25% of cases), or even the gastroduodenal artery (about 2% of cases), and may lie anterior to the cystic and common hepatic ducts. Knowledge of these variations is obviously important to the surgeon removing a gallbladder (*cholecystectomy*) and wanting to avoid "accidental" hemorrhage from an artery lacerated because variations in its position were not recognized and understood.

THE SPLEEN

The **spleen** has a firm connective tissue capsule and complex inner trabeculae traversing the interior of the organ. Abundant lymphocytes, macrophages, fibroblasts, and complex vascular networks are found in the organ's interior. Although the blood supply of the spleen and the GI tract are closely intertwined, the spleen does not relate functionally to the gastrointestinal tract, except that hemoglobin breakdown products are delivered to the liver through the splenic venous circulation. In the liver, these products are gluconurated and excreted as a major component of bile (bile pigments).

The spleen carries out several major functions: (1) *phagocytosis of foreign materials,* carried out by macrophages; (2) *erythrocyte removal,* where aged red cells are removed from the circulation (also carried out by macrophages); (3) *immune responses,* involving both T- and B-cell functions; (4) *hematopoiesis,* transiently occurring in the spleen of the fetus but not in postnatal life; and (5) *storage of erythrocytes and platelets,* both of which can be rapidly released into the circulation in cases of hemorrhage or coagulopathy (a kind of "autotransfusion"). Enlarged spleens, however, may sequester too many red cells and/or platelets, and removal of the spleen may be necessary to allow the patient to have normal amounts of circulating red cells and platelets.

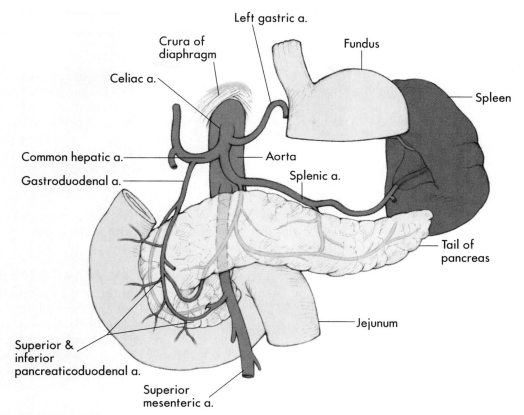

Figure 5-27 BLOOD SUPPLY TO THE PANCREAS, DUODENUM, AND SPLEEN, ANTERI-OR VIEW. Most of the body and pyloric antrum regions of the stomach have been removed to allow direct view of the underlying pancreas and aorta. The three branches of the celiac artery have distinct and important targets. The *common hepatic artery* supplies most of the arterial blood to the liver and gives off the important *gastroduodenal artery,* supplying much of the head of the pancreas and the duodenum. The *splenic artery* provides important arterial supply to the pancreas, spleen, and the greater curvature of the stomach. SEE ATLAS, FIGS. 5-54, 5-58, 5-62, 5-63

The spleen is not a vital organ and may be removed surgically in cases of trauma-induced hemorrhage, diseases that involve excessive red cell destruction in the spleen, and malignancies. Splenic injury is a frequent source of hemorrhage in abdominal or thoracic trauma. In development, the spleen is multilobed, and in most adult specimens, there is some suggestion of this (usually a serrated anterior edge).

Relations and Position of the Spleen

The shape of the spleen is variable, but in general it is a thickened disk, slightly curved, with a convex surface facing the diaphragm and a concave surface facing the fundus of the stomach. This concave surface is the *splenic hilum,* where vessels, nerves, and lymphatics enter and leave the spleen (Figure 5-25). The left *costodiaphragmatic recess* is interposed between the spleen and the lower ribs on the left side.

The spleen lies in the posterosuperior area of the left side of the abdomen, under cover of the left ninth, tenth, and eleventh ribs (Figure 5-26), and is not palpable unless it is enlarged. Its concave surface faces the stomach. The left kidney lies posterior to it, and the tail of the pancreas, within the lienorenal ligament, approaches and often contacts the splenic hilum.

Ligaments and Mesenteries of the Spleen

The spleen lies within the two leaflets of the dorsal mesentery. The double fold of peritoneum enclosing the spleen and extending to the posterior wall is the **lienorenal** (L. *lien,* spleen) **ligament,** so named because the point at which it originates from the posterior wall is over the left kidney (see Figure 5-25). This double fold encloses the spleen and then continues anteriorly to the greater curvature of the stomach as the **gastro-splenic ligament.** The splenic artery reaches the

THE SPLEEN

THE SPLEEN AND RIB FRACTURE

Although protected by the ribs, the spleen is frequently injured in trauma. In many cases, the force applied to the ribcage pushes the ribs inward, and they lacerate the spleen.

SURGICAL APPROACH FOR SPLENECTOMY

Surgical approach to the spleen may be anterior or posterior and involves careful ligation of the splenic branches of the splenic artery and the short gastric vessels.

Diagnostic imaging studies of the spleen include the splenoportogram, where dye is injected directly into the spleen and its subsequent uptake and circulation through splenic veins to the portal vein are viewed by x-ray.

CONSEQUENCES OF BEING WITHOUT A SPLEEN

Patients with sickle cell anemia usually have destroyed their own spleens by the time they are 4 to 5 years old because of repeated sickling of red cells in the splenic capillaries and subsequent infarction of the spleen. These patients, or any patient who has lost his/her spleen for any reason, has heightened vulnerability to infection, particularly from encapsulated bacteria (which are phagocytosed in the spleen). Prophylactic antibiotics are usually recommended for such patients whenever they have dental work or any other minor or major surgery.

ACCESSORY SPLEENS

There is (are) often one or more splenunculi or accessory spleen(s) within the gastrosplenic ligament (see later discussion).

ABDOMINAL SYMMETRY AND THE SPLEEN

When there are errors in the symmetry of abdominal-thoracic development, there may be an absence of the normal "left" side of the abdomen (in which cases no spleen is present); alternatively, there may be "left-sided" anatomy on *both* sides of the abdomen, with anatomic left lobes of the liver on both right and left. In such cases, there may be spleens on both the right and left sides of the abdomen, or even multiple spleens scattered across the upper abdominal cavity.

---

spleen by traveling through the lienorenal ligament; the short gastric and left gastroepiploic arteries travel in the gastrosplenic ligament (see next section).

Blood Supply of the Spleen

The spleen lies within the two leaflets of the dorsal mesentery and receives its blood supply from the **splenic artery,** a branch of the celiac artery (Figure 5-27; see also Figure 5-34). The tortuous splenic artery is embedded in the upper half of the pancreas, which it also supplies. It then reaches the splenic hilum by traveling in the lienorenal ligament. The splenic artery also supplies the stomach through the **short gastric arteries**. The **left gastroepiploic artery**, a branch of the splenic, reaches the greater omentum by traveling through the gastrosplenic ligament. This vessel supplies the greater omentum and much of the stomach tissue along its greater curvature.

The **splenic vein,** in contrast to the splenic artery, is rather straight. Like the splenic artery, it lies in the lienorenal ligament. It travels posterior to the pancreas and meets the superior mesenteric vein behind the head of the pancreas. The two unite to form the *portal vein* (see Figure 5-21).

THE PANCREAS

The **pancreas** is an exocrine gland insofar as it secretes substances into the lumen of the GI tract and an endocrine gland because of its production of insulin, glucagon, VIP, and other substances released into the bloodstream. Clusters of cells, the **pancreatic islets**, secrete the endocrine hormones (see p. 498).

The pancreas (Figure 5-28) is an elongated organ, 13 to 16 cm in length. It is draped over the vertebral column at the L1 vertebral level, approximately at the *transpyloric plane* (a horizontal line drawn through the pylorus at approximately L1-L2, Figure 5-29). The pancreas consists of several parts, shown in Table 5-5.

Developmental Anatomy of the Pancreas

The pancreas develops as two buds (dorsal and ventral) growing out of the second part of the duodenum. Each of these two originally has its own duct, emptying into the duodenum at separate points on the interior of the second part of the duodenum. The *greater (or major) duodenal papilla* represents the entrance of the ventral pancreatic bud duct and the *lesser duodenal papilla* that of the dorsal pancreatic bud duct.

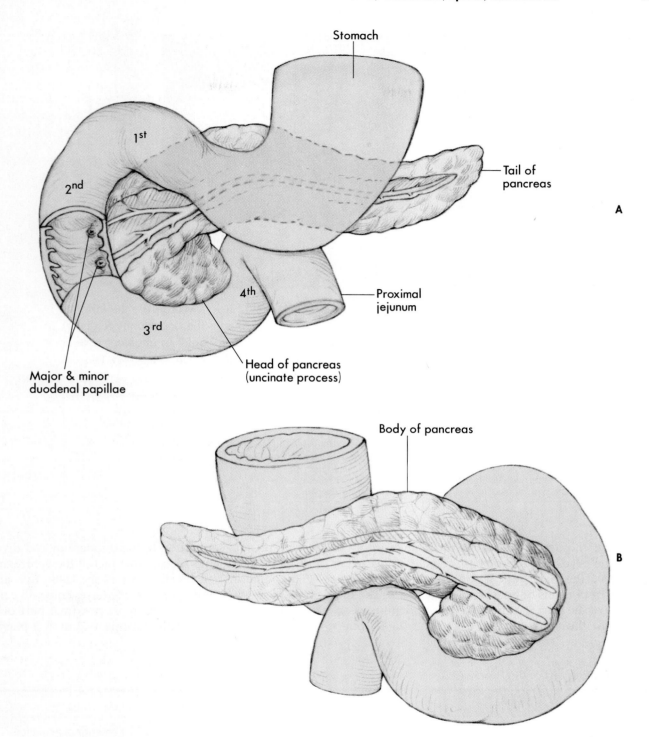

Figure 5-28 THE PANCREAS AND PANCREATIC DUCTS. Anterior (**A**) and posterior (**B**) view. The main pancreatic duct runs along the long axis of the pancreas, from left to right. Entering the head of the pancreas, the single duct divides into two, although the degree to which the upper duct (the accessory duct) is present varies a great deal. The lower of the two ducts is the *major pancreatic duct* and is consistently present. It ends by emptying into the second part of the duodenum and in so doing forming the major duodenal papilla. When an *accessory duct* is present, it empties via a minor duodenal papilla, usually about 2 to 4 cm proximal to the major papilla.   **SEE ATLAS, FIGS. 5-64, 5-65**

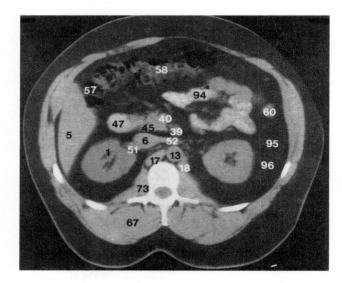

Figure 5-29   ABDOMINAL CT SCAN, L2 LEVEL. At the L2 level, we can see the kidneys and the body of the pancreas. A CT scan in this region provides the opportunity to detect small abnormalities within the posterior abdominal wall that would go undetected on a conventional x-ray. (From Weir J, Abrahams PH: *An imaging atlas of human anatomy,* London, 1992, Mosby.)   SEE ATLAS, FIG. 5-3

1 Right kidney	**40** Superior mesenteric vein	**60** Descending colon
5 Posterior segment of right lobe	**45** Uncinate process of head of pancreas	**67** Erector spinae muscle
6 Inferior vena cava	**47** Second part of duodenum	**73** Psoas major muscle
13 Aorta	**51** Right renal vein	**94** Ileum
17 Right crus of diaphragm	**52** Left renal vein	**95** Renal fascia
18 Left crus of diaphragm	**57** Right colis (hepatic) flexure	**96** Perirenal fat
39 Superior mesenteric artery	**58** Transverse colon	

The *ventral bud* gives rise to the uncinate process and part of the head of the pancreas. The *dorsal bud* forms the rest of the pancreas. The adult pancreatic duct forms from portions of both embryonic ducts. The first 2 to 3 cm of the duct (i.e., nearest the duodenum) is derived from the ventral bud's duct. The dorsal bud's duct loses its connection to the duodenum and diverts itself so that it empties into the duct of the ventral bud. This "hybrid" pancreatic duct is the definitive adult *pancreatic duct,* or *duct of Wirsung* (a seventeenth century German anatomist). The most proximal part of the dorsal bud's duct usually disappears, but, if it persists,

Table 5-5   Regions of the Pancreas

Region	Relations and Characteristic Features
Head	Sits within the curvature of the duodenum; portal vein forms posterior to head. The anterior pancreatico-duodenal vessels are anterior to the head, and the posterior pancreaticoduodenal vessels posterior to it.
Uncinate process	An inferior "tongue" of the head of the pancreas. It sweeps from right to left posterior to the superior mesenteric vessels.
Neck	Connects head and body; superior mesenteric vein is posterolateral to it, while gastroduodenal artery is anterior to it.
Body	In a retroperitoneal position, extending toward left upper quadrant. The aorta, superior mesenteric vessels, left crus of diaphragm, and upper pole of left kidney are posterior to it; forms posterior wall of lesser sac, which is just anterior to it.
Tail	Contained within leaflets of the lienorenal ligament and comes very near to hilum of spleen. Only part of pancreas that is intraperitoneal. Greatest density of islet cells, producing insulin and other hormones, is found in the pancreatic tail.

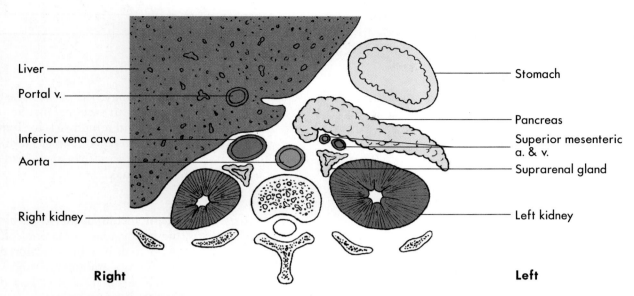

Liver
Portal v.
Inferior vena cava
Aorta
Right kidney

Stomach
Pancreas
Superior mesenteric a. & v.
Suprarenal gland
Left kidney

Right

Left

Figure 5-30 RELATIONSHIPS OF THE PANCREAS. This cross-section through the abdominal cavity at the level of the body of the pancreas is shown from the same vantage as a CT scan—that is, as though we are at the feet of the patient, who is lying on his back (supine). The patient's right and left are indicated. The two kidneys are not the same size because the left kidney lies somewhat more superior on the posterior abdominal wall than the right kidney, so only the upper pole of the right kidney is in the section while the midportion of the left kidney is in the section. The medial portion of the left suprarenal gland is also in view. The aorta lies almost directly anterior to the vertebral column, while the inferior vena cava lies to the right side of the vertebral column. The splenic artery and vein lie just posterior to the pancreas. The liver occupies much of the anterior part of the right side of the section.

it also may be patent and is known as the *accessory pancreatic duct* or *duct of Santorini* (a seventeenth century Italian anatomist). When an accessory pancreatic duct is present, its entry into the duodenum is marked by a *minor papilla*, some distance proximal to the entrance of the main pancreatic duct at the *major papilla*.

The **main pancreatic duct** (see Figure 5-28) normally unites with the common bile duct just outside or even within the duodenal wall. As a result, the secretions of both are deposited into the duodenum through the *ampulla of Vater* (hepatopancreatic ampulla). The ampulla has in its walls a prominent smooth muscle *sphincter of Oddi*.

The pancreas is originally a peritonealized organ (in the dorsal mesentery), but with the rotation of the stomach the pancreas "falls" against the posterior wall and becomes secondarily retroperitoneal (except for a small part of the tail remaining within the leaflets of the lienorenal ligament).

Blood Supply of the Pancreas

Pancreatic blood supply is via the **short gastric arteries** (for the pancreatic tail), the **splenic artery** (embed-

ded in the pancreas and supplying the body), and also the **superior and inferior pancreaticoduodenal arteries** (supplying the head, neck, and body) (Figure 5-34). The superior pancreaticoduodenal arteries are branches of the gastroduodenal artery, and the inferior pancreati-

Table 5-6 Endocrine Cells of the Pancreas

Cell Type	Substance(s) Secreted	Location of Cells
A(α_2)	Glucagon	More peripheral in islets
B(β)	Insulin	More central in islets
D(α_1)	Somatostatin, gastrin	More peripheral in islets; may inhibit glucagon release in adjacent cells
PP	Pancreatic polypeptide	In islets and through pancreatic tissue generally
D-1	VIP-like substance	In islets and through pancreatic tissue generally

CLINICAL ANATOMY OF

THE PANCREAS

PANCREATIC EXOCRINE SECRETIONS

Pancreatic secretions are very important in digestion. The solution produced contains various lytic enzymes, including lipases, trypsin, and amylase. Pancreatic fluid also contains large amounts of bicarbonate. When the pancreatic secretions reach the duodenum, they help neutralize the acid that was added upon passage through the stomach. Conveniently enough, the three groups of enzymes mentioned have maximum activity at a pH of 6.5 to 8.0.

PANCREATIC INNERVATION

Innervation probably plays a limited role in the digestive process. Vagus nerve stimulation causes an increase in exocrine secretions; sympathetic input increases the tone of muscle cells on the necks of secretory units and inhibits release of excretory secretions.

PANCREATIC STONES

The passage of stones through the biliary tree to the ampulla of Vater may ultimately occlude the pancreatic ducts also, producing the risk of autodigestion of pancreatic tissue by its own powerful enzymes.

THE PANCREAS AND SPLENECTOMY

The presence of the pancreatic tail in the pedicle of the spleen (the lienorenal ligament) makes possible injury of the pancreas during splenectomy.

PANCREATIC NEOPLASMS

Pancreatic endocrine cells may become neoplastic. If β-cells are involved, there is an excess of insulin (referred to as an insulinoma) and a high risk for hypoglycemia. If non-β-cells are involved, excess stimulation of acid-producing cells by gastrin may lead to gastric ulceration (glucagonoma).

DIABETES MELLITUS

Inadequate secretion of insulin leads to diabetes mellitus (L. *mellitus*, the honeystone, a material often found in association with coal; it is honey-colored—hence the reference to the large amounts of sugar in the urine of untreated diabetics). "Diabetes" (Gr. *diabetes*, a siphon) refers to the excessive urination found in this condition. Indeed, diabetes insipidus, a disorder resulting from pituitary injury, leads to massive urination but is unrelated to sugar metabolism.

ANNULAR PANCREAS

The annular pancreas is among the most common congenital pancreatic abnormalities. In this entity, the migration of the dorsal and ventral pancreatic ducts is abnormal, and the result is an obstructive "ring" of pancreatic tissue around the duodenum.

coduodenal arteries are branches of the superior mesenteric artery.

The *superior mesenteric* artery, after leaving the aorta at about L1, emerges between the pancreas and duodenum (see Figures 5-17, 5-27, and 5-30). Its inferior pancreaticoduodenal branch meets the superior pancreaticoduodenal branch of the gastroduodenal artery to supply most of the head and body of the pancreas. The superior mesenteric vessels normally lie anterior to the third part of the duodenum and posterior to the body of the pancreas.

The Endocrine Pancreas

The **islets of Langerhans** are clusters of endocrine cells scattered throughout the pancreas but especially in the tail. There are also scattered isolated endocrine cells found throughout the pancreas. Their characteristics are shown in Table 5-6. Small intestinal hormones, especially secretin and cholecystikinin, increase pancreatic exocrine secretions.

5.5

Esophagus, Stomach, and Lesser Sac

▶ The Esophagus

▶ The Stomach

▶ Formation of the Lesser Sac (Omental Bursa)

*T*he stomach's role in digestion is one of physical movement and churning, plus the release of powerful lytic enzymes and hydrochloric acid. It can expand to accommodate as much as 2 L of fluid. Delicate mechanisms protect the stomach from the cytolytic effects of its own acid and enzymatic secretions. Clinically, any irritation of intestinal lining resulting from excess gastric acidity is a *"peptic" ulcer*—whether it is in the stomach, duodenum, or esophagus.

THE ESOPHAGUS

The **esophagus** is a muscular cylinder consisting of an inner circular and outer longitudinal layer of muscle. The esophagus passes through a muscular sling in the diaphragm, positioned at vertebral level T10. It then turns to the left and enters the stomach at the *gastroesophageal junction* (where the *cardiac sphincter* is located) (see Figures 5-17 and 5-31). About 2 to 3 cm of esophagus is normally below the diaphragm.

The **cardiac sphincter** is a physiologic (but not a true anatomic) sphincter. That is, sphincteric function is demonstrable here, but no specialized muscular structure corresponding to it can be found. The "sphincter" effect is probably produced by a combination of (1) the esophageal musculature, (2) the diaphragmatic muscular sling, and (3) the angle at which the esophagus meets the stomach.

The upper third of the esophagus is largely *striated muscle,* the middle third is a *mixture,* and the lower third of the esophagus is nearly all *smooth muscle.* It has an *autonomic plexus,* in which sympathetic and parasympathetic axons take part. The walls of the esophagus also contain ganglion cells, especially in the lower third. The *vagus nerves* travel through the thorax into the abdomen as a plexus on the esophagus, on their way to the ab-

PRINCIPLES

The abdominal portions of the intestinal tract are considerably different from each other (stomach, duodenum, colon, etc), but there is a *common structural plan* which they all share. The *mucosa* lining the intestinal tract is modified in each area to reflect the functions carried out there. Endodermally derived epithelial cells line the gut and are important for selective absorption of ingested materials. Just external to the mucosa is loose connective tissue, the *submucosa,* containing lymphoid tissue and thin layers of smooth muscle. External to the submucosa is an inner circular and outer longitudinal layer of *smooth muscle* although they are not completely represented in all areas of the intestine. External to these muscle layers is the peritoneal covering known as the *serosa* (see Figure 5-41).

499

domen. As the stomach rotates, the left vagus becomes anterior and the right vagus posterior.

Throughout most of its course, the esophagus lacks a peritoneal covering, which, unfortunately, makes it easy for esophageal malignancies to spread into the adjacent mediastinal tissue. Complete surgical removal is often difficult or impossible.

Vascular Supply of the Esophagus

Arterial supply to the esophagus arises in the *inferior thyroid artery* (approximately the upper 15% to 20% of the esophagus), direct *aortic branches* and collaterals of the *bronchial arteries* (approximately the middle 70%), and branches of the *inferior phrenic* and *left gastric arteries* (approximately the lower 10% to 15%). **Venous drainage** is by the *inferior thyroid, azygos/hemiazygos ve-*

nous system, and the inferiormost part into the *left gastric vein.* This last connection is enlarged when a patient has portal hypertension, in which blood from the portal vein shunts through this connection to drain through esophageal veins to the IVC. The result is enlargement of the esophageal veins (*varices*), which are prone to serious and sometimes fatal hemorrhage into the lumen of the esophagus.

Nerve Supply of the Esophagus

The esophagus receives both sympathetic and parasympathetic (vagal) neural input. There are neural ganglion cells in the wall of the esophagus, especially in its lower third. Even though it is partially striated and partly smooth muscle, the esophagus must be capable of coordinated contractions (*peristalsis*).

CLINICAL ANATOMY OF

THE ESOPHAGUS

HIATUS HERNIA

When portions of the stomach protrude through the esophageal hiatus into the thorax, it is termed a hiatus hernia. The most common variety has the gastroesophageal junction itself herniated upward into the thorax, along with a part of the stomach (a "sliding" hernia); more rarely, the gastroesophageal junction remains in the abdomen, but a portion of adjacent stomach passes upward through the esophageal hiatus into the thorax ("paraesophageal hernia"). Sliding hernias outnumber the paraesophageal types 10:1; however, when hiatus hernias occur in women, the paraesophageal type is more common. Hiatus hernia can mimic the substernal pain of a myocardial infarction (MI or "heart attack"); an important difference is that pain of hiatus hernia is usually lessened by sitting up from a supine position, that of MI, however, is not.

GASTROESOPHAGEAL REFLUX

The esophageal mucosa may be irritated by excess reflux of gastric acid through an incompetent gastroesophageal sphincter. When this occurs chronically, the mucosa of the lower esophagus changes from its normal stratified squamous to columnar—an example of metaplasia.

ESOPHAGEAL VARICES

The small veins of the lower esophagus may become grossly enlarged (esophageal varices) in portal hypertension, when portal blood is under high pressure and is shunted through collateral routes of flow like the esophageal veins. They then may rupture with cough or other stress and hemorrhage profusely.

ACHALASIA

Achalasia (Gr. *akalasos*, relaxation) results from dysmotility (abnormal contractions) at the lower end of the esophagus. The affected part of the esophagus cannot participate in peristalsis. In time, the esophagus above this level hypertrophies and dilates. Patients with this condition demonstrate recurrent vomiting and, in time, even malnutrition. The intrinsic neurons in the affected part of the esophagus usually are absent, but it is unclear whether this is the cause or an effect of achalasia.

ESOPHAGEAL WEBS

Partial obstructions of the lumen of the esophagus by bands or webs of tissue also will produce difficulty swallowing (dysphagia) and/or vomiting. They may be dilated with a metal instrument or by inflation of a balloon placed within the narrowed segment, or they may need surgery.

THE STOMACH

The **stomach** functions as a chamber in which chemical and mechanical disruption of ingested foods takes place. Its position is quite variable, depending on how full it is. An adult stomach may hold 1200 to 2000 ml. The stomach consists of a *fundus* (the portion above the level of the gastroesophageal junction), a *cardia* (in the region of the junction), a *body,* and a *pylorus* (Gr. *pyloros,* gatekeeper), including an antrum, canal, and sphincter (Figure 5-31). Important external features of the stomach include the *greater curvature, lesser curvature, cardiac incisure,* and *angular incisure.* The characteristic internal foldings of the gastric mucosa are known as *rugae.* In the region of the pyloric antrum, the rugae are aligned and arranged parallel to the long axis of the stomach (see Figure 5-31). Much of the stomach is mobile, suspended in peritoneal sheaths. The anterior surface of the stomach is related to various components of the anterior abdominal wall. The posterior surface faces the lumen of the lesser sac. The right-hand margin (the lesser curvature), is attached to the two layers of the lesser omentum; the left-hand margin (the greater curvature) is attached to the greater omentum. The pylorus, however, is generally anchored to the posterior abdominal wall in the midline at the L1 to L2 vertebral level (Figure 5-32).

The Pyloric Sphincter and Pyloric Antrum

The **pyloric sphincter** is a circular thickened mass of muscle surrounding the area of transition from stomach to duodenum (see Figure 5-31). There is a large *pyloric vein,* visible in virtually all patients at surgery, that serves the surgeon as a marker of the exact location of the pylorus.

The **pyloric antrum** is a 5 to 6 cm long area of the stomach located just proximal to the pylorus. Externally, the proximal limit of the pyloric antrum is indicated by a shallow notch in the lesser curvature, the *angular incisure* (see Figure 5-31). The antrum is known chiefly as the location for most of the gastrin-producing cells (G-cells) of the gastric mucosa. On occasion, an antrectomy may be performed to treat severe hyperacidity causing inflammation and ulceration of the stomach mucosa.

Vasculature of the Stomach

Gastric vasculature is derived mainly from the **celiac artery** (Figures 5-33 and 5-34). The *splenic artery,* a branch of the celiac, divides into the *short gastric* and *left gastroepiploic arteries,* supplying some areas along the left side of the greater curvature. By contrast, the *gastroduodenal* and the *right gastroepiploic arteries,* supplying some areas near the pylorus and right side of the greater curvature, are branches of the **hepatic artery.** The *left gastric artery,* supplying the lesser curvature, is a direct branch of the **celiac artery.** The blood supply to the stomach is richly anastomotic. In one series, 60% to 70% of cadavers had a "posterior gastric artery" arising from the splenic artery and supplying the posterior surface along the greater curvature, although this occurrence is not often described.

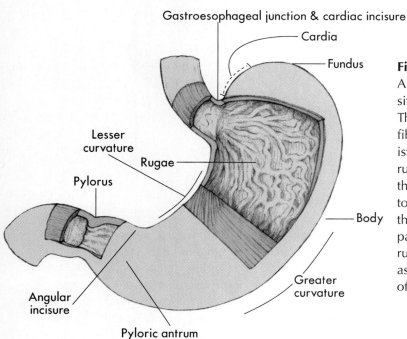

Figure 5-31 THE INTERIOR OF THE STOMACH. Anterior view. The gastroesophageal junction is the site of a physiologically significant sphincter activity. The wall of the body is made up of smooth muscle fibers running in different directions and a characteristic series of raised interior mucosal folds known as rugae. The pyloric valve is a true anatomic sphincter that controls flow of digested food from the stomach to the duodenum and prevents its reflux. Proximal to the pyloric valve, the rugae are linear and nearly parallel, in contrast to the criss-crossing pattern of rugae in the fundus and body. This region is known as the pyloric antrum and contains a preponderance of acid-secreting cells.

Labels on figure:
Gastroesophageal junction & cardiac incisure
Cardia
Fundus
Lesser curvature
Rugae
Pylorus
Body
Greater curvature
Angular incisure
Pyloric antrum

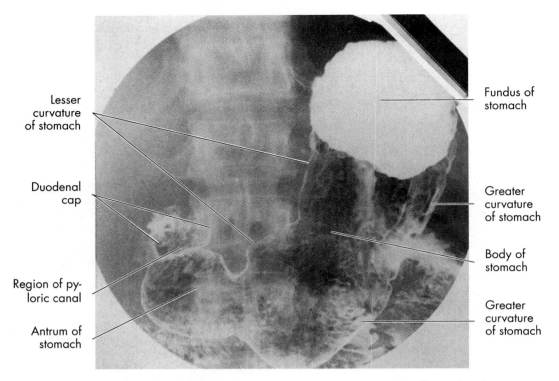

Lesser curvature of stomach

Duodenal cap

Region of py-loric canal

Antrum of stomach

Fundus of stomach

Greater curvature of stomach

Body of stomach

Greater curvature of stomach

Figure 5-32   BARIUM CONTRAST STUDY OF THE STOMACH. Swallowed radioopaque barium coats the walls of the stomach and makes them visible on x-ray. Contrast has accumulated in the fundus of the stomach. (From Weir J, Abrahams PH: *An imaging atlas of human anatomy,* London, 1992, Mosby.)   SEE ATLAS, FIGS. 5-50, 5-51

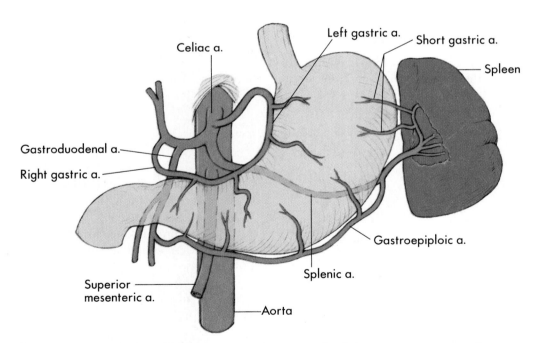

Celiac a.

Left gastric a.

Short gastric a.

Spleen

Gastroduodenal a.

Right gastric a.

Gastroepiploic a.

Splenic a.

Superior mesenteric a.

Aorta

Figure 5-33   BLOOD SUPPLY OF THE STOMACH. The left gastric artery runs between the leaflets of the lesser omentum and gives off several branches along the lesser curvature. Much of the body of the stomach is supplied by the left gastric and the left and right gastroepiploic arteries. The left gastroepiploic artery is a branch of the splenic artery, and the right gastroepiploic a branch of the gastroduodenal artery. The splenic artery itself provides a small number of important branches called short gastric arteries, supplying the upper greater curvature of the stomach by traveling through the gastrosplenic ligament.
SEE ATLAS, FIGS. 5-54, 5-74

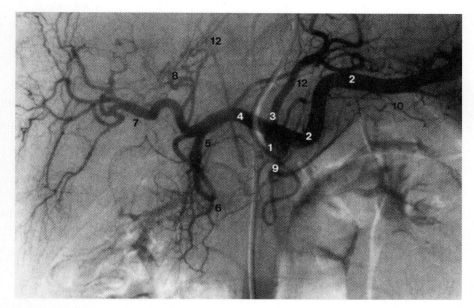

Figure 5-34 CELIAC ARTERIOGRAM. Here a small catheter has been threaded up the aorta so that its tip is positioned in the base of the celiac artery. Dye is then injected, and the x-ray taken. The film has been developed in a reverse fashion, so that the dye-injected vessels appear black. (From Weir J, Abrahams PH: *An imaging atlas of human anatomy,* London, 1992, Mosby.)

1 Tip of catheter in celiac trunk	**5** Gastroduodenal artery	**9** Dorsal pancreatic artery
2 Splenic artery	**6** Superior pancreaticoduodenal artery	**10** Left gastroepiploic artery
3 Left gastric artery	**7** Right hepatic artery	**12** Phrenic artery
4 Common hepatic artery	**8** Left hepatic artery	

Innervation of the Stomach

Sympathetic innervation reaches the stomach as a diffuse plexus on the arteries supplying the stomach. Its major roles are regulation of gastric vascular tone and response to painful stimuli. The two **parasympathetic vagus nerves** travel along the esophagus, and upon reaching the stomach they divide into (1) the *hepatic branches,* (2) the branches that will travel toward the *celiac ganglion* (but *do not synapse* in it) and later distribute to more distal parts of the gut and the pancreas and (3) the *gastric branches,* notable among which are the nerves of Latarjet (Figure 5-35), which distribute branches to the fundus, body, and pyloric region. The main bodies of these nerves of Latarjet, one derived from the left and the other from the right vagal trunk, travel along a course parallel to the lesser curvature. They are called the *anterior and posterior nerves of Latarjet,* however, because the rotation of the stomach has caused left to become anterior and right to become posterior (see later discussion on the nerves of Latarjet).

FORMATION OF THE LESSER SAC (OMENTAL BURSA)

The rotation of the stomach creates a space, known as the **lesser sac** or **omental bursa,** between the stomach and the posterior abdominal wall (Figures 5-36; see also Figure 5-25). This space is bounded anteriorly by the stomach and lesser omentum, superiorly by the liver, inferiorly by the greater omentum (and its fusion to the transverse colon), and to the left by the spleen and its ligaments. On the right, the lesser sac opens into the greater sac through the **epiploic foramen (of Winslow)** (Figure 5-37). The greater sac of the abdomen is all the remaining space within the peritoneal cavity. Table 5-7 further describes the perimeter of the epiploic foramen.

The use of the word "bursa" to describe this space is appropriate because this space allows for movements and changes of shape in the stomach (just as, for example, the deltoid bursa facilitates minimum-friction movements of the deltoid muscle with respect to the shoulder).

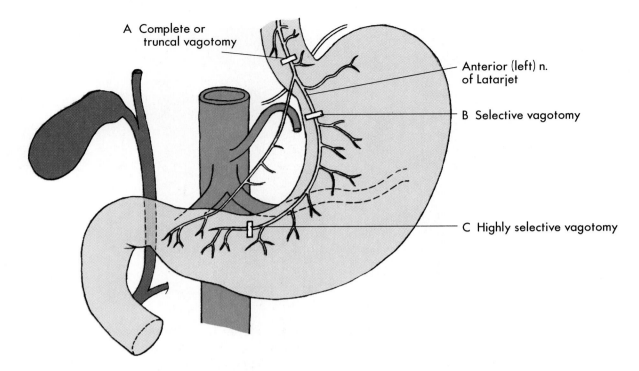

A Complete or
   truncal vagotomy

Anterior (left) n.
of Latarjet

B Selective vagotomy

C Highly selective vagotomy

Figure 5-35   INNERVATION OF THE STOMACH. The anterior of left vagus nerve branches into a nerve of Latarjet along the lesser curvature. A similar branch from the right vagus nerve lies on the posterior side of the stomach. Lesions at positions *A, B,* and *C* are examples of surgical interruptions of the vagus, performed to reduce stomach acidity to treat ulcers.   SEE ATLAS, FIG. 5-113

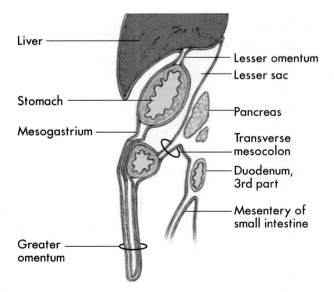

Liver

Lesser omentum
Lesser sac

Stomach

Pancreas

Mesogastrium

Transverse
mesocolon

Duodenum,
3rd part

Mesentery of
small intestine

Greater
omentum

Figure 5-36   THE GREATER OMENTUM. A parasagittal view through the posterior abdominal wall shows the relationships between the posterior wall, various abdominal viscera, and the layers of peritoneum that enclose them.

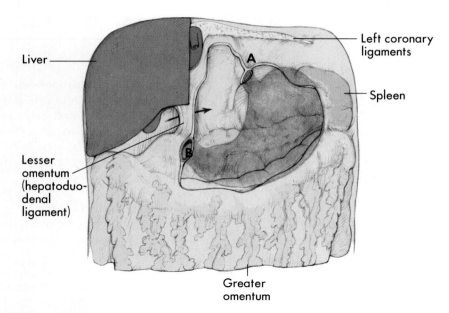

Liver — Left coronary ligaments — A — Spleen — Lesser omentum (hepatoduodenal ligament) — B — Greater omentum

Figure 5-37   THE BED OF THE STOMACH. The stomach has been removed by an incision at the gastroesophageal junction (*A*) and the pyloric sphincter (*B*). Most of the lesser omentum also has been removed, and incisions were made in the gastrosplenic ligament (separating the stomach from the spleen), and in the greater omentum just a centimeter or two distal to the greater curvature of the stomach. The extreme right-hand side of the lesser omentum (the hepatoduodenal ligament) has been left intact, and the *solid arrow* shows the position of the epiploic foramen (of Winslow). Removal of the stomach has revealed the lesser sac or omental bursa. The spleen, attached to the posterior wall by the lienorenal ligament and to the stomach by the gastrosplenic ligament, encloses the lesser sac and forms a cul-de-sac on the left. The sac can be entered only from the right side, through the foramen of Winslow.   Sᴇᴇ ATLAS, Fɪɢs. 5-39, 5-40, 5-47

Table 5-7   Borders of the Epiploic Foramen

Wall of Foramen	Component Structures
Anterior wall	Hepatoduodenal ligament (containing portal vein, common bile duct, proper hepatic artery), enclosed in lesser omentum
Superior wall	Caudate lobe of liver and coronary ligament of liver (right posterior leaflet)
Posterior wall	Pancreas (in inferior portion) and inferior vena cava (covered anteriorly by peritoneum)
Inferior wall	Attachment of transverse mesocolon to posterior wall of stomach; first part of duodenum

Gastric Development and Mesenteries

The stomach, like other parts of the gut, is enclosed in a double layer of peritoneum. The two peritoneal layers reflecting off the greater curvature of the stomach form the *gastrosplenic ligament*. The gastrosplenic ligament moves posteriorly to envelop the spleen in a similar fashion. A double layer of peritoneum reflects off the lesser curvature of the stomach and ascends to envelop the liver. This is the *lesser omentum* (see Figures 5-19 and 5-36).

More inferiorly, the double layer of peritoneum reflecting off the greater curvature evaginates anteriorly, and the resultant layer of peritoneum is known as the *greater omentum*. As this evagination enlarges, its inferior surface becomes attached tightly to the transverse colon. What results is a quadruple layer of peritoneum forming a "drape" over the underlying intestines. It is of variable size but often extends downward well into the pelvis (Figure 5-37; see also Figures 5-20 and 5-36).

THE STOMACH

GASTRIC ULCERS AND THEIR TREATMENT

The stomach is subject to ulceration through the effects of acid. The vagus nerves stimulate the release of acid. Drug therapy may be directed to reducing acid secretion (histamine blockers—cimetidine, ranitidine), or surgical therapy may remove branches of the vagus nerve or parts of the antrum itself (see later discussion).

ABNORMAL EMPTYING OF THE STOMACH

Too rapid emptying of the stomach (referred to picturesquely as the "dumping syndrome") follows many surgeries of the antrum or the vagi.

BLOOD SUPPLY TO THE STOMACH

As always, vascular variations are abundant. The celiac artery, for example, may arise in the thorax, requiring it to descend through the aortic hiatus to reach the stomach. Interruption of the blood supply to the stomach can lead to ischemia and mid-abdominal pain. The pattern of branching in the celiac artery (see Figure 5-34) itself is highly variable, especially in the branching of the common hepatic and gastroduodenal arteries.

SECRETIONS OF THE STOMACH

The stomach manufactures hydrochloric acid (from parietal cells), pepsinogen from chief cells (activated into pepsin in acid conditions—most active in peptide cleavage when pH is about 2.0), intrinsic factor (a substance that attaches to and helps in absorption of dietary vitamin B_{12}) from parietal cells, and mucus (from mucus neck cells, especially in body and fundus), which helps protect the stomach mucosa from autodigestion.

GASTRIC HORMONES

The stomach, like many other parts of the intestine, has populations of hormone-secreting cells. Those producing gastrin (G cells) are found in the pyloric region. Gastrin increases acid production and gastric motility. Other cells in this area produce vasoactive intestinal peptide, somatostatin, and indoleamine derivatives. In the body of the stomach, there are very small numbers of such cells.

SURGERY FOR SEVERE GASTRIC ULCERS

The Bilroth procedures are surgical techniques for treatment of severe ulcers. They involve removing the antrum and performing a vagotomy. The proximal part of the stomach may be reattached to the duodenum (Bilroth I) or to the jejunum (Bilroth II). In a Bilroth II procedure, the proximal duodenal segment is left as an elongated blind pouch (often described as a "Roux-en-Y").

Small Intestine

▶ The Duodenum

▶ The Jejunum and Ileum

▶ Lymphatic Drainage of the Small
Intestine

*T*he small intestine consists of three subsections, the duodenum, jejunum, and ileum (Figures 5-28, 5-38, 5-39). Although only about 25 cm in length, the **duodenum** is surely the "busiest" section of the intestine. It has complex relationships to the pancreas and receives hepatobiliary and pancreatic secretions. Its position in the abdomen is relatively fixed and predictable because most of it is retroperitoneal. Its secretions neutralize the acidity of gastric contents as they leave the stomach and enter the small intestine and allow for the digestive action of several powerful enzymes to take place. Beyond the duodenum, the remainder of the small intestine is specialized for absorption; in the **jejunum** and **ileum,** little further digestive activity occurs, but the mucosa of this part of the small intestine is thrown into folds that increase absorptive surface area.

THE DUODENUM

This segment of the small intestine is named the **duodenum** (L. *duodecim,* twelve) because it is 12 finger-breadths (about 10 inches, or 25 cm) long. Only the first and fourth parts of the duodenum are at least partially intraperitoneal; the rest is retroperitoneal. The duodenum is positioned over the vertebral column at the T12-L1 level and forms a C-shaped loop that is "open" to the left. The C is in reality almost a closed circle, because the fourth part of the duodenum drains into the jejunum at a level only 1 cm inferior to the pyloric sphincter, where the duodenum begins. In the duodenum, acidic stomach fluid is neutralized by mixture with pancreatic secretions. Biliary secretions also enter the intestine in the duodenum (Figure 5-39; see also Figure 5-35).

The lining of most of the duodenum is thrown into a series of semicircular folds, which are rigid and do not disappear if the duodenum is distended. These are known as the *plicae circulares* and are most prominent in the duodenum and jejunum, disappearing in the distal ileum (Figure 5-40). The walls of the duodenum contain (1) mucus-secreting cells and (2) endocrine cells secreting gastrin, VIP, somatostatin, and 5-hydroxytryptamine derivatives.

Structural Divisions of the Duodenum (Table 5-8)

The *first part of the duodenum* is partially retroperitoneal and continues distally past the pylorus. The *second part of the duodenum* is also called the descending part. Into it drain the ducts from both the liver and the pancreas. The *third part of the duodenum* ascends slightly as it passes from right to left. The *fourth part of the duodenum* ascends and lies anterior to L2. Where the duodenum becomes the jejunum, it is suspended from the posterior wall by a specialized peritoneal fold known as the *ligament of Treitz* (a suspensory ligament).

Blood Supply of the Duodenum

Blood supply is from branches (see Figure 5-27) of the *right gastric* or *gastroduodenal arteries* (to the first and second part) and from branches of the *gastroduodenal,*

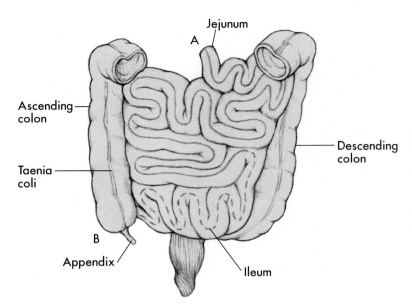

Figure 5-38   THE SMALL INTESTINE. Transverse colon has been removed to allow greater visibility of the small intestine. The part of the small intestine with the *solid line* along its long axis is the jejunum; that with the *dashed line* is the ileum. The jejunum commences at *A,* which is the junction with the duodenum; the ileum ends at *B,* which is the ileocecal junction.

SEE ATLAS, FIGS. 5-40, 5-75

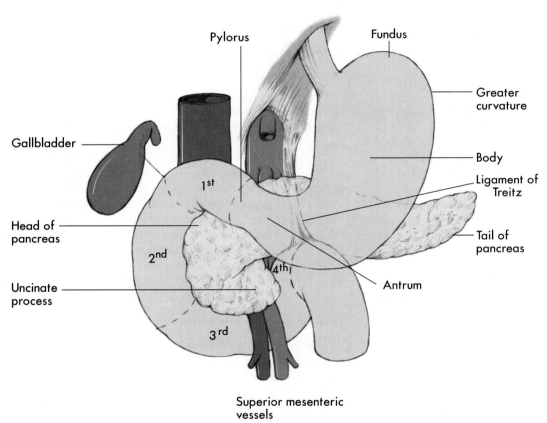

Figure 5-39   THE DUODENUM. The *first part* of the duodenum commences at the pylorus and runs mostly in a horizontal plane. The *second part* of the duodenum is mostly descending and receives the drainage of the pancreas and the biliary system. The *third part* of the duodenum once again is mostly horizontal, running from right to left approximately at vertebral level L3. The *fourth part* of the duodenum ascends and becomes continuous with the jejunum slightly to the left of the midline. Where it does, the retroperitoneal duodenum is continuous with the intraperitoneal jejunum. A thickened sling of peritoneum, the ligament of Treitz, supports the proximal part of the jejunum.

SEE ATLAS, FIGS. 5-58, 5-62, 5-63

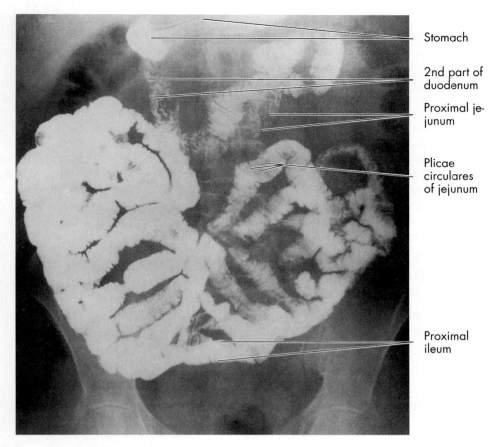

Stomach

2nd part of duodenum

Proximal je-junum

Plicae circulares of jejunum

Proximal ileum

Figure 5-40　THE SMALL INTESTINE, BARIUM STUDY. Dye has been swallowed by the patient, and it has then passed into the small intestine, where the characteristic plicae circulares of the mucosa are highlighted. (From Weir J, Abrahams PH: *An imaging atlas of human anatomy,* London, 1992, Mosby.)

Table 5-8　　Divisions of the Duodenum

Part	Length	To Its Left	To Its Right	Superior to It	Inferior to It	Anterior to It	Posterior to It
First	2.5 cm	Body of pancreas	Right kidney (partial)	Epiploic foramen; lesser omentum	Head of pancreas; free border of greater omentum	Fundus of gallbladder	Gastroduodenal artery; common bile duct
Second	10 cm	Head of pancreas, common bile duct	Right colic flexure, right kidney	Right lobe of liver	Right ureter, psoas major muscle	Transverse colon	Right kidney hilum, right ureter
Third	7 cm	(Runs in horizontal plane)	(Runs in horizontal plane)	Head and uncinate process of pancreas	Inferior mesenteric artery	Superior mesenteric vessels	Inferior vena cava, aorta, L3, hypogastric nerve
Fourth	3 cm	Left kidney, left ureter	Root of mesentery	Body of pancreas	Inferior mesenteric vessels	Transverse colon	Left sympathetic trunk, psoas major, left gonadal vessels

pancreaticoduodenal, and *gastroepiploic arteries* (second, third, and fourth part). **Venous drainage** is to the *superior mesenteric vein* and then to the *portal vein.*

Pathology of the Duodenum

The duodenal mucosa is subject to ulceration and erosion from the gastric acidic fluids (peptic ulceration) or from the powerful enzymes of the pancreatic juices. The duodenum may be externally obstructed by abnormalities of the pancreas, whether congenital (e.g., annular pancreas) or acquired (e.g., carcinoma of pancreatic head). The duodenum may be partially obstructed by webs or be obstructed because of a failure of the normal embryologic process of recanalization to occur.

THE JEJUNUM AND ILEUM

Together the jejunum and ileum are 7 to 10 m in length, while the duodenum is only about 25 cm (see Figure 5-38). Beyond the duodenum, the jejunum is approximately the proximal two fifths of the small intestine, and the ileum the distal three fifths. The **jejunum** (L. *jejunus,* empty or barren) is so named because the emptiness of the jejunum at death was thought by early physicians to be unique to this region of the gut. The **ileum** (Gr. *eileon,* twisted or convoluted) extends from the jejunum to the cecum. The major function of the jejunum and ileum is absorption, and mucosal folds increase the absorptive surface area (Figure 5-41). Table 5-9 shows some characteristics distinguishing the jejunum and ileum. Transition from one region to the other is gradual, however, and there is no clear point of change.

Both the jejunum and ileum are completely peritonealized (suspended by a sling of the Mesentery). The root of the Mesentery runs diagonally from the upper left to the lower right quadrant of the posterior abdominal wall. Within its leaflets pass many branches of the superior mesenteric vessels, lymphatics, and autonomic nerves of the small intestine (see Figure 5-18).

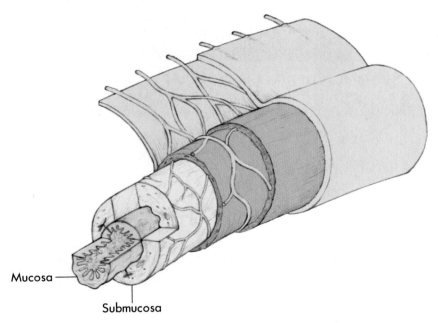

Mucosa

Submucosa

Figure 5-41   LAYERS OF THE INTESTINAL WALL. The lumen is typically thrown into a series of folds, to increase the amount of absorptive surface area. There is a thin layer of muscle just beneath the mucosa. Lymphatic nodules also are found just beneath the mucosa, especially in the ileum. Just external to this is a circular layer of smooth muscle. Just external to the circular smooth muscle is a plexus of nerve cells, axons, and blood vessels. Next is a longitudinal muscle layer, and external to it is yet another collection of neural and vascular elements. These axons represent the "intrinsic" plexus of the gut and are composed of (1) extrinsic branches of the vagus, sacral parasympathetic and sympathetic nerves, and (2) a rich intrinsic plexus of neurons and axons that have a very important role in regulating the contractility of the gut.

Table 5-9 The Jejunum and the Ileum

Feature	Jejunum	Ileum
Diameter	2-4 cm	2-3 cm
Wall	Thicker	Thinner
Vessels	Smaller number of arcades; longer vasa recta; poorer anastomoses	Larger number of arcades; shorter vasa recta; better anastomoses
Amount of fat	Less	More
Plicae	Numerous	Rudimentary
Peyer's patches	Few	Many

The terminal ileum is partially invaginated into the cecum (the **ileocecal valve**), forming a sort of "valve" that prevents reflux, although not with great efficiency (Figure 5-42). As the cecum fills with fecal material, the perimeter surrounding the opening into the ileum is compressed closed, so that filling of the cecum means increasing closure of the entrance back into the terminal ileum.

Vascular Supply of the Jejunum and Ileum

Blood supply to the small intestine is through the jejunal and ileal branches of the *superior mesenteric artery (SMA)*, forming arcades within the mesentery (Figure 5-43; see also Figure 5-17). Anastomotic connections are usually good. The superior mesenteric artery emerges from the aorta at the T12-L1 level. It passes anterior to the left renal vein, then travels forward anterior to the duodenum and posterior to the body of the pancreas. It then enters the mesentery and travels between its leaflets downward in the direction of the right lower quadrant. Branches of the superior mesenteric system anastomose proximally with branches of the celiac system (especially the superior pancreaticoduodenal artery) and distally with branches of the inferior mesenteric artery (especially the left colic artery).

Branches of the superior mesenteric artery (SMA). The first branch of the superior mesenteric artery (Figure 5-44; see also Figures 5-27 and 5-43), the *inferior pancreaticoduodenal artery,* emerges opposite the head of the pancreas and divides into an anterior and posterior branch, passing on either side of the pancreatic head. The *jejunal and ileal arteries* arise as a series of 8 to 12 branches along the left side of the superior mesenteric artery and supply the length of the small intestine by traveling toward it between the two leaflets of the Mesentery proper (see Table 5-9). The *middle colic artery* travels in the transverse mesocolon and anastomoses with the left and right colic arteries to each side of it. The *right colic artery* passes retroperitoneally in front of the psoas and the ureter to distribute to the ascending colon. The *Ileocolic artery* passes retroperitoneally toward the ileocecal junction and gives off anterior and posterior cecal, appendicular, and ileal branches. Anastomotic connections between various branches of the superior mesenteric are good; therefore slowly de-

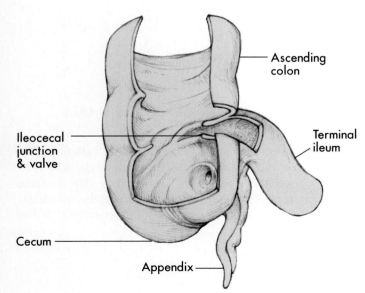

Ascending colon

Ileocecal junction & valve

Terminal ileum

Cecum

Appendix

Figure 5-42 THE ILEOCECAL JUNCTION. A detail of the ileocecal junction is presented. The terminal ileum "telescopes" into the first part of the large intestine (the cecum), so that when feces accumulate in the cecum, the pressure "pinches" the sides of the ileum together. This prevents feces from traveling in a retrograde direction, back into the small intestine. Also evident is the appendix, which is a thin cylindrical diverticulum emptying into the cecum 2 to 3 cm inferior to the ileocecal valve.

SEE ATLAS, FIGS. 5-76, 5-84

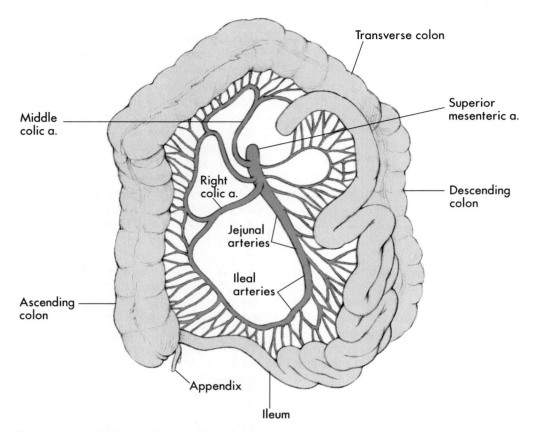

Figure 5-43   THE SUPERIOR MESENTERIC ARTERY. Shown here is that portion of the intestinal tract supplied with arterial blood by the superior mesenteric artery (SMA). The vessel emerges from the aorta at approximately L1 to L2 and gives off initial branches supplying the head of the pancreas (not shown). From its right side, there appear branches for the ileocecal region, the ascending colon (right colic artery), and the transverse colon (middle colic artery). From its left side, there is a variable number of branches for the jejunum and ileum.   SEE ATLAS, FIG. 5-88

veloping occlusions of one or another branch are usually well compensated by the collateral flow.

Distinction is made between the *mesenteric border* of the small bowel (i.e., that surface of the bowel closest to the Mesentery) and the *antimesenteric side* (opposite the Mesentery), which generally has a less good blood supply and may suffer more from ischemic events.

LYMPHATIC DRAINAGE OF THE SMALL INTESTINE

Lymphatic vessels travel within the leaflets of the mesentery and drain into the **cisterna chyli,** which in turn above the diaphragm drains into the **thoracic duct.** Lymph nodes are more abundant in the distal parts of the Mesentery, especially in the vicinity of the ileocecal valve.

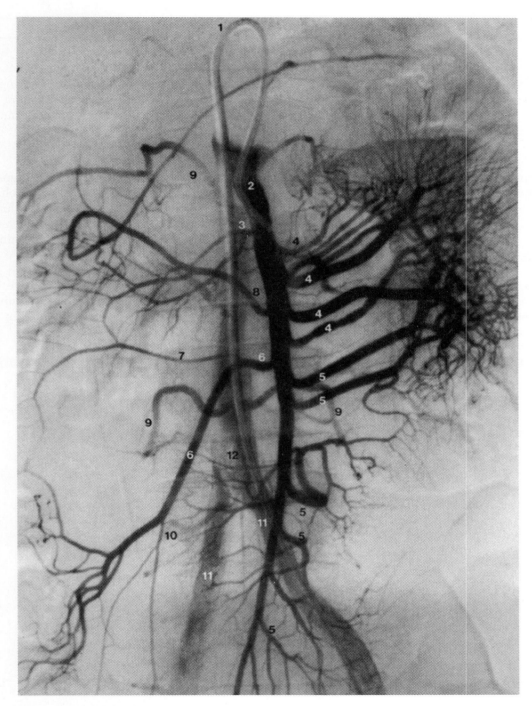

Figure 5-44   SUPERIOR MESENTERIC ARTERIOGRAM. Jejunal and ileal branches arise off the left side of the superior mesenteric artery and appendiceal and colic branches from the right side. (From Weir J, Abrahams PH: *An imaging atlas of human anatomy,* London, 1992, Mosby.)

1 Catheter with tip selectively in superior mesenteric artery	**5** Ileal branches of superior mesenteric artery	**10** Appendicular artery
2 Superior mesenteric artery	**6** Ileocolic artery	**11** Iliac artery
3 Inferior pancreaticoduodenal artery	**7** Right colic artery	**12** Aorta
4 Jejunal branches of superior mesenteric artery	**8** Middle colic artery	
	9 Lumbar arteries arising from abdominal aorta	

THE SMALL INTESTINE

MALROTATION OF THE GUT

If the intestines are malrotated, this implies that the return of the intestinal loops to the intestinal cavity was abnormal. In many cases, such a malrotation will produce no symptoms whatever; however, the chances are increased that an obstructive event will occur. The most common form of malrotation is the failure of the cecum to descend to the right lower quadrant, remaining instead in the right upper quadrant.

INTUSSUSCEPTION AND VOLVULUS

When one section of the small bowel "telescopes" into the adjacent section (intussusception), it can compromise the blood flow and lead to a partial or even complete obstruction of the intestine. Intussusception may also occur between the distal ileum and the colon. When there is an acquired twisting of the intestines around their mesenteric support (volvulus), the blood supply is compromised and the intestine is at risk to become necrotic.

DISEASES OF THE SMALL INTESTINE

There is a very low incidence of malignancy in the small intestine. Regional enteritis or Crohn's disease is one of the more frequent illnesses (abdominal pain, diarrhea, vomiting, weight loss), often requiring removal of large portions of the small intestine.

MESENTERIC ADENITIS

Mesenteric adenitis is a generic term for inflammation of the lymph nodes, which are so abundant in the mesentery of the small intestine. Its pain can mimic that of appendicitis.

5.7

Colon and Anorectal Region

▶ Form and Function of the Colon

▶ Peritoneal Reflections and the Colon

▶ The Cecum and Ascending Colon

▶ The Vermiform Appendix

▶ The Transverse Colon

▶ The Descending Colon

▶ The Sigmoid Colon

▶ The Anorectal Canal

▶ Innervation of the Intestine

*T*his region of the digestive tract is the site of a large share of the total pathology affecting the GI tract and is a frequent site of cancer in both men and women. The appendix, an outgrowth of the cecum, is alone one of the most frequently diseased organs in the body and one of the most common reasons for abdominal surgery (see Figure 5-42). A knowledge of the anatomy of the rectal canal is important for all physicians, for not only are there key structures within the rectum it-

self, but significant parts of the genitourinary systems in both male and female may be palpated through the walls of the rectum.

FORM AND FUNCTION OF THE COLON

The colon (Figure 5-45) is specialized principally for the reabsorption of water and electrolytes, not primarily for nutrient absorption. When portions of the colon are removed, patients are vulnerable to imbalances of

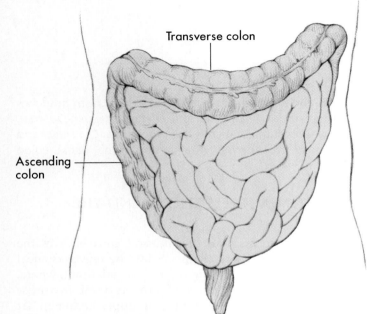

Transverse colon

Ascending colon

Figure 5-45 THE COLON, ANTERIOR VIEW. The colon commences in the right lower quadrant, where the ileocecal valve is located. From this point the ascending colon passes upward toward the right upper quadrant, where at the hepatic flexure it makes a sharp leftward turn to become the transverse colon. This travels across the upper abdomen toward the left upper quadrant, where at the splenic flexure the transverse colon becomes the descending colon (shielded by the small intestine). See Figure 5-48 for more details of the distal colon.

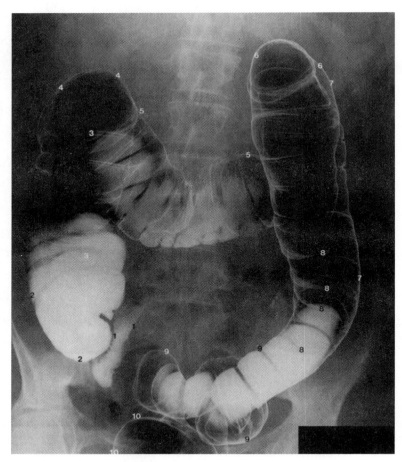

Figure 5-46 THE LARGE INTESTINE, BARIUM STUDY. Barium contrast material is placed into the rectum and large intestine through a barium enema, and in this study air has been injected as well, to distend the bowel and make its walls more visible. (From Weir J, Abrahams PH: *An imaging atlas of human anatomy,* London, 1992, Mosby.)

1 Terminal ileum	**5** Transverse portion of colon	**9** Sigmoid colon
2 Cecum	**6** Left colic (splenic) flexure of	**10** Rectum
3 Ascending portion of colon	colon	
4 Right colic (hepatic) flexure	**7** Descending portion of colon	
of colon	**8** Sacculations (haustra)	

both water and electrolytes (especially sodium). Some carbohydrate absorption does occur here, however. There is also important bacterial flora in the colon, some of which produce important substances (e.g., vitamin K) that are absorbed in the colon.

Colonic musculature is unique in that the external longitudinal coat is not continuous around the circumference of the colon. Instead, it is found in three longitudinal strips or bands, the **taenia coli.** The large bowel also is characterized by **haustra** (periodic sacculations of the mucosa; Figure 5-46) and by **appendices epiplioca** (polyp-like fatty appendages on the serosal surface of the colon; see Figure 5-48). The colon is divided into the *ascending, transverse, descending,* and *sigmoid portions.* Distal to this lies the *rectum.*

Blood supply of the colon is derived from branches of the *superior mesenteric* and *inferior mesenteric arteries,* as well as some branches from the *internal pudendal* and *internal iliac arteries,* which supply the distal colon (Figure 5-47).

PERITONEAL REFLECTIONS AND THE COLON

In most individuals, the *ileocecal junction* is in the right lower quadrant (Figure 5-48); the retroperitoneal *ascending colon* rises to the right upper quadrant, where, at the hepatic flexure, the intraperitoneal *transverse colon* begins, it courses across the upper abdomen. At the splenic flexure, in the left upper quadrant, the

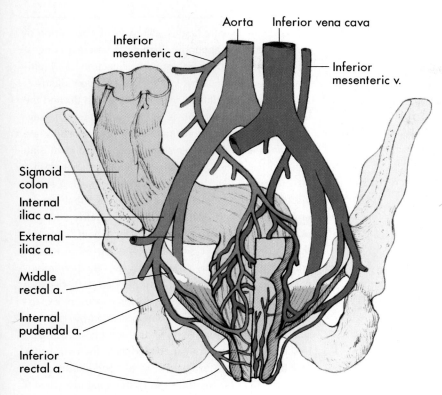

Figure 5-47 BLOOD SUPPLY OF THE REC-TUM. This coronal section shows a posterior view of the pelvis. The sigmoid colon approaches the midline from the left side and is continuous with the rectum. The superior rectal artery and vein arise from the inferior mesenteric artery and vein (draining to the portal vein). The middle rectal vein drains to the internal iliac vein, and the inferior rectal vein to the internal pudendal vein (both the internal pudendal and internal iliac veins drain to the vena cava). The rectal canal is a common site for portocaval shunting of blood, leading to hemorrhoids.

SEE ATLAS, FIG. 5-89

retroperitoneal *descending colon* begins; it continues into the left lower quadrant. Here the intraperitoneal *sigmoid colon* begins; it is of quite variable shape, length, and position. It may loop upward as high as the stomach or remain entirely in the lower abdomen and pelvis. The sigmoid colon then continues into the *rectum.*

THE CECUM AND ASCENDING COLON

The large intestine begins with the **cecum** (blind sac) and continues in a cranial direction as the **ascending colon** (see Figures 5-42 and 5-48). The ileocecal valve marks the connection between the ileum and colon and is positioned several centimeters above the base of the cecum. In fact, the *appendix* opens into the cecum at a

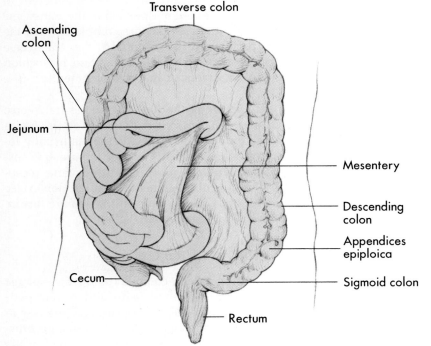

Figure 5-48 THE DISTAL COLON. The small intestine has been folded to the right, revealing the transverse, descending, and sigmoid colon. The descending colon is retroperitoneal, but the transverse and sigmoid are intraperitoneal. SEE ATLAS, FIG. 5-5

point inferior to the position where the ileum enters the cecum. The *ileocecal valve* (see Figure 5-42) is simply that part of the ileum that "telescopes" into the cecum. As the cecum fills with feces, the opening into the ileum is pinched closed and reflux of feces from cecum back into the ileum is minimized. Blood supply to the cecum is from the *ileocolic artery* (a vessel derived from the superior mesenteric artery) (see Figures 5-17 and 5-43).

Unlike the rest of the ascending colon, the *cecum* is intraperitoneal and relatively mobile, at least early in life. In most individuals, the cecum will become progressively more fixed to the posterior wall as life progresses. The remainder of the ascending colon is retroperitoneal and lies anterior to the psoas major, quadratus lumborum, gonadal vessels, ureter, and right kidney as it ascends. It is supplied with blood mainly by the *right colic artery,* with accessory branches from the *ileocolic* and *middle colic arteries.* The vessel circling around the inner perimeter of the ascending, transverse, and descending parts of the colon is the *marginal artery* (see Figure 5-43).

The *hepatic flexure* lies just under the right lobe of the liver and represents the transition of the ascending colon into the transverse colon. It is suspended by a mesenteric sling attached to the undersurface of the right lobe of the liver and to the gallbladder.

THE VERMIFORM APPENDIX

The **appendix** connects to the cecum below the level of the ileocecal valve. The appendix is a vestigial appendage of the digestive system. The position of the root of the appendix is always indicated by the point where the three taenia converge and meet on the inferomedial border of the cecum (see Figure 5-42). Taenia coli are not found on the appendix itself. The submucosa of the appendix contains large quantities of lymphoid tissue. The position of the appendix may be retrocecal (i.e., behind the cecum—about 65%), pelvic (located more inferiorly, lying against the levator ani muscle—about 30%), or in a variety of other positions. Knowledge of these variations is important to the surgeon removing the appendix through a small incision with limited visibility in the abdomen.

THE TRANSVERSE COLON

The **transverse mesocolon** extends across the upper abdominal cavity from the hepatic flexure to the splenic flexure (see Figure 5-46). It is positioned anteriorly, away from the posterior abdominal wall, in the region of the pancreas and the third part of the duodenum (see Figure 5-36). The transverse colon is supplied with blood by the *middle colic artery,* a branch of the superior mesenteric artery. The left side of the transverse mesocolon contains few blood vessels and for that rea-

PRINCIPLES ■

Appendicitis usually begins with a fecal obstruction of the lumen of the appendix, leading to vascular congestion, ischemia, bacterial growth, infection, and ultimately perforation. The initial pain of appendicitis is usually mild and diffuse and is experienced around the umbilical area. The pain is felt there because the segments of the spinal cord innervating the appendix are the same as those innervating the periumbilical skin (about T10). Our belief is that irritation originating in a visceral organ like the appendix delivers such a strong visceral sensory signal to the spinal cord that nearby groups of somatic sensory axons are activated. In a manner reminiscent of "phantom limb pain," stimulation of these somatic sensory axons causes an experience of pain in the area they innervate—the periumbilical region. This is an example of *referred pain,* because stimulation of visceral sensory axons causes an experience "referred" to the skin area innervated by the same spinal cord segments. As long as the process is limited to direct irritation of the appendix itself, the pain is diffuse and moderate in severity. When perforation of the appendix occurs, pus spills out of the appendix, directly irritating the parietal peritoneum of the abdominal wall, and sharp pain is felt, localized to the abdominal wall, usually the right lower quadrant (RLQ).

son is a favored route for surgical access to the lesser sac and the pancreas. The greater omentum, a derivative of the dorsal mesogastrium, becomes adherent to the superior surface of the midportion of the transverse mesocolon. When these events are complete, then, the "sling" of peritoneum surrounding the transverse colon in reality consists of the transverse mesocolon and the adherent layers of the greater omentum (see Figure 5-36).

The *splenic flexure* is the junction of the transverse colon and the descending colon, in the left upper quadrant of the abdomen. The splenic flexure is usually located 4 to 6 cm superior to the hepatic flexure. It is suspended by a specialized part of the transverse mesocolon, the phrenicocolic ligament, to the undersurface of the diaphragm. Located deep to the splenic flexure are the left kidney and left adrenal glands.

THE DESCENDING COLON

The **descending colon** commences at the splenic flexure (see Figures 5-18 and 5-46) and is retroperitoneal. The descending colon is positioned anterior to the left kidney, quadratus lumborum, psoas major muscles, ureter, and gonadal vessels. The distal half of the transverse colon, the descending colon, and all of the gut distal to it receive their parasympathetic innervation from the *sacral plexus,* whereas the intestine proximal to this point receives parasympathetic innervation from the *vagus nerve.*

THE SIGMOID COLON

The **sigmoid colon** is intraperitoneal and is of extremely variable size and shape (but often S-shaped; hence its name). It may be short and confined to the pelvis or may be much longer and extend upward to the region of the liver (see Figure 5-46). It is a storage organ for feces, from which most water has been reabsorbed. The mesentery of the sigmoid colon arises from the posterior wall at a point anterior to the external iliac vessels on the left. Vascular supply is from the *inferior mesenteric artery,* arising at the L2-L3 level and supplying the descending and sigmoid colon. Its major branches are the *left colic,* a *sigmoid arterial arcade, rectosigmoid,* and *superior rectal arteries.*

THE ANORECTAL CANAL

The **rectum** (L. straight, in contrast to sigmoid) extends from the sigmoid colon to the anus (defined as commencing at the level of the puborectalis muscle). Part of the rectum is within the abdominopelvic cavity, and part is inferior to it. It is 12 to 15 cm in length (see Figure 5-47). The rectum lacks haustra, appendices epiploica, and taenia coli. Only the proximal 50% to 60% of the rectum is covered by peritoneum. Although the rectum too can function as a storage area for feces, its distension creates a greater sense of urgency than is

true for the sigmoid colon. Like the rest of the GI tract, the wall of the rectum has intrinsic smooth musculature. In addition, the rectum passes through several layers of extrinsic striated muscle, some of which form distinct *sphincters* around the recum and anus.

The transition from rectum to anal canal is not a sharply defined line but a zone of change. Fundamentally, the rectum is endodermally derived, but the anal canal has some proximal regions of endodermally derived lining and distal regions that are ectodermally derived. Table 5-10 highlights some of the similarities and differences of the rectum and anus.

The beginning of the anus is marked by the point where the *puborectalis muscle* (a portion of the levator ani muscle) attaches to the external wall (i.e., where it blends with the deep portion of the external anal sphincter). The *sphincter ani internus* is an extension of the intrinsic longitudinal smooth muscle of the gut in general. It extends down as far as the white line, in the midpoint of the anal wall. The *sphincter ani externus* has three parts (subcutaneous, superficial, and deep): (1) the most inferior portion, the subcutaneous, is attached to the perineal body and extends laterally and superiorly to partially enclose the superficial portion, (2) the superficial portion is the thinnest of the three and attaches anteriorly to the perineal body and posteriorly to the coccyx—the only bony attachment of the external and sphincter, and (3) the deep portion, positioned most superiorly, surrounds the distal end of the rectum and the proximal anal canal. The external sphincter mediates voluntary continence. The *pudendal nerve* innervates the entire muscle.

The rectum receives blood from the *superior rectal*

Table 5-10   The Rectum and the Anus

Characteristic	Rectal Canal	Anal Canal
Epithelium	All columnar (endodermal)	Columnar as far distal as white line (see below in table); squamous below the white line (see pp. 566-567).
Epithelial specializations	Rectal ampulla in its lower third	Anal columns are 4-6 cm long longitudinal ridges in upper anal canal.
		Crescentic folds of mucosa, the anal valves, connect these columns at their bases.
		Anal sinuses are grooves between columns. The anal crypts are the parts of the sinuses behind the anal valves. Anal glands, in the rectal submucosa, empty into the anal crypts.
		Lower end of the anal columns constitute the pectinate line.
		Midway down the distal anal mucosa is the white line, marking the distal end of the internal sphincter and the beginning of squamous epithelium.
Innervation of mucosa	Autonomic (mostly unconscious)	*Above white line:* autonomic nerves *Below white line:* somatic (from pudendal)
Arterial supply	From inferior mesenteric artery	*Above white line:* from inferior mesenteric and iliac arteries *Below white line:* from internal pudendal artery
Venous drainage	To portal system	*Above white line:* to portal system *Below white line:* to IVC

THE LARGE INTESTINE

ULCERATIVE COLITIS

Ulcerative colitis involves chronic inflammation and destruction of the colonic mucosa, resulting in chronic diarrhea and abdominal pain.

CONGENITAL MEGACOLON

Congenital megacolon results from absence of the autonomic plexus and subsequent poor contractility of colonic musculature. The denervated area causes a functional obstruction, and the bowel proximal to it enlarges.

DIVERTICULOSIS

Diverticulosis (numerous small sacculations of the colonic wall, eventually becoming inflamed and rupturing) affects an increasing number of people of advancing age.

VOLVULUS

Intraperitoneal parts of the large intestine also may become twisted around the mesentery and "kinked"—volvulus.

PORTOCAVAL ANASTOMOSES

The anorectal canal is another region in which venous blood destined for the portal vein (superior rectal vein) can be diverted into vena caval flow (through the middle and inferior rectals). This forms hemorrhoids, by a process similar to that resulting in esophageal varices. It should be remembered, however, that most cases of hemorrhoids are *not* indicative of portal hypertension but are simply a reflection of inherent weakness and distension in the walls of the rectal veins.

INFECTION IN THE ANAL CANAL

The anal canal is a frequent site of abscesses. These can cause enlarging areas of necrosis and, if untreated, even form fistulae (abnormal connections) with the vagina, bladder, or peritoneal cavity.

THE RECTAL EXAMINATION

Through the anal wall, palpation of the posterior surface of the prostate, the posterior vaginal wall, and the coccyx is possible.

---

artery (from the inferior mesenteric artery) and the *middle rectal artery* (from the internal iliac artery). The anus receives blood from the *inferior rectal artery* (a branch of the internal pudendal artery). Venous blood returns to the portal system (via the *superior rectal veins*) and to the vena cava (through the *middle rectal* and *inferior rectal veins*). There is a rectal *submucous venous plexus* in which venous blood from all these sources can mingle (see Figure 5-47).

INNERVATION OF THE INTESTINE

The intestinal tract in general has a great deal of intrinsic contractility and can function in the absence of extrinsic innervation (although its function will not be entirely normal). The **parasympathetic system** in general promotes digestive activity (through increased peristalsis, relaxation of sphincters, production of digestive mucus and enzymes). The **sympathetic input** is generally antagonistic (contraction of sphincters, decreased muscular activity), although much of its effect may be as a result of changes in blood flow. In the ascending colon, movement is complex and usually results in the forward and backward propulsion of contents. This presumably promotes mixing (and therefore softening) of the contents and tends to keep them con-

fined to the ascending colon until new material enters from the ileum. In the other parts of the colon, movement is simpler and promotes forward movement of fecal contents.

Parasympathetic Nerves

The vagus nerve is responsible for parasympathetic innervation of the gut as far distal as the midpoint of the transverse colon (see Figures 5-25 and 6-44). Distal to this point, the sacral parasympathetic system takes over (derived from spinal cord segments S2 to S4). In the parasympathetic system, a small number of the intrinsic neurons constitutes the postganglionic portion of the connection (remember that there must be a preganglionic and postganglionic neuron in an autonomic motor pathway). We recognize these and other intrinsic neurons histologically as the myenteric plexus (also called Auerbach's and Meissner's plexus of the gut wall) (see Figure 5-41).

Sympathetic Nerves

The sympathetic axons for the ascending and transverse colon arise in the celiac and mesenteric ganglia, having received preganglionic input from the greater and lesser splanchnic nerves, originating mostly in T9 to T12 level of the cord. They travel along with the vasculature supplying the gut. Sympathetic nerves for the descending colon and beyond arise in the lumbar chain ganglia and accompany branches of the inferior mesenteric artery to reach the colon. These ganglia receive their preganglionic input from cord levels L1 to L3.

Enteric Nerves

In recent years, we have come to recognize increasingly the existence of a set of neurons, ganglia, and axons that are wholly confined within the abdominal wall. These nerves, called the *enteric nervous system,* are clearly different from the sympathetic and parasympathetic influences on the gut; in fact, these nerves may act on the gut through their influence on enteric nerves. The neurons of the enteric nervous system are located in the small clusters of ganglia in the gut wall (Meissner's and Auerbach's plexus). The transmitters used by enteric neurons differ from those in the CNS or in the conventional autonomic system. They are peptides like glycine and substance P and nucleotides like adenosine triphosphate (ATP). We know very little about how they work or how to influence them pharmacologically. Some better understood diseases, such as aganglioniosis of the colon (Hirschspung's disease), are best understood as abnormalities of these enteric neurons.

5.8

Kidneys and Suprarenal Glands

▶ General Functions of the Kidneys

▶ Position and Structural Features of the Kidneys

▶ The Collecting System

▶ The Ureteropelvic Junction

▶ Vascular Supply to the Kidneys

▶ The Suprarenal (Adrenal) Glands

*T*he urinary system is usually described as having an *"upper"* portion—the kidneys and ureters, and a *"lower"* portion—the bladder and urethra. The **kidneys** are vital organs and are partially protected by the ribcage. The embryonic development of the kidney is very complex, and, in fact, the embryo has unique and transient excretory organs of its own that form and disappear before birth. Aside from the responsibility for urinary excretion, the kidneys are also central to acid–base regulation, electrolyte balance, calcium homeostasis, and regulation of blood pressure. The **adrenal** (or **suprarenal**) glands sit atop the kidneys and often share a blood supply with them (Figure 5-49).

GENERAL FUNCTIONS OF THE KIDNEYS

The kidneys receive up to 25% of the total cardiac output (that is, the volume of blood pumped by the heart per unit time—usually expressed in liters per minute). The main function of the kidneys is to produce a glomerular filtrate of the blood (ultimately called urine). Then, in a series of tubules within the kidney, reabsorption of the desired amounts of water, electrolytes, and other solutes takes place. This keeps the body in good *metabolic* and *acid–base status*. In particular, organic acids and nitrogenous wastes are excreted. In addition, a number of *drugs* are actively metabolized in the kidney. *Blood pressure* is directly regulated by the renin-angiotensin enzymes, produced

within the kidney. The kidney monitors its own blood flow as an indication of the need for raising or lowering blood pressure by way of these enzymes. Salt reabsorption also influences blood pressure. In addition, the kidney produces a series of hormonelike substances that influence *red blood cell production* and activates an inactive form of Vitamin D, which in turn increases *calcium absorption* from the gut.

POSITION AND STRUCTURAL FEATURES OF THE KIDNEYS

The kidneys are paired ovoid organs located retroperitoneally on the posterior abdominal wall (see Figure 5-49). The left kidney is positioned slightly more superior than the right. The eleventh and twelfth left ribs cover the upper pole of the left kidney on its posterior surface, and the twelfth rib covers the upper pole of the right kidney (Figure 5-50). The kidneys are flattened ovoids positioned at a 45 degree angle. Both are embedded in large amounts of fat. Each kidney is a flattened ovoid with a *hilus* facing medially. At this hilus, the *vessels* enter and leave the kidney, and the *ureter* exits here too.

Internally, the kidney has an outer *cortex* (crust) and inner *medulla*. Histologically, the cortex consists of thousands of *glomeruli* (filtering units) and the medulla of highly convoluted *tubules* that ultimately empty urine into the drainage system (the renal pelvis then

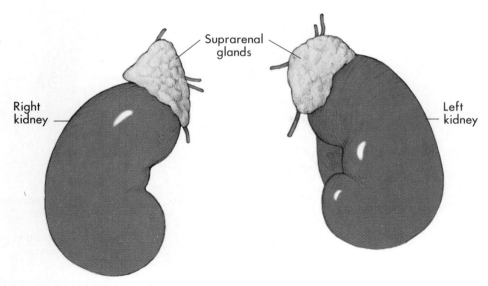

Figure 5-49   THE KIDNEYS AND ADRENAL GLANDS, ANTERIOR VIEW. The gland on the left is more rounded, while that on the right is more in the shape of a three-cornered-hat. The three potential sources of blood supply for each gland are shown here and in Figure 5-54.

the ureter). The selective reabsorption and secretion of materials takes place in the glomerular and tubular systems.

On its anterior surface, the *right kidney* is related to the adrenal gland superiorly, the liver over much of its anterior surface, the duodenum at its hilus, and the hepatic flexure of the colon on its inferior surface. The *left kidney* is related to the spleen superolaterally, the stomach superiorly, the body of the pancreas at its hilus, and the jejunum inferiorly. Posteriorly, both kidneys rest on the quadratus lumborum and psoas muscles. The kidneys are protected to some degree posteriorly by the overlying lower ribs (Figure 5-51).

The kidney has a true *capsule* closely adherent to its surface. The *transversalis layer of fascia* splits at the lateral border of the kidney into two leaflets that enclose the kidney (forming "Gerota's capsule"). Fat within these two leaflets is the *perineal fat*. Fat external to this layer, found mostly posteriorly, is the *pararenal fat* (see Figure 5-51).

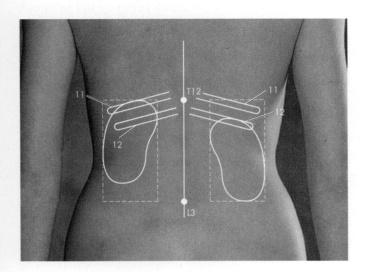

Figure 5-50   POSITION OF THE KIDNEYS AND THE POSTERIOR ABDOMINAL WALL. The left kidney is positioned slightly superior to the right with respect to the posterior body wall. The upper pole of the left kidney is crossed by the eleventh and twelfth ribs, while the upper pole of the right kidney is crossed by only the twelfth rib.

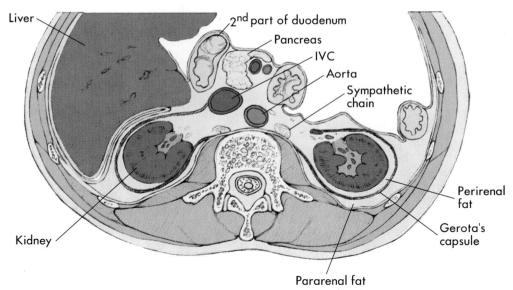

Liver — 2nd part of duodenum — Pancreas — IVC — Aorta — Sympathetic chain — Perirenal fat — Gerota's capsule — Kidney — Pararenal fat

Figure 5-51   THE KIDNEYS. Transverse section at approximately L2, through the middle of the two kidneys. Separate layers of fat are found between the surface of the kidney and the renal capsule (the *perirenal fat*) and between the renal capsule and the transversalis fascia (*pararenal fat*). The renal capsule itself is a special extension of the transversalis fascia.   SEE ATLAS, FIGS. 5-96, 5-100

THE COLLECTING SYSTEM

Each kidney is organized radially with its *hilus* lying along its medial border and several *lobules,* extending radially, manufacturing urine. Urine accumulates at the *papilla* of the lobule and first drains into the *minor calyx,* thence to a *major calyx,* and finally into the *renal pelvis* of each kidney (Figures 5-52 and 5-53). The ureter meets the renal pelvis at the *ureteropelvic junction.*

The *ureters* connect the kidney to the bladder. They are muscular tubes with a peristaltic motion promoting the movement of urine from kidney to bladder (even if you stood on your head all day your bladder would still fill!). The ureters exit the renal hilus posteriorly and travel along the posterior abdominal wall and sacrum (see Figure 6-60). Along their course they pass anterior to the common iliac arteries, then posteroinferior to the uterine arteries in the female and the ductus deferens in the male.

THE URETEROPELVIC JUNCTION

The ureteropelvic junction (UPJ) (see Figure 5-52) is a common site for obstruction of urinary flow. There is no sphincteric or otherwise specialized musculature present at the UPJ. In the normal state, the UPJ does not cause any blockage to flow but is a point of natural narrowing in the ureter (other naturally narrow points are found at the pelvic brim and the entrance to the bladder). Pathologic obstruction at the UPJ also may be caused by external compression (e.g., tumor, anomalous vessels). UPJ obstructions may lead to dilation of the renal calyces (hydronephrosis) and consequent pressure on the renal parenchyma. In the worst cases, this pressure may even destroy the functional renal tissue.

A chronically obstructed UPJ may lead to an occult infection in the renal pelvis. The infection will periodically "seed" the lower ureter and bladder, producing what initially seem to be innocuous recurrent bladder infections in the patient. Such recurrent bladder infections, however, always should alert one to the possibility of a UPJ obstruction (or other anomaly in the upper urinary tract).

VASCULAR SUPPLY TO THE KIDNEYS

The **left** and **right renal arteries** (branching at L1-L2) give important branches to the suprarenal glands as well as the kidneys (Figure 5-54). The renal artery on each side enters the anterior half of the renal hilus and divides into lobular branches (Figure 5-55). The right renal artery is longer than the left, and it passes behind the IVC. In about 20% of individuals, there is an anomalous (although not necessarily abnormal) arterial pattern. The most frequently seen is a *polar artery*—a separate vessel traveling from the aorta to the lower pole of the kidney and representing a persistent embryologic artery. This reminds us that the fetal kidney had 10 to

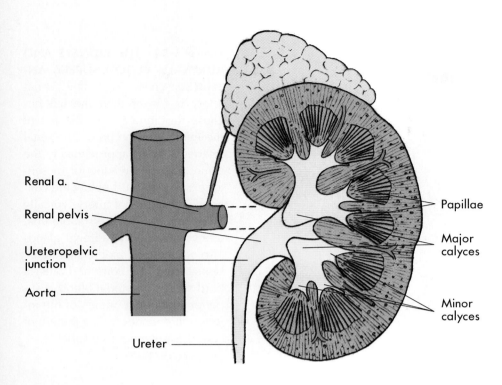

Renal a.

Renal pelvis

Ureteropelvic
junction

Aorta

Ureter

Papillae

Major
calyces

Minor
calyces

**Figure 5-52   URINARY COLLEC-
TION IN THE KIDNEY.** Parasagittal
cut through the kidney showing
the papillae, calyces, and renal
pelvis.   SEE ATLAS, FIGS. 5-94, 5-99

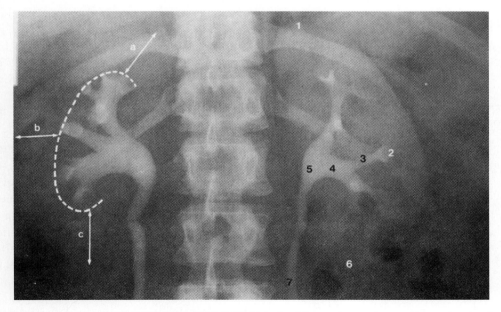

Figure 5-53   AN INTRAVENOUS PYELOGRAM. In this study, an intravenous dye is chosen for its property of being taken up by the kidneys and excreted in the urine. This creates an image of the collecting system within the kidneys, the ureters, and the bladder.
This study is known as an intravenous pyelogram. *a,* Upper pole cortex of right kidney; *b,*
central cortex of right kidney; *c,* lower pole cortex of right kidney; *1,* upper pole of left
kidney; *2,* renal papilla; *3,* minor calyx; *4,* major calyx; *5,* renal pelvis; *6,* lower pole of
left kidney; *7,* left ureter. (From Weir J, Abrahams PH: *An imaging atlas of human anatomy,*
London, 1992, Mosby.)   SEE ATLAS, FIGS. 5-6, 5-93, 5-95

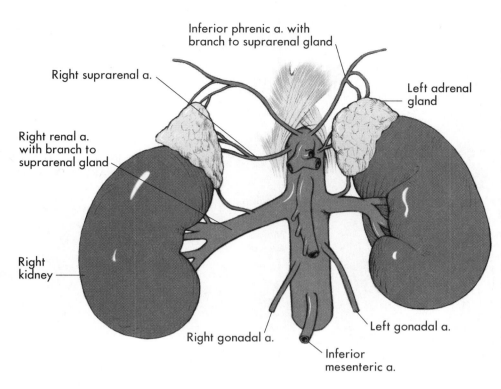

Inferior phrenic a. with
branch to suprarenal gland

Right suprarenal a.

Right renal a.
with branch to
suprarenal gland

Right
kidney

Left adrenal
gland

Right gonadal a.

Left gonadal a.

Inferior
mesenteric a.

Figure 5-54   THE KIDNEYS AND ADRENALS, BLOOD SUPPLY, ANTERIOR VIEW. The right renal artery is longer than the left because the aorta lies to the left of the midline of the body. The renal arteries arise at approximately the same level as the superior mesenteric artery and just below the celiac axis. Each renal artery typically gives off an inferior suprarenal artery as well. The adrenal glands also get a direct middle suprarenal branch from the aorta and often a third source of arterial blood, a superior suprarenal branch of the inferior phrenic artery. The pattern of supply is tremendously variable.

SEE ATLAS, FIGS. 5-92, 5-103

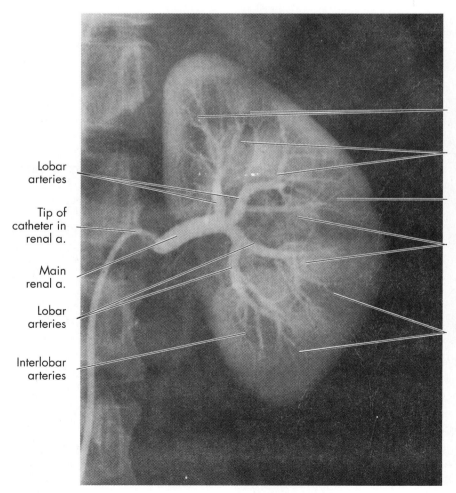

Lobar
arteries

Tip of
catheter in
renal a.

Main
renal a.

Lobar
arteries

Interlobar
arteries

Arcuate
arteries

Interlobar
arteries

Arcuate
arteries

Interlobar
arteries

Arcuate
arteries

Figure 5-55   A RENAL ARTERIOGRAM. Tip of a catheter is placed in the entrance to the left renal artery, and dye is injected. The subsequent x-ray reveals the branching arterial pattern within the kidney. If a tumor or other space-occupying mass were present, its position could be inferred from the distortion it would produce in the position of the arteries within the kidney. (From Weir J, Abrahams PH: *An imaging atlas of human anatomy,* London, 1992, Mosby.)

SEE ATLAS, FIG. 5-102

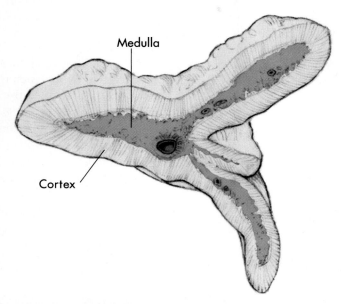

Medulla

Cortex

Figure 5-56 THE ADRENAL GLAND, CROSS-SECTION. Note the outer cortex, where steroid hormone biosynthesis takes place, and central medulla, where epinephrine (and to a small degree norepinephrine) are released into the bloodstream, under the regulation of incoming axonal stimulation.

12 distinct lobules, each with a separate blood supply. The **left renal vein** is longer than the **right renal vein** and usually receives the left gonadal vein (blood from the right gonadal vein drains directly to the inferior vena cava). Crossing the midline, the left renal vein passes anterior to the aorta. At the renal hilus, the renal veins are positioned anterior to the renal arteries.

THE SUPRARENAL (ADRENAL) GLANDS

The **right adrenal gland** is pyramid-shaped, while the **left adrenal gland** is more like a curved disk. Each gland is embedded in fat and firmly fixed to the upper surface of the kidney. The right adrenal gland lies just posterior and lateral to the IVC. The left adrenal gland is in the lower posterior wall of the lesser sac, just lateral to the aorta and is in contact anteriorly with the pancreas and the splenic artery (see Figure 5-49).

The adrenal glands have a *cortex* (Figure 5-56) where are synthesized a variety of endocrine steroid products including mineralocorticoids (salt-regulating), gluco-corticoids (regulating stress responses, glucose mobilization, and overall metabolism), and sex hormones (which in the male are the major source of estrogenic hormones). The *medulla* or central area of each adrenal gland is innervated by small splanchnic nerves from the thorax, and in response the medullary chromaffin cells release epinephrine into the circulation.

The adrenals usually share part of their **arterial blood supply** with the kidney. There is in most of us an independent left and right suprarenal artery arising directly from the aorta; a branch from this vessel supplies the renal hilus as well. Branches of the renal arteries and inferior phrenic arteries often supply branches to the adrenals. The paired inferior phrenic arteries are the most superior intraabdominal branches of the aorta. They ramify on the undersurface of the hemidiaphragm and supply that muscle on each side. Adrenal **venous drainage** is much more constant and predictable than the arterial supply. The right adrenal vein drains into the IVC, and the left adrenal vein drains into the left renal vein.

THE KIDNEYS AND SUPRARENAL GLANDS

THE KIDNEYS AND BLOOD PRESSURE

Whenever there is diminished blood flow through the kidney, the kidney interprets it as a sign of lowered blood pressure and "up-regulates" the production of a renin, which stimulates production of angiotensin (a vasoconstrictor), and increases the release of aldosterone (which retains sodium, increases total body fluid, and thereby increases blood pressure).

FACTORS INFLUENCING BLOOD FLOW TO THE KIDNEY

There are numerous potential sources of diminished renal blood flow—poor cardiac function (bad pump), obstruction of renal artery and/or vein (often a part of arteriosclerosis, or a space-occupying lesion in the abdomen), dehydration (starvation, heat, or prolonged vomiting), or coarctation of the aorta, to name a few.

ABNORMALITIES OF THE ADRENAL MEDULLA

Inappropriate growth and metabolic activity in the adrenal medulla produces a pheochromocytoma, where high levels of epinephrine or norepinephrine are released into the blood, raising blood pressure and causing a number of other symptoms.

ADRENAL STEROIDS

Abnormalities in steroid production in the adrenal may lead to wide-reaching changes in growth and metabolism. Examples are:

- *Hyperaldosteronism:* Excess aldosterone, leading to obesity, hypertension, polydipsia (excess water intake)
- *Excess cortisol:* High levels of glucocorticoids, leading to obesity, muscle wasting, altered body shape, and psychosis
- *Virilizing/feminizing lesions:* Produce abnormal levels of sex hormones or their active intermediaries; produces early onset or exaggeration of secondary sexual changes and may be congenital or acquired

5.9

Posterior Wall and Diaphragm

- ▶ General Structure of the Posterior Abdominal Wall
- ▶ The Diaphragm and Relationships
- ▶ Innervation and Blood Supply of the Diaphragm
- ▶ Structures Traversing the Diaphragm
- ▶ The Lumbar Plexus
- ▶ The Abdominal Aorta and its Branches
- ▶ Venous Drainage of the Abdominal Wall

*T*he posterior abdominal wall is the framework on which all of the intraabdominal viscera are positioned. It is also a continuation of the body wall as a whole, and comparisons with the anterior abdominal and thoracic walls always should be remembered. The diaphragm is of obvious major importance in respiration, abdominal pressure regulation, and body movement. On the surface of the abdominal wall we see the components of the lumbar plexus, the first of two major plexuses that innervate the hip region and lower limb.

GENERAL STRUCTURE OF THE POSTERIOR ABDOMINAL WALL

The posterior abdominal wall is formed by the *diaphragm,* the *vertebral column,* the *psoas major,* the *quadratus lumborum,* and the upper edge of the *iliac crest.* The quadratus lumborum muscle constitutes the majority of the soft-tissue "bridge" filling the gap between the twelfth rib superiorly and the iliac crest inferiorly on each side.

Lateral to the quadratus lumborum, the posterior wall is formed by the *lumbodorsal fascia.* This fascia originates as a single layer from the vertebral transverse processes, splits laterally to enclose the various subcomponents of the erector spinae, and lateral to this reforms into a single fascial layer. To this single layer of the lumbodorsal fascia attach the fasciae of the internal

oblique and transversus muscles. The external oblique muscle has a free posterior edge and therefore does not attach to the lumbodorsal fascia.

THE DIAPHRAGM AND RELATIONSHIPS

The **diaphragm** is a large and complex muscle separating the abdominal cavity from the thoracic cavity (Figure 5-57). There is a tendinous *central tendon* (of connective tissue but not musculature) and a *peripheral area* of striated muscle surrounding that. Most of the muscle is innervated by the *phrenic nerve,* but there are supplemental sensory innervations by *intercostal nerves* to the most peripheral portions of the diaphragm.

Posteriorly, the diaphragm forms thickened tendinous arches over the psoas major and the quadratus lumborum as each passes posterior to the diaphragm. The portion arching over the psoas is the *medial arcuate ligament,* and that arching over the quadratus lumborum is the *lateral arcuate ligament.* They are called ligaments because the connective tissue forming these specialized arches is especially thick and easily palpable.

Anteriorly, specialized sternal fibers of the diaphragm arise on the posterior part of the sternum and blend into the central tendon. Similar slips of muscle arise from the cartilage of the costal angle and run inward to blend into the central tendon.

The **diaphragmatic crura** (see Figure 5-26) are two

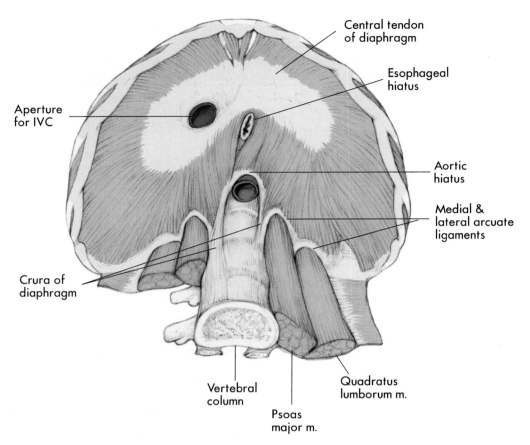

Central tendon
of diaphragm

Esophageal
hiatus

Aperture
for IVC

Aortic
hiatus

Medial &
lateral arcuate
ligaments

Crura of
diaphragm

Vertebral
column

Psoas
major m.

Quadratus
lumborum m.

Figure 5-57   THE DIAPHRAGM, INFERIOR VIEW. Pictured are the three major structures passing through or behind the diaphragm—the esophagus, the inferior vena cava (IVC), and the aorta. The medial and lateral arcuate ligaments are draped across the psoas major and quadratus lumborum muscles on each side, respectively. Consult the text for the full list of structures that pass from thorax to abdomen through various parts of the diaphragm. The lumbocostal angle is a potential spot for herniation of abdominal contents upward into the left side of the chest.   SEE ATLAS, FIGS. 5-121, 5-124

large muscular arches that pass along the lateral sides of the upper lumbar vertebrae, attaching to the anterior longitudinal ligaments. The right crus extends down alongside L1, L2, and L3. The left crus extends downward slightly less far, to L1 and L2. The crura together form the *aortic hiatus,* arching over the aorta as it passes from thorax to abdomen.

INNERVATION AND BLOOD SUPPLY OF THE DIAPHRAGM

Innervation of the diaphragm is primarily from C4, with inconstant help from C3 and C5. This combination of axons is the **phrenic nerve.** The phrenic nerve also carries sensory and autonomic axons because it is a typical spinal nerve. Blood supply is from **internal thoracic, inferior epigastric,** and **intercostal arteries,** and the **aorta** itself, through its inferior phrenic arteries.

STRUCTURES TRAVERSING THE DIAPHRAGM

The diaphragm has special relations to the major structures passing between abdomen and pelvis, and with the muscles of the posterior wall. There is a posterior hiatus for the *aorta,* formed by the arching of the two diaphragmatic crura over the aorta at T12. There is a similar muscular "sling" for the *esophagus,* opposite vertebral level T10. Third, there is an aperture for the *inferior vena cava* opposite the vertebral level T8. Table 5-11 details the many structures traversing the diaphragm.

THE LUMBAR PLEXUS

The lumbar plexus (Table 5-12) supplies innervation to the abdominal wall and part of the region of the pelvis. It comprises the anterior primary rami of spinal

Table 5-11 Structures Traversing the Diaphragm

Structure	Relationship to Diaphragm
Aorta	Through the aortic hiatus, surrounded by the two crura of the diaphragm at the level of vertebra T12
Esophagus	Through a muscular sling in the diaphragm at T10
Inferior vena cava	Through an aperture in the central tendon at the level of T8
Vagus nerves	As a plexus along with the esophagus
Sympathetic chains	Pass under medial arcuate ligament along with psoas major
Splanchnic nerves	Pass beneath crurae of the diaphragm in the aortic hiatus
Azygos-hemiazygos veins	May pass through aortic hiatus or beneath medial arcuate ligament
Thoracic duct	Forms from the cisterna chyli and lumbar trunks; passes through aortic hiatus
Phrenic nerve	The right phrenic nerve traverses the central tendon (or sometimes the IVC orifice) and ramifies on the inferior surface of the diaphragm; the left phrenic nerve penetrates the muscular part of the diaphragm, anterior to the central tendon, and ramifies on the inferior diaphragmatic surface

nerves T12 to L4 (L4 joins with L5 to form the **lumbosacral trunk,** a group of axons communicating to the sacral plexus). Several roots of the lumbar plexus are embedded in the psoas major muscle. As branches of this plexus extend laterally, they are incorporated into the posterolateral abdominal wall, running in a plane between the transversus abdominus and the internal oblique muscles (see Figure 5-59).

The Individual Nerves

The **iliohypogastric nerve** (T12-L1) supplies motor axons to the internal oblique and transversus and has a cutaneous branch to the pubic region. It lies lateral to the psoas major. The **ilioinguinal nerve** (T12-L1) may be fused to the iliohypogastric. It runs a similar course, supplies the transversus and internal oblique, and is cutaneous to the scrotum/labia and the base of the penis/clitoris. A terminal branch goes through the superficial inguinal ring.

The **genitofemoral nerve** (L1-L2) runs within the psoas major. The *genital branch* is motor to the cremaster muscle and travels in the spermatic cord. The *femoral branch* is cutaneous to the medial thigh. Both branches take part in the cremasteric reflex (see p. 469). The **lateral femoral cutaneous nerve** (L2-L3) runs laterally in the fascia of the iliacus and passes beneath the inguinal ligament in the vicinity of the anterior superior spine. It is a cutaneous nerve to the lateral thigh and may be compressed by tight clothing or prolonged sitting with the hips flexed.

The **femoral nerve** (L2-L4) is the major nerve to the anterior thigh (both cutaneous and muscular branches). It passes beneath the inguinal ligament just lateral to the psoas and breaks up into numerous branches. The **obturator nerve** (L2-L4) is the major nerve to the medi-

al compartment of the thigh. It lies medial to the psoas major in the posterior abdominal wall and leaves the pelvis by passing through the obturator foramen.

The **lumbosacral trunk** (L4-L5) lies medial to the psoas major and passes anterior to the sacral promon-

PRINCIPLES

The abdominal cavity is bounded both superiorly and inferiorly by complex muscular sheets that are capable of contraction, changing the pressure within the abdominal cavity (Figure 5-58). Each also features a number of apertures through which pass portions of the digestive tube and other important structures. The *respiratory diaphragm* (between the thorax and abdomen) is attached around the lower perimeter of the thoracic cage and over the upper lumbar vertebral column. It is also attached by thickened tendinous arches over the quadratus lumborum and psoas major muscles (the medial and lateral arcuate ligaments). The aorta, esophagus, inferior vena cava, sympathetic chains, splanchnic nerves, and thoracic duct pass through or posterior to the diaphragm, between abdomen and thorax. The *pelvic diaphragm* is also a muscular sling, whose contraction also increases pressure within the abdominal cavity. It too has central apertures, for the anal canal, vagina, and urethra, and is attached to a thickened tendinous arch (the arcus tendineus), which lies on the medial surface of the obturator internus muscle (see Chapter 6). Contraction of both the pelvic and "respiratory" diaphragms is important in activities such as defecation, urination, and parturition (childbirth) because each results from an increase in pressure within the abdominal cavity.

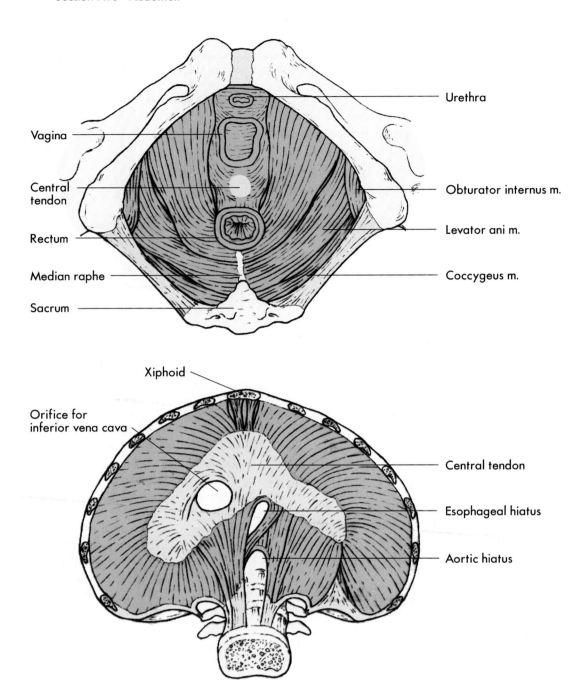

Urethra

Vagina

Central tendon

Rectum

Median raphe

Sacrum

Obturator internus m.

Levator ani m.

Coccygeus m.

Xiphoid

Orifice for inferior vena cava

Central tendon

Esophageal hiatus

Aortic hiatus

Figure 5-58   THE THORACIC AND PELVIC DIAPHRAGMS. This figure points out the similarities of the diaphragm separating the abdomen and thorax and the diaphragm found at the inferior end of the pelvis. Each has arched ligaments of connective tissue that attach part of the perimeter of the muscle to the body wall; each is perforated by several important structures; and each contributes to a variety of functions by contracting and flattening itself, changing the capacity and the pressure within the abdominopelvic cavity.

Table 5-12   The Lumbar Plexus

Nerve	Muscles Innervated	Cutaneous Area Supplied
Iliohypogastric nerve (T12–L1)	Internal oblique, transversus abdominus, external oblique	Cutaneous to pubic region
Ilioinguinal nerve (T12–L1)	Internal oblique, transversus abdominus, external oblique	Cutaneous to scrotum/labia, penis/clitoris
Genitofemoral nerve (L1–L2)	Cremaster	Cutaneous to medial thigh
Lateral femoral cutaneous nerve (L2–L3)	None	Cutaneous to lateral thigh
Femoral nerve (L2–L4)	Anterior compartment of thigh	Cutaneous to anterior thigh
Obturator nerve (L2–L4)	Medial compartment of thigh	Mid-portion of medial thigh
Lumbosacral trunk (L4–L5)	Contributes to sacral plexus, common peroneal and tibial portions of the sciatic nerve	

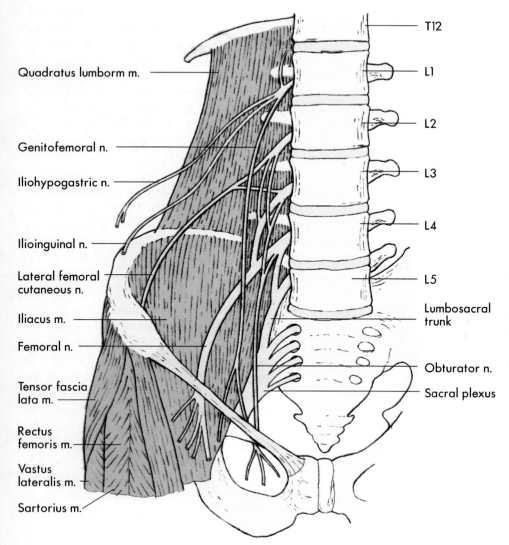

Figure 5-59 THE LUMBO-SACRAL PLEXUS. The lumbar plexus is the major source of innervation for the anterolateral body wall and anteromedial thigh, while the sacral plexus innervates the internal pelvic viscera, the gluteal region, the posterior thigh, and all of the leg and foot.

SEE ATLAS, FIGS. 5-116, 5-118, 5-119

Table 5-13   Bracnches of The Abdominal Aorta

Unpaired, to Viscera	Paired, to Viscera	To Body Wall
Celiac artery (trunk) (Figure 5-34)	Middle suprarenal	Inferior phrenic (paired)
Superior mesenteric	Renal	Lumbar arteries (paired)
Inferior mesenteric	Gonadal	Median sacral (unpaired)

tory to enter the pelvis and the sacral plexus. It is destined to contribute to both the common peroneal and tibial portions of the **sciatic nerve,** the largest peripheral nerve in the body.

THE ABDOMINAL AORTA AND ITS BRANCHES

The **abdominal aorta** begins at level of T12 to L1 and descends along the posterior wall slightly to the left of the midline. It terminates by dividing into two *common iliac arteries,* at about L4. Along the posterior abdominal wall, the aorta gives off numerous branches, which may be grouped into (1) unpaired branches to viscera, (2) paired branches to viscera, and (3) paired branches to the body wall. These are listed in Table 5-13.

VENOUS DRAINAGE OF THE ABDOMINAL WALL

The **left renal vein** passes anterior to the aorta at approximately L2; as the aorta bifurcates, its common iliac branches lie anterior to the comparable venous branches (see Figures 5-12 and 5-60). The body of the pancreas, as it is "draped" over the vertebral column, is separated from the aorta by the left renal vein as well. Pulsations of the abdominal aorta are easily palpated by a hand placed just above the umbilicus, exerting gentle pressure in a posterior direction.

The **inferior vena cava (IVC)** forms from the confluence of the *left* and *right common iliac veins,* at about L4 to L5. It drains blood to the right atrium from all of the body below the diaphragm. It normally lies slightly to

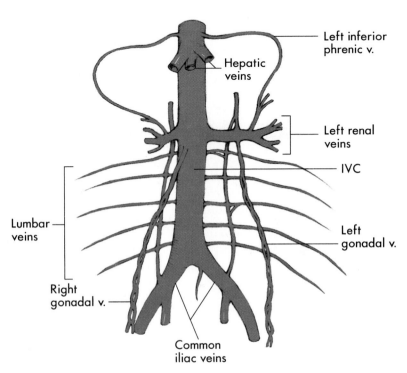

Figure 5-60   VEINS OF THE POSTERIOR ABDOMINAL WALL. Like the thorax, the abdominal wall is segmental, although there are no ribs to emphasize the point. There are five pairs of lumbar veins, comparable in every way to the intercostal vessels of the thorax. The lumbar veins arise in the anterolateral body wall and drain blood posteriorly and directly into the IVC. On each side there is a vertical ascending lumbar vein, which passes behind the diaphragm and connects with the azygos (on the right) or hemiazygos (on the left) system of veins in the thorax. The inferior phrenic veins drain blood from the inferior surface of the diaphragm, and empty, at least in part, into the renal veins. They also connect superiorly with the superior epigastric veins, which drain into the internal thoracic and eventually into the subclavian veins on each side. Recall that the gonadal veins (testicular or ovarian) drain into the IVC on the right and the renal vein on the left.

SEE ATLAS, FIGS. 5-8, 5-92, 5-104, 5-108, 5-109

THE POSTERIOR ABDOMINAL WALL

DIAPHRAGMATIC HERNIAS (SEE FIGURE 5-7)

The diaphragm is subject to congenital and acquired defects (that is, perforations in the substance of the diaphragm), which if severe enough may permit intestines to pass into the thoracic cavity. Congenital diaphragmatic hernias are most common on the left, at the angle between the costal and lumbar portions of the diaphragm (Bochdalek hernias). They cause death through the inhibitory effect they have on lung development and not through any direct effect on the diaphragm (thus, the embryonic time at which the herniation occurs becomes more crucial than exactly how much or which parts of the intestine are herniated into the chest). Less commonly, hernias may occur at the region of the xiphoid (Morgagni hernias).

HIATUS HERNIAS

Hiatus hernias occur when the upper portions of the stomach herniate superiorly through the esophageal hiatus (see section on esophagus).

the right of the vertebral column. In the lower abdominal wall, it is crossed obliquely by the root of the Mesentery (see Figure 5-18).

The *tributaries of the IVC* are the common iliac veins, the gonadal veins, the renal veins, the suprarenal veins, the inferior phrenic veins, and the hepatic veins. Note that the major veins from the GI tract drain to the portal venous system and deliver blood to the liver. Thereafter this blood drains into the hepatic veins and thence to the IVC.

Large blood clots (*thrombi*) from either the lower limbs or the pelvic plexus may lodge in the IVC and significantly obstruct it. In such cases, the collateral routes for blood flow will be called into service (the epigastric veins of the anterior abdominal wall, lateral thoracic veins, thoracoepigastric vein, internal thoracic vein, and intercostal veins, to name just a few).

5.10 ▶ Systems Review and Surface Anatomy of the Abdomen

▶ Musculoskeletal Anatomy of the Abdomen

▶ Arterial Supply of the Abdomen

▶ Venous Drainage of the Abdomen

▶ Lymphatic Drainage of the Abdomen

▶ Innervation of the Abdomen

▶ Surface Anatomy of the Abdomen

MUSCULOSKELETAL ANATOMY OF THE ABDOMEN

The skeletal structures involved in the formation of the abdomen are the lower four or five **ribs** and **costal margin,** the **xiphoid process** of the sternum, the five **lumbar vertebrae,** the **sacrum,** and the **hip bones.** The **diaphragm** forms the superior limit of the abdominal cavity, and much of the anterolateral wall is formed by the layers of the abdominal wall. An important specialized area of the abdominal wall is the **inguinal canal,** which in the male marks the area where the testis descends from the abdominal wall into the scrotum. As the testis descends, it is accompanied by several concentric layers of the muscle and fascia composing the abdominal wall. The location of the inguinal canal subjects it to high levels of pressure, because of gravity and to the movements of the intestinal viscera.

The pelvic diaphragm (see Figure 5-58) forms the lower limit of the abdominal cavity, providing a barrier to prevent contents from leaving the abdominal cavity. It is also capable of contraction, to increase intraabdominal pressure.

ARTERIAL SUPPLY OF THE ABDOMEN

The abdominal wall is supplied with blood by the **lower intercostal arteries,** which extend beyond the ends of the lower ribs and travel across the anterior abdominal wall toward the midline. In the posterior abdominal wall, the four or five **lumbar arteries** (see Figure 5-44), segmental branches off the abdominal aorta, provide blood supply.

The organs within the abdominal cavity and those embedded in its wall are supplied by branches of the abdominal aorta. The aorta has three distinct types of branches within the abdomen: (1) **unpaired branches to viscera** (the celiac, superior mesenteric, and inferior mesenteric arteries, see Figures 5-34 and 5-44), (2) **paired visceral branches** (the suprarenal, renal, and gonadal arteries), and (3) **paired branches to the body wall** (the inferior phrenic and lumbar arteries). The median sacral artery is a single midline vessel supplying the tissue covering the anterior surface of the sacrum. It arises from the bifurcation of the aorta, at the L4 vertebral level.

Arterial supply of the abdomen has anastomoses with vessels in the thorax, pelvis, and lower limbs. From above, the **internal thoracic artery** ends by dividing into the **musculophrenic artery** (to the diaphragm) and the **superior epigastric artery,** which descends on the deep surface of the rectus abdominus muscle and anastomoses with the **inferior epigastric artery.** The inferior and superior epigastric arteries both anastomose with branches of the lower intercostal arteries as they course around the abdominal wall toward the anterior midline.

Within the abdominal cavity, there are rich anastomoses between the arteries supplying the digestive tract. The celiac and superior mesenteric arteries anastomose through branches that supply the head of the pancreas—specifically through the **superior pancreaticoduodenal artery** (from the celiac) and the **inferior pancreaticoduodenal artery** (from the superior mesenteric artery). The superior and inferior mesenteric arteries anastomose through the **middle colic branch** (of the superior mesenteric) and the **left colic branch** (of the inferior mesenteric). In fact, there is a **marginal artery** that supplies blood to the ascending, transverse, and descending colon. It courses along the convex side of the colon, about 2 to 3 cm from it. This marginal artery is fed by both the superior and inferior mesenteric arteries, and is a source of collateral flow for the entire colon if any single vessel supplying it becomes interrupted (see Figure 5-17).

The **gonadal arteries (ovarian** or **testicular)** arise from the aorta at the L2 level, reminding us that the gonads took their embryologic origin from this part of the abdominal wall and later undergo considerable migration inferiorly. They appear to "drag" their blood supply with them as they migrate, accounting for the long intraabdominal course of the gonadal vessels.

VENOUS DRAINAGE OF THE ABDOMEN

Venous drainage of the abdomen also falls into two major groups: the drainage of the abdominal wall and the drainage of the abdominal viscera. The *abdominal wall* is drained by intercostal, lumbar, and epigastric veins. The **intercostal veins** drain to the azygos and hemiazygos systems, passing posterior to the diaphragm as they do. The **lumbar veins,** especially the lower two or three, drain directly to the inferior vena cava. The anterior abdominal wall is drained by the **superior epigastric veins,** which drain upward to the internal thoracic and ultimately to the subclavian veins, and the **inferior epigastric veins,** which drain inferiorly to the external iliac veins and ultimately to the inferior vena cava.

The *abdominal viscera* are drained by a set of veins that converge in the upper abdomen to form the **hepatic portal vein.** The portal vein is formed by the union of the **splenic** and **superior mesenteric veins,** with the inferior mesenteric vein usually draining into the splenic vein. Blood in the portal vein arose in the capillary beds of the intestinal tract and will pass into the capillary beds of the liver. The passage of blood from one set of capillaries into another set of capillaries, before returning to the heart, is what defines a portal system. From the liver, blood passes through the short hepatic veins into the inferior vena cava.

LYMPHATIC DRAINAGE OF THE ABDOMEN

The abdominal wall drains inferiorly to the inguinal region and superiorly to the sternal and anterior wall nodes. Internally, the abdominal viscera drain to nodes located along the abdominal aorta, and for the most part the drainage of a particular organ corresponds to the arterial supply to that organ. The one seeming exception is the gonads, whose lymphatic drainage is to nodes along the aorta in the vicinity of the renal arteries because the embryologic origin of the gonads is from that region of the posterior abdominal wall.

INNERVATION OF THE ABDOMEN

The abdominal wall is innervated by distal branches of the **intercostal nerves T8 to L12.** These nerves innervate the muscles of the abdominal wall in these regions and the skin overlying these areas. The T12 segment supplies axons to both the iliohypogastric and iliohypogastric nerves. The **iliohypogastric nerve** innervates the area just above the pubic symphysis, and the **ilioinguinal nerve** traverses the inguinal canal to innervate the skin at the base of the upper scrotum/labium majus and the skin in the upper medial thigh.

The tissue layers of the spermatic cord are derived from the layers of the lower abdominal wall and are innervated by branches of the upper lumbar nerves. In particular, the **genitofemoral nerve** (from L1 to L2) innervates the *cremaster muscle,* a derivative of the internal oblique muscle of the abdominal wall.

Innervation of the lining of the abdominal cavity (i.e., the peritoneal membrane) varies by region. The inner lining of the body wall, from posterior to anterior, is innervated by branches of the intercostal nerves. The peritoneum covering the inferior surface of the diaphragm also is innervated by the phrenic nerve. The peritoneal layers enclosing the abdominal viscera are innervated by sensory axons accompanying the parasympathetic and sympathetic motor axons supplying those organs.

The motor innervation of the *abdominal viscera* is by sympathetic and parasympathetic axons. The **sympathetic** supply originates in the T6 to T12 segments of the spinal cord. These preganglionic axons collect into the *greater, lesser,* and *least splanchnic nerves,* which course medially away from the sympathetic chain, pass from thorax to abdomen by coursing posterior to the diaphragm, and synapse in one of several ganglia located along the abdominal aorta. Most prominent among these is the *celiac ganglion;* the other ganglia are the *superior mesenteric, inferior mesenteric,* and *aorticorenal.* From each of these ganglia, postganglionic axons arise and follow arterial branches traveling from the aorta to the various regions of the digestive tracts (from lower esophagus to rectum) via the celiac, superior, and inferior mesenteric arteries and their branches. Generally, the sympathetic input reduces peristaltic activity and inhibits the digestive process.

Parasympathetic supply to the abdomen is via the *vagus nerve*, innervating the GI tract from the esophagus to the mid-transverse colon, and via the *sacral parasympathetics* (the pelvic nerve) for points distal to the mid-transverse colon. In each instance, the nerves reaching the wall of the intestine are preganglionic; they synapse on mural ganglia in the wall of the intestine, and from these small clusters of neurons originate short postganglionic axons that directly innervate the intestine. In general, parasympathetic input increases digestive activity, promoting peristalsis and relaxing gastrointestinal sphincters. Both sympathetic and parasympathetic nerves reach the intraperitoneal parts of the GI tract by traveling within the two leaflets of the mesentery supporting that part of the gut (e.g., mesojejunum, mesogastrium, mesocolon).

SURFACE ANATOMY OF THE ABDOMEN

The boundaries of the abdomen are the **costal** margin superiorly, the **pubis** and **inguinal ligaments** inferiorly, and the lumbar **vertebral column** posteriorly. The two sides of the abdominal wall meet in the anterior midline in a vertical fibrous cord, the linea alba (see Figure 5-5). In a slender person, the vertical linea alba may be seen easily, extending from the xiphoid process to the pubis. Just lateral to the linea alba, on both sides of the abdomen, lies the vertical–band–like rectus abdominus muscle, also extending from the xiphoid process to the pubis. The lateral borders of the rectus femoris (known as the linea semilunaris) also are visible in the slender subject (see Figure 5-6). Three or sometimes four horizontal tendinous inscriptions are visible on the rectus abdominus muscle, extending from the linea alba to the **linea semilunaris**. Usually two of the inscriptions are above the level of the umbilicus and the remainder below it.

Complex nomenclatures have been devised to describe particular regions on the anterior abdominal wall, but the one in most common use is the simple division of the abdominal wall into four quadrants, with the umbilicus as the central point. These are known as the *right upper quadrant (RUQ), left lower quadrant (LLQ),* and so on. These terms may be used, for example, to describe the location of pain or of an abnormal mass in the abdominal wall. Other important landmarks in the abdominal wall include the transpyloric plane, a horizontal line passing through the pyloric sphincter at approximately the L1 vertebral level. Many structures in the abdomen are mobile and cannot be expected to remain in a given position. However, the pylorus and proximal duodenum are fixed to the posterior wall and remain a consistent point of reference for the localization of other structures: the **epigastric region**, an area located just beneath the xiphoid process, and the **suprapubic region**, a small expanse of skin lying just superior to the pubis. **McBurney's point** is located about two thirds of the way along an imaginary line extending from the pubic symphysis to the anterior superior iliac spine of the pelvis. In the majority of patients, this marks the location of the appendix.

The anterior abdominal region of most clinical importance is the **inguinal region**. The inguinal canal is located 1 to 2 cm superior to the **inguinal ligament** and is parallel to it. It is particularly important in the male because it accommodates passage of the testis from the abdominal wall into the scrotum, accompanied by coverings derived from several layers of the abdominal wall. At the medial end of the inguinal canal is the **superficial** or **external inguinal ring**, the crescentlike edge of which is concave inferomedially. It is palpable on physical examination of a slender male.

The posterior abdominal wall also has some interesting and important landmarks. The **crests of the ilia** form bony arcs in the lower back. A horizontal line connecting the crests of the two ilia cross the vertebral column at the level of L4 and this simple relationship is used routinely by those performing spinal taps. Locating the L4 vertebra makes it possible to be sure that the needle can be inserted into the correct intervertebral space (usually L4-L5 or L5-S1). Inserting the spinal needle into the interior of the vertebral canal is safe at this level because the spinal cord itself ends at approximately the level of the L2 vertebra. The lower two ribs on the left side overly the **kidney**, while on the right only the twelfth rib overlies the superior pole of the kidney. The left kidney is positioned slightly higher than the right. Ribs 9 through 11 on the left overlie the **spleen**.

It is important to emphasize the difference between the **thoracic cavity** and the **thoracic cage**, and the implications of this arrangement for the abdominal viscera. The thoracic cage extends inferiorly and partially protects much of the abdominal viscera, including the spleen, stomach, liver, and kidneys. These organs are in the abdominal cavity because they are inferior to the diaphragm.

5.11 ◀ case studies
Abdomen

■ CASE 1

A 37-YEAR-OLD FEMALE WITH A CHEST WALL MASS

A 37-year-old woman had noted for several months a growing, firm, brownish-colored mass about 1 cm in diameter on the lower part of her ribcage on the left, 2 to 3 cm inferior to the lateral margin of her breast. It was not painful at rest but had increasingly been abraded by her clothing, leading to recurrent bleeding and signs of inflammation. She consulted with her physician, and the physician recommended excision and laboratory diagnosis of the mass. The patient inquired about what method of pain relief would be used, because she was very fearful of the pain that might be involved in excision of the mass. The patient also was against the idea of "going to sleep" and having to stay overnight in the hospital to accomplish removal of the mass. The physician reassured her that the pain involved could be eliminated and that the removal could be accomplished without need for general anesthesia.

Questions

1. What method of pain relief would you recommend for this patient?
2. How and where is pain relief of this sort provided for the patient?

■ CASE 2

A 49-YEAR-OLD MALE WITH LOWER ABDOMINAL PAIN

A 49-year old male experienced a sharp pain in the lower part of his abdomen on the right. The pain was exacerbated during lifting and other forceful exertions but vanished when he rested. His physician noted a palpable swelling slightly above and lateral to the pubic tubercle on the right and recommended rest for several weeks. He ignored the pain initially, however, and economic necessity forced him to continue to work as a carpenter. Several weeks later, he once again experienced a sharp pain in the abdomen, but this time it was unrelenting and was accompanied by fever and sweating. Over the next several hours, he vomited repeatedly, and his abdomen felt firm. He again visited his physician, where a distended abdomen and an extremely tender lower abdominal wall on the right were observed. His right scrotal sac was extremely painful to the touch. His white cell count was high, consistent with infection, and measurement of blood chemistry revealed that he was acidotic (blood pH abnormally low), indicating tissue inflammation. He was taken to the operating room.

Questions

1. What caused the earlier lower abdominal pain associated with exertion but relieved at rest?
2. What complication may have caused the pain to become constant and to be associated with fever and other signs of infection?

■ CASE 3

A 12-YEAR-OLD GIRL WITH BLOODY STOOLS

A 12-year-old girl noted blood on the tissue she used after having a bowel movement. She felt that it might somehow be connected to the onset of menses, which for her had begun just 1 month earlier. She did not mention this bleeding to her parents, but, when it continued for several weeks, she decided to tell her parents about it. She reported to them and to the physician that the blood was not always present, was sometimes present in large amounts, and was never associated with pain. She had no fever, sweating, chills, or other sign of infection, but several days later she developed vomiting and abdominal distension. An imaging study was performed, and she was subsequently taken to the operating room.

Questions

1. What caused the painless rectal bleeding in this patient?
2. Why did the anatomy of her disease change abruptly and produce signs of intestinal obstruction?

■ CASE 4

A 75-YEAR-OLD MAN WITH VOMITING, LETHARGY AND JAUNDICE

A 75-year-old man in good general health noted some episodic vomiting and diarrhea but felt it was nothing more than a reflection of his busy life, with travel and irregular meals and sleep. However, he also noted progressive weakness and loss of his usual energy. He began to be more concerned when he realized that he had lost 8 pounds and observed a mild yellowing of his sclerae. On visiting a physician, he recalled that he had been having more frequent bowel movements and that they were light in color and seemed to be very greasy and foul-smelling. Several blood tests and imaging studies confirmed the diagnosis.

Questions

1. What signs arouse suspicion that this is more than a nonspecific gastroenteritis?
2. How can the yellowish discoloration of sclerae and the fatty stools be explained by one lesion or disease process?

■ CASE 5

A 50-YEAR-OLD WITH STRESS AND ABDOMINAL PAIN

A 50-year-old executive was constantly plagued with epigastric pain, vomiting, and weight loss. She was increasingly intolerant of various types of foods and lost sleep because of pain and increasingly frequent vomiting as well. On a recent visit to her physician, it was discovered that she was slightly anemic (her red blood cell count was low), although her menses had ceased 7 years earlier. Her physician recommended use of antacids and other medications to lower gastric acidity, but the symptoms continued and even worsened. Because her problems were interrupting her family and work life, she agreed to a surgical procedure.

Questions

1. What sort of surgical procedure would be recommended, and what is the anatomic-physiologic basis for the surgery?

■ CASE 6

A 2-WEEK-OLD CHILD WITH VOMITING

A newborn male child was taken home from the hospital by his parents and was seemingly normal for about 2 weeks, but after that began to vomit increasingly often. The vomiting was worst after feeding, and, on the advice of their pediatrician, the parents tried to give smaller and more frequent feedings, but this did not help the situation. There was no history of diarrhea. On visiting the pediatrician again, the parents reported that the vomiting seemed very forceful and clearly was not simply the regurgitation of a small amount of the food the child had ingested at feeding. The physician inquired about the color of the vomitus, and the parents stated that it was pale yellow to whitish and was not greenish. Physical examination of the child quickly disclosed the source of the problem, and a surgical procedure was scheduled.

Questions

1. What accounts for the "projectile" nature of the vomiting?
2. What is the significance of the observation that the vomitus was not greenish in color?

■ CASE 7

A 9-YEAR-OLD GIRL WITH A "SORE TUMMY"

A 9-year-old awoke in the middle of the night and complained to her father and mother that her "tummy hurt," especially around her umbilicus. The pain was not sharp or stabbing, and her abdomen was only slightly tender to the touch. Her parents gave her some antacids and she went back to sleep. At about 6 AM she awoke once again, and this time was crying with the sharpness and severity of the pain. The pain now was not paraumbilical, seemed located in the right lower quadrant, and was severe, not mild or moderate. Touching her abdomen, especially in the right lower area, caused excruciating pain, and she demonstrated rebound tenderness—that is, when the examiner's hand was pressed gently into the abdominal wall and then released quickly, there was a quick and intense pain in that area. Her fever was now 103° F, and her eyes seemed glassy and shining. She was nauseated and refused food or drink. She was moaning softly and found it necessary to lie down in a "curled-up" position to get at least a little relief from the pain. She was taken to the emergency room, and blood tests showed a very high white blood cell count. Her mother objected when the physician on duty said that she needed to perform a rectal examination on the little girl, but eventually the mother understood its importance. With the diagnosis confirmed, surgery was performed.

Questions

1. What disease process is at work here, and what is the usual therapy for it?
2. Why was the little girl's pain initially milder and periumbilical?
3. Why is the later pain very sharp and localized in the right lower quadrant?
4. Why would a process such as this cause nausea and vomiting?
5. What is the importance of the rectal examination in this case?

■ *CASE 8*

STAB WOUNDS IN THE ABDOMINAL WALL OF A 19-YEAR-OLD MAN

A 19-year-old man was involved in an altercation in a bar, and was brought to an emergency room for treatment. His opponent evidently had stabbed him several times in the back and sides. The patient, on arrival at the ER, was in some pain but seemed otherwise stable. There was a moderate amount of blood in his urine. He had several stab wounds over the lower ribs and on each side of the posterior abdominal wall. It was decided to observe him overnight in the hospital. He awoke at about 3 AM with a distended abdomen, very painful to the touch, and was vomiting blood-tinged material. His blood count showed that his hematocrit had fallen from 35% (when he had first arrived at the ER) to 17%. He was taken immediately to surgery.

Questions

1. What accounted for the blood in his urine on arrival at the ER?
2. What abdominal structures are vulnerable to a penetrating stab wound near the kidney?
3. What single stab wound might be able to produce all of these symptoms and signs?

■ *CASE 9*

A NEWBORN BABY WITH DIFFICULTY BREATHING

A term baby, weighing 3600 g (8 lb), underwent a normal birth and seemed healthy for the first several minutes. She then began to show very labored breathing, with deep retractions and an accelerated respiratory rate. She lost her initial pink color and became progressively dark and ashen. Her level of alertness also began to deteriorate. When the intern examined the patient, he seemed to hear the baby's heartbeat stronger on the right side of the chest than on the left but was reluctant to report this to his supervisors. The baby seemed to have much better movement of air on the right side of the chest than on the left. Another strange finding that impressed the intern was the flatness of the baby's abdomen, almost to the point where it appeared "scooped-out." A chest x-ray was taken, and the diagnosis was confirmed. Surgery was performed, and, although the baby experienced some improvement over the first postoperative week, she then became progressively sicker and eventually died about three weeks later.

Questions

1. What accounts for the shift of the heartbeat to the left side of the chest and the stronger breath sounds on the right side of the chest than the left?
2. Why is the abdominal wall flattened?
3. What is the developmental error that produces this major congenital defect?
4. Why do many such patients die even when the anatomic abnormalities are corrected?

▌ *CASE 1*

1. Excision of masses of this sort are perfect opportunities for use of local or regional anesthesia. The use of regional anesthesia is desirable for a number of reasons—it does not require overnight hospitalization, it avoids the small but real risks attendant to general anesthesia, it minimizes the risk of systemic spread of the anesthetic agent, and it reduces the expense associated with minor surgical procedures of this kind.

2. Regional anesthesia for a procedure like this would be administered by injecting a local anesthetic such as lidocaine into the tissues near the intercostal nerve(s) innervating the skin regions in which the mass is located. The anesthetic usually is injected into the posterior thoracic wall, along the inferior margin of the ribs in the selected interspaces, meaning that distal to the area where the anesthetic is injected, the tissues (including the skin) will be numb and painfree. For example, if this mass is located in the skin overlying the seventh intercostal space, the anesthetic is injected posteriorly, just inferior to the seventh rib. It also will be necessary to anesthetize the fifth, sixth, eighth, and ninth intercostal nerves, in an identical fashion, in recognition of the fact that there is overlap of nerve branches into the tissues of one to two intercostal spaces on each side of the intercostal space where the lesion is located.

▌ *CASE 2*

1. This patient has all the signs of an inguinal hernia, in which forceful exertion, leading to an increase in intraabdominal pressure, would force intestinal contents to herniate into the inguinal region.

2. Later, when the patient began to have signs of systemic infection, the most reasonable surmise is that a portion of his intestine has herniated much further into the inguinal canal and has become trapped within that hernia sac so that the blood supply to that portion of the intestine is interrupted. This is known as *incarceration of the hernia.* This leads to tissue injury and necrosis of that portion of the intestine. Injury to the intestine in this way leads to an obstruction proximal to the interruption, leading to abdominal distension and vomiting. As the necrotic intestinal segment becomes inflamed, white cells increase and fever increases as part of the normal response to inflammation. In the operating room, the surgeon will attempt to remove the loop of intestine from the inguinal canal, and, if necessary, remove the segment of bowel that has been injured by lack of blood supply. Recall that the surgeon will locate the inferior epigastric vessels when exploring the inguinal region (see Figure 5-10), knowing that if the herniated portion of intestine passes lateral to those vessels, the hernia is a *congenital hernia* (meaning that the hernia retraces the descent of the testis). If the hernia is medial to the inferior epigastric vessels, it is an *acquired hernia,* not retracing the path of testicular migration, but instead pushing directly forward through the weakened tissues of the lower anterior abdominal wall.

▌ *CASE 3*

1. *Meckel's diverticulum* is a remnant of the vitelline duct (connection of definitive gut with primary yolk sac). It reminds us of the fact that during the sixth to tenth weeks of gestation, much of the intestinal tract of the embryo herniates through the umbilicus to the outside of the body as a part of normal development. It is found about 30 to 35 cm proximal to the ileocecal junction. Present in about 2% to 3% of adults, a Meckel's diverticulum may be lined with ectopic gastric mucosa, produce HCl, and lead to bleeding caused by irritation of the mucosa of the ileum (to which the diverticulum is connected).

2. In this patient, the abrupt worsening of her condition was caused by a *volvulus,* or twisting of the adjacent intestinal loops around the diverticulum, which serves as a sort of tether around which the rotation occurs. This compromises the blood flow to the intestine and produces symptoms of an obstruction. The Meckel's diverticulum may be a simple strand of tissue or may be enlarged and actually contain a portion of the intestine itself.

■ *CASE 4*

1. This patient almost certainly is suffering from a *tumor in the head of his pancreas,* enlarging to the point that it is obstructing both the common bile duct and the pancreatic duct. The obstructed common bile duct prevents bile from reaching the interior of the intestine, meaning that the stool will be unusually light in color and that the patient will have difficulty absorbing fats. The blockage of pancreatic enzyme delivery to the intestine also promotes fat malabsorption and limits the digestion of carbohydrates and proteins as well. Over 80% of pancreatic cancers are found in the head region. *Benign pancreatic cysts* also may form. Neither surgical nor medical treatments of pancreatic cancer are very successful, and the mortality rate from this disease is high. This sort of tumor is one of many illustrations of how a relatively small lesion can cause major symptoms and even be life-threatening.

2. *Jaundice* is the accumulation of a yellow pigment, bilirubin, and can appear in the sclerae of the eyes as well as beneath the skin. The fatty stools suggest a deficiency of lipase enzymes manufactured in the pancreas. A tumor in the head of the pancreas can enlarge and obstruct both the bile duct and pancreatic duct.

■ *CASE 5*

1. Some version of a *vagotomy* (see Figure 5-35) often is performed to diminish gastric acidity (because vagal innervation promotes acid secretion by parietal cells). A *complete vagotomy* (sectioning the vagus nerves completely on the surface of the esophagus) diminishes acid production but produces adverse side effects on gastric emptying and pancreatic, hepatic, and proximal large bowel function. When all of the branches of the nerves of Latarjet including the antral branches, are cut, but branches to pancreas, liver, and distal bowel are spared, it is termed a *selective vagotomy.* When the antral branches of the nerves of Latarjet are spared, but their other branches are cut, it is a *highly selective vagotomy,* aimed at diminishing HCl production in the body and fundus but preserving the innervation of the antrum (and avoiding problems in gastric emptying). Any procedure that affects gastric emptying may necessitate a surgical change in the gastric outlet.

■ *CASE 6*

1. Projectile vomiting means that vomitus is expelled from the mouth with considerable force. It is caused by the complete or near-complete obstruction of the pylorus, so that gastric contents accumulate and are forcibly propelled with contraction of the stomach musculature and the striated muscles of the anterior abdominal wall.

2. This child suffers from *pyloric stenosis,* an excessive thickening of the pyloric sphincter. The vomitus in these situations is not greenish because the obstruction is proximal to the point where bile enters the intestine. Enlargement of the pyloric outlet is indicated in this sort of case. The surgery is performed by making a partial-thickness incision in the wall of the pyloric sphincter, allowing the diameter of the lumen of the pylorus to enlarge. Oddly, this condition is most common in first-born male white children.

■ *CASE 7*

1. The diagnosis is *acute appendicitis,* and the therapy in virtually every case is surgical removal of the inflamed appendix and attention to any ancillary injury that has resulted from the injury to the appendix.

2. Her pain was initially paraumbilical because the appendix is innervated by a segment of the spinal cord that also provides sensory innervation to the skin at and around the umbilicus. Evidently the pathologic process in the appendix itself cannot cause a conscious sense of pain, presumably because the nerves there do not usually cause conscious sensations. This is a classic example of *referred pain,* where a pathologic process in one area (in this case the appendix) can cause painful sensations in an area of skin that is innervated by the same segment of the spinal cord (even though there is no pathologic process afoot in the umbilicus itself).

3. The right lower quadrant pain began when the inflamed appendix burst, and its inflammatory pus contacted the parietal peritoneum lining the anterior abdominal wall (or perhaps when the swollen and inflamed appendix simply came into contact with the anterior abdominal wall). The parietal peritoneum is richly innervated and very sensitive to various stimuli. Rebound tenderness probably results from the stretching force that deep palpation of the abdominal wall produces.

4. A variety of abnormal processes in the digestive tract cause the normal peristaltic muscular activity to cease, so that the gut becomes immobile (an ileus) along all or part of its course. When this occurs, gas and liquid can build up in the digestive tube, causing it to distend and eventually leading to vomiting. When infections are the course of appendicitis, there also may be toxins, produced by the bacteria, that produce nausea and vomiting.

5. If an inflamed appendix is in a very low position, extending downward into the pelvis, it may not be accessible by ordinary palpation and examination of the anterior abdominal wall. In such cases, a digital rectal examination may allow the examiner to detect the location of the inflamed appendix.

■ *CASE 8*

1. The history and finding of *hematuria* (blood in the urine) suggests that the kidney on one or both sides has been stabbed, causing blood to leak into the urine. The kidneys are both positioned internal to the lower ribs (the twelfth alone on the right side and the eleventh and twelfth on the left side).

2. A review of the relationships of the kidneys will reveal that the liver, hepatic flexure, and duodenum lie anterior to the right kidney, while the spleen, stomach, pancreas, and jejunum lie anterior to the left kidney.

3. A single penetrating wound of the upper half of the left kidney would injure the kidney itself as well as the stomach and spleen. Continued bleeding of the spleen can cause blood to spill into the abdominal cavity, making it tense and painful to the touch. Vomiting of blood would result from the penetrating wound of the stomach.

■ *CASE 9*

1. In this case of *congenital diaphragmatic hernia* (see Figure 5-7), a major share of the intestinal tract has herniated through a diaphragmatic defect into the left pleural cavity. The presence of these intestinal loops in the chest shifts the mediastinum (and thus the heart) to the right and tends to compress whatever left lung tissue may be present, so that little aeration of the left lung occurs.

2. The abdominal wall is flattened, or *scaphoid*, because a significant share of the intestinal contents has herniated into the chest.

3. The diaphragm forms by the fusion of a series of tissue primordia, and, when the fusion of two or more of these primordia is incomplete, a defect will persist. The most common location for such a defect is on the left side, along the posterior border of the diaphragm.

4. If this developmental error occurs early in development, the intestinal loops will occupy the chest cavity for many months and prevent the lung on that side of the chest from developing normally. If the defect occurs early in development, even surgical replacement of the intestines into the abdomen will not stabilize the patient because the left lung in particular and to a lesser degree the right lung will be *hypoplastic*, or dwarfed, and not sufficient to the task of providing effective respiration for the patient. If the defect occurs later in development, the lung on the left will have developed enough to allow it to carry out respiration successfully when the intestines are surgically replaced in the abdomen.

SECTION SIX

Pelvis and Perineum

▶ **6.1** Bony Pelvis

▶ **6.2** Perineum

▶ **6.3** Pelvic Vasculature and Nerve Supply

▶ **6.4** Urinary System

▶ **6.5** Pelvic Viscera in the Female

▶ **6.6** Pelvic Viscera in the Male

▶ **6.7** Systems Review and Surface Anatomy of the Pelvis and Perineum

▶ **6.8** Case Studies: Pelvis and Perineum

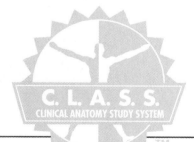

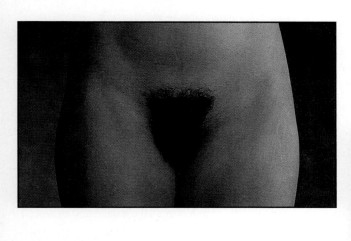
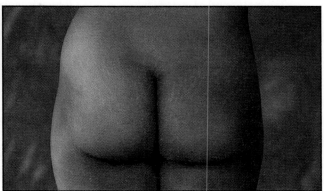
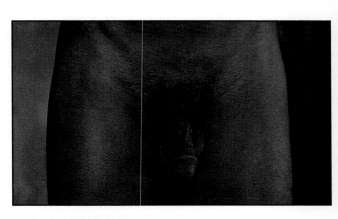
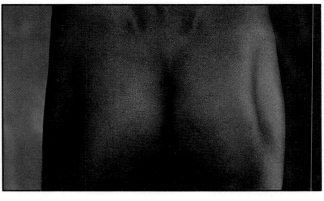

6.1

section six.one

Bony Pelvis

▶ Bones of the Pelvis

▶ Ligaments and Joints of the Pelvis

▶ Greater and Lesser Sciatic Foramina

▶ Sexual Dimorphism in Pelvic Shape

▶ Pelvic Interior

▶ Peritoneum, Pelvic Fascia, and Pelvic Viscera

The three-dimensional relationships of structures in the pelvis are difficult to visualize. The bony **pelvis** is a funnel-shaped structure made up of several individual bones. The superior aperture leading into the pelvis (the **pelvic inlet**) is wider than the inferior aperture leading out of the pelvis (the **pelvic outlet**). The pelvic inlet is the space surrounded by the broad wings of the ilia, the sacrum, and the pubic symphysis (Figure 6-1). The pelvic outlet is the space outlined by the paired inferior pubic rami, the ischia, the ischial spines, and the coccyx. The pelvis is often considered to consist of (1) a *greater pelvis* (or *"false" pelvis*), which is the space surrounded by the upper portions of the iliac bones and the upper part of the sacrum posteriorly (see Figure 6-1, *B* and *C*), and (2) a *lesser pelvis* (or *"true" pelvis*) more deeply placed and surrounded by the margins of the obturator foramen, the ischial spines, and the lower portion of the sacrum (see Figure 6-1). The *arcuate line* of the ilium (see below) marks a rough boundary between the greater and lesser pelves. The lesser pelvis contains the true structures of the pelvis, including the internal genitalia and the bladder, while the greater pelvis is in reality the lower portion of the abdominal cavity.

There are two important muscular diaphragms in the lower part of the pelvis, the **urogenital** and the **pelvic diaphragms** (see Figures 6-14 and 6-17). These close off the pelvic outlet and form a barrier (with appropriate perforations) between visceral contents of the pelvis (e.g., bladder, urethra, vagina, anus) and the ex-

terior. The pelvis also is the outlet for structures connecting the trunk and lower limbs (e.g., obturator nerve and vessels, sciatic nerve, gluteal vessels), just as the axilla is a zone of transition between the upper limb and the thorax and neck. A fuller description of these muscular diaphragms follows.

BONES OF THE PELVIS

The two *innominate bones* (or "hip" bones), the *sacrum,* and the *coccyx* (Figure 6-2) comprise the pelvis. The innominate bone is composed of the *ilium, ischium,* and *pubis.* Its *lateral* or *exterior surface* (Figure 6-3) consists of (1) an upper area, the lateral surface of the ilium, (2) a central depressed socket, the *acetabulum,* where the head of the femur articulates with the hip bone, and (3) a lower region, in which curved rami of the pubis and ischium unite to form a circular aperture surrounding the *obturator foramen.* On the *medial* or *interior surface* of the superior half of the pelvis is found (1) superiorly, the *iliac fossa,* a shallow depression in the ilium (see Figure 6-2), (2) a posterior roughened articular surface, facing medially, for the sacroiliac joint, and (3) inferiorly, the medial surface of the bony ring surrounding the *obturator foramen.*

The **ilium** (see Figure 6-3) consists of an upper fan-shaped segment, or *ala* (wing) and an inferior *body.* The *arcuate line* is the curved bony ridge on the interior surface of the ilium, dividing the iliac fossa from the lower portion of the ilium. The curved upper edge of the ilium is known as the *iliac crest.* The *anterior superior*

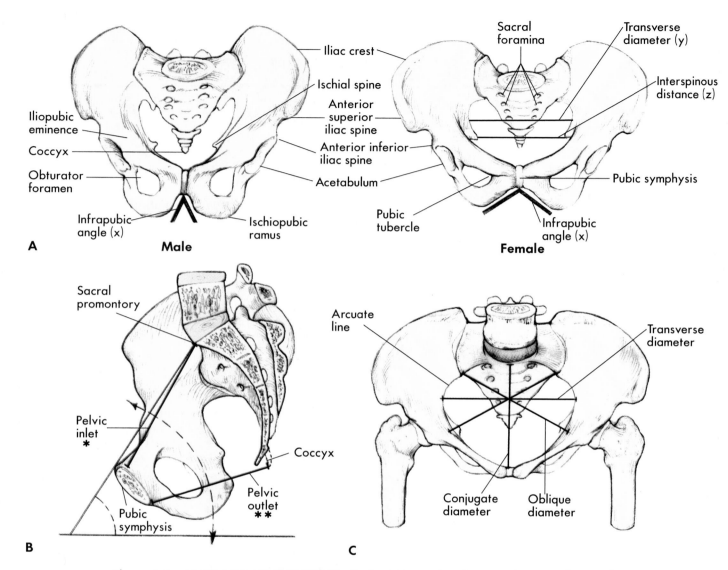

Figure 6-1   MALE AND FEMALE PELVIS. A, In this anterior view can be seen the gender differences in the infrapubic angle (*x*), the transverse diameter of the pelvic inlet (*y*), and the distance between ischial spines (*z*), one of the important dimensions of the pelvic outlet. **B,** A midsagittal view of the sacrum and right hip bone. The obstetrical conjugate (*) is the distance between the sacral promontory and the pubic symphysis; the inferior outlet (**) is the distance, in the midsagittal plane, between the pubic symphysis and the coccyx. **C,** An anterosuperior view of the pelvis. Marked are the transverse, oblique, and conjugate diameters. They are measured at the level of the arcuate line, separating the true and false pelves.

Iliac spine (ASIS) is not a spine at all but a smooth raised prominence at the anterior end of the iliac crest. To it attach the inguinal ligament and the sartorius muscle. The *anterior inferior iliac spine* lies along the anterior edge of the ilium, just inferior to the ASIS, and is an attachment for the rectus femoris muscle. At the posterior end of the iliac crest is the *posterior superior iliac spine*

which lies lateral to the articular surface for the sacroiliac joint (see Figure 6-2).

The **ischium** (see Figures 6-1 and 6-2) consists of a thick posteriorly directed *tuberosity*, from which radiates (1) an upwardly directed bony process forming part of the posterior perimeter of the obturator foramen and (2) a lower bony process fusing with the pubis to

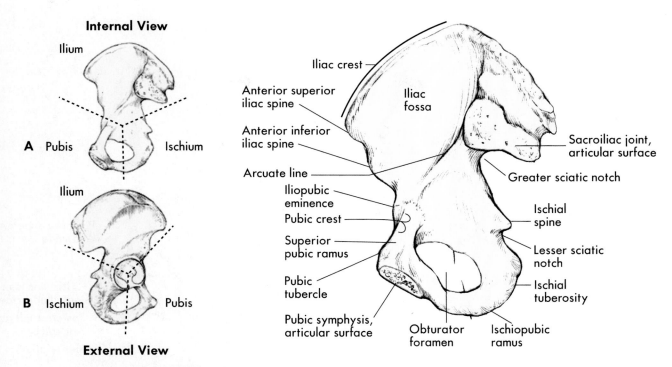

Internal View

Ilium

A Pubis   Ischium

Ilium

B Ischium   Pubis

External View

Iliac crest

Anterior superior iliac spine

Anterior inferior iliac spine

Arcuate line

Iliopubic eminence

Pubic crest

Superior pubic ramus

Pubic tubercle

Pubic symphysis, articular surface

Iliac fossa

Sacroiliac joint, articular surface

Greater sciatic notch

Ischial spine

Lesser sciatic notch

Ischial tuberosity

Obturator foramen

Ischiopubic ramus

Figure 6-2   INTERIOR OF THE HIP BONE. Note how in the natural position of the hip bone, the anterior superior spine, and the pubic tubercle are in the same vertical plane. Recognize that the pelvic canal is at a ~45 degree angle, not in a vertical plane. **A** and **B** show the internal and external views of the hip bone and the portions made up by the ilium, ischium, and pubis. SEE ATLAS, FIG. 6-4

complete the lower perimeter of the obturator foramen. This portion of the bony ring (see Figure 6-3) surrounding the obturator foramen is called the *ischiopubic ramus* to connote its dual origin. From the posterior margin of the ischium, 2 to 3 cm superior to the ischial tuberosity, protrudes the *ischial spine*. The sacrospinous ligament attaches to it. The inwardly curved bony edge (see Figures 6-2 and 6-3) connecting the ischial tuberosity to the ischial spine is the *lesser sciatic notch;* through it pass the pudendal vessels and nerves and the tendon of the obturator internus muscle (see Figure 6-8). A similar but larger curved bony ridge extends upward from the ischial spine to the articular surface of the sacroiliac joint; through this *greater sciatic notch* pass the sciatic nerve, gluteal vessels, and piriformis muscle.

The **pubis** is a V-shaped bone, with the apex of the V pointing medially (see Figures 6-2 and 6-3). The two pubic bones meet medially in the midline to form the *pubic symphysis.* The pubic symphysis consists of a fibrocartilaginous disk between the opposed pubic articular surfaces surrounded by strong ligaments (see following discussion). From the pubis there radiates laterally a superior and an inferior pubic ramus. The *superior pubic ramus* unites with the ilium and forms the superior bony strut partially surrounding the obturator foramen. The *inferior pubic ramus* joins a process from

the ischium to form the *ischiopubic ramus,* which serves as the inferior perimeter for the obturator foramen. The *pubic tubercle* is a small superiorly directed elevation (see Figures 6-2 and 6-3) about 1 to 2 cm lateral to the pubic symphysis; the medial end of the inguinal ligament attaches to the pubic tubercle, and the rectus abdominus attaches to it from above.

The **acetabulum** is a deep bony socket (see Figure 6-3) facing anteroinferolaterally and set in the innominate bone. The head of the femur articulates with the pelvis in the acetabulum. It is formed by parts of the ilium, ischium, and pubis, though not to equal degrees. The Y-shaped line of fusion of the three bones is often visible in the floor of the socket (see Figure 6-2). The raised circumferential perimeter of the acetabulum is interrupted inferiorly, forming the *acetabular notch*. This notch in life is spanned by the *transverse acetabular ligament*. The ligamentum teres of the femur appearing to "emerge" from the femoral head, attaches to the edges of the acetabular notch. An important part of the blood supply to the head of the femur travels with the ligamentum teres (see Figure 7-1, *C* and *D*), and injury to the ligament can interrupt this blood supply and jeopardize the head of the femur.

The **obturator foramen** is an ovoid aperture surrounded by a continuous rim of bone, derived from the

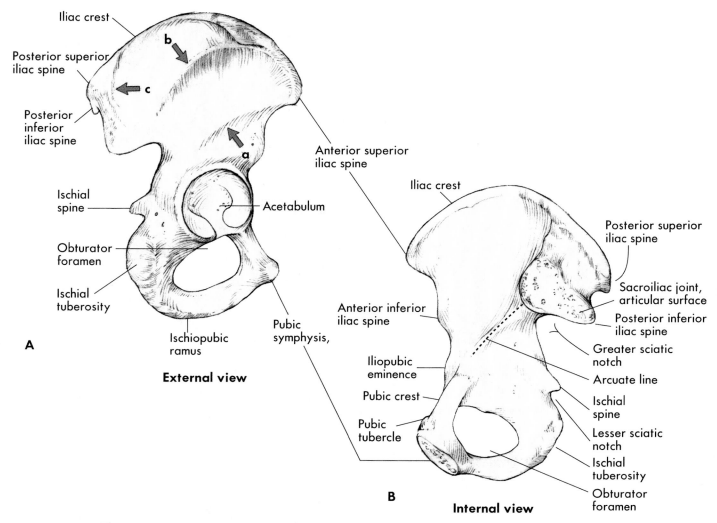

A

Iliac crest

Posterior superior iliac spine

Posterior inferior iliac spine

Ischial spine

Obturator foramen

Ischial tuberosity

Ischiopubic ramus

Acetabulum

Anterior superior iliac spine

Pubic symphysis,

External view

Iliac crest

Posterior superior iliac spine

Sacroiliac joint, articular surface

Posterior inferior iliac spine

Greater sciatic notch

Arcuate line

Ischial spine

Lesser sciatic notch

Ischial tuberosity

Obturator foramen

Anterior inferior iliac spine

Iliopubic eminence

Pubic crest

Pubic tubercle

B

Internal view

Figure 6-3   INNOMINATE (HIP) BONE. A, On the *lateral surface* of the hip bone are the acetabulum, posterior gluteal line (*c*), anterior gluteal line (*b*), and inferior gluteal line (*a*). **B,** On the *medial surface,* the linea terminalis (terminal line) is important because it marks the separation of the true pelvis (inferior to it) and the false pelvis (superior to it). The linea terminalis comprises the arcuate line, pubic crest, and pubic tubercle.

pubis and ischium (see Figure 6-3). The obturator foramen is filled in life by a tough obturator membrane, except for a small superomedial gap through which pass the obturator nerve and vessels.

The **sacrum** is the fusion of five sacral vertebrae, separate in embryonic life. The fusion of these vertebrae yields a bony shield, shaped like a curved inverted triangle (Figure 6-4). Pairs of anterior and posterior *sacral foramina*, located on the anterior and posterior surface of the sacrum, permit the exit of segmental nerves (anterior and posterior divisions). These foramina are analogous to the intervertebral foramina of the cervical, thoracic, and lumbar areas of the vertebral column. At the caudal end of the sacrum is a midline aperture, the *sacral hiatus* (Figure 6-5), which can be

used for injection of anesthetic material to numb the lower sacral segments.

The **coccyx** is a rudimentary tail, and forms from the fusion of two to four coccygeal vertebrae (see Figure 6-4). In mammals with long tails it can consist of dozens of individual vertebrae.

It is important to remember that the pelvis, although "funnel-like" in shape, is not positioned like an ordinary funnel, with the wide portion facing upwards and the spout inferiorly. Instead, the anterior superior spines lie directly superior to the pubic symphysis, so that the upper brim of the pelvis is *inclined forward at a ~50 degree angle* (when the person is standing in the anatomic position) (see Figure 6-1, *B* and *C*). This has consequences for some of the important organs in the

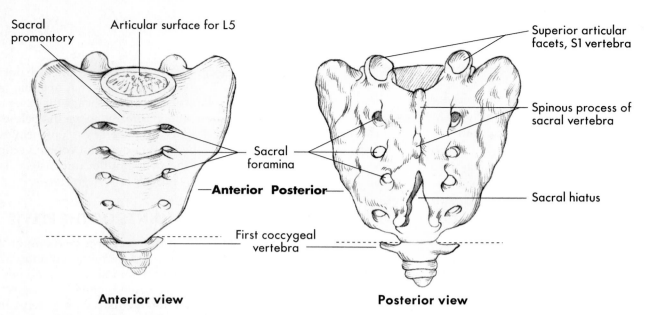

Anterior view　　　　　**Posterior view**

Figure 6-4　SACRUM AND COCCYX. Anterior and posterior sacral foramina for each segment together represent the equivalent of the intervertebral foramina found between adjacent separate vertebrae (e.g., lumbar, thoracic, cervical). The sacral promontory can interfere with delivery of the baby's head during childbirth. The coccyx represents the fusion of two to four individual coccygeal vertebrae. The Co1 vertebra articulates with the sacrum (*dashed lines*).

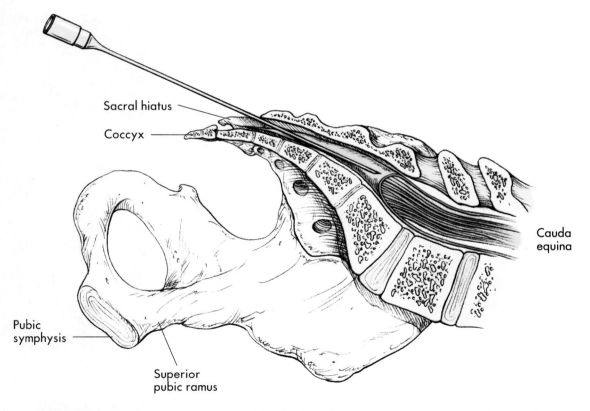

Figure 6-5　SACRAL ANESTHESIA. Midsagittal section through the sacrum, with a needle inserted through the sacral hiatus so that anesthetic material may bathe the lower sacral nerve roots. This technique allows anesthesia of the involved nerve roots without any necessity to provide full general anesthesia.

Human pelves exhibit some variation in shape and size apart from the major differences between male and female (Figure 6-6). A *gynecoid pelvis* (found in ~50% of women) features vertical pelvic walls with a transverse diameter greater than the anteroposterior diameter. An *android pelvis* has inwardly sloping walls, and, although the measurements of the pelvic inlet do not differ greatly from the gynecoid pelvis, the pelvic outlet is considerably more narrow. It is found in ~20% of women. A pelvis in which the transverse diameter is very much greater than the anteroposterior dimension is a *platypelloid pelvis.* It is rare in general but more frequent in whites than in Blacks or Asians. An *anthropoid pelvis* has an anteroposterior dimension greater than the transverse. It has a higher incidence in Black women. Knowledge of these shapes can predict certain difficulties in the passage of the baby's head during birth.

pelvis. As an example, the rectum and anus are not vertical, but tilted forward, while the anal opening is directed somewhat posteriorly. This means that the pelvic organs are not positioned directly above the pelvic and urogenital diaphragms, and the stress on them is reduced. Similarly, the urethra does not course vertically downward to exit the pelvic outlet but instead is inclined *anteriorly at a 45-degree to 50-degree angle.*

LIGAMENTS AND JOINTS OF THE PELVIS

Several strong ligaments connect portions of each hip bone to the sacrum and vertebral column. These ligaments provide strength, and also form the perimeter of some important named pelvic passages and spaces. The **sacroiliac ligaments** are extremely strong (Figures 6-7 and 6-8), and pass directly anterior and posterior to the *sacroiliac joint.* They bind the vertebral column (by way of the sacrum) to the pelvis and, by extension, the lower limb. This joint is of prime importance in transmitting force from the lower limb and pelvis to the vertebral column.

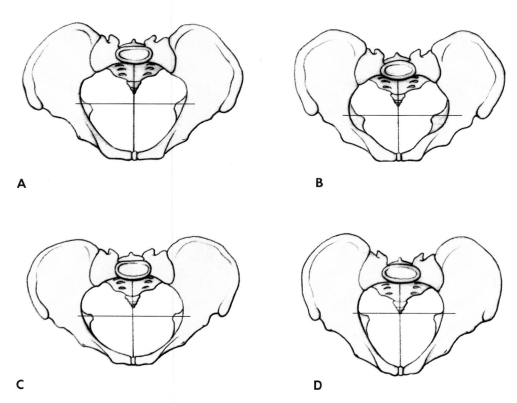

A

B

C

D

Figure 6-6   VARIATIONS IN PELVIC SHAPE. Four variations in pelvic shape. The intersecting horizontal (transverse diameter) and vertical (anteroposterior diameter) lines drawn through each help illustrate the variation in dimensions of the pelvic inlet. **A,** Gynecoid (typical female) shape. **B,** Android (typical male) shape. **C,** Platypelloid shape (overly wide). **D,** Anthropoid shape (overly narrow).

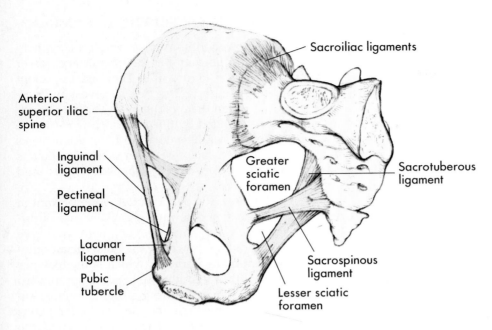

Anterior superior iliac spine

Inguinal ligament

Pectineal ligament

Lacunar ligament

Pubic tubercle

Sacroiliac ligaments

Greater sciatic foramen

Sacrotuberous ligament

Sacrospinous ligament

Lesser sciatic foramen

Figure 6-7 PELVIC LIGAMENTS, INTERNAL VIEW FROM SUPERIOR. Most of the important ligaments of the pelvis and sacrum, including the sacroiliac ligaments, inguinal ligament, lacunar ligament, sacrotuberous ligament, and sacrospinous ligament are visible here. SEE ATLAS, FIG. 7-37

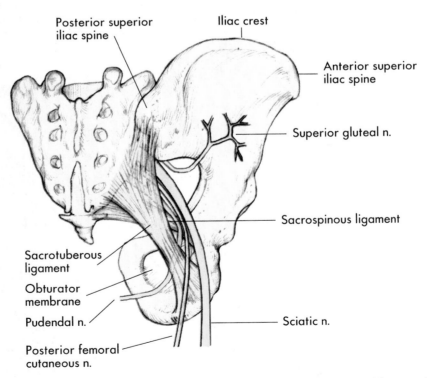

Posterior superior iliac spine

Iliac crest

Anterior superior iliac spine

Superior gluteal n.

Sacrospinous ligament

Sacrotuberous ligament

Obturator membrane

Pudendal n.

Sciatic n.

Posterior femoral cutaneous n.

Figure 6-8 PELVIC LIGAMENTS, EXTERNAL VIEW FROM POSTERIOR. Visible are the sacrotuberous and sacrospinous ligaments, as well as the sciatic, superior gluteal, posterior femoral cutaneous, and pudendal nerves. SEE ATLAS, FIG. 7-37

The body of vertebra L5 articulates (see Figures 6-1 and 6-4) directly with an upward-facing articular surface on the sacrum (forming the *lumbosacral joint*). The **iliolumbar ligaments** (Figure 6-9) connect the transverse processes of L5 to the iliac crests on each side. Some inferior fibers of this ligament attach to the lateral margin of the sacrum, and are recognized as the **lumbosacral ligament.**

The pubic symphysis (see Figures 6-1 and 6-9) consists of a fibrocartilaginous disk, joining the two pubic bones, surrounded by ligaments. This disk softens and the joint becomes more mobile during pregnancy. Note that such fibrocartilaginous joints occur in the midline of the body in other areas than the pubis—for example, the mental symphysis of the mandible, and the intervertebral disks.

The **sacrospinous ligaments** on each side connect the ischial spine (see Figures 6-8 and 6-9) to the lateral side of the sacrum. The **sacrotuberous ligaments** on each side connect the lower sacrum and coccyx to the ischial tuberosity.

GREATER AND LESSER SCIATIC FORAMINA

The sacrospinous and sacrotuberous ligaments help to create and form borders for the **greater** and **lesser sciatic foramina** (see Figure 6-7). They are important for the numerous important muscles, nerves, and vessels that pass through them (Table 6-1). The greater sciatic foramen is bounded by the *greater sciatic notch,* the upper lateral border of the *sacrum,* and the *sacrotuberous* and *sacrospinous ligaments.* The lesser sciatic foramen is bounded by the *lesser sciatic notch, sacrospinous,* and *sacrotuberous ligaments* (see Figure 6-7).

The dimensions of the pelvic outlet are important in obstetrics because they determine the likely ease or difficulty with which a vaginal delivery will occur (see Figure 6-6). In practice, however, the obstetrician relies most on the **conjugate diameter,** which is the distance between the sacral promontory and pubic symphysis, as palpated and estimated during a digital vaginal examination (see section on surface anatomy of the pelvis at the end of this chapter). The widest part of the baby's head is the **biparietal diameter,** or line extend-

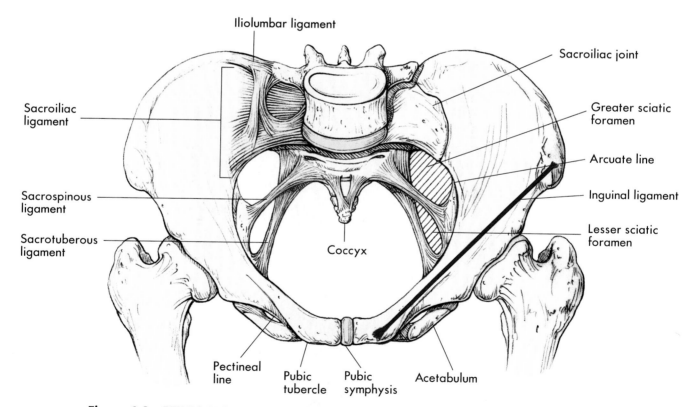

Figure 6-9   PELVIC LIGAMENTS, SUPEROANTERIOR VIEW. These important ligaments give the pelvis its strength.   SEE ATLAS, FIG. 6-6

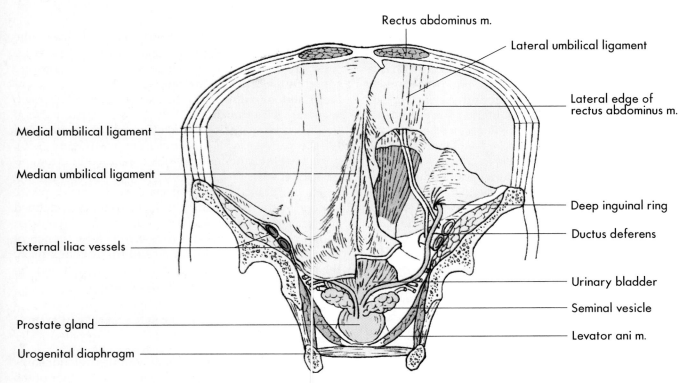

Rectus abdominus m.

Lateral umbilical ligament

Lateral edge of
rectus abdominus m.

Medial umbilical ligament

Median umbilical ligament

Deep inguinal ring

Ductus deferens

External iliac vessels

Urinary bladder

Seminal vesicle

Prostate gland

Levator ani m.

Urogenital diaphragm

Figure 6-10   THE THREE UMBILICAL LIGAMENTS.

ing from one parietal bone to the other. This fetal dimension should not be larger than the diagonal conjugate in the mother, if vaginal delivery is to succeed.

SEXUAL DIMORPHISM IN PELVIC SHAPE

Males and females typically have differently shaped pelves (see Figures 6-1, A, and 6-6). The female pelvis is more cylindrical (i.e., with parallel walls), while the male tends to have funnel-like, inwardly sloping walls. In most cases, these specializations in the shape of the female pelvis accommodate the passage of the infant's head (the largest part of the term baby), although the overall dimensions of the female pelvis may be smaller than those of the male.

Some other features (see Figure 6-6) that distinguish the male and female pelves are (1) the *infrapubic angle*, which is wider in the female than the male; (2) the *pubic tubercles*, which are more widely separated in the female than the male; (3) the upward-facing *articular surface of the sacrum*, intended to articulate with the body of L5, which is a larger fraction of the sacral width in the male than in the female; and (4) the *greater sciatic notch*, which is much wider in the female than in the male.

In the female or **gynecoid pelvis** (see Figure 6-6), an imaginary line connecting the two ischial spines divides the pelvic outlet into two nearly equal subparts, anterior and posterior. In the male or **android pelvis**, the line divides the pelvic outlet into a large anterior

area and a much smaller posterior part. Rarer pelvic variations include (1) the **platypelloid pelvis,** very wide from side to side and flattened in the anteroposterior plane, and (2) the **anthropoid pelvis,** very narrow from side to side and elongated in the anteroposterior plane.

PELVIC INTERIOR

Posteriorly, the pelvic wall (see Figures 6-4 and 6-9) is made up mostly of the anterior surface of the *sacrum*

Table 6-1   Greater and Lesser Sciatic Foramina

Structures Traversing the Greater Sciatic Foramen	Structures Traversing the Lesser Sciatic Foramen
Piriformis muscle	Tendon of obturator internus
Superior gluteal vessels and nerve	Nerve to obturator internus
Inferior gluteal vessels and nerve	Internal pudendal vessels
Internal pudendal vessels	Pudendal nerve
Pudendal nerve	
Sciatic nerve	
Posterior femoral cutaneous nerve	
Nerve to obturator internus	
Nerve to quadratus femoris	

and the flanking *iliac fossae*. It is lined by the *peritoneum*, and just external to it the *endopelvic fascia* (a continuation of transversalis fascia of the abdominal wall). Embedded in the posterior wall of the abdomen, coursing downward into the pelvis, are found the *iliac vessels,* the *inferior vena cava* and its tributaries, the *sympathetic chains,* the *hypogastric plexus,* the *lumbosacral plexus,* and the *iliacus* and *psoas major muscles* (see Figures 6-20, 6-40, 6-43). These vessels and nerves continue inferiorly from the abdomen into the posterior wall of the pelvis.

Anteriorly, the abdominal wall ends at the level of the inguinal ligaments (see Figures 6-9 and 7-2). The *femoral canals* are inferior extensions of the endopelvic fascia, and lie between the inguinal ligament and the superior surface of the superior pubic ramus. Lateral to the femoral canals lie the *femoral vein, femoral artery,* and *femoral nerve.* Normally, there are no specific contents in the femoral canals, but when femoral herniation of intestinal contents occurs, it is most often in this area. Inferior to this, the peritoneum continues downward over the inner surface of the pubic symphysis, to form the lining of the anterior pelvic wall.

The *umbilical vessels,* remnant of the *urachus,* and the *inferior epigastric vessels* may all be seen just external to

the peritoneal covering in the transversalis fascia on the inside surface of the anterior abdominal wall (see Figures 5-9, 1-32, and 1-33). Three specific structures are found in the endopelvic/transversalis fascia of the anterior abdominal wall: (1) the *median umbilical ligament,* remnant of the urachus, (2) the paired *medial umbilical ligaments,* remnants of the fetal umbilical arteries, and (3) the paired *lateral umbilical ligaments* (Figure 6-10), peritoneal folds under which lie the paired inferior epigastric vessels.

The peritoneal drape reflects over the major pelvic viscera in the pelvic floor to form some well-defined spaces. The female has a *vesico-uterine recess* (between bladder and uterus) and a *recto-uterine fossa* (pouch of Douglas—between uterus and rectum). By comparison, the male has only a space between the bladder and the rectum (*vesico-rectal fossa*) (see Figure 6-25).

PERITONEUM, PELVIC FASCIA, AND PELVIC VISCERA

The peritoneum forms some complex relationships with the uterus, oviducts, and ovaries in the floor of the female pelvis (Figure 6-11). The portion of the peri-

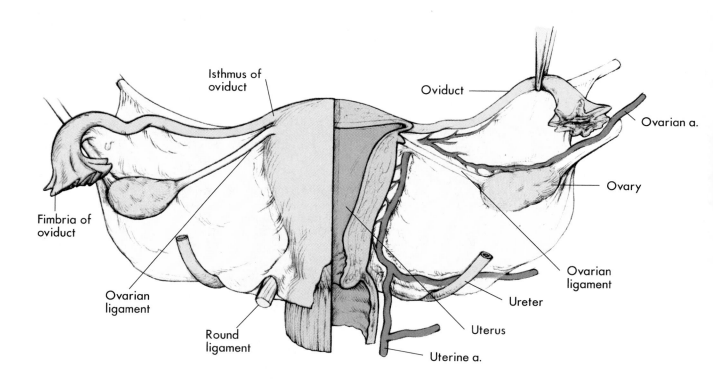

Figure 6-11   FEMALE INTERNAL GENITALIA. Viewing the ovaries and uterus from the posterior aspect, the structures that lie lateral to the uterus can be seen, enclosed within the two layers of the broad ligament. The structures are shown intact on the left side and revealed by removing the posterior leaflet of the broad ligament on the right.
SEE ATLAS, FIG. 6-1

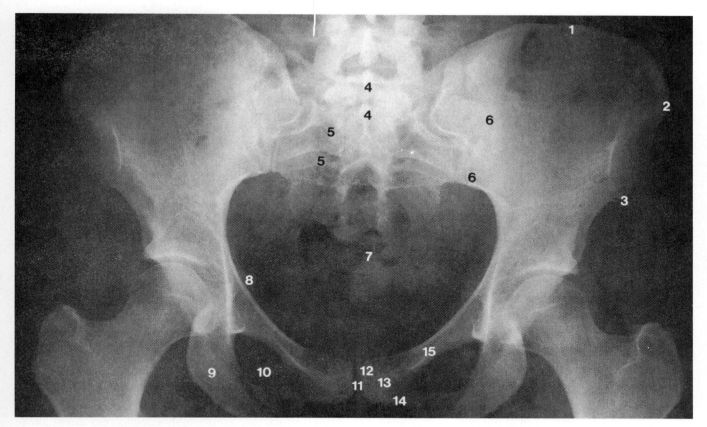

Figure 6-12   X-RAY OF PELVIS. Anteroposterior x-ray of the pelvis is used most frequently to evaluate the pelvis for possible traumatic fracture. Many anatomic structures are identifiable on such films. (From Weir J, Abrahams PH: *An imaging atlas of human anatomy,* London, 1992, Mosby.)

1 Iliac crest	**9** Ischial tuberosity
2 Anterior superior spine	**10** Obturator foramen
3 Anterior inferior spine	**11** Pubic symphysis
4 Sacral promontory	**12** Medial end of pubis
5 Anterior sacral foramina	**13** Pubic tubercle
6 Sacroiliac joint	**14** Ischial ramus
7 Coccyx	**15** Pectineal line
8 Arcuate line or entrance to true pelvis	

toneum covering the anterior and posterior surface of the uterus is called the *mesometrium.* The anterior and posterior layers of peritoneum extend laterally off of the surface of the uterus on the left and right sides. They drape themselves over the oviducts to form the *mesosalpinx.* The special posterior reflection of the mesosalpinx that encloses the ovary is termed the *mesovarium.* Collectively, this set of special peritoneal reflections is called the **broad ligament.** The *infundibulopelvic ligament* is a thickened region of the peritoneum extending inward from the lateral pelvic wall to a point near the infundibulum of the oviduct (see Figure 6-11). Within it are enclosed the ovarian artery, vein, and nerves.

The *endopelvic fascia* lies just external to the peritoneum (see Figure 6-55). It also has some thickened portions, which seem to give support to major pelvic organs. For example, the *uterosacral ligaments* connect the lateral wall of the sacrum with the uterine cervix; the *transverse cervical ligaments* (or *cardinal ligaments*) connect the upper vagina and cervix to the lateral pelvic wall. The *round ligaments* of the uterus and ovary, also found embedded in the endopelvic fascia, are remnants of the gubernacular processes, which guide testicular and ovarian migration early in embryonic life (see Figure 6-11).

THE PELVIS

A-P PELVIC X-RAY (FIGURE 6-12)

The anteroposterior x-ray of the pelvis is used to evaluate patients for possible traumatic fracture in the case of auto accidents or other traumatic forces applied to the pelvis. Fractures of the pelvis may cause injury to any of the organs surrounded by the bones of the pelvis, including the bladder and the reproductive organs. This x-ray view is also useful in evaluating the acetabular fossae and the status of the hip joints.

MECHANISMS OF PELVIC FRACTURE

Since the pelvis is a solid bony ring, it often responds to traumatic forces by suffering fracture in two places—one where the force is directly applied to the pelvis and the second—180 degrees opposite that. When examining a patient with pelvic trauma, it is wise to look for these secondary fractures.

THE PELVIS AND GAIT

The pelvis plays an active role in gait, or walking. The femoral heads articulate with the acetabulum on each side, and as one and then the other femur strides forward, the pelvis must "rock" from side-to-side. Viewed from above, then, the pelvis appears to rotate its right side anteriorly when the right lower limb strides forward, and the left side of the pelvis moves forward when the left lower limb swings forward. In addition to these movements, the pelvis as a whole slides in an alternating fashion to the left and right, as part of bringing the weight of the body over the planted foot. If this did not occur, the body would fall toward the side opposite the planted foot.

If the hip joints should become less mobile, as a result of arthritis for example, then the head of the femur will not rotate easily within the acetabulum. This could result in a limitation on the length of the stride and/or pain accompanying gait.

THE PELVIS AND REGIONAL ANESTHESIA

Regional anesthetic blocks of the pudendal nerves may be achieved by injecting local agents into the vicinity of the female's ischial spines, bathing the pudendal nerves as they wrap around the spine. This type of anesthesia is useful in childbirth and in surgical procedures on the perineum because effective pain control can be achieved without subjecting the patients to general anesthesia and forcing them to become unconscious.

Another widely used anesthetic technique is the **caudal block** (see Figure 6-5), in which anesthetic material is injected into the lower part of the sacral canal, where it can bathe the lower sacral nerve roots, providing anesthesia to the perianal areas. This technique can be very useful in minor surgical procedures involving perianal abscesses and anal fistulas.

6.2 ▸ section six.two
Perineum

- ▸ Boundaries of the Perineum
- ▸ Pelvic Diaphragm
- ▸ Urogenital Diaphragm
- ▸ Ischiorectal Fossa
- ▸ Anus and Anal Canal
- ▸ Arterial Supply of the Anorectal Region
- ▸ Venous Drainage of the Anorectal Region

- ▸ Innervation of the Anorectal Region
- ▸ Female External Genitalia
- ▸ Male External Genitalia
- ▸ Vascular and Lymphatic Supply of the Perineum
- ▸ Somatic Innervation of the Perineum
- ▸ Autonomic Innervation of the Perineum

The perineum is a region (Figure 6-13) like the axilla or the posterior fossa, and not a single discrete structure. Its basic configuration is that of a muscular sheet or barrier through which pass the urethra, vagina, uterus/cervix, and rectum/anus. Although always described as a flattened diamondlike area, when a person is standing the perineum consists of two sharply sloping walls bounding a narrow horizontal space through which pass the viscera mentioned above. When the person is supine, and the thighs are moved laterally, however, the perineum assumes the familiar flattened diamond shaped region seen in textbooks.

BOUNDARIES OF THE PERINEUM

The **perineum** is a diamond-shaped area (but see previously) with the *pubic symphysis* at the anterior corner and the *coccyx* at the posterior corner (see Figure 6-13). The paired ischial tuberosities form the right- and left-hand corners of the diamond. An imaginary horizontal line connecting the two ischial tuberosities defines the *urogenital triangle* (lying anterior) and the *anal triangle* (lying posterior). On each side, the *ischiopubic*

ramus extends forward from the ischial tuberosity to the pubic symphysis, forming the two sloped sides of the urogenital triangle. A similar pair of structures extending backward from the ischial tuberosities to the coccyx, the *sacrotuberous ligaments,* form most of the sides of the anal triangle. The line forming the posterior margin of the urogenital diaphragm passes through the *perineal body,* a hard knot of connective tissue located in the midline, between the *anal opening* and the *bulb of the penis* (or *vagina* in the female). Another thickened connective structure is the *anococcygeal raphe,* a narrow midline cord connecting the anus and coccyx.

When muscular and ligamentous structures are added to the bony pelvis, an incomplete barrier across the pelvic outlet is created (Figure 6-14; see also Figures 6-15 and 6-16). This **pelvic diaphragm** has defined apertures to allow the passage of certain structures, just as there were defined apertures and passages in the respiratory diaphragm (see Figure 5-43) and between abdomen and thorax (the aortic hiatus, esophageal hiatus, etc.). These muscular and ligamentous structures serve to support the abdominal and pelvic viscera and play active roles in urination, defecation, and childbirth as well.

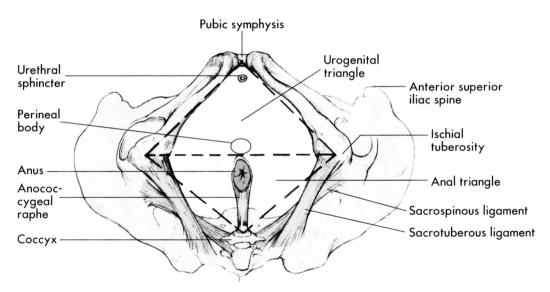

Figure 6-13   UROGENITAL AND ANAL TRIANGLES. The perineum is a diamond-shaped region. It is bordered by the two ischiopubic rami and the two sacrotuberous ligaments (some authors define the posterior margins of this region to be an imaginary line, on each side, extending from the ischial tuberosity to the coccyx). A horizontal line connecting the two ischial tuberosities divides the perineum into the anterior urogenital triangle and the posterior anal triangle. At the midpoint of this line is found the perineal body, just anterior to the anal canal.   SEE ATLAS, FIG. 6-39

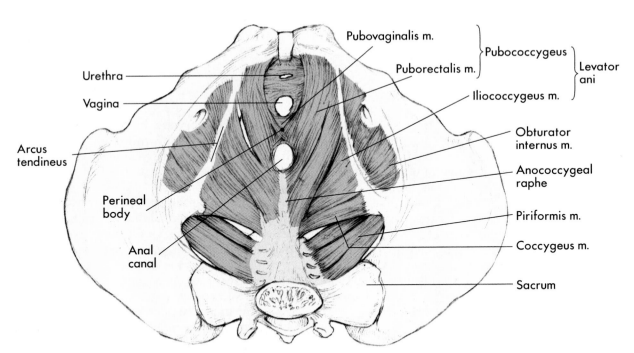

Figure 6-14   PELVIC DIAPHRAGM, SUPERIOR VIEW, FEMALE. All of the viscera have been removed to reveal muscles forming the pelvic floor, with apertures for the rectum/anus, vagina, and urethra. The most medial and largest muscle in this area is the *pubococcygeus*, with its subdivisions *puborectalis* and *pubovaginalis* shown as well. Further posterior, on each side, is the *iliococcygeus* muscle. The posterior margin of this muscle is at the level of the sacrospinous ligament, with which the *coccygeus* muscle is often blended. Iliococcygeus is also unique in originating from the ischial spine and along the fibrous *arcus tendineus*, on the medial surface of the obturator internus muscle. The piriformis muscle appears to "fill in" the gap between the posterior edge of coccygeus and the sacrum but is not a true pelvic floor muscle.   SEE ATLAS, FIG. 6-1

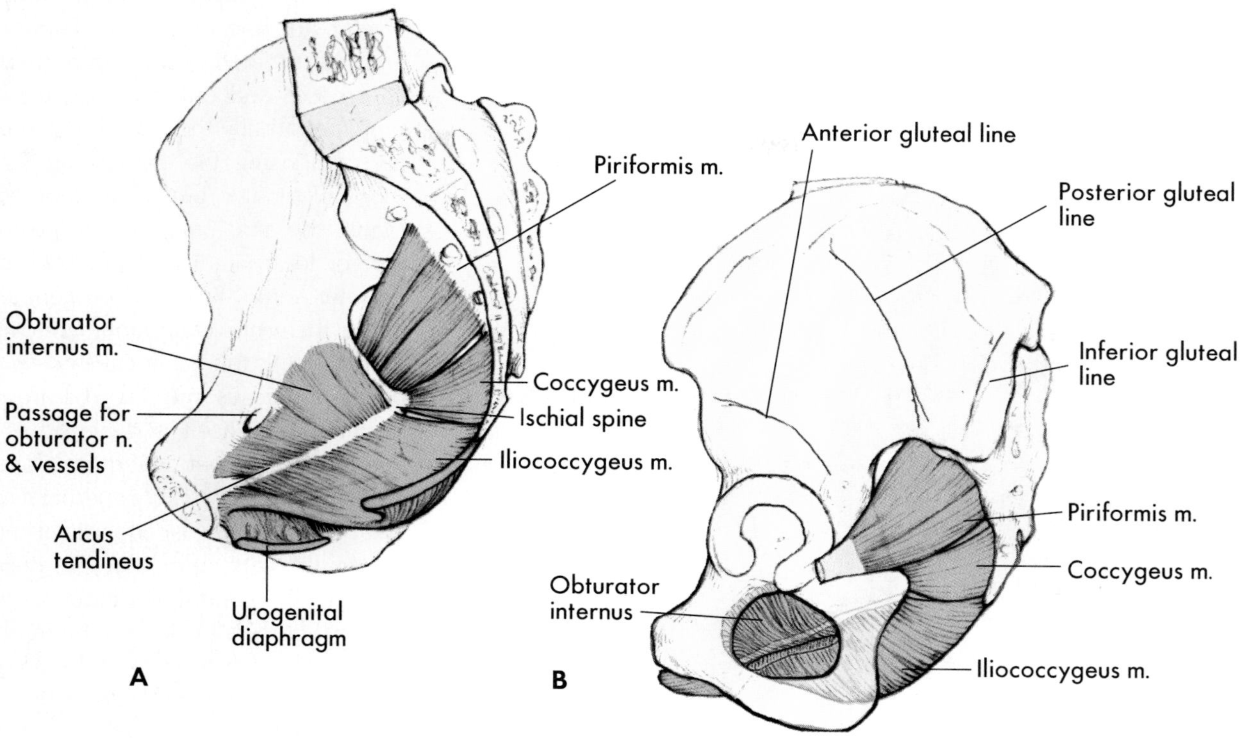

Figure 6-15 PELVIC AND UROGENITAL DIAPHRAGMS. Internal view of the right hemipelvis and an external view of the left hemipelvis. It is as though the intact pelvis had been split in the midsagittal plane and the two halves separated. **A,** In the *internal view,* the piriformis, obturator internus, and obturator foramen are labeled. Note the arcus tendineus, extending from the inner surface of the pubic symphysis anteriorly to the ischial spine posteriorly. Anteriorly, note the deep transverse perineal muscle, and the anterior recess of the ischiorectal fossa that lies between it and the iliococcygeus. **B,** On the *lateral or external view,* the posterior half of the bony ring surrounding the obturator foramen has been removed. The portion of obturator internus inferior to the arcus tendineus has also been removed to reveal the inferior surface of the iliococcygeus muscle. SEE ATLAS, FIGS. 6-31, 6-32, 6-33

PELVIC DIAPHRAGM

The **pelvic diaphragm** is a composite muscle, including the *coccygeus* and *levator ani muscles* (see Figures 6-14 and 6-15; Table 6-2). The levator ani, in turn, is composed of *iliococcygeus* and *pubococcygeus. Puborectalis, pubovaginalis,* or *levator prostatae* are specialized parts of pubococcygeus that are distinct enough functionally to merit individual description. These muscles all originate from areas of bone or ligament on the inner surface of the lateral pelvic wall. The line of origin extends from the pubis to the ischial spine and includes a thickened obturator fascia along the medial surface of the obturator internus muscle (the *arcus tendineus*). Muscle fibers then course medially and fuse in the midline with the fibers from the comparison muscle on the other side.

This midline region of muscle fusion extends from the pubis anteriorly to the coccyx posteriorly, with several perforations. The *urethral* and *vaginal orifices* pass through this region anteriorly, and the *anal orifice* lies more posteriorly (Figures 6-15 and 6-16). Between the anal orifice and the vagina (or the anal orifice and bulb of the penis in the male) is found the *perineal body* (see preceding). The anal orifice and the coccyx are joined by the thickened *anococcygeal raphe.*

PRINCIPLES

In humans, with our upright posture, the floor of the pelvis becomes important in supporting the organs of the pelvis and abdomen and preventing them from sliding out of the pelvic cavity. In quadripedal animals, the muscles of the pelvic floor have only a minor supportive function and instead are important in defecation, urination, and the "wagging" of the tail.

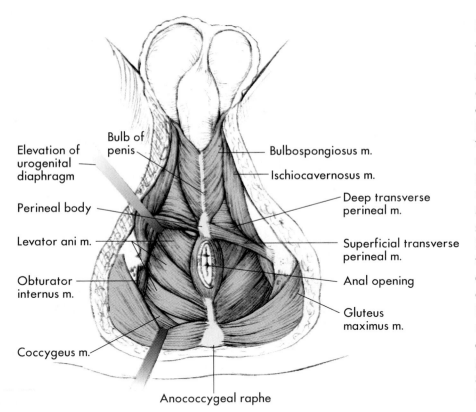

Figure 6-16 MALE UROGENITAL DIAPHRAGM, INFERIOR VIEW. Note the levator ani, the urogenital diaphragm, and the striated musculature (ischiocavernosus and bulbospongiosus) covering proximally the three erectile bodies comprising the penis. Labeled in the anal triangle are the anococcygeal raphe, the anal opening, the posterior part of levator ani and the coccygeus muscle. Anteriorly, in the urogenital triangle, the urogenital diaphragm can be seen deep to the ischiocavernosus and bulbospongiosus muscles. The urogenital diaphragm itself is made up of the deep transverse perineal muscle and its covering fasciae. The superficial perineal muscle lies just superficial to the urogenital diaphragm, along its posterior edge. The central tendinous point or perineal body is located in the midline, along the posterior edge of the urogenital diaphragm. SEE ATLAS, FIG. 6-43

Image labels: Elevation of urogenital diaphragm; Perineal body; Levator ani m.; Obturator internus m.; Coccygeus m.; Bulb of penis; Bulbospongiosus m.; Ischiocavernosus m.; Deep transverse perineal m.; Superficial transverse perineal m.; Anal opening; Gluteus maximus m.; Anococcygeal raphe

The schematic on p. 565 shows the components of the pelvic diaphragm and the sometimes confusing nomenclature used to describe them.

Together, the muscles of the pelvic diaphragm incompletely close the space surrounded by the ischiopubic rami, ischial tuberosities, and the coccyx. Each muscle of the pelvic diaphragm originates laterally, from the medial surface of bone and/or fascia surrounding the true pelvis. Each attaches to viscera or linear fascial thickenings in the midline. Posteriorly, the coccyx and anococcygeal raphe are the points of attachment for muscles comprising levator ani. Anteriorly, there is not

Table 6-2 Muscles of the Pelvic Diaphragm

Muscle	Origin	Insertion	Innervation	Comments
Pubococcygeus	Back of body of pubis and obturator fascia (with small gap near pubic symphysis)	To coccyx, anococcygeal raphe	Branches of S3 to S4; Branch from pudendal nerve	Each muscle separated from its partner by a narrow slot, the genital hiatus
Puborectalis	Back of pubic symphysis	To coccyx, anococcygeal raphe; many fibers blend with external anal sphincter	Branches of S3 to S4; Branch from pudendal nerve	Just lateral to pubovaginalis/levator prostate; surrounds at anorectal junction and pulls it anteriorly
Pubovaginalis (female only)	Back of body of pubis; run nearest midline	Close to vaginal walls, then to perineal body	Branches of S3 to S4; Branch from pudendal nerve	Fibers attach to perineal body posteriorly
Levator prostatae (male only)	Back of body of pubis; run nearest midline	Close to prostatic capsule, then to perineal body	Branches of S3 to S4; Branch from pudendal nerve	Fibers attach to perineal body posteriorly
Iliococcygeus	Arcus tendineus and ischial spine	To coccyx, anococcygeal raphe	Branches of S3 to S4; Branch from pudendal nerve	Also blends with anal wall; aids in "tail-wagging"
Coccygeus	Ischial spine and sacrospinous ligament	Coccyx and lower sacral margin	Branches of S4 to S5	Does not attach to muscles or fascia of pelvic floor Main "tail-wagger"

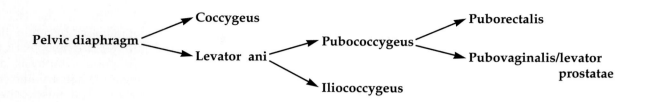

such closure in the midline. Instead, there is a longitudinal *genital hiatus* that allows the urethra (in both sexes) and additionally the vagina (females) to reach the perineum.

Levator ani is positioned so that it resembles a kind of "hammock" in the pelvic floor (see Figure 6-17). The levator ani helps to maintain anorectal angle (the rectum is normally "flexed" anterior on the anus). It also elevates the anal sphincter and lower anal canal upward during defecation.

Inferior to the anterior part of the levator ani, the urethra and/or vagina must pass through a second flat sheet of muscle and fascia, the urogenital diaphragm.

UROGENITAL DIAPHRAGM

The urogenital (UG) diaphragm is composed of the *deep transverse perineal muscle* and its covering fascia (see Figures 6-16 and 6-17). This muscle connects the two ischiopubic rami and is shaped like a triangle. In

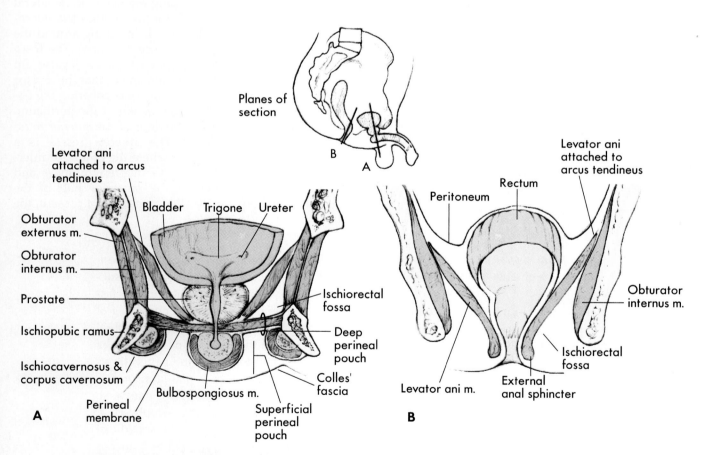

Figure 6-17 FLOOR OF THE MALE PELVIS. The *inset* shows the planes of the two coronal sections. **A,** Plane through the prostate gland. Note the passage of the urethra as it exits the bladder, traverses the prostate, and enters the bulb of the penis. **B,** The plane of section has passed posterior to the urogenital diaphragm; therefore, it does not appear in the section. There is no urogenital diaphragm to form its floor. The rectum and anal canal now occupy the center of the section. The attachment of the levator ani to the arcus tendineus, on the medial surface of obturator internus, is clearly shown.

Few subjects produce as much frustration and confusion in the minds of students than the complexities of fascial and muscle layers in the abdominal and pelvic regions. The abdomen is the simpler of the two. It features, from outside inward, the skin, the superficial layer of the superficial fascia (Camper's), the deep layer of the superficial fascia (Scarpa's), the investing fascia of the abdominal wall muscles, the transversalis fascia, and the peritoneal membrane. In the pelvis and perineum, many of these layers are continued.

In the perineum, the deep and superficial layers of the urogenital diaphragm are simply examples of the investing fascia found in virtually all muscles of the body wall. The deep layer of the superficial fascia of the perineum (Colles' fascia) is a continuation of the deep layer of the superficial fascia of the abdomen. This superficial perineal fascia extends as far posterior as the posterior edge of the urogenital diaphragm, where it is tightly anchored. It encloses the superficial transverse perineal muscle as well, and extends downward into the scrotum as the dartos layer. Rupture of the penile urethra usually results from a fall astride a firm object (like the rail of a fence on which a young boy has decided to try to walk). Urinary extravasation extends into the scrotum and upward into the abdominal wall but does not extend posteriorly beyond the UG diaphragm because the fascia is anchored there.

By contrast, injury to the membranous urethra, if strictly confined to the deep perineal pouch, causes leakage of urine only within the deep perineal pouch.

most individuals, the muscle tissue in the UG diaphragm is thin or even absent, replaced by a thin plate of connective tissue (see Figure 6-32). The apex of the triangle is just posterior to the pubic symphysis, and the base of the triangle is along an imaginary line connecting the two ischial tuberosities. The muscle, therefore, has a free posterior edge. The posterior free border of the UG diaphragm is not a straight line, as often shown in drawings. In reality it is a sweeping curve, concave posteriorly, extending posterolaterally from perineal body to the ischial tuberosities on each side. Its relationship to the external genitalia in the female and male is described in more detail following.

ISCHIORECTAL FOSSA

The ischiorectal fossa contains much fat (Figure 6-19), which at body temperature is semiliquid. The ischiorectal fossa (Figures 6-17 and 6-19) is a triangular space filled with fat, lying inferolateral to the *levator ani* muscle, which forms its sloping medial wall. Its lateral wall, more nearly vertical, is formed by the *obturator internus muscle* (a broad flat muscle attaching around the medial perimeter of the obturator foramen). The fossa extends superiorly to the point where the levator ani and obturator internus meet (remember that the levator ani takes partial origin from the fascia covering the obturator internus). In the anterior half of the perineum, the UG diaphragm forms the floor of the *anterior recess* of the ischiorectal fossa. The anterior recess is a cul-de-sac anteriorly, ending where the obturator internus, levator ani, and the UG diaphragm meet and blend with each other. In the posterior half of the perineum, where the UG diaphragm is not present, the

Figure 6-18   LAYERS OF THE UROGENITAL DIAPHRAGM. Each view is from the superior aspect, and view *1* is the deepest (i.e., with all overlying structures removed). In successive views, more superficial structures are added on layer-by-layer. *1,* The superior fascial layer, enclosing the deep perineal pouch. *2,* The deep perineal pouch, consisting of the deep traverse perineal muscle, sphincter urethrae muscle, and the bulbourethral glands (male only). It also contains the membranous part of the urethra and branches of the pudendal nerves and internal pudendal vessels destined to supply the penis/clitoris and erectile bodies in the superficial perineal pouch. *3,* The inferior fascial layer or perineal membrane. It is attached to the ischiopubic rami laterally, to the deep transverse perineal muscle posteriorly, and has a small gap anteriorly, near the pubic symphysis. *4,* The superficial perineal pouch, enclosed by the perineal membrane and the superficial fascia. It contains the erectile structures and their covering muscles, as well as branches of the pudendal nerves and internal pudendal vessels. *5,* The deep layer of the superficial fascia (or Colles' fascia), which is the inferior limit of the superficial perineal pouch. Anteriorly, it is continuous with the deep layer of the superficial fascia of the abdominal wall and the thin fascial layer of the penis/clitoris; laterally, it is attached to the ischiopubic ramus; posteriorly, it encloses the superficial transverse perineal muscle and is firmly attached to the posterior margin of the deep transverse perineal muscle and the perineal membrane. In the lower right is a sagittal section of the male perineum. Numbers 1 to 5 indicate the levels shown in the five other drawings in this figure.

**Layers of the Urogenital Diaphragm
(viewed from above)**

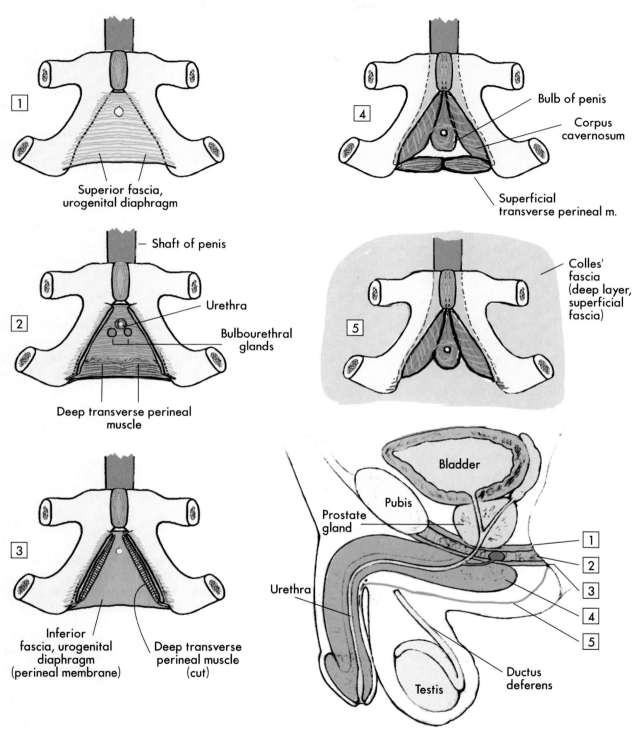

1

Superior fascia,
urogenital diaphragm

2

Shaft of penis

Urethra

Bulbourethral
glands

Deep transverse perineal
muscle

3

Inferior
fascia, urogenital
diaphragm
(perineal membrane)

Deep transverse
perineal muscle
(cut)

4

Bulb of penis

Corpus
cavernosum

Superficial
transverse perineal m.

5

Colles'
fascia
(deep layer,
superficial
fascia)

Bladder

Pubis

Prostate
gland

Urethra

1
2
3
4
5

Ductus
deferens

Testis

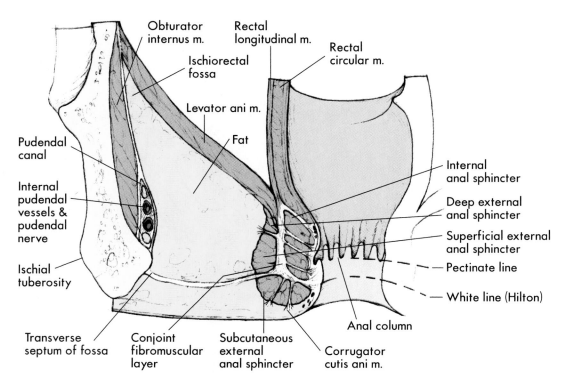

Figure 6-19   CORONAL SECTION OF THE RECTUM AND ANUS. Note that the smooth muscle of the rectal wall ends as the internal anal sphincter, while the striated external anal sphincter has three subdivisions—the deep, superficial, and subcutaneous. The levator ani muscle blends into the wall of the rectum at the level of the external anal sphincters. The pectinate line on the rectal wall marks the end of the pure columnar epithelium of the rectal mucosa, and the white line marks the beginning of pure stratified squamous epithelium. Between the two lines the epithelium is a blend of the two. Note the obturator internus muscle, on the lateral wall of the ischiorectal fossa, and the pudendal structures contained within its pudendal canal. Corrugator cutis ani is a set of fibromuscular strands extending from the conjoint fibromuscular layer of the perianal skin, "puckering" the latter.   **SEE ATLAS, FIG. 6-40**

fat of the ischiorectal fossa is continuous inferiorly with the fatty tissue of the perineum and the anterior gluteal region.

In the lateral wall of the ischiorectal fossa are the *pudendal nerve* and *internal pudendal vessels,* traveling in a tunnel of obturator internus fascia known as the *pudendal (Alcock's) canal.* The *inferior rectal vessels* (branches of the internal pudendal artery and vein) and *inferior rectal nerves* (branches of the pudendal nerve) traverse the fatty space from the pudendal canal to the region of the external anal sphincter, which they supply.

ANUS AND ANAL CANAL

The **anal canal** is at the distal end of the digestive tube and is about 4 to 5 cm long (see Figure 6-19). The intrinsic muscle of the distal rectum and anus is smooth muscle. The *levator ani,* a striated muscle, ap-

proaches the anal canal from above and lateral and blends into the striated *external anal sphincter muscle.* The transition from rectum to anus is marked by the point where the *puborectalis muscle* (a portion of the levator ani muscle) blends with the deep portion of the *external anal sphincter* (see following). The levator ani also forms the medial wall of the ischiorectal fossa.

The *internal anal sphincter* is an extension of the longitudinal smooth muscle of the gut in general. It extends down as far as the white line (see following section and table). The *external anal sphincter* (see Figure 6-19) is striated muscle. The vertical *conjoint fibromuscular layer* separates the external and internal sphincters.

The most inferior portion of the external anal sphincter, the *subcutaneous,* is attached to the anococcygeal raphe and perineal body. It also extends laterally and superior to partially enclose the superficial portion of the external sphincter. The *superficial portion* is immediately superior to the subcutaneous and is the thinnest of the three. The *deep portion,* positioned further superiorly, surrounds the distal end of the rectum and the proximal anal canal. The external sphincter mediates voluntary continence. The *pudendal nerve* innervates the entire muscle (i.e., all three portions of the external sphincter). The *levator ani/puborectalis muscles* approach and blend into the wall of the anal canal just superior to the deep portion of the external sphincter (see Figure 6-19).

Defecation is accomplished through voluntary relaxation of the striated muscle sphincters of the anus and simultaneous contraction of muscles of the abdominal wall and the diaphragm (*the Valsalva maneuver*).

The upper third of the anal canal is lined entirely by *columnar epithelium,* the lower third by *stratified squamous epithelium,* and the middle third by a *mixture of the two epithelia* (see Figure 6-19). A ring of small raised crescents of mucosa (known as the *pectinate line*) on the inside of the anal canal marks the end of pure columnar epithelium in the upper third of the anal canal. One or two cm further inferior to the pectinate line is the white line. The *white line* marks the inferior limit of the internal anal sphincter, a thickened portion of the smooth muscle lining the gut. Inferior to the white line, the lining of the anal canal is entirely stratified squamous. Table 6-3 contrasts the features of the rectum and the anal canal.

ARTERIAL SUPPLY OF THE ANORECTAL REGION

The rectum receives arterial blood (Figures 6-20 and 6-39) from the *superior rectal artery* (a branch of the inferior mesenteric artery) and the *middle rectal artery* (a branch of the internal iliac artery). The anus receives blood from the *inferior rectal artery* (a branch of the internal pudendal artery). These vessels anastomose freely with each other in the substance of the rectal wall.

VENOUS DRAINAGE OF THE ANORECTAL REGION

The upper third of the external surface of the rectum (see Figure 6-19) is covered by peritoneum, but the lower two thirds is below the level of peritoneum (hence not considered to be in the abdominal cavity). A rich blood supply is found within the walls of the rectal canal. The *internal rectal venous plexus* lies just deep to the epithelium and internal to the rectal muscular coats. It forms the longitudinal anal columns of the upper rectal canal (see Figures 5-35 and 6-19). The *external rectal venous plexus* lies outside the rectal muscular coats, and communicates with the internal plexus. Dilations of the veins in the internal plexus can cause them to protrude into the rectal canal, where they are subject to mechanical injury and bleeding (Figure 6-21).

Table 6-3 Rectum and Anal Canal (see Figures 6-19 and 6-21)

Characteristic of	Rectal Canal	Anal Canal
Epithelium	All columnar (endodermal)	Columnar as far distal as pectinate line (see below); squamous below the white line (see below); mixed columnar/squamous between pectinate and white lines
Epithelial specializations	Rectal ampulla in its lower third	Anal columns are 4 to 6 cm long longitudinal ridges in upper anal canal; columns are created by the underlying rectal veins Anal valves, horizontal crescentic folds of mucosa, connect the anal columns at their bases Anal sinuses are grooves between columns; the anal crypts are the parts of the sinuses behind the anal valves; anal glands, in the rectal submucosa, empty into the anal crypts Lower end of the anal columns constitute the pectinate line (see above) Midway down the distal anal mucosa is the white line (see above), marking the distal end of the internal sphincter and the beginning of the squamous epithelium
Innervation of mucosa	Autonomic (mostly unconscious)	Above white line: autonomic Below white line: somatic (from pudendal)
Arterial supply	From inferior mesenteric artery	Above white line: from inferior mesenteric and iliac arteries Below white line: from internal pudendal artery
Venous drainage	To portal system	Above white line: to portal system Below white line: to IVC

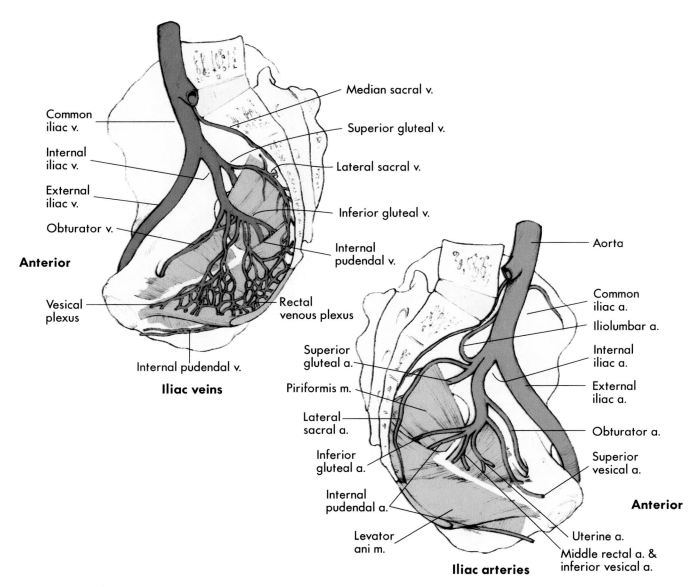

Figure 6-20   ILIAC ARTERY AND VEIN. The common iliac artery divides into an external and internal iliac branch. The internal iliac artery, in turn, divides into an anterior and posterior trunk. The internal iliac vein has many tributaries, which follow the branching pattern of the artery in general. We recognize a vesical and rectal venous plexus because there is such variation in the dense venous drainage from these structures.
SEE ATLAS, FIGS. 6-2, 6-18, 6-37, 6-38

There is also a division between rectal venous blood draining to the hepatic *portal circulation* (mostly from the superior rectal veins, tributaries of the inferior mesenteric vein) and anal venous blood draining to the *systemic circulation* from the internal iliac veins (via the middle and inferior rectal veins), draining to the *inferior*

vena cava. Dilation of the superior rectal veins (internal hemorrhoids) might occur in cases of hepatic injury, where blood flow in the portal vein is impeded. The blood, unable to flow easily into the liver, causes dilations in the tributaries of the portal vein, such as the superior rectal veins (see Figures 5-35 and 6-21). Collater-

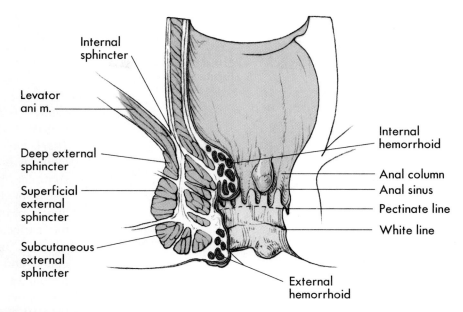

Internal sphincter

Levator ani m.

Deep external sphincter

Superficial external sphincter

Subcutaneous external sphincter

Internal hemorrhoid

Anal column

Anal sinus

Pectinate line

White line

External hemorrhoid

Figure 6-21   INTERNAL AND EXTERNAL HEMORRHOIDS. When venous flow in the superior rectal veins is obstructed, capillaries high in the rectal mucosa become dilated and protude into the lumen of the rectal canal (*internal hemorrhoids*). Because they are innervated by sensory axons accompanying autonomic nerves, this swelling and irritation generally is painless. By contrast, swelling in the capillaries of the inferior rectal veins is painful because the sensory axons innervating the mucosa here accompany somatic nerves (*external hemorrhoids*).

al blood flow also causes tributaries of the inferior vena cava, such as the middle and inferior rectal veins, to dilate as well and cause further hemorrhoids to form.

INNERVATION OF THE ANORECTAL REGION

The *internal anal sphincter* is innervated by the ordinary autonomic innervation of the gut as a whole. The *external anal sphincter* is innervated by the inferior rectal branches of the pudendal nerve (Figure 6-22) and by some small branches from the sacral plexus. The *mucosa* is innervated by autonomic nerves above the white line and by cutaneous branches of the inferior rectal nerves below the white line (see Figure 6-21).

FEMALE EXTERNAL GENITALIA

In the female perineum (Figures 6-22 and 6-23) there is a sizable subcutaneous fat pad just inferior to the pubis, causing a raised skin eminence called the *mons pubis*. The labia majora and labia minora, clitoris, and vestibule comprise the **vulva.** The *labia majora* (singular,

labium majus) are a pair of raised, thickened curvilinear skin folds lying just lateral to the *labia minora* (singular, *labium minus*).

The two labia majora meet each other at a *posterior* and *anterior commissure.* The labia majora contain fat and are covered with hair. The *round ligaments* from each side of the uterus terminate in the labia majora. Each labium majus has at its base a *greater vestibular gland* (Bartholin's gland) (Figure 6-24). These glands secrete a lubricant fluid into the vaginal lumen. The orifices of the greater vestibular glands open on the posterior walls of the labia minora (see following). These glands are homologues of the bulbourethral glands of the male.

Lying just medial to and partially covered by the labia majora are two smaller skin folds known as the *labia minora* (see Figures 6-23 to 6-25). The labia minora surround the *vestibule* or entrance to the vagina (sometimes called the vaginal introitus). The *urethral* and *vaginal outlets* pass through the vestibule, and some minor vestibular glands empty here too. The labia minora meet superiorly in the midline, where each divides into two slips. The slips passing superi-

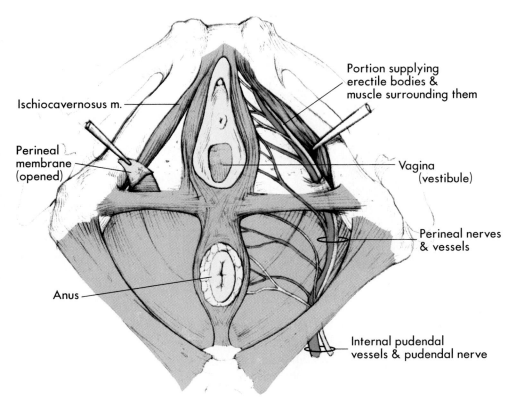

Ischiocavernosus m.

Perineal membrane (opened)

Anus

Portion supplying erectile bodies & muscle surrounding them

Vagina (vestibule)

Perineal nerves & vessels

Internal pudendal vessels & pudendal nerve

Figure 6-22 FEMALE PERINEUM, SUPERFICIAL DISSECTION. Here the female perineum is partially dissected to show the inferior layer of the fascia of the urogenital diaphragm, otherwise known as the perineal membrane, and on the opposite side the course and distribution of pudendal vessels and nerves in the perineal region.
SEE ATLAS, FIGS. 6-5, 6-41

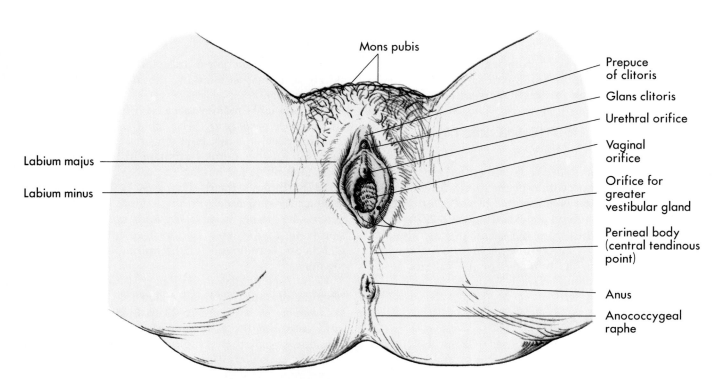

Mons pubis

Prepuce of clitoris

Glans clitoris

Urethral orifice

Vaginal orifice

Orifice for greater vestibular gland

Perineal body (central tendinous point)

Anus

Anococcygeal raphe

Labium majus

Labium minus

Figure 6-23   EXTERNAL GENITALIA OF THE FEMALE. The labia majora flank the labia minora, and the urethral and vaginal orifices are seen between the labia minora.

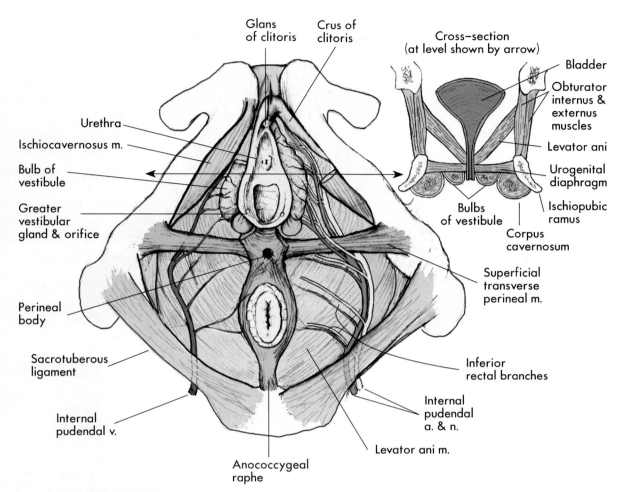

Figure 6-24   FEMALE PERINEUM, DEEPER DISSECTION. Erectile bodies are present in the superficial pouch. The pudendal arteries and veins are shown, each on one side of the perineum. The glans and frenulum of the clitoris are also shown here. The striated ischiocavernosus muscle surrounds the proximal part of each corpora cavernosa, where they are attached firmly to the medial sides of the ischiopubic rami.   SEE ATLAS, FIG. 6-47

or to the clitoris meet in the midline to form the *prepuce of the clitoris* (Figure 6-27). The slips passing inferior to the clitoris meet to form the *frenulum of the clitoris* (see Figures 6-24 and 6-27). Further posteriorly and inferiorly, the labia minora blend with the perineal skin by forming narrow folds, the *fourchettes*. Before insertion of a speculum for a vaginal examination one should note that there is a thin membrane joining the inferior ends of the labia minora and partially covering the entrance to the vestibule. Note that this is not the same as the *hymen* (*Gr. hymen,* a thin membrane, and also Hymen, son of Bacchus and Venus, and the god of marriage), which is a membra-

nous partial covering of the vaginal outlet positioned internal to this membrane.

The **clitoris** is made up of two masses of erectile tissue that joint to lie side-by-side in the midline (see Figures 6-24 and 6-27). These paired erectile masses are known as the *corpora cavernos* (Figures 6-27 and 6-28). Each has a *crus*, a tapering cylindrical projection by which it is firmly attached to the ischiopubic ramus. Each crus is composed of erectile tissue covered by a thin striated muscle, the *ischiocavernosus.* There is also a midline free portion, which, by joining with the similar structure from the other side, forms the glans of the clitoris. The *glans* is suspended from the pubic sym-

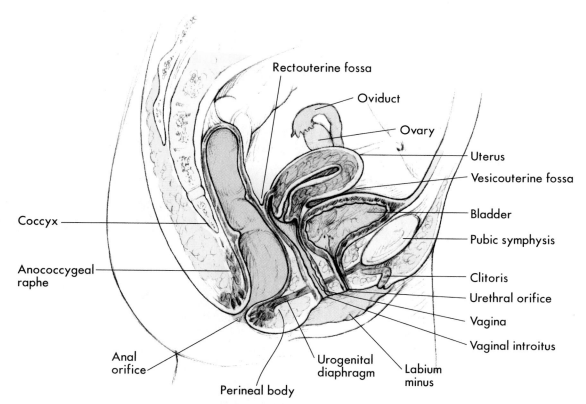

Figure 6-25   FEMALE PELVIC FLOOR, MIDSAGITTAL VIEW. The anterior limit of the perineal area is the pubic symphysis, and the posterior limit the coccyx. Just anterior to the anal canal is the perineal body, an important landmark and point of attachment for several perineal muscles, ligaments, and organs. The anterior parts of the two corpora cavernosa are seen as the clitoris, lying just inferior to the pubic symphysis. Note that the urethral orifice is about halfway between the clitoris and the vaginal opening. The peritoneal membrane, covering the superior surfaces of the organs located in the pelvis, forms two special areas, the vesicouterine fossa, and the rectouterine fossa (or pouch of Douglas).
SEE ATLAS, FIGS. 6-11, 6-12, 6-21

physis by a *suspensory ligament* (see Figure 6-27). The clitoris shares many similarities with the penis, but remember that it differs as well, primarily in that the urethra is not incorporated into the clitoris.

The *urethral outlet* is a small aperture (see Figures 6-25 and 6-27) located 2 to 3 cm inferoposterior to the clitoris. It is also located immediately superior to the vaginal orifice. There are small paraurethral glands (Skene's glands) surrounding the urethral orifice, and draining into it.

Urogenital Diaphragm in the Female

The urogenital diaphragm (see Figures 6-22 and 6-25) is composed of the *deep transverse perineal muscle*, the *sphincter urethrae muscle* (a modified part of deep transverse perineal muscle), and their covering *fasciae*. These muscles and their fasciae form a triangular barri-

er connecting the two inferior pubic rami, as far posterior as the ischial tuberosities. The fascia on the deep (i.e., internal) surface of the muscles is the superior fascia. The fascia on the superficial (i.e., external) surface is the inferior fascia. This latter fascia is also known as the *perineal membrane* (see Figure 6-18). It is useful to remember that when a patient is standing upright, the urogenital diaphragm is angled at ~45 degrees, although it is often pictured diagrammatically as a horizontal sheet of muscle and fascia (see Figure 6-1, *B* and *C*).

The two fascial layers described previously and their contents form the *deep perineal pouch*. In the tissue external (i.e., inferior) to the deep perineal pouch (see Figures 6-24 and 6-25), the space between the perineal membrane and the deep layer of the superficial fascia (Colles' fascia) is the *superficial perineal pouch*. It contains the erectile bodies and associated muscles, the

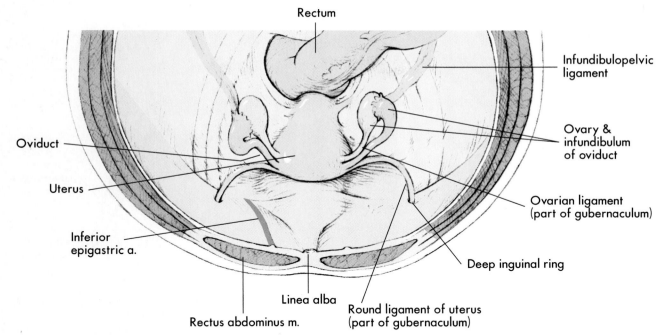

Rectum

Infundibulopelvic ligament

Ovary & infundibulum of oviduct

Oviduct

Ovarian ligament (part of gubernaculum)

Uterus

Inferior epigastric a.

Deep inguinal ring

Linea alba

Rectus abdominus m.

Round ligament of uterus (part of gubernaculum)

Figure 6-26 FEMALE PELVIC VISCERA, SUPERIOR VIEW. The uterus is positioned in the center of the area. The round ligaments are fibrous cords that traverse the inguinal canal and terminate in the labia majora. They are comparable to the spermatic cord in the male. From this aspect can be seen how the ovaries lie in a plane posterior to the uterus. The ovarian ligament that joins the ovary to the lateral wall of the uterus is in fact the proximal part of the embryologic gubernacular ligament, which also gives rise to the round ligament of the uterus. The ovarian vessels reach the ovary enclosed in a fold of peritoneum, the suspensory ligament of the ovary (or infundibulopelvic ligament).
SEE ATLAS, FIG. 6-9

greater vestibular glands, and the perineal body, as detailed in Table 6-4.

The inferior layer of fascia covering the deep perineal pouch can be subdivided into other layers of fascia (see Figure 6-32). A sublayer of inferior fascia is known as the *deep investing fascia* (Galludet's) and extends distally around the erectile bodies (two corpora cavernosi in both male and female, the paired vestibular bulbs in the female, and, in the male, the midline corpus spongiosum) (see Figure 6-27). *Buck's fascia* is also continuous with the inferior fascia of the UG diaphragm and lies just external to and is tightly attached to the *tunica albuginea,* the thick fibrous coat surrounding the shafts of the erectile bodies themselves.

In the perineum, the *deep layer of the superficial fascia* (see Figure 6-32) is called *Colles' fascia* (comparable to Scarpa's fascia of the anterior abdominal wall). This fascia is external to the deep investing fascia. The *rectovesical fascia (Denonvillier's fascia)* is a prominent band of fascia separating the anterior wall of the rectum and anal canal from the posterior surface of the prostate or uterus. It is a downward extension of the endopelvic fascia but does not extend fully downward to the perineal skin.

MALE EXTERNAL GENITALIA

The penis is the male phallus, analogous to the clitoris (see Figures 6-27 and 6-28 and Table 6-5). It is composed of three erectile bodies not two as in the clitoris. The penis is described as having (1) a *bulb* and *paired crurae,* attached firmly to the urogenital diaphragm and in the superficial pouch, (2) a *body,* the portion extending away from the perineal region (see Table 6-5), and (3) a distal head or glans.

The skin surrounding the penis is thin and pliable. There is little or no subcutaneous tissue or fat. The scrotal subcutaneous tissue is similarly lacking in fat, and skin lies directly atop the superficial layer of the superficial fascia (equivalent to Camper's fascia in the abdomen). The *prepuce* or *foreskin* is a collar of integument attached to the penis at the base of the glans (Figure 6-29, *B*). It is often removed as a religious-cultural practice called circumcision (Figure 6-30). There is little evidence to suggest either a health benefit or risk from circumcision.

The *bulbourethral glands (Cowper's glands)* are found (see Figure 6-18) within the urogenital diaphragm (in the male only) and have ducts entering the spongy (pe-

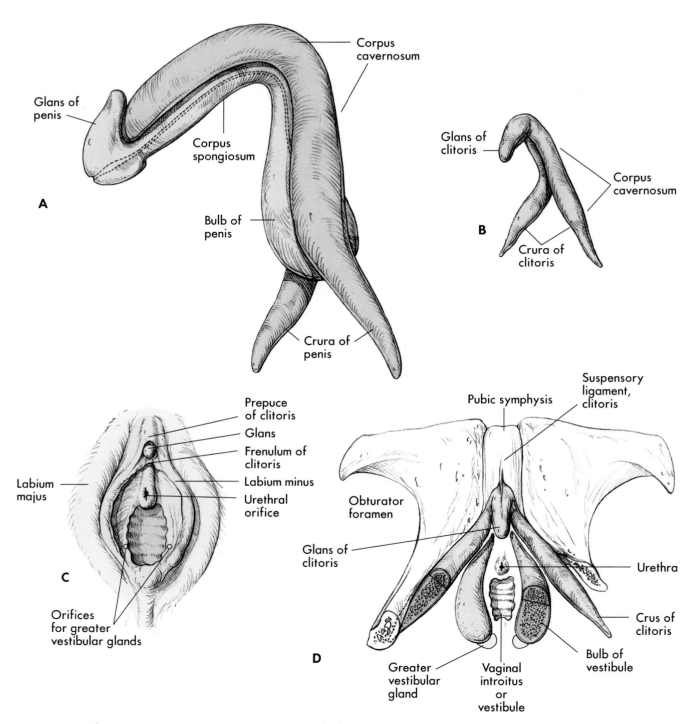

Figure 6-27   PENIS AND CLITORIS. Both the penis and clitoris (**A** and **B**) are composed of a pair of corpora cavernosa, but the penis in addition is composed of a midline corpus spongiosum. **C,** Frenulum and prepuce of the clitoris are extensions of the labia minora. **D,** Relationship of the corpora cavernosa and bulbs of the vestibule are shown.

See Atlas, Figs. 6-44, 6-46, 6-48

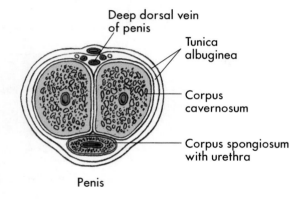

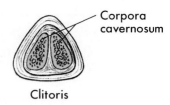

Figure 6-28 PENIS AND CLITORIS, CROSS-SECTION.
Note the paired corpora cavernosa, the ventral single corpus spongiosum, and the deep and superficial vessels located on the dorsum of the penis. In addition there are helicine (helix-like) arteries within the erectile structures. The urethra is suspended within the corpus spongiosum.

nile) part of the urethra. There is no structure in the deep pouch of the female homologous to the male bulbourethral glands (but the greater vestibular glands, located in the walls of the vagina [see Figure 6-24] can be considered homologous in the female).

Urogenital Diaphragm in the Male

Fascial arrangements in the male are identical to those in the female—there is a *deep* and *superficial perineal pouch*, limited by distinct fascial layers. The con-

tents are different in the two sexes, although they are analogous to each other (see Table 6-6).

The *deep perineal pouch* (Figures 6-31 and 6-32; see also Figure 6-18) is structurally the same in the male as in the female (consisting of the deep transverse perineal muscle, the sphincter urethrae, and their fascial coverings). However, in the male, the *bulbourethral glands* are also contained within this layer (although their ducts leave this layer and empty into the penile portion of the urethra) (see Figure 6-33).

The *superficial perineal pouch* (see Figures 6-16, 6-17, and 6-31, *B*) contains the bulb of the penis and its enclosed urethra, the bulbospongiosus muscle, the perineal body, the superficial transverse perineal muscle, and, more laterally, the corpus cavernosum and ischiocavernosus muscle. It is continuous with a comparable space in the abdominal wall (in the space just beneath the superficial fascia), as well as with similar superficial spaces in the scrotum and penis. The superficial pouch is limited posteriorly by the firm attachment of the deep layer of the superficial fascia to the posterior edge of the urogenital diaphragm. If the urethra is torn and urine dissects into the superficial pouch, it can travel upward to the anterior abdominal wall or into the subcutaneous parts of the scrotum or testis. Usually, however, it cannot dissect backward past the posterior margin of the urogenital diaphragm.

The *corpus cavernosum* (see Figures 6-29 and 6-31) in both the penis and the clitoris has a crus that attaches to the ischiopubic ramus on each side. The free portion of the corpus cavernosum of the male is much larger than in the female. Like the female, the crus of the cavernosum is covered first by the tunica albuginea, Buck's fascia, and then by the ischiocavernosus muscle.

The *corpus spongiosum* (see Figure 6-27) is a large single midline body of erectile tissue, composed of a bulb (attached to the urogenital diaphragm) and a freely suspended shaft. The shaft joins with the free portions of the two corpora cavernosi to form the body of the penis.

Table 6-4   External Genitalia of the Female

Name of Structure(s)	Description
Corpora cavernosa	Paired erectile structures forming the substance of the clitoris
Ischiocavernosus muscles	Muscles covering the portion of the corpora cavernosa attached to the ischiopubic rami
Vestibular bulbs	Masses of erectile tissue flanking the external half of the vagina
Bulbospongiosus (bulbocavernosus)	Muscle covering the vestibular bulbs
Superficial transverse perineal muscle	Thin rectangular muscle passing between ischiopubic rami and attaching to the perineal body in the midline
Perineal body	Body located between vaginal orifice and anus; serves as an anchor for many of the muscles and connective tissue structures of the perineum

Table 6-5   External Genitalia of the Male

Name of Structure(s)	Description
Corpora cavernosa	Paired structures forming the substance of the upper two thirds of the penis
Ischiocavernosus muscles	Muscles covering the portion of the corpora cavernosa attached to the ischiopubic rami
Corpus spongiosum and bulb of the penis	Bulb of the penis is a mass of erectile tissue lying in midline, just inferior to the UG diaphragm; traversed by urethra; extends outward as the cylindrical erectile mass in the ventral part of the shaft of the penis, containing the urethra; the bulb and the midline extension are the corpus spongiosum
Bulbospongiosus (or bulbocavernosus)	Muscle covering the bulb of the penis
Superficial transverse perineal muscle	Thin rectangular muscle passing between ischiopubic ramus laterally and attaching to the perineal body in the midline
Perineal body	Body serves as an anchor for many of the muscles and connective tissue structures of the perineum

The *bulb of the penis* (to be exact, of the *corpus spongiosum*) is covered by a tunica albuginea, Buck's fascia, and then by the *bulbospongiosus* (also called *bulbocavernosus) muscle* (see Figures 6-31 and 6-32). This muscle helps to compress the bulb of the penis and expel urine from the urethra. It also contracts rhythmically (and involuntarily) during ejaculation. This is a good example of a striated muscle that can be under voluntary or involuntary regulation, depending on the circumstances.

Each of the three erectile bodies of the penis has a thick coating, the *tunica albuginea* (see Figure 6-29, *A*). Especially in the two corpora cavernosa, the tunica is strong and helps maintain turgidity during erection (by preventing venous return of blood from the distended erectile body).

Within the corpus spongiosum is the **urethra.** The urethra (Figure 6-33) has a *prostatic part,* a *membranous part* (lying within the urogenital diaphragm), and a *penile* or *spongiose part* within the corpus spongiosum. Because the urethra must not be compressed completely, even during erection (in order that semen may pass through it during ejaculation), the corpus spongiosum does not become as rigid as the corpora cavernosa during erection.

VASCULAR AND LYMPHATIC SUPPLY OF THE PERINEUM

Vascular supply to the perineum is essential for the erectile function of the clitoris and penis as well as the general nourishment of the tissues present. The vaginal artery, a branch of the internal iliac artery, is an important source of blood to the female perineum, and the internal pudendal arteries are an important source of arterial blood in both sexes.

The *tunica albuginea* plays a role in erection by tightly surrounding the corpora cavernosa and spongiosum to "trap" the increased blood flow within the erectile tissue, presumably by compressing thin-walled veins in the periphery of these bodies.

Lymphatic drainage of the penis and scrotum is directed to the inguinal area (Figure 6-34) while that of the testis is directed to the posterior abdominal wall. Similarly, in the female, lymphatic drainage from the labia and clitoris is directed to the inguinal region, while that from the ovaries and uterus is directed to the posterior abdominal wall. In general, the lymphatic drainage of an organ follows the arterial supply to that organ.

SOMATIC INNERVATION OF THE PERINEUM

The major nerve of the perineum is the **pudendal nerve** (S2 to S4) (see Figures 6-22 and 6-24). Among the important structures it supplies are the external anal sphincter, the urethral sphincter, the striated muscle jackets of the erectile tissues (ischiocavernosus and bulbospongiosus), and the scrotum/labia majora. It is also the sensory nerve supply to the vaginal canal and the labia (Figure 6-35) and comparable structures in the male (root of the scrotum and penis).

Other nerves involved in the innervation of this area are the **genital branch of the genitofemoral** and the **ilioinguinal,** both of which innervate small areas at the base of the scrotum or labia.

AUTONOMIC INNERVATION OF THE PERINEUM

Autonomic innervation of the external genitalia is crucial to normal function. **Sympathetic nerves** (postganglionic) reach the perineum (Figure 6-36) on blood vessels and by the hypogastric nerve. Their role is

Text continued on p. 584.

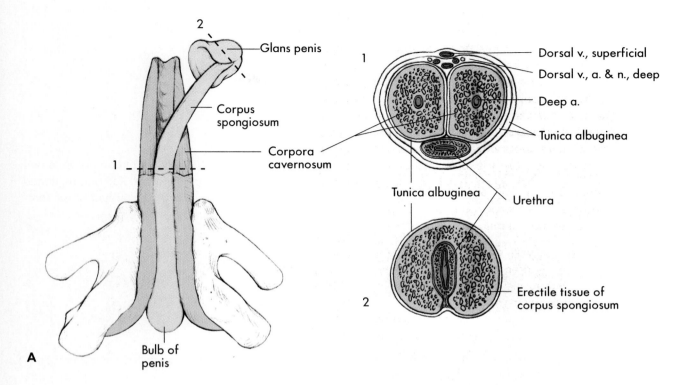

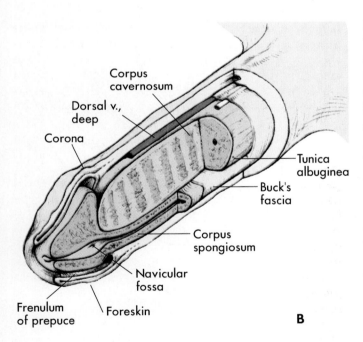

Figure 6-29 ERECTILE BODIES AND STRUCTURE OF THE PENIS. A, The erectile body attached to each is- chiopubic ramus is a corpus cavernosum, which extends forward to join its partner from the opposite side. Togeth- er they form the paired elongated dorsolateral erectile bodies making up the majority of the substance of the shaft of the penis (cross-section at *1*). The cross-section at *2* shows that at this point the penis is made up solely of the corpus spongiosum because the two corpora caver- nosa end just behind the glans. The thick and strong tu- nica albuginea surrounds each of the three erectile bod- ies independently and then forms a second lamina encir- cling all three and binding them together. **B,** Interiors of two of the erectile structures of the penis—the corpus spongiosum and the left side corpus cavernosum—and the foreskin that covers the glans of the penis. There is a small dilation, the navicular fossa, just proximal to the end of the urethra. In the center of the corpus caver- nosum is found a helicine or deep artery, which is the source of increased blood flow occurring during erec- tions. The skin on the shaft of the penis extends distally beyond the base of the glans and forms a two-layered flexible structure known as the foreskin.

SEE ATLAS, FIG. 6-45

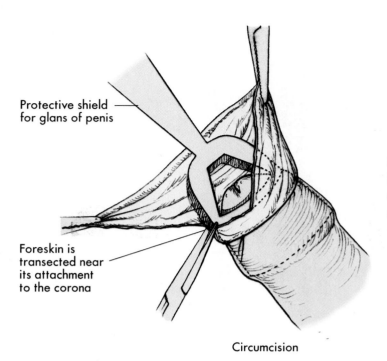

Protective shield for glans of penis

Foreskin is transected near its attachment to the corona

Circumcision

Figure 6-30   CIRCUMCISION. In circumcision, a bell is fitted over the glans penis, a circular ring tightened external to the foreskin, and the distal half of the foreskin incised and removed.

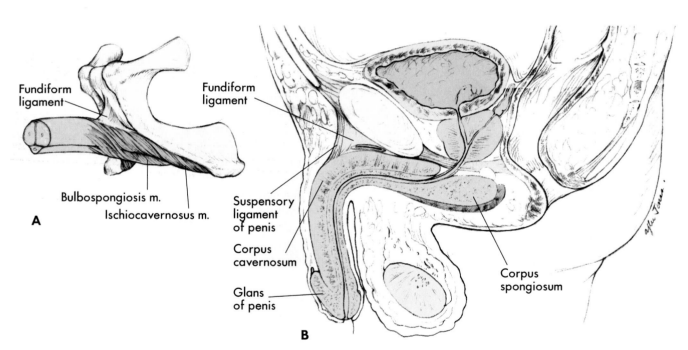

Fundiform ligament

Bulbospongiosis m.

Ischiocavernosus m.

A

Fundiform ligament

Suspensory ligament of penis

Corpus cavernosum

Glans of penis

Corpus spongiosum

B

Figure 6-31   STRUCTURE OF THE PENIS. A, Oblique view of the base of the penis showing the ischiocavernosus and bulbospongiosus muscles and how far distally along the penis they extend. Shown also is the fundiform ligament, attaching the dorsal surface of the penis to the pubic symphysis. Another ligament, anterior to the fundiform ligament, is the suspensory ligament of the penis. It is a downward extension of the linea alba. **B,** Midsagittal section through the male pelvis showing both the fundiform and suspensory ligaments as well as many other pelvic viscera.   SEE ATLAS, FIG. 6-24

Table 6-6   Contents of Perineal Pouches by Gender

Perineal Pouches	Female Perineum	Male Perineum
Deep pouch	Part of vagina Dorsal nerves of clitoris Part of urethra Sphincter urethrae Deep transverse perineal muscle Internal pudendal vessels	Bulbourethral glands Part of urethra Sphincter urethrae Deep transverse perineal muscle Internal pudendal vessels
Superficial pouch	Greater vestibular glands Bulbospongiosus Ischiocavernosus Corpus cavernosum Superior transverse perineal muscle Perineal body Perineal branch of pudendal nerve	Bulb of penis Bulbospongiosus Ischiocavernosus Corpus cavernosum Superior transverse perineal muscle Perineal body Perineal branch of pudendal nerve

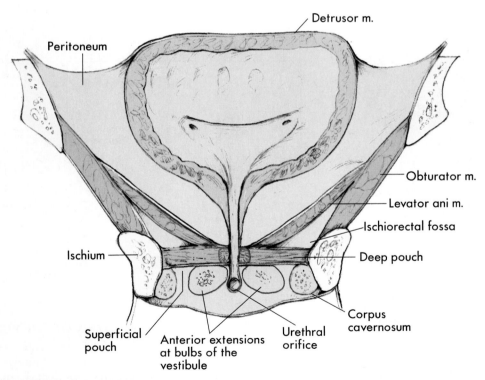

Figure 6-32 BLADDER NECK IN THE FEMALE, CORONAL SECTION. Coronal section through the mid-portion of the female pelvis, where the urethra passes through the urogenital diaphragm. SEE ATLAS, FIG. 6-19

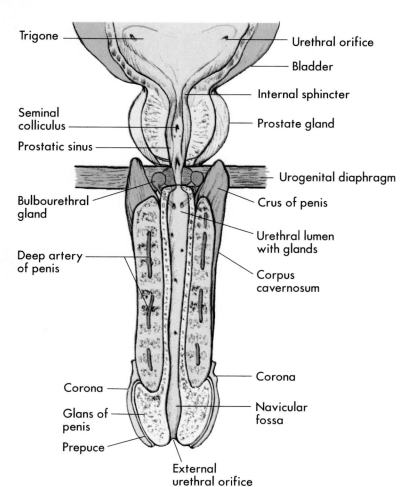

Trigone
Urethral orifice
Bladder
Internal sphincter
Seminal colliculus
Prostate gland
Prostatic sinus
Urogenital diaphragm
Bulbourethral gland
Crus of penis
Urethral lumen with glands
Deep artery of penis
Corpus cavernosum
Corona
Corona
Navicular fossa
Glans of penis
Prepuce
External urethral orifice

Figure 6-33 COURSE OF THE MALE URETHRA. This longitudinal view involves a horizontal section through the penis, following the plane of the urethra. The entire length of the urethra can be seen. To the left and the right of the urethra and its surrounding corpus spongiosum are the corpora cavernosa, also incised longitudinally so that their interiors may be seen. The interior of the bladder may be seen, with its two ureteral orifices outlining the bladder trigone. Next the urethra continues through the center of the prostate gland. In the prostatic urethra can be seen the seminal colliculus, and the ejaculatory duct orifices lying to either side of it. As the urethra enters the penis, the orifices of the bulbourethral glands may be seen emptying into it. Further along the interior of the penile urethra can be seen the orifices of several poorly understood urethral glands.

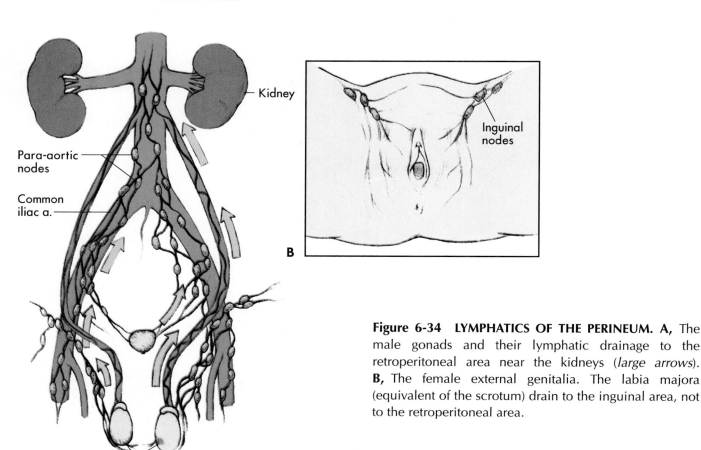

Kidney
Para-aortic nodes
Common iliac a.
Inguinal nodes
Testis
A
B

Figure 6-34 LYMPHATICS OF THE PERINEUM. A, The male gonads and their lymphatic drainage to the retroperitoneal area near the kidneys (*large arrows*). **B,** The female external genitalia. The labia majora (equivalent of the scrotum) drain to the inguinal area, not to the retroperitoneal area.

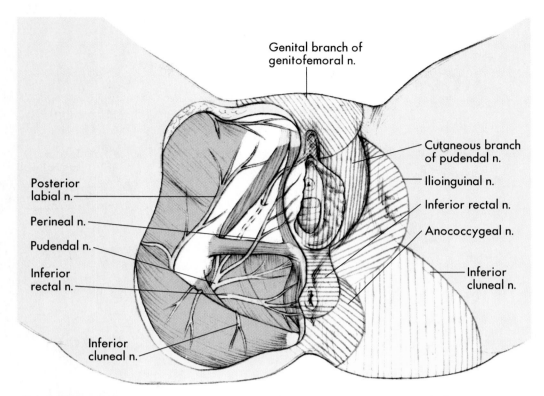

Figure 6-35 CUTANEOUS INNERVATION OF THE FEMALE PERINEUM. The perineum is dissected on the right side and intact on the left, with the distribution of various cutaneous nerves shown.

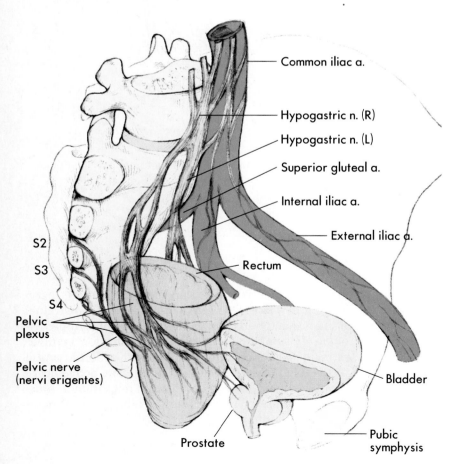

Figure 6-36 PELVIC PLEXUS. This midsagittal view shows the bladder, prostate, and rectum and the plexus of autonomic axons that surrounds them (the pelvic plexus). The *sympathetic axons* arise from the two hypogastric nerves (or plexuses), which descend from the bifurcation of the aorta down into the pelvis. The *parasympathetic axons* arise in the roots of S2 to S4 and are shown here collecting into a loosely organized structure known as the pelvic nerve or nervi erigentes. Both the sympathetic and parasympathetic components of the pelvic plexus carry sensory axons with them, but the particular role played by one subgroup of axons vs. another is not understood. <small>**SEE ATLAS, FIG. 6-34**</small>

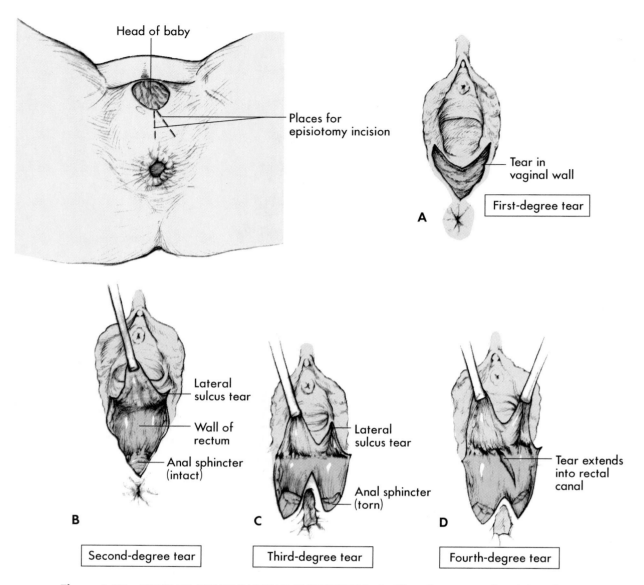

Figure 6-37   VAGINAL TEARS DURING CHILDBIRTH. A, *First-degree tear,* involving skin or mucosa only. **B,** *Second-degree tear,* involving skin/mucosa, superficial fascia, and the superficial transverse perineal muscle. **C,** *Third-degree tear,* involving those structures in second-degree tears plus the external anal sphincter. **D,** *Fourth-degree tear,* involving all of the above, with the laceration extending into the interior of the anal/rectal canal.

mainly as a regulator of blood flow and to cause contraction of smooth muscle in the vas deferens and seminal vesicle during ejaculation.

Parasympathetic nerves (preganglionic) (see Figure 6-36) are derived from the *pelvic splanchnic nerves* (S2 to S4). Their main function in the perineum is the vasoregulatory mechanism of the erectile tissues. Classical thought gives full responsibility for erection to parasympathetic nerves (hence the classic alternate term for the pelvic splanchnic nerves is nervi "erigentes"), but more recent studies have shown dual mechanisms for erection, involving the parasympathetic and/or sympathetic nerves. Since erection involves an increase in blood flow to the erectile bodies and a decrease in the egress of blood from them, active nerve impulses would have to act through relaxation of muscular sphincters or by inhibition of other neurons regulating vascular tone.

THE PERINEUM

BARTHOLIN'S GLANDS (THE GREATER VESTIBULAR GLANDS)

Bartholin's glands (see Figure 6-24) may be infected repeatedly and require corrective surgery. When they are infected they produce painful swelling in the entrance to the vagina and may produce discharge as well.

EPISIOTOMY

An episiotomy is the purposeful incision of the posterior vaginal wall downward toward the perineal body, with the goal of enlarging the birth canal for easier passage of a large baby. These incisions are repaired after birth and are made when there is high risk of a spontaneous tear, which may extend uncontrolled into the rectal mucosa (Figure 6-37). Childbirth may tear the perineal body. Because so many muscles of the area are anchored to it, injury to the perineal body may seriously disturb urination, defecation, sexual activity, and the like.

PERINEAL BODY

The importance of the perineal body is its central location in the perineum (see Figure 6-23), where it serves as a point of attachment for muscles (transverse perineal muscles, sphincter urethrae) and for the other ligamentous structures that support the perineum (the anococcygeal raphe, etc.). Childbirth puts great stresses on the perineal body in the female, and in both genders repeated straining in defecation can weaken it as well.

PROLAPSE AND THE PERINEUM (FIGURE 6-38)

If the perineum is weakened, one great risk is prolapse—the phenomenon in which pelvic organs "sag" at levels lower than normal and in the extreme can protrude outward through the perineal barrier. The urethra and bladder can prolapse downward through a weakened urogenital diaphragm, the cervix and uterus can prolapse through a stretched and weakened vaginal canal, and the rectum can prolapse through the anus. Surgical repair of these problems is difficult and not always successful.

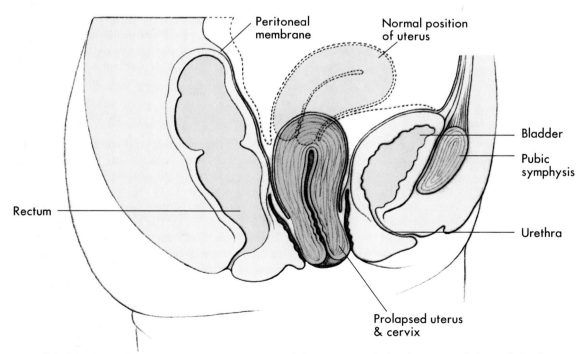

Figure 6-38 PROLAPSE OF THE UTERUS. If the urogenital diaphragm and the pelvic diaphragms are weakened, or if the ligaments in the endopelvic fascia that support the uterus are damaged, one consequence may be prolapse of the uterus downward into the vaginal canal.

6.3

section six.three

Pelvic Vasculature and Nerve Supply

▶ Arterial Supply to the Pelvis

▶ Venous Drainage of the Pelvis

▶ Nerve Supply of the Pelvis

The inferior ends of the iliac vessels pass from interior to exterior through certain defined spaces and apertures in the floor of the pelvis (see Figures 6-20 and 6-39). Many of their branches remain within the pelvis and supply the viscera present there. Others penetrate the levator ani and leave the pelvis to supply blood to the lower limb (Table 6-7). The lumbosacral plexus (see Figure 6-40) takes shape on the medial surface of the levator ani muscle. Like the iliac vessels, some branches of the lumbosacral plexus supply structures in the pelvis, and other branches supply structures in the lower limb (Table 6-8).

ARTERIAL SUPPLY TO THE PELVIS

The *internal iliac artery* (Figure 6-39) is the major vascular source to the pelvic structures. The abdominal aorta bifurcates at L4 into the two *common iliac arteries,* each of which is 5 to 6 cm long. Anterior to the sacroiliac joint, these vessels in turn bifurcate into the *internal* and *external iliac arteries.* Just before this bifurcation, the common iliac on each side is crossed anteriorly by the ureter.

The *external* and *internal iliac veins* (see Figure 6-20) unite to form a *common iliac vein,* which joins its counterpart from the opposite side to form the *inferior vena cava* (IVC) at L4-L5. The location of these vessels is similar to the corresponding arterial vessels but generally posterior to the arteries and slightly to the right. The

IVC is, of course, on the right side of the vertebral column, and the aorta on the left.

The internal iliac artery is divided into an anterior and posterior trunk, each of which has several branches. The *anterior trunk* of the internal iliac artery supplies structures of the pelvic wall, perineal region, and the pelvic viscera (see Figure 6-20). It courses downward along the wall of the pelvis in the direction of the ischial spine. The *posterior trunk* supplies branches to body wall structures, and *no* branches to viscera.

VENOUS DRAINAGE OF THE PELVIS

There is a complex and quite varied pelvic venous plexus (see Figure 6-20) with branches accompanying most of the named arteries. One large component of this plexus surrounds the lower rectum, while another major collection of veins surrounds the prostate (male) (see Figure 6-64) or the uterovaginal junction (female). Variation is quite common. The chief clinical significance of the pelvic veins is their potential for forming thrombi, which can break loose and flow upward to cause obstruction in the lungs. This phenomenon is especially likely to occur in the bedridden or immobile patient.

NERVE SUPPLY OF THE PELVIS

The **lumbosacral plexus** is an imprecise term often applied to the entirety of innervation of the pelvis and

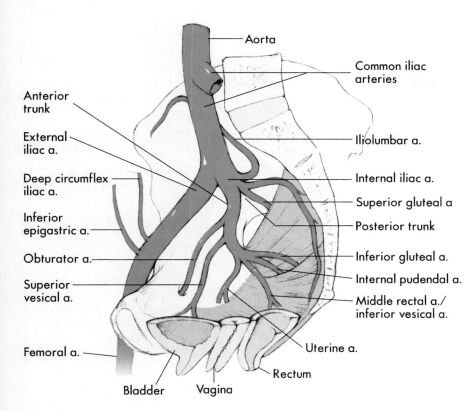

Aorta

Common iliac
arteries

Anterior
trunk

External
iliac a.

Deep circumflex
iliac a.

Inferior
epigastric a.

Obturator a.

Superior
vesical a.

Femoral a.

Iliolumbar a.

Internal iliac a.

Superior gluteal a

Posterior trunk

Inferior gluteal a.

Internal pudendal a.

Middle rectal a./
inferior vesical a.

Uterine a.

Rectum

Bladder   Vagina

Figure 6-39 BRANCHES OF THE COMMON ILIAC ARTERY. The common iliac artery divides into an internal and external branch. The internal iliac artery supplies the gluteal and internal pelvic structures, while the external iliac artery continues inferiorly as the femoral artery, major blood supply to the entire lower limb.
Sᴇᴇ ATLAS, Fɪɢꜱ. 6-35, 6-37

lower limb (Figure 6-40). The *lumbar plexus* proper consists of branches from T12 to L4. The sacral plexus proper consists of neural inputs from L4 to S4 and innervates the pelvis and lower extremity. The lumbar plexus innervates the anterolateral body wall in the lower abdomen, the inguinal and scrotal regions, and a small area of the thigh. The *sacral plexus* innervates the pelvic viscera, gluteal regions, perineum, and some portions of the proximal thigh.

In addition to the somatic motor and sensory axons of the lumbar and sacral plexuses, there are also *sacral parasympathetic axons* (see Figure 6-44), arising in segments S2 to S4. Only cranial nerves III, VII, IX, and X and these sacral segments contain preganglionic parasympathetic axons. These sacral parasympathetic axons separate from the rest of the sacral plexus and form an indistinct structure known as the *pelvic splanchnic nerve* or *nervi erigentes* (nerve of erection).

Branches of the Sacral Plexus

The **sacral plexus** consists of the descending *lumbosacral trunk* (from the lumbar plexus) and the *anterior primary rami of S1 to S4* (Table 6-8).

Like the brachial plexus, the sacral plexus may be described by its roots, trunks, divisions, and terminal branches (see Figure 6-40). The trunks divide into anterior and posterior divisions, on the anterior surface of

piriformis muscle. These divisions produce the following nerves, the most important of which are discussed in detail.

The **sciatic nerve** (L4 to S3), the largest peripheral nerve in the body (Figure 6-41), divides into the *common peroneal* and *tibial nerves*. It exits the pelvis through the greater sciatic foramen inferior to piriformis and lies deep to the gluteus maximus. It then runs down the mid-region of the posterior thigh. Above the knee, the *common peroneal branch* separates and wraps around the neck of the fibula, where the nerve is vulnerable to injury. The common peroneal branch then innervates lateral and anterior leg muscles and skin and superficial structures of the anterolateral leg and dorsum of the foot.

The **tibial nerve** is the larger of the two components of the sciatic nerve. It separates from the common peroneal nerve just above the knee and continues inferiorly as the muscular nerve to the posterior calf muscles, the muscles of the sole of the foot, and a cutaneous nerve to the medial thigh, heel, and sole of the foot.

The **lumbar plexus** has been described in the section on the posterior abdominal wall.

The point at which the common peroneal and tibial components unite (see Figure 6-41) to form the sciatic nerve is variable. Most commonly, it occurs proximally, and the united sciatic nerve emerges inferior to the piriformis to enter the gluteal region. In other cases the

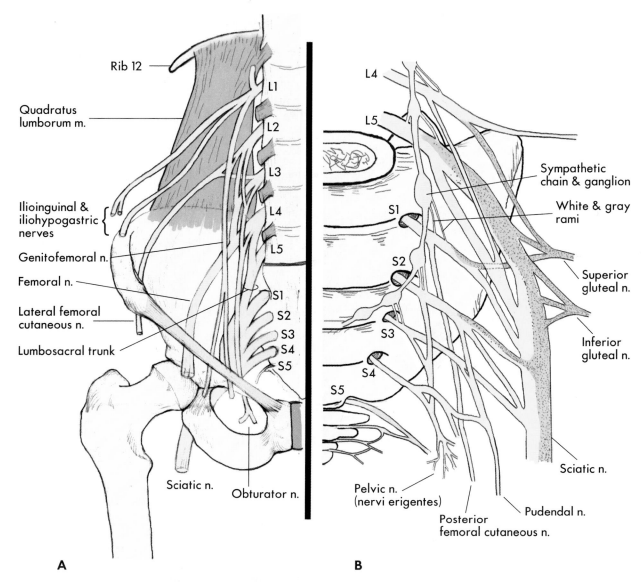

Figure 6-40 LUMBOSACRAL PLEXUS. A, The lumbar and sacral plexuses are shown here as a continuum of nerve fibers emerging from vertebral levels L1 to S5. The lumbar plexus is directed at innervation of the lower anterolateral abdominal wall and the inguinal canal. The sacral plexus innervates pelvic organs and continues outside the pelvis to supply the posterior thigh and nearly all of the lower limb below the knee. **B,** This schematic drawing of the sacral plexus illustrates formation of its major branches and the distribution of anterior and posterior division branches in them. SEE ATLAS, FIG. 6-36

union of the two is delayed; in these cases, the tibial nerve emerges inferior to the piriformis, and the common peroneal either pierces this muscle or lies superior to it. In such cases they unite to form the sciatic nerve in the gluteal region, or even more distally in the posterior thigh.

The **superior gluteal nerve** (L4 to S1) traverses greater sciatic foramen superior to piriformis (see Figures 6-8 and 6-41). It innervates gluteus medius and minimus and tensor fascia lata; its branches ramify in the plane between the gluteus medius and the gluteus minimus muscles. Injury to this nerve produces the Trendelenburg sign. The *Trendelenburg sign* occurs

when, during walking, one foot is planted and the other elevated. As this occurs, the pelvis on the side opposite to the planted foot "sags" or "droops." The cause for this is the paralysis or weakness of the gluteus medius and minimus on the planted side and the consequent inability to produce hip joint abduction on the same side as the planted foot. When hip abduction of the planted limb is accomplished, it helps to maintain the position of the opposite limb off the ground.

The **inferior gluteal nerve** (L5 to S2) traverses greater sciatic foramen and emerges inferior to piriformis (see Figures 6-8 and 6-41). It supplies the gluteus maximus, providing major abductor and extensor

Table 6-7   Branches of the Internal Iliac Artery

Branch	Course	Supplies
BRANCHES OF THE ANTERIOR TRUNK		
Inferior gluteal artery	Passes between S1 to S2 or S2 to S3, then between piriformis and coccygeus.	Gluteal muscles and upper posterior thigh.
Internal pudendal artery	Passes between piriformis and coccygeus and leaves pelvis through greater sciatic foramen. Curves around ischial spine to enter pelvis through lesser sciatic foramen (Figure 6-42).	Perineal area (UG diaphragm, corpus spongiosum, corpora cavernosa, penis); also supplies distal end of rectum and anus.
Obturator artery	Descends medial to psoas, then exits pelvis through obturator foramen. Divides into anterior and posterior branch over the adductor brevis muscle in thigh.	Supplies muscles in adductor group (medial thigh); in most, supplies acetabulum and in ~30% gives rise to inferior epigastric artery.
Superior vesical artery	Branches from internal iliac and travels medially to bladder; distal to bladder, the remnant of the umbilical artery travels from the bladder toward the umbilicus.	Supplies upper surface of bladder.
Uterine artery	Travels inferiorly and medially on surface of levator ani, crosses anterior to the ureter. Branches descend alongside vagina and ascend as high as uterine isthmus.	Most of uterine body and upper portion of vagina.
Middle rectal/inferior vesical artery	One is often a branch of the other. Departs anterior branch and travels medially.	*Middle rectal* artery supplies lower rectum, prostate, and seminal vesicles; *inferior, vesical* artery supplies neck of bladder, prostate, and seminal vesicle.
BRANCHES OF THE POSTERIOR TRUNK		
Iliolumbar artery	Emerges posteriorly, then turns laterally; divides into an iliac and a lumbar branch.	Supplies branches to the pelvic wall, representing a lower "segmental" artery to the body wall.
Lateral sacral artery	Enters the anterior first or second sacral foramen, then exits the sacrum through the posterior sacral foramen.	Supplies the interior of the sacral canal, also supplies skin over the sacrum.
Superior gluteal artery	Leaves the pelvis above the piriformis, through the greater sciatic foramen. Usually passes between the lumbosacral trunk and the anterior ramus of S1 as it leaves the interior of the pelvis.	Supplies branches to the gluteal region, with one branch just deep to gluteus maximus and one deep to gluteus medius.

force to the hip. The **pudendal nerve** (S2 to S4) exits the greater sciatic foramen, wraps around sacrospinous ligament, and reenters the pelvis through the lesser sciatic foramen. It travels forward in the ischiorectal fossa within the *pudendal (Alcock's) canal* (see Figures 6-8 and 6-19). Major branches are inferior rectal nerves, labial/scrotal nerves, and perineal nerves (to the urogenital diaphragm). This nerve is the major source of innervation to the perineum and external genitalia.

The **posterior femoral cutaneous nerve** (S1 to S2) exits the greater sciatic foramen below piriformis (see Figure 6-41). It provides the major cutaneous innervation to posterior thigh, with some small branches descending further into the leg. The sacral plexus also gives rise to a group of preganglionic parasympathetic axons, mostly from cord segments S2 to S4. They are described following.

Table 6-8   Branches of the Sacral Plexus

From Anterior Divisions	From Posterior Divisions
Nerve to quadratus femoris/inferior gemellus	Nerve to piriformis
Nerve to obturator internus/superior gemellus	Superior gluteal nerve
Posterior femoral cutaneous nerve*	Inferior gluteal nerve
Tibial nerve	Posterior femoral cutaneous nerve*
Pudendal nerve	Common peroneal nerve
Pelvic splanchnic nerves	Perforating cutaneous nerve
Nerve to levator ani/coccygeus	—

*Both divisions contribute to this nerve.

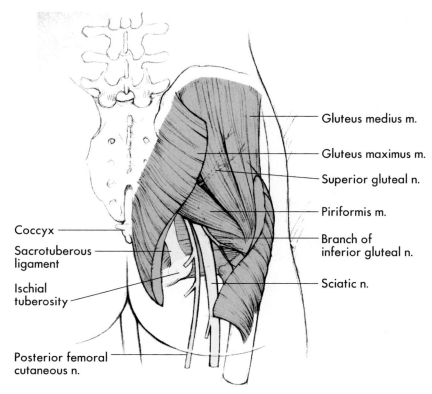

Gluteus medius m.

Gluteus maximus m.

Superior gluteal n.

Piriformis m.

Branch of
inferior gluteal n.

Sciatic n.

Coccyx

Sacrotuberous
ligament

Ischial
tuberosity

Posterior femoral
cutaneous n.

Figure 6-41   POSTERIOR BRANCHES OF THE SACRAL PLEXUS. Here are shown the principal posterior branches of the sacral plexus: the superior gluteal nerve, the inferior gluteal nerve, the posterior femoral cutaneous nerve, and the sciatic nerve.

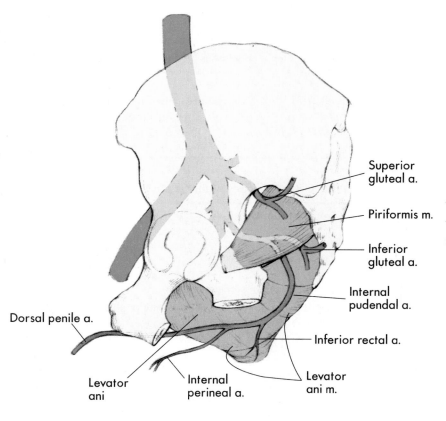

Superior
gluteal a.

Piriformis m.

Inferior
gluteal a.

Internal
pudendal a.

Inferior rectal a.

Levator
ani m.

Dorsal penile a.

Levator
ani

Internal
perineal a.

Figure 6-42   INTERNAL PUDENDAL ARTERY. Lateral view of several branches of the internal iliac artery shows their relationship lateral to the piriformis and levator ani muscles.

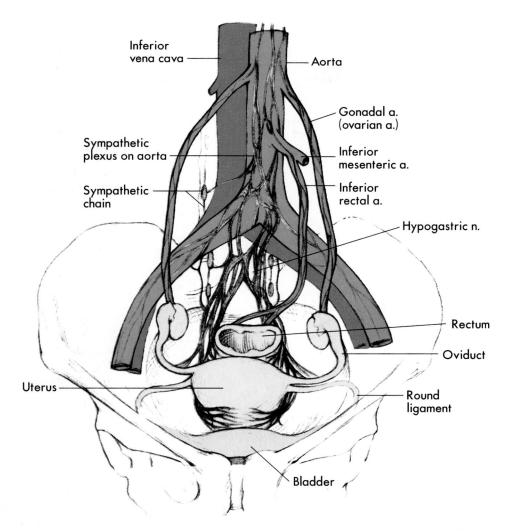

Figure 6-43 SYMPATHETIC NERVES IN THE PELVIS. These nerves arise from two sources: *first,* from the plexus of sympathetic axons traveling on the aorta and forming the hypogastric nerve (or plexus), and, *second,* via the branches of the sympathetic chain that join the segmental spinal nerves, forming the sacral plexus, whose branches innervate the pelvic organs. There does not appear to be any clear functional difference in the sympathetic axons arising in one source vs. those arising in the other. It is known, however, that the majority of sensory axons innervating the pelvic viscera returns to the spinal cord by traveling with sympathetic axons arising in gray rami and accompanying branches of the sacral plexus that innervate the pelvic viscera. SEE ATLAS, FIG. 6-42

Pelvic Autonomic Nerves

Sympathetic axons (see Figures 6-36 and 6-43) reach the pelvis by two routes: (1) as postganglionic axons from the superior and inferior hypogastric nerves (or plexus), which represents a continuation of the sympathetic plexus on the aorta, and (2) as sympathetic axons forming part of the branches of the sacral plexus innervating the pelvic organs. It is not clear whether these two sources of supply represent different functions or why there should be two different sources. Sympathet-

ic input produces constriction of the bladder neck, blocking the flow of urine, but it also promotes the expulsion of semen from the male genital structures during ejaculation. By contrast, sympathetic input probably inhibits uterine contraction, proving again that it is the nature of the receptors on the target tissue that determines the effect of innervation in each organ, not the incoming axons themselves.

The **superior hypogastric nerve (or plexus)** arises at the bifurcation of the aorta and is composed of (1) *postganglionic sympathetic axons* from the lumbar sympa-

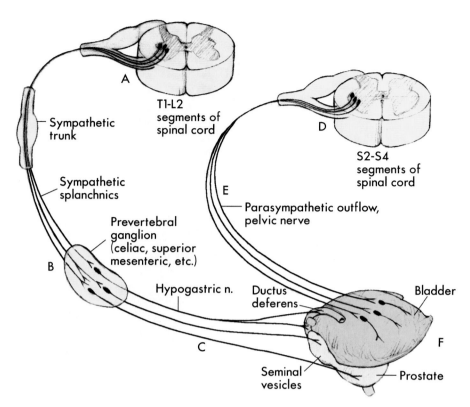

Figure 6-44   AUTONOMIC INNERVATION OF THE BLADDER. The sympathetic innervation begins with preganglionic axons arising in the lower thoracic spinal cord (*A*) in the intermediolateral cell column. These axons must synapse in a peripheral ganglion, and it is from the neurons of those ganglia that the axons actually innervating the intended target tissues arise. For pelvic viscera, preganglionic axons travel as part of the group of splanchnic nerves (greater, lesser, least) that separate from the segmental thoracic nerves and descend along the posterior thoracic wall to enter the abdomen. Here they synapse in one of the large prevertebral ganglia (*B*) along the aorta (e.g., the celiac, superior mesenteric, renal, etc.). Postganglionic axons arising in these ganglia distribute themselves along the arterial branches of the abdominal aorta, and, in addition, a portion of them continues inferiorly to descend from the bifurcation of the aorta into the pelvis and the hypogastric nerve (or plexus) (*C*). Parasympathetic innervation begins with preganglionic axons arising in spinal cord segments S2 to S4 (*D*). These axons travel in the pelvic nerve (*E*) to small groups of neurons embedded in the walls of target organs. Here the preganglionic axons synapse, and the small neurons give rise to postganglionic axons (*F*), which actually innervate the muscle or glands in that organ.

thetic ganglia (therefore analogous to gray rami), (2) some branches from the *aortic sympathetic plexus* (which arise in the inferior mesenteric ganglion and are also postganglionic), and (3) an oft-forgotten but nonetheless important group of *sensory axons* from the pelvic viscera. The superior hypogastric nerve passes inferiorly in front of the sacral promontory, where it divides into two *inferior hypogastric nerves* or *plexuses* (which contain the same assortment of axons as the superior nerve). These nerves innervate the bladder, the smooth

muscle of the male ejaculatory pathway, and parts of the ureter.

Sacral preganglionic **parasympathetic axons** arise in sacral cord segments S2 to S4 and depart the roots of these segments to form the loosely aggregated *pelvic nerve* or *nervi erigentes* on each side (see Figures 6-36 and 6-44). This nerve travels across the pelvic floor (mostly on the levator ani muscle) and distributes axons to intramural ganglia in the lower rectum, bladder wall and neck, the erectile tissue of the phallus, the

THE PELVIC NERVES AND VESSELS

SURGERY ON THE PELVIC FLOOR

Surgical procedures involving the pelvic viscera place autonomic nerves in jeopardy, especially considering that the nerves are small, diffuse in organization, and hard to identify at operation. The nerves converge on the lower rectum and bladder neck, and surgical injury to them may affect urinary continence, anal continence, erection, or ejaculation.

THROMBOPHLEBITIS OF PELVIC VEINS

The pelvic veins are common sites of thrombophlebitis, an *inflammatory condition* of clots in veins. These clots can embolize to the lungs.

CAUDAL ANESTHETIC BLOCK (SEE FIGURE 6-5)

A caudal block is anesthesia produced by injecting anesthetic into the *sacral hiatus* and numbing the sacral nerve roots, affecting the perineal area especially. *Surgery* on perineal structures is sometimes done with this anesthetic technique.

PRESACRAL NEURECTOMY

In certain cases of intractable pain, a surgical division of the hypogastric nerve will help alleviate symptoms (see Figures 6-36 and 6-43). It must be remembered, however, that urinary and/or sexual function will likely be permanently altered by such a procedure.

UMBILICAL ARTERY

After birth is accomplished, the umbilical artery becomes obstructed with clot and over the course of days to weeks is permanently obliterated. Sick neonates, however, often require arterial cannulation, and the umbilical artery is a convenient and easy site in which to place an arterial catheter. The cut end of the vessel is located in the umbilical stump, and a catheter is placed into it and threaded upstream into the common iliac artery or higher up into the aorta itself.

ARTERIAL GRAFTS

Certain arteriosclerotic diseases characteristically involve the iliac vessels and their larger branches. Because of this, surgical placement of *shunts* and *bypass grafts* in the region of the *iliac arteries* is a fairly common procedure for the vascular surgeon. Segments of native vessels or synthetic materials such as Dacron or Goretex are used for such arterial grafts.

---

uterus and ovaries, and as far proximal as the mid-transverse colon. The smooth muscular walls of the bladder and rectum receive important parasympathetic innervation from spinal cord segments S2 to S4. This innervation is key to promoting expulsion of contents (e.g., urine, feces) from these structures. By contrast, the uterus, which has a thick smooth muscle wall, is not under the control of these parasympathetic nerves. This difference derives from the particular receptors expressed on the surfaces of cells in these particular organs. Male genital organs, like the seminal vesicles, ductus deferens, and prostate gland, are similarly not under parasympathetic control. The one exception to this statement is the well-known role of parasympathetic nerves in producing erection in the penis or clitoris.

Parasympathetic axons in the pelvic splanchnics are *preganglionic*, destined to synapse in neurons arranged in small clusters within the walls (see Figure 6-44) of the urinary or reproductive viscera they supply (the intramural ganglia). The *postganglionic axons* emanating from these ganglia, therefore, are very short in comparison to the postganglionic axons characteristic of sympathetic nerves.

Both sympathetic and parasympathetic axons carry with them *sensory axons*, which relay information back to the spinal cord and brain. For example, the presence of large amounts of urine in the bladder is detected by these axons, and the information relayed to the spinal cord and brain. As a result, the sense of bladder fullness is appreciated, and the mechanisms for bladder emptying are set in motion (in this particular tissue, sensory axons in the parasympathetic nerves seem to be most important). Unlike the parasympathetic and sympathetic motor nerves, which involve two neurons, sensory signals are conveyed from the periphery to the spinal cord by single neurons, typical of sensory neurons in other areas of the body. The peripheral and central processes of these sensory nerves extend all the way from the tissues they innervate to the spinal cord dorsal horn and have their cell bodies in dorsal root ganglia just as with somatic sensory axons.

6.4 ▶ section six.four
Urinary System

▶ Ureter

▶ Surfaces and Position of the Urinary Bladder

▶ Structure of the Urinary Bladder

▶ Neurovascular Supply of the Urinary Bladder

▶ Functional Regulation in the Genitourinary System

Within the pelvic cavity are found the reproductive and important urinary viscera. The differences between the sexes are obvious and important, but the common embryologic origin of many seemingly different structures should not be forgotten. The interior of the pelvis is a difficult place to dissect and is no less difficult when it comes to surgical exposure in the living patient. The positions of different pelvic structures are not obvious, and three-dimensional relations are not easy to picture. Sectional imaging techniques have been especially helpful in detecting disease processes in the interior of the pelvis, which is not accessible by ordinary physical examination.

The abdominal and pelvic portions of the urinary system consist of the *kidneys, ureters,* and the *urinary bladder.* Distal to the bladder, urine flows through the *urethra* to reach the exterior.

URETER

The ureter is usually 25 to 30 cm in length and slightly longer on the left than the right (remember the left kidney is usually a bit more superior on the posterior abdominal wall). The ureter is composed of an *inner longitudinal* and *outer circular smooth muscle* layer. Superiorly, this musculature blends smoothly with that of the renal pelvis. The ureter demonstrates important peristaltic activity, necessary for the propulsion of urine from kidney to bladder.

As it leaves the hilus of the kidney, the ureter is in a posterior position with respect to the renal vessels (Fig-

ure 6-45). Descending on the medial border of the psoas major muscle, the ureter passes posterior to the gonadal vessels and then descends further and passes anterior to the common iliac vessels. *In the male,* the ureter travels down the posterior pelvic wall, then passes toward the midline to reach the posterior surface of the bladder. As it does, it passes posterior and inferior (see Figure 6-46) to the ductus deferens. *In the female,* the ureter similarly courses down the posterior pelvic wall, and, as it turns medially to approach the bladder (see Figure 6-45), it passes posterior and inferior to the uterine artery. After doing this it runs for a time along the vagino-cervical junction before entering the bladder. The proximity of the ureter in the female to the uterine artery is an important surgical relationship (Figure 6-46) because the ureters may be ligated accidentally during surgery to remove the uterus (hysterectomy) when the uterine arteries are being isolated and ligated (tied off).

Where the ureter originates, from the renal pelvis, there is a tendency for narrowing of the ureter to occur and obstruction of urine flow to take place. This region is known as the *ureteropelvic junction* (UPJ) (Figure 6-47). In addition to the UPJ, there are further normal points of ureteral narrowing (1) where the ureters cross the iliac vessels and (2) at the entrance to the bladder. Each of these is potentially a point of obstruction.

The ureter is innervated successively by small branches from the sympathetic chain, extending from T12 to the sacral region. There are also parasympathetic axons present and a small number of intrinsic ganglia

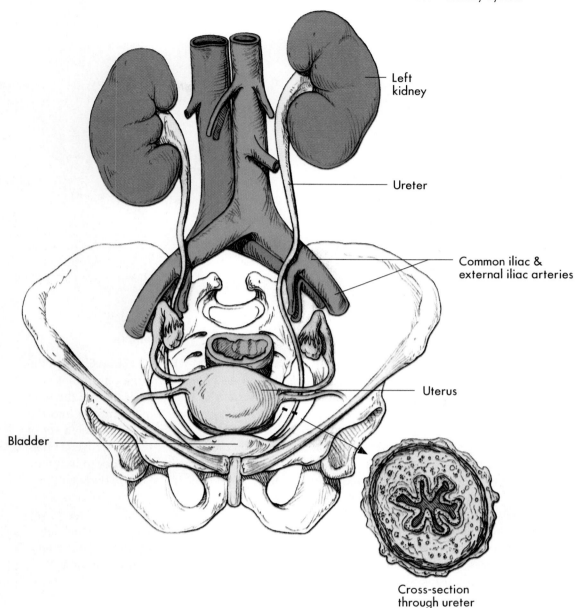

Left
kidney

Ureter

Common iliac &
external iliac arteries

Uterus

Bladder

Cross-section
through ureter

Figure 6-45 DESCENT OF THE URETER INTO THE PELVIS. The ureter exits the antero-medial margin of the kidney, then descends in the retroperitoneal fascia covering the psoas major. It crosses anterior to the common iliac artery, usually at or near the point where they divide into internal and external branches. Further inferior it passes anterior to the genitofemoral nerve but posterior to the gonadal vessels. In the pelvis it descends along the margin of the greater sciatic notch, then turns medially to enter the base of the bladder. Just before entering the bladder wall it loops posterior to the ductus deferens (in the male) or the uterine artery (in the female).

in the wall of the ureter. This innervation is largely motor (though the completely denervated ureter still has a considerable degree of contractility). Abundant sensory innervation is also present. Blood supply to the ureter arises from a series of sources, including small branches from the renal arteries, abdominal aorta, gonadal, iliac, and vesical arteries.

SURFACES AND POSITION OF THE URINARY BLADDER

The urinary bladder (Figure 6-48) is a muscular organ which, when full, can extend up well above the level of the pubic symphysis, holding as much as a liter of urine (it can distend still further in pathologic conditions). The urinary bladder lies wholly outside the peri-

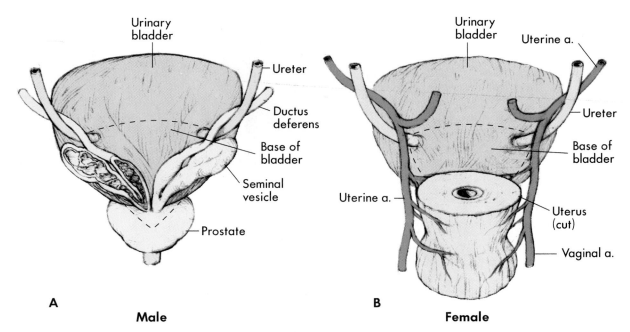

A   Male

B   Female

Figure 6-46   POSTERIOR SURFACE OF THE BLADDER IN MALE AND FEMALE. A, In the male, the seminal vesicles and ductus deferens on each side converge on a point near the neck of the bladder, just above the prostate gland. The ductus deferens and the duct of the seminal vesicle here unite to form the ejaculatory duct, which empties into the lumen of the prostatic urethra. The interior of the seminal vesicle is a convoluted set of coiled tubules, shown by the longitudinal section on the left side. The ureter has a characteristic relationship to the ductus deferens, "looping" posterior and inferior to it as they both approach the posterior bladder surface. **B,** In the female, most of the body and fundus of the uterus have been removed to afford a clear view of the posterior surface of the bladder. The ureters approach the posterior surface of the bladder in much the same way as in the male, but it is the uterine artery that is related to the ureter as the ductus deferens is in the male—that is, the ureter loops posterior and inferior to the uterine artery. Note how the uterine artery gives rise to vaginal branches that descend along the side of the vagina. The *dashed lines* outline the bladder trigone.

toneum although a layer of peritoneum is in contact with the superior surface of the bladder. The urinary bladder is a urine reservoir whose shape varies with its degree of fullness. It has a narrow *neck*, which descends to the urogenital diaphragm, where it unites with the urethra. *In the male*, the neck lies just superior to the prostate, and *in the female* it lies just anterior to the middle third of the vagina.

Superior to the neck is the *body* of the bladder, which is roughly in the shape of an inverted triangle. The superior surface of the bladder faces upward and is covered by peritoneum. The *apex* of the bladder is its most anterior point on the superior surface, where the bladder was attached to the *urachus* (see Figure 6-48) in fetal life. In the adult state, this is represented by the *median umbilical ligament,* which is seen as an unpaired midline ridge of tissue on the interior surface of the anterior abdominal wall, connecting the bladder apex to the um-

bilicus (see Figure 6-10). The *anterolateral surfaces* of the bladder are "cradled" in a space "supported" on each side by the two superior and inferior pubic rami.

The posteroinferior surface of the bladder is called the base. The *base* of the bladder (see Figure 6-48) is nearly vertical, faces posteriorly, and resembles an inverted triangle in shape. The two ureters enter the bladder wall at positions corresponding to two of the "corners" of the base of this triangle. The third point of the triangle is positioned inferiorly, where the bladder outlet joins the urethra. *In the female*, the base of the bladder is in contact with the anterior surface of the vagina and *in the male* with the seminal vesicle and ejaculatory ducts. Although other parts of the bladder change position and/or shape in correspondence to bladder fullness, the base remains in a similar orientation regardless of bladder fullness.

When empty, the bladder has a narrow, elongated

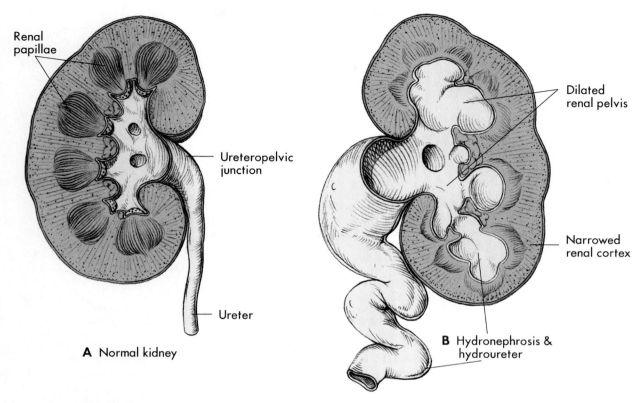

Figure 6-47 HYDROURETER AND HYDRONEPHROSIS. A, Normal kidney and ureter. **B,** Situation of distal obstruction to the flow of urine, so that the ureter and the renal pelvis are dilated, conditions known as hydroureter and hydronephrosis. With time these conditions lead to irreversible destruction of the kidney tissue.

shape, aligned along a superoinferior axis parallel to the anterior body wall. The midline anterior surface of the empty bladder rests against the pubic symphysis and the internal surface of the urogenital diaphragm. When full, the bladder expands to a nearly spherical shape and appears to "tip" forward, its superior surface now facing anterior and resting on the levator ani, pudendal cleft (space between the labia), and pubic symphysis.

STRUCTURE OF THE URINARY BLADDER

The wall of the bladder is made up of thick smooth muscle running in several planes. This muscle is called the *detrusor*. The presence of this muscle in the bladder wall creates a series of irregular thickened ridges on the interior wall of the bladder (Figure 6-50). These are known collectively as the *bladder trabeculae*.

While most of the interior of the bladder is trabeculated, at the trigone the mucosal lining is smooth. The

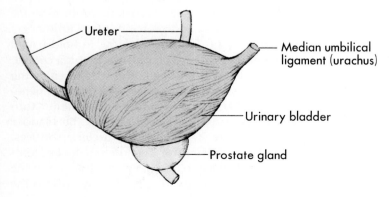

Figure 6-48 BLADDER AND PROSTATE, ANTERO-LATERAL VIEW. The bladder is a muscular organ with a flattened surface facing superiorly. The left and right sides of the bladder converge on a midline fibrous cord, the median umbilical ligament. The two ureters approach the bladder posterolaterally and travel a short distance within its wall before emptying into the bladder interior. The urethra exits from the inferior aspect of the bladder, rather like the neck of a funnel. The proximal part of the urethra is surrounded by the prostate gland.

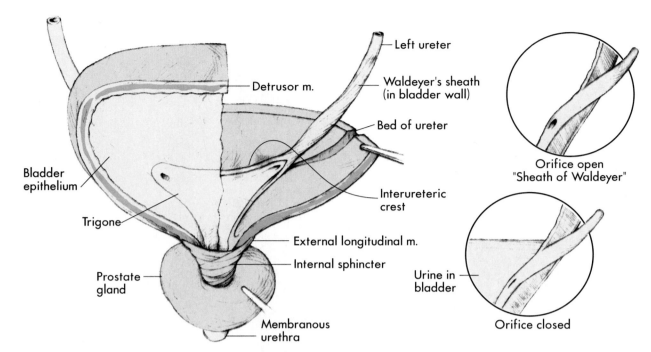

Figure 6-49   DETAILED VIEW OF THE BLADDER WALL. Entrance of the ureters into the bladder wall and how these arrangements help minimize the risk of reflux of urine from the interior of the bladder back up into the ureters. The two *inserts* show how the ureter courses at a shallow angle through the wall of the bladder, so that the point where the ureters enter the bladder wall is not in line with the orifice of the ureter as it empties into the bladder interior. When the bladder is full and there is distension of the bladder wall, the tendency is for the intraluminal portion of the ureter to be compressed. This prevents the reflux of urine when the bladder musculature is contracting and urine is intended to flow outward through the urethra. This course of the ureter in the bladder wall is called the "sheath of Waldeyer." The triangular area of the bladder interior outlined by the two ureteral orifices and the origin of the urethra is the trigone. In the trigonal region, the ordinary smooth muscle of the bladder wall is present, but internal to it is a triangular region of additional smooth muscle created as a continuation of the musculature of the ureters.

trigone is the triangular smooth mucosal region outlined by imaginary lines linking the orifices of the two ureters and the urethra. Along the upper side of the trigone, the mucosa is raised, forming a roughly horizontal line connecting the two ureteral orifices (see Figure 6-49). This is known as the *interureteric crest*.

Just deep to the trigonal mucosa is a specialized layer of trigonal smooth muscle. The trigonal musculature (see Figure 6-49) contracts differently than the detrusor muscle. While the detrusor muscle lies within the body of the entire bladder and is innervated by parasympathetic nerves, the trigonal smooth muscle is located only in the trigonal area and is innervated instead by sympathetic nerves.

Smooth musculature extends downward from the trigone to encircle the bladder neck and urethra (in

part). This extension of bladder smooth muscle is called the *vesical sphincter* (see following). It extends inferiorly, *in the male*, to a point slightly above the orifices of the ejaculatory ducts in the prostatic urethra. *In the female* it is rudimentary and probably plays little or no role in *continence* (Old French, *continere*, to hold back). Muscular control of urinary continence is still a controversial issue in clinical anatomy. The ureters enter the bladder at the corners of the trigone. The ureters penetrate the external wall of the bladder and actually "tunnel" some distance before emerging into the bladder interior (see Figure 6-49) at the ureteric orifices. This arrangement allows for the ureters to be compressed during distension and active contraction of the detrusor, preventing reflux of urine backward into the ureter.

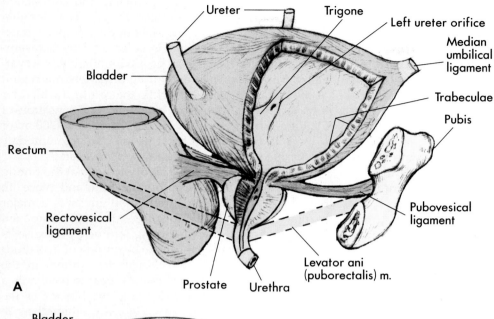

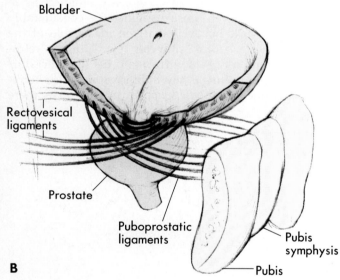

Figure 6-50 LIGAMENTOUS SUPPORTS OF THE BLAD-DER AND RECTUM. A, Two of the more important muscular supports for the bladder and rectum. Both are specialized regions of the endopelvic fascia. It is believed that these pubovesical and rectovesical ligaments play a significant role in preventing the prolapse of the rectum and to a lesser degree the bladder/prostate. The ligaments usually contain some muscle fibers too. **B,** More detail of the supportive ligaments for the male bladder, prostate, and rectum. See Figure 6-55 for further information about comparable ligaments in the female.

The neck of the male bladder penetrates the prostate gland and continues as the *prostatic urethra.* As the urethra passes through the urogenital diaphragm, a thickened and circular *sphincter urethrae* (sometimes called the *external urethral sphincter*) forms a collar around the urethra (see Figures 6-32 and 6-64). This sphincter represents a specialization of the deep transverse perineal muscle. This striated muscle sphincter is under voluntary control and probably represents the best and most important mechanism to maintain urinary continence, in both sexes.

Several ligamentous structures within the endopelvic fascia attach the neck and base of the bladder to the interior of the pelvic wall. Most notable are the *puboprostatic* and the *pubovesical ligaments.* These ligaments are important in maintaining the position of the

bladder with respect to the urogenital diaphragm and the levator ani muscle (Figure 6-50). When these ligaments are damaged, the bladder may "sink" to an abnormally low position, and continence may be affected.

NEUROVASCULAR SUPPLY OF THE URINARY BLADDER

The *superior and inferior vesical arteries,* branches of the anterior trunk of the internal iliac artery, provide most of the blood supply to the bladder (see Figures 6-20 and 6-39). At its neck, small branches of the uterine and vaginal arteries also help. Veins from the surface of the bladder converge on the *prostatic plexus* and, in turn, drain to the internal iliac veins (see Figure 6-64). In the female this is referred to as the *vesical plexus.*

The *parasympathetic nerve supply* to the detrusor is derived from cord segments S2 to S4 and reaches the neck of the bladder by traveling in the pelvic splanchnic nerves. These nerves stimulate contraction of detrusor and inhibit the vesical sphincter. Axons carrying *sympathetic innervation* are derived from T10 to L2 and synapse in paraaortic sympathetic ganglia. Postganglionic sympathetic axons are concentrated in the trigonal region. Since sympathetic innervation produces the strong muscle contractions that accompany ejaculation, it makes sense that similar sympathetic innervation causes the trigonal and bladder neck muscles to contract, preventing reflux ejaculation of semen into the bladder (see Figures 6-44 and 6-49).

Painful stimuli originating in the bladder (from overdistension, stones, etc.), are carried predominantly by sensory nerves accompanying the parasympathetic axons. Based on observations in people with various spinal cord and sympathetic chain injuries, it seems that the pathway for pain detection is different than the one mediating the sense of bladder fullness. Thus the spinal cord may be partially divided to achieve pain control, but the conscious sense of bladder fullness remain intact.

FUNCTIONAL REGULATION IN THE GENITOURINARY SYSTEM

Urination or micturition (L., *micturitius*, to make water; French, *urina*, or urine) is a process that results from relaxation of bladder sphincters and contraction of the bladder detrusor muscles as well as abdominal wall muscles (Figure 6-51). Most of the bladder's musculature (i.e., the detrusor) is innervated by parasympathetic nerves. The trigone is predominantly innervated by sympathetic nerves. During urination, this region of the bladder must relax while the rest of the bladder muscle (i.e., the detrusor) contracts. The sensation of bladder fullness generally occurs when 200 to 300 ml of urine is in the bladder. Most people can accommodate up to 800 to 900 ml when necessary, however.

Urinary continence is the ability to control the timing of urination until the appropriate time and place. In both sexes, the external urethral sphincter is a major regulator of urinary continence. Also the levator ani likely plays a role in maintaining continence because its relaxation occurs just before the beginning of urination.

The *smooth muscle vesical sphincter** differs in the male and female bladder. *Females* appear to have only a rudimentary smooth muscle vesical sphincter at the bladder neck (see Figure 6-49). In *males*, where the size of the vesical smooth muscle sphincter is considerably greater, it is now believed that the major role of the smooth muscle vesical sphincter is to prevent retrograde ejaculation of semen (i.e., into the bladder) during orgasm. In the male, this sphincter may also be referred to as the *preprostatic sphincter.* In both sexes, there

---

*Previously described as the "internal sphincter."

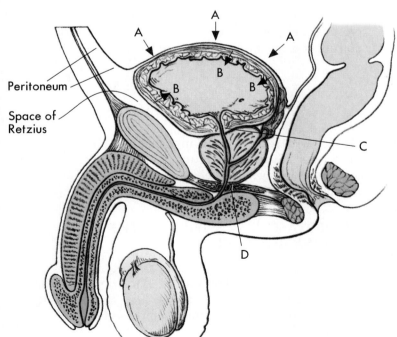

Peritoneum

Space of Retzius

Figure 6-51 MECHANISMS OF URINATION. Contraction of the abdominal wall muscles puts pressure on the bladder (*A*), by increasing the pressure within the peritoneal cavity. The detrusor muscle (*B*) of the bladder wall also contracts, under the direction of parasympathetic nerves. Smooth muscles in the bladder neck (*C*), as well as striated muscles in the sphincter urethrae (*D*), must relax to allow the urine to flow.
SEE ATLAS, FIG. 6-8

Urine is produced in the kidneys and passes through the ureters to reach the bladder. The ureter is capable of a kind of peristaltic contraction that ensures that urine flows to the bladder even if the patient is supine (or even upside down). The basic mechanism in urination is a spinal reflex, where increasing fullness of the bladder triggers sensory axons in the wall of the bladder. These sensory axons deliver a signal to neurons in the sacral spinal cord, which in response stimulate contraction of the detrusor muscle of the bladder wall (through parasympathetic nerves). Simultaneously, sympathetic and somatic motor nerves are activated to relax the sphincters of the bladder and urethra and to activate adjacent muscles involved in the act of urination (see Figure 6-51).

The bladder itself, when containing 200 to 300 ml of urine, provokes this spinal reflex emptying mechanism. The brain, however, alters the threshold for this reflex (allowing the bladder to become fuller), and, in addition, conscious CNS mechanisms can regulate urination. Thus when children learn to be "potty-trained," or when a family pet is "house-broken," the CNS has been trained to override these spinal reflexes to allow urination only when appropriate.

If the sensory nerves from the bladder are damaged, but motor innervation is intact (as in syphilis), the bladder wall will distend abnormally because the normal signal to empty is not delivered. When there is spinal cord injury, both the sensory and motor nerves are damaged. The bladder may at first distend abnormally, and the walls become very thin (a neurogenic bladder). Often, as time passes, the denervated bladder begins to shrink and later becomes small and hypertrophic.

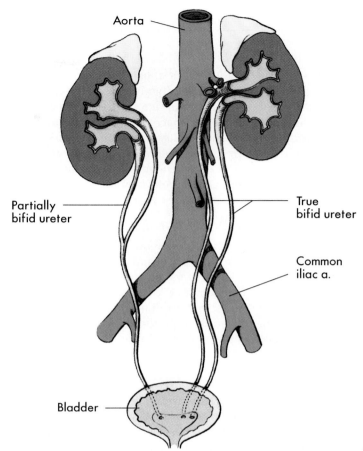

Figure 6-52 DEVELOPMENTAL ERRORS IN THE URETERS. Here the right kidney gives rise to a partially bifid ureter—where there are two separate origins from within the kidney, but distally, at the level of the bladder, all have fused into a single ureter. On the left is a true bifid ureter, where two ureters originate from different parts of the kidney and remain separate throughout, entering the bladder by different orifices.

is evidence that the smooth muscle vesical sphincter relaxes reflexively when the detrusor begins to contract. Fibromuscular extensions of the smooth muscle sphincter help fix the bladder with respect to the pubis and rectum.

The *striated muscle sphincter*[†] of the urethra is the

major regulator of urinary flow in the female, while in the male both the striated and smooth muscle sphincters play important roles (see Figures 6-32, 6-49, and 6-64). The sphincter is under the control of the pudendal nerve and is another example of a muscle that can be regulated at either the conscious or the unconscious level.

[†]Previously described as the "external sphincter."

THE URINARY SYSTEM

SPACE OF RETZIUS (SEE FIGURE 6-51)

There is a wide area of endopelvic fascial tissue between the anterosuperior surface of the bladder and the skin. This space is the space of Retzius. It is a useful extraperitoneal surgical approach to the prostate and the bladder (recovery from abdominal surgery is made more complicated whenever the peritoneal cavity must be entered, and therefore extraperitoneal approaches are desirable).

CATHETERIZATION OF THE BLADDER

When a patient is unable to empty his or her bladder, it is common for physicians to carry out a catheterization. This is usually accomplished by threading a soft catheter up the urethra to the interior of the bladder, but, if that approach is not possible, a needle may be passed through the anterior abdominal wall just above the pubic symphysis (suprapubic catheterization).

ASPIRATION OF URINE FROM THE BLADDER

When circumstances warrant, a suprapubic bladder tap is undertaken to obtain a urine specimen. In this procedure, a needle is inserted in the midline over the superior edge of the pubic symphysis and into the lumen of the bladder. Because of the fat in the space of Retzius (see preceding), such a procedure should not penetrate the peritoneum. Few vessels and no important nerves are in the anterior midline, so no injury to these structures should occur either.

STONES (LITHIASIS) IN THE URINARY SYSTEM

Stones may form in the kidney, ureters, and the bladder. All cause obstruction and recurrent infection as well as considerable pain. When a stone lodges in the upper portion of the ureter, pain is referred to the back. If the stone is lower in the ureter, pain is referred to the perineal region or to the groin. Spasm of the ureteric musculature, with or without the presence of a stone, is referred to *as renal colic.* In fact, ureteral or vesical stones are rarer in the United States, but more common in the Middle East, possibly due to different dietary preferences.

URETERAL ANOMALIES (FIGURE 6-52)

Duplication of the ureter, or other developmental anomalies, are not uncommon, and many are asymptomatic. They may, however, produce difficulty in the flow of urine into the bladder and predispose to retention of urine in the ureters and kidneys and subsequent increased risk of infection.

SPINAL CORD INJURIES AND URINATION (SEE FIGURE 6-44)

Any injury to the lower spinal cord, involving S2 to S4, will disrupt bladder emptying. Because the denervated detrusor cannot contract firmly enough (relying now only on its intrinsic contractility) to cause the bladder to empty, sequestration of urine may lead to flaccid dilation of the bladder, sometimes to very impressive proportions. Note that sensory denervation must also be present to allow the bladder to reach such size without causing pain (a neurogenic bladder).

HORSESHOE KIDNEY (FIGURE 6-53)

One of the more common errors of kidney development is the horseshoe kidney, where there is a continuous loop of kidney tissue connecting the right and left kidneys, forming a sling over the anterior surface of the aorta and IVC. It may be undetected through life, or may cause obstruction to arterial flow and come to the attention of the physician and patient.

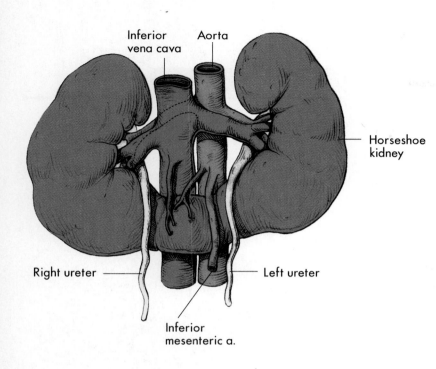

Inferior
vena cava

Aorta

Horseshoe
kidney

Right ureter

Left ureter

Inferior
mesenteric a.

Figure 6-53 HORSESHOE KIDNEY. Horseshoe kidney is one of the more common anomalies of kidney formation. In this condition the two kidneys are joined by a bridge of tissue lying anterior to the inferior vena cava and aorta. It may or may not be symptomatic.

Pelvic Viscera in the Female

▶ Peritoneal and Fascial Structures in the Female Pelvis

▶ Ovaries

▶ Oviducts

▶ Uterus

▶ Vagina

▶ Urethra

PERITONEAL AND FASCIAL STRUCTURES IN THE FEMALE PELVIS

The peritoneal reflections over the female internal genitalia have been described and include the *rectouterine fossa* (of Douglas) and the anterior *vesicouterine fossa* (see Figure 6-25). The part of the peritoneum that drapes over the fundus of the uterus and downward onto its anterior and posterior sides is the **broad ligament.** Within the leaflets of the broad ligament (and its specialized subareas) lie the vessels and nerves supplying the female reproductive viscera. These specialized regions of the broad ligament include the *mesosalpinx* (enclosing the oviduct), *mesovarium* (enclosing the ovary), and *mesometrium* (enclosing the body of the uterus).

The *endopelvic fascia* (equivalent to transversalis fascia of abdominal wall) is specialized and thickened to form the *uterosacral* and *transverse cervical* (or cardinal) *ligaments,* each of which helps to support the uterus (see Figure 6-55).

OVARIES

The ovaries are ovoid glands (see Figures 6-11 and 6-54) about $3 \times 1.5 \times 1.5$ cm, and are enclosed by a specialized reflection of the posterior leaflet of the broad ligament, the **mesovarium** (Figure 6-55). The ovaries are densely cellular organs, in which are found the *primary oogonia* (see Figure 6-54), derived from primitive germ cells. These cells are arrested in the process of meiotic division, and only a small fraction of these will

ever go on to mature into *oocytes*. Oogonia mature constantly throughout reproductive life. The increased rate of chromosomal abnormalities in pregnancies in women in their older reproductive years may result from the long period (often decades) between the first and second meiotic divisions. The many ovarian cells that are not oogonia take part in the maturation of the ovarian follicle by serving as nutritive and hormone-secreting cells.

The ovary has a somewhat denser outer *cortex* and a looser central *medulla* in which many larger veins may be seen. The surface of the ovary has a *tunica albuginea,* comparable to a similar layer in the testis but not as thick or strong. The external ovarian covering of peritoneum is cuboidal in early life and becomes progressively flattened. It is peritoneum and is continuous with the rest of the pelvic peritoneum, but nonetheless is named separately as the *germinal epithelium* (see Figure 6-54).

An *infundibulopelvic ligament* (a distinct fold of the broad ligament) connects the lateral pelvic wall to the lateral end of the oviduct (the infundibulum) and in so doing also stabilizes the position of the ovary as well (see Figures 6-11 and 6-26). This ligament attaches to the lateral pole of the ovary and contains within its folds the ovarian vessels as well as lymphatics and nerves.

Within the leaflets of the broad ligament is found also the *ovarian ligament,* which extends from the medial pole of the ovary to the side of the uterus (see Figures 6-11 and 6-54). This ligament is continued inferior-

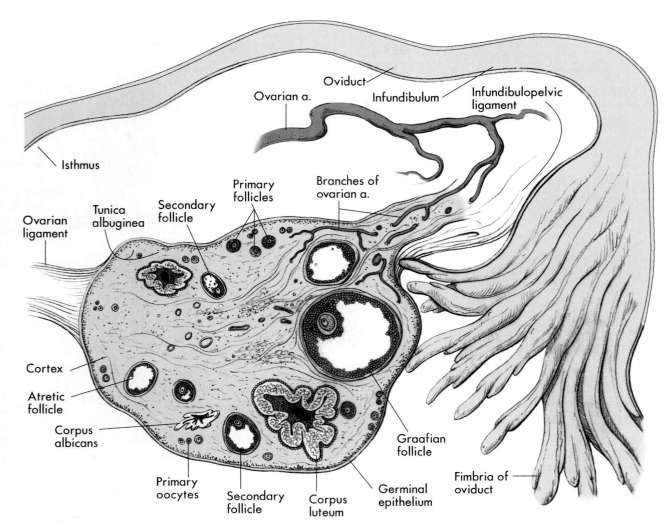

Figure 6-54 INTERNAL STRUCTURE OF THE OVARY. Cross-section through the ovary showing follicles in various stages of maturation or deterioration. The peritoneal covering of the ovary is highly modified, so that it is a cuboidal layer known as the germinal epithelium.

ly as the *round ligament of the uterus*, which passes from the lateral side of the uterus to the abdominal wall and finally through the inguinal canal to the labia majora. The ovarian and round ligaments, then, are the embryologic derivatives of the gubernaculum.

The left and right *ovarian arteries*, having originated from the aorta at the L1 to L2 level, run inferiorly in the posterior abdominal wall (see Figure 6-43). When they reach the pelvis, they turn medially and travel within the infundibulopelvic ligament to reach the ovaries (Figure 6-56). Small terminal branches of the uterine arteries also supply the ovary, approaching it from its medial side. The *left ovarian vein* travels in the same peritoneal fold, ascends the posterior abdominal wall, and drains to the left renal vein, which then drains to the inferior vena cava (see Figure 5-31). The *right ovari-*

an vein, however, usually drains directly to the inferior vena cava.

OVIDUCTS

The **oviducts** or **Fallopian tubes** (Gustavo Fallopio, 16th century Italian anatomist) are two tubes extending laterally from the upper lateral uterine surface (see Figures 6-11 and 6-26) to the vicinity of the ovary on each side. The terminal end of each is a set of elongated "fingers" or **fimbriae,** which lie near the ovary. Fimbriae sweep to and fro and help guide the ovum from the surface of the ovary into the oviduct. The portion of the oviduct opening to the peritoneal cavity is the **infundibulum** (L., funnel). The opposite end of the oviduct, opening into the uterus, is the **isthmus.** The

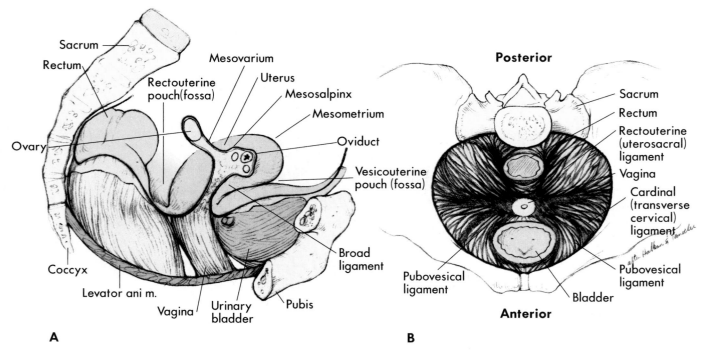

A

B

Figure 6-55 FEMALE INTERNAL GENITALIA. A, Parasagittal view through the female pelvic viscera, approximately 3 to 4 cm lateral to the midline on the right. This view shows the anterior and posterior layers of the broad ligament and how they enclose the oviduct and ovary. That portion of the broad ligament that surrounds the ovary is the mesovarium; that surrounding the oviduct is the mesosalpinx. More medially, the broad ligament covers the body and fundus of the uterus (where it is known as the mesometrium). **B,** The thickenings in the endopelvic fascia serve to stabilize and support the pelvic viscera. The transverse cervical (cardinal) ligaments approach the side of the uterus in the lower portion of the broad ligament. The uterosacral ligament has fibers running predominantly in an anteroposterior direction, stabilizing the uterus, and pubovesical ligaments connecting the pubis to the bladder. SEE ATLAS, FIG. 6-23

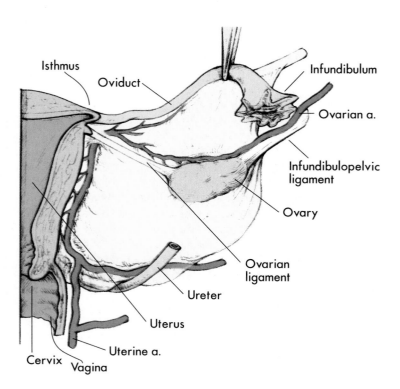

Figure 6-56 BLOOD SUPPLY TO THE UTERUS AND VAGINA. The ovarian and uterine arteries (and veins) approach the uterus and vagina from the lateral side, lying deep to the posterior layer of the peritoneum. The ovarian artery lies within the infundibulopelvic ligament. The two arteries anastomose liberally along the lateral margin of the uterus and vagina.

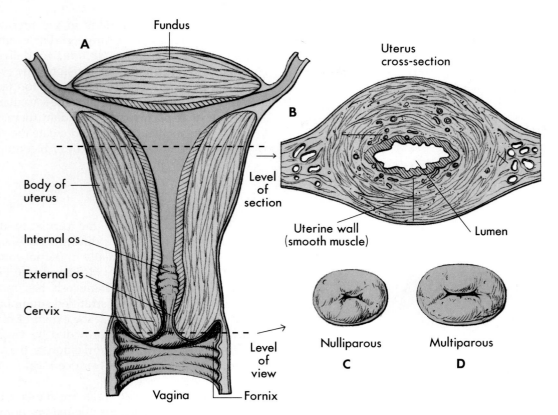

Figure 6-57   UTERUS AND CERVIX.   A, Longitudinal section through the uterus, showing its major regions. **B,** Transverse section through the upper uterus (see dashed line). **C,** Appearance of the cervix as seen from inferiorly in a *nulliparous* (not having given birth) woman. **D,** Cervix in a *multiparous* (having given birth more than once) woman.

SEE ATLAS, FIGS. 6-13, 6-16

oviduct is muscular and lined with cilia, which beat synchronously to help move the ovum toward the uterus.

Blood supply is from the *ovarian* and *uterine arteries. Autonomic nerves,* both sympathetic and parasympathetic, reach the oviducts, but their role is unclear. There are also numerous *sensory axons.*

UTERUS

The uterus is a muscular organ with a cervix, body, and fundus (the uterine area above the level of the isthmus). The *cervix* or *neck* (see Figures 6-11, 6-25 and 6-57) is the portion of the uterus protruding into the upper vagina and can be visualized on direct vaginal examination. The upper end of the cervix joins the *body* or *corpus* of the uterus at the *internal os* (L., opening or mouth). The *external os* (part visible from exterior) is the inferior end of the cervix. The annular space separating the upper vaginal wall from the exterior of the cervix is the *fornix* (see Figure 6-57). The anterior and posterior portions of the fornix are the

largest although in fact it is a continuous circular space.

At the level of the cervix, the uterus is surrounded by specialized thickenings of the endopelvic fascia—the *uterosacral ligaments* posteriorly, the *transverse cervical ligaments* laterally, and the *pubovesical ligaments* anteriorly (see Figure 6-55, *B*). The urinary bladder also provides some support anteriorly.

In its normal position, the uterus is said to be *anteflexed* (forward angulation of the uterine body on the cervix) and *anteverted* (forward angulation of cervical canal on the vagina). The uterus may assume abnormal positions (retroflexion, retroversion), which can have an influence on the ability to carry a pregnancy successfully to term or may be involved in painful menstrual periods (Figure 6-58).

Blood supply is through the *uterine arteries,* which pass anterior to the ureter in the transverse cervical ligament (see Figures 6-46 and 6-56). During hysterectomy, special care must be taken that the ureters are not themselves tied off or otherwise obstructed as the uterine arteries are ligated (a necessary part of removal of the uterus). The density of blood supply and the extent

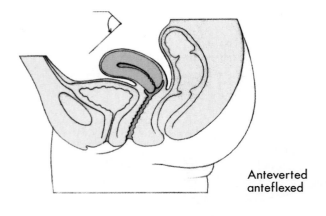

Anteverted
anteflexed

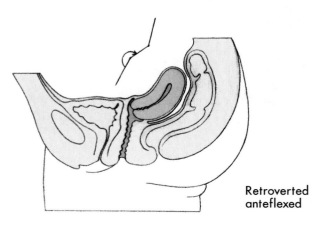

Retroverted
anteflexed

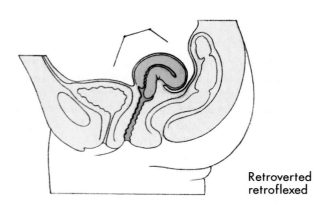

Retroverted
retroflexed

Figure 6-58 POSITIONS OF THE UTERUS. The "version" of the uterus refers to the angle between the vagina and the cervix, while the "flexion" refers to the angle between the cervix and the body of the uterus. The normal position is anteverted and anteflexed, but other combinations of version and flexion are possible. These abnormal positions tend to be associated with higher incidences of difficulty in carrying a pregnancy.

of anastomotic connections in the uterine wall are quite important to the surgeon. For example, when performing a cesarian section, to deliver a child through an abdominal incision, the obstetrician avoids placing the uterine incision too far lateral in the wall of the uterus because the vascular supply of the uterus is particularly abundant there. Placing an incision in such an area would create the risk of difficulty with hemostasis (control of bleeding) after the operation is completed.

VAGINA

The vagina connects the cervix to the outside space. It is a muscular cylinder whose anterior and posterior walls are normally in partial collapse, making its "lumen" actually H-shaped (see Figures 6-11 and 6-25). The vaginal mucosa has many mucus glands and is otherwise stratified squamous epithelium. There is debate about the extent of mucus secretion during intercourse provided by vaginal glands themselves, versus the lubrication of the vagina produced by the secretions from cervical mucus glands from above.

The lateral vaginal walls are flanked by the two bulbs of the vestibule, erectile masses homologous to the bulb of the penis in the male (see Figure 6-24). These become engorged with blood during sexual excitation. The bulbs of the vestibule are surrounded by the bulbospongiosus muscle.

Blood supply to the vagina (see Figures 6-46 and 6-56) is via the vaginal branches of the uterine artery and smaller branches from the internal pudendal and internal iliac arteries.

URETHRA

The female urethra is short (~4 cm) and corresponds roughly to the spongy (penile) and membranous portions of the male urethra (see Figures 6-25 and 6-59). Numerous paraurethral glands empty into it near its distal end. As in the male, the female urethra passes through the urogenital diaphragm and is here surrounded by the external urethral sphincter. In the female particularly, this sphincter is the most important means of maintaining urinary continence.

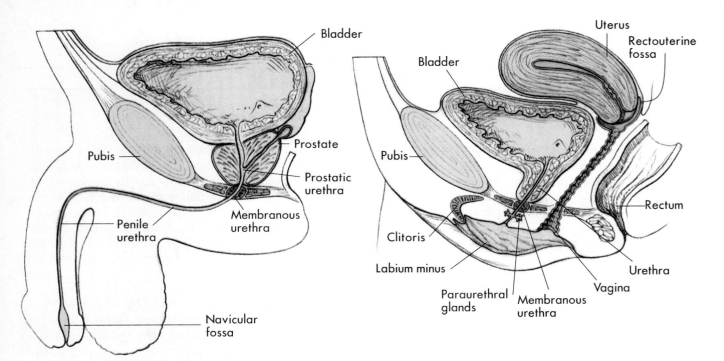

Figure 6-59   MALE AND FEMALE URETHRAE. The male urethra is composed of prostatic, membranous, and spongiose or penile segments. In the female the urethra is short, 3 to 4 cm in length. It receives drainage from several small glands distal to the urogenital diaphragm and is often said to be the equivalent of the membranous and spongy (penile) portions described in the male. In fact the homology between the two is poor.

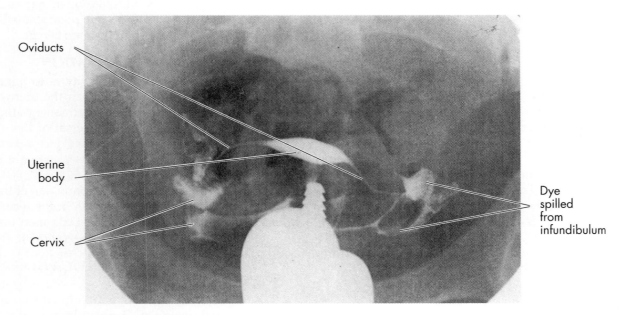

Figure 6-60   HYSTEROSALPINGOGRAM. A hysterosalpingogram involves the injection of a dye substance into the uterus and the retrograde filling of the oviducts. The dye usually spills out of the infundibular end of the oviduct into the abdominal cavity. Such studies are used as part of an evaluation for female infertility, to verify patency of the oviducts. Scarring and closure of the oviducts is an unfortunately frequent complication of recurrent infections with various sexually transmitted diseases, which spread from the vaginal region retrograde to infect the uterus and oviducts, causing scarring and closure of the oviducts. (From Weir J, Abrahams PH: *An imaging atlas of human anatomy,* London, 1992, Mosby.)

THE FEMALE PELVIC VISCERA

OVIDUCTS AND STDS

Sexually transmitted disease (STDs), especially gonorrhea, can spread from the vaginal area to the oviducts and produce pelvic inflammatory disease (PID), often producing sterility through scarring of the oviducts, so that they no longer will allow the passage of a fertilized ovum. The patency of the oviduct can be studied with a hysterosalpingogram, where dye material is injected into the lumen of the uterus and allowed to pass laterally into the oviducts (Figure 6-60).

PREGNANT UTERUS (FIGURE 6-61)

The pregnant uterus assumes massive proportions and poses a considerable potential threat to other organs and tissues in the abdominal and pelvic cavities. A term (the 38th week of pregnancy or beyond), the fundus of the uterus can reach as high as the xiphoid process. Among other things, the large uterus can (1) impede venous return, leading to edema of the lower limbs, hemorrhoids, and thrombophlebitis; (2) compress renal blood flow, compromising kidney function; and (3) interfere with normal bladder emptying or disturb urinary continence.

CERVIX AND PREGNANCY (SEE FIGURE 6-57)

Changes in the texture and appearance of the external os of the cervix appear early in pregnancy. If a woman has borne no children (i.e., is nulliparous), the external os is more or less circular. After vaginal delivery, the external os is a flattened horizontal aperture with thickened anterior and posterior lips.

PUDENDAL BLOCK

The ischial spine can be palpated through the lateral vaginal wall. This is used to guide placement of a long needle in the vicinity of the ischial spine, so that local anesthetic may be injected. This will bathe the pudendal nerve (which wraps around the ischial spine) and effectively anesthetize the perineal area (used for childbirth—the "pudendal block").

CULDOSCOPY (SEE FIGURE 6-59)

The posterior part of the fornix (the circular space just lateral to the uterine cervix) is separated from the peritoneal cavity only by the thin floor of the rectouterine fossa. Samples of fluid in the peritoneal cavity (present in infections) may be removed by passing a needle through the posterior fornix up into the rectouterine fossa.

STRESS INCONTINENCE

Women are particularly prone to stress incontinence of urine in their later years. This is "leakage" of urine during coughing or any activity increasing intraabdominal pressure and may be due to dysfunction of the sphincter or to progressive laxity in ligaments of the bladder. Surgical intervention can involve creation of a fascial sling to be looped under the bladder neck in an attempt to prevent uncontrolled emptying of the bladder.

CERVICAL EPITHELIUM AND THE PAP SMEAR

Small samples of the epithelium of the external os are removed by gentle scraping and studied under the microscope for any cellular changes suspicious for malignancy or other pathology. This is the Pap test (for Dr. Papinicolau, who developed it) and is recommended as a regular screening procedure for women as they age.

SMOOTH MUSCLE TUMORS (FIBROIDS) OF THE UTERUS (FIGURE 6-62)

The uterine smooth musculature can hypertrophy to form leiomyomas or fibroids, often necessitating surgical removal because of the painful menstrual bleeding they cause. These tumors are benign.

STERILIZATION BY TUBAL LIGATION

One method of achieving sterility is to ligate the oviducts so that no ovum can reach the uterus. The operation should be considered permanent although there is growing success with reversal of these ligations in women who wish to conceive once again.

ECTOPIC PREGNANCY

An ectopic pregnancy is the implantation of the fertilized ovum somewhere other than in the interior of the uterus. In Figure 6-62, the most common form of ectopic pregnancy—in the oviduct—is shown.

IMAGING OF THE FEMALE PELVIC VISCERA (FIGURE 6-63)

Ultrasonography is a common technique for evaluating the female genitalia. The bladder is easy to visualize because the urine it contains reflects sound waves differently than the surrounding tissues.

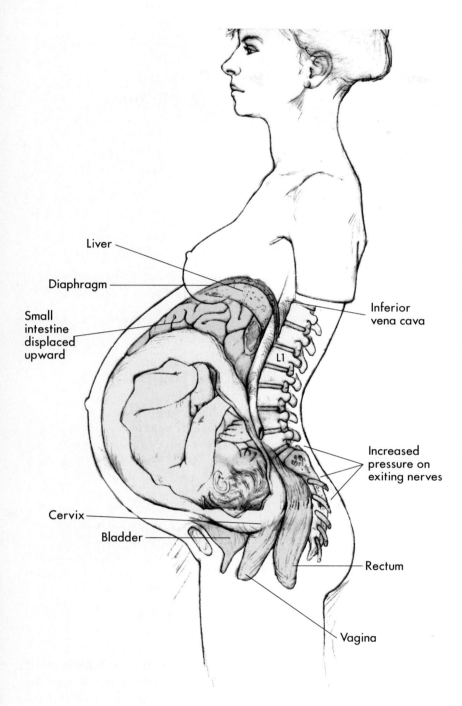

Liver

Diaphragm

Small
intestine
displaced
upward

Inferior
vena cava

L1

Increased
pressure on
exiting nerves

Cervix

Bladder

Rectum

Vagina

Figure 6-61   FETUS IN UTERO. This illustration shows the impressive degree to which the pregnant uterus displaces other abdominopelvic structures and puts pressure on important regions such as the pelvic diaphragm and the respiratory diaphragm. Venous return from pelvic and lower limb structures is made more difficult by pressure on the inferior vena cava, and women commonly develop hemorrhoids and varicose veins in the lower limbs. Breathing may be difficult due to pressure on the diaphragm and the inability to depress it fully to permit filling of the lungs. Back and lower limb pain is common because of pressure on exiting nerves of the lumbar and sacral plexuses.

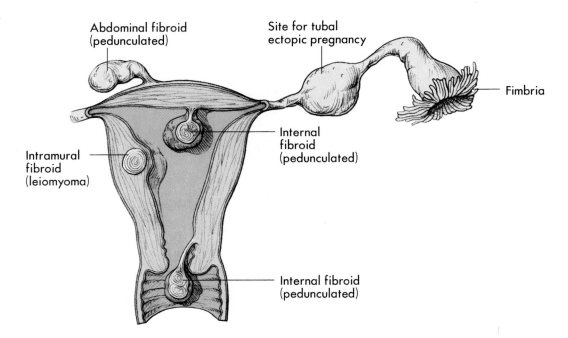

Abdominal fibroid
(pedunculated)

Site for tubal
ectopic pregnancy

Fimbria

Internal
fibroid
(pedunculated)

Intramural
fibroid
(leiomyoma)

Internal fibroid
(pedunculated)

Figure 6-62   ECTOPIC PREGNANCIES AND UTERINE FIBROMAS. The most common location of an ectopic pregnancy is in the oviduct. It is characterized by an abnormal degree of bleeding and pain in early pregnancy, lowered levels of the hormones that normally rise significantly as a confirmation of pregnancy, and inevitably a spontaneous abortion in the first or second trimester. Benign tumors of uterine smooth muscle are known as leiomyomas or fibroids, and they may occur in a variety of locations, as shown here. They generally produce abnormal pain and bleeding with menstruation, but they are not a risk for transformation into cancer. Depending on their location, they may interfere with pregnancy.

Uterus

Urinary
bladder

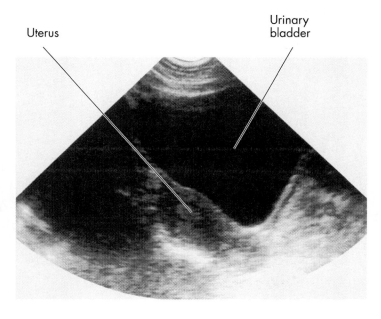

Figure 6-63   ULTRASOUND OF BLADDER AND UTERUS. This is a parasagittal ultrasound through the female pelvis, outlining the urinary bladder and the uterus. Ultrasound is a very useful technique because it is noninvasive, and to date there is no evidence of any injury associated with sound waves. Studies like this are routinely used to evaluate pregnancies. The success of the technique requires the bladder to be filled with liquid because the liquid transmits the sound waves more accurately to the transducer placed on the patient's lower abdomen. (From Weir J, Abrahams PH: *An imaging atlas of human anatomy,* London, 1992, Mosby.)

Pelvic Viscera in the Male

▶ Ductus Deferens   ▶ Penis

▶ Prostate Gland   ▶ Urethra

▶ Seminal Vesicles   ▶ Erection and Ejaculation

DUCTUS DEFERENS

The **ductus deferens** originates at the epididymis, then ascends in the scrotum to traverse the inguinal canal and reach the posterolateral abdominal wall (see Figures 5-13 and 6-65). The ductus travels around the abdominal wall and approaches the base of the bladder posteriorly. In doing so, it passes anterior and superior to the ureters.

In actuality, the ductus is destined to enter the prostatic urethra. Near the base of the prostate, the ductus expands into a swollen bulb or *ampulla.* Within 1 cm of the prostatic urethra (see Figure 6-64), the ductus is joined by the duct of the seminal vesicle, and together they form the **ejaculatory duct,** draining the secretions of the seminal vesicle and the testis together into the prostatic urethra.

PROSTATE GLAND

The **prostate** is a spherical gland, traversed by the urethra, and positioned just inferior to the neck of the bladder (see Figures 6-17, 6-31, 6-33 and 6-64). It lies just superior to the levator ani and urogenital diaphragm. It is composed of a pair of small *median lobes,* surrounding the urethra and positioned deep within the gland. Superficial to these are the *lateral* and *posterior lobes,* on both left and right, which in fact cover the median lobes. None of these lobes is clearly demarcated by a fissure, as is the case with the liver or lungs, and therefore are difficult to demonstrate by dissection. Connective tissue septa may be visualized microscopically, however. The *capsule* surrounding the prostate contains a rich venous plexus and a dense accumulation of autonomic nerves, many of which are destined for the perineum.

Prostatic secretions reach the urethra through the **prostatic ducts,** a series of 20 to 30 small apertures in the posterior wall of the prostatic urethra (see Figure 6-32) near the *urethral crest* (see Figure 6-64). Prostatic secretions are rich in prostaglandins, citrate, prostate specific antigen (PSA), and acid phosphatase, all of which can be used as a plasma marker for prostatic hyperactivity.

SEMINAL VESICLES

The **seminal vesicles** lie on the posterior surface of the bladder base (see Figure 6-70) and empty into the urethra with the ductus deferens as the **ejaculatory ducts.** The seminal vesicles are coiled tubules, which are 12 to 15 cm long if uncoiled. A smooth muscle coat surrounds the seminal vesicles and contracts during ejaculation to help deposit seminal vesicular secretions in the urethra. They may be imaged through a vesiculo-

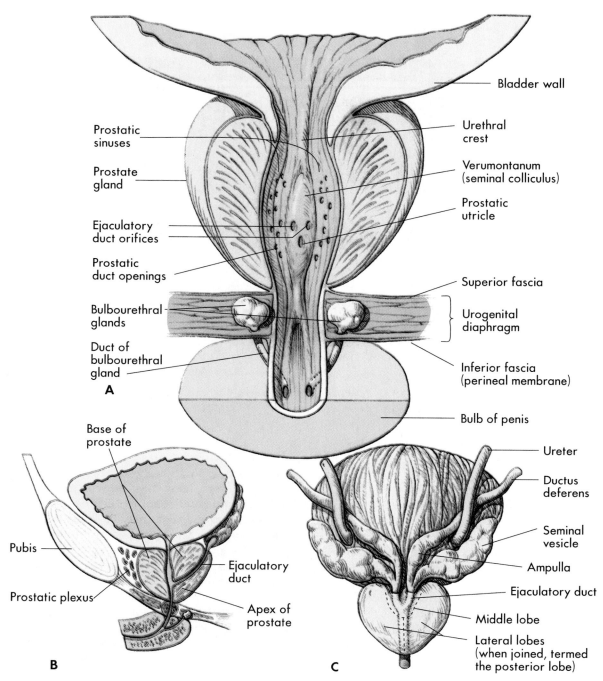

Bladder wall

Prostatic sinuses

Prostate gland

Ejaculatory duct orifices

Prostatic duct openings

Bulbourethral glands

Duct of bulbourethral gland

A

Urethral crest

Verumontanum (seminal colliculus)

Prostatic utricle

Superior fascia

Urogenital diaphragm

Inferior fascia (perineal membrane)

Bulb of penis

Base of prostate

Pubis

Prostatic plexus

B

Ejaculatory duct

Apex of prostate

Ureter

Ductus deferens

Seminal vesicle

Ampulla

Ejaculatory duct

Middle lobe

Lateral lobes (when joined, termed the posterior lobe)

C

Figure 6-64   PROSTATE GLAND. A, Anterior view of the prostate with an incision made along the vertical midline, to reveal the lumen of the urethra as it traverses the prostate. The urethral crest runs the length of the prostatic urethra, and at its midpoint the verumontanum marks the site of the seminal colliculus and the orifices of the two ejaculatory ducts. The 15 to 25 prostate ducts on each side open alongside the urethral crest. **B,** Midsagittal section through the prostate gland, revealing its relationships with the urethra and ejaculatory ducts. **C,** Posterior view of the prostate, showing the relationships of the seminal vesicles, ureters, and ductus deferens. Palpation of the posterior surface reveals a shallow groove separating the right and left portions of the posterior lobe of the prostate gland.   SEE ATLAS, FIGS. 6-20, 6-25, 6-26, 6-27, 6-28

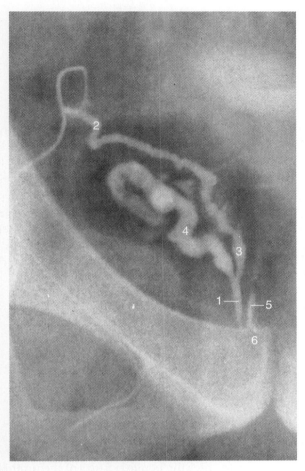

Figure 6-65   SEMINAL VESICULOGRAM. This is a seminal vesiculogram, where dye is injected into the male urethra and fills the seminal vesicles, ejaculatory duct, and ductus deferens by retrograde flow. This study might be used to evaluate abnormalities in sexual function, fertility, or urination. (From Weir J, Abrahams PH: *An imaging atlas of human anatomy*, London, 1992, Mosby.)

1	Right ejaculatory duct	**4**	Seminal vesicle
2	Ductus deferens (vas deferens)	**5**	Left ejaculatory duct
3	Ampulla of ductus deferens	**6**	Position of seminal colliculus

gram (Figure 6-65). The duct of the seminal vesicle joins with the end ductus deferens on each side to form the ejaculatory duct. The **ejaculatory ducts** are ~2 cm long and empty into the prostatic urethra (see Figure 6-64) through a pair of slitlike openings situated at the apex of the seminal colliculus in the prostatic urethra (see next section).

PENIS

The penis has been described on pp. 575 to 578 and Table 6-6 (see Figures 6-16, 6-17 and 6-31). Briefly, it

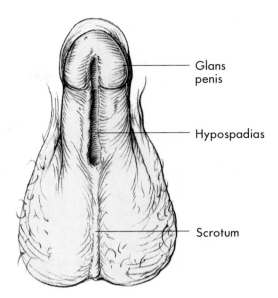

Figure 6-66   HYPOSPADIAS. Hypospadias is a developmental failure of the urethra to close on its ventral surface, so that there is a groove along the ventral surface of the penis. It is benign when present only to a minor degree, but more extensive cases require surgery.

consists of a *corpus spongiosum,* made up of a midline erectile mass, the *bulb,* attached to the inferior surface of the UG diaphragm, and its outward extension into the shaft of the penis, and two *corpora cavernosa,* erectile cylinders anchored laterally to the ischiopubic rami and extending forward to join the extension of the corpus spongiosum to form the shaft of the penis. At its distal end, the corpus spongiosum expands into a rounded shieldlike mass known as the *glans* of the penis. The shafts of the two corpora cavernosa make contact with the proximal side of this structure. All three erectile structures are surrounded individually by a thick tunica albuginea and are further enclosed by a layer of the tunic that surrounds them all. Both the corpus spongiosum and the two corpora cavernosa are covered proximally with striated muscle—the *bulbospongiosus* and *bulbocavernosus muscles,* respectively (see Figure 6-16).

URETHRA

The male urethra is from 18 to 20 cm in total length (see Figures 6-31 and 6-33). Of its three portions, only the first and part of the second sections are analogous to urethral structures in the female, while the third and longest part of the male urethra (the penile or spongiose) is developmentally analogous instead to the labia minora in the female.

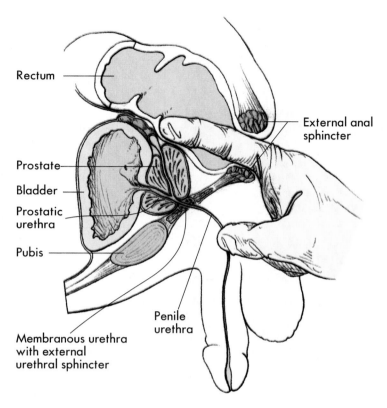

Rectum

External anal
sphincter

Prostate

Bladder

Prostatic
urethra

Pubis

Penile
urethra

Membranous urethra
with external
urethral sphincter

Figure 6-67 PALPATION OF THE PROSTATE GLAND. This diagram shows the technique of the rectal examination, where the finger inserted in the rectum allows palpation of the posterior surface of the prostate gland. Benign prostatic enlargement usually occurs in the median lobe and compresses the urethra so that urination is interrupted and slowed. In time the bladder enlarges and reflux of urine into the ureters is made more likely, posing risk of kidney infection (see Figure 6-47).

The *prostatic urethra* commences at the bladder neck and is about 3 cm long. As it passes through the center of the prostate gland, there is a longitudinal raised *urethral crest* on its posterior luminal surface (see Figures 6-32 and 6-64). Flanking the urethral crest on each side are depressions or grooves called the *prostatic sinuses,* in the floors of which are the small *prostatic ducts.* On the apex of the urethral crest is a circular elevation known as the *seminal colliculus* or *verumontanum* (see Figure 6-64) (L., mountain ridge). The *prostatic utricle* is a single depression in the center of the seminal colliculus and is thought by some to be a remnant of paramesonephric ducts in the male (i.e., developmentally analogous to the uterus). The prostatic utricle is about 5 to 6 mm long and projects backward into the substance of the prostate gland. It is near the prostatic utricle that the two ejaculatory ducts open, emptying the secretions of the ductus deferens (i.e., sperm, plus some fluid) and the seminal vesicles into the urethra.

The next section of the urethra, the *membranous urethra* is within the urogenital diaphragm and is only 1 to 2 cm long (see Figure 6-64). It derives its name from an alternate name for the urogenital diaphragm, the *urogenital membrane.* The external urethral sphincter (a special portion of the deep transverse perineal muscle) surrounds the urethra here. The membranous urethra

is also the site of a significant curvature in the urethra, as it prepares to enter the penile portion of the urethra.

The *penile (spongiose) urethra* begins within the bulb of the penis. The penile urethra is about 15 cm in length (see Figure 6-32). The ducts of the bulbourethral glands enter the urethra in the bulb of the penis. Small accessory glands located all along the penile urethra also deposit secretions into the urethra as part of the ejaculate. At the end of the penis, the urethra dilates into a *navicular fossa.*

ERECTION AND EJACULATION

Erection is the process whereby more blood enters the erectile bodies than leaves them, and, as a consequence, they engorge with blood, becoming larger and firmer. This process occurs both in males and females as a part of sexual arousal. In the female the process involves the clitoris and bulbs of the vestibule, while in the male it involves the three erectile bodies comprising the penis.

Neural signals start the process by increasing the flow of blood into the erectile structures. As the ingress of blood exceeds the egress, the erectile structures enlarge. As this proceeds, the thin-walled veins in the erectile bodies that would carry blood away are com-

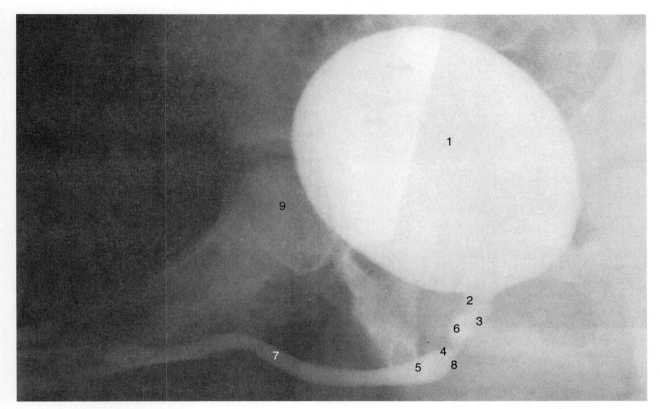

Figure 6-68 VOIDING CYSTOURETHROGRAM. A voiding cystourethrogram is a study in which dye substance is placed in the bladder, and an x-ray taken as the bladder empties. The dye outlines the urethra as it passes outward and might reveal an obstruction caused by lesions such as prostatic hypertrophy or urethral valves. (From Weir J, Abrahams PH: *An imaging atlas of human anatomy,* London, 1992, Mosby.)

1	Contrast in urinary bladder	**6**	Seminal colliculus (verumontanum)
2	Neck of urinary bladder	**7**	Penile urethra
3	Prostatic urethra	**8**	External sphincter
4	Membranous urethra	**9**	Head of femur
5	Urethra in bulb of penis		

pressed, adding to the tendency for blood to accumulate in the erectile tissues. As erection subsides, the autonomic nervous system diminishes the amount of arterial blood being delivered into the erectile tissues, allowing the veins to open once more and blood to leave the erectile tissues. This process is known as *detumescence.* Sacral parasympathetic nerves are classically described as being necessary for normal erections to occur, although more recently evidence has developed that erection may be mediated by a separate set of sympathetic nerves.

Ejaculation is a physiological and psychological event, the physical manifestation of which *in the male* is the expulsion of semen from the urethra. *In the female,* there is a comparable series of muscular processes and psychological reactions, although the goal is not, of course, to move gametes out of the body, as is the case in the male.

Semen is composed in part of sperm, formed in the testis, and traveling through the ductular system to reach the urethra. Additional liquid is added to the semen from the seminal vesicles, prostate, and bulbourethral glands. When sexual arousal in the male reaches its peak, neural signals cause rhythmic and involuntary contractions of the smooth muscle of the ductus deferens, seminal vesicles, and prostatic capsule (see Figure 6-29). In addition, the vesical sphincter closes off the bladder neck and prevents reflux ejaculation. The semen is deposited into the prostatic urethra, where the second phase of ejaculation begins. In this,

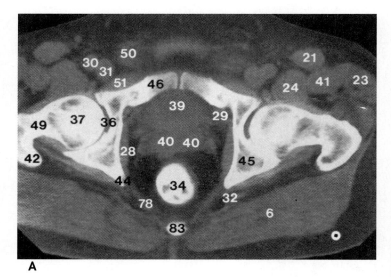

A

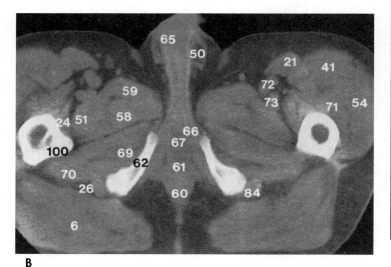

B

Figure 6-69   CT SCANS OF THE PELVIS. Transverse CT scans through the male pelvis at the level of the pubic symphysis **(A),** and the level of the superficial perineal pouch **(B).** Scans such as these are very valuable in the detection and treatment of disease in the pelvis and perineum because these areas are difficult to approach with conventional physical exam and x-ray techniques. (From Weir J, Abrahams PH: *An imaging atlas of human anatomy,* London, Mosby, 1992.)

6 Gluteus maximus muscle	**51** Pectineus muscle
21 Sartorius muscle	**54** Vastus lateralis muscle
23 Tensor fasciae latae muscle	**58** Adductor brevis muscle
24 Iliopsoas muscle	**59** Adductor longus muscle
26 Sciatic nerve	**60** Anal canal
28 Obturator internus muscle	**61** Membranous urethra
29 Obturator artery and vein	**62** Inferior ramus of pubis
30 Femoral artery	**65** Corpus cavernosum
31 Femoral vein	**66** Crus of corpus cavernosum
32 Inferior gluteal artery and vein	**67** Bulb of penis
34 Rectum	**69** Adductor magnus muscle
36 Acetabulum	**70** Quadratus femoris muscle
37 Head of femur	**71** Vastus intermedius muscle
39 Bladder	**72** Superficial femoral artery
40 Seminal vesicle	**73** Profunda femoris artery
41 Rectus femoris muscle	**78** Sacropinous ligament
42 Greater trochanter	**83** Coccyx
44 Ischial spine	**84** Semitendinosus muscle
45 Ischium	**100** Lesser trochanter of femur
46 Superior ramus of pubis	
49 Neck of femur	
50 Spermatic cord	

the striated muscles of the bulbospongiosus contract rhythmically and expel the semen from the penis.

Certain elements of sexual function may be intact even in those individuals who have suffered a complete transection of the spinal cord. Thus without any neural contact with the brain (and thus no conscious sensation), a man may produce an ejaculation (with or without an erection), through appropriate tactile stimulation of the genitalia. This shows that local spinal cord reflex activities are sufficient to mediate an ejaculation.

Ejaculation and emission are used more or less interchangeably to describe the movement of semen out of the male genitalia, although the derivation of the words would suggest that the former is the more ap-

propriate choice, because it suggests the forceful aspect of the movement (L. *jaculatus,* to throw out or dart out, vs. L. *emissio,* to send out). In certain physiologic dysfunctions, an individual may be able to move semen from the ductus deferens to the prostatic urethra but be unable to expel it from the penis; in such individuals, it would appear that the contribution of striated muscle to ejaculation is impaired. Conversely, in *reflux ejaculation,* semen is deposited into the prostatic urethra, but much or all of it passes upward into the bladder instead of distally out the urethra, despite normal contractions of the striated muscles of the bulbospongiosus. The smooth muscle sphincter in the neck of the male bladder is thought to prevent this from occurring.

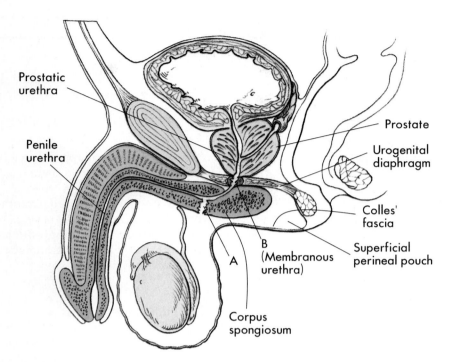

Figure 6-70 TRAUMATIC URETHRAL RUPTURE. Corpus spongiosum and the urethra (*A*) have been ruptured (usually by a forceful blow to the perineum, such as falling astride a fence rail), and urine has extravasated into the superficial perineal pouch. It is limited posteriorly by the attachment of Colles' fascia to the posterior margin of the urogenital diaphragm. The urine can spread upward into the superficial layers of the lower abdominal wall, a space that is continuous with the superficial perineal pouch. Rupture of the membranous urethra (*B*) would not permit urine to spread within the superficial perineal pouch.

There is no widely agreed-upon language, however, to describe the two separate phases of this process, as described in the preceding discussion.

Disorders in erection are of obvious significance in sexual dysfunctions, but they may (and do) exist quite apart from any inability to move semen through the genital ducts. In the majority of cases they are caused by either (1) psychological barriers to normal sexual function and/or (2) circulatory abnormalities preventing the normal changes in blood flow to the erectile bodies that result in an erection. Such impotence is a not infrequent side-effect of the use of certain medications to combat high blood pressure because such medications work by inhibiting sympathetic nerve activity and are unfortunately not specific to just the heart and vasculature. Current research in male sexual dysfunction has uncovered an increasing number of physical causes for erectile and ejaculatory problems, although psychological factors are usually interwoven as well. New vasoregulatory drugs, sometimes injected locally into the penis, are being employed to treat these problems more frequently now than in the past.

Female sexual dysfunctions are still more likely to be ascribed primarily to psychological causes, although further understanding of the physical basis of female sexual function may well uncover a greater number of treatable anatomic or physiologic problems in women as well.

CLINICAL ANATOMY OF

THE MALE PELVIC VISCERA

HYPOSPADIAS (SEE FIGURE 6-66)

Hypospadias is a developmental abnormality in which the opening at the tip of the penis extends abnormally along the ventral surface (i.e., undersurface) of the penis. Epispadius is a much rarer error involving a linear fissure on the dorsal side of the penis.

CHORDEE OF THE PENIS

Chordee is the abnormal curvature of the penis so that it is concave inferiorly and often accompanies hypospadias.

PROSTATE GLAND (FIGURE 6-67)

The prostate is examined most often through a digital rectal examination where the posterior surface of the prostate can be palpated directly through the anterior rectal wall.

Surgery involving the prostatic capsule can harm the nerves within it and cause impotence or urinary incompetence. For this reason, much prostate surgery is performed transurethrally (through a cystoscope passed up the urethra).

Numerous connections between the prostatic venous plexus and the vertebral venous plexus help explain the tendency of prostatic malignancies to spread to bone.

The median lobe of the prostate is predisposed to benign enlargement and subsequent urinary obstruction in older males. The posterior lobes are more predisposed to malignant enlargement.

Pubertal testosterone produces a proliferation in prostatic glands and ducts. Beyond age 45, the prostate begins a process of involution in some men, but in others is subject to benign enlargement.

PHIMOSIS OF THE PENIS

Phimosis is the inability fully to retract the foreskin around the glans of the penis. It requires surgical correction.

POSTERIOR URETHRAL VALVES

The bladder neck may be obstructed by posterior urethral valves—which are in reality persistent strands of embryonic tissue obstructing the flow of urine from bladder into urethra. Recurrent bladder and kidney infections often result, placing the kidney in danger. Urethral valves are virtually confined to males and present in infancy as poor urine output and poor urine stream.

VOIDING CYSTOURETHROGRAM (FIGURE 6-68)

When a patient appears to have obstructions to the flow of urine or when there has been trauma possibly involving the urethra, then a voiding cystourethrogram may be performed. Contrast material is injected into the bladder and several x-rays taken (or the process observed through fluoroscopy) during urination. Any anatomic or traumatic abnormalities will be demonstrated in this way.

PRIAPISM

Individuals suffering from sickle cell anemia are prone to a congestion of sickled (structurally deformed) red blood cells in various small capillary beds throughout the body. When this occurs in the erectile tissues, it can produce an unrelenting and very painful erection known as priapism.

VASECTOMY

The ductus deferens is ligated in the upper scrotum as a means of producing sterility in the male. Although the procedure should be considered permanent, in fact there is a reasonable probability of reanastomosing the ductus deferens and producing fertility. However, the success of this procedure declines in proportion to the time since the vasectomy was performed.

IMAGING THE MALE PELVIS (FIGURE 6-69)

Computed tomography (CT) images have revolutionized the field of noninvasive detection of disease in the pelvic area. Physical examination techniques do not allow direct examination of most pelvic viscera, and the examiner must depend on accurate interpretation of the complex cross-sectional images to detect disease in its earlier stages.

TRAUMATIC INJURY TO THE MALE URETHRA (FIGURE 6-70)

Traumatic injury to the perineum frequently injures or even ruptures the urethra. Depending on the site of the injury, the urine (and blood associated with the injury) can dissect through the tissue spaces in the perineum. A rupture in the membranous urethra, if truly

THE MALE PELVIC VISCERA (Continued)

isolated to that area, would cause urine/blood to spread only within the urogenital diaphragm. Much more common is rupture of the penile or spongiose urethra, causing the urine and blood to dissect posteriorly to the posterior end of the UG diaphragm (where the fascia of the superficial pouch is firmly attached) and anteriorly into the lower abdominal wall because the superficial pouch is continuous with the superficial fascia of the abdomen.

IMAGING THE SEMINAL VESICLES (SEE FIGURE 6-65)

Injection of contrast material into the urethra can fill the seminal vesicles by retrograde flow, and an x-ray may then be taken. Abnormal growths, dilations, or other structural changes may be identified in this fashion.

Systems Review and Surface Anatomy of the Pelvis and Perineum

▶ Skeletal Anatomy

▶ Muscular Anatomy

▶ Arterial Supply

▶ Venous Drainage

▶ Lymphatic Drainage

▶ Innervation of the Pelvis and Perineum

▶ Physical Examination and Surface Anatomy of the Pelvis and Perineum

SKELETAL ANATOMY

The skeletal structure of the pelvis and perineum is dominated by one structure—the pelvis, consisting of the two hip bones and the sacrum/coccyx (see Figures 6-1, *A*, 6-2, and 6-6). The rigidity of the pelvis is ensured by the fibrocartilaginous pubic symphysis (see Figure 6-9)—a joint that can soften and relax during pregnancy in anticipation of childbirth. The powerful sacroiliac joints transmit force between the vertebral column and the lower limb (see Figure 6-9). Mobility is at a minimum at these joints.

Although not strictly a skeletal structure, the perineal body is an extremely important landmark (see Figure 6-16) in the perineum because so many structures seem to attach to it. It lies between the anal opening and the urethra in the midsagittal plane.

MUSCULAR ANATOMY

Muscles attached to the outer surface of the pelvis either ascend to form part of the abdominal wall or descend to attach to the thigh and leg. This latter group of muscles, then, is designed to help stabilize ("balance") the body over the lower limbs and to provide motive force for walking and running.

Most muscles attaching in the inner surface of the pelvis form parts of the pelvic or urogenital diaphragms (see Figure 6-15), while a smaller number leave the pelvis to descend into the lower limb (e.g., obturator internus, iliacus). The pelvic diaphragm serves as a support for pelvic viscera, as well as taking an active role in urination, defecation, etc. Remember that the change from four-legged to two-legged posture puts considerable new pressure on certain regions of the body, such as the pelvic diaphragm and the inguinal canal. In both male and female there is a special set of perineal muscles, covering the erectile structures and playing a role in their erection. In the male, the smooth muscle dartos tunic helps to regulate testicular temperature, as does the striated cremaster muscle, drawing the testis closer to the superficial inguinal ring.

Many of the organs found in the pelvis are made up to a large degree of smooth and/or striated muscle. The bladder is essentially a muscular bag, which enlarges to store urine and then contracts to help expel it from the body. The uterus is a thick-walled muscular receptacle in which the fetus develops. The uterine smooth muscle, although distended by fetal enlargement over nine months, contracts importantly ("labor") to cause expulsion of the baby from the uterus. The rectum is a cylindrical chamber with an inner smooth muscle lining and an exterior complex sheath of striated muscles, especially the external anal sphincter (see Figure 6-19). The smooth muscle of the rectal wall takes part in the peristaltic movements common to all of the gut, while the striated sphincters regulate the passage of feces from the rectum to appropriate times and places. All of these actions (urination, parturition (childbirth), and defecation) are aided by contraction of the abdominal wall musculature (especially the anterior muscles), which contract and increase intraabdominal pressure, further forcing the contents out of the bladder, uterus, or rectum (see Figure 6-51).

ARTERIAL SUPPLY

All of the arterial vessels supplying the pelvis and perineum are branches of the aorta or of its branches. The great majority of vessels supplying the pelvic regions are branches of the internal iliac artery (see Figure 6-20). Its anterior and posterior trunks supply the pelvic interior, the perineum, the gluteal region, and the medial thigh. Major exceptions are the gonadal arteries, which arise not from the internal iliac but from the aorta itself in the upper posterior abdominal wall. These vessels descend along a lengthy course to reach the pelvis. The external iliac artery supplies a small number of arteries to the anterior part of the pelvis, including regions around the obturator membrane. The major role of the external iliac artery, however, is to continue onward into the thigh and leg to become the major blood supply to the lower limb.

The urogenital diaphragm lies deep in the pelvis, and the terminal branches of the internal pudendal arteries (see Figures 6-24 and 6-42) course through the substance of the diaphragm, after traveling in the pudendal canal on the medial surface of the obturator internus. Branches of the internal pudendal artery then descend through the diaphragm to supply the erectile structures in the superficial perineal pouch, while the continuation of the internal pudendal arteries moves further anteriorly to become the dorsal arteries of the penis/clitoris.

VENOUS DRAINAGE

Venous drainage of the pelvis is through the complex pelvic venous plexus, which is a set of vessels draining the bladder, reproductive organs, and rectum in a very variable manner. These veins converge on the internal iliac vein (see Figure 6-20), which drains into the inferior vena cava and returns blood to the right atrium. By contrast, the superior rectal vein drains blood to the portal venous system. Anastomoses between these superior rectal veins (see Figure 5-35) and the middle and inferior rectal veins (draining ultimately to the inferior vena cava) set the stage for the development of dilated superior mucosal veins in the rectum (hemorrhoids) when, for example, liver disease causes resistance to blood flow through the portal vein (to which the superior rectal vein drains). It should be emphasized, however, that the majority of hemorrhoid cases result not from obstruction to flow in the superior rectal veins but from generalized weakness in the walls of rectal veins.

Often neglected are the segmental veins for the lumbar areas of the posterior abdominal wall. These vessels are linked to each other by the ascending lumbar veins (see Figure 1-38), which drain superiorly into the azygos and accessory hemiazygos veins in the posterior thoracic wall.

LYMPHATIC DRAINAGE

The most important distinction to be made about lymphatic drainage of the pelvis (see Figure 6-34) is that drainage of the gonads is directed to the upper posterior abdominal wall and that of the remainder of the perineal areas is directed to the deep and superficial inguinal nodes. This has enormous implications for the detection of infection or malignancy that has originated in the testis or ovary, when contrasted with infection or malignancy that has originated in the perianal or perineal regions.

INNERVATION OF THE PELVIS AND PERINEUM

The pelvis and perineal area is richly innervated with somatic, autonomic, and sensory nerves. The somatic nerves are branches of the sacral plexus (see Figure 6-40) and supply the striated muscles on the external surface of the pelvis and those contained within it (e.g., the pelvic diaphragm, the piriformis, etc.). The striated muscles of the perineal region (transverse perineal muscles, muscles covering erectile bodies) are all innervated by the pudendal nerve. The lower end of the digestive tract is also innervated by the pudendal nerve (see Figure 6-22). The internal pelvic wall muscles (levator ani, coccygeus, piriformis, obturator internus) are innervated by small branches of the sacral plexus. Gluteal muscles are innervated by the superior and inferior gluteal nerves, which also are branches of the sacral plexus. The anterolateral thigh muscles, by contrast, are innervated by the largest branch of the lumbar plexus, the femoral nerve (see Figure 6-40). The posterior thigh is innervated by the sciatic nerve of the sacral plexus (see Figure 6-40) and the medial thigh by the obturator nerve, a branch of the lumbar plexus.

Both parasympathetic and sympathetic innervation are rich and important in the pelvis and perineum. Sympathetic input is largely derived from the hypogastric nerve (see Figure 6-44) and is directed at the smooth musculature of the male reproductive tract (ductus deferens, seminal vesicle, trigonal region of the bladder). The ganglia from which the sympathetic axons have arisen are located along the aorta. Parasympathetic input (see Figure 6-36) is confined almost entirely to the pelvic nerve (S2 to S4) and is directed at the urinary bladder as well as to the erectile structures of the perineum. In the bladder, the parasympathetic nerves stimulate contraction of the muscular wall of the bladder (the detrusor muscle), while in the erectile structures the parasympathetic axons cause erection, presumably through regulation of blood flow.

Sensory axons accompany both the sympathetic and parasympathetic nerves into the pelvis and perineum. Their cell bodies are in the dorsal root ganglia of the lower lumbar and upper sacral axons. Reflexes involving pelvic structures do exist, and they resemble the more familiar reflexes of the patellar tendon, biceps tendon, etc. An example is in the urinary bladder, which sends a message of fullness to the spinal cord level through sensory nerves accompanying the pelvic nerve. This sensory signal stimulates parasympathetic outflow from the spinal cord, causing the detrusor muscle to contract, and at the same time influences both sympathetic and somatic nerves, so that sphincter muscles in the path of the urine can relax. The sensory "information" from pelvic organs is not so much consciously appreciated as is sensory information from, for example, the surface of the nose or the tip of the finger. Sensory axons innervating visceral structures have been called visceral sensory axons to represent this functional distinction from somatic axons although the anatomic pattern is the same as in somatic sensory axons. At the spinal cord level, visceral sensory axons have the capability of stimulating certain somatic sensory pathways so that a stimulus originating in an organ, such as the ureter or bladder, can cause feeling in a part of the body surface innervated with somatic sensory axons arising in the same spinal cord level as the visceral sensory axons innervating the bladder. When this "cross-talk" occurs, the patient feels intense sensations in the area of the body supplied by the somatic sensory axons, even though the actual source of the neural "signal" is in the organ innervated by the visceral sensory nerves. It is known as "referred pain" and can be useful to the clinician. An example is the periumbilical pain felt by the patient whose appendix is inflamed, or the sharp groin pain felt when a stone is passed in the ureter.

Although it is harder to appreciate, there is a pattern of dermatomal (segmental) cutaneous innervation in the pelvic and perineal regions, just as there is in the trunk. The lowest spinal cord segments, S4 and S5, innervate successively wider concentric circular regions around the anus (Figure 6-71).

PHYSICAL EXAMINATION AND SURFACE ANATOMY OF THE PELVIS AND PERINEUM
Male Pelvis and Perineum

Physical examination of the pelvic and perineal regions demands special sensitivity to the feelings of the patient and a respect for his or her dignity and privacy. Physicians may become accustomed to examination techniques that are unfamiliar to the patient and are likely to make him or her uncomfortable. Examination will be much more informative and successful for all concerned if these principles are kept in mind.

In comparison to other regions of the body, palpation of internal organs and structures in the pelvic region is relatively difficult. In the male, the most frequently examined area of the pelvis and perineum is the inguinal canal and testes. When palpating the inguinal region, the patient must be relaxed and comfortable, because contraction of muscles in the area may prevent accurate detection of a hernia or other abnormal structure. The inguinal ligament should be visualized extending from the anterosuperior iliac spine to the pubic tubercle. About 2 to 3 cm lateral to its medial end, and just above the plane of the ligament, is the location of the superficial inguinal ring. By placing the index finger on the base of the scrotum and gently pressing upward toward the superficial ring, the examining finger can be placed in a position to palpate any herniation present at this ring. It may be possible to palpate the firm cylindrical spermatic cord as it emerges from the ring. When the patient is asked to cough while the examining finger stays in this position, the increased intraabdominal pressure associated with the cough will cause any herniated peritoneum to "bulge" outward, where it will be felt by the fingertip. Although it is possible to categorize inguinal hernias as direct (those passing medial to the inferior epigastric vessels) and indirect (those following the course of the spermatic cord, passing lateral to the inferior epigastric vessels), in practice it may not be easy to make this distinction by physical examination alone (see Figure 5-11, *A* and *B*). When no hernia is present, and the patient is not overly obese, the edges of the superficial inguinal ring can be felt quite easily.

Examination of this area should continue with the palpation of the spermatic cord in the upper part of the

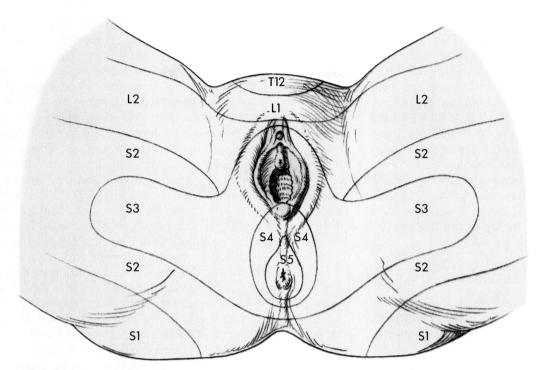

Figure 6-71 **DERMATOMES IN THE PELVIC REGION.** The perineal region is shown in the lithotomy position (i.e., that used for childbirth, and for many medical examinations of the genitalia). The pattern of cutaneous innervation is that of a series of concentric areas with the anal region as its focus.

scrotum and then palpation of the testis (see Figure 5-13). It is possible to feel the solid elongated mass of the epididymis on the posterior surface of the testis, and the remaining surface of the testis should be smooth and nontender. Malignancies of the testis are among the most common malignancies in young men, and men should practice self-examination on a regular basis every bit as much as breast self-examination should be practiced by women. In male children, confirmation of the descent of the testis into the scrotum is important because failure to descend places the ultimate fertility of the individual in jeopardy. Undescended testes also have a much increased incidence of malignancy. Palpation of the region above the testis will often detect a tortuous mass of vessels—the varicocoele—which represents enlargement and coiling of veins of the pampiniform plexus, presumably brought about by impeded venous return. Varicocoeles are more common on the left than the right side. Recall that the testicular veins drain upward to the inferior vena cava (right side) or the left renal vein (left side); this gravitational pressure presumably adds to the tendency for varicocoeles to form. They frequently contribute to infertility in the male, perhaps because of changes in the temperature at which the testis is maintained.

Another important component of the male examination is the palpation of inguinal lymph nodes (see Figure 6-34). Enlargement and tenderness of these nodes can suggest a wide variety of conditions, ranging from a past history of inflammations in the bladder, perianal region, prostate, or lower limb, to a malignancy such as lymphoma or Hodgkin's disease.

The cremasteric reflex involves gentle stimulation of the skin on the upper medial thigh, with resultant elevation of the testis toward the root of the scrotum. This may be a protective reflex or may be a means of controlling testicular temperature. The muscle mediating this reflex is the cremaster, a prolongation of the internal oblique of the abdominal wall, innervated by the genital branch of the genitofemoral nerve. The sensory innervation of the medial thigh is through the femoral branch of the genitofemoral nerve. Both nerves are derived from cord segments L1 and L2.

The other major component of the male pelvis and perineal examination is the rectal examination (see Figure 6-67). For the examination to yield useful information, the patient must be relaxed. Using adequate lubricant gel, a gloved index finger is inserted past the anal sphincter into the lower rectum, or rectal ampulla. About 2 cm above the sphincter, a groove can be palpated that marks the end of the internal sphincter and the point at which the levator ani inserts into the rectal wall. By directing the finger anteriorly, the posterior surface of the prostate gland can be palpated, which will have a shallow midline groove separating the two lateral lobes of the gland. Enlargement or tenderness of the prostate may be detected, and, in appropriate situations, the gland can be "massaged," causing some prostatic secretions to be deposited into the urethra, from which they can be collected for laboratory analysis. By sweeping the finger laterally, the ischial spines may be palpated and the sacrospinous ligaments identified as they sweep posteriorly toward the sacrum. In the posterior midline, the tip of the coccyx can be felt through the rectal wall.

Female Pelvis and Perineum

The inguinal region in the female is not subject to the same risk of herniation as in the male. When hernias in this region do occur (as a result of increased intraabdominal pressure, as in pregnancy), they are most often femoral hernias—herniation inferior to the inguinal ligament (see Figure 7-4, *A*). Detection of inguinal lymph node enlargement, however, is just as important in the female as in the male.

Examination of the female genitalia is best performed with the patient in the supine position (on her back), with thighs spread apart to improve access to the perineal area. Many examining tables have stirrups or other supports to position the lower limbs of the patient correctly. The female external genitalia, occupying the urogenital triangle, are described by the nonanatomic term vulva. The fat-filled eminence just superior to the pubic symphysis in the female is known as the mons pubis. Also of interest is the pattern of hair growth in the female as opposed to the male. In the female, pubic hair grows on the surface of the labia majora and upward to form a distinct horizontal upper border just above the pubis. This pattern of hair growth is known as the female escutcheon ("shield") and differs from the hair pattern in the male, where hair grows on the scrotum and extends upward in the shape of a triangle with its apex at the umbilicus (the male escutcheon). The hair extending upward from the scrotum to the umbilicus is not pubic hair, however, but similar to ordinary body hair found on the chest or the thighs.

In the normal female, the labia majora flank the entrance to the vagina (see Figure 6-23). They are gently curved linear fat-filled masses of tissue, extending from the perineal body posteriorly to the region superior to the clitoris, where the two labia join in an anterior commissure. The bulbs of the vestibule (see Figure 6-24) lie beneath the surface along most of the length of the labia majora. The vestibular glands are located at the

posterior end of each vestibular bulb. The labia majora have no hair growing on their medial sides, but their lateral sides are covered with hair.

The examiner next gently separates the labia majora, revealing the labia minora, slender raised vertical elevations of tissue running along the inner surface of the labia majora. The space between the two labia minora is the entrance to the vaginal canal, known as the vestibule or "vaginal introitus." The anterior end of each labium minor splits around the clitoris to form a commissure superior to it and the frenulum of the clitoris inferiorly (see Figure 6-27). At the posterior end of each labium minor, on its medial surface, are found the orifices of the greater vestibular glands, emptying into the vestibule. Separating the labia minora allows inspection of the vaginal walls and, superior to them, the orifice of the urethra. Cannulation of the urethral orifice with a soft flexible catheter is commonly performed, to drain the bladder of urine if there is an obstruction within the bladder, or if the patient is unconscious and unable to urinate normally. Above the urethral orifice is the clitoris (see Figure 6-27). On the surface the clitoris appears to be a small cylindrical protrusion, but most of the substance of the clitoris lies more deeply, as a pair of elongated erectile bodies, attached to the ischiopubic ramus on each side.

To inspect the full length of the vagina, it is necessary to insert a speculum into the vaginal canal. The speculum gently spreads the walls of the vagina apart, so that the interior of the vagina may be examined. Also, the speculum allows visual inspection of the uterine cervix. The examiner's finger is passed upward in the vaginal canal until the cervix is reached. The cervix should be firm, mobile, and not painful to the touch. Color and consistency changes in the cervix are one of the earliest physical manifestations of pregnancy (although today early detection of pregnancy is performed by simple tests of urine). In addition, by placing a finger in the vaginal canal and palpating posterior to identify the sacral promontory, and at the same time identifying the position of the pubis on the external surface of the abdominal wall (using the thumb of the examining hand) a rough estimate of the A-P diameter of the pelvis can be obtained (the obstetric or diagonal conjugate—see Figure 6-1, *B* and *C*).

It is also possible to palpate the vaginal fornix, a thin space that surrounds the cervix (see Figure 6-57). With appropriate instruments, samples of tissue may be removed from vagina or cervix, or other special procedures performed. For example, placement of intrauterine devices (IUDs) is carried out by separating the vaginal walls with a speculum and placing the IUD through the cervix into the uterine interior.

Bimanual examination allows the examiner to palpate the ovary, uterus, and nearby structures of the broad ligament between ovary and uterus. These struc-

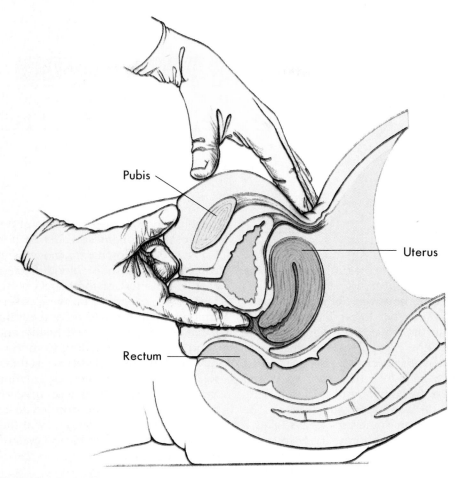

Figure 6-72   BIMANUAL EXAMINATION. By placing one hand on the lower abdominal wall and a finger of the other hand within the vaginal canal, the examiner can gently palpate structures by placing them between the two hands. Here the cervix is being palpated. By moving the hands more laterally, the ovaries can be palpated with this procedure.

tures are known as the uterine adnexa. With one or two fingers in the vagina, the examiner uses his or her other hand to press downward on the midline abdominal wall just superior to the pubic symphysis (Figure 6-72). With the other hand the examiner's fingers gently elevate the cervix. This permits the examiner to feel the uterus between the fingers in the vaginal canal and the fingers of the hand on the lower abdominal wall. By moving the fingers in the vagina somewhat laterally and simultaneously pressing on the abdomen to one side of the midline, it is possible to palpate the ovary and the other structures within the broad ligament.

Such an examination can detect ovarian masses or other abnormal growths adjacent to the uterus.

Palpating in a posterior direction within the vagina allows examination of the perineal body. Inflammation, perhaps present as a result of a recent traumatic vaginal delivery, produces severe pain when pressure is placed on the perineal body. By placing the index finger in the vagina and the middle finger in the rectum, the examiner can palpate the cervix, especially its posterior part, and assess the lower rectum and posterior vaginal wall for abnormal growths or tenderness. This technique is known as the rectovaginal examination.

■ CASE 1

BACK PAIN AND THE DELIVERY OF A BABY

A 27-year-old woman was pregnant for the first time and anxiously awaited the delivery of her first child. As the pregnancy progressed, however, the woman began to notice increased pain in her lower back and even had trouble bending at the waist, owing to the sharpness of the pain she would experience in the lower back. She informed her obstetrician that she had had back pain off and on her job over the past 3 years and that she had even seen the company physician 2 years ago when the back pain was particularly severe. The obstetrician was able to locate some back x-rays taken 2 years earlier, and a vertebral abnormality helped explain the patient's current problems and was important in planning the upcoming delivery of the patient's child. She described to the patient an abnormality called spondylolisthesis and said that it might make necessary a cesarian delivery.

Questions

1. What is *spondylolisthesis,* and its related condition, *spondylolysis?*
2. What abnormalities in vertebral structure result from this condition?
3. What influence does spondylolisthesis have on the birth process?

■ CASE 2

PERINEAL INJURY DURING CHILDBIRTH

A 16-year-old female had reached full term of her pregnancy, and the process of labor and delivery began. She had not sought medical care during the pregnancy and in fact had concealed the fact of her pregnancy from her parents (from whom she was estranged) and all but a few friends her own age. She planned to deliver the baby at a friend's home and then give it up for adoption. As the baby moved further through the birth canal, the young woman began to experience increasing pain, some of it stabbing and quite severe. As the baby's head first became visible, there was a sudden downward movement of the head and a considerable gush of blood from the vagina of the mother. The rest of the baby's body emerged quickly. Her young friends, who were observing the birth and trying to help her, tied off and cut the umbilical cord of the baby. The baby cried lustily and seemed to be in good health. The bleeding from the mother continued, however, and her friends were unable to see precisely where the bleeding was originating. It became clear that the young mother was appearing more pale and becoming dizzy. They decided to call 911, and emergency attendants started an IV at the scene, packed the vagina to dampen the bleeding, and took her to a local emergency room.

Questions

1. What sudden event allowed the baby's head to descend rapidly and caused the bleeding?
2. What anatomic structures are involved in the lacerations occuring in vaginal childbirth?
3. What potential complications can follow from an uncontrolled tear of the perineum such as occurred in this case?

■ CASE 3

ANESTHESIA FOR CHILDBIRTH

A 29-year-old mother of three was expecting her fourth child and was very fearful of the pain associated with the passage of the child through the birth canal during a vaginal delivery. She did not wish to undergo general anesthesia and have a cesarian section because she did not want any postoperative scars and wished to be awake for the first moments after her baby was born. She asked her obstetrician if any alternatives were available. The obstetrician explained to her patient that there were several alternatives to provide pain relief that would involve injection of local anesthetic in the perineal area.

Questions

1. What single nerve is most responsible for the painful sensations that accompany natural childbirth?
2. Where is that nerve most accessible to treatment with a local anesthetic?
3. What landmarks should the obstetrician use to deliver the local anesthetic accurately?

■ CASE 4

URINARY ABNORMALITY IN A 3-MONTH OLD BOY

A healthy newborn boy seemed normal in every way, but his mother became convinced over the first few weeks of his life that he did not urinate normally. He was able to produce urine, but it dribbled out of his penis, rather than forming a normal stream. Sometimes his lower abdomen seemed to her to be distended. At 3 months of age he developed a fever and seemed very listless. His pediatrician performed an examination, ordered several laboratory tests, and discovered to the surprise of all that the young boy had a urinary tract infection. After ordering antibiotics as treatment, he explained to the mother that it would be necessary to perform some further diagnostic tests on the boy's urinary tract, to see if a structural abnormality was present. After the tests confirmed the pediatrician's suspicions, the mother was told that the boy's bladder and ureters were enlarged and that his bladder outlet was obstructed. She was also advised that an operation would be required because the abnormality posed a serious threat to the boy's kidneys (see Figure 6-47).

Questions

1. What are posterior urethral valves and how do they threaten the entire urinary system?
2. What mechanisms normally prevent urine from "refluxing" from bladder into the ureters?
3. Why are the kidneys threatened by such an abnormality?

■ CASE 5

A 59-YEAR OLD WOMAN WITH UTERINE CANCER

A 59-year-old woman had not had any visits to the gynecologist since her menopause 10 years earlier and was surprised when she began to have some irregular vaginal bleeding and pain in the lower abdomen. She visited a physician, who determined that she had a cancerous lesion in the wall of her uterus and recommended a hysterectomy (removal of the uterus). The

operation was performed, and all seemingly went well. About 2 months later, however, the patient had recurrent fevers and was determined to have a bacterial infection. An ultrasound study of her abdomen showed that the pelvis of her left kidney was distended with fluid and that the kidney tissue was thinned as a result of the distension of the renal pelvis. A second surgical procedure was required to correct the problem.

Questions

1. What steps must be taken to separate the uterus from surrounding structures before it is removed?
2. What occurred in this procedure that led to injury to the kidney?
3. What repair procedures may be applied in this situation?

■ CASE 6

A TRAUMATIC INJURY TO THE PERINEUM

An 8-year-old boy was out riding his bike and crashed into an oncoming car. His hips slid forward off of the bicycle seat and he sustained a very forceful "straddle" injury as his legs went on either side of the strut extending from the seat to the front wheel strut. The injury was very painful, and he was taken to the emergency room. The physicians there noted that his scrotum was tense and swollen, and the skin seemed dark in color. The discoloration also extended upward over the lower part of the anterior abdominal wall. On further examination they noted that the subcutaneous discoloration also extended posterior from the scrotum but seemed to end as a rather sharp horizontal line connecting the two ischial tuberosities. It was further noted that as he attempted to pass urine there was great pain, and the resultant few drops of urine were blood-tinged. The physicians informed his parents that they suspected an injury to his urethra, with spillage of urine and blood accounting for the discolored regions noted beneath the skin.

Questions

1. What is the course of the male urethra as it leaves the bladder and eventually opens at the distal end of the penis?
2. What portion of the urethra has been injured, and what is the nature of the injury?
3. What accounts for the discoloration beneath the skin in several areas, and particularly what explains the seeming barriers beneath the skin, beyond which the subcutaneous fluid did not extend?

■ CASE 1

1. *Spondylolysis* is a condition in which the region between the superior and inferior articular facets, on the posterior arch of the L5 vertebra, is damaged or missing. This region is known as the pars interarticularis, and, when it is absent or only partially developed on both sides of the vertebra, the entire neural arch of the L5 vertebra may separate from the body of the vertebra. In such cases the anterior part of the L5 vertebra, the body, may slide anteriorly on the sacrum. This creates a irregularity in the anterior margin of the vertebral column, such that L5 and the overlying L4 and L3 protrude forward. This anterior displacement is known as *spondylolisthesis.*
2. In the case of spondylolisthesis, the absence of the pars interarticularis on each side of L5 causes the body to slide forward and the neural arch to remain in a posterior position, separated from the body.
3. In childbirth, the conjugate diameter is the distance between the sacral promontory and the pubic symphysis and is an important limiting dimension in the passage of the baby's head through the birth canal. In cases of spondylolisthesis, the body of L5 may protrude forward, causing the distance between it and the pubic symphysis to be actually less than that between the sacral promontory and the pubis, and pose a significant obstruction to passage of the baby's head. In such cases, a cesarian delivery (i.e., delivery of the baby through an abdominal incision in the mother) may be required.

■ CASE 2

1. The passage of the baby's head through the birth canal puts great stress on the musculature of the lower uterine wall and, in the terminal stages of delivery, stretches the vaginal wall to a diameter of 10 cm or more (Figure 6-73). In an uncontrolled delivery, such as occurred here, there is increased risk that the baby's head will produce a sudden tear in the wall of the vagina, causing a sudden decompression of the baby's head and a rapid descent. The vaginal tear can extend for a considerable distance, in the most extreme cases into the wall of the rectum.
2. Vaginal tears are graded 1 through 4 by obstetricians, the least serious involving the local vaginal wall only and the most serious involving the vaginal wall and a continuous tear throughout the anal sphincter into the rectal wall (grade 4). Serious tears may become infected, due to the presence of bowel organisms, although neither the vagina nor the rectum is an aseptic area and healing is never under completely sterile conditions. In a controlled delivery, the obstetrician can slow the passage of the fetal head and minimize tearing. Also the obstetrician can perform an episiotomy, or a planned incision through the vaginal wall, in order to prevent a larger tear from occurring during a precipitous delivery. If a tear involves the perineal body of the perineum, then other important structures (e.g., the transverse perineal muscles, the levator ani) are weakened as well. Repair of a vaginal tear or of an episiotomy incision should always include the perineal body (if it has been injured) so that the perineum will not be subject to laxity and weakness (see Figure 6-37).
3. As discussed, unrepaired injury to the perineal body weakens the whole perineum and causes dysfunction in the levator ani and transverse perineal muscles. This can lead to prolapse (abnormal downward "saging" or even "telescoping" of these organs through the pelvic diaphragm) of the rectum, cervix, or urinary bladder, each of which is supported by the pelvic diaphragm and depends on its tautness to keep these organs in their normal position (see Figure 6-38). Disturbances in the pelvic diaphragm may also tend to make the affected woman incontinent of urine, because the mechanism of urinary continence depends in part on the support of the female urethra as it traverses the urogenital and pelvic diaphragms.

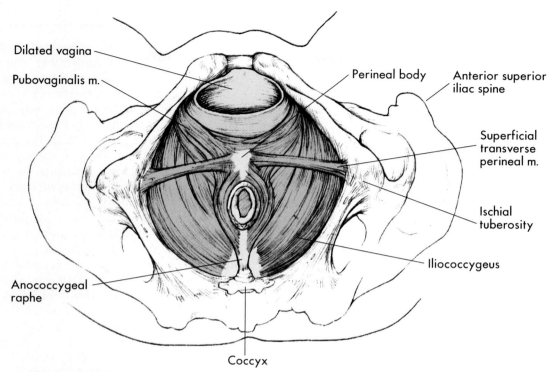

Dilated vagina

Pubovaginalis m.

Perineal body

Anterior superior iliac spine

Superficial transverse perineal m.

Ischial tuberosity

Iliococcygeus

Anococcygeal raphe

Coccyx

Figure 6-73 PELVIC DIAPHRAGM AND CHILDBIRTH. The levator ani is stretched to many times its normal width, and the walls of the vagina have also dilated to permit passage of the baby's head.

■ CASE 3

1. The process of childbirth puts considerable stretch on the walls of the uterus, the walls of the vagina, the pelvic and urogenital diaphragms, and the labia minora and majora. The one nerve that is responsible for providing sensory innervation to these areas is the pudendal nerve. It is derived from sacral spinal cord segments S2, S3, and S4. In addition to providing sensory innervation to these areas, it also provides motor innervation to most of the striated muscles in the perineal area.

2. The pudendal nerve originates deep within the pelvis and there is not easily accessible to administration of a local anesthetic. It wraps itself around the ischial spine of the pelvis and then turns anteriorly to run in the urogenital diaphragm. Along its course, it gives off several branches to the skin of the perianal area, the labia, and clitoral areas in the female. It would not be practical to attempt to anesthetize each of these individual cutaneous branches. The only practical point where the pudendal nerve can be bathed in a local anesthetic is as it wraps itself around the ischial spine.

3. Delivering the local anesthetic to the pudendal nerve at the ischial spine begins with the physician gently inserting a finger into the vaginal canal and palpating laterally until the ischial spine is felt. Leaving that hand in place to mark the position of the spine, the physician then uses the other hand to insert a long needle through the wall of the vagina in the direction of the ischial spine. The needle has a circular metal cuff a short distance back from the tip of the needle. The purpose of this arrangement is to enable the physician to insert the needle tip through the sacrospinous ligament so that the opening at the end of the needle lies in between the sacrospinous and sacrotuberous ligaments in the plane where the pudendal nerve and vessels wrap around the ischial spine. The circular cuff on the needle prevents the needle from going too far, through both the sacrospinous and sacrotuberous ligaments. Once the needle is properly placed, the anesthetic solution is infused, bathing the pudendal nerve and producing anesthesia in the perineal area.

■ *CASE 4*

1. Posterior urethral valves are small abnormal growths of tissue at the bladder neck that obstruct the normal flow of urine from bladder into urethra. They are found in males almost exclusively and cause the retention of urine in the bladder and an increase of pressure within it as well (see Figure 6-47).

2. Even when there is residual urine in the bladder, the ureter is arranged in such a way that the urine normally does not flow backward into the ureters. This is accomplished because the distal portion of the ureter runs for a short distance through the wall of the bladder (and parallel to it) before it opens into the lumen of the bladder in the bladder trigone. This short segment of the ureter, coursing within the wall of the bladder, is normally compressed as the bladder fills with urine, preventing the reflux of urine into the ureters. Active compression of the bladder, during contraction of the detrusor muscle, also produces compression of the ureter as it traverses the bladder wall. This anatomic arrangement is known as the sheath of Waldeyer (see Figure 6-49).

3. Eventually such a situation leads to reflux of urine backward into the ureters, causing them to become dilated and tortuous (hydroureter—see Figure 6-47). The reflux of urine then progresses further proximally into the renal calyces (hydronephrosis). Over time such a situation leads to dilation of the calyces and injury to the functioning kidney tissue, ultimately threatening the very survival of the kidney.

■ *CASE 5*

1. The uterus is of course connected to the oviducts, which extend laterally from either side of the upper uterine wall, and these must be severed and left behind, along with the ovaries (in a radical hysterectomy, however, these too are removed). Next the ovarian/round ligaments and infundibulopelvic ligaments are isolated and divided. The ovarian vessels are within the latter. Further inferior, also between the leaflets of the broad ligaments, are the uterine arteries, embedded in the thickened fascia of the transverse cervical ligament. The ureter passes across this area at the base of the broad ligament and arches over the internal iliac arteries, from which the uterine artery arises (see Figure 6-56).

2. In the performance of an abdominal hysterectomy, the ligation ("tying off") of the uterine arteries places the ureters in jeopardy of being accidentally included in the sutures with which the surgeon secures the uterine arteries. This results in the flow of urine through the ureter being interrupted, and the urine produced by the kidney on that side accumulates in the ureter, distends it and the renal pelvis above it, and ultimately poses a threat to the kidney tissue itself on that side (see Figure 6-47).

3. The obvious goal in repairing this error would be to remove the ureter from the surgical ligation surrounding the uterine artery, free it, and reestablish urine flow. However, if the ureter is no longer patent, even when removed from the accidental ligation, then it may need to be transected above and below the area of obstruction and reanastomosed. If this is not effective, then more elaborate solutions may be required, such as anastomosing the proximal segment of the ureter on the affected side to the unaffected ureter on the opposite side.

■ *CASE 6*

1. The male urethra begins at the bladder neck and passes inferiorly to traverse the prostate gland (during which passage it is known as the prostatic urethra). Beyond this it traverses the urogenital diaphragm, where it is known as the membranous urethra. Finally, it enters the bulb of the corpus spongiosum and then travels distally toward the end of the penis. Throughout this course it is known as the penile or spongiose urethra. The prostatic urethra receives secretions from the prostate and also receives the fluids from the ductus deferens and seminal vesicles. The membranous urethra receives the secretions of the bulbourethral glands.

2. The urethra has been injured in its penile or cavernous portion that is distal to the urogenital diaphragm. In this area the urethra lies within the cylindrical erectile mass known as the corpus spongiosum (see Figure 6-70).

3. The injury allows urine, mixed with blood (accounting for its discoloration), to leak into the superficial perineal pouch. It is this tissue space, with its complex borders and attachments, which explains the seemingly unusual pattern of the discolored area beneath the skin. Posteriorly, the superficial perineal pouch ends where the Colles' fascia attaches firmly to the posterior border of the urogenital diaphragm. Anteriorly, the superficial perineal pouch extends freely up into the superficial fascia of the lower anterior abdominal wall. Laterally, the superficial pouch is limited by the ischiopubic rami, the two corpora cavernosa, and the ischiocavernosus muscles surrounding them.

SECTION SEVEN

Lower Limb

▶ **7.1** Anteromedial Thigh

▶ **7.2** Gluteal Region

▶ **7.3** Posterior Thigh and Knee

▶ **7.4** Leg and Ankle Joint

▶ **7.5** Foot

▶ **7.6** Systems Review and
         Surface Anatomy of
         the Lower Limb

▶ **7.7** Case Studies: Lower Limb

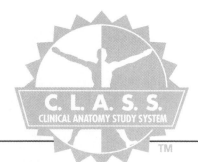

C. L. A. S. S.
CLINICAL ANATOMY STUDY SYSTEM
TM

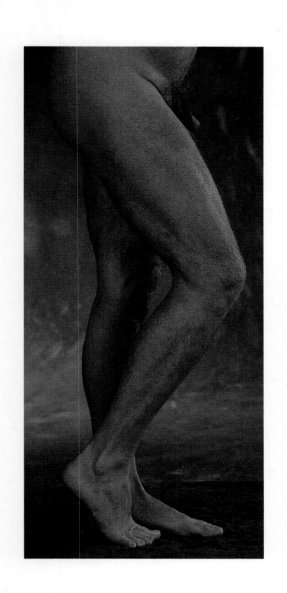
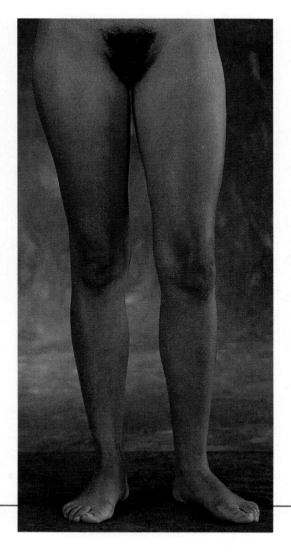

7.1

section seven.one

Anteromedial Thigh

▶ Femur

▶ Hip Joint

▶ Fascia Lata

▶ Muscle Compartments of the Thigh

▶ Anterior Thigh

▶ Medial Thigh

The anterior and medial portions of the thigh (Figure 7-1) are usually considered together because they have a common embryologic origin and because they often cooperate in the performance of movements. The anterior thigh and its muscles are embryologically analogous to the posterior part of the arm (e.g., the triceps muscles), a situation that results from the different directions in which the upper and lower limbs rotate early in the first trimester of development (laterally and medially, respectively). The first key structure in the anteromedial thigh is the **femur** (see Figure 7-2), which forms the axis of the thigh and articulates with both the pelvis and the knee. The **hip joint** represents the articulation of the entire lower limb with the pelvic girdle. Another key region is the **femoral triangle,** the outlines of which are formed by the adductor longus and sartorius muscles and the inguinal ligament (see Figures 7-19 and 7-20). Within the boundaries of the femoral triangle lie the most important vessels and nerves of the anterior thigh. The **femoral nerve** and **vessels** are the most important neurovascular supply to the anterior thigh (see Figure 7-20); the **obturator nerve** and **vessels** are the key neurovascular supply to the medial thigh (see Figure 7-26).

FEMUR

The femur has at its superior end a rounded **head,** supported by a thick **neck** that connects it to the **shaft** of the femur (Figure 7-2). A large **greater trochanter** (Gr., ball or runner) protrudes laterally from the upper shaft of the femur, and a small **lesser trochanter** pro-

trudes medially. Many muscles of the gluteal region attach to the greater trochanter. A few centimeters inferior to the greater trochanter, on the posterolateral surface of the femur, is the **gluteal tuberosity** to which attach the more inferior fibers of the gluteus maximus as well as some of the most superior fibers of the adductor magnus. The lesser trochanter is the point of insertion for the important iliopsoas muscle (see Figures 7-2 and 7-21).

A roughened *intertrochanteric crest* runs on the posterior surface of the femur, connecting the greater and lesser trochanters (see Figure 7-2). A shallow *intertrochanteric fossa* also is present between the crest and the neck of the femur. Several small gluteal-region muscles attach along the crest and to parts of the fossa.

From the superior end of the posterior surface of the shaft, two curved ridges converge toward the midline of the femur and meet about one third of the way down the shaft to form a single vertically raised ridge, the *linea aspera* (L. *asperitas*, roughened) (see Figure 7-2). Several adductor and extensor hip muscles attach here, as do the medial and lateral intermuscular septae of the thigh. More inferiorly, the linea aspera separates into medial and lateral supracondylar lines, which diverge and end just above the medial and lateral femoral condyles, respectively (see Figure 7-2). Superiorly, the linea aspera inclines laterally and ends in the gluteal tuberosity.

The inferior end of the femur is notable for its two condyles (Gr. *kondylos*, a knuckle). The **lateral** and **medial femoral condyle** are bridged to each other anteriorly, but on the posterior surface of the femur they

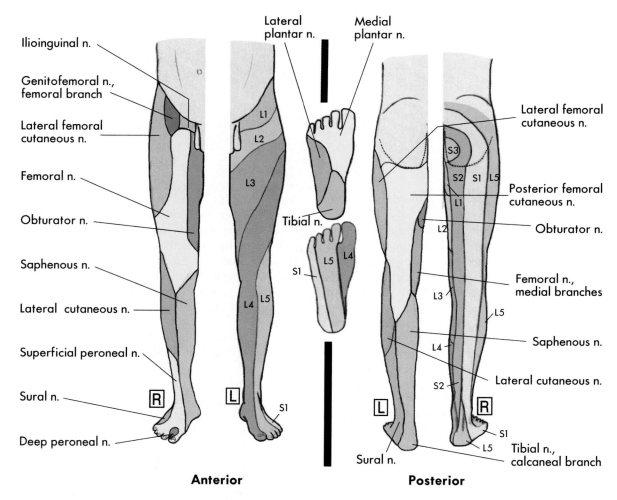

Lateral plantar n.

Medial plantar n.

Ilioinguinal n.

Genitofemoral n., femoral branch

Lateral femoral cutaneous n.

Femoral n.

Obturator n.

Saphenous n.

Lateral cutaneous n.

Superficial peroneal n.

Sural n.

Deep peroneal n.

Lateral femoral cutaneous n.

Posterior femoral cutaneous n.

Obturator n.

Femoral n., medial branches

Saphenous n.

Lateral cutaneous n.

Tibial n., calcaneal branch

Tibial n.

Sural n.

L1
L2
L3
L4
L5
S1

S3
S2 S1 L5
L1
L2
L3
L4
S2
S1
L5

S1 L5 L4

R   L   L   R

Anterior   **Posterior**

Figure 7-1   LOWER LIMB, ANTERIOR AND POSTERIOR VIEWS. Branches of cutaneous nerves are shown on one side and dermatomes are shown on the other. *Inset* shows dermatomes on the sole of the foot.   SEE ATLAS, FIG. 7-35

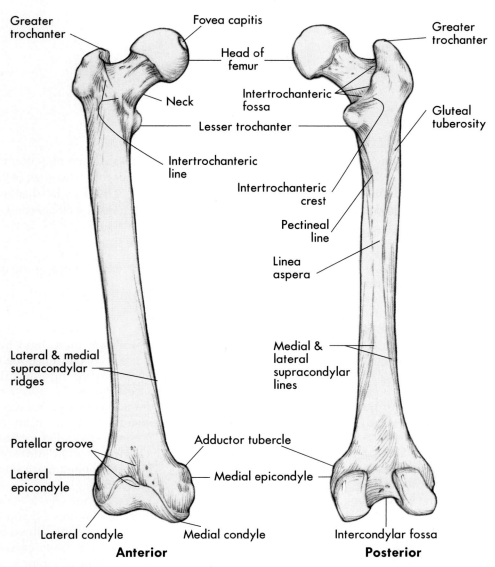

Greater trochanter

Fovea capitis

Head of femur

Neck

Intertrochanteric fossa

Lesser trochanter

Intertrochanteric line

Greater trochanter

Gluteal tuberosity

Intertrochanteric crest

Pectineal line

Linea aspera

Lateral & medial supracondylar ridges

Medial & lateral supracondylar lines

Patellar groove

Adductor tubercle

Lateral epicondyle

Medial epicondyle

Lateral condyle

Medial condyle

Intercondylar fossa

Anterior

Posterior

Figure 7-2   FEMUR. Anterior and posterior views of the right femur.
SEE ATLAS, FIGS. 7-15, 7-16

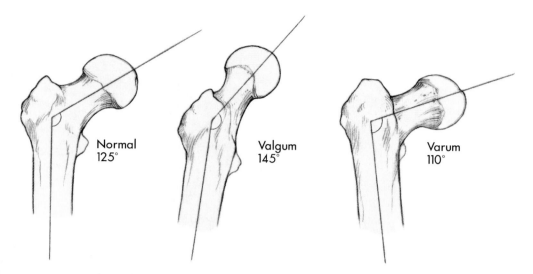

Figure 7-3   VARIATIONS IN THE ANGLE OF THE FEMORAL NECK. The femoral shaft and neck normally intersect at an angle of about 125 degrees. When this angle is abnormally large (about 145 degrees), the shaft of the femur is displaced laterally, and *coxa varum* ("bowleggedness") results. When the angle of the femoral shaft and neck is too small (about 110 degrees), the femoral shaft is displaced medially, and *coxa valgum* ("knock-kneedness") results.

are separated by a deep *intercondylar fossa* (see Figure 7-2). On the anterior surface of the distal femur, there is a shallow depression for articulation with the patella (see Figure 7-41). Inferiorly and posteriorly, each condyle has an articular surface for the tibia. The medial condyle has a "longer" articular surface for the tibia (in the anteroposterior direction), enabling the femur to rotate medially during full extension of the knee joint (see Figure 7-45) (see Chapter 7.3 on the knee).

The neck and shaft of the femur normally connect at an angle of about 125 degrees (Figure 7-3). However, this angle of inclination is about 140 degrees in early childhood and diminishes to less than 120 degrees in old age. The inward angulation of the femoral shafts makes it possible for the knees to be closer together than are the two hip joints. Smaller angles of inclination (i.e., making the neck and shaft of the femur more nearly perpendicular) increase the weight-bearing stress on the femoral neck and make fractures of it more likely. This contributes to the increased incidence of hip fracture in the elderly.

The shaft of the femur is convex anteriorly, so that an imaginary line drawn from the midpoint of the femoral head (i.e., the center of the hip joint) downward through the midpoint of the knee joint does *not* pass through the center of the femoral shaft but is instead *posterior* to it, especially in the lower two thirds of the thigh (Figure 7-4). This arrangement is important in understanding the action of some muscles inserting on the femur: although they insert on the posterior surface of the femur, they nonetheless can be medial rotators of the thigh because the axis of rotation of the thigh pass-

es posterior to the femur along some of its length (see Table 7-3).

HIP JOINT

Portions of the ilium, pubis, and ischium combine on the lateral surface of the hip bone to form the **acetabulum,** or socket of the hip joint (L. *acetabulum,* a vinegar cup) (see Figures 7-5 and 7-8). It is further deepened by the fibrocartilaginous *acetabular labrum,* a rim of tissue extending outward from the margin of the acetabulum. There is a small discontinuity in the inferior aspect of the bony rim of the joint socket (the acetabular notch), which is spanned by the *transverse acetabular ligament* (Figure 7-5).

The femoral head fits into the acetabulum in a ball-and-socket fashion (see Figures 7-5 and 7-6). As with all synovial joints, the joint cavity is lined by *synovial membrane,* covered closely by a *fibrous capsule.* The synovial cavity in the interior of the hip joint is continuous with the *iliac bursal sac,* a membranous sac separating the anterior surface of the hip joint capsule from the overlying tendon of iliacus/psoas.

Ligaments of the Hip Joint

The hip joint is reinforced by ligaments anteriorly and posteriorly. The ligaments pass from the pelvis to the femur in a spiral fashion that allows for a considerable degree of flexion of the hip but stringently limits extension (to only 10 to 20 degrees past the neutral position). These ligaments form a sort of continuum encir-

Figure 7-4   FEMUR, MEDIAL VIEW. The vertical axis for rotation of the thigh lies posterior to much of the femoral shaft.

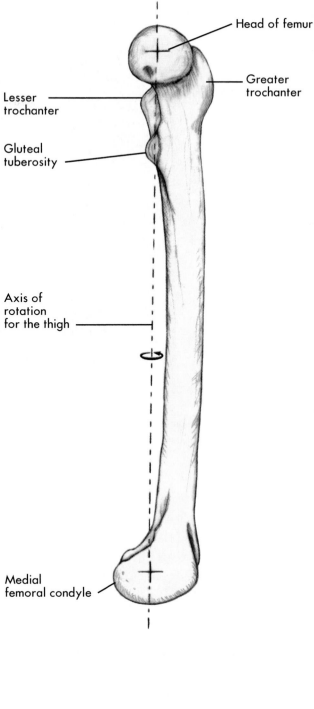

Figure 7-5 HEAD OF THE FEMUR IN THE ACETABULUM. Note the individual ligaments surrounding the capsule of the hip joint and the ligamentum teres of the femur in which an important blood supply reaches the head of the femur.

SEE ATLAS, FIGS. 7-70, 7-71, 7-77

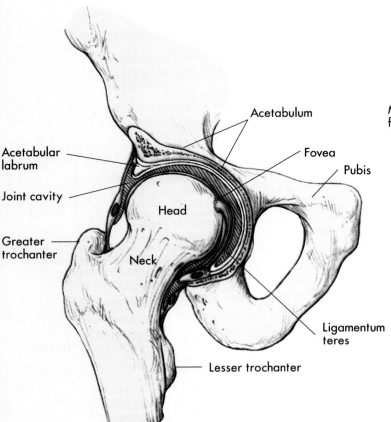

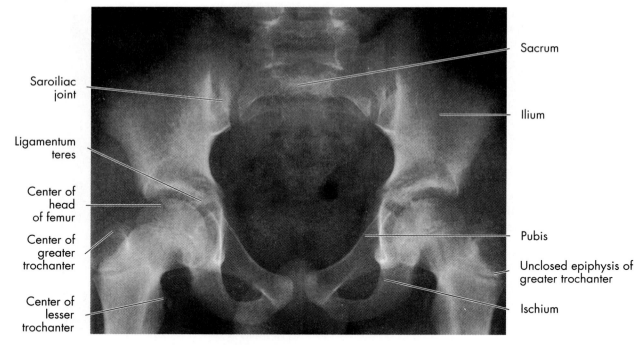

Figure 7-6   ANTEROPOSTERIOR X-RAY OF HIP JOINTS OF 14-YEAR-OLD. Epiphyseal plates are not fully ossified (and therefore lucent) at the greater and lesser trochanters and at the sacroiliac joint. (From Weir J, Abrahams PH: *an imaging atlas of human anatomy,* London, 1992, Mosby.)

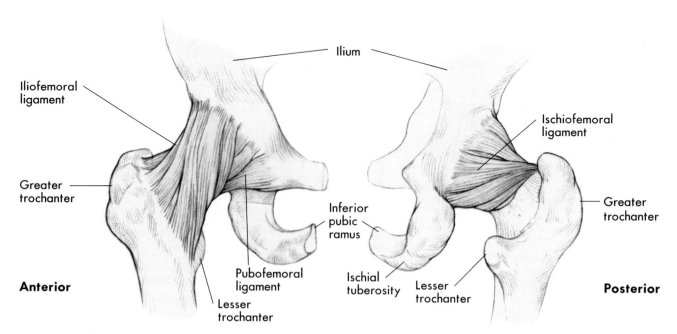

Figure 7-7   LIGAMENTS OF THE HIP JOINT. The three principal hip joint ligaments are arranged in a continuum that surrounds the joint. The iliofemoral ligament is especially important in limiting the extension of the hip. SEE ATLAS, FIGS. 7-72, 7-75

cling the joint but are separately named as the **iliofemoral, ischiofemoral,** and **pubofemoral ligaments** (Figure 7-7). The ligaments attach to the femur along the intertrochanteric line anteriorly and the midpoint of the femoral neck posteriorly (Table 7-1).

The **ligamentum teres** (ligamentum capitis femoris) arises from the transverse acetabular ligament (Figure 7-8) and inserts into the fovea capitus (L. *fovea*, a small pit or depression) in the head of the femur (see Figure 7-5). Important small blood vessels supplying blood to the epiphyseal region of the head of the femur usually travel with this ligament (Figure 7-9), meaning that injury to this ligament may make the epiphysis ischemic (in about 80% of the population, in others, this small vessel is not crucial). This is known as *avascular necrosis of the femoral head* and usually results in permanent disturbance to the head of the femur and to proper functioning of the hip joint.

Relations and Movements of the Hip Joint

In comparison to the shoulder joint, the hip joint is deeper and more heavily reinforced with ligaments and muscles and allows less mobility. It is designed to bear weight and transmit stress from the lower limb to the vertebral column. Anteriorly, the hip joint is cov-

Table 7-1   Ligaments of the Hip Joint

Ligament	Pelvic Attachment	Femoral Attachment	Comments
Iliofemoral ligament	Anterior inferior iliac spine	Intertrochanteric line	Thinned centrally, but thickened at both edges so that it looks like an inverted "Y"; the tendon of iliopsoas overlies the central thinned area of this ligament
Pubofemoral ligament	Superior pubic ramus and obturator membrane	Joint capsule, and to adjacent iliofemoral ligament	Limits abduction, prevents dislocation
Ischiofemoral ligament	Posterior acetabular rim, ischium	Posterior neck of femur	Spiraled to allow flexion but not extension

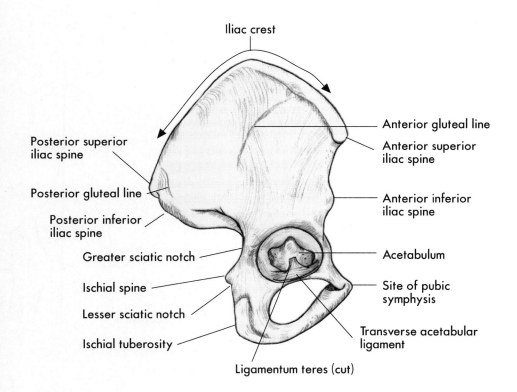

Iliac crest

Posterior superior iliac spine

Posterior gluteal line

Posterior inferior iliac spine

Greater sciatic notch

Ischial spine

Lesser sciatic notch

Ischial tuberosity

Ligamentum teres (cut)

Anterior gluteal line

Anterior superior iliac spine

Anterior inferior iliac spine

Acetabulum

Site of pubic symphysis

Transverse acetabular ligament

Figure 7-8   ACETABULUM AND LATERAL SURFACE OF THE HIP BONE.
SEE ATLAS, FIGS. 7-4, 7-26

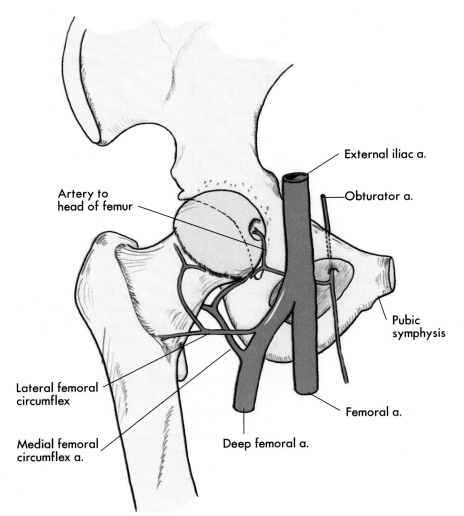

Artery to
head of femur

External iliac a.

Obturator a.

Lateral femoral
circumflex

Medial femoral
circumflex a.

Deep femoral a.

Femoral a.

Pubic
symphysis

Figure 7-9 BLOOD SUPPLY TO THE HEAD OF THE FEMUR. Branches of the medial and lateral femoral circumflex arteries supply the femoral head as well as the obturator artery, from which a small branch often travels with the ligamentum teres to reach the head of the femur.   SEE ATLAS, FIG. 7-73

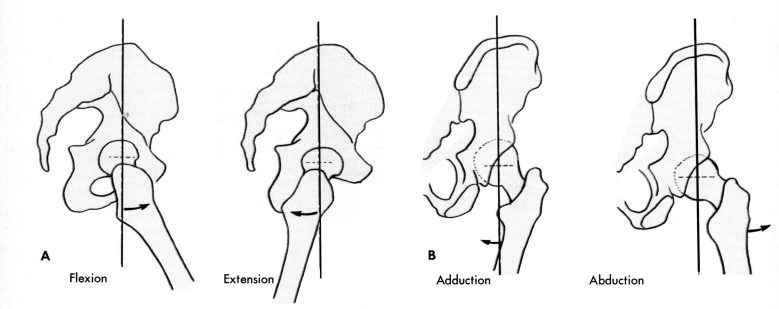

A   Flexion   Extension

B   Adduction   Abduction

Figure 7-10   HIP MOVEMENTS, FOUR VIEWS. A, Lateral view. **B,** Anterior view.

ered by *pectineus muscle* medially and the *tendons of psoas major* and *iliacus* muscles more laterally. Just anterior to these are the femoral vessels and nerve. Laterally, the joint is covered by the *rectus femoris*, the *iliotibial tract*, and the *gluteus minimus muscles*. Posteriorly, the joint capsule is overlain by the two *obturator muscles* (externus and internus) and the two *gemellus muscles* (superior and inferior). The obturator externus tendon lies inferior to the joint. Portions of the pectineus muscle also sweep along the inferior surface of the joint.

The hip joint allows flexion, extension, abduction, adduction, rotation, and a sequential combination of them all, circumduction (Figure 7-10). Flexion can occur over a wide range of movement, as much as 150 degrees, but extension is much more limited, owing primarily to the tautness of the iliofemoral ligament when extension exceeds 10 to 15 degrees. *Flexion* of the hip is accomplished mainly by the iliopsoas, rectus femoris, and sartorius muscles. The femoral nerve mediates this motion (except for the psoas). *Extension* is

■

PRINCIPLES

The **pelvic** and **shoulder girdles** share certain structural similarities, despite their obviously different functional rules. Embryologic studies suggest that in most vertebrates there are *posterior elements* (from the posterior half of the limb bud) and *anterior elements* (from the anterior half of the limb bud). In the pelvis, the *ilium,* a posterior element, joins the girdle to the vertebral column. In the upper limb, the posterior element, the *scapula,* has no attachment to the vertebral column, but the *clavicle* (an anterior element), articulates with the trunk.

In the pelvic girdle, the ilium is a constant feature in more vertebrates, serving to attach the lower limb to the vertebral column. The pubis is well-developed in mammals and fused across the midline in most, but in birds it is smaller and there is no symphysis. Presumably this corresponds to the demands of egg-laying in birds. The ischium is large in mammals with long tails, where it helps support the muscles of these tails.

The upper limb or pectoral girdle of other vertebrates may consist of a scapula, a clavicle, a very large coracoid bone, and a number of other bones not present in humans (the "wishbone" of birds). In man the coracoid exists only as a small remnant fused to the scapula proper.

The clavicle is generally large in mammals who use great strength to climb or gather food; in cows and sea mammals, by contrast, the clavicle is small or absent altogether.

■

PRINCIPLES

When standing upright, the *center of gravity* (or line of force) representing the weight of the body passes anterior to the vertebral column and through the midpoint of the pelvis. It goes through the center of the acetabulum. This means that when standing, there must be considerable static contraction of the extensor muscles of the vertebral column to prevent the body from falling forward (because much of the weight of the thorax and abdomen is anterior to the center of gravity). This extensor force might cause the sacrum to swing in a posterior direction were it not for the sacrospinous and sacrotuberous ligaments, which stabilize the position of the sacrum with respect to the pelvis.

The *sacroiliac joints* are the most important site of the transmission of force from lower limb to vertebral column (through the sacrum, which is part of the vertebral column). Because the sacrum and ilium are not aligned in a vertical axis, the ligaments reinforcing this joint must be very strong. The *iliolumbar ligaments,* extending from the transverse processes of L5 to the ilium, also help prevent the vertebral column from moving posteriorly with respect to the ilium.

carried out by the hamstrings and the gluteus maximus, innervated by the sciatic and inferior gluteal nerves. For ordinary extension, as in unlabored walking, the hamstrings are sufficient, but in forceful extension of the hip, as in climbing stairs, the gluteus maximus is necessary. *Adduction* is performed by the medial thigh muscles, innervated by the obturator nerve. *Abduction* is performed by the lateral gluteal muscles, innervated by the superior gluteal nerve. Lateral rotation is described on pp. 667, 672 and Table 7-9, and medial rotation on p. 661.

Blood Supply to the Hip Joint

Blood supply to the proximal femur and part of its epiphysis is from the **medial and lateral femoral circumflex arteries** (see pp. 658 and 668 for a description of these vessels) (see Figure 7-9 and 7-11). In about 80% of us, an *artery of the ligamentum teres* also is present. This vessel arises from the obturator artery and enters the femoral head by traveling along with the ligamentum teres (see later discussion).

Branches of the *medial femoral circumflex, lateral femoral circumflex, first perforating,* and *inferior gluteal arteries* combine to form a **cruciate anastomosis** (see Figure 7-33) near the ischial tuberosity, just deep to the lower edge of the gluteus maximus, on the posterior aspect of the hip joint. This anastomosis allows blood to reach

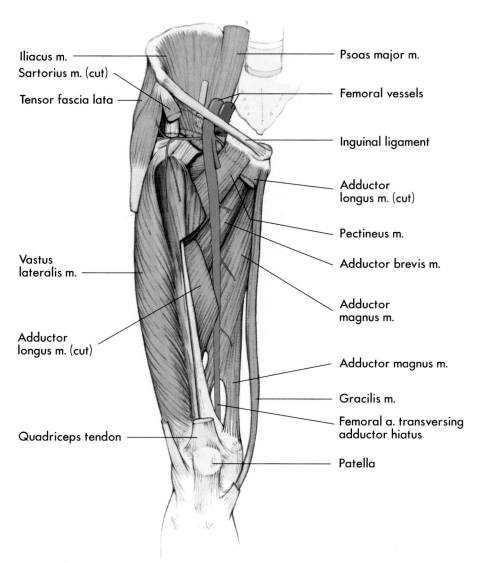

Iliacus m.

Sartorius m. (cut)

Tensor fascia lata

Vastus lateralis m.

Adductor longus m. (cut)

Quadriceps tendon

Psoas major m.

Femoral vessels

Inguinal ligament

Adductor longus m. (cut)

Pectineus m.

Adductor brevis m.

Adductor magnus m.

Adductor magnus m.

Gracilis m.

Femoral a. transversing adductor hiatus

Patella

Figure 7-11 COURSE OF THE FEMORAL ARTERY IN THE ANTERIOR THIGH. The femoral artery branches into a deep femoral artery and two circumflex arteries, a medial and a lateral. **SEE ATLAS, FIG. 7-18**

the lower limb in those cases where the femoral artery is partially or totally obstructed.

Innervation of the Hip Joint

The hip joint is innervated by branches of the anterior division of the **obturator nerve,** branches of the **femoral nerve,** and small branches of the **nerve to quadratus femoris** (from the sacral plexus). Spinal cord segments L4, L5, and S1 are represented.

FASCIA LATA

The deep fascia of the thigh is the fascia lata (see Figures 7-13 and 7-16). Superiorly, this fascia attaches to the sacrotuberous ligament, the sacrum and coccyx, the iliac crest, the inguinal ligament, and the medial side of the pubis. Inferiorly, it blends with the condyles of the femur and tibia, as well as the head of the fibula.

The fascia lata is especially thick laterally, where it

forms the *iliotibial tract/iliotibial band* (Figure 7-13). At its upper end, the iliotibial tract is firmly attached to the gluteus maximus and the tensor fascia lata muscles. These two muscles can "pull" on the iliotibial band from a posterosuperior and anterosuperior angle, respectively. The iliotibial tract extends inferiorly to attach to the lateral tibial surface (although it lies on the lateral side of the thigh and knee, it does not attach to the fibula). Several muscles (e.g., vastus lateralis, biceps femoris) attach to the iliotibial tract along its course in the lateral thigh.

MUSCLE COMPARTMENTS OF THE THIGH

One thick and prominent and two thinner fascial septa (Figures 7-14 and 7-15) extend from the fascia lata inward to attach to the femur. The first is the thick **lateral intermuscular septum,** separating the anterior and posterior compartments of the thigh. It descends to attach to the linea aspera on the posterior aspect of the

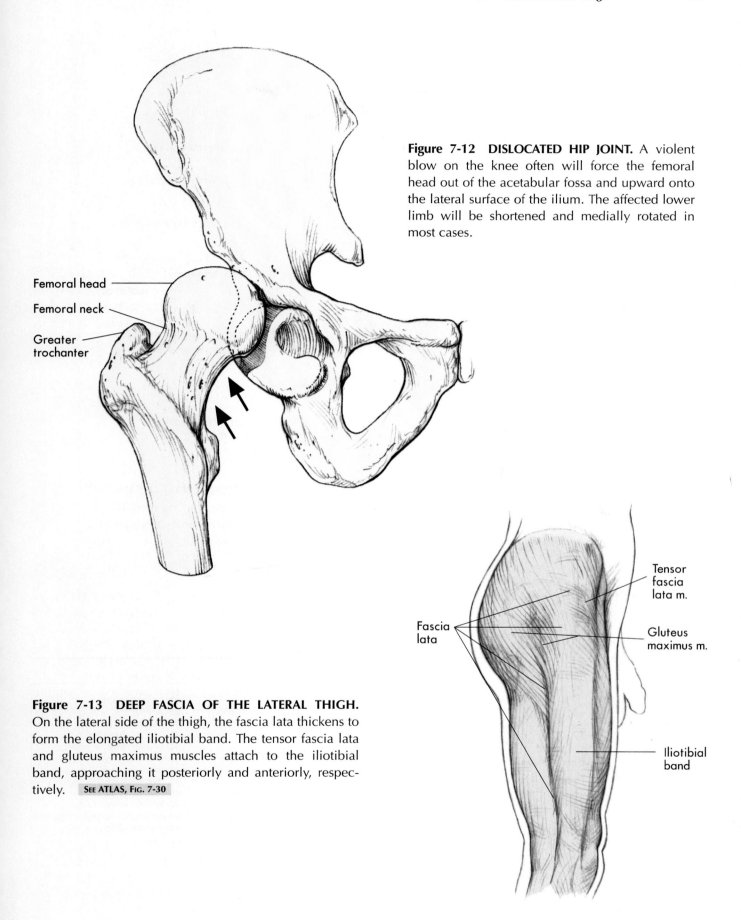

Figure 7-12 DISLOCATED HIP JOINT. A violent blow on the knee often will force the femoral head out of the acetabular fossa and upward onto the lateral surface of the ilium. The affected lower limb will be shortened and medially rotated in most cases.

Femoral head

Femoral neck

Greater trochanter

Tensor fascia lata m.

Gluteus maximus m.

Fascia lata

Iliotibial band

Figure 7-13 DEEP FASCIA OF THE LATERAL THIGH. On the lateral side of the thigh, the fascia lata thickens to form the elongated iliotibial band. The tensor fascia lata and gluteus maximus muscles attach to the iliotibial band, approaching it posteriorly and anteriorly, respectively. SEE ATLAS, FIG. 7-30

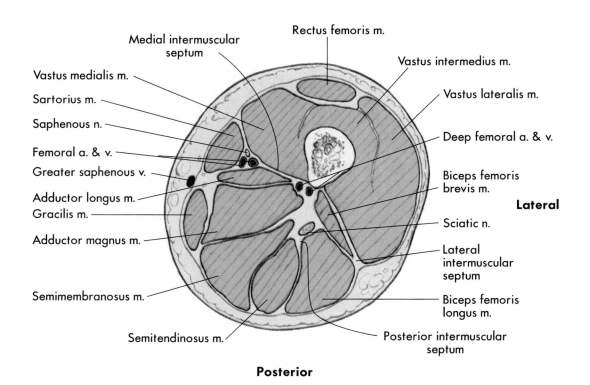

Rectus femoris m.

Medial intermuscular septum

Vastus intermedius m.

Vastus medialis m.

Vastus lateralis m.

Sartorius m.

Saphenous n.

Deep femoral a. & v.

Femoral a. & v.

Greater saphenous v.

Biceps femoris brevis m.

Lateral

Adductor longus m.

Gracilis m.

Sciatic n.

Adductor magnus m.

Lateral intermuscular septum

Semimembranosus m.

Biceps femoris longus m.

Semitendinosus m.

Posterior intermuscular septum

Posterior

**Figure 7-14   CROSS-SECTION THROUGH LEFT LOWER THIGH, VIEWED FROM THE IN-
FERIOR ASPECT.** There are three muscular compartments: anterior, posterior, and medial.
This section must be in the lower portion of the thigh because it is below the level where
the pectineus and adductor brevis would be included.   SEE ATLAS, FIGS. 7-2, 7-14

1 Gracilis muscle	**14** Femoral vein	**38** Ischioanal fossa
2 Adductor longus muscle	**15** Great (long) saphenous vein	**39** Prostate
3 Adductor brevis muscle	**17** Lateral intermuscular septum	**40** Anal canal
4 Adductor magnus muscle	**18** Sciatic nerve	**41** Ischial tuberosity
5 Semitendinosus muscle	**19** Femur	**42** Inferior ramus of pubis
7 Semimembranosus muscle	**31** Femoral nerve	**43** Pubic symphysis
8 Biceps femoris muscle	**32** Iliopsoas muscle	**44** Spermatic cord
9 Sartorius muscle	**33** Pectineus muscle	**45** Iliotibial tract
10 Rectus femoris muscle	**34** Obturator externus muscle	**46** Neck of femur
11 Vastus intermedius muscle	**35** Quadratus femoris muscle	**47** Intertrochanteric ridge
12 Vastus lateralis muscle	**36** Obturator internus muscle	**61** Superficial femoral artery
13 Femoral artery	**37** Levator ani muscle	**62** Superficial femoral vein

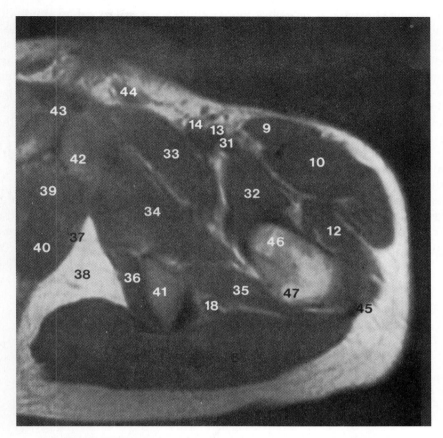

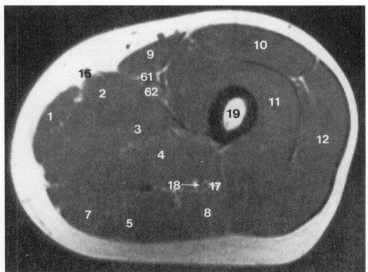

Figure 7-15 **MRI CROSS-SECTIONS OF THIGH AND HIP JOINT.** (From Weir J, and Abrahams PH: *An imaging atlas of human anatomy,* London, 1992, Mosby.) See opposite page for legend box. SEE ATLAS, FIGS. 7-2, 7-76

femur. The vastus lateralis and biceps femoris attach to this lateral septum. The second or **medial intermuscular septum** lies on the medial side of the thigh and also descends to attach to the linea aspera. It separates the anterior and medial (adductor) muscle groups. Embedded in this medial septum are the femoral vessels, deep femoral vessels, and certain branches of the femoral nerve. The third or **posterior septum** is a sometimes incomplete fascial process, extending posteriorly from the femur, partially separating the medial and posterior muscle groups of the thigh. In it is embedded the important sciatic nerve.

These connective tissue septae, then, divide the thigh into **three compartments**—an *anterior,* a *posterior,* and a *medial* (or adductor). To a degree, each of these compartments and its muscles are supplied by a particular artery and nerve (Figure 7-14): the *anterior compartment* with its femoral nerve and vessels, the *medial compartment* with its obturator nerve and vessels, and the *posterior compartment* with its sciatic nerve and perforat-

ing branches of femoral vessels. There is no substantial lateral or abductor compartment of the thigh because two of the muscles that would be included in it—the gluteus minimus and medius—do not extend below the level of the greater trochanter. The third muscle that would be in this "compartment," the tensor fascia lata, does not extend as a muscle far into the thigh but instead is represented there by the iliotibial band, into the superior end of which it inserts (see Figure 7-13). The superior gluteal nerve would be the nerve of this fourth "lateral compartment" of the thigh, if we recognized such a compartment.

ANTERIOR THIGH

The elongated gap between the inguinal ligament and the superior pubic ramus transmits the femoral artery, vein, and nerve, the iliacus and tendon of the psoas major, and other structures (see Figure 7-20). The femoral nerve, artery, and vein are in a constant lateral-

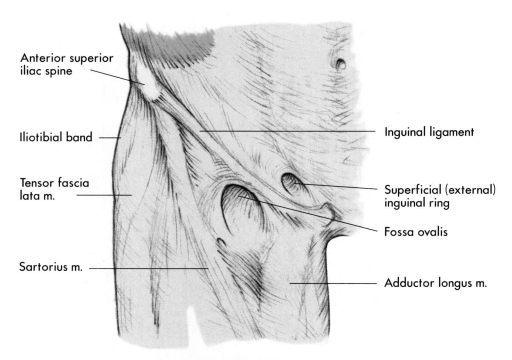

Figure 7-16 FASCIA OF THE UPPER ANTERIOR THIGH. The inguinal ligament extends from the anterior superior spine to the pubic tubercle. Deep fascia of the anterior thigh (the fascia lata) is continuous with the inguinal ligament, representing the lower border of the external oblique muscle. The external inguinal ring, actually formed mainly from the fascia of the external oblique muscle, is shown here near the medial end of the inguinal ligament. The fossa ovalis is a semicircular depression in the deep fascia of the anterior thigh through which passes the greater saphenous vein as it drains into the femoral vein. The contour of the sartorius muscle produces a diagonal elevation in the superficial fascia, and a similar contour of tensor fascia lata also is visible. SEE ATLAS, FIG. 7-11

to-medial relationship in the femoral region. This is an important relationship to remember, because these vessels often are used for intravenous cannulation or blood sampling in an emergency. A knowledge of anatomy should enable one to locate these vessels accurately, even if the patient has no pulse.

The Superficial Fascia and Great Saphenous Vein

The **fascia lata** is the deep or investing fascia of this and all other parts of the thigh (Figure 7-16). The muscles of the anterior thigh, the femoral vessels, and the femoral nerve all are positioned deep to the fascia lata. The **superficial fascia** of the thigh lies external to this and is most prominent medially. One thickened area, the **cribriform fascia,** overlies the saphenous opening.

The **great saphenous vein** (Figures 7-17 and 7-18) originates on the dorsum of the foot and passes anterior to the medial malleous, up the medial side of the leg, and into the superficial fascia of the medial thigh.

About 6 to 8 cm below the inguinal ligament, the great saphenous vein descends through the superficial fascia (where it is known as the *cribiform fascia*) and drains into the femoral vein through an aperture in the fascia lata known variously as the saphenous opening, saphenous hiatus, or fossa ovalis. In the upper limb, the homolog of the great saphenous vein is the cephalic vein.

Femoral Triangle

The *medial edge of the sartorius,* the *medial edge of adductor longus,* and the *inguinal ligament* (as the base of this inverted triangle) form the perimeters of the **femoral triangle** (Figures 7-19 and 7-20). Within the boundaries of this triangle are found the femoral artery, the femoral vein, and the several branches of the femoral nerve. The floor of the triangle is made up, from medial to lateral, of the *pectineus,* the *tendon of the psoas major,* and the *iliacus muscles* (also known as the iliopsoas). The fascia lata (deep fascia of the thigh) covers the triangle superficially (see previous discussion).

CLINICAL ANATOMY OF
THE HIP JOINT

DISLOCATION OF THE HIP

The hip is most easily dislocated (i.e., femoral head dislodged from the acetabulum) when the hip is flexed and medially rotated. Unfortunately, this is almost exactly the position in which we sit while riding in a car, and a collision results in forceful impact of the knee with the dashboard. This force, applied to the thigh, often results in traumatic dislocation of the hip upward, adjacent to the outer surface of the ilium (see Figure 7-12).

SURGICAL REPLACEMENT OF THE HIP

Traumatic and/or arthritic destruction of the interior of the hip joint can be so advanced that mobility is reduced to a minimum or the pain of standing or walking is unbearable. For such patients, the upper end of the femur and the acetabular socket may be replaced with Teflon or other inert materials and the patient provided with a vastly improved degree of mobility and relief of pain.

TRAUMATIC FRACTURES OF THE HIP

The neck of the femur is prone to fracture, even when traumatic force is applied to the feet and ankle and not the hip itself. When the foot is firmly planted and the knee locked, the force of a blow is transmitted

superiorly and may result in fracture of the femoral neck.

Especially with advancing age and osteoporosis, the femoral neck becomes more and more vulnerable to fracture. Such events have a tendency to recur, and it is commonplace today for the entire upper end and head of the femur to be replaced with a metal or plastic prosthesis. Degenerative arthritis (with diminishing capacity for hip movement) also is a good reason to consider total hip replacement.

INTERRUPTION OF BLOOD SUPPLY TO THE FEMORAL HEAD

The head of the femur depends, to varying degrees in different individuals, on blood flow through the delicate artery of the ligamentum teres, arising from the obturator artery. When the femoral head undergoes necrosis caused by interruption of blood supply (avascular necrosis) in a child, the femoral head can be compressed and flattened, leading to slippage of the femoral head along the epiphyseal plate connecting the neck and head of the femur. It is most frequent in children 3 to 9 years of age, and the most common presenting symptom is pain over the hip joint, although the pain commonly also radiates down the thigh as far as the knee.

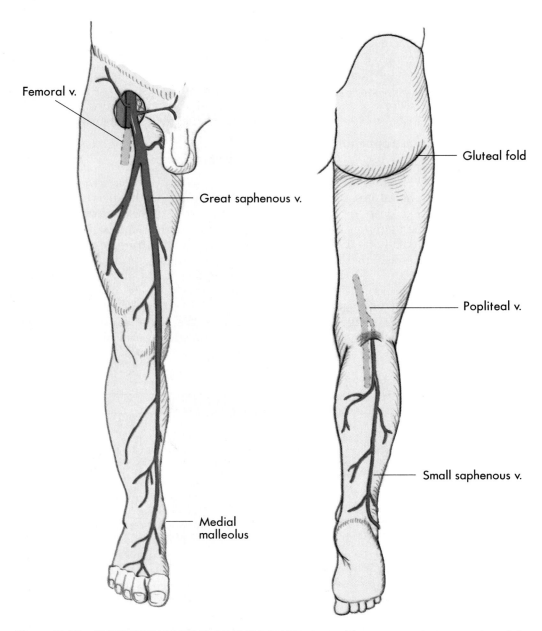

Figure 7-17   SUPERFICIAL VEINS OF THE LOWER LIMB. The great saphenous vein originates on the medial side of the foot, ascends anterior to the medial malleolus along the
medial aspect of the leg and knee, and penetrates the superficial fascia of the upper thigh
to join with the femoral vein. The small saphenous vein originates on the lateral side of
the foot, ascends in the posterior midline of the leg, and penetrates the superficial fascia
to join the popliteal vein.   See Atlas, Figs . 7-6, 7-38, 7-43

The *profunda femoris* or *deep femoral artery* arises in
the femoral triangle (see Figure 7-9). The triangle ends
where the femoral vessels enter the adductor canal (see
later discussion).

Femoral Sheath

The **femoral sheath** is a downward extension of the
abdominal transversalis fascia through the gap between the inguinal ligament and the superior pubic
ramus. It is in the shape of a funnel, with its inferiorly
directed lower end fusing with the fascia of the femoral
vessels. This "sheath" is a tangle of connective tissue
filaments in which the femoral vessels and femoral
canal are embedded. The fascia is arrayed in such a
way that *three compartments* in the femoral sheath are
defined: the **lateral compartment,** containing the

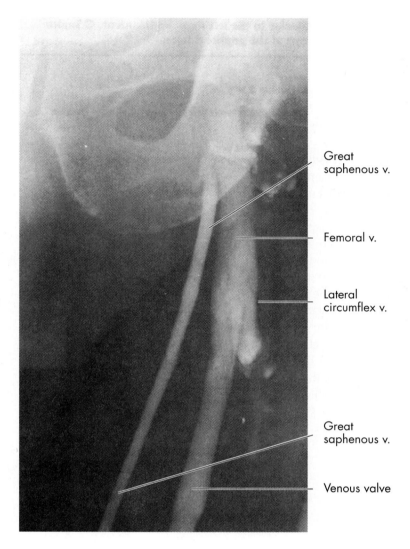

Great
saphenous v.

Femoral v.

Lateral
circumflex v.

Great
saphenous v.

Venous valve

Figure 7-18 X-RAY OF SAPHENOUS AND FEMORAL VEINS. When dye is injected into the veins of the foot, it is conveyed superiorly through both the deep and superficial sets of veins (represented by the femoral and great saphenous veins, respectively). (From Weir J, Abrahams PH: *An imaging atlas of human anatomy,* London, 1992, Mosby.)
SEE ATLAS, FIG . 7-6

femoral artery; the **intermediate compartment,** containing the femoral vein; and the **medial compartment,** also called the **femoral canal,** which normally contains no discrete structures other than a lymph node or two. The medial boundary of the femoral canal is the *lacunar ligament*. This thickened rim, part of the inguinal ligament, forms the medial edge of the femoral canal and is palpable on physical examination. This apparent space also is known as the **femoral ring** (Figure 7-20).

The tendons of the psoas major and pectineus are directly posterior to the femoral sheath (Figures 7-21). The fascia lata (deep fascia of the thigh; attaches superiorly to the inguinal ligament) lies just anterior to the femoral sheath. Just medial to the femoral sheath (specifically to the femoral canal) is the lacunar ligament, a triangular reflection of the medial end of the inguinal ligament onto the upper surface of the superior

pubic ramus. The femoral nerve lies just lateral to the femoral sheath.

Muscles of the Anterior Thigh

The superficial group of muscles in the anterior thigh (see Figures 7-19 and 7-22) are primarily flexors of the hip and extensors of the knee. They are described more completely in Table 7-2. **Rectus femoris** and the three vastus muscles (**vastus medialis, intermedius, and lateralis**) are referred to as the **quadriceps.** These muscles lie in a more superficial position of the anterior thigh. Rectus femoris originates from the anterior inferior iliac spine, and the remaining three vastus muscles originate from the shaft of the femur (Figure 7-23). Note that the three vastus muscles cross only the knee joint, because they pass from the shaft of the femur to the tibia, but the rectus femoris, passing from the ante-

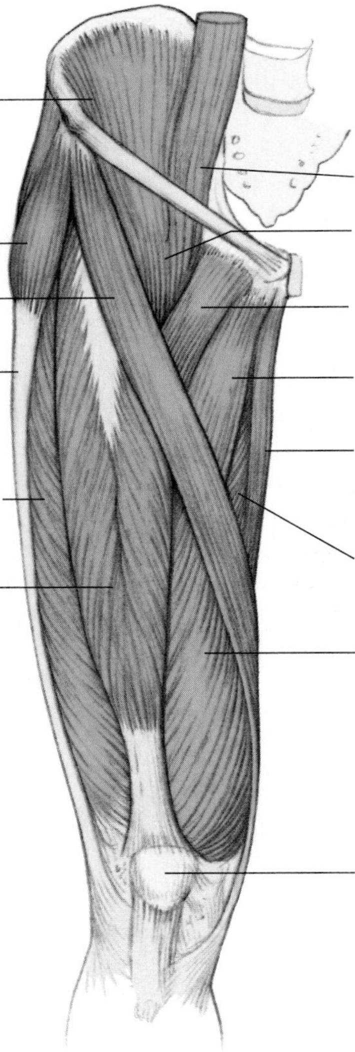

**Figure 7-19   ANTERIOR THIGH MUSCLES, SU-
PERFICIAL VIEW.** The thigh extends from the
inguinal ligament to the knee. Coursing diagonally from lateral to medial as it descends is
the sartorius muscle. Sharing with it an origin
from the anterior superior spine is the tensor
fascia lata muscle, continuing inferiorly as the
iliotibial band. Between the iliotibial band and
the sartorius is the massive quadriceps, composed of the vastus medialis, rectus femoris,
and vastus lateralis. Medial to the sartorius is
the adductor group, composed of the pectineus, adductor longus, and gracilis. The iliopsoas muscle descends from the abdomen into
the anterior thigh deep to the middle portion of
the inguinal ligament.

SEE ATLAS, FIGS. 7-12, 7-17, 7-21

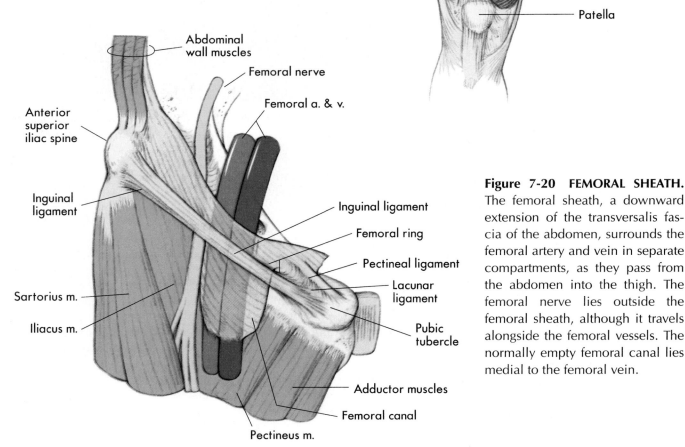

Iliacus m.
Psoas major m.
Tensor fascia lata
Iliopsoas m.
Sartorius m.
Pectineus m.
Iliotibial band
Adductor longus m.
Gracilis m.
Vastus lateralis m.
Adductor magnus m.
Rectus femoris m.
Vastus medialis m.
Patella

Abdominal wall muscles
Femoral nerve
Anterior superior iliac spine
Femoral a. & v.
Inguinal ligament
Inguinal ligament
Femoral ring
Pectineal ligament
Lacunar ligament
Sartorius m.
Iliacus m.
Pubic tubercle
Adductor muscles
Femoral canal
Pectineus m.

Figure 7-20   FEMORAL SHEATH.
The femoral sheath, a downward
extension of the transversalis fascia of the abdomen, surrounds the
femoral artery and vein in separate
compartments, as they pass from
the abdomen into the thigh. The
femoral nerve lies outside the
femoral sheath, although it travels
alongside the femoral vessels. The
normally empty femoral canal lies
medial to the femoral vein.

Figure 7-21 ILIOPSOAS MUSCLE. The iliacus and psoas major have different origins but unite distally to form a common insertion into the lesser trochanter of the femur. The iliacus originates from the concave surface of the inner ilium, while the psoas major originates from the bodies and transverse processes of vertebrae T12 to L4. Together they pass deep to the lateral half of the inguinal ligament, lying lateral to the femoral artery. The femoral nerve often is embedded in the anterior fascia of the iliopsoas tendon. The quadratus lumborum, along with the psoas major, creates part of the posterior abdominal wall.

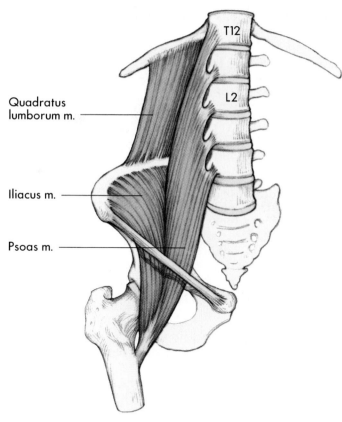

Quadratus lumborum m.

Iliacus m.

Psoas m.

T12

L2

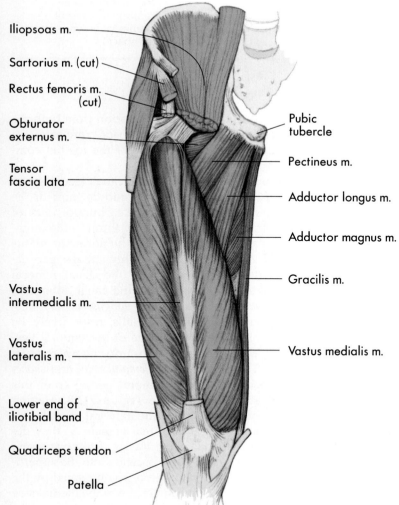

Iliopsoas m.

Sartorius m. (cut)

Rectus femoris m. (cut)

Obturator externus m.

Tensor fascia lata

Vastus intermedialis m.

Vastus lateralis m.

Lower end of iliotibial band

Quadriceps tendon

Patella

Pubic tubercle

Pectineus m.

Adductor longus m.

Adductor magnus m.

Gracilis m.

Vastus medialis m.

Figure 7-22 ANTERIOR THIGH MUSCLES, DEEPER VIEW. The tensor fascia lata, iliopsoas, and sartorius have been removed, showing the origin of the rectus femoris from the anterior inferior iliac spine. The gracilis lies along the medial border of the thigh. With the iliopsoas removed, we can see the obturator externus muscle, anteriorly covering the obturator foramen of the pelvis. The adductor muscles and pectineus originate from the medial ends of the pubic and ischial rami and descend inferolaterally to insert on the femur.

Table 7-2   Muscles of the Anterior Compartment

Muscle	Attachments	Innervation	Action(s)
Iliacus	Iliac fossa/sacrum to lesser trochanter	Femoral nerve (L2-L4)	Hip flexion
Psoas major	Vertebrae T12-L4 to lesser trochanter	Lumbar plexus (L2-L5)	Hip flexion, medial rotation of thigh
Pectineus (also considered part of medial muscle group)	Pectineal line of pubis, pubic tubercle to lesser trochanter and bone medial to it	Femoral and obturator nerves	Flexes and adducts hip
Sartorius	Anterior superior spine to upper medial tibia	Femoral nerve (L2-L4)	Flexes, abducts, laterally rotates hip; flexes knee (as in sitting with legs crossed)
Rectus femoris	Anterior inferior spine to patellar tendon and tibial tuberosity (also has small reflected head to lip of acetabulum)	Femoral nerve (L2-L4)	Hip flexion, knee extension
Vastus lateralis; vastus medialis; vastus intermedius	Proximal femur to patellar tendon and tibial tuberosity	Femoral nerve (L2-L4)	Knee extension
Articularis genu*	Lower anterior femoral shaft to synovial membrane of knee joint	Femoral nerve (L2-L4)	Retracts knee joint synovium upward during knee extension (to prevent entrapment of synovium in joint space)

*Often appears to be a part of vastus intermedius.

rior inferior spine of the pelvis to the tibia, crosses the hip and weakly extends it. The **sartorius muscle** is also in the more superficial part of the muscular compartment of the anterior thigh. It also crosses both the hip and knee joint, because it passes from the anterior superior spine of the pelvis to the medial side of the tibia (see Figure 7-20). The **articularis genu** (see Figure 7-23) is a small muscle in the distal anterior thigh, originating on the distal shaft of the femur and attaching to the synovial sheath of the knee joint.

The floor of the femoral triangle (see p. 651) is made up of the deep group of three anterior thigh muscles—the *iliacus, psoas major,* and *pectineus.* The **iliacus** and **psoas major** (see Figures 7-20 and 7-21) cross the superior pubic ramus lateral to the femoral nerve and join to form a single tendon as they descend and attach to the lesser trochanter of the femur. A subiliac bursa separates this common tendon from the hip joint, over which it passes. The *femoral nerve* lies in a shallow groove between the iliacus and psoas major before they fuse into their common tendon, and the *femoral artery* lies directly anterior to the psoas muscle. The **pectineus** is a flattened muscle lying medial to the psoas major and lateral to the adductor longus. It arises from the pubis and inserts on the femur just inferior to the lesser trochanter. The capsule of the hip joint is deep to the lateral half of the pectineus, and the femoral vein overlies its lateral border. Pectineus is truly a "borderline"

muscle, sometimes receiving innervation from both the *femoral nerve* (the nerve of the anterior compartment) and the *obturator nerve* (the nerve of the medial compartment).

The **adductor (or subsartorial) canal** (see Figures 7-11 and 7-26) is a passage in the middle third of the thigh. It commences at the apex (i.e., inferior end) of the femoral triangle, leads inferiorly through the medial thigh musculature, and ends at the adductor hiatus (see Figure 7-26), a small and roughly circular gap between the adductor magnus and the distal femoral shaft. The *sartorius muscle* covers the canal anteriorly, while *vastus medialis* and *adductor longus/magnus muscles* form its lateral and medial walls, respectively. Its principal role is to permit passage of the femoral vessels between the anterior and posterior compartments of the thigh. The *femoral artery, femoral vein,* and *saphenous nerve* (a branch of the femoral nerve) enter this canal at its superior end (see Figure 7-20). Having reached the posterior thigh, the femoral vessels are henceforth known as the **popliteal vessels,** as they descend posterior to the knee into the leg. After traversing the canal, the saphenous nerve ascends into the superficial fascia of the leg. Hereafter it is accompanied by the great saphenous vein as it courses down the medial side of the leg. The saphenous nerve supplies cutaneous innervation (see Figure 7-1) to the medial leg, ankle, and foot (the other femoral nerve branch entering the ad-

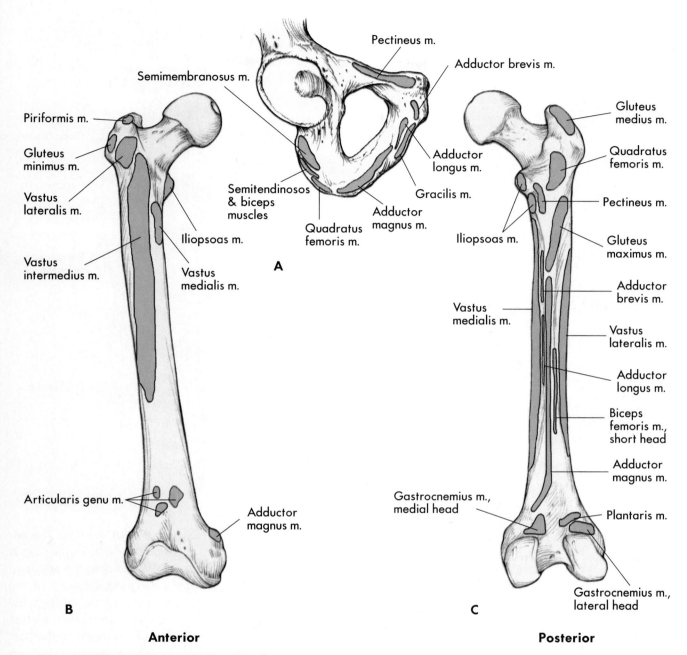

Figure 7-23 ATTACHMENTS OF SEVERAL THIGH MUSCLES. A, Part of the hip bone, with attachments for several muscles of the medial and posterior compartments. **B** and **C,** Muscle attachments onto the anterior and posterior surfaces of the femur.
SEE ATLAS, FIGS . 7-15, 7-16, 7-26, 7-27

ductor canal is the nerve to vastus medialis, but it terminates within the canal, unlike the saphenous nerve).

Vascular Supply of the Anterior Thigh

The major arterial supply to the anterior thigh is the **femoral artery** (see Figures 7-9, 7-11, and 7-24). The femoral artery emerges from beneath the inguinal ligament approximately midway between the anterior superior spine and the pubic tubercle. It crosses directly anterior to the capsule of the hip joint, and, distally, passes into the adductor canal, bounded by the vastus medialis, adductor longus, and sartorius muscles (see previous discussion).

Before becoming the femoral artery, the vessel is known as the **external iliac artery.** Immediately proximal to the inguinal ligament, it gives rise to (1) the important **inferior epigastric artery,** lateral to which the ductus deferens passes (see Chapter 5), and (2) the **deep iliac circumflex artery**, which travels laterally in

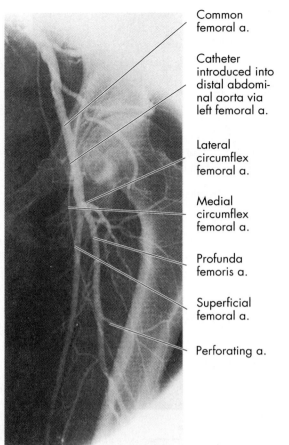

Common femoral a.

Catheter introduced into distal abdominal aorta via left femoral a.

Lateral circumflex femoral a.

Medial circumflex femoral a.

Profunda femoris a.

Superficial femoral a.

Perforating a.

Figure 7-24   X-RAY ARTERIOGRAM OF THE FEMORAL ARTERIES. The femoral artery has been injected with dye and the subsequent filling of distal branches is shown on x-ray. (From Weir J, Abrahams PH: *An imaging atlas of human anatomy,* London, 1992, Mosby.)   **SEE ATLAS, FIG . 7-2**

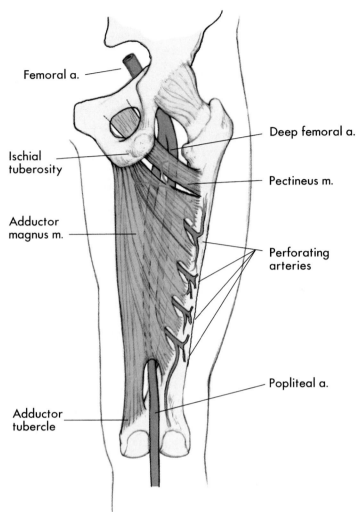

Femoral a.

Ischial tuberosity

Adductor magnus m.

Adductor tubercle

Deep femoral a.

Pectineus m.

Perforating arteries

Popliteal a.

Figure 7-25   RIGHT THIGH, POSTERIOR VIEW. The adductor magnus originates from the ischiopubic ramus and inserts along the linea aspera and onto the adductor tubercle of the femur. Along the medial border of the femur, about four perforating arteries pass through the substance of the adductor magnus and other medial compartment muscles and bring blood supply to the posterior compartment. These perforating vessels arise from the deep femoral artery, a branch of the femoral artery in the upper thigh, on the anterior side. Distally, the femoral artery passes through the adductor hiatus, a gap between the portion attaching to the adductor tubercle and the portion attaching to the femoral shaft.   **SEE ATLAS, FIG . 7-70**

the transversalis fascial layer toward the anterior superior spine, where it anastomoses with several other vessels.

The femoral artery emerges from beneath the inguinal ligament (see Figure 7-20). For its first 2 to 3 cm it is enclosed in the lateral compartment of the femoral sheath; thereafter it courses distally within the femoral triangle and enters the adductor canal, under cover of the sartorius muscle. While in the femoral triangle, the femoral artery rests posteriorly on the psoas major, and the femoral vein and nerve are medial and lateral to it, respectively.

Important branches of the femoral artery (see Figure 7-11) are the *medial* and *lateral circumflex femoral arteries*

and the *deep femoral artery (profunda femoris).** The circumflex femoral arteries may arise directly from the femoral artery or from the deep femoral artery. The circumflex vessels produce many branches that participate in anastomoses near the iliac spines, the gluteal region, and the knee. In particular, the anastomosis of branches of the inferior gluteal artery, medial and later-

---

*In clinical medicine and in older anatomy texts, the custom is to refer to what we call the femoral artery as the "common femoral artery." The profunda femoris arises from this, and the remaining continuation of the femoral artery is known as the "superficial femoral" artery, not simply the femoral.

Table 7-3   Muscles of the Medial (Adductor) Compartment

Muscle	Attachments	Innervation	Action
Pectineus	Pectineal line of pubis, pubic tubercle to lesser trochanter, and bone medial to it	Femoral and obturator nerves (L2 to L4)	Flexes and adducts hip
Adductor magnus*	Ischial tuberosity and ramus to adductor tubercle and lower linea aspera; has adductor hiatus at inferior end	Obturator and tibial nerves (tibial nerve for that portion arising from ischial tuberosity; obturator nerve for that portion arising from ischiopubic ramus)	Adducts and flexes hip; probably rotates thigh medially as well
Adductor longus	Area near to pubic symphysis to mid linea aspera	Obturator nerve (L2 to L4)	Adducts, flexes hip; ? medial rotation
Adductor brevis	Inferior pubic ramus to upper linea aspera and lesser trochanter	Obturator nerve (L2 to L4)	Adducts and flexes hip
Gracilis	Ischiopubic ramus to medial upper tibia, below condyle (inserts with sartorius and semitendinosus—"pes anserinus")	Obturator nerve (L2 to L4)	Adducts hip; also flexes and medially rotates knee

*The upper fibers of the adductor magnus are sometimes recognized separately as adductor minimus.

al femoral circumflex arteries, and first perforating artery is positioned posteriorly, near the ischial tuberosity, where it is known as the *cruciate anastomosis* (see Figure 7-33).

The **deep femoral artery** originates from the lateral side of the femoral artery, about 3 to 4 cm distal to the inguinal ligament. It then passes behind the femoral vein, traveling toward the medial side of the femur. Passing between the adductor longus and magnus, it descends alongside the femoral shaft. During this descent it gives off several (usually three or four) perforating arteries that penetrate the medial and posterior fascial septae and are the major blood supply to the posterior thigh (Figure 7-25). Unlike the anterior and medial compartments of the thigh, the posterior compartment has no major blood supply of its own and depends heavily on these perforating arteries.

Femoral Nerve

The **femoral nerve** (see Figure 7-20) is derived from the lumbar plexus (cord segments L2 to L4) and descends along the lower lumbar vertebral column embedded in the psoas major muscle. Passing inferior to the inguinal ligament, it breaks up quickly into a large number of individual branches to all the anterior thigh muscles and to the anterolateral skin of the thigh. It also supplies the hip joint, through its branch to the pectineus.

The femoral nerve has one notable distal branch, the **saphenous nerve** (see Figure 7-14). The saphenous nerve is a cutaneous nerve, innervating no striated muscles (however, as a mixed nerve, it does contain both sensory and motor axons—the motor innervation being for sweat glands, hair arrector muscles, and vascular smooth muscle). The saphenous nerve is one of only two branches of the femoral nerve that accompany it and the femoral vessels into the adductor canal. The saphenous nerve does not, however, traverse the canal to emerge in the popliteal fossa. Instead, it leaves the adductor canal medially and supplies cutaneous innervation of the medial leg, ankle, and foot.

MEDIAL THIGH

The medial thigh compartment contains the most important adductors of the hip (many of which rotate the thigh as well), the obturator nerve, and the obturator vessels. It extends from the medial region of the pelvis inferiorly to the level of the upper tibia.

Muscles of the Medial Thigh

In general these muscles (Table 7-3) originate from the ischiopubic ramus and superior pubic ramus (see Figure 7-23) and attach to the upper posterior femur along the *linea aspera* and supracondylar line. Only one medial thigh muscle, the gracilis, crosses both the hip and knee joints, attaching inferiorly to the tibia.

The **adductor longus** and **pectineus muscles** (Figure 7-26) are in a single plane, anterior to the other medial compartment muscles (see Figures 7-22 and 7-25). They cover the adductor brevis. The adductor longus serves as medial border of the femoral triangle, and the pectineus is part of its floor.

The **adductor brevis** (see Figure 7-26) is the key

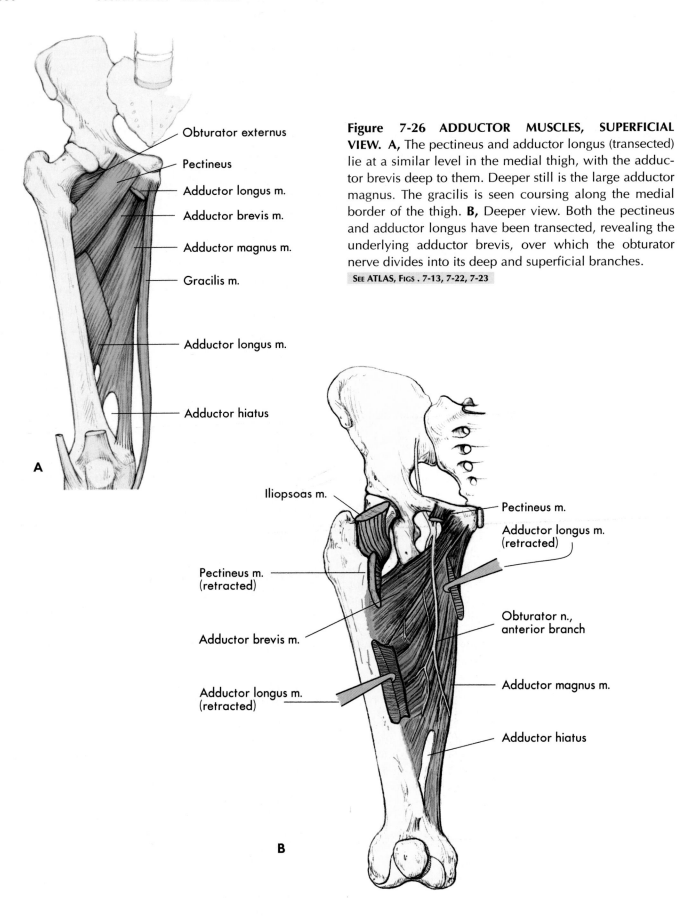

Obturator externus

Pectineus

Adductor longus m.

Adductor brevis m.

Adductor magnus m.

Gracilis m.

Adductor longus m.

Adductor hiatus

A

Figure 7-26 ADDUCTOR MUSCLES, SUPERFICIAL VIEW. A, The pectineus and adductor longus (transected) lie at a similar level in the medial thigh, with the adductor brevis deep to them. Deeper still is the large adductor magnus. The gracilis is seen coursing along the medial border of the thigh. **B,** Deeper view. Both the pectineus and adductor longus have been transected, revealing the underlying adductor brevis, over which the obturator nerve divides into its deep and superficial branches.
SEE ATLAS, FIGS . 7-13, 7-22, 7-23

Iliopsoas m.

Pectineus m.

Adductor longus m.
(retracted)

Pectineus m.
(retracted)

Adductor brevis m.

Obturator n.,
anterior branch

Adductor longus m.
(retracted)

Adductor magnus m.

Adductor hiatus

B

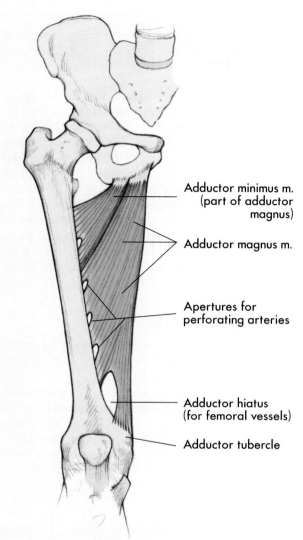

Figure 7-27 ADDUCTOR MAGNUS, ANTERIOR VIEW. The origin of the adductor magnus from the ischiopubic ramus is clearly seen here. The upper fibers of the adductor magnus are sometimes recognized separately as the adductor minimus.

muscle for understanding the arrangement of muscles in the medial thigh compartment. The adductor brevis originates on the ischiopubic ramus and descends inferomedially to attach to the upper linea aspera and lesser trochanter. It lies in a plane deep to the adductor longus and pectineus but superficial to the adductor magnus. Both the obturator vessels and nerve divide into anterior and posterior branches that lie superficial and deep, respectively, to the adductor brevis.

The **adductor magnus muscle** (Figure 7-27) lies deep to the adductor brevis and is by far the largest of the medial compartment muscles. It has two heads. The *first head*, originating from the ischial tuberosity and attaching inferiorly to the adductor tubercle, resembles a hamstring muscle (i.e., a hip extensor) and is innervat-

Table 7-4 Targets of the Obturator Nerve

Anterior Division	Posterior Division
Adductor longus	Obturator externus
Adductor brevis	Adductor brevis
Gracilis	Adductor magnus (part)
Pectineus*	Knee joint
Hip joint	Branches to popliteal artery
Medial thigh skin	

*More commonly innervated by femoral nerve; about 10% innervated by both.

ed by the tibial nerve. It is sometimes recognized separately as the adductor minimus. The *second head* originates from the ischial ramus and attaches to the linea aspera. It is innervated by the obturator nerve, more closely resembling the other adductor muscles.

The **gracilis** is medial to the adductor brevis and is positioned at approximately the same posterior plane as the adductor magnus (see Figure 7-26). In addition to their role as adductors, many of the muscles of the medial compartment can produce rotation of the thigh (see Table 7-3).

Neurovascular Supply of the Medial Thigh

The **obturator nerve** (see Figure 7-26) is a branch of the lumbar plexus, composed of axons arising in L2, L3, and L4. It exits the pelvis through the obturator foramen and enters the medial compartment of the thigh. It divides into an *anterior* and *posterior branch* on the deep and superficial sides of the adductor brevis muscle (Table 7-4).

The obturator nerve seldom undergoes any isolated injury of clinical significance. It is possible to selectively anesthetize this nerve with an injection of local anesthetic near its exit from the obturator foramen. An **accessory obturator nerve** is present in 5% to 10% of individuals. When present, it arises from cord segments L3 to L4 and descends through the pelvis to innervate the pectineus, ultimately linking with the anterior branch of the obturator nerve.

Medial Rotation of the Thigh

Medial rotation of the thigh occurs along the central axis of the thigh, which is *not* the same as the shaft of the femur (see Figure 7-4). Since the axis of the thigh is posterior to the femur along much of its course, muscles connecting the hip bone to the posterior surface of the femur may still serve as *medial rotators*, although this may seem counterintuitive. Many of the adductor muscles (adductor longus, adductor magnus) are medial rotators (see Table 7-3).

THE ANTEROMEDIAL THIGH

ATHLETIC INJURIES TO THE ANTEROMEDIAL THIGH

A hip pointer is a bruise or hematoma along the iliac crest, especially in the region where the sartorius originates.

"Charley-horse" is a less specific term, referring to a hematoma within a muscle, usually as a result of a forceful impact. They occur often in the quadriceps.

CANNULATION OF FEMORAL VESSELS

Insertion of catheters into either the arterial or the deep venous system is often performed by percutaneous placement of the catheter in either the femoral artery or vein and subsequent threading of the catheter upward toward the heart. Knowledge of anatomy of these vessels in relation to anatomic landmarks in the inguinal region is of obvious importance.

FEMORAL AND INGUINAL HERNIAS

Herniation of intestinal contents can occur through either the femoral canal or the obturator foramen. The former is among the more frequent causes of intestinal herniation in women, whereas inguinal hernias predominate in men. Obturator hernias are rare in either sex. When femoral herniation of intestinal contents occurs, hemorrhage or inflammatory exudate also may track downward into the thigh along the path of the femoral sheath.

PSOAS ABSCESS

The psoas major muscle originates in the upper posterior abdominal wall and inserts inferiorly on the lesser trochanter. In the abdomen, its fascial covering is the medial arcuate ligament, which extends inferiorly as a loose fascial covering of the muscle as it travels into the thigh. Infectious material may work its way into the space between the muscle and its fascia. Having done this, it may track all the way down into the upper thigh and present in the patient as a painful swelling in the groin or upper thigh. This is a psoas abscess and always should be considered when a patient has a swelling in the upper anterior thigh. Tuberculosis is one of the more common pathogens for psoas abscesses.

GREAT SAPHENOUS VEIN

The great saphenous vein often is used as a source for vascular grafts, especially for coronary bypass surgery.

There are usually numerous valves in the greater saphenous vein. Some authors have attempted to correlate the risk for varicose veins (pooling of venous blood in the legs and feet with subsequent venous dilation) with the absence of great saphenous vein valves in some individuals.

Gluteal Region

- Skeletal Anatomy of the Gluteal Region
- Large Muscles of the Gluteal Region
- Smaller Muscles of the Gluteal Region
- Vessels of the Gluteal Region
- Sacral Plexus and the Gluteal Region

The gluteal region includes the muscles, vessels, nerves, and connective tissues overlying the posterior aspect of the hip joint (see Figure 7-1). It contain muscles that form the contour of the buttocks and whose main function involves abduction and extension of the hip joint, important in gait and maintenance of posture. The large **gluteus maximus** muscle dominates the gluteal region, but there are at least nine additional muscles deep to gluteus maximus. The smaller **piriformis muscle** is the structural point of reference to which we relate most of the other structures in the region (see Figures 7-29, 7-33, and 7-34). The gluteus maximus muscle is of immense significance in walking, serving as an extensor of the hip joint. In addition, the gluteal muscles are centrally involved in maintaining a successful upright posture. The gluteal muscles also carry out abduction and lateral rotation of the femur with respect to the pelvis. Deep to the covering muscles are nerves, arteries, and veins that supply the gluteal area itself and also extend inferiorly into the posterior thigh. The very important sciatic nerve exits the pelvis here and begins its extensive journey through the lower limb.

SKELETAL ANATOMY OF THE GLUTEAL REGION

Underlying the gluteal region are the posterior surfaces of the pelvis and hip joint (see Figures 7-8 and 7-30). The **sacrum** and **coccyx** form a solid bony strut in the midline. The medial border of the hip bone consists of two curved surfaces whose concave surfaces, the **greater sciatic notch** and the lesser sciatic **notch,** face laterally. Where the two meet is found the **ischial spine,** which also serves as the lateral attachment of the **sacrospinous ligament.** At the inferior end of the lesser sciatic notch is the **ischial tuberosity,** the superior attachment of the hamstring muscles, and part of the adductor magnus muscle. The hip bone is joined to the sacrum through three strong ligaments: (1) the heavily reinforced **sacroiliac ligaments;** (2) the **sacrotuberous ligament,** uniting the ischial tuberosity and the lateral margin of the sacrum; and (3) the **sacrospinous ligament,** uniting the lateral margin of the sacrum and the ischial spine. Deep fascia covering the gluteal region reflects posteriorly from the margin of the iliotibial band.

LARGE MUSCLES OF THE GLUTEAL REGION

The gluteal muscles (maximus, medius, and minimus; Table 7-5) all originate, at least in part, from the outer surface of the ilium. Its outer surface is divided into three areas by the inferior, anterior, and posterior gluteal lines (see Figure 7-8), which course from the iliac crest irregularly downward to the root of the ilium. These three lines demarcate the *anterior, middle,* and *posterior fossae of the ilium.*

The **gluteus maximus muscle** (Figure 7-28) is the principal forceful extensor of the hip. It is especially

Table 7-5   Muscles of the Gluteal Region

Muscle	Attachments	Innervation	Action(s)
Gluteus maximus	Posterior iliac fossa, sacrum, and sacrotuberous ligament to gluteal tuberosity and iliotibial tract	Inferior gluteal nerve (L5, S1-S2)	Hip extension, abduction
Gluteus medius	Middle iliac fossa to greater trochanter	Superior gluteal nerve (L4-L5, S1)	Hip abduction
Gluteus minimus	Middle iliac fossa to greater trochanter	Superior gluteal nerve (L4-L5, S1)	Hip abduction
Piriformis	Inner sacrum and sacroiliac joint to greater trochanter	Nerve to piriformis (S1-S2)	Lateral rotation
Obturator externus	Outside perimeter of obturator foramen to intertrochanteric fossa	Obturator nerve (L3-L4)	Lateral rotation
Obturator internus	Inside margin of obturator foramen perimeter to greater trochanter	Nerve to obturator internus (L5-S2)	Lateral rotation
Gemellus superior	Upper part of lesser sciatic notch to greater trochanter	Nerve to obturator internus (L5-S2)	Lateral rotation
Gemellus inferior	Lower part of lesser sciatic notch to greater trochanter	Nerve to quadratus femoris (L4 to S1)	Lateral rotation
Quadratus femoris	Ischial tuberosity to greater trochanter	Nerve to quadratus femoris (L4-S1)	Lateral rotation
Tensor fascia lata	Superior iliac crest to iliotibial band (and lateral tibia)	Superior gluteal nerve (L4-S1)	Flex or extend knee

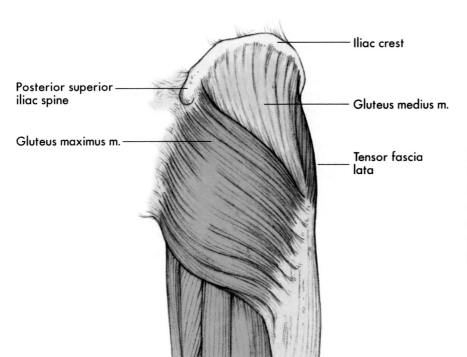

Posterior superior iliac spine

Gluteus maximus m.

Iliac crest

Gluteus medius m.

Tensor fascia lata

Figure 7-28 GLUTEAL REGION, SUPERFICIAL EXPOSURE. The gluteus maximus muscle originates along the sacrum and sacrotuberous ligament and extends laterally to insert on the gluteal tuberosity and iliotibial tract.

SEE ATLAS, FIG. 7-28

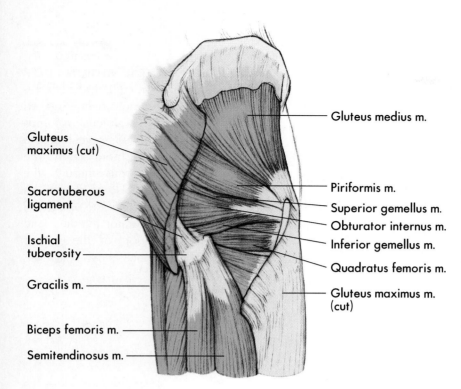

Gluteus medius m.

Gluteus maximus (cut)

Sacrotuberous ligament

Ischial tuberosity

Gracilis m.

Biceps femoris m.

Semitendinosus m.

Piriformis m.

Superior gemellus m.

Obturator internus m.

Inferior gemellus m.

Quadratus femoris m.

Gluteus maximus m. (cut)

Figure 7-29 GLUTEAL REGION, INTER-MEDIATE LAYER. The central two thirds of the gluteus maximus has been removed, revealing some of the short rotator muscles of the gluteal region. The piriformis is a key landmark muscle used as a reference for the position of other structures. The obturator internus lies just inferior to the piriformis, flanked by the superior and inferior gemellus muscles. More inferior still is the quadratus femoris muscle. Just lateral to the lower edge of the medial portion of the cut gluteus maximus muscle is the sacrotuberous ligament, to which the gluteus maximus attaches. **SEE ATLAS, FIG. 7-29**

important in walking, where a powerful thrust off the trailing foot is required (e.g., when going up stairs). In unlabored walking, by contrast, the gluteus maximus is not required for hip extension, and the hamstring muscles suffice. The gluteus maximus is a roughly quadrangular muscle that covers the entire gluteal region. Its lower margin helps define the **gluteal fold** (see Figure 7-17), marking the upper limit of the posterior thigh. The gluteus medius is visible above its superior border. The gluteus maximus originates from the sacrotuberous ligament, the back of the sacrum and coccyx, and the posterior iliac fossa on the outer surface of the ilium. The gluteus maximus passes inferolaterally over the ischial tuberosity, separated from it by a large bursal sac. Its strong flattened tendon inserts into the upper posterior border of the iliotibial band and the gluteal tuberosity. It is innervated by the inferior gluteal nerve. In addition to being a strong hip extensor, the gluteus maximus works in synchrony with the tensor fascia lata to regulate the "tautness" of the iliotibial band (see preceding section on "fascia lata").

The **gluteus medius** (Figure 7-29) and **gluteus minimus** (Figure 7-30) **muscles** link the iliac fossa and femur in a generally superoinferior direction, with the gluteus medius partially overlying the gluteus minimus. The gluteus medius originates from the middle third of the outer surface of the ilium (the middle iliac fossa), and the gluteus minimus originates from the lateral third of the outer surface of the ilium (the anterior iliac fossa). Each inserts on the greater trochanter, and the gluteus minimus also inserts on a part of the hip joint capsule. Both muscles are hip abductors. They are important in gait because they carry out abduction of the hip joint for the planted foot. This permits the opposite side of the pelvis (and the entire lower limb on that side) to be elevated and swing forward unimpeded. When these muscles do not function, then the side opposite the planted foot sags (Figure 7-31), and the patient must tilt his or her trunk toward the side of the planted foot as a compensation (the Trendelenburg sign) (see following for a further discussion of gait and the lower limbs).

The **tensor fascia lata muscle** arises along the anterior border of the iliac crest, from the anterior superior spine 4 to 5 cm posterior along the iliac crest, and inserts into the iliotibial band. It lies superficial to the anterior third of the gluteus medius. It approaches the iliotibial band from the superoanterior aspect. Its pull is "balanced" by the pull of the gluteus maximus, which attaches the iliotibial band from the superoposterior aspect. Together they exert a strong force on the iliotibial band. The iliotibial band lies lateral to the greater trochanter of the femur, and, because the iliotibial band is maintained under some tension, it helps to prevent lateral hip dislocation (see Figure 7-36).

SMALLER MUSCLES OF THE GLUTEAL REGION

The **piriformis** (see Figures 7-29 and 7-30) deserves special mention because it is a landmark for many structures in the gluteal region. It has a broad origin

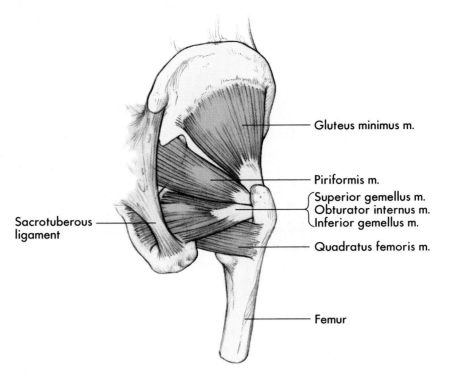

Gluteus minimus m.

Piriformis m.

Superior gemellus m.
Obturator internus m.
Inferior gemellus m.

Quadratus femoris m.

Sacrotuberous ligament

Femur

Figure 7-30 GLUTEAL REGION, DEEP LAYER. The gluteus medius has been removed to reveal the more deeply placed gluteus minimus. The gluteus maximus also has been removed, revealing the sacrotuberous ligament more clearly. The passage of the piriformis through the greater sciatic notch also is shown, as well as the convergence of the piriformis, gluteus minimus, obturator internus, and gemelli on the region of the greater trochanter of the femur. SEE ATLAS, FIG. 7-31

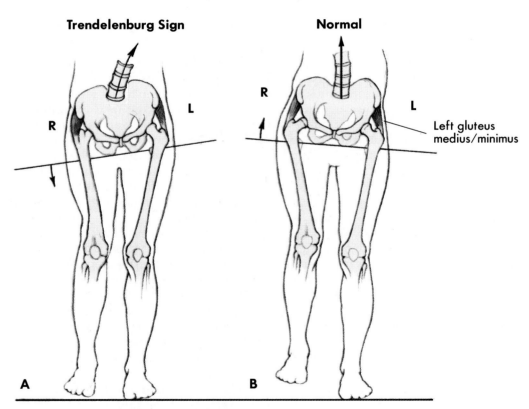

Trendelenburg Sign

R

L

Normal

R

L

Left gluteus medius/minimus

A

B

Figure 7-31 TRENDELENBURG SIGN. When the gluteus medius and minimus are injured on one side, gait is notably affected. These abductors of the femur are instrumental in preventing the elevated limb from dragging along the floor during walking. **A,** Positive Trendelenburg sign occurs when the right foot is off the ground and the left gluteus medius/minimus is damaged; then the pelvis tilts or "sags" to the right. To compensate for this and to maintain balance, the vertebral column tilts markedly to the left. **B,** In a normal gait, when the right foot is off the ground, the pelvis is prevented from sagging to the right (i.e., right side lower than left) by contraction of the left gluteus medius/minimus. The vertebral column can thus remain in a near-vertical orientation.

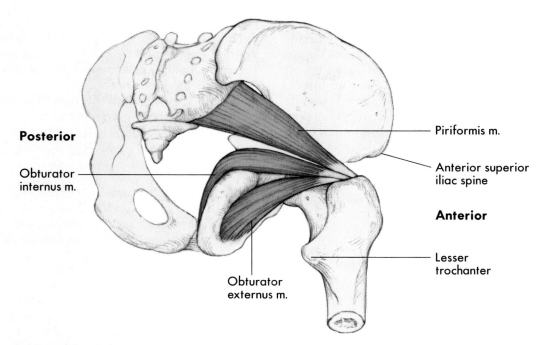

Posterior

Obturator
internus m.

Obturator
externus m.

Piriformis m.

Anterior superior
iliac spine

Anterior

Lesser
trochanter

Figure 7-32   SHORT ROTATORS OF THE HIP JOINT. The pelvis has been tilted anteriorly, so that in this view from the posterior it is possible to see both the obturator internus and obturator externus. The latter originates from the anterior perimeter of the obturator foramen and is hidden from view by the obturator internus in the anterior-posterior axis. The obturator internus originates from the posterior perimeter of the obturator foramen.
SEE ATLAS, FIG. 7-34

from the inner surface of the middle third of the sacrum and narrows as it moves laterally and traverses the greater sciatic foramen, inserting as a tendon on the upper greater trochanter of the femur. It passes directly over the posterior surface of the hip joint. Most structures leaving the pelvis to enter the gluteal region (e.g., sciatic nerve, posterior femoral cutaneous nerve, gemellus muscles) travel inferior to the piriformis; only the superior gluteal vessels and nerves exit superior to the piriformis.

Deep to the gluteus maximus, and moving from superior to inferior, the first of the remaining deep gluteal muscles is the **superior gemellus** (see Figure 7-29). It originates from the upper part of the lesser sciatic notch and passes laterally, attaching to the tendon of the obturator internus, which in turn attaches to the upper medial side of the greater trochanter. The **obturator internus muscle** originates from the interior surface of the rim of the obturator foramen of the pelvis. It emerges through the lesser sciatic notch and narrows as it does so. Both the superior and inferior gemellus muscles attach to the obturator internus tendon firmly, one on its superior and one on its inferior side, as all three muscles pass further laterally toward the femur. The **inferior gemellus muscle** originates from the lower

part of the lesser sciatic notch, passes through the lesser sciatic foramen, and blends with the tendon of the obturator internus. Together, as they cross the gluteal region, these three muscles and their tendons lie directly posterior to the capsule of the hip joint.

Originating from the ischial tuberosity and lying just inferior and slightly deep to the plane of the inferior gemellus is the **quadratus femoris muscle** (see Figure 7-30). It attaches laterally to the posterior surface of the greater trochanter. Directly inferior to it is the superior margin of the adductor magnus muscle. The quadratus femoris is quadrangular in shape.

The gemelli, obturator internus, and quadratus femoris are functionally a group of muscles known as the **short rotators of the hip** (Figures 7-33 and 7-34). They pass over the posterior surface of the hip joint capsule and help reinforce the joint. Because they are muscles, they act like ligaments whose tension can be adjusted to help prevent posterior dislocation of the head of the femur from the acetabulum. They are described functionally as *lateral rotators*, especially the quadratus femoris, because of their position. Their dual role as muscles and joint reinforcers makes them analogous to the rotator cuff of the shoulder joint.

The **obturator externus muscle** is deep to the obturator internus and usually not visible without removal of the obturator internus and the gemelli. The obturator externus originates from the external surface of the rim of the obturator foramen. It narrows as it passes laterally, deep to the obturator internus and just inferior to the hip joint capsule and inserts on the intertrochanteric fossa, near the base of the greater trochanter. Although its course is parallel to that of the obturator internus, it does not traverse the lesser sciatic notch, because the obturator externus is always external to the pelvis and therefore need not leave its interior. It is innervated by the *obturator nerve,* not a branch of the sacral plexus as is true for the other muscles in this region.

VESSELS OF THE GLUTEAL REGION

The **superior gluteal artery,** a branch of the posterior division of the internal iliac artery, exits the pelvis through the greater sciatic foramen above the upper edge of the piriformis (Figure 7-33). It divides into two branches, a *superficial branch* just deep to the gluteus maximus, and a *deep branch* deep to the gluteus medius. This latter branch supplies both the gluteus minimus and tensor fascia lata.

The **inferior gluteal artery** exits the greater sciatic foramen below the lower edge of the piriformis (see Figure 7-33). It travels and branches deep to the gluteus maximus. Over the ischial tuberosity, it contributes to the **cruciate anastomosis,** along with the *medial and lateral femoral circumflex arteries* (branches of the femoral

artery) and the *first perforating branch of the profunda femoris.* One inferior branch of the inferior gluteal artery descends into the posterior thigh along with the posterior femoral cutaneous nerve, and a second accompanies the sciatic nerve.

Venous drainage of these regions is through veins accompanying these arterial branches.

SACRAL PLEXUS AND THE GLUTEAL REGION

The **inferior gluteal nerve** supplies the gluteus maximus, and the **superior gluteal nerve** supplies the other two gluteal muscles and the tensor fascia lata. Both the inferior and superior gluteal nerves travel along with the arteries of the same name.

The **sciatic nerve** is the largest and most significant nerve of the lower limb and the largest peripheral nerve in the entire body. It has two subcomponents, the tibial and common peroneal nerves, each of which is very large in its own right. The sciatic nerve exits the pelvis through the greater sciatic foramen inferior to the piriformis and lies deep to the gluteus maximus. It then runs down the midregion of the posterior thigh, innervating muscles in the posterior thigh and calf. Just above the knee (but with some variation—see later discussion), the **common peroneal branch** separates and wraps around the neck of the fibula, where the nerve is especially vulnerable to injury. The common peroneal branch then innervates lateral and anterior leg muscles and skin and superficial structures of the anterolateral

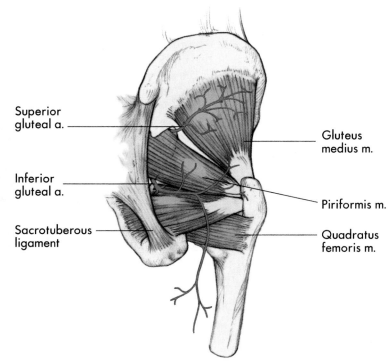

Figure 7-33   VESSELS OF THE GLUTEAL REGION. Branches of the inferior gluteal vessels help form the cruciate anastomosis, lying posterior to the hip joint. The first perforating artery and femoral circumflex arteries also take part.
SEE ATLAS, FIG. 7-32

Superior gluteal a.

Inferior gluteal a.

Sacrotuberous ligament

Gluteus medius m.

Piriformis m.

Quadratus femoris m.

THE GLUTEAL REGION

ILIOTIBIAL BAND

The iliotibial band serves to bind the lateral surface of the thigh and especially to reinforce the upper portion of the femur to prevent lateral dislocation of the hip.

HIP DISLOCATION

Hip dislocation may be *congenital* or *acquired.* In the newborn, the femoral head is dislocated upward into the iliac fossa (large depressed area on lateral surface of ilium). This lessens full mobility of the joint and may be detected as shortening of the limb on that side. Dislocation of the hip in this manner also makes the gluteus medius and minimus unable to contract effectively (because they are shortened) and seriously impairs posture and gait.

INJECTIONS AND ASPIRATIONS

Intramuscular injection into the buttocks is aimed at the upper outer quadrant to avoid harming the sciatic nerve (and other neurovascular structures in the medial and inferior parts of the gluteal region) with the injected material.

Aspiration of joint fluid is usually performed by inserting a needle through the anterior joint capsule by entering the skin 1 to 2 cm inferior to the inguinal ligament. Nearby structures that must be avoided include the femoral vessels and nerve.

When vascular cannulation of the femoral vessels is being attempted, care must be exercised not to puncture the joint capsule and produce an arthritis or osteomyelitis.

Figure 7-34 ORIGIN OF THE SCIATIC NERVE. Two variations in the point at which the tibial and common peroneal nerves unite are shown here.

SEE ATLAS, FIG. 7-33

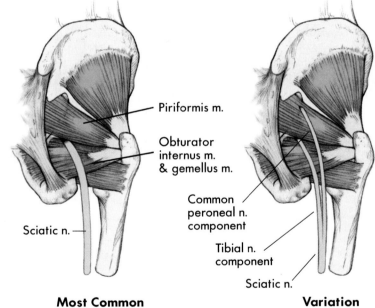

Piriformis m.

Obturator internus m. & gemellus m.

Common peroneal n. component

Tibial n. component

Sciatic n.

Sciatic n.

Most Common

Variation

leg and dorsum of the foot. The **tibial nerve** is the larger of the two components of the sciatic. After separating from the common peroneal above the knee, the tibial nerve continues inferiorly as the muscular nerve to the posterior leg muscles and the muscles of the sole of the foot and as a cutaneous nerve to the medial thigh, heel, and sole of the foot. The sciatic nerve innervates no structures in the gluteal region itself.

The point at which the common peroneal and tibial

components come together to form the united sciatic nerve is also variable (Figure 7-34). Most commonly, the union occurs just beyond the sacral foramina, and the completed sciatic nerve emerges inferior to the piriformis to enter the gluteal region. In other individuals, the joining of the two is delayed; in such cases, the tibial component emerges inferior to the piriformis, and the common peroneal component either pierces the piriformis or lies superior to it. In these cases of delayed

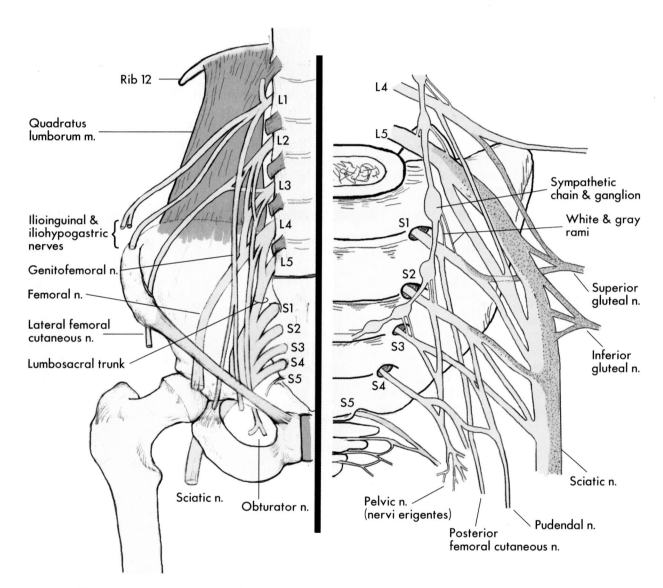

Figure 7-35   LUMBAR AND SACRAL PLEXUS. The sacral plexus innervates pelvic organs and continues outside the pelvis to supply the posterior thigh and nearly all of the lower limb below the knee. On the right is a diagrammatic view of the sacral plexus.

Table 7-6 The Sacral Plexus and the Lower Limb

From Anterior Divisions	From Posterior Divisions
Nerve to quadratus femoris/inferior gemellus	Nerve to piriformis
Nerve to obturator internus/superior gemellus	Superior gluteal nerve
Posterior femoral cutaneous nerve*	Inferior gluteal nerve
Tibial nerve	Posterior femoral cutaneous nerve*
Pudendal nerve	Common peroneal nerve
Pelvic splanchnic nerves— sensory and parasympathetic	Perforating cutaneous
Nerve to levator ani/coccygeus muscles	

*Both divisions contribute to this nerve.

unification, the sciatic nerve is unified lower in the gluteal region or even in the posterior thigh.

The **posterior femoral cutaneous nerve** (S1 to S3) emerges inferior to the piriformis and courses down the posterior thigh in a path parallel to that of the sciatic, embedded in the fascia lata. It is the cutaneous nerve for the posterior thigh, skin over the popliteal fossa, and a wedge-shaped area of skin of the posterior calf.

The **lumbar plexus** has been described in the section on the posterior abdominal wall. The **sacral plexus** (Figure 7-35) consists of the descending lumbosacral trunk (from the lumbar plexus) and the anterior primary rami of S1 to S4.

Like the brachial plexus, the sacral plexus may be described by its roots, trunks, divisions, and terminal branches. The trunks divide into *anterior and posterior divisions,* from which the named terminal branches originate. These divisions produce the branches shown in Table 7-6, which we identify as the sacral plexus.

Posterior Thigh and Knee

▶ Distal End of the Femur

▶ Posterior Thigh

▶ Knee

The muscles of the posterior thigh are commonly known as the "hamstrings" and are among the most commonly injured in athletics and other activities involving considerable force and exertion. The hamstrings lead directly to the knee, which is the most complex and the most highly stressed joint of any in the body. It is poorly designed to absorb force and bear weight but does allow mobility and flexibility. Ligaments, cartilages, and menisci are damaged in literally tens of thousands of people every year. Athletes of today develop increased muscle mass (with or without steroids), which puts disproportionate stress on the structural elements of the knee. Increasingly, the development of osteoarthritic changes in the knees is seriously impairing the mobility of older individuals who have engaged in vigorous athletic activity when younger. On the positive side, great strides have been made in the development of prosthetic devices to replace worn or destroyed parts.

DISTAL END OF THE FEMUR

Understanding the attachments of muscles and their actions requires knowledge of the femoral anatomy (see Figure 7-2). The femur has a prominent *head, anatomical neck,* and a long *shaft.* At the base of the neck are the *greater and lesser trochanters* with an intervening fossa. Many gluteal muscles attach to the femur in this area. At its distal end, the femur terminates as two *condyles,*

medial and lateral, between which there is a deep *intercondylar fossa.* The medial condyle projects somewhat further distally than the lateral condyle. The region immediately superior to each of these condyles is the *epicondyle.* Immediately proximal to each of the epicondyles is a *supracondylar ridge* or line. On the posterior surface of the shaft is a raised vertical ridge, the *linea aspera,* to which attach several large muscles in the adductor group. The femur is normally bowed anteriorly to a slight degree. Because the articulation of the femur with the pelvis is relatively lateral to the midline, the shafts of both femurs are directed medially as they extend inferiorly. As a result, the knees lie more squarely underneath the center of gravity in the standing position.

The medial and lateral condyles articulate with smooth surfaces on the upper surface of the tibia—the **medial and lateral tibial plateaus.** The medial condyle is larger, and there is a "longer" articular surface on the medial tibial plateau. Thus when the lateral condyle has reached its full degree of extension, the medial condyle can slide still further. Assuming that the knee is "locked" in extension (anteroposterior slippage of the femur and tibia is prevented by the cruciate ligaments), this produces a rotation of the femoral shaft medially as full knee *extension* is achieved. Conversely, before knee *flexion* can take place, the medial rotation of the femur must be undone, by lateral rotation. This is precisely what the popliteus muscle does—produce a small degree of lateral femoral rotation at the beginning of flexion of the knee.

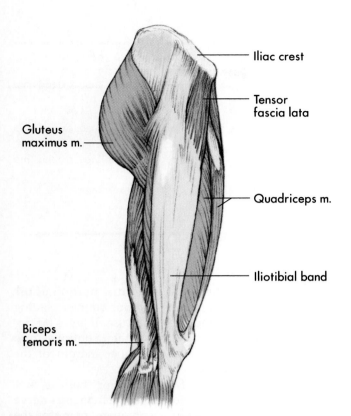

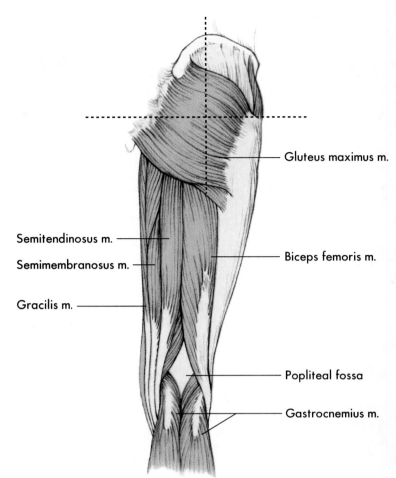

Figure 7-36 ILIOTIBIAL BAND (OR TRACT). All of the fascia lata (superficial fascia) of the thigh has been removed except for the specialized thick elongated portion known as the iliotibial band or tract. The insertion of the tensor fascia lata and gluteus maximus into the band is clearly seen here. Distally, the iliotibial band attaches to the lateral surface of the tibia, anterior to the fibular head. SEE ATLAS, FIG. 7-28

POSTERIOR THIGH
Muscles of the Posterior Thigh

The various muscles of the thigh are encircled by the **fascia lata** or deep fascia. Laterally, this fascia is especially thickened to form the **iliotibial band** or **tract** (Figure 7-36). It attaches to the lateral tibial condyle inferiorly. The gluteus maximus muscle inserts on this band from the posterior side and the smaller tensor fascia lata inserts on it from the anterior side at a comparable angle. These two muscles thus exert complementary "pulls" on the iliotibial band and help maintain its lateral position. Because it crosses the knee joint, the iliotibial band can aid in both flexion and extension of the knee, depending on the position of the knee when the movement starts. The iliotibial band, with its superiorly attached muscles, represents the "lateral muscle group" of the thigh, to complement the posterior, medial, and anterior groups.

Figure 7-37 POSTERIOR THIGH, SUPERFICIAL VIEW. The iliotibial band courses along the lateral margin of the thigh, and the gracilis muscle courses along the medial border. The gluteus maximus covers the gluteal region and the upper thigh. The biceps femoris descends toward the knee, where it turns laterally to insert on the head of the fibula. The semimembranosus and semitendinosus also descend in the posterior thigh, but instead turn medially to insert on the tibia and as part of the pes anserinus ("goose's foot"). The facing edges of these two muscles form the upper sides of the diamond-shaped popliteal fossa. SEE ATLAS, FIGS. 7-36, 7-39

The posterior thigh muscles (Figure 7-37 and Table 7-7), or **hamstrings,** act on both hip and knee. The **biceps femoris** lies on the lateral side of the posterior compartment of the thigh, and the **semimembranosus** and **semitendinosus muscles** lie on the medial side. As they approach the popliteal region, the biceps moves further laterally to help define the diamond shape of the popliteal fossa. On the medial side, the semimem-

Table 7-7   Muscles of the Posterior Thigh

Muscle	Attachments	Innervation	Actions
Semimembranosus	Ischial tuberosity to medial tibial condyle, also forms oblique popliteal ligament	Tibial nerve (L5 to S1)	Flexes knee, extends hip
Semitendinosus	Ischial tuberosity to medial tibial condyle	Tibial nerve (L5 to S1)	Flexes knee, extends hip
Biceps femoris (long head)	Ischial tuberosity to lateral fibula	Tibial nerve (L5 to S1)	Flexes knee, extends hip
Biceps femoris (short head)	Linea aspera and lateral supracondylar ridge to lateral fibula	Common peroneal nerve (L5 to S1)	Flexes knee

branosus has become flattened and broad, and lies deep to the semitendinosus, which at this point has narrowed into a cordlike structure lying superficial to the semimembranosus. These two muscles form the superior medial boundary of the popliteal fossa as they cross the knee posteriorly to insert on the tibia (Figure 7-38). Thus semimembranosus, lying deep to the semitendinosus, should insert more proximally on the tibia than does semitendinosus.

The **pes anserinus** (goose's foot) (Figure 7-39) is the common point at which three thigh muscles attach to the medial side of the tibia below the condyle. The three muscles (supplied by three different nerves) are the **gracilis** (obturator nerve), **sartorius** (femoral nerve), and **semitendinosus** (tibial nerve). The semimembranosus attaches more proximally on the upper rim of the medial tibial condyle, while the muscles of the pes anserinus attach more distally on the medial side of the tibial medial condyle. The medial collateral ligament of the knee also attaches to the tibia near the pes anserinus.

Neurovascular Supply of the Posterior Thigh

The **sciatic nerve** passes out of the gluteal region and in the upper thigh lies between the upper fibers of the adductor magnus and the biceps femoris. It then travels distally down the midportion of the thigh. The sciatic nerve innervates the *hip joint* (from its posterior aspect, while the anterior division of the obturator nerve also innervates the hip), the *biceps femoris*, the *semitendinosus*, the *semimembranosus*, and the *ischial head of the adductor magnus* (the obturator nerve innervates the rest).

Reaching the popliteal fossa, the **common peroneal portion of the sciatic nerve** separates and diverges laterally along the inferior border of the biceps femoris. In so doing it lies just superficial to the lateral head of the gastrocnemius. It continues onward to wrap laterally

around the neck of the fibula. The **tibial portion of the sciatic nerve** continues on an inferior course, passing through the center of the popliteal fossa. It gives off numerous branches within the fossa, then continues into the leg by passing deep to the upper margin of the soleus muscle.

Cutaneous innervation of the posterior thigh is supplied mostly by the **posterior femoral cutaneous nerve** (also known as the "posterior cutaneous nerve of the thigh"), derived from the upper two or three sacral segments of the spinal cord.

The **perforating branches of the profunda femoris,** which penetrate the medial intramuscular septum separating the anterior from the posterior compartment, are the major blood supply to the posterior thigh. There are usually three such perforating vessels plus the termination of the profunda femoris, which serves as a fourth "branch." In the popliteal fossa, the **popliteal artery** (continuation of the femoral artery; see Figure 7-25) enters the popliteal fossa by passing out of the distal end of the aperture in the adductor magnus muscle. A **popliteal vein** accompanies the artery and continues superiorly as the femoral vein.

KNEE

The knee joint is the articulation of the femur, patella, and tibia (Figure 7-40). The fibula is not involved in this articulation. The knee allows for flexion and extension, and for rotation when the knee is already flexed (but not if the knee is fully extended).

The knee joint has maximal flexibility but lacks strength (and is therefore highly vulnerable to traumatic injury). In development, three separate joints ultimately become continuous with each other and form the single large knee joint. The individual joints are (1) between the patella and the femur and (2 and 3) the articulations of the medial and lateral femoral condyles with the upward-facing surfaces of the tibia. These lat-

Figure 7-38 POSTERIOR THIGH, DEEP-ER VIEW. With the biceps and semitendinosus transected, the posterior surface of the semimembranosus is visible, as well as the posterior side of the adductor magnus. The gluteus maximus also has been transected, revealing the gluteus medius and the short rotators of the hip. Clearly seen is the ischial tuberosity, common origin for the hamstring muscles.

S‌ee Atlas, Fig. 7-36

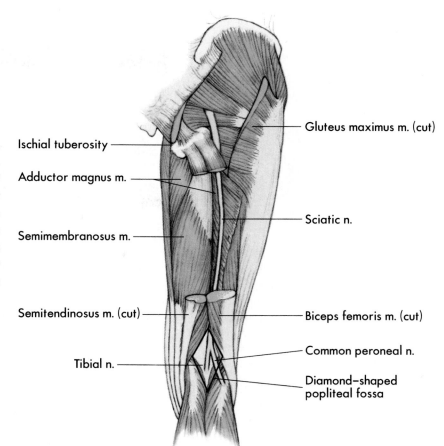

Ischial tuberosity

Adductor magnus m.

Semimembranosus m.

Semitendinosus m. (cut)

Tibial n.

Gluteus maximus m. (cut)

Sciatic n.

Biceps femoris m. (cut)

Common peroneal n.

Diamond–shaped popliteal fossa

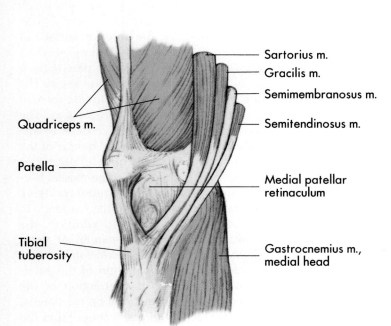

Quadriceps m.

Patella

Tibial tuberosity

Sartorius m.

Gracilis m.

Semimembranosus m.

Semitendinosus m.

Medial patellar retinaculum

Gastrocnemius m., medial head

Figure 7-39 PES ANSERINUS. The pes anserinus, or "goose's foot," is the common insertion of three thigh muscles onto the medial surface of the medial condyle of the tibia. The semitendinosus, gracilis, and sartorius (from posterior to anterior) muscles attach here. The semimembranosus attaches independently, 1 to 2 cm superior to the pes anserinus but also on the medial tibial condyle. S‌ee Atlas, Fig. 7-84

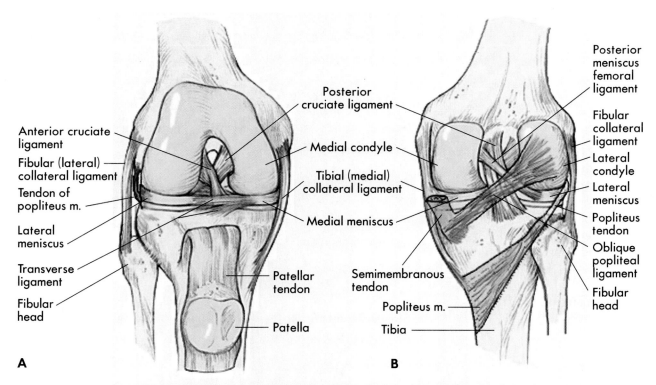

Figure 7-40   KNEE JOINT OPENED, ANTERIOR AND POSTERIOR VIEW. A, Anterior view of the knee joint, opened by folding the patella and patellar tendon inferiorly. On the *lateral side* is the fibular collateral ligament, separated by the popliteus tendon from the lateral meniscus. On the *medial side,* the tibial collateral ligament is attached to the medial meniscus. The anterior and posterior cruciate ligaments are seen between the femoral condyles. **B,** Posterior view of the opened knee joint, with a more complete view of the posterior cruciate ligament. Also shown is the posterior meniscofemoral ligament.

SEE ATLAS, FIGS. 7-82, 7-83, 7-86

ter two joints are, in reality, one continuous joint space. However, the movements of the lateral and medial femoral condyles are sufficiently different to justify considering them as two separate joints.

Patellofemoral Joint

The **patella** is the largest sesamoid bone in the body. It is an inverted triangle (see Figure 7-40) and has a curved upper margin to which attach the quadriceps muscles and their tendons. Its lower margin, where the patellar tendon is attached, forms a very wide-angled V. Because it "elevates" the quadriceps tendon off the surface of the distal femur, the patella increases the mechanical advantage of the quadriceps in producing knee extension.

The patella's *anterior surface is roughened* and is attached to the quadriceps tendon superiorly and the patellar ligament inferiorly. The *posterior surface is smooth* and distinguished by a broad, vertical midline ridge. This raised ridge "fits" into the **patellar groove**

(also called the **"trochlea"**) on the anterior surface of the distal femur between the condyles (Figure 7-41).

The quadriceps muscle approaches the patella from above and from its lateral side at an oblique angle. The tendon extending from the patella to the tibial tuberosity, by contrast, is aligned along the vertical axis. The natural tendency, then, would be for the patella to dislocate in a lateral direction, but the lateral border of the trochlea (part of the lateral femoral condyle) protrudes anteriorly farther (i.e., is "higher") than the medial border of the trochlea (part of the medial femoral condyle). This higher elevation helps discourage the tendency to lateral dislocation (see Figure 7-41). In addition, the vastus medialis muscle inserts on the patella all along its medial edge (whereas the vastus lateralis inserts to a greater degree along the superior margin of the patella). This means that the effect of contraction of the quadriceps is to exert a medialward pull on the patella, also helping to discourage lateral dislocation. From the lateral and medial sides of the patella, a *lateral* and *medial patellar retinaculum* extends to the lateral and medi-

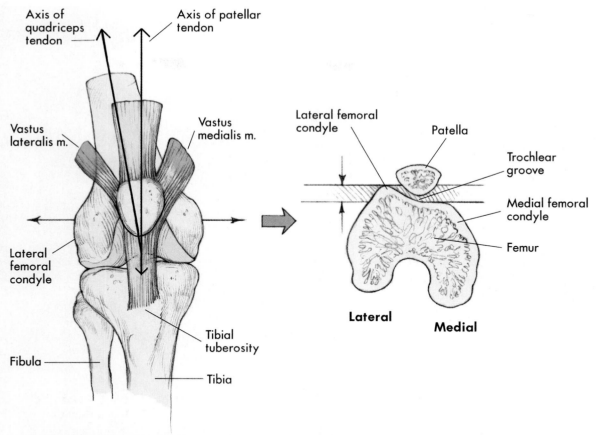

Figure 7-41   PATELLOFEMORAL JOINT. The patella slides longitudinally in the patellar groove (trochlea), flanked by the medial and lateral femoral condyles. The greater elevation of the lateral femoral condyle and the insertion of the vastus medialis low along the side of the patella help counteract the natural tendency of the patella to dislocate laterally (see text).   SEE ATLAS, FIGS. 7-78, 7-80

al sides of the knee joint, blending with the joint capsule. The collateral ligaments lie just external to these retinacula and blend with them.

The relationship of the patella and femur varies with knee position. It does not always lie directly anterior to the gap between femur and tibia. This patellar groove of the femur is flanked by the medial and lateral condyles of the distal femur (Figure 7-42). The patella slides in this groove as the knee is flexed and extended. In *full extension,* the patella moves superiorly with the contraction of the quadriceps and lies just anterior to the most superior part of the femoral condyles. In *full flexion* of the knee, the quadriceps muscle relaxes and the patella descends so that it is positioned anterior to the gap between the tibia and femur.

A *synovial membrane* lines the entire joint cavity. It has several extensions outside of the knee cavity proper, most prominent among which is the *suprapatellar bursa,* immediately posterior to the quadriceps tendon (Figure 7-43). The interior of this and several other bur-

sae is usually (but not always) continuous with the cavity of the knee joint. The suprapatellar bursa is a favored place for the aspiration (collection of fluid through a slender needle) of synovial fluid (to help in diagnosing inflammatory conditions or to relieve swelling). This is performed by inserting a needle along either the lateral or medial margin of the patella and withdrawing fluid. There is usually also a small subcutaneous *prepatellar bursa,* lying anterior and somewhat superior to the patella. Inflammation of the prepatellar bursa, producing pain and limitation of motion, is known as "housemaid's knee."

A normal variant (but less than 5%) of patellar structure is the *bipartite patella,* in which the two normal ossification centers do not fuse. So, if a patient injures his knee and an x-ray is ordered, the bipartite patella may be confused with a fracture of the patella. Normally, the edges of the two segments of a bipartite patella will be smoother than the edges of two freshly fractured patellar fragments.

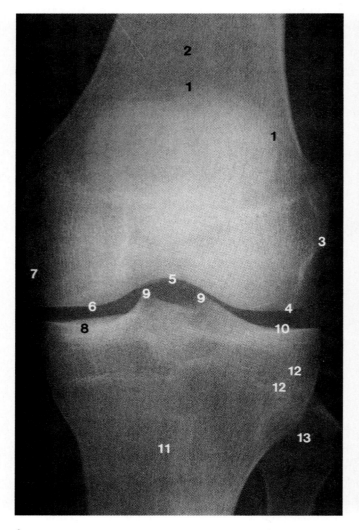

A

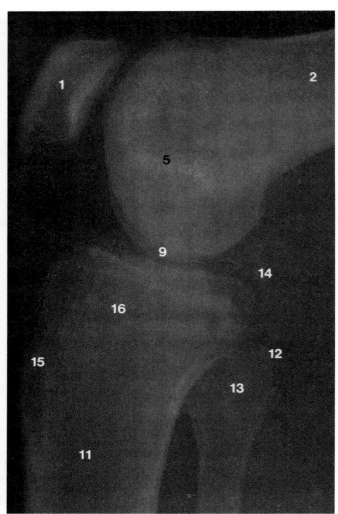

B

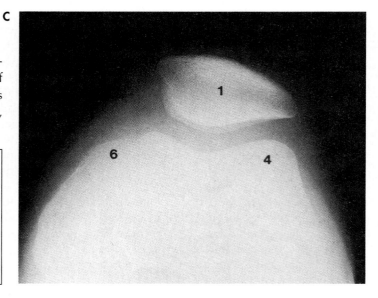

C

Figure 7-42   X-RAYS OF THE KNEE JOINT. A, Antero-posterior projection. **B,** Lateral projection. **C,** View of the patellofemoral articulation. (From Weir J, Abrahams PH: *An imaging atlas of human anatomy,* London, 1992, Mosby.)

1 Patella	10 Lateral condyle of tibia
2 Femur	11 Tibia
3 Lateral epicondyle of femur	12 Apex (styloid process) of
4 Lateral condyle of femur	fibula
5 Intercondylar fossa	13 Head of fibula
6 Medial condyle of femur	14 Fabella
7 Medial epicondyle of femur	15 Tuberosity of tibia
8 Medial condyle of tibia	16 Epiphyseal line
9 Tubercles of intercondylar	
eminence	

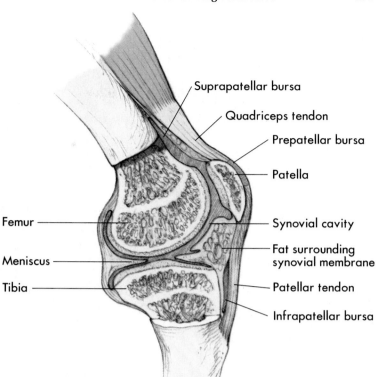

Suprapatellar bursa

Quadriceps tendon

Prepatellar bursa

Patella

Femur

Synovial cavity

Fat surrounding synovial membrane

Meniscus

Tibia

Patellar tendon

Infrapatellar bursa

Figure 7-43 SAGITTAL SECTION, KNEE JOINT. Note the continuity between the synovial cavity in the interior of the knee joint (articular cavity) and the suprapatellar bursa. The infrapatellar bursa is not continuous with the joint interior but is identical to the suprapatellar bursa in other respects—it is a fluid-filled space lined with synovium. An inflamed prepatellar bursa is the source of "housemaid's knee." SEE ATLAS, FIG. 7-79

The Interior of the Knee Joint and Ligaments

Most authorities describe two joints within the knee—the first *between the femoral condyles and the tibial condyles,* and the second *between the patella and the femur*—although the interior of the knee joint is one continuous (although intricate) synovial space.

The interior of the knee joint (see Figure 7-40) is complex. There is hyaline cartilage on the facing surfaces of both the tibia and femur. The hyaline cartilage of the femoral condyles extends around anteriorly to line the patellar groove on the anterior surface of the femur. There is also cartilage on the posterior surface of the patella, where it "slides" within the patellar groove.

In both the lateral and medial compartments of the joint is a C-shaped flattened cartilaginous **meniscus** (Figure 7-44), loosely attached to the superior surface of the tibial plateau. The menisci and some of the surrounding upward-facing surface of the *tibia,* covered with hyaline cartilage, constitute the **articular surface** for both the medial and lateral compartments of the knee joint. The menisci are important in weight-bearing and minimize friction when the tibia and femur move with respect to each other. Both menisci are wedge-shaped when cut in cross-section, with their broader edge facing outward. On both the lateral and medial sides, the femoral condyle can move with respect to the meniscus, but the femoral condyles and menisci can move together as a unit with respect to the tibia. Thus we recognize a *suprameniscal* (i.e., above the meniscus) *compartment* and an *inframeniscal compartment* in the knee joint. On viewing the tibial plateau from above, the medial articular surface appears longer (along the anteroposterior axis) than the articular surface on the lateral compartment of the joint.

The shape of the medial meniscus is a less sharply curved C than that of the lateral meniscus. The "ends" or "tips" of the Cs of both menisci are anchored to the *tibial intercondylar area* (Figure 7-44). The anterior convex margins of both menisci (but not their anterior "tips") are attached to each other by a **transverse ligament** (see Figure 7-44); no comparable ligament is found posteriorly. This transverse ligament passes anterior to the tibial attachment of the anterior cruciate ligament, which in turn lies anterior to the most medial and anterior portions of the menisci as they attach to the tibia (Table 7-8). The outer curved border of each meniscus is attached to the outer margin of the tibial plateau by *coronary ligaments.*

At its midpoint, the outer margin of the medial meniscus is firmly attached to the internal surface of the **tibial collateral ligament** (see Figure 7-40). By contrast, the lateral meniscus is not attached to the nearby **fibular collateral ligament.** The tendon of popliteus (see Figure 7-40) courses across the posterior surface of the knee joint from the medial side of the tibia to attach to the lateral femoral condyle. It separates the lateral meniscus from the fibular collateral ligament. From the posterior convex surface of the lateral meniscus, there arises a narrow **posterior meniscofemoral ligament,** sweeping across the posterior surface of the knee joint, just lateral to the posterior cruciate ligament, to attach to the medial femoral condyle. This ligament passes just posterior to the posterior cruciate ligament and is deep to the popliteus.

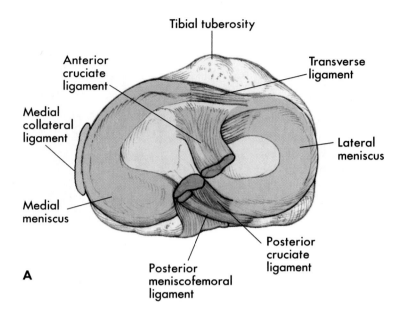

Tibial tuberosity

Anterior cruciate ligament

Transverse ligament

Medial collateral ligament

Lateral meniscus

Medial meniscus

Posterior cruciate ligament

Posterior meniscofemoral ligament

A

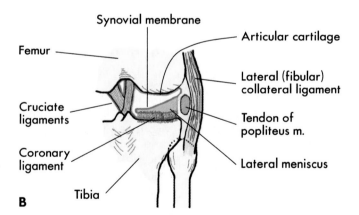

Synovial membrane

Articular cartilage

Femur

Lateral (fibular) collateral ligament

Cruciate ligaments

Tendon of popliteus m.

Coronary ligament

Lateral meniscus

Tibia

B

Figure 7-44   SUPERIOR END OF THE RIGHT TIBIA. A, The femur is removed, showing the superior (articular) end of the right tibia. On the medial side is the gently curved medial meniscus, and, on the lateral side, the more tightly curved lateral meniscus. The anterior end of the medial meniscus is anchored to the surface of the tibia by the transverse ligament. The cut ends of both the anterior and posterior cruciate ligaments are shown, as well and the meniscofemoral ligaments. **B,** This view of the lateral side of the knee illustrates how the lateral meniscus is attached to the tibial plateau by the coronary ligaments. It is enclosed by synovial membrane, continuous with the general synovial lining of the joint space.   SEE ATLAS, FIG. 7-87

Table 7-8 Ligaments of the Knee Joint

Ligament	Attachments	Features/Functions
Medial (tibial) collateral	Medial femoral condyle to tibia near pes anserinus; also attaches to medial meniscus	A flattened sheet; prevents excessive adduction of knee
Lateral (fibular) collateral	Lateral femoral condyle to anterolateral fibular head; not attached to lateral meniscus	A rounded cord; on deep surface, separated from lateral meniscus by popliteus tendon; on superficial surface, covered by biceps
Patellar	Inferior margin patellar to tibial tuberosity	Blends with lateral and medial patellar retinacula on lateral and medial sides
Medial meniscus	Medial surface attached to medial collateral ligament; coronary ligaments attach perimeter to medial tibial plateau	Roughly C-shaped (a semicircle); makes the tibial condyle more concave; has a relatively good blood supply
Lateral meniscus	By coronary ligaments, to lateral tibial plateau	More nearly circular than medial meniscus; both ends attached to intercondylar area of tibia; posterior end gives rise to posterior meniscofemoral ligament (see below in this table)
Anterior cruciate	Medial surface of lateral femoral condyle to anterior intercondylar area of tibia	Prevents excessive posterior movement of femur on tibia; limits anterior movement of tibia on femur when knee is extended; ligament is lax when knee is flexed; has relatively poor blood supply
Posterior cruciate	Lateral surface of medial femoral condyle to posterior intercondylar area of tibia	Prevents excessive anterior movement of femur on tibia; passes posteromedial to the anterior cruciate ligament; ligament is lax when knee is extended
Oblique popliteal	From tendon of semimembranosus to lateral femoral condyle	Forms major part of floor of popliteal fossa
Arcuate popliteal	From head of fibula upward to (1) the posterior intercondylar area of tibia and (2) lateral femoral condyle	Lies just external to popliteus tendon
Iliotibial tract	Superiorly attaches to iliac crest; inferiorly, blends with lateral patellar retinaculum and lateral condyle of tibia	Reinforces joint laterally
Transverse	Connects anterior ends of medial and lateral menisci to each other	May be absent in 20% to 30% of individuals
Posterior meniscofemoral	From posterior limb of lateral meniscus to medial femoral condyle; lies posterior to posterior cruciate ligament	Helps anchor the lateral meniscus in place
Tendon of popliteus	Posteromedial surface of tibia to posterior surface of lateral femoral condyle	Separates fibular collateral ligament from lateral meniscus

Several important ligaments are placed deep within the interior of the knee joint and are designated *intracapsular ligaments*. The femur and tibia are directly attached to each other by the cruciate ligaments, which connect the intercondylar area of the tibia with the condyles of the femur. The cruciate ligaments provide stability to the knee joint and are located in the center of the knee joint space (but not truly within the joint). The synovial membrane is closely applied to the surfaces of the ligaments so that the ligaments are surrounded by synovial membrane, but the ligaments remain outside the true joint space. The **anterior cruciate ligament** extends from the anterior tibial intercondylar area to the medial surface of the lateral condyle of the femur. It passes anterolateral to the posterior cruciate ligament. The **posterior cruciate ligament** extends from the posterior tibial intercondylar area to the lateral surface of the medial condyle of the femur.

The anterior cruciate ligament prevents excessive anterior "sliding" of the tibia with respect to the femur; the posterior cruciate ligament prevents excessive posterior "sliding" of the tibia on the femur. The anterior cruciate ligament in particular plays a role in extension of the knee joint. As knee extension progresses, the anterior ligament becomes progressively taut. This tautness prevents any anterior-posterior slippage but also serves to anchor the lateral femoral condyle (to which it is attached) and cause it to become the axis for the medial rotation the femur subsequently will undergo.

Several other important ligaments are classified as *extracapsular* (i.e., not within the knee joint). Often overlooked is the **patellar tendon,** which covers the anterior aspect of the knee joint and contains a large sesamoid bone—the patella. It attaches inferiorly to the tibial tuberosity. The **collateral ligaments** (tibial and fibular, or medial and lateral) reinforce the medial and lateral aspects of the knee joint.

The **fibular (lateral) collateral ligament** is cordlike and very strong, so is seldom damaged. It connects the lateral femoral condyle with the anterior surface of the fibular head. The femoral attachment of the ligament is just superior to the insertion of the popliteus on the lateral femoral condyle. The popliteus extends laterally from the medial surface of the tibia and across the posterior surface of the knee, to attach to the posterolateral surface of the lateral femoral condyle. The tendon of the popliteus muscle is interposed between the fibular collateral ligament and the lateral meniscus, preventing an attachment between them. The biceps femoris, attaching to the fibular head, also covers the fibular collateral ligament externally. The *lateral patellar retinaculum* extends from the inferolateral border of the quadriceps to the tibial tuberosity, reinforcing the anterolateral "gap" between the lateral surface of the patella and the fibular collateral ligament.

The **tibial (medial) collateral ligament** is sheetlike and weaker than the fibular ligament. As a result, it is more often damaged. It attaches proximally to the medial femoral condyle, just below the adductor tubercle, and passes downward as a broad sheet attaching distally to the tibia in an area just posterior to the pes anserinus. As it travels downward, the inner surface of the tibial collateral ligament is attached to the medial meniscus in the interior of the knee joint.

The semimembranosus muscle passes deep to the medial collateral ligament, just superior to its attachment to the tibia. Posteriorly, the knee joint is further reinforced by the **oblique popliteal ligament,** an outgrowth of the semimembranosus muscle that extends across the joint surface. It passes from medial to lateral, attaching to the posterior surface of the lateral femoral condyle. It forms part of the floor of the popliteal region. The **arcuate popliteal ligament** attaches to the fibular head and has separate slips that extend to the lateral femoral condyle and the tibia. Its fibers lie just superficial to popliteus, with which it also blends.

The **pes anserinus** (semitendinosus, gracilis, and sartorius muscles) passes just superficial to the tibial collateral ligament as it terminates on the medial tibial surface. In addition, a flattened fibrous sheet arises from the quadriceps tendon and passes forward to attach to the medial border of the patella and inferiorly to attach to the tibial tuberosity. This **medial patellar retinaculum** reinforces the medial side of the knee, lying between the patellar tendon and the tibial collateral ligament.

Movements of the Knee

The flexion-extension movement of the knee is not a simple hinge motion. As the knee passes through its degrees of flexion and extensions, the imaginary mediolateral axis through which the movement occurs shifts up and down on the femur. As full extension is reached, the femur rotates medially with respect to the tibia (assuming the leg and foot are fixed on the ground and therefore may not rotate themselves). Medial rotation occurs because during full knee extension, the medial condyle of the femur slides further to the posterior than does the lateral condyle of the femur (Figure 7-45). This occurs because (1) the cruciate ligaments prevent anterior-posterior slippage of the femur on the tibia and (2) the medial compartment of the knee joint is larger than the lateral compartment. The natural consequence of this difference between the joint "spaces" of the medial and lateral condyles and their movements is medial rotation of the femur.

With the foot planted on the ground and the knee fully extended, the knee is said to be "locked" in such a way that muscles of the thigh and leg can relax for short periods of time without making the joint too unstable.

If the knee joint were a perfect hinge (i.e., the mediolateral axis for flexion-extension would stay in the same place throughout the full range of motion), the collateral ligaments would have equal length and tension whether the knee was flexed, extended, or in the neutral position. However, the distal attachments of the collateral ligaments are posterior to the midline; thus, when the knee is flexed, the ligaments are lax, and in extension they are taut. Laxity of the collateral ligaments in flexion (Figure 7-46) is the major reason rotation of the knee is permitted only if the knee is already flexed (and can't occur in the fully extended knee). The rotation occurring at the end of knee extension is described as a femoral movement because the usual situation is one in which the foot and leg are planted on the ground (and therefore immobile). Remember, however, that if the femur were immobile and the leg and foot mobile, then as knee extension occurred the leg and

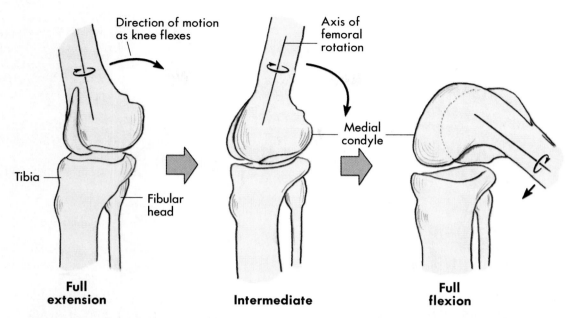

Figure 7-45   ROTATION AT THE KNEE. In moving from the fully extended to the flexed position, the femur initially rotates laterally on the tibia, thanks to the action of the popliteus muscle. The medial condyle of the femur moves in an anterior direction at the start of knee flexion. The greater degree of movement exhibited by the medial femoral condyle is made possible because the medial articular surface with the tibia is larger than the comparable articular surface between the femoral lateral condyle and the tibia.

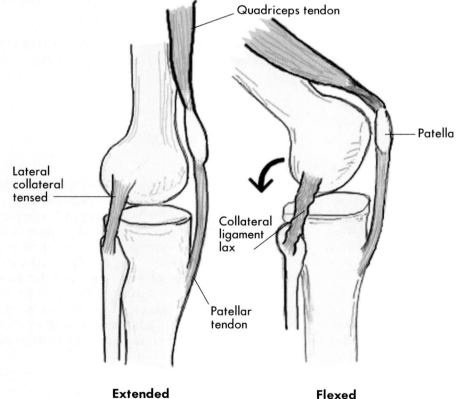

Figure 7-46   KNEE LIGAMENTS IN FLEXION AND EXTENSION. Rotation of the knee is allowed only in flexion because in extension the collateral ligaments are taut and do not allow rotation.   SEE ATLAS, FIG. 7-85

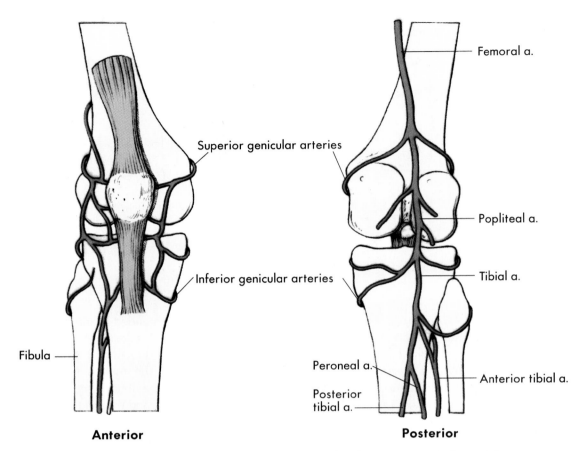

Figure 7-47   BLOOD SUPPLY TO THE KNEE JOINT. Rich anastomosis, derived from several branches of the femoral and popliteal arteries, supplies the knee with blood.
SEE ATLAS, FIG. 7-41

foot would rotate laterally with respect to the femur. In either case, the popliteus muscle is responsible for this initial lateral femoral rotation (or "unlocking" of the extended knee) because it passes across the posterior surface of the knee joint, from the tibial medial condyle to the femoral lateral condyle.

Neurovascular Supply of the Knee

The knee joint receives branches from the **femoral, popliteal,** and **lateral femoral circumflex arteries** (Figures 7-47 and 7-48). The blood supply is rich and re-dundant. Innervation of the knee is from the nearby somatic branches. There is no particular autonomic innervation of the knee, save that accompanying blood vessels. Knees whose nerve supply is injured (e.g., from diabetic neuropathy or advanced syphilis) are subject to severe arthritic damage (because the patient has no sensation of pain and does not protect the inflamed knee from further injury). When syphilis was more widespread, especially tertiary syphilis, such arthritic joints were not uncommon (they were called "Charcot joints," after the famous French neurologist).

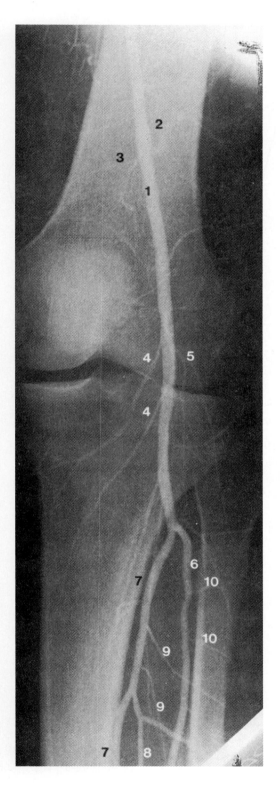

Figure 7-48 X-RAY ARTERIOGRAM OF THE POPLITEAL ARTERIES. (From Weir J, Abrahams PH: *An imaging atlas of human anatomy,* London, 1992, Mosby.)

1	Popliteal artery	**6**	Anterior tibial artery
2	Superior lateral genicular artery	**7**	Posterior tibial artery
3	Superior medial genicular artery	**8**	Peroneal artery
4	Inferior medial genicular artery	**9**	Muscular branches of posterior tibial artery
5	Inferior lateral genicular artery	**10**	Muscular branches of anterior tibial artery

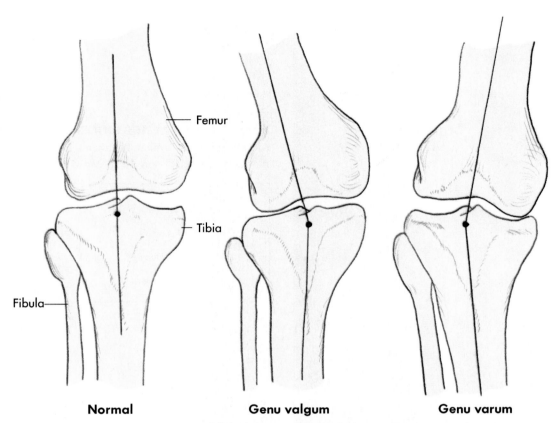

Normal   **Genu valgum**   **Genu varum**

Figure 7-49   VALGUS AND VARUS DEFORMITIES AT THE KNEE JOINT. A valgus deformity is one in which the distal element of a joint (here the tibia) is deviated laterally (away from the midline). A varus deformity is one in which the distal element of a joint is deviated medially (toward the midline).

THE KNEE

KNEE INJURIES

The knee is one of the most frequently injured joints. Violent sports or accidents that involve traumatic blows to the lateral side of the knee and leg are especially dangerous. Forces resulting from a direct blow and involving a twisting motion (e.g., when cleated athletic shoes are planted in artificial turf and a twisting force occurs) are likely to produce damage to the menisci (especially the medial meniscus). Knee joints from which menisci must be removed suffer no loss of mobility; however, the articular surfaces of the tibia and femur undergo serious inflammatory reactions and permanent destructive injury.

The medial meniscus suffers injury far more frequently than the lateral; the reasons for this are not clear. Meniscal tears cannot heal unless they are near the outer margin because this is the only area with enough blood supply to permit repair. In the large majority of injuries, the injured part of the meniscus must be removed.

Violent abduction and twisting (as with a planted foot) often injures the medial collateral ligament, the medial meniscus, and the anterior cruciate ligament.

Injuries to the collateral ligaments will produce abnormal mobility of the leg in the mediolateral plane. Rupture of the cruciate ligaments allows the leg to slide forward or backward to an abnormal degree with respect to the femur (the "drawer sign").

The knee joint has an extensive set of bursal sacs, most of which are continuous with the synovial space within the joint itself. Bursal sacs provide a certain amount of "cushioning" for the knee joint, especially where structures move and friction might cause inflammation. Immediately after a serious knee injury, the swelling and/or bleeding into the joint (producing an effusion) may make determination of normal or abnormal mobility impossible. Swelling and effusion in the prepatellar bursa is "housemaid's knee."

Herniation of a part of the knee synovial membrane through the joint capsule and into the popliteal fossa creates a firm swelling known as a popliteal cyst (or "Baker's cyst"). Pain can be serious, and mobility limited.

ARTHROSOCOPY OF THE KNEE

The most direct way to examine a patient's knee joint is to look inside it with a fiberoptic arthroscope. Arthroscopy is increasingly common and allows surgical repair of many injuries without the need for general anesthesia and a stay in the hospital.

VALGUS AND VARUS DEFORMITIES (FIGURE 7-49)

The terms *valgus* and *varus deformity* are used to refer to the knee and other joints of the lower limb. A varus deformity means that the distal component of a joint is deviated toward the midline. For example, a varus deformity of the knee means one is "bow-legged"—the leg is diverted medially. In contrast, a valgus deformity means that the distal member of a joint is deviated away from the midline (i.e., "knock-kneed"). These two terms, when applied to deformities of the hip area, describe abnormalities in the angle between the femoral shaft and neck. In fact, a valgus deformity of the knee is often accompanied by a varus deformity of the hip, as a means of maintaining the center of gravity over the foot.

OSGOOD-SCHLATTER DISEASE

Osgood-Schlatter disease involves disruption of the epiphyseal plate found at the tibial tuberosity, where the patellar tendon inserts into the tibia. It is a source of chronic recurrent pain, especially in young athletes.

HAMSTRING INJURIES

Forceful contraction of the long muscles in the posterior thigh—the hamstring—can lead to small tears within the muscles and subsequent hemorrhaging. This causes strong pain and an inability to use the muscle in its normal fashion. Like many other muscle injuries, repair is confounded by the fact that continued use of the muscle causes pain and limits function.

7.4

section seven.four

Leg and Ankle Joint

▶ Popliteal Fossa

▶ Tibia

▶ Fibula

▶ Tibiofibular Articulations

▶ Fascial Compartments of the Leg

▶ Ankle

The leg is divided into **posterior** and **anterolateral muscular compartments,** each of which is supplied by different nerves and vessels. The **tibia** is the principal bony element, with the **fibula** involved very little in the knee articulation but playing a more important role in the ankle joint. As was the case with the forearm, many large and powerful muscles have their bellies in the leg but insert onto structures in the foot. This means that there will be important **fibrous retinacula** that bind the tendons in place. The leg is a frequent and important site of traumatic injury. Movements at the ankle joint are flexion (or "plantar-flexion") and extension (which is also referred to as "dorsiflexion"). Only negligible amounts of side-to-side or rotary movements are allowed at the talocrural joint. Other important motions of which the foot is capable (e.g., inversion, eversion) are carried out at other joints.

POPLITEAL FOSSA

The popliteal fossa lies behind the knee. It is diamond-shaped, bounded inferiorly by the two heads of the *gastrocnemius* (Figure 7-50) and superiorly by the *hamstring tendons*—the biceps femoris (lateral side) and the margins of the semitendinosus and semimembranosus (medial side). When the knee is fully flexed, the diamond-shaped fossa is nothing more than a narrow slit. The fascia lata (deep fascia of thigh) forms a superficial roof over the fossa.

In the superficial tissues over the popliteal fossa are found the distal end of the posterior femoral cutaneous nerve, the sural nerve, and the small saphenous vein.

The small (or lesser) saphenous vein (see Figure 7-17) arises along the posterolateral aspect of the ankle, travels in the superficial fascia to the back of the knee, and pierces the fascia lata to drain into the popliteal vein. More deeply positioned are the terminal branches of the sciatic nerve (common peroneal and tibial) and the popliteal artery (continuation of the femoral artery).

The deepest portion of the fossa is formed by the posterior aspect of the knee joint, the plantaris muscle, the popliteus muscle, and the oblique popliteal ligament.

Muscles of the Popliteal Fossa

The hamstring muscles have been described in Section 7-3. The **gastrocnemius muscle** arises by two heads, one from the posterior surface of each of the femoral epicondyles. The muscle bellies of these two heads move toward each other and meet in the midline to form the complete gastrocnemius muscle, and they also form the lower border of the popliteal fossa. Further distally, the muscle ends by becoming a major part of the tendo calcaneus (Achilles tendon) (see Figure 7-50). Note that the gastrocnemius crosses (and therefore acts on) two joints, the knee and the ankle.

The **plantaris** is a small muscle arising from the lateral femoral epicondyle, just superior to the attachment of the lateral head of the gastrocnemius (see Figure 7-55). The muscle rapidly narrows to form a slender tendon, which travels distally in the posterior compartment of the leg just deep to the gastrocnemius. Because it is so slender, it is often mistaken for a nerve (the "fool's nerve"). The **soleus muscle,** a very significant

688

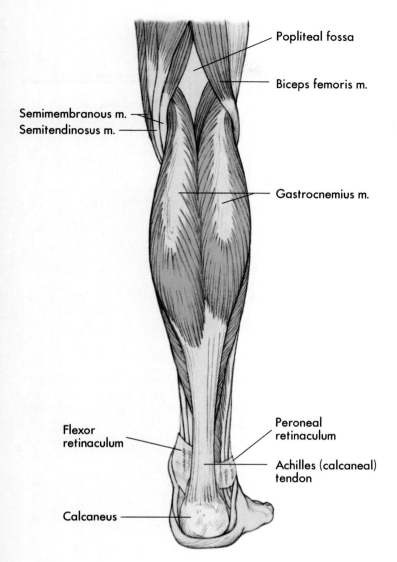

Popliteal fossa

Biceps femoris m.

Semimembranous m.
Semitendinosus m.

Gastrocnemius m.

Flexor
retinaculum

Peroneal
retinaculum

Achilles (calcaneal)
tendon

Calcaneus

Figure 7-50   RIGHT LEG MUSCLES, POSTERIOR VIEW (SUPERFICIAL LAYER). The two heads of the gastrocnemius originate from the lateral and medial femoral condyles, then join to terminate in the tendo calcaneus ("Achilles tendon"). The two heads of the gastrocnemius, along with the biceps femoris and the semimembranosus, form the perimeter of the diamond-shaped popliteal fossa.

SEE ATLAS, FIG. 7-44

part of the posterior leg, is described later in this section. The **popliteus** is a triangular muscle passing from the posterior surface of the lateral femoral condyle to the proximal posterior surface of the medial tibia. It forms part of the floor of the popliteal fossa.

Nerves of the Popliteal Fossa

The **sciatic nerve** may divide into its two major derivative branches anywhere in the posterior thigh but most often does so as it approaches the popliteal fossa (Figure 7-58). The **tibial nerve** (L4 to S3), larger of the two branches of the sciatic, appears to be a direct continuation of the sciatic. In the distal part of the popliteal fossa, the tibial nerve gives off a *medial sural cutaneous* branch, which is cutaneous to the posterior leg. Within the popliteal fossa, the tibial nerve is always superficial to the popliteal vessels and runs deep to the soleus muscle in the leg. The tibial nerve is deep

within the leg and therefore less vulnerable to traumatic injuries. It may be injured, however, in cases of deep laceration.

The **common peroneal nerve** (L4 to S2), having separated from the sciatic, travels just deep to the medial edge of the biceps femoris (which is the superolateral "edge" of the popliteal fossa). Here it emits a *lateral sural cutaneous branch,* which usually joins with the medial sural cutaneous branch of the tibial nerve to form the definitive **sural nerve.** The common peroneal nerve moves laterally and inferiorly in the popliteal fossa, then passes lateral to the neck of the fibula. One usually can palpate the common peroneal nerve by rolling it against the neck of the fibula. The nerve is covered by the peroneus longus tendon as it wraps around the fibular neck. Shortly after wrapping around the fibular neck, the nerve divides into a *deep peroneal nerve* (traveling in the anterior muscular compartment in the leg) and a *superficial peroneal nerve* (traveling between the

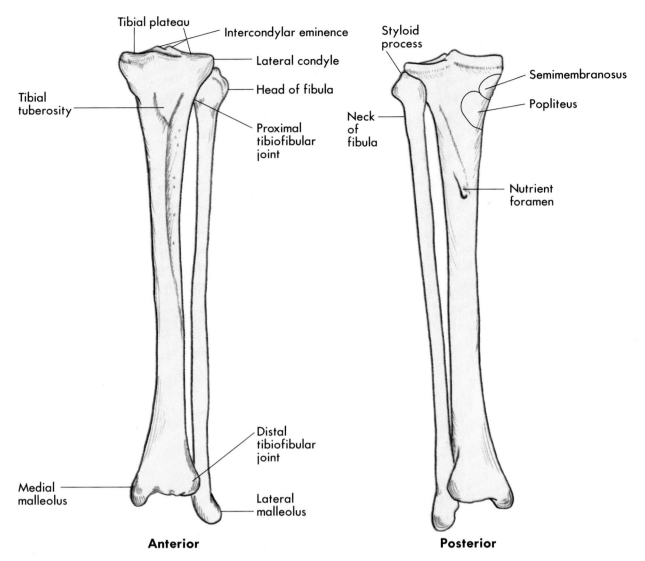

Figure 7-51   TIBIA AND FIBULA, ANTERIOR AND POSTERIOR VIEWS.
SEE ATLAS, FIGS. 7-45, 7-65, 7-69

peroneus longus and brevis in the lateral compartment). Distally, the superficial lateral nerve pierces the fascia and enters the anterior muscular compartment of the leg. The sural nerve is a cutaneous nerve innervating the posterior surface of the leg and part of the lateral side of the foot.

The neck of the fibula (around which the common peroneal nerve passes) is commonly injured in external trauma. Injury to the peroneal nerve at this point leads to weakness of anterolateral leg muscles and resultant "foot drop."

Vessels of the Popliteal Fossa

The **popliteal artery** is the continuation of the femoral artery, after the latter emerges from the adduc-

tor canal (see Figure 7-48). It gives off several genicular branches (to the knee joint) and continues inferiorly as the posterior tibial artery (see Figure 7-57). The **popliteal vein** forms from tributaries of the posterior and anterior tibial veins. Within the fossa it receives the small saphenous vein.

TIBIA

The tibia is the larger and stronger of the two bones in the leg (Figure 7-51). It has a flattened upper end with two prominent *condyles,* each of which has an articular surface facing the corresponding condyle of the femur. In the center of the upper tibial surface are bony prominences and depressions, to which attach the cruciate ligaments and the menisci of the knee joint.

Approximately 5 to 6 cm inferior to the proximal end of the tibia, and in the anterior midline, is the *tibial tuberosity*, where the patellar tendon inserts. On the lateral side of the upper end of the tibia is a depression for the articulation with the fibular head. On the medial side are specialized areas for the attachment of the tendons of the pes anserinus (semitendinosus, gracilis, and sartorius) and, a bit more posteriorly, the tibial collateral ligament. The semimembranosus attaches on the posterior rim of the tibial plateau, and the popliteus attaches somewhat more inferiorly on the posterior tibial shaft. The midshaft of the tibia becomes progressively more triangular, with a sharp edge facing anteriorly and very near the surface of the skin (the "shin").

The distal end of the tibia ends as a flattened horizontal face with a prominent bony protuberance, the *medial malleolus*. This forms part of the ankle mortise. To the medial malleolus is attached the deltoid ligament, and the long flexor tendons of the posterior leg pass beneath the medial malleolus to reach the sole of the foot.

FIBULA

The fibula is a slender bone whose upper head plays no part in the knee joint (see Figure 7-51). Atop the head is a small prominence of *styloid process*, to which the biceps femoris muscle attaches. The *neck*, lying just inferior to the head, is crossed laterally by the common peroneal nerve. At the fibula's lower end is the *lateral malleolus*, completing the ankle mortise, into which fits the talus. The lateral malleolus protrudes further inferior than the medial malleolus, the result of which is that there is a lesser degree of ankle eversion than inversion.

The fibula is fractured most often just above its lateral malleolus or at its neck. This latter injury location can involve the common peroneal nerve, leading to dysfunction of the anterolateral muscles and "foot drop."

TIBIOFIBULAR ARTICULATIONS

The **superior tibiofibular joint** (Figure 7-52) involves the head of the fibula fitting into a shallow de-

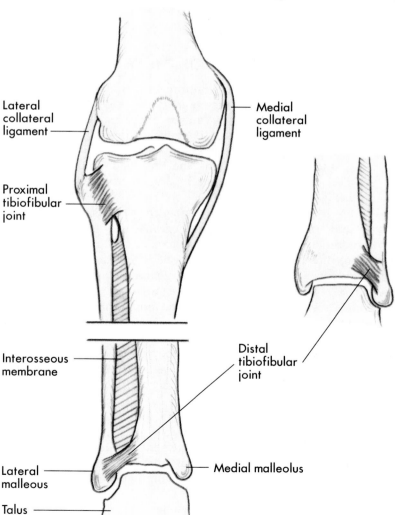

Figure 7-52 TIBIOFIBULAR JOINTS.
See Atlas, Fig. 7-88

Lateral collateral ligament

Medial collateral ligament

Proximal tibiofibular joint

Interosseous membrane

Distal tibiofibular joint

Lateral malleous

Medial malleolus

Talus

pression in the side of the lateral tibial condyle. It is a standard synovial joint reinforced by ligaments.

The *interosseous membrane* connects the shafts of the two bones. It divides the leg into a posterior and anterior compartment. It has a large hiatus at its upper end through which travel the *anterior tibial vessels.* They are joined by the *deep peroneal nerve,* which reaches the anterior compartment not by traversing this hiatus, but by winding around the neck of the fibula. At the lower end of the interosseous membrane there is a second smaller hiatus, through which passes the *perforating branch* of the peroneal artery.

The **inferior tibiofibular joint** (Figure 7-52) is formed by the lateral side of the distal tibial shaft and a small raised area on the distal fibula just above the malleolus. It is not a synovial joint, but rather a fibrous joint heavily reinforced by ligaments.

Note that the tibia and fibula do not undergo any movement comparable to the supination/pronation seen between the ulna and radius. Whereas supination/pronation allows for changes in the position of the palm, similar changes in the position of the sole of the foot take place at the transverse tarsal joints.

FASCIAL COMPARTMENTS OF THE LEG

A thick layer of deep fascia, continuous with the fascia lata of the thigh, encircles the tibia, fibula, and all of the muscles of the three compartments of the leg (Figures 7-53 and 7-54). The fascia is attached directly to the tibia but is tethered to the fibula by an anterior and posterior intermuscular septum. The tibia and fibula are further joined to each other by the interosseous membrane (see earlier discussion).

The leg is divided by fascial septae into **posterior, lateral,** and **anterior compartments.** Because they have a common nerve supply, the anterior and lateral compartments often are considered to be one. The posterior compartment is further divided into a superficial and deep area.

Although each compartment of the leg—anterior, lateral, and posterior—has a specialized vascular and nerve supply, the nerves and vessels are sometimes not physically within the compartment they supply (e.g., the lateral compartment is supplied by the peroneal artery, which lies in the posterior compartment).

Posterior Compartment of the Leg

Muscles of the posterior compartment of the leg. In addition to the more superficial muscles already mentioned (gastrocnemius, plantaris, popliteus), there are others that arise more deeply in the leg and insert onto the foot, acting only on the ankle joint (Table 7-9). All are innervated by the tibial nerve.

The **soleus** (Figure 7-55) is a myoglobin-rich muscle specialized for more sustained contractions ("red" muscle), while the **gastrocnemius muscle** (see Figure 7-50) is a myoglobin-poor muscle specialized for "fast-twitch" activities ("white" muscle) but is more rapidly fatigued. These two muscles are the only ones really effective in raising the heel off the ground, although there are other muscles that are ankle flexors per se.

A complex venous plexus is located deep to these muscles, especially the soleus, and the muscular action of the soleus plays an important part in the venous return of blood from the lower extremities. A fairly common variation (3% to 5% of individuals) is the finding of a **fabella,** a small sesamoid bone located in the lateral head of the gastrocnemius.

The tendons of the **flexor digitorum longus** (FDL) and **tibialis posterior** (Figure 7-56) cross each other in the lower leg. Note also that the muscle belly of the FDL lies on the medial side of the leg, although its insertions are on the lateral side of the foot. Similarly, the muscle belly of the **flexor hallucis longus** originates laterally in the leg but inserts on the most medial toe, the first.

The **tendo calcaneus** (Achilles tendon) inserts into the posterior surface of the calcaneus. The tendon is about 15 cm long and is the common point of insertion for many of the posterior leg muscles (see Table 7-9). The tendon fibers are laid down in a spiral fashion, endowing the tendon with considerable elastic recoil when stretched. Animals such as kangaroos use this to advantage to make their locomotion maximally powerful. There is a *bursa* between the most distal part of the tendon and the posterior surface of the calcaneus.

The two heads of the gastrocnemius and the soleus are sometimes called the *triceps surae.* The muscles fuse distally as they end in the tendo calcaneus.

Vessels and nerves of the posterior compartment of the leg. The **posterior tibial artery** is the continuation of the popliteal artery (Figure 7-57). After the **anterior tibial artery** arises and passes into the anterior compartment by traversing the interosseous membrane, the posterior tibial artery begins at the soleus muscle (by passing deep to its upper margin) and ends at the flexor retinaculum. It travels deep to the soleus and just superficial to the tibialis posterior and FDL. Its terminal branches are the medial and lateral plantar arteries. As the posterior tibial artery passes posterior to the medial malleolus, its pulse may be palpated.

The **peroneal artery** is a branch of the posterior tibial (see Figure 7-65). It arises about 2 to 3 cm inferior to the fibular head and first courses laterally. It then begins to descend down the leg, lying just posterior to the fibula in a small space between the tibialis posterior and flexor hallucis longus. It then passes posterior to the distal tibiofibular joint and ends as a series of calcaneal branches. A perforating branch traverses a small hiatus

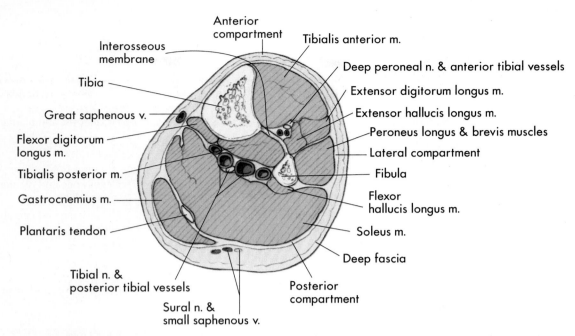

Figure 7-53 **CROSS-SECTION THROUGH MID-LEG.** Displayed in the manner used for clinical cross-sectional imaging (e.g., CT scans, MRI), this is a view of the left leg from below. The tibia and fibula are joined by an interosseous membrane separating the anterior and posterior compartments. The tendons of the peroneus longus and brevis represent the lateral compartment. SEE ATLAS, FIGS. 7-42, 7-60

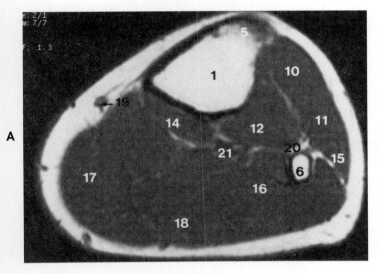

Figure 7-54 **MRI OF THE LEG. A,** Cross-section approximately 10 cm below the knee. **B,** Cross-section of the mid-leg. (From Weir J, Abrahams PH: *An imaging atlas of human anatomy,* London, 1992, Mosby.)

SEE ATLAS, FIGS. 7-3, 7-42, 7-60

1 Tibia	**18** Lateral head of gastrocnemius muscle
5 Tuberosity of tibia	**19** Great (long) saphenous vein
6 Fibula	
10 Tibialis anterior muscle	**20** Anterior tibial artery
11 Extensor digitorum longus muscle	**21** Posterior tibial artery
12 Tibialis posterior muscle	**22** Flexor digitorum longus muscle
13 Extensor hallucis longus muscle	**25** Peroneus brevis muscle
14 Popliteus muscle	**26** Interosseous membrane
15 Peroneus longus muscle	**27** Small saphenous vein
16 Soleus muscle	
17 Medial head of gastrocnemius muscle	

Table 7-9   Muscles of the Posterior Leg

Muscle	Attachments	Innervation	Action(s)
Gastrocnemius	Posterior femoral condyles to calcaneal tendon	Tibial nerve	Flexes knee and plantar flexes foot
Soleus	Upper tibia (along soleal line) and fibula to calcaneal tendon	Tibial nerve	Plantar flexes foot
Plantaris	Posterior lateral femoral condyle to calcaneal tendon	Tibial nerve	Flexes knee and plantar flexes foot (weakly)
Popliteus	Posterior lateral femoral condyle to posterior medial tibia	Tibial nerve	Flexes knee and laterally rotates femur
Flexor hallucis longus	Distal fibula, interosseous membrane to distal phalanx of first toe	Tibial nerve	Flexes toe
Tibialis posterior	Mid-posterior tibia, interosseous membrane, and fibula to navicular and medial cuneiform	Tibial nerve	Plantar flexes and inverts foot
Flexor digitorum longus	Mid-posterior tibia to distal phalanges of toes 2-5	Tibial nerve	Flexes toes

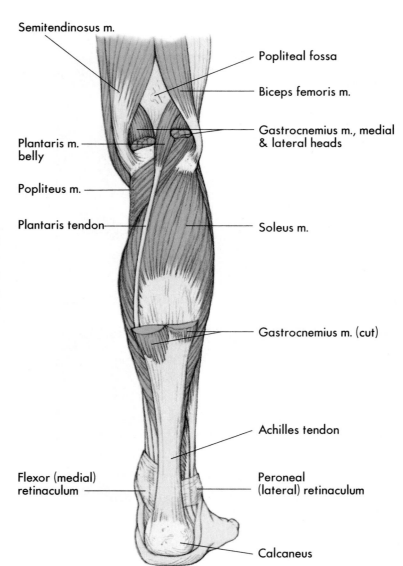

Figure 7-55   RIGHT LEG MUSCLES, POSTERIOR VIEW (MIDDLE LAYER). The two heads of gastrocnemius have been transected, revealing the popliteus, plantaris, and soleus muscles underneath. Most of plantaris is tendinous, and it terminates in the tendo calcaneus.
Sᴇᴇ ATLAS, Fɪɢs. 7-40, 7-46, 7-81

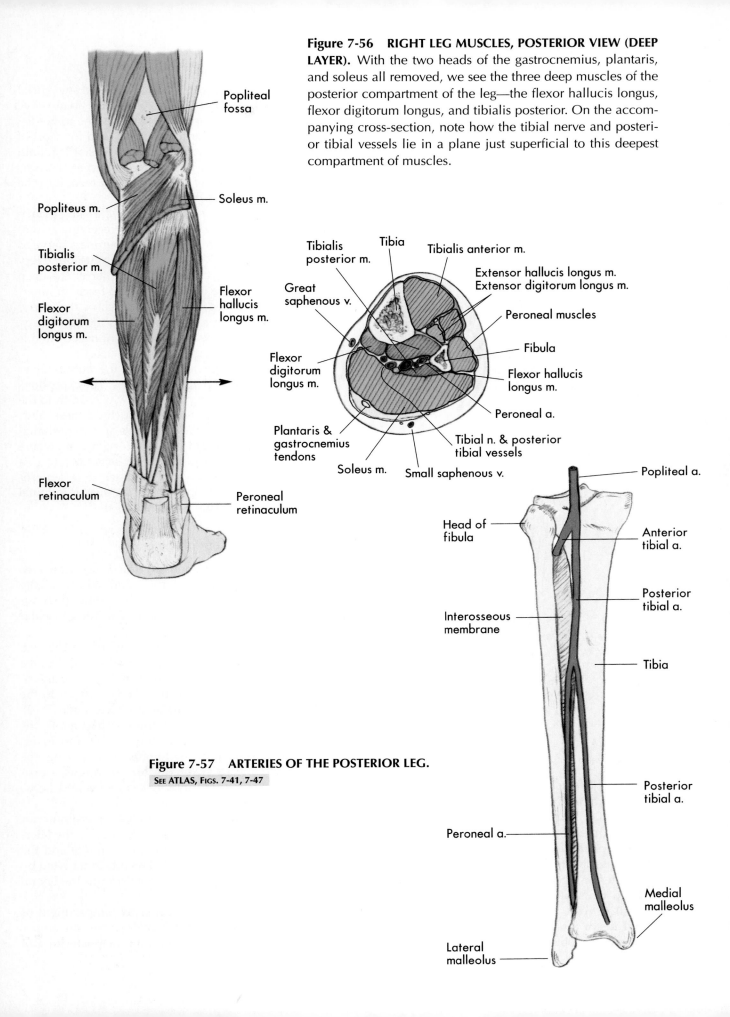

Popliteal fossa

Popliteus m.

Tibialis posterior m.

Flexor digitorum longus m.

Flexor retinaculum

Soleus m.

Flexor hallucis longus m.

Peroneal retinaculum

Figure 7-56 RIGHT LEG MUSCLES, POSTERIOR VIEW (DEEP LAYER). With the two heads of the gastrocnemius, plantaris, and soleus all removed, we see the three deep muscles of the posterior compartment of the leg—the flexor hallucis longus, flexor digitorum longus, and tibialis posterior. On the accompanying cross-section, note how the tibial nerve and posterior tibial vessels lie in a plane just superficial to this deepest compartment of muscles.

Tibialis posterior m.

Tibia

Tibialis anterior m.

Extensor hallucis longus m.
Extensor digitorum longus m.

Great saphenous v.

Peroneal muscles

Fibula

Flexor digitorum longus m.

Flexor hallucis longus m.

Peroneal a.

Plantaris & gastrocnemius tendons

Tibial n. & posterior tibial vessels

Soleus m.

Small saphenous v.

Figure 7-57 ARTERIES OF THE POSTERIOR LEG.
See ATLAS, Figs. 7-41, 7-47

Head of fibula

Interosseous membrane

Peroneal a.

Lateral malleolus

Popliteal a.

Anterior tibial a.

Posterior tibial a.

Tibia

Posterior tibial a.

Medial malleolus

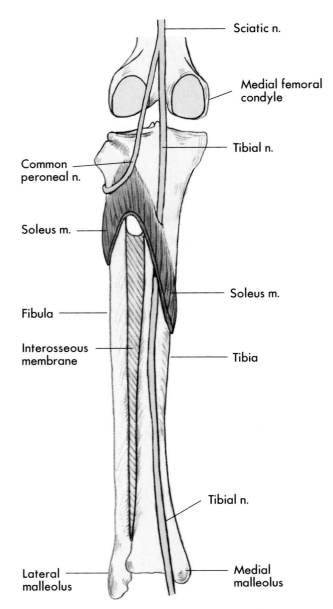

Figure 7-58   NERVES OF THE POSTERIOR LEG.
See Atlas, Figs. 7-41, 7-47

posterior tibial artery, deep to the soleus and superficial to the tibialis posterior (Figure 7-58). The tibial nerve lies medial to the posterior tibial artery in the upper leg but soon crosses posterior to the artery and for most of its course is lateral to the artery. In the distal leg, both the tibial nerve and the posterior tibial artery become progressively more superficial, lying just medial to the tendo calcaneus.

The **sural nerve** is a superficial nerve arising principally from the tibial nerve but usually receiving a communicating branch from the common peroneal nerve as well. It is initially deep to the gastrocnemius, but every one fourth of the way down the leg it pierces the deep fascia and comes to lie in the superficial fascia. It innervates the posterior leg and a small area of the lateral side of the foot. When a nerve biopsy is indicated (e.g., with demyelinating disease), a section of nerve often is removed from the sural nerve.

Lymphatic drainage for most of the entire lower limb is to the superficial inguinal nodes. The exceptions are the heel and the posterior thigh, which drain to the deep inguinal nodes. Distinctions such as these have importance in monitoring the possible spread of malignancies (e.g., melanoma) from their origin somewhere on the skin as they spread to deeper structures (e.g., a melanoma at the heel may not metastasize to superficial lymph nodes, and inspection of the deeper inguinal nodes is necessary to rule out metastasis).

Anterior Compartment of the Leg

The anterior compartment of the leg is the area bounded anteriorly by deep fascia and skin, medially by the shaft of the tibia, posteriorly by the interosseous membrane, and laterally by the anterior intermuscular septum.

Muscles of the anterior compartment of the leg. The anterior leg muscles (Figure 7-59) attach to the area between the tibia and fibula anteriorly, and pass inferiorly beneath the extensor retinaculum to attach to the tarsals, metatarsals, and phalanges (see Table 7-10). There are three large muscles in this compartment—the **tibialis anterior,** important in dorsiflexion and inversion; the **extensor hallucis longus,** dorsiflexing the great toe; and the **extensor digitorum longus,** dorsiflexing toes two through five. Attachments and nerve supply are detailed in Table 7-10.

The **peroneus tertius,** also located in the anterior compartment, is anatomically more related to the lateral muscle group (in that it connects the fibula and the base of metatarsal five). Nonetheless it is innervated by the *deep peroneal nerve* and passes *anterior* to the lateral malleolus.

Vessels and nerves of the anterior compartment of the leg. The popliteal artery divides near the upper edge of the interosseous septum into the **posterior and**

in the distal part of the interosseous membrane to reach the anterior compartment and anastomose with branches of the anterior tibial artery.

The **small saphenous vein** commences at the dorsolateral foot, passes posterior to the lateral malleolus, ascends the posterior leg in the superficial fascia, perforates the deep fascia of the popliteal area, and drains into the popliteal vein.

The **tibial nerve** (not the "posterior tibial," because there is no "anterior tibial nerve") travels alongside the

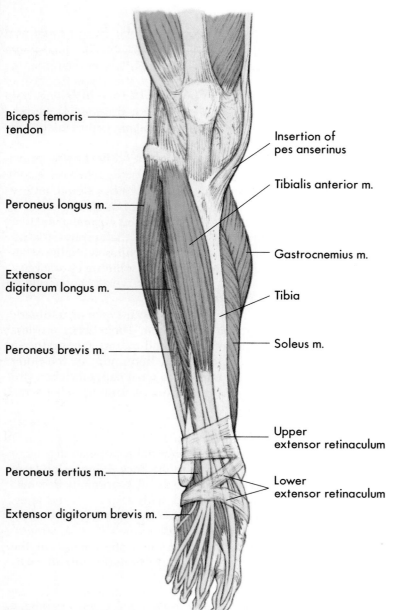

Biceps femoris tendon

Peroneus longus m.

Extensor digitorum longus m.

Peroneus brevis m.

Peroneus tertius m.

Extensor digitorum brevis m.

Insertion of pes anserinus

Tibialis anterior m.

Gastrocnemius m.

Tibia

Soleus m.

Upper extensor retinaculum

Lower extensor retinaculum

Figure 7-59 RIGHT LEG MUSCLES, ANTERIOR VIEW. The tibia lies very close to the surface along the anteromedial border of the leg. In the *anterior compartment* are the tibialis anterior, extensor digitorum longus, and extensor hallucis longus (mostly hidden by the previous two muscles). The peroneus longus and brevis course down the lateral margin of the leg.

SEE ATLAS, FIG. 7-63

Table 7-10   Anterolateral Leg Muscles

Muscle	Attachments	Innervation	Actions
Tibialis anterior	Anterior tibia and interosseous membrane to base of first metatarsal and medial cuneiform	Deep peroneal	Dorsiflexion of ankle and inversion of foot
Extensor hallucis longus	Anterior fibula to base of distal phalanx of first toe	Deep peroneal	Extends great toe
Extensor digitorum longus	Tibia and fibula to distal phalanges of toes 2-5	Deep peroneal	Extends toes
Peroneus tertius	Anterior distal fibula to base of fifth metatarsal	Deep peroneal	Dorsiflexes and everts
Peroneus longus	Proximal fibula to medial cuneiform and base of first metatarsal	Superficial peroneal	Flexion and eversion
Peroneus brevis	Distal fibula to base of metatarsal 5	Superficial peroneal	Flexion and eversion

*The peroneus tertius is absent in some individuals.

THE LEG

SHIN SPLINTS

Shin splints are small tears in the periosteal membrane covering the tibia. They can be the location of considerable swelling and pain. They are generally produced by traumatic injury or by excessive exercise involving repeated forceful landings on the ground.

INJURIES TO THE ANTEROLATERAL COMPARTMENT

All of the muscles in the anterior and lateral compartments might be injured with a traumatic blow to the lateral leg, damaging the common peroneal nerve (which innervates them all). The most noticeable deficits to result from such an injury would be a weakness in extension (dorsiflexion) of the ankle and a dragging of the toes ("foot-drop") in walking.

COMPARTMENT SYNDROMES

One of the most feared complications to traumatic injury of the leg is a compartment syndrome. Because the fascial enclosures of the three compartments are so strong, hemorrhage, major tissue injury, and edema within one or another of these compartments can cause pressure to build up and literally choke off the blood flow. If this occurs, structures distal to the injury may become ischemic and permanently injured. When the leg has been injured, the pressures within the compartments should be closely monitored (including the use of direct manometry) and a fasciotomy (i.e., incision in the fascia) performed to relieve pressure, if indicated.

RUPTURE OF THE PLANTARIS TENDON

Sudden rupture of the plantaris tendon is a common source of severe pain in athletes.

FRACTURES INVOLVING THE EPIPHYSEAL PLATE

Any childhood fractures of the tibia, fibula, or any other long bone are more dangerous if they involve the epiphyseal plate. The continued normal growth of the bone may be jeopardized if the epiphysis is involved, whereas diaphyseal fractures will almost always heal with realignment and splinting or casting.

GREENSTICK FRACTURES

Greenstick fractures are special types of traumatic fractures occurring in children. Their bones are less brittle than those of adults, and trauma can produce a fracture but not disrupt the continuity of the outer cortex of the bone (similar to what happens when you break a tender branch from a sapling—hence the name "greenstick").

TIBIAL TORSION

Tibial torsion is the abnormal rotational alignment of the tibia with respect to the knee. Progressing from childhood into adulthood, the tibia normally becomes slightly externally rotated with respect to the knee. Many parents, seeing the frequent "in-toeing" characteristic of infants and toddlers, believe that surgery may be needed to correct tibial alignment, but the condition nearly always corrects itself without medical intervention.

---

anterior tibial arteries. The anterior tibial courses inferiorly in the leg, lying just anterior to the interosseous membrane and on the medial side of the fibula. It crosses the ankle joint and continues on to the dorsum of the foot, just superficial to the talus and navicular bones, as the *dorsalis pedis artery*. The anterior tibial artery supplies important branches to the malleoli and the ankle joint. It is joined by a *perforating branch* from the peroneal artery in the vicinity of the ankle joint.

The **common peroneal nerve** wraps itself around the neck of the fibula, passing deep to the peroneus longus as it does so. Shortly thereafter it divides into its deep and superficial branches. The **deep branch of the common peroneal nerve** joins the anterior tibial artery in the upper leg and accompanies it downward toward the foot. After dividing away from the common nerve, the deep peroneal passes deep to extensor digitorum longus and takes a position along the lateral side of the anterior tibial artery. It innervates the anterior compartment muscles (see Table 7-10) and sends branches to the ankle joint as well. It accompanies the dorsalis pedis artery onto the dorsum of the foot. It also innervates a small area of skin at the base of the second and great toes.

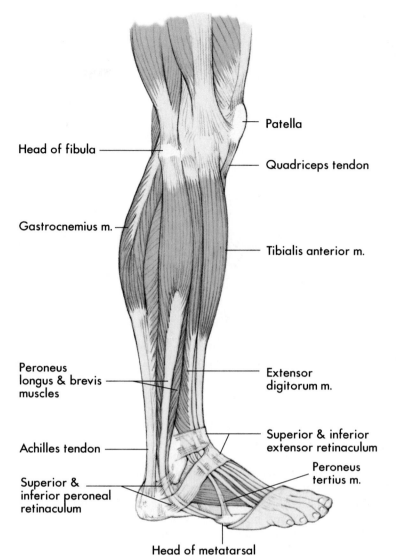

Figure 7-60 RIGHT LEG MUSCLES, LATERAL VIEW. Peroneus longus and brevis originate from the lateral fibula and course down the lateral margin of the leg. The peroneus longus passes along the sole of the foot by traversing a groove in the undersurface of the cuboid bone and more medially attaches to the base of the first metatarsal bone and the medial cuneiform. The peroneus brevis and peroneus tertius attach to the base of the fifth metatarsal. At the ankle, the long extensor tendons are enclosed by the extensor retinaculum, while the tendons of the peroneus longus and brevis are enclosed by the peroneal retinaculum.

SEE ATLAS, FIGS. 7-67, 7-68

Labels on figure:
- Head of fibula
- Patella
- Quadriceps tendon
- Gastrocnemius m.
- Tibialis anterior m.
- Peroneus longus & brevis muscles
- Extensor digitorum m.
- Achilles tendon
- Superior & inferior extensor retinaculum
- Peroneus tertius m.
- Superior & inferior peroneal retinaculum
- Head of metatarsal

Lateral Compartment of the Leg

The lateral compartment is quite small and is surrounded by the anterior intermuscular septum, the shaft of the fibula, the posterior intermuscular septum, and the deep fascia and skin.

Muscles of the lateral compartment of the leg. The lateral leg muscles attach to the fibula and interosseous membrane, then pass inferiorly posterior to the lateral malleolus, to attach to certain metatarsal and tarsal bones (see Table 7-10). These two muscles are the **peroneus longus** and **peroneus brevis** (Figure 7-60).

Tendons of the lateral compartment muscles do not pass beneath the extensor retinaculum but instead are prevented from "bowstringing" by the **superior** and **inferior peroneal retinacula**, located on the lateral side of the foot.

Vessels and nerves of the lateral compartment of the leg. The **peroneal artery** is unique in that it sup-plies structures within the peroneal compartment but does not itself occupy that compartment. This vessel arises 2 to 3 cm inferior to the origin of the posterior tibial artery (see preceding section on posterior tibial artery), of which it is a branch. It travels downward in the leg, lying just posterior to the interosseous membrane.

The **common peroneal nerve** wraps itself around the neck of the fibula, passing deep to the peroneus longus as it does so. Shortly thereafter it divides into its deep and superficial branches. The **superficial branch of the peroneal nerve** passes inferiorly along the medial edge of the peroneus longus and then penetrates the deep fascia about two thirds of the way down the leg. It supplies the peroneus longus and brevis (the peroneus tertius is supplied by the deep peroneal) and considerable cutaneous areas of the lateral leg, the dorsum of the foot, and the base of the lateral toes.

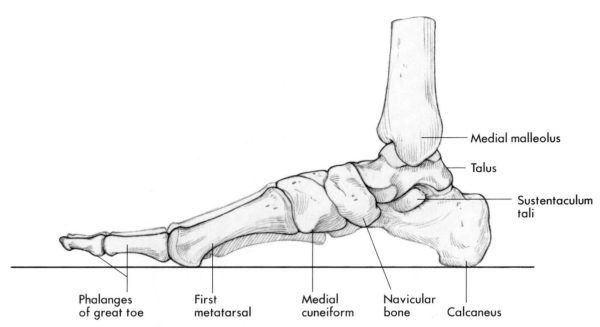

Figure 7-61   MEDIAL VIEW OF ANKLE AND BONES OF THE FOOT. The medial longitudinal arch of the foot is formed by the first metatarsal, medial cuneiform, navicular bone, talus, and calcaneus.   SEE ATLAS, FIGS. 7-57, 7-101

ANKLE

The ankle is the joint between (1) the **malleoli** of the tibia and fibula, which combine to form a mortise (Old French, *mortaise*, joined, fixed in), and (2) the **talus**, a tarsal bone that fits into this mortise (Figures 7-61 and 7-62). The portion of the talus (see discussion on tarsal bones) facing upward is convex superiorly (known as the **trochlea**). A *posterior tibiofibular ligament* connects the distal tibia and the lateral malleolus posteriorly, and deepens the mortise into which the talus fits.

The **lateral malleolus** is a bony distal extension of the fibula, and the **medial malleolus** is a similar extension of the tibia (but does not extend as far distally as the lateral malleolus).

Ligaments of the Ankle Joint

The **deltoid ligament** (Figure 7-63) extends from the medial malleolus to the sustentaculum tali of the calcaneus, the navicular bone, and the spring (plantar calcaneonavicular) ligament. The subdivisions of the deltoid ligament are the (1) *tibiotalar,* (2) *tibiocalcaneal,* and (3) *tibionavicular.* The tendons of the flexor digitorum longus and tibialis posterior lie just external to the deltoid ligament.

The *anterior* and *posterior talofibular ligaments* connect the fibula to different areas on the talus. Further inferiorly, a slender *calcaneofibular ligament* provides some lateral reinforcement for the ankle joint. These three ligaments constitute the **lateral ligament of the ankle joint** and are crossed externally by the tendons of the peroneus longus and brevis.

The **flexor retinaculum** connects the medial malleolus to the calcaneus and plantar aponeurosis posteroinferiorly. From anterior to posterior, the structures passing beneath it are: the tibialis posterior, flexor digitorum longus, posterior tibial vessels, tibial nerve, and flexor hallucis longus. This passage is also called the *tarsal tunnel,* and compression and pressure can produce a tarsal tunnel syndrome comparable to the carpal tunnel syndrome of the wrist.

Figure 7-62   X-RAYS OF THE ANKLE, ANTERIOR AND LATERAL VIEWS. (From Weir J, Abrahams PH: *An imaging atlas of human anatomy,* London, 1992, Mosby.)

1 Fibula	**9** Navicular
2 Lateral malleolus of fibula	**10** Cuboid
3 Lateral tubercle of talus	**11** Lateral cuneiform
4 Medial tubercle of talus	**12** Tuberosity of base of fifth metatarsal
5 Talus	**13** Tibia
6 Head of talus	**14** Medial malleolus of tibia
7 Calcaneus	**15** Region of inferior tibiofibular joint
8 Sustentaculum tali of calcaneus	

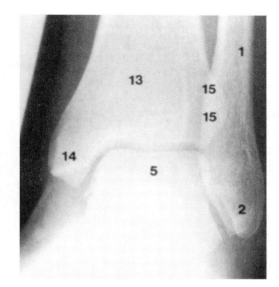

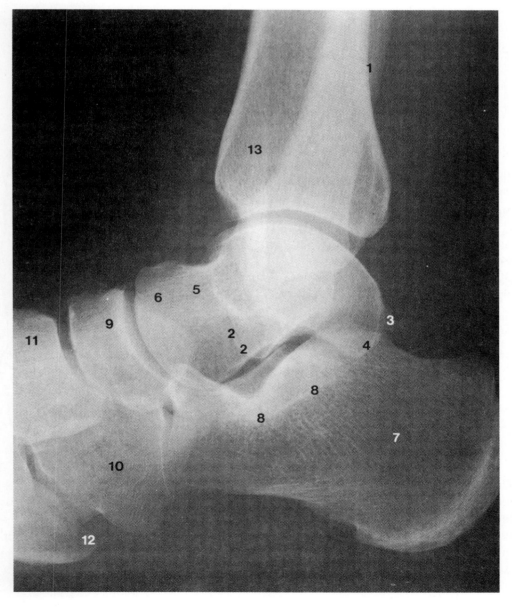

Figure 7-63 DELTOID LIGAMENT. The deltoid ligament attaches the medial malleolus of the tibia to several underlying bones. It consists of anterior tibiotalar, tibionavicular, tibiocalcaneal, and posterior tibiotalar portions.

SEE ATLAS, FIGS. 7-49, 7-94

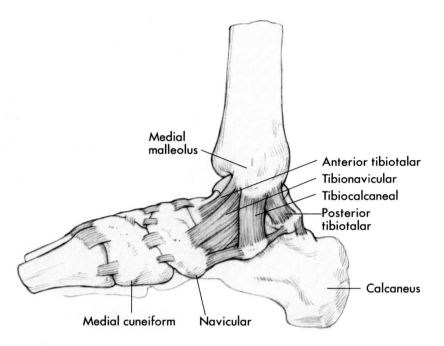

Figure 7-64 TENDONS AT THE ANKLE. Anterior to the talus are the tibialis anterior, extensor hallucis longus, and extensor digitorum longus tendons, as well as the peroneus tertius tendon. On the lateral side of the ankle, posterior to the lateral malleolus, are the peroneus longus and brevis tendons. On the medial side are, from anterior to posterior, the tibialis posterior, flexor digitorum longus, and flexor hallucis longus tendons. The Achilles tendon is seen attaching to the posterior surface of the calcaneus.

SEE ATLAS, FIGS. 7-49, 7-96

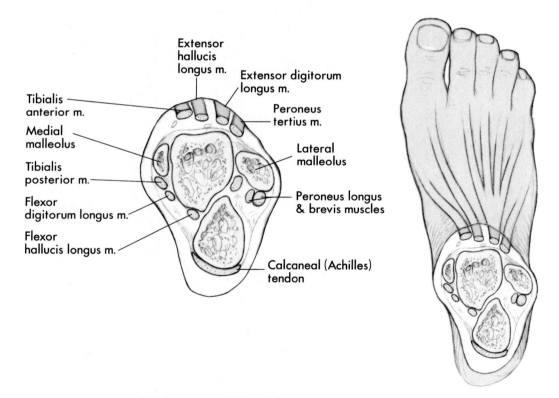

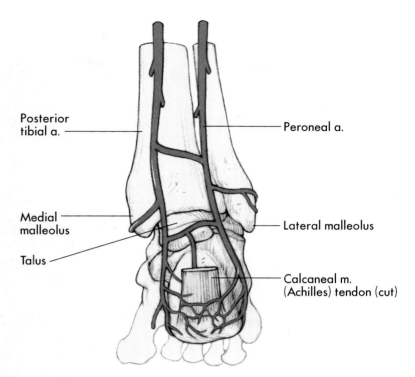

Figure 7-65   BLOOD SUPPLY TO THE ANKLE. The posterior tibial and peroneal arteries descend in the posterior compartment of the leg, supplying the posterior compartment and contributing to a vascular anastomosis around the ankle joint. The peroneal artery supplies a perforating branch that passes through a gap in the interosseous membrane to reach the lateral compartment, in which branches of the vessel ramify to supply the peroneal muscles.

Important structures cross the ankle joint on all sides (Figure 7-64). Anteriorly are the tendons of the tibialis anterior, the extensor hallucis longus, the anterior tibial vessels, the deep peroneal nerve, the extensor digitorum longus, and the peroneus tertius. Posteromedially, from anterior to posterior, are the tibialis posterior, flexor digitorum longus, posterior tibial vessels, tibial nerve, and flexor hallucis longus. Posterolaterally are the tendons of the peroneus longus and brevis (Figure 7-60).

Movements at the Ankle Joint

This joint is nearly a pure hinge allowing only flexion (or plantar flexion) and extension (confusingly, also called dorsiflexion). The ligaments of the ankle are at maximal tension in extension (dorsiflexion) and are relaxed in flexion. Because nearly all forceful movements involving this joint (e.g., jumping, climbing) begin from the dorsiflexed position, it is advantageous to have the ligaments tense and the joint maximally stable.

Although *inversion* (turning the sole of the foot to face medially) and *eversion* (turning the sole of the foot to face laterally) may seem to be analogous to pronation and supination of the upper limb, in fact inversion and eversion occur at joints within the foot and not at the ankle or leg. Chapter 7-5 contains a discussion of these unique movements of the foot.

THE ANKLE

NERVE ENTRAPMENTS

As with the upper limb, nerve entrapments may occur at various sites.

- Lateral femoral cutaneous nerve: Compressed by tight clothing at inguinal ligament.
- Common peroneal nerve: Pressure at neck of fibula (e.g., cast applied too tightly).
- Deep peroneal nerve: Excess exercise leading to muscle injury and edema in the anterior compartment of the leg.
- Tibial nerve: The tibial nerve may be compressed in the vicinity of the medial malleolus (called "tarsal tunnel syndrome"). This occurs when there is swelling of the synovial sheaths and/or the deltoid ligament, extending from the medial malleolus to the calcaneus. These fascial structures surround nerves and vessels of the posterior compartment of the leg as they pass beneath the medial malleolus.

VASCULAR GRAFTS IN THE LOWER LIMB

Arterial bypass surgery in the leg and thigh is now commonplace (although not always successful). It is made necessary by the prevalence of obstructive vascular diseases in the lower limbs. Relief is obtained when a grafted segment of vessel is put in place to allow blood to get past the obstruction in the native artery. Common places for such bypasses are the femoral arteries, popliteal arteries, and anterior tibial arteries.

THROMBOPHLEBITIS

The legs are common sites for clots to become infected (thrombophlebitis) and pose a risk of systemic infection. Immobilized patients and those who have suffered traumatic lower-limb injury are at high risk. The clots themselves are always a danger in that they may break loose, drift upward, and cause a pulmonary embolism.

SEVERE FRACTURE OF THE LEG (FIGURE 7-66)

A fracture of the lower end of the leg that involves both the lateral and medial malleolus is a Pott's fracture and is highly likely to result in dislocation of the talus from the ankle mortise. Isolated lateral (the more common) or medial malleolar fracture is less likely to destabilize the joint.

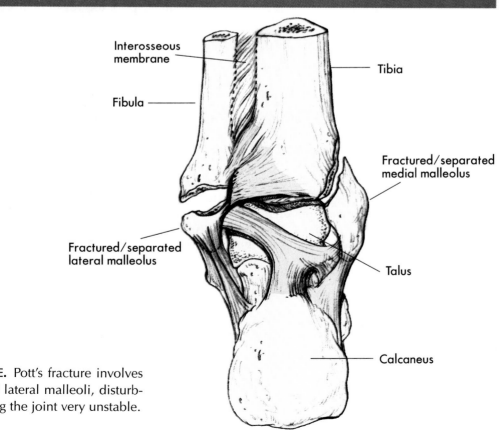

Interosseous membrane

Fibula

Tibia

Fractured/separated medial malleolus

Fractured/separated lateral malleolus

Talus

Calcaneus

Figure 7-66   POTT'S FRACTURE. Pott's fracture involves damage to both the medial and lateral malleoli, disturbing the ankle mortise and making the joint very unstable.

SEE ATLAS, FIG. 7-93

7.5

section seven.five

Foot

▶ Bones of the Foot

▶ Major Ligaments of the Foot

▶ Plantar Aponeurosis

▶ Arches of the Foot

▶ Subtalar Joints

▶ Transverse Tarsal Joint

▶ Distal Joints of the Foot

▶ Movements of the Foot

▶ Dynamics of the Foot and Gait

▶ Dorsum of the Foot

▶ Sole of the Foot

▶ Nerves of the Foot

For all of its complexity and importance, the human foot is surely one of the most neglected subjects in the typical medical curriculum. Its muscular anatomy is every bit as complex as that of the hand, but, because of the limited functional repertoire of the foot, we do not delve as deeply into the details of these arrangements as we do with the hand. The patterns of innervation and blood supply are essentially similar to those of the hand but just different enough to make it unwise to assume one understands the foot simply by having learned the anatomy of the hand! The foot and ankle are involved in many work-related and athletic injuries and are the cause of an increasing number of visits to the doctor or hospital. Podiatry is a growing specialty area and provides to patients a full range of medical and surgical treatments for their foot-related problems.

The portion of the foot facing the ground is the **plantar surface;** that facing superiorly is the **dorsal surface.** In a manner analogous to the hand, the foot consists of 7 tarsal bones, 5 metatarsals, and 14 phalanges. The **hindfoot** comprises the talus and calcaneus; the **midfoot** comprises the navicular, cuboid, and three cuneiform (L. *cunei,* a wedge) bones; the **forefoot** includes the metatarsals and phalanges.

BONES OF THE FOOT

The tarsal bones are analogous to the carpal bones at the wrist, although there are many differences in the individual bones and their arrangement (Figure 7-67). The tarsals can be grouped into (1) a **dorsal group** (talus and calcaneus); (2) a **middle single bone** (the navicular); and (3) a **ventral group** (cuneiforms and cuboid) (Table 7-11). Most of the tarsal bones are united to each other by synovial joints, permitting various degrees of intertarsal motion. An exception to this generalization is the fibrous union of the navicular and cuboid bones, which allows little motion.

The **talus** articulates with the distal ends of the tibia and fibula, forming the medial and lateral malleoli, respectively. The joint between the three bones is called the *talocrural joint* (see p. 700 in Chapter 7-4). The talus (see Figures 7-61 and 7-62) consists of an upper *body,* which participates in the talocrural joint, a *neck,* and a lower *head,* a ball-like extension that articulates with the calcaneus and navicular bones (see later discussion). The **calcaneus** (Figures 7-61 and 7-63) is a strong blocklike bone that forms the heel of the foot and articulates by two separate rounded surfaces with the talus above. The space between these two articular surfaces is the *sulcus calcanei.* There is also an articular surface

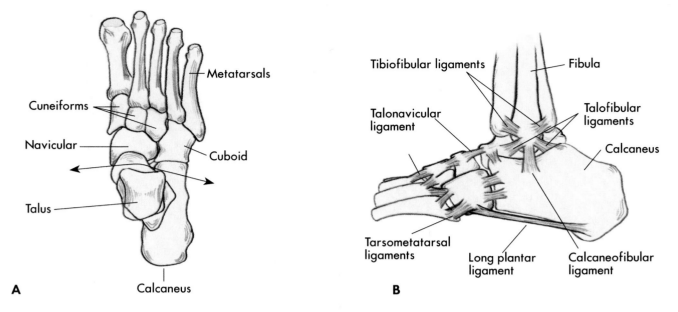

Figure 7-67   BONES AND LIGAMENTS OF THE FOOT. A, Talar and metatarsal bones, superior view. **B,** Ligaments of the foot, lateral view. The arrow in **A** indicates the position of the transverse tarsal joint.   See ATLAS, Fig. 7-97

Table 7-11   The Tarsal Bones

Name	Components and Attachments	Comments
DORSAL GROUP		
Talus	Articulates with ankle mortise superiorly and calcaneus inferiorly. The body is that portion suspended between the malleoli; the anterior head articulates with the navicular, and the neck connects the two areas.	Transmits weight from body to calcaneus; inferior surface forms the subtalar joint; has posterior groove for the flexor hallucis longus.
Calcaneus	The tendo calcaneus attaches to the posterior third; the upper surface of the middle third articulates with the talus; the anterior surface articulates with the cuboid. There are ligamentous attachments to navicular bone, cuboid bone, and the lateral and medial malleoli above.	Anterior two thirds supports talus; posterior third protrudes as "heel bone." The lateral surface is subcutaneous and palpable and is crossed by the tendons of the peroneus longus and brevis; from the medial surface protrudes the sustentaculum tali, a bony shelf supporting part of the talus.
MIDDLE BONE		
Navicular	Articulates with the talus posteriorly and the cuneiform bones anteriorly; has ligamentous attachments to calcaneus.	Lies on medial side of the foot anterior to the talus. The tibialis posterior inserts into a tuberosity on its medial side.
VENTRAL GROUP		
Cuboid	Articulates anteriorly with metatarsals 4 and 5, posteriorly with calcaneus, and medially with lateral cuneiform.	Has deep groove on its inferior surface for passage of peroneus longus tendon.
Medial cuneiform	Articulates with navicular posteriorly and base of metatarsal 1 anteriorly.	Receives tendons of tibialis anterior and peroneus longus.
Middle cuneiform	Articulates with navicular posteriorly and base of metatarsal 2 anteriorly.	Shortest of the three cuneiforms; has strong ligamentous attachments.
Lateral cuneiform	Articulates with navicular posteriorly and base of metatarsals 2-4 anteriorly; has posterolateral articulation with cuboid.	Has strong ligamentous attachments to other cuneiforms and cuboid.

anteriorly for the cuboid bone. On the medial border of the calcaneus is the *sustentaculum tali* (see Figure 7-67), a bony shelf that helps support the talus. The flexor hallucis longus tendon fills a groove on the inferior surface of the sustentaculum. The posterior surface of the calcaneus is smooth in its upper half for a bursa that lies between it and the tendo calcaneus. The tendon inserts on the middle portion of the posterior surface.

The **navicular bone** (see Figures 7-61, 7-62, and 7-68) is a curved thickened rectangular bone, facing the head of the talus posteriorly and the cuneiform bones anteriorly. There is a prominent tubercle on the medial side for attachment of the tibialis posterior.

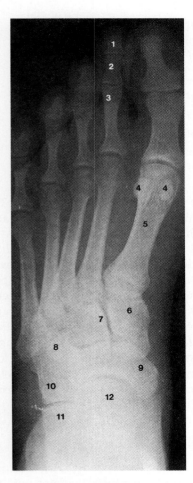

Figure 7-68   X-RAY OF THE DORSUM OF THE FOOT. (From Weir J, Abrahams PH: *An imaging atlas of human anatomy,* London, 1992, Mosby.) SEE ATLAS, FIG. 7-99

1 Distal phalanx	7 Intermediate cuneiform
2 Middle phalanx	(2nd)
3 Proximal phalanx	8 Lateral cuneiform (3rd)
4 Sesamoid bones in flexor	9 Navicular
hallucis brevis	10 Cuboid
5 Metatarsal, great toe	11 Calcaneus
6 Medial cuneiform (1st)	12 Talus (head)

The **cuboid bone** (Figures 7-67 and 7-68) lies lateral and anterior to the navicular. It articulates with the calcaneus posteriorly and the fourth and fifth metatarsal bones anteriorly. The peroneus longus grooves its inferior surface. Anterior to the navicular bone and lateral to the cuboid are the **three cuneiform bones,** the medial, intermediate, and lateral, all wedge-shaped and lying just posterior to the first, second, and third metatarsal bones, respectively (see Figures 7-61, 7-67, and 7-68).

There are five **metatarsal bones** (see Figure 7-67), each with a proximal base and a distal head. The base of the fifth metatarsal is an attachment for the peroneus brevis. There are 14 **phalanges,** two for the great toe and three for each of the other four digits of the foot.

MAJOR LIGAMENTS OF THE FOOT

The major ligaments connecting the lateral and medial malleoli to the tarsal bones are described in Section 7-4. Following is a description of the major ligaments linking the tarsal and metatarsal bones to each other.

The **plantar calcaneonavicular (spring)** (Figure 7-69) ligament extends from the sustentaculum tali (a medial bony shelf of the calcaneus) to the navicular bone. It supports the overlying talus and forms part of the socket for the head of the talus (i.e., forms part of the talocalcaneonavicular joint—see later discussion).

The **bifurcate ligament** (see Figure 7-69) has two parts, a *calcaneonavicular* and a *calcaneocuboid.* Note that the calcaneonavicular part of the bifurcate ligament is not the same as the spring ligament (which is also essentially a calcaneonavicular ligament). The bifurcate ligament is more dorsal and laterally placed than the spring ligament, which is located more inferiorly.

The **long plantar ligament** (see Figure 7-69) extends from the inferior surface of the calcaneus forward to the cuboid and bases of metatarsals 2 to 5. It passes over and encloses the tendon of the peroneus longus, to attach to the medial cuneiform and the base of the first metatarsal.

PLANTAR APONEUROSIS

The **plantar aponeurosis** (or fascia) (Figure 7-70) is a thick fibrous sheet analogous to the palmar fascia. It connects the undersurface of the calcaneus to the heads of the metatarsals.

ARCHES OF THE FOOT

The tarsal and metatarsal bones are arranged so as to form *horizontal arches* that add to the weight-bearing capabilities and resiliency of the foot. The **first horizontal arch** extends across the cuboid and three cuneiform bones, and more distally there is a **second horizontal arch** across the heads of the metatarsals.

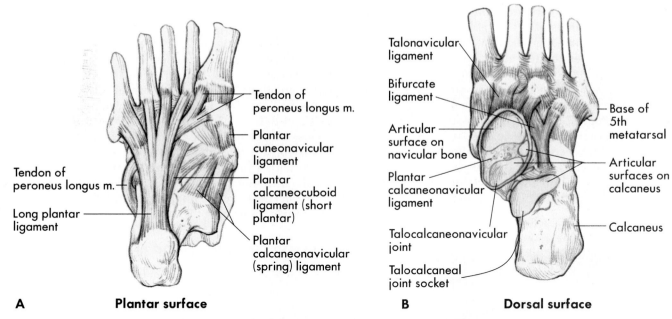

Figure 7-69 DORSAL AND PLANTAR LIGAMENTS OF THE FOOT. A, Plantar ligaments of the foot, including the long plantar, short plantar, and spring ligaments. **B,** Carpal bones with the talus removed, showing the rounded socket in which it articulates (the talocalcaneonavicular joint). The bifurcate and talonavicular ligaments help stabilize the bones forming this articulation.   SEE ATLAS, FIGS. 7-57, 7-58, 7-98

There is also a pair of *longitudinal arches,* formed by the tarsal and metatarsal bones. The **medial longitudinal arch** (Figure 7-61) is higher than the lateral and consists of the calcaneus, talar head, navicular, cuneiforms,

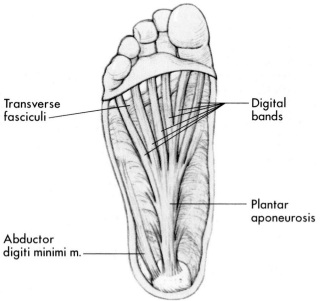

Figure 7-70   SUPERFICIAL FASCIA OF THE SOLE OF THE FOOT. The plantar aponeurosis is a specialization of the superficial fascia. It displays longitudinal fibers and transverse fibers at the level of the metatarsal heads.

SEE ATLAS, FIG. 7-48

and head of the medial three metatarsals. The head of the talus is the keystone of the arch. The **lateral longitudinal arch** (Figure 7-67) consists of the calcaneus, cuboid, and metatarsals. Both arches lend a resilient quality to the foot when weight is removed from it (e.g., when leaping off the ground) and help absorb the shock when landing forcefully on the feet. The *long plantar ligament* is most important in preserving the longitudinal arches. The *tibialis anterior* (see Figure 7-76), inserting into the first metatarsal and medial cuneiform, helps to strengthen the medial longitudinal arch. The *peroneus longus* (see Figures 7-69 and 7-81), crossing from lateral to medial, also supports the medial arch.

SUBTALAR JOINTS

The term *subtalar joints* refers to the complex joint by which the head of the talus articulates with underlying structures. Inversion and eversion are the principal movements carried out at this joint. The subtalar joint consists of two major components, the talocalcaneal joint and the talocalcaneonavicular joint (Figure 7-72).

Talocalcaneal Joint

There is a convex articular area on the upper surface of the *calcaneus* that faces a concave articular area on the undersurface of the *talus.* There are reinforcing ligaments laterally and medially and within the joint as

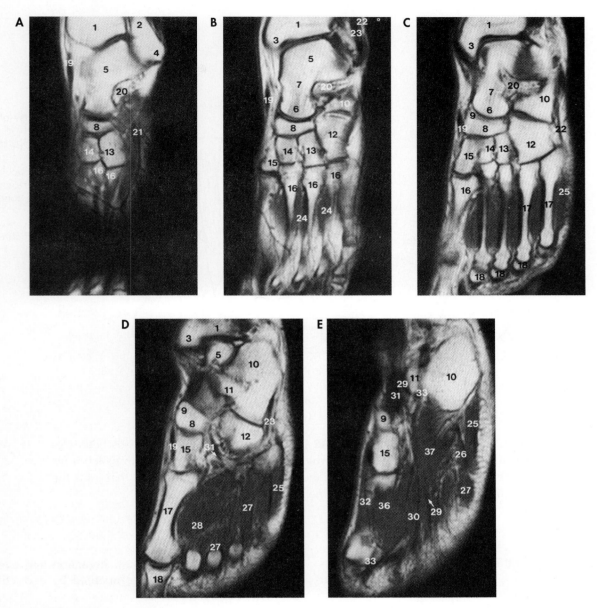

Figure 7-71   MRI OF FOOT AND ANKLE. A through **E,** Oblique axial MR images (T$_1$-weighted). (From Weir J Abrahams PH: *An imaging atlas of human anatomy,* London, 1992, Mosby.)   **See Atlas, Fig. 7-101**

1 Tibia	**16** Base of metatarsal
2 Fibula	**17** Shaft of metatarsal
3 Medial malleolus	**18** Base of proximal phalanx
4 Lateral malleolus	**19** Tendon of tibialis anterior muscle
5 Talus	**20** Tarsal sinus
6 Head of talus	**21** Extensor digitorum brevis muscle
7 Neck of talus	**22** Tendon of peroneus brevis muscle
8 Navicular	**23** Tendon of peroneus longus muscle
9 Tuberosity of talus	**24** Dorsal interossei muscle
10 Calcaneus	**25** Abductor digiti minimi muscle
11 Sustentaculum tali	**26** Flexor digiti minimi muscle
12 Cuboid	**27** Opponens digiti minimi muscle
13 Lateral cuneiform	**28** Adductor hallucis muscle
14 Intermediate cuneiform	**29** Tendon of flexor digitorum longus muscle
15 Medial cuneiform	

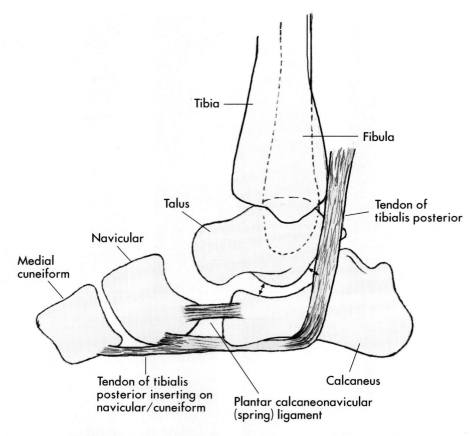

Tibia

Fibula

Talus

Tendon of tibialis posterior

Navicular

Medial cuneiform

Tendon of tibialis posterior inserting on navicular/cuneiform

Plantar calcaneonavicular (spring) ligament

Calcaneus

Figure 7-72   TALOCALCANEONAVICULAR JOINT. The head of the talus has been elevated slightly to show the surfaces with which it articulates. The socket into which it fits is formed by parts of the navicular bone, the calcaneus, and the ligament that joins the two, the calcaneonavicular ("spring") ligament.   SEE ATLAS, FIG. 7-90, 7-106

well. This is known as the **talocalcaneal joint** and is located posteriorly (see Figure 7-69). The talocalcaneal joint allows for a side-to-side gliding movement but not much inversion or eversion.

Talocalcaneonavicular Joint

In this joint, located more anterior than the talocalcaneal joint, the rounded head of the *talus* fits into a concave "socket" that is formed by parts of the *calcaneus* and the *navicular bone*, joined by the superior surface of the *spring ligament* (plantar calcaneonavicular ligament). The spring ligament (on its plantar side), bifurcate ligament (on its lateral side), and talonavicular ligament (on its dorsal side) all contribute to the reinforcement and stabilization of this joint. The **talocalcaneonavicular joint** (Figure 7-72) is unique in that the articular surface into which the head of the talus fits is made up largely of the superior surface of the spring ligament. The talocalcaneonavicular joint allows some side-to-side motion and a considerable fraction of the

inversion-eversion movement. Inversion and eversion at this joint always are accompanied by adduction or abduction of the forefoot.

TRANSVERSE TARSAL JOINT

This joint comprises the talonavicular and calcaneocuboid joints. It is in fact two separate joints aligned horizontally. The **talonavicular joint** is in fact part of the talocalcaneonavicular joint as described previously. The **calcaneocuboid joint,** joining the anterior surface of the calcaneus with the posterior surface of the cuboid, lies in the same transverse plane as the talocalcaneonavicular joint. The short and long plantar ligaments reinforce these joints on their plantar surfaces (Figure 7-69). Transection across these two joints is one standard method for surgical amputation of the foot. The transverse tarsal joint often is said to be specialized for inversion and eversion, but in fact its range of motion is limited, and many believe it contributes no more to these motions than do several other intertarsal joints.

PRINCIPLES

■ With the upper limbs dangling loosely at the sides, the upright posture of the body (i.e., standing at rest on one's feet) causes the center of gravity to pass through the two hip joints. The anterior (iliofemoral) ligaments prevent the trunk from flexing forward on the pelvis, and the iliopsoas muscles and pubofemoral ligaments prevent the trunk from hyperextending on the pelvis. The knees are maintained in a slight degree of hyperextension. The cruciate ligaments and the posterior portion of the knee joint capsule resist any further degree of hyperextension, and no muscular activity is required to keep the knee in this position. The center of gravity passes anterior to the ankle joints, requiring the posterior leg muscles to maintain a moderate state of contraction to prevent the body from collapsing forward as a result of excessive extension (dorsiflexion) of the ankles. The soleus muscle, biochemically specialized for slow sustained contractions, performs this role admirably. On the soles of the feet, the arches are maintained by the intrinsic structure of the bones in the lateral and medial arches and the presence of the plantar calcaneonavicular ("spring") and long plantar ligaments.

DISTAL JOINTS OF THE FOOT

The distal tarsals, metatarsals, and phalanges are joined to each other by many ligaments. Unlike the hand, where the thumb is not included in joints between metacarpals and phalanges, in the foot the first toe is included in such joints. This is a major factor in the extraordinary independence and mobility of the thumb, and the absence of such capabilities in the great toe.

MOVEMENTS OF THE FOOT

Inversion is the elevation of the medial edge of the foot in relation to the lateral edge, and *eversion* is the opposite movement. Inversion and eversion take place mainly at the transverse tarsal and talocalcaneonavicular joints. To perform inversion and eversion, the talus remains fixed in position, enclosed by the medial and lateral malleoli, and all the remaining bones of the foot move (Figure 7-73). By contrast, *flexion/extension* of the ankle involves the unified movement of the bones of the foot, including the talus, in relation to the tibia and fibula. Inversion and eversion are what allow us to walk on uneven surfaces, because the sole of the foot is not restricted to the horizontal plane. Inversion is limit-

PRINCIPLES

■ The human capability of upright posture (i.e., standing on the hindlimbs) frees the upper limbs for use in manipulation of objects rather than for providing support for the body, as is the case in most other mammals.

The *human foot* possesses several structural specializations that contribute to human posture and locomotion. The *tarsals, metatarsals,* and *phalanges* all are in contact with the ground during gait. The numerous small joints between these bones, particularly those between the tarsal bones, give the foot the ability to accommodate to uneven surfaces underfoot and allow us to walk on inclined surfaces as well. When standing still for prolonged periods, we subtly shift our weight back and forth from the balls to the heels of the foot, using the long leg flexor muscles to do so. The *longitudinal arch* of the foot, necessary to transfer the weight of the overlying body to the ball and heel of the foot, is maintained by the plantar calcaneonavicular ("spring") ligament. If the arch fails, the weight of the body is transmitted through the head of the talus directly to the underlying bones and then to the ground. The arch is no longer used to distribute this weight over the entire foot. This predisposes to injury to the talus, calcaneus, and other nearby bones. At rest, while standing on both feet, there is some flattening of the longitudinal arches. When a forceful "pushing-off" from the ground is begun (as in taking a step or jumping), considerable force is placed on the head of the first metatarsal bone and the heel.

The lower limbs are of obvious importance in *locomotion* or *gait*. Humans, along with marsupials and other slow-footed mammals, support their weight by planting the phalanges, metatarsals, and even some of the tarsal bones directly on the ground. By contrast, animals that are fleet typically contact the ground only on their phalanges (e.g., felines, canines, rabbits, deer). In humans, the position of the toes makes true opposability very difficult, although humans deprived of their arms or hands have made remarkable adjustments and learned to use their feet for many sophisticated functions normally carried out by the hands (e.g., manipulation of eating utensils, writing instruments).

---

ed by the tension of the peroneus muscle tendons and the interosseous ligaments of the subtalar joint. Eversion is limited by the tension of both tibialis muscles, the lateral malleolus, and the deltoid ligament.

Remember that inversion and eversion are not comparable to pronation and supination in the forearm,

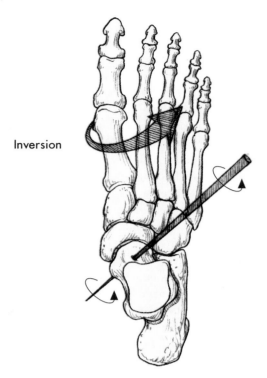

Inversion

Figure 7-73   MOVEMENTS IN THE TARSAL BONES. In-version and eversion occur around an imaginary slanted axis through the head of the talus. Inversion and eversion are compound movements involving intertarsal joints and metatarsal bones.   SEE ATLAS, FIG. 7-103

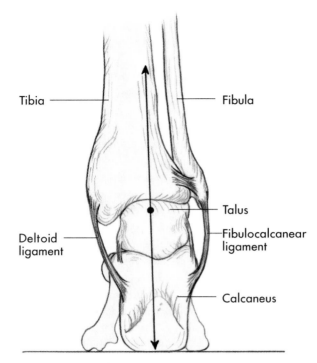

Tibia — Fibula

Talus

Deltoid ligament — Fibulocalcanear ligament

Calcaneus

Figure 7-74   WEIGHT BEARING AT THE ANKLE JOINT. SEE ATLAS, FIGS. 7-89, 7-90, 7-91

even though both result in turning of the plantar (or palmar) surface of the foot (or hand) in the mediolateral plane.

DYNAMICS OF THE FOOT AND GAIT

When one is standing upright, the weight of the body is borne on the heel (Figure 7-74) and the row of metatarsal heads. When one is walking, the foot being advanced first strikes the ground with its heel. There-after, the lateral edge of the foot and finally the heads of the metatarsals make contact with the ground. The various arches and ligaments serve the purpose of dis-tributing weight, so that no one area is unduly stressed.

Gait is the alternating forward and backward move-ments of the two limbs (Figure 7-75). As the limb on one side is moved forward, it leaves the *stance phase* and enters the swing phase. During the *swing phase,* the foot is off the ground and advancing through a semicir-cular arc in the parasagittal plane. When this foot reaches its farthest point in advance of the body, the

swing phase is terminated and the stance phase begins.

At the beginning of the swing phase, the limb ad-vances forward through *flexion* of the hip joint. If gait is unlabored, the limb may swing forward simply be-cause it follows the advancing body. If walking in-volves effort, the gluteus maximus becomes involved (as in climbing stairs or walking at a brisk pace). While the foot is planted in the stance phase, the femur goes through a motion of *extension* with respect to the hip joint. At the beginning of the swing phase, the femur is *medially rotated* with respect to the pelvis (although it is the pelvis that tilts, rather than it being a motion of the femur per se). As the swing phase proceeds, the femur undergoes *lateral rotation* relative to the pelvis. Third, because the body has been planted over the limb in the stance phase, it follows that as the swing phase begins, the center of gravity has shifted and the femur and pelvis are in a position of *adduction.* As the swing phase proceeds and the body's weight shifts over the oppo-site foot, the femur and pelvis go through a process of *abduction.* Thus gait involves the three cardinal pairs of motions at the hip joint—**flexion/extension, medial ro-tation/lateral rotation,** and finally **adduction/abduc-tion.**

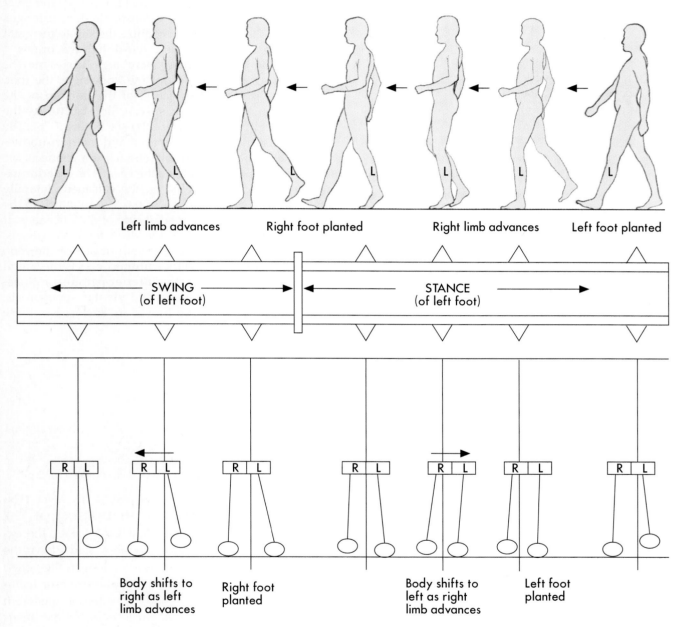

Left limb advances Right foot planted Right limb advances Left foot planted

SWING (of left foot)

STANCE (of left foot)

R L   R L   R L   R L   R L   R L   R L

Body shifts to right as left limb advances

Right foot planted

Body shifts to left as right limb advances

Left foot planted

Figure 7-75 MECHANICS OF GAIT. The upper series of illustrations shows one cycle of gait, beginning on the far right with the left foot being planted on the ground, for the beginning of the stance phase, the right lower limb swinging forward until it plants on the ground, and the left foot beginning its swing phase. The lower series of illustrations shows how the pelvis moves from side to side so that the weight of the body stays centered over the planted foot.

PRINCIPLES

■ Comparing ourselves with our primate relatives, we see that upright posture and walking on two lower limbs (**bipedal locomotion**) depend on certain special musculoskeletal arrangements in the lower limbs. First, the pelvis and lower limb must allow support of the entire body on one limb (while the other is lifted off the ground, as in walking or running). The gluteus medius and minimus function as extensors in most other primates, but in humans they serve as hip abductors, a motion crucial in allowing support of the body weight on the planted abductors, allowing support of the body weight on the planted limb while the other limb is off the ground in the swing phase of gait. Second, the hip joint must allow a wide range of flexion-extension, so that one lower limb may swing in front of and behind the body during gait. As mentioned previously, the gluteus medius and minimus allow humans greater degrees of abduction than in other mammals. Humans also possess the ability to extend their hips more extensively than other primates, very important for striding forward off the planted foot during walking.

DORSUM OF THE FOOT
Muscles of the Dorsum of the Foot

Only one muscle is found on the dorsum, the **extensor digitorum brevis** (Figures 7-76 and 7-77), extending from the calcaneus to the proximal phalanx of the great toe and the tendons of the extensor digitorum longus for toes two to five. Some recognize the slip to the great toe as a separate muscle, the **extensor hallucis brevis.**

The tendons of the anterolateral leg muscles may be seen through the thin skin of the dorsum of the foot. The otherwise thin deep fascia of the dorsum of the foot thickens to form two specialized structures—the extensor and peroneal retinacula (see Figure 7-76). The extensor retinaculum has superior and inferior subdivisions. The **superior extensor retinaculum** connects the distal ends of the fibula and the tibia. The **inferior extensor retinaculum** begins on the calcaneus laterally and arches over the dorsum of the foot to attach to the tibial malleolus and the medial side of the calcaneus. It surrounds or covers all of the deep tendons, vessels, and major nerves on the anterior surface of the foot. The **superior peroneal retinaculum** connects the lateral malleolus and calcaneus; the **inferior peroneal retinaculum** connects the calcaneus and plantar aponeurosis. The peroneus longus and brevis are enclosed in these retinacula.

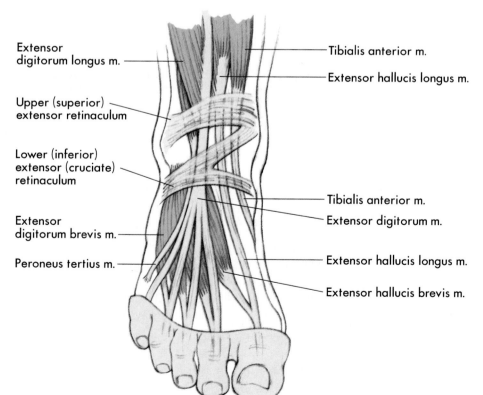

Extensor digitorum longus m.

Upper (superior) extensor retinaculum

Lower (inferior) extensor (cruciate) retinaculum

Extensor digitorum brevis m.

Peroneus tertius m.

Tibialis anterior m.

Extensor hallucis longus m.

Tibialis anterior m.

Extensor digitorum m.

Extensor hallucis longus m.

Extensor hallucis brevis m.

Figure 7-76 MUSCLES AND TENDONS ON THE DORSUM OF THE FOOT, SUPERFICIAL VIEW. The extensor retinaculum binds down the long extensor tendons as they cross the ankle joint. The extensor hallucis brevis and extensor digitorum brevis originate from the calcaneus and extend forward to insert on the extensor sheaths of the great toe and remaining four digits, respectively. SEE ATLAS, FIGS. 7-64, 7-66

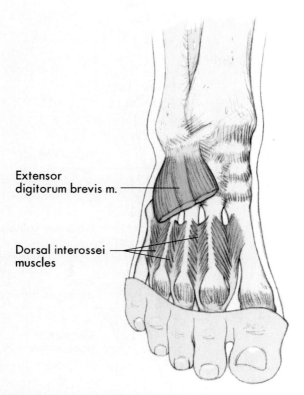

Figure 7-77 MUSCLES AND TENDONS OF THE DORSUM OF THE FOOT, DEEP VIEW. Here the extensor digitorum brevis has been transected, revealing the dorsal interosseous muscles, at the level of the metatarsal bones. SEE ATLAS, FIG. 7-56

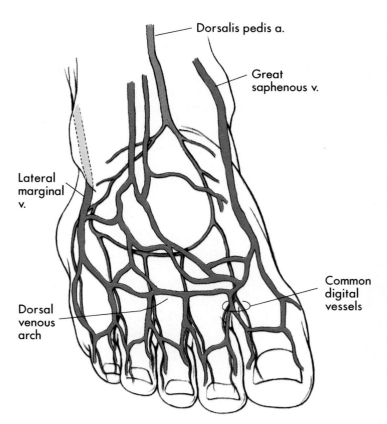

Figure 7-78 ARTERIAL SUPPLY TO THE DORSUM OF THE FOOT. SEE ATLAS, FIG. 7-61

Vessels on the Dorsum of the Foot

The **anterior tibial artery** becomes the dorsalis pedis (Figure 7-78) at the level of the ankle (talocrural) joint. The **dorsalis pedis** is the major source of the digital arterial branches to the toes and is palpable on the dorsum of the foot.

SOLE OF THE FOOT

The sole of the foot is generally similar to the palm of the hand, but there are important differences: (1) the great toe and little toe are not specialized to the degree that is true for the thumb and fifth finger (i.e., there is no opponens muscle), (2) the longitudinal axis of the foot is the second digit not the third digit as it is in the hand, and (3) the foot has a quadratus plantae muscle with no equivalent in the hand.

The sole or plantar surface of the foot contacts the ground and is centrally important in gait, posture, and weight-bearing. The foot usually rests on the ground at three points—the posterior *heel,* the eminence or *ball at the base of the great toe,* and a similar "ball" region at the

base of the fifth toe—forming a tripod for support. The plantar surface of the foot is protected from injury by the thick and strong plantar aponeurosis, extending from the heel forward to the balls of the feet.

Muscles of the Sole of the Foot

The individual muscles of the sole of the foot are conventionally described in four layers, interspersed with the long tendons of muscles originating in the posterior and lateral compartments of the leg (Figures 7-79 through 7-82). Table 7-12 lists these muscles and their attachments, innervations, and functions.

Functionally, however, it is easier and quite useful to think of the foot muscles as lateral, central, and medial.

The **lateral group** includes the abductor digiti minimi and flexor digiti minimi brevis. These insert on the base of the proximal phalanx of toe number five, and they abduct and flex the fifth toe.

The **central group** includes the flexor digitorum brevis, flexor digitorum longus, flexor hallucis longus, flexor accessorius (quadratus plantae), lumbricals, ad-

Figure 7-79 MUSCLES OF SOLE OF FOOT, LAYER ONE. The most superficial layer contains the abductor hallucis, flexor digitorum brevis, and abductor digiti minimi muscles. Also visible, at a deeper layer, is part of the flexor digiti minimi. **SEE ATLAS, FIG. 7-50**

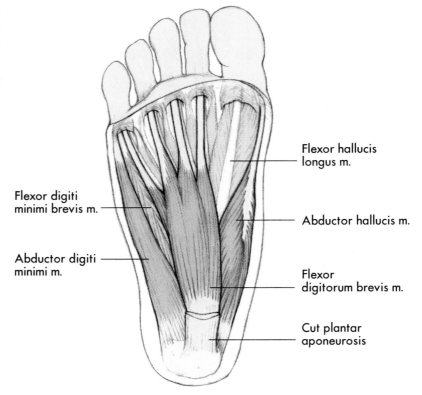

Flexor hallucis longus m.

Flexor digiti minimi brevis m.

Abductor hallucis m.

Abductor digiti minimi m.

Flexor digitorum brevis m.

Cut plantar aponeurosis

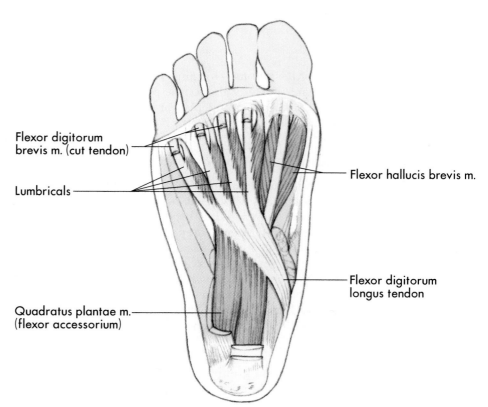

Flexor digitorum brevis m. (cut tendon)

Lumbricals

Flexor hallucis brevis m.

Flexor digitorum longus tendon

Quadratus plantae m. (flexor accessorium)

Figure 7-80 MUSCLES OF THE SOLE OF FOOT, LAYER TWO. Visible are the tendons of the flexor digitorum longus and the fibers of the quadratus plantae, which insert into it posterolaterally. The lumbricals arise from the medial side of each of the flexor digitorum longus tendons. Part of the flexor hallucis brevis also is visible.

SEE ATLAS, FIGS. 7-52, 7-53

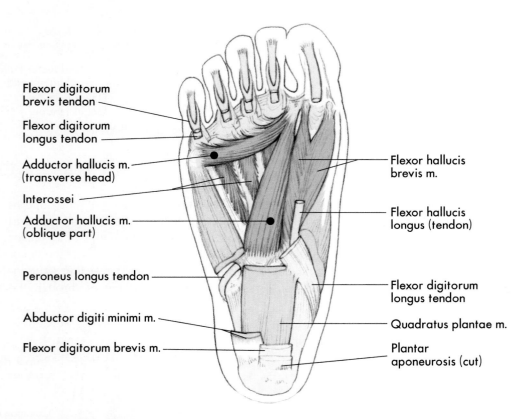

Flexor digitorum
brevis tendon

Flexor digitorum
longus tendon

Adductor hallucis m.
(transverse head)

Interossei

Adductor hallucis m.
(oblique part)

Peroneus longus tendon

Abductor digiti minimi m.

Flexor digitorum brevis m.

Flexor hallucis
brevis m.

Flexor hallucis
longus (tendon)

Flexor digitorum
longus tendon

Quadratus plantae m.

Plantar
aponeurosis (cut)

Figure 7-81 **MUSCLES OF THE SOLE OF FOOT, LAYERS THREE AND FOUR.** The flexor hallucis brevis, adductor hallucis, and flexor digiti minimi occupy the third layer, and the plantar and dorsal interossei the fourth layer. Also visible are the peroneus longus tendon, traveling medially across the deepest level of the sole, and the tendons of the flexor digitorum brevis, splitting to allow passage of the flexor digitorum longus tendons to attach to the distal phalanx. SEE ATLAS, FIGS. 7-54, 7-55

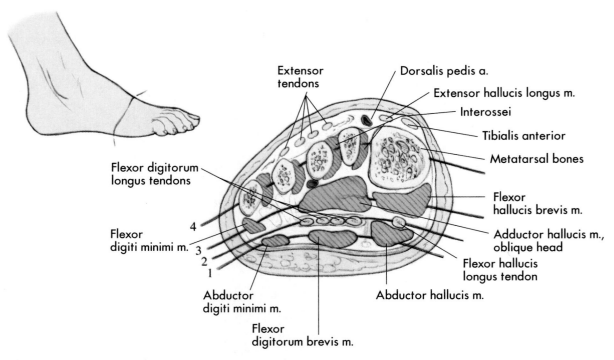

Extensor
tendons

Dorsalis pedis a.

Extensor hallucis longus m.

Interossei

Tibialis anterior

Metatarsal bones

Flexor digitorum
longus tendons

Flexor
digiti minimi m.

4

3

2

1

Flexor
hallucis brevis m.

Adductor hallucis m.,
oblique head

Flexor hallucis
longus tendon

Abductor hallucis m.

Abductor
digiti minimi m.

Flexor
digitorum brevis m.

Figure 7-82   TRANSVERSE SECTION THROUGH THE FOOT. Layer one (*1*), most superficial, is indicated by the line passing through the abductor hallucis, flexor digitorum brevis, and abductor digiti minimi muscles. Layer two (*2*) contains the tendons of the flexor digitorum longus, quadratus plantae, and lumbricals. Layer three (*3*) consists of the flexor hallucis brevis, adductor hallucis, and flexor digiti minimi muscles. Layer four (*4*) contains the dorsal and plantar interosseous muscles, and the line passes through the metatarsal bones of digits 1 to 5.

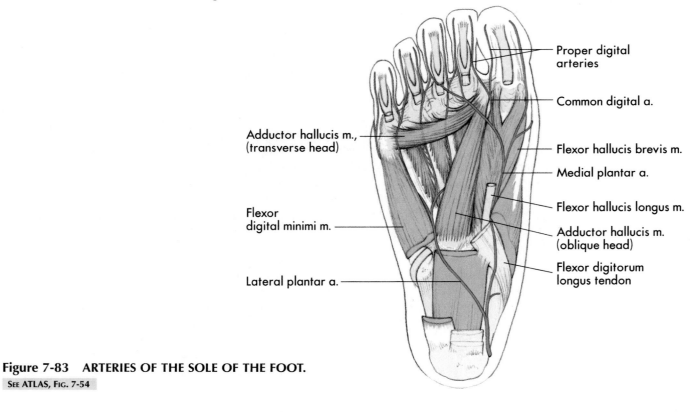

Proper digital
arteries

Common digital a.

Adductor hallucis m.,
(transverse head)

Flexor hallucis brevis m.

Medial plantar a.

Flexor
digital minimi m.

Flexor hallucis longus m.

Adductor hallucis m.
(oblique head)

Flexor digitorum
longus tendon

Lateral plantar a.

Figure 7-83   ARTERIES OF THE SOLE OF THE FOOT.
See Atlas, Fig. 7-54

Table 7-12   Plantar Muscles of the Foot

Muscle	Attachments	Innervation	Actions
FIRST LAYER			
Abductor hallucis	Calcaneus, flexor retinaculum to base of proximal phalanx of first toe	Medial plantar (S2-S3)	Abducts great toe
Flexor digitorum brevis	Calcaneus to sides of middle phalanges of toes 2-5	Medial plantar (S2-S3)	Flexes toes 2-5-[+4]
Abductor digiti minimi	Calcaneus to fifth toe proximal phalanx	Lateral plantar (S2-S3)	Abducts fifth toe
SECOND LAYER (LONG POSTERIOR LEG FLEXOR TENDONS ALSO HERE)			
Quadratus plantae	Calcaneus to tendons of flexor digitorum longus	Lateral plantar (S2-S3)	Stabilizes long flexor and flexes toes
Lumbricals	Tendons of FDL to extensor hood, toes 2-5	Lateral plantar (except first—medial plantar)	Flexes proximal, extends distal interphalangeal joints
THIRD LAYER			
Flexor hallucis brevis	Cuneiform/cuboid to base of proximal phalanx of great toe	Medial plantar (S2-S3)	Flexes toe
Adductor hallucis (two heads— oblique and transverse)	Oblique head: bases of metatarsals 2-4 to base of first toe proximal phalanx		
	Transverse head: metatarso-phalangeal joints of toes 3-5 to base of first toe proximal phalanx	Lateral plantar (S2-S3)	Abducts first toe
Flexor digiti minimi (flexor digiti minimi brevis)	Base of metatarsal 5 to first phalanx of fifth toe	Lateral plantar (S2-S3)	Flexes toe
FOURTH LAYER			
Interossei (dorsal)	Adjacent sides of metatarsals to proximal phalanges and extensor sheaths of toes	Lateral plantar (S2-S3)	Abducts
Interossei (plantar)	Adjacent sides of metatarsals to proximal phalanges and extensor sheaths of toes	Lateral plantar (S2-S3)	Adducts
	Tendons of peroneus longus and tibialis posterior		

ductor hallucis, and interossei. As a group, these muscles attach to the middle and distal phalanges of toes two to five; some of them flex the toes, and others extend the interphalangeal joints while flexing the metatarsophalangeal joints (interossei and lumbricals).

The **medial group** includes the abductor hallucis, flexor hallucis brevis, and adductor hallucis. As a group these insert on the proximal phalanx of toe one and flex and abduct it. Their main significance functionally is to maintain the longitudinal medial arch of the foot.

As in the hand, the **long flexor muscle tendons** insert on the distal phalanx by passing through an aperture in the slips of the flexor digitorum brevis.

The **tibialis posterior** and **peroneus longus tendons** travel at the level of the deepest intrinsic foot muscles. Each is important in maintaining the longitudinal arches of the foot and plays a role in inversion and eversion.

BLOOD SUPPLY OF THE SOLE OF THE FOOT

Blood supply to the sole of foot is from the **posterior tibial artery** via the medial and lateral plantar arteries; most supply is from the **medial plantar artery** (Figure 7-83). The deep vascular arch is found at the level of the heads of the metatarsals.

PRINCIPLES

■ The motor and sensory nerve supply to the lower limb is arranged in such a way that evaluation of certain reflexes and areas of sensation can give very helpful clues to the possibility of segmental nerve injury often found in the lower spine as a result of disk disease. The following chart presents these relationships:

Region	Nerve Segments	Functions/Muscles
Hip joint	L4-L5, S1	Extension of gluteal muscles, hamstrings
	L2–L4	Flexion of iliopsoas, anterior thigh muscles
Knee	L2–L4	Extension of quadriceps
	L5–S1	Flexion of gastrocnemius
Ankle	L4–L5	Extension (dorsiflexion) of anterior leg muscles
	S1–S2	Flexion of posterior leg muscles
Foot	L4–L5	Inversion of tibialis posterior
	L5–S1	Eversion of tibialis anterior, peroneals

In general, lumbar segments supply the anterior surface of the lower limb, and sacral segments supply the posterior surface.

Figure 7-84 METATARSUS ADDUCTUS. Excessive medial deviation of the first metatarsal (*A*) and resultant lateral deviation at the first metatarsophalangeal joint (*B*) results in "bunions."

NERVES OF THE FOOT

The **medial and lateral plantar nerves** travel between the first and second muscle layers; the deep component of the lateral plantar nerve lies between the third and fourth layers. The *lateral plantar artery* has a similar main branch between layers one and two and a deep arch between layers three and four.

The **lateral plantar nerve** is comparable to the ulnar nerve of the hand; it supplies the skin over the lateral one and one half digits and innervates the quadratus plantae, abductor and digiti minimi V, all the interossei, the adductor hallucis, and three of the lumbricals.

The **medial plantar nerve** is comparable to the median nerve of the hand. It innervates the skin over the medial three and one half digits and innervates the abductor hallucis, flexor digitorum brevis, flexor hallucis brevis, and first lumbrical.

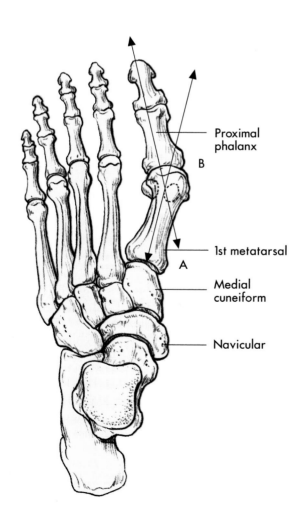

- Proximal phalanx
- B
- 1st metatarsal
- A
- Medial cuneiform
- Navicular

THE FOOT

COMPLICATIONS OF DECREASED CIRCULATION

The foot is subject to ulceration secondary to marginal blood perfusion exacerbated in small vessel diseases such as diabetes mellitus.

COMMON FOOT DEFORMITIES

Hallux valgus (bunions) is a progressively worsening medial deviation of the great toe. The deformity is at the metatarsophalangeal joint (Figure 7-84).

Pes planus (flat feet) is a common disorder resulting from laxity of the ligaments and fasciae on the sole of the foot.

Clubfoot (talipes equinovarus) is a condition in which the foot is inverted, the ankle flexed, and the forefoot adducted. Involves subtalar joint, affects 1 per 1000 live births, with males at 75% and females 25%.

COMMON FOOT INJURIES

Stress fractures are injuries to metatarsals as a result of long marches, as in military training.

Ankle sprain is a traumatic injury that does not cause dislocation or displacement of normal anatomic relationships. In the ankle, it is most common in the region of the talofibular and talocalcaneal ligaments.

LYMPHANGIOGRAPHY

When there is concern about malignancy in the lymph nodes of the groin or pelvic area, dye may be injected into the dorsum of the foot, where lymphatics will transport this material to the regions in question. On x-ray, the lymph nodes will be outlined by the dye, and their size and number can be studied. Today, this kind of study is being replaced by axial imaging (CT or MRI), which requires no dye injection.

▶ Musculoskeletal System

▶ Vascular Supply of the Lower Limb

▶ Lymphatic Drainage of the Lower Limb

▶ Innervation of the Lower Limb

▶ Surface Anatomy and Physical Examination of the Lower Limb

MUSCULOSKELETAL SYSTEM

The skeletal system of the lower limb is specialized for strength because it must bear the weight of the body above it, and for mobility, because gait occurs through the bones and joints of the lower limb. The **pelvic girdle,** consisting of the ilium, ischium, pubis, and sacrum, constitutes a solid ring of bone (see Figure 7-6). The many large muscles of the thigh attach to various parts of the pelvis, as do the large muscles of the abdominal wall. The solid bony ring of the pelvis allows for stability of the entire trunk even if one lower limb is lifted off the ground and the opposite limb sustains the entire weight of the body.

The **hip joint** is a heavily reinforced and supported joint. The articulation between the femoral head and the acetabulum is a deep ball-and-socket joint (see Figure 7-6) and dislocates only with extreme force. Despite its emphasis on strength, it provides for considerable mobility, including flexion, extension, abduction, adduction, and lateral and medial rotation (see Figure 7-10). The three strong ligaments of the hip joint (Figure 7-7), the *ischiofemoral, iliofemoral,* and *pubofemoral,* are arranged in a spiral fashion that allows for considerable flexion of the joint but only limited extension. The arrangement of the joint itself plus these surrounding ligaments provide most of the reinforcement for the joint. This distinguishes it from the comparable joint in the upper limb, the glenohumeral, where the rotator cuff muscles are as important in support of the joint stability as are the geometry of the joint or its surrounding ligaments.

The **knee joint** is specialized for mobility but lacks strength and is therefore injured much more often than is the hip joint. When the knee is in full extension, the angle between the femur and tibia slightly exceeds 180 degrees, and the ligaments supporting the knee become taut (the *medial* and *lateral collateral ligaments,* and the *cruciate ligaments*) (see Figure 7-46). This arrangement allows us to maintain a stable upright posture without continuous contraction of the muscles supporting the knee. Were this arrangement not present, the quadriceps muscles would have to be in continuous contraction, counteracting the tendency for the knee to collapse in flexion because of the weight of the body above it. When the knee is in this upright "locked" position, the femur has rotated medially with respect to the tibia to such a degree that the medial femoral condyle lies posterior to the lateral femoral condyle. When the extended knee is to be flexed, the popliteus muscle must rotate the femur laterally on the tibia before the actual flexion of the joint can begin.

The knee joint is subject to a great variety of traumatic injuries, usually occurring in two kinds of situations: (1) when a blow of considerable force is delivered to the side of the knee (usually the lateral side and occurring in a sport such as football or soccer) and (2) when the foot is planted firmly on the ground and a twisting force is applied to the knee (occurring in a sport such as skiing, or in football, where the foot is planted because the athlete is wearing shoes with cleats). Twisting forces such as these jeopardize the cruciate ligaments especially (see Figure 7-40). The menisci (see Figure 7-44) may be chronically injured by arthritis involving the knee but also may undergo acute injury if they are "pinched" between the condyles of the tibia and femur when a violent stress is applied to the knee.

The distal segment of the lower limb (i.e., the **leg**) is in many ways not comparable to the corresponding segment of the upper limb (i.e., the forearm). Although each contains two bones, in the leg both bones take part significantly in the articulation with the ankle, whereas in the arm the radius alone articulates with the carpal bones. Second, the unique movement of supination-pronation has no equivalent in the leg. The movement that results in the plantar surface of the foot facing laterally or medially takes place at a compound joint in the tarsal bones, not between the tibia and fibula—but the movement resulting in the palm of the hand facing laterally or medially does take place at the radioulnar joints, and not in joints between the carpal bones. In comparison with the radiocarpal joint, the ankle joint has limited mobility and significant strength. Flexion and extension are the only motions allowed at the ankle joint, unlike the radiocarpal or wrist joint, where a wide range of movements is allowed.

In the analysis of the intrinsic musculature and movements of the foot, the second digit is the axis around which the abduction-adduction movements occur. This differs from the hand, where the third digit is the central structure around which movements of the digits occur.

The *upper limb girdle* (scapula proper and coracoid) differs considerably from the *lower limb girdle* (pelvis, consisting of fused ilium, ischium, and pubis). The clavicle is not technically part of the upper limb girdle because it does not articulate directly with the humerus. Both the humerus and femur articulate with the limb girdle in a socket-type structure, shallow in

the case of the upper limb (*glenoid fossa*) and deeper in the case of the lower limb (*acetabulum*). Because of differential rotation of the limbs, the *anterior and posterior compartment muscles* end up on opposite sides of the upper and lower limbs (e.g., the quadriceps are posterior compartment muscles on the anterior surface of the thigh, while the triceps are posterior compartment muscles on the posterior surface of the arm).

Each limb has an *abductor group of muscles,* the well-developed deltoid in the case of the upper limb and the less-well-developed tensor fascia lata and gluteal muscles in the case of the lower limb.

The lower limb has a prominent group of *adductor muscles* (brevis, magnus, longus, and pectineus) extending from the pelvis to the femur. In the upper limb, by contrast, only the coracobrachialis muscle can be considered comparable to the thigh adductors, but the pectoralis major and latissimus dorsi muscles assume the bulk of the adduction role for the upper limb.

Both the thigh and arm have a single principal *artery,* the femoral and brachial, respectively. Each has a *deep branch,* which in the thigh provides the great majority of the blood supply, while in the arm most of the blood supply is from the brachial artery proper, not its deep branch.

The leg and forearm each consists of two parallel *bones,* the tibia/fibula and the radius/ulna. In each case, only one of the bones is principally involved in the mid-limb articulation (the ulna for the elbow; the tibia for the knee). The radius and ulna can move with respect to each other (supination and pronation), while the fibula and tibia are essentially welded together and do not supinate or pronate. At the distal ends of these segments, the radius alone articulates with the wrist, while both fibula and tibia articulate at the ankle.

The *wrist and ankle bones* are built on a similar plan, but in the wrist mobility is emphasized and in the ankle strength is emphasized. Changing the direction of the palm is accomplished through the pronation and supination carried out at the radioulnar joints. Inversion and eversion of the sole of the foot produce sweeping movements of the foot, so that the sole faces laterally or medially, and are sometimes compared with pronation and supination in the upper limb. However, these movements occur within the tarsal bones, while the carpal and metacarpal bones of the hand do not allow the twisting movements possible in the tarsal bones of the foot during inversion and eversion. The intercarpal joints of the wrist allow much less motion than do the comparable intertarsal joints of the foot.

Both the hand and foot consist of *five digits,* but in the hand the thumb has considerable independence from the other four digits, while in the foot the five digits are essentially parallel, and the great toe and second toe share the burden of supporting the weight of the body during the stage when the body "pushes off" of its trailing foot. The opposability of the thumb is what gives the hand much of its unique range of capabilities.

VASCULAR SUPPLY OF THE LOWER LIMB

A single main artery, the femoral (see Figures 7-20 and 7-11), delivers blood to most of the thigh and all of the lower limb distal to the knee. The anterior compartment of the thigh contains the **femoral artery,** which has important circumflex branches that contribute to an anastomosis around the hip joint. The **superior and inferior gluteal arteries,** branches of the internal iliac artery, supply blood to the gluteal region and also contribute to this anastomosis (see Figure 7-33). The most significant branch of the femoral artery is the **deep femoral artery** (profunda femoris), which runs deep in the anterior compartment and gives off a series of three or four perforating arteries that penetrate the adductor magnus and become the major blood supply to the posterior compartment of the thigh (see Figure 7-25). The **obturator artery,** arising in the interior of the pelvis, supplies blood to the medial compartment of the thigh and terminates by contributing branches to the anastomosis around the knee.

In the lower thigh, the femoral artery passes through the adductor hiatus in the adductor magnus to become the **popliteal artery,** traveling vertically along the floor of the popliteal fossa. Entering the posterior compartment of the leg, the popliteal artery gives off an anterior tibial and posterior tibial branch (see Figure 7-57). The anterior tibial artery passes between the neck of the fibula and tibia, through a small gap in the interosseous membrane. The vessel then passes between the two origins of the tibialis anterior into the anterior compartment and descends in the leg between the tibialis anterior and the extensor digitorum longus. Distally, this vessel passes beneath the extensor retinaculum onto the dorsum of the foot and becomes known as the **dorsalis pedis** (see Figure 7-78). The anterior tibial artery provides anastomotic branches around both the knee and ankle joints (see Figure 7-65).

The **posterior tibial artery,** the apparent continuation of the popliteal artery, travels distally in a plane between the deep (flexor hallucis longus, flexor digitorum longus, tibialis posterior) and superficial (plantaris, gastrocnemius, soleus) groups of muscles. It terminates on the sole of the foot as the **medial and lateral plantar arteries** (see Figure 7-83). The large peroneal branch (see Figure 7-65) of the posterior tibial artery descends between the fibula and flexor hallucis longus muscle, providing perforating branches into the lateral (peroneal) compartment. The lateral compartment of the leg has no major independent arterial supply.

Venous drainage of the lower limb is by two broad groups of vessels, the superficial and deep veins. The **superficial veins** are in the superficial fascia. The two most important are the great saphenous vein and the small saphenous vein (see Figure 7-17). The **great saphenous vein** commences on the dorsum of the foot and crosses the ankle just anterior to the medial malleolus. It then travels up the medial thigh, passes medial to the medial femoral condyle, and ascends in the medial thigh to penetrate the superficial fascia at the fossa ovalis, in the upper medial thigh. The great saphenous vein then passes through the **saphenous opening** to drain into the femoral vein. The **small saphenous vein** originates on the lateral side of the heel and ascends in the superficial fascia of the posterior side of the leg. Just above the upper margin of the gastrocnemius, the small saphenous vein penetrates the fascia to drain into the **popliteal vein.**

Deep venous drainage is represented by veins accompanying the major named arteries (see previous discussion). As is true in the upper limb, the veins accompanying major arteries often are multiple, meaning that there may be two or three separate veins accompanying the major arteries. In such cases, the veins are known collectively as **venae comitantes.** The major deep venous drainage of the lower limb converges on the **femoral vein,** which passes beneath the inguinal ligament to drain into the **external iliac vein.** Deep venous drainage of the gluteal region flows through the **superior and inferior gluteal veins** and drains into the **internal iliac** venous system. Both the deep and superficial veins of the lower limb possess many valves. A significant part of the force moving the flow of deep venous blood upward into the pelvis is provided by the contraction of the striated muscles of the lower limbs. During periods of immobility (e.g., hospitalization, bedrest) this mechanism is not in effect, and fluid may pool in the lower limb veins and diffuse out into the tissues of the lower limb, causing swelling or *edema*. Prolonged superficial venous distension leads to their tortuous swelling, known as *varicose veins*.

LYMPHATIC DRAINAGE OF THE LOWER LIMB

As in other parts of the body, deep lymphatic drainage in general follows the course of arterial blood supply to a given region. However, lymphatic drainage in the superficial fascia and skin tends to follow the *greater saphenous vein* (if on the posteromedial aspect of the lower limb) or the *small saphenous vein* (if on the anterolateral leg and foot). Lymphatic drainage along the greater saphenous vein drains to the superficial inguinal nodes; that accompanying the small saphenous vein drains into the popliteal nodes.

In the lower limb, the most important elements of the lymphatic system are the **superficial** and **deep inguinal lymph nodes.** Virtually all lower limb lymph drainage passes through the inguinal nodes. Swelling in the superficial inguinal nodes indicates disease in the scrotal/labial region or the perianal region. Swelling in the deep inguinal nodes suggests disease in the lower limbs.

INNERVATION OF THE LOWER LIMB

The **cutaneous innervation** of the lower limbs is represented as a series of dermatomes (see Figure 7-1), or regions of skin that receive their major innervation from given segments of the spinal cord. The lower limb is innervated by cord segments L2 to S3. As with the upper limb, the outward growth of the lower limb during development distorts the relationship of these segments so that they are no longer adjacent to each other in a simple pattern. Segments L4, L5, and S1 are represented most distally, at the level of the ankle and foot, while L2 to L3 and S2 to S3 are located more proximally (see Figure 7-1).

The **deep innervation** of the lower limb is the responsibility of the gluteal, femoral, obturator, and sciatic nerves. The **superior and inferior gluteal nerves** are branches of the sacral plexus, entering the gluteal region through the greater sciatic notch. They innervate the gluteal muscles and the tensor fascia lata. The small rotators of the gluteal area are innervated by small direct branches from the upper sacral segments. The **femoral nerve** (see Figure 7-20) derives from the lumbar plexus and enters the thigh anteriorly lying lateral to the femoral sheath. At the level of the inguinal ligament it has already broken up into several branches, which supply the anterior and lateral thigh muscles. Its most important distal continuation is the saphenous nerve, which supplies cutaneous innervation to the medial aspect of the leg. The **obturator nerve** accompanies the obturator artery, entering the medial compartment of the thigh, and innervates the medial muscle group. It also supplies the skin of the medial thigh.

The **sciatic nerve** (see Figure 7-34) is the largest and most important nerve supply to the lower limb. It emerges inferior to the piriformis and descends in the posterior thigh just deep to the hamstring muscles. It passes vertically into the popliteal fossa, branching into a common peroneal and tibial branch. The **common peroneal nerve** wraps around the neck of the fibula and divides into the superficial and deep peroneal nerves. The **tibial nerve** descends in the posterior compartment in the plane between the superficial and deep muscle groups. Accompanying the posterior tibial artery, it then passes posterior to the medial malleolus and distributes to the sole of the foot as the **medial and lateral plantar nerves.**

Branches of the major nerves supply the skin of the lower limb as follows: the *obturator nerve* supplies the medial thigh; the *lateral femoral cutaneous nerve* supplies the lateral thigh; cutaneous branches of the *femoral nerve* supply the anterior thigh, and the *posterior femoral cutaneous nerve* supplies the posterior thigh. The *saphenous nerve* (branch of the femoral) supplies the medial leg and foot; cutaneous branches of the *superficial and deep peroneal nerves* innervate the anterolateral leg and dorsum of foot; the *sural nerve* innervates the posterior leg and lateral side of the foot; and the *tibial nerve* innervates the posterior leg and sole of the foot.

SURFACE ANATOMY AND PHYSICAL EXAMINATION OF THE LOWER LIMB

Several important musculoskeletal landmarks are palpable in the lower limb (Figure 7-85). On the lateral surface of the upper end of the thigh, the **greater trochanter** of the femur is palpable and can be felt moving from posterior to anterior as the femur medially rotates in full extension of the knee. It lies just deep to the upper end of the iliotibial band. At the superior end of the thigh, the **anterior superior spine (ASIS)** of the ilium and the **pubic tubercle** can be palpated, as can the **inguinal ligament,** which extends inferomedially between the ASIS and the pubic tubercle. The pulsations of the femoral artery may be felt, just deep to the inguinal ligament, approximately halfway between the ASIS and the pubic tubercle. The femoral vein lies parallel to the femoral artery, approximately 1 cm medial to it. At the distal end of the femur, the *medial and lateral femoral condyles* are easily palpable. Anterior to the distal end of the femur is the **patella,** separated from the lateral and medial condyles on each side by a shallow groove. Distal to the patella, the **patellar tendon** can be felt inserting on the **tibial tuberosity,** a prominence on the anterior edge of the tibial tuberosity about 2 to 3 cm inferior to the inferior edge of the patella. On the lateral side of the upper leg is the **head of the fibula;** immediately below this is the neck of the fibula. The common peroneal nerve, passing from posterior to anterior in the upper leg, wraps around the neck of the fibula, just below the fibular head. Distal to the fibular neck, the bone is not easily palpable because it is covered by the peroneal muscles. The anterior edge of the tibia is palpable as a sharpened bony edge just beneath the skin. Lateral to it is the anterior muscle group, and medial is the flattened anteromedial surface of the tibia, or the "shin." At the distal end of the tibia is the rounded **medial malleolus,** protruding medially on the side of the ankle. A comparable prominence on the lateral side of the ankle is the **lateral malleolus,** a prominence on the distal end of the fibula that actually extends further inferiorly than does the medial malleolus. Along the lateral margin of the foot, the base of the fifth metatarsal bone is palpable as a rounded eminence. The **Achilles tendon** may be felt on the posterior aspect of the ankle joint, inserting firmly into the

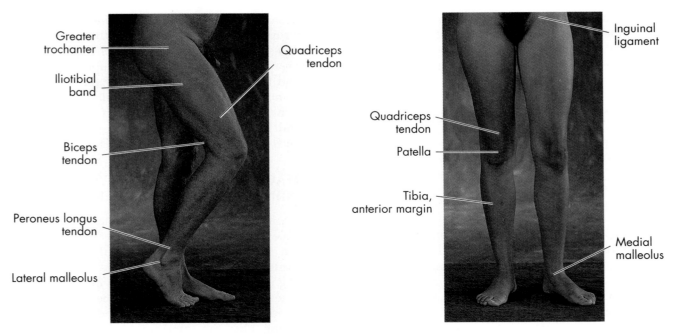

Figure 7-85   SURFACE ANATOMY OF THE LOWER LIMB.

posterior aspect of the **calcaneus.** The portion of the sole of the foot underlying the calcaneus is the heel of the foot; that underlying the heads of the metatarsal bones is the ball of the foot.

Pulses may be palpated at several points in the lower limb. As mentioned previously, the *femoral arterial pulse* is easily palpable beneath the midpoint of the inguinal ligament. The *popliteal artery,* although apparently accessible in the middle of the popliteal fossa, is in fact not easy to palpate and not commonly used to assess pulse in physical diagnosis. Two pulses, by contrast, are readily palpable at the ankle. The *dorsalis pedis,* the continuation of the anterior tibial artery, is located just lateral to the tendon of the tibialis anterior as it crosses the ankle joint. It travels distally just beneath the skin for several centimeters along the dorsum of the foot. The *posterior tibial artery* descends in the posterior compartment of the leg and crosses posterior to the medial malleolus to enter the sole of the foot. It is palpated by placing a finger lightly on the skin about 1 cm posterior to the medial malleolus and slightly inferior to it.

Testing of muscular reflexes in the lower limb is a frequent part of a physical examination, especially when damage to particular nerves is suspected, often as a result of herniated intervertebral disks. Tapping on the *patellar tendon* tests the integrity of the quadriceps muscle, which mediates extension of the knee. This motion is controlled principally by spinal cord segments L2 to L4, and damage to this reflex suggests injury to these nerves. Tapping on the *Achilles tendon* produces flexion (plantar flexion) of the ankle, brought

about by several muscles—soleus, gastrocnemius, and the deep muscles of the posterior compartment prominent among them. This movement is controlled by spinal cord segments L5 to S1.

The **cremaster reflex** is an example of a superficial reflex, in contrast to the deep tendon reflexes described previously. Stroking the skin of the medial thigh produces contraction of the cremaster muscle and elevation of the testis. It is a superficial reflex because the stimulus is not forceful tapping on a tendon but activation of sensory receptors in the skin and superficial fascia. Stroking the skin on the sole of the foot, moving from heel toward the toes, normally causes a flexion of the great toe. When there is injury to the brain, upward movement of the great toe (extension; known as the **Babinski reflex**) often results. This is an example of a pathologic reflex, one not present unless a lesion is present.

Several surface landmarks in the lower limb are important in clinical medicine. Localizing the **femoral vessels** beneath the midpoint of the inguinal ligament is useful in obtaining blood samples or cannulating vessels, especially in emergencies. The reliable location of the **great saphenous vein** just anterior to the medial malleolus of the ankle leads to its frequent use as a site for cannulation of a vein for blood sampling or delivery of medications. Surgical "cutdowns" (exposure of the vein through an incision in the skin and dissection down to the vein) are often employed, especially in emergencies.

Intramuscular injections frequently are given in the buttocks, and it is important to safely inject the medication into the gluteus maximus muscle and to avoid injuring nearby nerves or vessels with the injection. To ensure this, the gluteal region is visualized as divided into four quadrants, and injections are delivered into the *upper outer quadrant*. This minimizes the risk of affecting the sciatic nerve, the superior and inferior gluteal nerves, and the gluteal vessels.

7.7

Lower Limb

■ *CASE 1*

A SEEMINGLY SIMPLE SLIP AND FALL IN AN ELDERLY WOMAN

A 77-year-old woman slipped on the stairs as she was coming down to breakfast in the morning. She felt a loud "pop" when she fell and was in extreme pain afterward. Her children attempted to help her to her feet, but she could bear no weight on the right lower limb and needed to lie down for relief. She was taken to the emergency room, where it was noted that the right lower limb was shorter than the left, laterally rotated, and very painful when any passive motion of the hip was attempted. The hip area was tender to palpation from all sides. An x-ray of the pelvis showed that the right greater trochanter was higher than the left, and the contour of the upper femur was not smooth and symmetric compared with the normal femur on the left. A lateral pelvic film showed that there was a clean break through the neck of the femur, and that the fragment of the neck still connected to the shaft of the femur had slid anterior to the head and the attached fragment of the femoral neck. Doctors advised the patient that a hip replacement was necessary, because if the hip were allowed to heal without surgical intervention, it might heal in misalignment or fail to heal altogether.

Questions

1. Where has the fracture occurred, and why is the position of the whole lower limb changed as a result?
2. What factors make these injuries more common in the elderly?
3. What is involved in a hip replacement surgery, and why is it recommended?

■ *CASE 2*

A SORE BACK WITH PROGRESSIVE COMPLICATIONS

A 45-year-old construction foreman began to feel pain in his back and found that at the end of the work-day he was forced to lie down. The pain first appeared several weeks earlier diffusely in the small of his back. More recently, however, the pain had spread down the back of his right leg. On the same side, he noted that his foot often scraped against the ground while he was walking. He went to the company physician, who at first advised rest, heat to his back, and gentle exercise (e.g., walking, leg lifts while lying on his back). The leg lifts in particular actually were quite painful, however, and he stopped doing them. A few weeks later he went to a neurologist, who performed a careful examination of his sensory and motor function in the lower limbs. The neurologist discovered that the patient had sensory loss on the dorsum of the lateral side of his foot and leg, a weakness in dorsiflexion of the ankle on the right, and the absence of an ankle jerk reflex (tested by tapping the reflex hammer on the Achilles tendon (tendo calcaneus) on the right. She recommended that the patient have an MRI scan of his lower back.

Questions

1. What sort of injury produces these symptoms?
2. Why were the symptoms made worse by the leg-lift exercise?
3. What is the specific location of the injury, and how do the symptoms indicate this?
4. What does the physician hope to accomplish with the MRI scan?

■ *CASE 3*

A SEASON-ENDING INJURY FOR A YOUNG FOOTBALL PLAYER

A 17-year-old young man, 6 feet 3 inches and 240 pounds, had a promising career in football and already had received offers of football scholarships to many excellent colleges and universities. One night, during a game, he was blocked illegally by another player, who threw his upper body across the posterolateral aspect of the young man's legs. To make matters worse, his feet were firmly planted in the ground at the time he was struck by the other player. He lay on the ground in pain, and the trainer rushed to his side. His leg seemed to be abnormally positioned, so that the knee was in effect deviated inward—as in genu valgum ("knock-knees"). Any attempt to move his knee was very painful, but the trainer noted that it seemed possible to bring about excessive anterior movement of the tibia with respect to the femur. The young man was taken to the sidelines, the knee was immobilized and packed in ice, and he sat out the rest of the game. In the next several days he visited a physician, who gave him the disappointing news that this football season was over, and that his whole lifetime ambition to play football might be in jeopardy.

Questions

1. What structures in the knee have been injured, and how does the history of the injury help us understand how the damage was done?
2. Why does a blow from the lateral side of the knee produce especially serious injuries?
3. What are the most common techniques used to assay the damage in the knee, and how are they carried out?

▐ CASE 4

LOCALIZED SWELLING IN THE LEG

A 22-year-old male was playing soccer and was kicked very hard along the anterolateral side of his left leg. He attempted to keep playing, but soon had to retire because of the pain. He showered and changed to street clothes, and as he left the locker room, he noted a seeming numbness in the left foot. By the time he got home, the pain in his leg was increasing, and when he dressed for bed he noticed that the color of his left foot was somewhat darkened. In the middle of the night the pain was so severe that he had to go to the emergency room. There it was noted that the anterolateral surface of the left leg was now swollen and very hard, in addition to being tender. The temperature of his left foot was notably less than that of the right, and the dorsalis

pedis pulse was absent. The patient then could not dorsiflex (i.e., extend) the toes on the left side, and when attempting to walk he dragged his left foot when swinging it forward (i.e., foot drop). X-rays showed no fracture of any bone in the lower limb on either side. The physicians advised him that surgical intervention was necessary and even urgent.

Questions

1. How can this constellation of symptoms occur if there has been no fracture of bone?
2. How might one monitor the progression of symptoms in cases such as this?
3. What surgical procedure is performed to relieve the symptoms?

▐ CASE 5

A FORCEFUL SKIING INJURY

A 32-year-old man was skiing, and, while moving downhill at moderate speed, he planted his left ski in anticipation of a jump turn. The left ski tip caught in the snow, however, and as a result he severely twisted his left ankle, so that his left foot was overeverted and the leg actually rotated with respect to the foot. There was a cracking noise when the accident occurred, and the swelling and pain were almost immediate and very strong. In the emergency clinic, after the patient was given some pain medication, it was possible to demonstrate anterior and lateral displacement of the talus, some small irregular densities just inferior to the medial malleolus, and a continued ability to evert and invert the foot far past the normal range of these movements.

Questions

1. What sort of fracture seems to have occurred in this patient?
2. What accounts for the small densities seen near the medial malleolus?
3. What steps must be taken to ensure proper healing and repair of this injury?

ANSWERS AND EXPLANATIONS

▐ CASE 1

1. This injury has fractured the neck of the femur, just beneath the base of the femoral head, and the two fragments have separated. The force of placing weight on the fractured femur tends to push the shaft and attached part of the neck superiorly, so

that it partially overrides the head of the femur in the acetabulum. The upward thrust of the femoral shaft narrows the angle of inclination of the femoral neck, and the limb is laterally rotated because the short rotators of the hip (obturator, gemellus muscles, quadratus femoris) are stronger than the medial rotators.

2. Postmenopausal women in particular and the elderly in general have more "brittle" bones—osteoporosis—because of a diminished mineral content in the bones.

3. Fractures such as this, especially if they involve that part of the femoral neck inside the capsule of the hip joint (intracapsular), are highly likely to damage the blood supply to the femoral head and make healing impossible even if the bone fragments are aligned. The blood supply to the head of the femur involves the branches of the medial and lateral femoral circumflex arteries and the small branch of the obturator artery that travels along the ligament of the head of the femur to reach the femoral head. Because of this and other clinical considerations, a hip replacement or prosthesis often is chosen. In these procedures, the hip joint is approached posteriorly, and the head and part of the femoral neck are removed altogether. A strong metallic ball, attached to a long metal spike, is placed so that the metal ball replaces the femoral head, and the metal spike is anchored deep within the shaft of the femur. If indicated, a smooth metallic cup can be positioned to replace the acetabulum (if it too has been traumatized or damaged severely by arthritis).

■ *CASE 2*

1. Although the symptoms are in the lower leg, the lesion is most likely to be in the vertebral canal. This is because the combination of sensory and motor deficits, the time course of the onset of the disease, and the changes in symptoms associated with certain positions and movements fit best into that source of pathology. We must ask ourselves where the lesion is most likely located, based on the observed symptoms. There is no single peripheral nerve that will produce weakness in ankle flexion and extension and at the same time produce the focal and limited sensory loss described here. The time course of the illness suggests a slow onset, rather than something acute such as a hemorrhage. The worsening of symptoms with position or exercise suggests something more than a local disease process confined to the leg or foot. This set of symptoms is typical of a herniated disk, where the posterolateral protrusion of the disk puts pressure on nerve roots exiting the vertebral canal through the intervertebral foramen at the same level. The affected muscles are not innervated by a common single peripheral nerve, but their dysfunction is consistent with an injury to the spinal nerves arising at the L5 and S1 segments.

2. A leg-lift exercise (i.e., extension of the thigh, with extended knee) puts additional stretch on the nerve roots exiting the vertebral canal and typically worsens the symptoms of a herniated disk.

3. Sensory loss on the lateral side of the leg and foot, a foot drop (the dragging of the affected foot during walking), and the weakness in ankle dorsiflexion suggest a lesion affecting the L5 and S1 nerve roots. The involved disks are most likely the L4-L5 and L5-S1 disks. The seeming disparity between the nerve roots and disks is explained by the anatomy of exiting nerve roots in the lower vertebral column. Because axons on this part of the vertebral canal descend at a sharp angle and exit through the upper part of the corresponding intervertebral foramen, herniated disks usually affect the nerve roots exiting one intervertebral foramen below the level of the herniated disk. Thus, in this case, the L5-S1 disk, which might be expected when herniated to affect the L5 nerve root, instead affects the S1 nerve root.

4. The most informative diagnostic study for a herniated disk is the MRI or CT scan, both cross-sectional images with the ability to identify small herniations and to reveal considerable detail about soft tissue abnormalities as well.

■ *CASE 3*

1. A blow to the posterolateral aspect of the knee puts a very forceful momentary valgus stress on the knee (deviating in a medial direction, as in "knock-knees"). The medial collateral ligament is stretched, often to the point of tearing the medial meniscus, which is attached to the inner surface of the medial collateral ligament. When the blow is especially severe, the anterior cruciate ligament (ACL) also may be torn or ruptured. The lateral side of the knee joint is the focus of forceful blows much more often than any other part of the knee. Blows here put a stretch on the medial collateral ligament, and because this ligament is firmly attached to the medial meniscus, the two often are injured in tandem. Rupture of the ACL deeply destabilizes the knee and requires surgical repair (if the tear is complete) and a prolonged period of rest and recovery.

2. The aforementioned attachment of the medial meniscus to the medial collateral ligament means that both often are injured together. The lateral collateral ligament is not connected to the lateral meniscus; the tendon of the popliteus muscle intervenes between the two.

3. Physical examination of the knee after an injury of this sort would be of limited value initially, because there is such a large degree of swelling and pain. When the initial inflammation has subsided a bit, however, one could palpate the knee, move the knee through a variety of motions, and elicit tenderness

and pain, usually in the area overlying the torn ligaments or cartilages. In the case of an ACL tear, the tibia will move forward with respect to the femur to an abnormal degree (the "drawer sign"). In the past 10 to 15 years, knee arthroscopy has become the standard for the evaluation of internal knee-joint injuries. A flexible fiberoptic tube is inserted into the interior of the joint, and in addition to inspection of injuries, fragments of cartilage and certain other repair procedures can be accomplished through the arthroscope, obviating the need for more invasive surgery, which would require prolonged recuperation.

■ CASE 4

1. This is a classic case of compartment syndrome, where an injury (in this case a forceful blow, leading to hemorrhage from the anterior tibial artery), causes pressure to build up within a fascial compartment, in this case the anterior fascial compartment of the leg. With arterial bleeding, the pressure reaches levels high enough to produce compression injuries of other structures in the anterior compartment and to inhibit the flow of blood distal to the point of injury. Common signs helpful in evaluating the progression of the condition are the pulse, the temperature of the tissues distal to the compression, and any loss of motor function in muscles whose blood supply and/or innervation is susceptible to compression. In this case, the inability to dorsiflex the toes and foot drop were telling signs that the compression was worsening.

2. Physicians can monitor the progression of these injuries by placing a thin needle connected to a pressure transducer into the interior of the fascial space and following changes in the pressure within.

3. If pressure within such compartments does not subside, the patient can be treated by creating a surgical opening in the fascial membranes enclosing the compartment and dissipating the pressure within.

■ CASE 5

1. To produce such an unstable ankle joint requires a serious traumatic force on the joint. The ankle is, when normal, a strong mortise, with the fibular lateral malleolus and the tibial medial malleolus straddling the talus. The intact ankle joint can move in only one plane—through flexion and extension. To produce eversion and inversion as described previously suggests that the lateral and medial malleolus have been fractured and displaced, allowing the underlying foot a greater range of motion.

2. When great stress is placed on ligaments, they are often so strong that they can pull small fragments of bone away from the bone to which they attach. In this case, the small bony fragments represent fragments of the medial malleolus pulled loose when the tibiocalcaneal (deltoid) ligament underwent very forceful stretching during the twisting accident.

3. In injuries of this kind, the goal is to stabilize the joint in a position as close to normal as possible and allow natural healing to occur over several weeks or even months. This sometimes can be accomplished (1) simply by manipulating the patient in such a way that the fragments are aligned, or (2) by placing metallic screws in the bone fragments, uniting them once again. A second major concern in the healing of such an injury is the arthritis that may take place, leading to permanent scarring of the joint surfaces and a subsequent loss of mobility and/or significant pain associated with motion of the joint in the future.

Glossary

This glossary provides the *Nomina Anatomica (NA)* equivalents for many of the English terms used in the text. Items that differ only by the adjectives in the list to the right are often given in stem form only. Thus, 'nervus gluteus' is included but not 'nervus gluteus inferior' or 'nervus gluteus superior'.

right/left: dexter/sinister
medial/lateral: medialis/lateralis
anterior/posterior: anterior/posterior
superior/inferior: superior/inferior
external/internal: externus/internus
superficial/deep: superficialis/profundus

ENGLISH	NOMINA ANATOMICA
A	
abdomen	–abdomen
acetabulum	–acetabulum
Achilles tendon	–tendo calcaneus
acromion	–acromion
adenoid	–tonsilla pharyngealis
ala of sacrum	–ala sacralis
ampulla	
of rectum	–ampulla recti
of uterine tube	–ampulla tubae uterinae
of vas deferens	–ampulla ductus deferentis
of Vater	–ampulla hepatopancreatica
anastomosis	–vas anastomoticum
angle, subcostal	–angulus infrasternalis
annulus fibrosus	–annulus fibrosus
ansa cervicalis	–ansa cervicalis
subclavia	–ansa subclavia
antrum	–antrum
maxillary	–sinus maxillarius
of stomach	–antrum pyloricum
anus	–anus
aorta	–aorta
abdominal	–aorta abdominalis
arch	–arcus aortae
bifurcation	–bifurcatio aortae
sinus	–sinus aortae
thoracic	
ascending	–pars ascendens aortae
descending	–pars descendens aortae
apex	–apex
aponeurosis	–aponeurosis
bicipital	–aponeurosis musculi bicipitis brachii
epicranial	–galea aponeurotica
palatine	–aponeurosis palatina
palmar	–aponeurosis palmaris
plantar	–aponeurosis plantaris
apparatus, lacrimal	–apparatus lacrimalis
appendage, atrial	–auricula
appendix	–appendix vermiformis
epiploicae	–appendices epiploicae
vermiform	–appendix vermiformis

ENGLISH	NOMINA ANATOMICA
arachnoid mater	–arachnoid mater
granulations	–granulationes arachnoideales
arch	–arcus
aortic	–arcus aortae
anterior, of atlas	–arcus anterior atlantis
of azygos vein	–arcus venae azygos
dorsal venous, of foot	–arcus venosus dorsalis pedis
dorsal venous, of hand	–rete venosus dorsalis manus
neural	–arcus vertebrae
palmar, arterial, of hand	–arcus palmaris
planter	–arcus plantaris
posterior, of atlas	–arcus posterior atlantis
tendinous, of levator ani	–arcus tendineus, m. levator ani
vertebral (neural)	–arcus vertebralis
area, bare of liver	–area nuda
arm	–brachium
arteriole	–arteriola
artery	–arteria
auricular, posterior	–a. auricularis posterior
axillary	–a. axillaris
basilar	–a. basilaris
brachial	–a. brachialis
carotid	
common	–a. carotis communis
external	–a. carotis externa
internal	–a. carotis interna
cecal	–a. caecalis
celiac	–truncus coeliacus
cerebral, middle	–a. cerebri media
cervical	
deep	–a. cervicalis profunda
transverse	–a. transversa cervicis
circumflex branch of right coronary	–ramus circumflexus
femoral	–a. circumflexa femoris
humeral	–a. circumflexa humeri
scapular	–a. circumflexa scapulae
colic	
left	–a. colica sinistra
middle	–a. colica media
right	–a. colica dextra
collateral	–a. collateralis

Reprinted from Gosling JA, Harris PF, Humpherson JR, Whitmore I, Willan PLT: *Human anatomy: text and colour atlas*, London, 1990, Gower.

ENGLISH	NOMINA ANATOMICA
artery (*cont.*)	
communicating	–a. communicans
coronary	–a. coronaria
cystic	–a. cystica
deep	
of clitoris	–a. profunda clitoridis
of penis	–a. profunda penis
digital	–aa. digitales
dorsal	
of clitoris	–a. dorsalis clitoridis
of penis	–a. dorsalis penis
dorsalis pedis	–a. dorsalis pedis
epigastric	–a. epigastrica
facial	–a. facialis
femoral	–a. femoralis
gastric	–a. gastrica
gastroduodenal	–a. gastroduodenalis
gastroepiploic	–a. gastro-omentalis
gluteal	–a. glutealis
hepatic	–a. hepatica communis
ileal	–aa. ileales
ileocolic	–a. ileocolica
iliac	
common	–a. iliaca communis
external	–a. iliaca externa
internal	–a. iliaca interna
intercostal	–aa. intercostales
anterior	–rami intercostales anteriores
posterior	–aa. intercostales posteriores
interosseous, common	–a. interossea communis
interventricular	
anterior	–ramus interventricularis anterior
inferior	–ramus interventricularis posterior
jejunal	–aa. jejunales
lingual	–a. lingualis
lumbar	–aa. lumbales
marginal, of heart	–ramus marginalis dexter
maxillary	–a. maxillaris
meningeal, middle	–a. meningea media
mesenteric	–a. mesenterica
metacarpal	–aa. metacarpales
metatarsal	–aa. metatarsales
musculophrenic	–a. musculophrenica
nutrient	–a. nutrica
obturator	–a. obturatoria
abnormal obturator	–a. obturatoria accessoria
occipital	–a. occipitalis
ophthalmic	–a. ophthalmica
ovarian	–a. ovarica
pancreaticoduodenal	–a. pancreaticoduodenalis
peroneal	–a. fibularis
pharyngeal, ascending	–a. pharyngea ascendens
phrenic, inferior	–a. phrenica inferior
plantar	–a. plantaris
popliteal	–a. poplitea
profunda	
brachii	–a. profunda brachii
femoris	–a. profunda femoris
pudenal	
external	–aa. pudendae externae
internal	–a. pudenda interna
pulmonary	–a. pulmonalis
radial	–a. radialis
rectal	–a. rectalis
renal	–a. renalis
retinal, central	–a. centralis retinae
sacral, median	–a. sacralis mediana
sigmoid	–aa. sigmoideae
splenic	–a. splenica
subclavian	–a. subclavia
subscapular	–rami subscapulares
suprarenal	–a. suprarenalis
suprascapular	–a. suprascapularis

ENGLISH	NOMINA ANATOMICA
temporal, superficial	–a. temporalis superficialis
testicular	–a. testicularis
thoracic	
internal	–a. thoracica interna
lateral	–a. thoracica lateralis
superior	–a. thoracica superior
thoracoacromial	–a. thoracoacromialis
thyrocervical	–a. thyrocervicalis
thyroid	–a. thyroidea
tibial	–a. tibialis
ulnar	–a. ulnaris
umbilical, obliterated	–a. umbilicalis, pars occlusa
uterine	–a. uterina
vertebral	–a. vertebralis
vesical	–a. vesicalis
articulation (joint)	–articulatio
atlas vertebra	–atlas
atrial appendage	–auricula
atrioventricular	
bundle	–fasciculus atrioventricularis
groove	–sulcus coronarius
orifice	–ostium atrioventriculare
atrium of heart	–atrium cordis
autonomic nervous system	–systema nervosum autonomicum
axilla	–axilla
axis vertebra	–axis
axon	–axon

B

base	–basis
of cranium	–basis cranii
of heart	–basis cordis
of lung	–basis pulmonis
bifurcation	–bifurcatio
bladder	–vesica
gall	–vesica biliaris
urinary	–vesica urinaria
blood vessels	
body	–corpus
border	–margo
branch	–ramus
breast	–mamma
areola	–areola mammae
glandular elements	–glandula mammaria
lactiferous duct	–ductus lactiferi
nipple	–papilla mammaria
bronchopulmonary segments	–segmenta bronchopulmonalia
bronchus	–bronchus
main, principal	–bronchus principalis
bulb	
of penis	–bulbus penis
of vestibule	–bulbus vestibuli
bundle of His (atrioventricular)	–fasciculus atrioventricularis
bundle branch	–crus
bursa	–bursa synovialis
infrapatellar	–bursa infrapatellaris
olecranon	–bursa subcutanea olecrani
omental	–bursa omentalis
prepatellar	–bursa subcutanea prepatellaris
semimembranosus	–bursa musculi semimembranosi
subacromial	–bursa subacromialis
subscapular	–bursa subtendinea musculi subscapularis
suprapatellar	–bursa suprapatellaris
buttock	–regio glutealis

C

calcaneum	–calcaneus
calf	–sura
calices	–calices renales
canal	

ENGLISH	NOMINA ANATOMICA
canal (*cont.*)	
anal	–canalis analis
carotid	–canalis caroticus
carpal	–canalis carpi
cervical	–canalis cervicis uteri
femoral	–canalis femoralis
hypoglossal	–canalis hypoglossi
inguinal	–canalis inguinalis
nasolacrimal	–canalis nasolacrimalis
obturator	–canalis obturatorius
optic	–canalis opticus
pudendal	–canalis pudendalis
pyloric	–canalis pyloricus
subsartorial	–canalis adductorius
vertebral	–canalis vertebralis
capillaries	–vasa capillare
capitate bone	–os capitatum
capsule, articular	–capsula articularis
carina	–carina tracheae
carpal bones	–ossa carpi
carpus	–carpus
cartilage	
articular	–cartilago articularis
arytenoid	–cartilago arytenoidea
costal	–cartilago costalis
cricoid	–cartilago cricoidea
elastic	–cartilago elastica
fibrocartilage	–cartilago fibrosa
hyaline	–cartilago hyalina
thyroid	–cartilago thyroidea
tracheal	–cartilagines trachealis
cauda equina	–cauda equina
cavity	
abdominal	–cavitas abdominale
nasal	–cavitas nasi
pelvis	–cavitas pelvis
pericardial	–cavitas pericardialis
peritoneal	–cavitas peritonealis
pleural	–cavitas pleuralis
thorax	–cavitas thoracis
uterine	–cavitas uteri
cecum	–caecum
cerebellum	–cerebellum
cerebrospinal fluid	–liquor cerebrospinalis
cerebrum	–cerebrum
cervix, uterine	–cervix uteri
chordae tendineae	–chordae tendineae
circle of Willis	–circulus arteriosus cerebri
cisterna chyli	–cisterna chyli
clavicle	–clavicula
clitoris	–clitoris
clivus	–clivus
coccyx	–os coccygis
colliculus, seminal	–colliculus seminalis
colon	–colon
ascending	–colon ascendens
descending	–colon descendens
sigmoid	–colon sigmoideum
transverse	–colon transversum
column	
anal	–columna anales
vertebral	–columna vertebrales
cervical	–vertebrae cervicales
coccygeal	–vertebrae coccygeae
lumbar	–vertebrae lumbales
sacral	–vertebrae sacrales (os sacrum)
thoracic	–vertebrae thoracicae
colliculus, seminal	–colliculus seminalis
concha, nasal	–concha nasalis
conducting system of heart	–systema conducens cordis
condyle	
femoral	–condylus femoris
tibial	–condylus tibiae

ENGLISH	NOMINA ANATOMICA
conjunctiva	–tunica conjunctiva
connective tissue	–textus connectivus
cord	
of brachial plexus	–plexus brachialis
lateral	–fasciculus lateralis
medial	–fasciculus medialis
posterior	–fasciculus posterior
spermatic	–funiculus spermaticus
spinal	–medulla spinalis
cornea	–cornea
corpus	
cavernosum	–corpus cavernosum
spongiosum	–corpus spongiosum
cranium	–cranium
crest	
sacral	–crista sacralis
urethral	–crista urethralis
crista	–crista
galli	–crista galli
terminalis	–crista terminalis
crus	
of clitoris	–crus clitoridis
of diaphragm	–crus partis lumbalis diaphragmatis
of penis	–crus penis
cuboid bone	–os cuboideum
cuneiform bone	–os cuneiforme
curve, curvature	–curvatura gastrica
cusp	–cuspis
of aortic valve	–valvula semilunares
of mitral valve	–cuspis valvula mitrealis
of pulmonary	–valvula semilunaris
of tricuspid valve	–cuspis valvula tricuspidalis

D

dens	–dens axis
dermatomes	–dermatomi
diaphragm	–diaphragma (thoraco-abdominale)
pelvic	–diaphragma pelvis
urogential	–diaphragma urogenitale
diaphragma sellae	–diaphragma sellae
digits	
of hand (fingers)	–digiti manus
of foot (toes)	–digiti pedis
disk	
articular cartilage	–discus articularis
intervertebral	–discus intervertebralis
diverticulum, ileal (Meckel's)	–diverticulum ilei
dorsum	
of foot	–dorsum pedis
of hand	–dorsum manus
duct	
bile	–ductus choledochus
cystic	–ductus cysticus
efferent of testis	–ductuli efferentes testis
ejaculatory	–ductus ejaculatorius
hepatic	–ductus hepaticus
nasolacrimal	–ductus nasolacrimalis
pancreatic	–ductus pancreaticus
accessory	–ductus pancreaticus accessorius
thoracic	–ductus thoracicus
ductus	
arteriosus	–ductus arteriosus
deferens	–ductus deferens
duodenum	–duodenum
papilla	–papilla duodeni
dura mater	–dura mater

E

ear	–auris
external	–auris externa
eminence	

ENGLISH	NOMINA ANATOMICA
eminence (*cont.*)	
hypothenar	–eminentia hypothenar
iliopectineal	–eminentia iliopubica
intercondylar	–eminentia intercondylaris
thenar	–eminentia thenar
enlargement	
cervical	–intumescentia cervicalis
lumbosacral	–intumescentia lumbosacralis
epicondyle	–epicondylus
epidermis	–epidermis
epididymis	–epididymis
epiglottis	–epiglottis
epiphysis	–epiphysis
esophagus	–oesophagus
ethmoid bone	–os ethmoidale
eyeball	–bulbus oculi
eyelashes	–cilia
eyelid	–palpebra

F

ENGLISH	NOMINA ANATOMICA
face	–facies
muscles	–mm. faciales
nerve	–n. facialis
falx cerebri	–falx cerebri
fascia	–fascia
bulbi	–vagina bulbi
cremasteric	–fascia cremasterica
deep	–fascia profunda
dorsum of foot	–fascia dorsalis pedis
leg	–fascia cruris
iliac	–fascia iliaca
investing	–fascia cervicalis: lamina superficialis
lata	–fascia lata
lumbar	–fascia thoracolumbalis
neck	–fascia cervicalis
obturator	–fascia obturatoria
pelvic	–fascia pelvis
penile	–fascia penis
pharyngobasilar	–fascia pharyngobasilaris
pretracheal	–fascia cervicalis: lamina pretrachealis
prevertebral	–fascia cervicalis: lamina prevertebralis
renal	–fascia renalis
spermatic	–fascia spermatica
superficial	–fascia superficialis
thoracolumbar (lumbar)	–fascia thoracolumbalis
transversalis	–fascia transversalis
fat	
perinephric	–corpus adiposum pararenale
femur	–femur
fiber	–fibra
fibrocartilage	–cartilago fibrosa
filum terminale	–filum terminale
fimbriae	–fimbriae tubae
fingers	–digiti manus
index	–index
little	–digitus minimus
middle	–digitus medius
ring	–digitus annularis
fissure	–fissura
of liver	
for ligamentum teres	–fissura ligamenti teretis
for ligamentum venosum	–fissura ligamenti venosi
of lung	
horizontal	–fissura horizontalis
oblique	–fissura obliqua
orbital	–fissura orbitalis
palpebral	–rima palpebrarum
flexure	
duodenojejunal	–flexura duodenojejunalis
colic	–flexura coli
floor	
pelvic	–diaphragma pelvis

ENGLISH	NOMINA ANATOMICA
fold	
aryepiglottic	–plica aryepiglottica
horizontal, of rectum	–plicae transversae recti
peritoneal	–plica peritonealis
vestibular	–plica vestibularis
vocal	–plica vocalis
foot	–pes
dorsal surface	–dorsum pedis
sole	–planta pedis
foramen	
epiploic	–foramen omentale
intervertebral	–foramen intervertebrale
jugular	–foramen jugulare
lacerum	–foramen lacerum
magnum	–foramen magnum
nutrient	–foramen nutriens
obturator	–foramen obturatum
ovale	–foramen ovale
rotundum	–foramen rotundum
sacral	–foramina sacralia
sciatic	–foramen ischiadicum
spinosum	–foramen spinosum
transversarium	–foramen transversarium
forearm	–antebrachium
fornix, vaginal	–fornix vaginae
fossa	
acetabular	–fossa acetabuli
cranial	–fossa cranii
cubital	–fossa cubitalis
glenoid	–cavitas glenoidalis
infraspinous	–fossa infraspinatus
infratemporal	–fossa infratemporalis
intersigmoid	–recessus intersigmoideus
ischiorectal	–fossa ischioanalis
lacrimal	–fossa sacci lacrimalis
navicular	–fossa navicularis urethrae
ovalis	–fossa ovalis
ovarian	–fossa ovarica
paraduodenal	–recessus duodenalis
peritoneal	–fossae peritonealis
popliteal	–fossa poplitea
pterygopalatine	–fossa pterygopalatina
retrocecal	–recessus retrocaecalis
subscapular	–fossa subscapularis
supraspinous	–fossa supraspinatis
temporal	–fossa temporalis
of temporal bone	–fossa mandibularis
fourchette	–commisura labiorum posterior
frenulum	–frenulum
frontal bone	–os frontale
fundus	–fundus

G

ENGLISH	NOMINA ANATOMICA
gallbladder	–vesica bilaris
ganglion	
ciliary	–ganglion ciliae
otic	–ganglion oticum
parasympathetic	–ganglion parasympathicum
pterygopalatine	–ganglion pterygopalatinum
stellate	–ganglion cervicothoracicum
submandibular	–ganglion submandibulare
sympathetic	–ganglion sympathicum
thoracic	–ganglia thoracica
genitalia, external	–organa genitalia externa
female	–organa genitalia feminina externa
male	–organa genitalia masculina externa
girdle	
pectoral	–cingulum pectorale
pelvic	–cingulum membri inferioris
gland	–glandula
bulbourethral	–glandula bulbourethralis
greater vestibular	–glandula vestibularis major

ENGLISH	NOMINA ANATOMICA
gland (*cont.*)	
lacrimal	–glandula lacrimalis
parathyroid	–glandula parathyroidea
parotid	–glandula parotidea
prostate	–prostata
sublingual	–glandula sublingualis
submandibular	–glandula submandibularis
suprarenal	–glandula suprarenalis
thyroid	–glandula thyroidea
glans	
of clitoris	–glans clitoridis
of penis	–glans penis
groove	
atrioventricular	–sulcus coronarius
in liver for inferior vena cava	–sulcus venae cavae
subcostal	–sulcus costae
gutters	
paracolic	–sulci paracolici

H

ENGLISH	NOMINA ANATOMICA
hamate bone	–os hamatum
hamulus	
of hamate	–hamulus ossis hamati
of pterygoid	–hamulus pterygoideus
hand	–manus
dorsal surface	–dorsum manus
palm of	–palma manus
haustrations	–haustra
head	–caput
of rib	–caput costae
heart	–cor
conducting system	–systema conducens cordis
hemisphere, cerebral	–hemispherium cerebralis
hiatus semilunaris	–hiatus semilunaris
hilum	–hilum
hindbrain	–rhombencephalon
hip bone	–os coxae
humerus	–humerus
hyoid bone	–os hyoideum

I

ENGLISH	NOMINA ANATOMICA
ileum	–ileum
ilium	–os ilii
impression	
cardiac, of left lung	–impressio cardiaca
incisura angularis	–incisura angularis
infundibulum	
of right ventricle	–conus arteriosus
inlet	
thoracic	–apertura thoracica superior
pelvic	–apertura pelvis superior
intestine	
large	–intestinum crassum
small	–intestinum tenue
ischium	–os ischii

J

ENGLISH	NOMINA ANATOMICA
jejunum	–jejunum
joint	
acromioclavicular	–articulatio acromioclavicularis
ankle	–articulatio talocruris
atlantoaxial	–articulatio atlantoaxialis
atlantooccipital	–articulatio atlantooccipitalis
calcaneocuboid	–articulatio calcaneocuboidea
carpometacarpal	–articulationes carpometacarpales
cartilaginous	–articulationes cartilaginea
elbow	–articulatio cubiti
fibrous	–articulationes fibrosae
foot	–articulationes pedis
hand	–articulationes manus

ENGLISH	NOMINA ANATOMICA
hip	–articulatio coxae
intercarpal	–articulationes intercarpales
intermetacarpal	–articulationes intermetacarpales
intermetatarsal	–articulationes intermetatarsales
interphalangeal	–articulationes interphalangeales
knee	–articulatio genus
lumbosacral	–articulo lumbosacralis
manubriosternal	–symphysis manubriosternalis
metacarpophalangeal	–articulationes metacarpophalangeales
metatarsophalangeal	–articulationes metatarsophalangeales
midcarpal	–articulatio mediocarpalis
radiocarpal	–articulatio radiocarpalis
radioulnar	–articulatio radioulnaris
sacrococcygeal	–articulatio sacrococcygea
sacroiliac	–articulatio sacroiliaca
shoulder (glenohumeral)	–articulatio humeri
sternoclavicular	–articulatio sternoclavicularis
subtalar	–articulatio subtalaris
synovial	–articulationes synoviales
talocalcaneal	–articulatio subtalaris
talocalcaneonavicular	–articulatio talocalcaneonavicularis
tarsal	–articulatio tarsi
tarsometatarsal	–articulationes tarsometatarsales
temporomandibular	–articulatio temporomandibularis
wrist	–articulatio radiocarpalis

K

ENGLISH	NOMINA ANATOMICA
kidney	–ren

L

ENGLISH	NOMINA ANATOMICA
labia	
majora	–labia majora pudendi
minora	–labia minora pudendi
labrum	
acetabular	–labrum acetabulare
glenoid	–labrum glenoidale
lacunae (venous) of	
superior sagittal sinus	–lacunae laterales
lamina, vertebral	–lamina arcus vertebrae
laryngopharynx	–pars laryngea pharyngis
larynx	–larynx
leg	–crus
ligament	–ligamentum
annular, of radius	–ligamentum annulare radii
arcuate	
of diaphragm	–ligamentum arcuatum diaphragmatis
of knee	–ligamentum popliteum arcuatum
arteriosum	–ligamentum arteriosum
atlantooccipital	–ligamentum altantooccipitale
broad, of uterus	–ligamentum latum uteri
calcaneofibular	–ligamentum calcaneofibulare
calcaneonavicular, 'spring' plantare	–ligamentum calcaneonaviculare
capsular	–ligamenta capsularia
collateral	–ligamentum collaterale
coracoacromial	–ligamentum coracoacromial
coracoclavicular	–ligamentum coracoclaviculare
coronary	–ligamentum coronarium
costoclavicular	–ligamentum costoclaviculare
cricothyroid	–ligamentum cricothyroideum medianum
cruciate of atlas	–ligamentum cruciforme atlantis
deltoid of ankle	–ligamentum mediale
denticulate	–ligamentum denticulatum
extracapsular	–ligamenta extracapsularia
falciform	–ligamentum falciforme hepatis
gastrosplenic	–ligamentum gastrosplenicum
glenohumeral	–ligamenta glenohumeralia
iliofemoral	–ligamentum iliofemorale
iliolumbar	–ligamentum iliolumbale
inguinal	–ligamentum inguinale

ENGLISH	NOMINA ANATOMICA	ENGLISH	NOMINA ANATOMICA
ligament (*cont.*)		urethral	–ostium urethrae
intercarpal	–ligamenta intercarpalia	Meckel's diverticulum	–diverticulum ilei
interosseous, sacroiliac	–ligamenta sacroiliaca interossea	mediastinum	–mediastinum
intracapsular	–ligamenta intracapsularia	medulla oblongata	–medulla oblongata
ischiofemoral	–ligamentum ischiofemorale	membrane	
lacunar	–ligamentum lacunare	aryepiglottic	–membrana quadrangularis
lienorenal	–ligamentum splenorenale	atlantooccipital	–membranum atlantooccipitale
longitudinal	–ligamentum longitudinale	cricovocal (cricothyroid)	–conus elasticus
meniscofemoral	–ligamentum meniscofemorale	intercostal	
metatarsal, deep transverse	–ligamentum metatarsale transversum profundum	anterior	–membrana intercostalis externa
		posterior	–membrana intercostalis interna
nuchae	–ligamentum nuchae	interosseous	
oblique popliteal	–ligamentum popliteum obliquum	radioulnar	–membrana interossea antebrachii
palpebral	–ligamentum palpebrale	tibiofibular	–membrana interossea cruris
patellar	–ligamentum patellae	perineal	–membrana perinei
pisohamate	–ligamentum pisohamatum	suprapleural	–membrana suprapleuralis
pisometacarpal	–ligamentum pisometacarpale	synovial	–membrana synovialis
plantar	–ligamenta tarsi plantaria	thyrohyoid	–membrana thyrohyoidea
pubofemoral	–ligamentum pubofemorale	meninges	–meninges
puboprostatic	–ligamentum puboprostaticum	meniscus	–meniscus
pulmonary	–ligamentum pulmonale	mesentery	–mesenterium
round		mesoappendix	–mesoappendix
of liver	–ligamentum teres hepatis	mesocolon	
of ovary	–ligamentum ovarii proprium	sigmoid	–mesocolon sigmoideum
of uterus	–ligamentum teres uteri	transverse	–mesocolon transversum
sacroiliac	–ligamenta sacroilaca	mesovarium	–mesovarium
sacrospinous	–ligamentum sacrospinale	metacarpal bones	–ossa metacarpi
sacrotuberous	–ligamentum sacrotuberale	metacarpus	–metacarpus
scapular, transverse	–ligamentum transversum scapulae	metatarsal bones	–ossa metatarsi
'spring'	–ligamentum calcaneonaviculare	moderator band	–trabecula septomarginalis
plantare		mons pubis	–mons pubis
stylohyoid	–ligamentum stylohyoideum	mouth	–cavitas oris
talofibular	–ligamentum talofibulare	muscle	–musculus
teres		abductor	
of hip joint	–ligamentum capitis femoris	digiti minimi	–m. abductor digiti minimi
of liver	–ligamentum teres hepatis	hallucis	–m. abductor hallucis
tibiofibular	–ligamentum tibiofibulare	pollicis brevis	–m. abductor pollicis brevis
triangular	–ligamentum triangulare	pollicis longus	–m. abductor pollicis longus
venosum	–ligamentum venosum	adductor	
limb, lower	–membrum inferius	brevis	–m. adductor brevis
foot	–pes	hallucis	–m. adductor hallucis
dorsum	–dorsum pedis	longus	–m. adductor longus
sole	–planta pedis	magnus	–m. adductor magnus
leg	–crus	pollicis	–m. adductor pollicis
thigh	–femur	anconeus	–m. anconeus
limb, upper	–membrum superius	auricular	–mm. auriculares
line, arcuate	–linea arcuata	biceps brachii	–m. biceps brachii
linea		biceps femoris	–m. biceps femoris
alba	–linea alba	bipennate	–m. bipennatus
semilunaris	–linea semilunaris	brachialis	–m. brachialis
lingula, of left lung	–lingula pulmonis sinistri	brachioradialis	–m. brachioradialis
liver	–hepar	buccinator	–m. buccinator
lobe	–lobus	bulbospongiosus	–m. bulbospongiosus
caudate	–lobus caudatus	cardiac	–m. cardiacus striatus
quadrate	–lobus quadratus	ciliary	–m. ciliaris
lunate bone	–os lunatum	coccygeus	–m. coccygeus
lung	–pulmo	compressor nares	–m. nasalis: pars transversum
lymphatic vessel	–vasa lymphatica	constrictor of pharynx	–m. constrictor pharyngis
		coracobrachialis	–m. coracobrachialis
		cremaster	–m. cremaster
M		cricoarytenoid	–m. cricoarytenoideus
malleolus	–malleolus	cricothyroid	–m. cricothyroideus
mandible	–mandibula	dartos	–m. dartos
manubrium	–manubrium sterni	deltoid	–m. deltoideus
margin, costal	–arcus costalis	depressor anguli oris	–m. depressor angulioris
mater		depressor labii inferioris	–m. depressor labii inferioris
arachnoid	–arachnoid mater	detrusor	–m. detrusor vesicae
dura	–dura mater	digastric	–m. digastricus
pia	–pia mater	dilator nares	–m. nasalis: pars alaris
maxilla	–maxilla	dilator pupillae	–m. dilator pupillae
meatus		erector spinae	–m. erector spine
acoustic	–meatus acusticus	extensor	
nasal	–meatus nasi	carpi radialis brevis	–m. extensor carpi radialis brevis

ENGLISH	NOMINA ANATOMICA	ENGLISH	NOMINA ANATOMICA
muscle (*cont.*)		occipitofrontalis	—m. occipitofrontalis
carpi radialis longus	—m. extensor carpi radialis longus	omohyoid	—m. omohyoideus
carpi ulnaris	—m. extensor carpi ulnaris	opponens digiti minimi	—m. opponens digiti minimi
digiti minimi	—m. extensor digiti minimi	opponens pollicis	—m. opponens pollicis
digitorum	—m. extensor extensor digitorum	orbicularis oculi	—m. orbicularis oculi
brevis	—m. extensor digitorum brevis	orbicularis oris	—m. orbicularis oris
longus	—m. extensor digitorum longus	palatoglossus	—m. palatoglossus
hallucis brevis	—m. extensor hallucis brevis	palatopharyngeus	—m. palatopharyngeus
hallucis longus	—m. extensor hallucis longus	palmaris brevis	—m. palmaris brevis
indicis	—m. extensor indicis	palmaris longus	—m. palmaris longus
pollicis brevis	—m. extensor pollicis brevis	papillary	—mm. papillares
pollicis longus	—m. extensor pollicis longus	pectinati	—mm. pectinati
extraocular	—mm. bulbi oculi	pectineus	—m. pectineus
of facial expression	—mm. faciales	pectoralis major	—m. pectoralis major
flexor		pectoralis minor	—m. pectoralis minor
accessorius	—m. quadratus plantae	peroneus	
carpi radialis	—m. flexor carpi radialis	brevis	—m. peroneus brevis
carpi ulnaris	—m. flexor carpi ulnaris	longus	—m. peroneus longus
digiti minimi	—m. flexor digiti minimi	tertius	—m. peroneus tertius
digiti minimi brevis	—m. flexor digiti minimi brevis	pharyngeal	—tunica muscularis pharyngis
digitorum		piriformis	—m. piriformis
brevis	—m. flexor digitorum brevis	plantaris	—m. plantaris
longus	—m. flexor digitorum longus	platysma	—m. platysma
profundus	—m. flexor digitorum profundus	popliteus	—m. popliteus
superficialis	—m. flexor digitorum superficialis	pronator quadratus	—m. pronator quadratus
hallucis brevis	—m. flexor hallucis brevis	pronator teres	—m. pronator teres
hallucis longus	—m. flexor hallucis longus	psoas major	—m. psoas major
pollicis brevis	—m. flexor pollicis brevis	psoas minor	—m. psoas minor
pollicis longus	—m. flexor pollicis longus	pterygoid	—m. pterygoideus
gastrocnemius	—m. gastrocnemius	pubococcygeus	—m. pubococcygeus
gemelli	—mm. gemelli	pyramidalis	—m. pyramidalis
genioglossus	—m. genioglossus	quadratus femoris	—m. quadratus femoris
geniohyoid	—m. geniohyoideus	quadratus lumborum	—m. quadratus lumborum
gluteus		quadriceps femoris	—m. quadriceps femoris
maximus	—m. gluteus maximus	rectus	
medius	—m. gluteus medius	abdominis	—m. rectus abdominis
minimus	—m. gluteus minimus	of eye	—mm. recti bulbi
gracilis	—m. gracilis	femoris	—m. rectus femoris
hyoglossus	—m. hyoglossus	rhomboid major	—m. rhomboideus major
iliacus	—m. iliacus	rhomboid minor	—m. rhomboideus minor
iliococcygeus	—m. iliococcygeus	salpingopharyngeus	—m. salpingopharyngeus
iliopsoas	—m. iliopsoas	sartorius	—m. sartorius
infrahyoid	—mm. infrahyoidei	scalenus	
infraspinatus	—m. infraspinatus	anterior	—m. scalenus anterior
interarytenoid	—m. arytenoideus	medius	—m. scalenus medius
intercostal		posterior	—m. scalenus posterior
external	—mm. intercostales externi	semimembranosus	—m. semimembranosus
innermost	—mm. intercostales intimi	semitendinosus	—m. semitendinosus
internal	—mm. intercostales interni	serratus	
interosseous	—mm. interossei dorsales	anterior	—m. serratus anterior
dorsal	—mm. interossei plantares	posterior	
plantar	—mm. interossei palmares	inferior	—m. serratus posterior inferior
palmar	—m. ischiocavernosus	superior	—m. serratus posterior superior
ischiocavernosus	—mm. laryngis	skeletal	—textus muscularis striatus skeletalis
laryngeal, intrinsic	—m. latissimus dorsi	smooth	—textus muscularis nonstriatus
latissimus dorsi		soleus	—m. soleus
levator	—m. levator ani	sphincter	
ani	—m. levator veli palatini	anal	
palati	—m. levator palpebrae superioris	external	—m. sphincter ani externus
palpebrae superioris	—m. levator scapulae	deep part	—pars profunda
scapulae	—mm. lumbricales	subcutaneous part	—pars subcutanea
lumbrical	—m. masseter	superficial part	—pars superficialis
masseter	—m. mentalis	internal	—m. sphincter ani internus
mentalis	—m. multipennatus	pupillae	—m. sphincter pupillae
multipennate	—m. mylohyoideus	urethral	—m. sphincter urethrae
mylohyoid		splenius capitis	—m. splenius capitis
oblique		splenius cervicis	—m. splenius cervicis
external	—m. obliquus externus abdominis	sternohyoid	—m. sternohyoideus
inferior	—m. obliquus inferior	sternomastoid	—m. sternocleidomastoideus
internal	—m. obliquus internus abdominis	sternothyroid	—m. sternothyroideus
superior	—m. obliquus superior	styloglossus	—m. styloglossus
obturator externus	—m. obturator externus	stylohyoid	—m. stylohyoideus
obturator internus	—m. obturator externus	stylopharyngeus	—m. stylopharyngeus

ENGLISH	NOMINA ANATOMICA	ENGLISH	NOMINA ANATOMICA
muscle (*cont.*)		interosseus	–n. interosseus
subscapularis	–m. subscapularis	lacrimal	–n. lacrimalis
supinator	–m. supinator	laryngeal	
supraspinatus	–m. supraspinatus	recurrent	–n. laryngeus recurrens
temporalis	–m. temporalis	superior	–n. laryngeus superior
tensor fasciae latae	–m. tensor fasciae latae	lingual	–n. lingualis
tensor palati	–m. tensor veli palatini	long thoracic (serratus anterior)	–n. thoracicus longus
teres major	–m. teres major	lumbar	–nn. lumbales
teres minor	–m. teres minor	mandibular (V3)	–n. mandibularis
thyroarytenoid	–m. thyroarytenoideus	masseteric	–n. massetericus
thyrohyoid	–m. thyrohyoideus	maxillary (V2)	–n. maxillaris
tibialis anterior	–m. tibialis anterior	median	–n. medianus
tibialis posterior	–m. tibialis posterior	musculocutaneous	–n. musculocutaneus
transversospinal	–mm. transversospinales	mylohyoid	–n. mylohyoideus
transversus abdominis	–m. transversus abdominis	nasociliary	–n. nasociliaris
transversus thoracis	–m. transversus thoracis	nasopalatine	–n. nasopalatini
trapezius	–m. trapezius	obturator	–n. obturatorius
triceps brachii	–m. triceps brachii	occipital	
unipennate	–m. unipennatus	greater	–n. occipitalis major
uvular	–m. uvulae	lesser	–n. occipitalis minor
vastus		oculomotor (III)	–n. oculomotorius
intermedius	–m. vastus intermedius	olfactory (I)	–nn. olfactorii
lateralis	–m. vastus lateralis	ophthalmic (V1)	–n. ophthalmicus
medialis	–m. vastus medialis	optic (II)	–n. opticus
voluntary striated	–textus muscularis striatus skeletalis	palatine	
zygomaticus major	–m. zygomaticus major	greater	–n. palatinus major
zygomaticus minor	–m. zygomaticus minor	lesser	–nn. palatini minores
myocardium	–m. myocardium	pectoral	–n. pectoralis
		perineal	–nn. perineales
		peroneal	
N		common	–n. fibularis communis
nasopharynx	–pars nasalis pharyngis	deep	–n. fibularis profundus
neck	–cervix, collum	superficial	–n. fibularis superficialis
of femur	–collum femoris	phrenic	–n. phrenicus
of humerus		plantar	–n. plantaris
anatomic	–collum anatomicum	of pterygoid canal	–n. canalis pterygoidei
surgical	–collum chirurgicum	pudenal	–n. pudendus
of radius	–collum radii	to quadratus femoris	–n. musculi quadrati femoris
of uterus	–cervix uteri	radial	–n. radialis
nerve	–nervus	rectal inferior	–nn. rectales inferiores
abducens (VI)	–n. abducens	sacral	–nn. sacrales
accessory (XI)	–n. accessorius	saphenous	–n. saphenus
alveolar	–n. alveolaris	sciatic	–n. ischiadicus
auricular, great	–n. auricularis magnus	spinal	–nn. spinales
auriculotemporal	–n. auriculotemporalis	anterior rami	–rami anteriores
autonomic	–systema nervosum autonomicum	posterior rami	–rami posteriores
axillary	–n. axillaris	splanchnic	–n. splanchnicus
buccal	–n. buccalis	pelvic	–nn. pelvici splanchnici
cervical, transverse	–n. transversus colli	subcostal	–n. subcostalis
chorda tympani	–chorda tympani	subscapular	–nn. subscapularis
ciliary	–nn. ciliares	supraclavicular	–nn. supraclaviculares
coccygeal	–n. coccygeus	supraorbital	–n. supraorbitalis
cranial	–nn. craniales	suprascapular	–n. suprascapularis
cutaneous		supratrochlear	–n. supratrochlearis
of thigh	–n. cutaneous femoris	sural	–n. suralis
antebrachial	–n. cutaneous antebrachial	temporal, deep	–nn. temporales profundi
brachial	–n. cutaneous brachii	thoracic, long	–n. thoracicus longus
digital	–nn. digitales	thoracodorsal	–n. thoracodorsalis
dorsal		tibial	–n. tibialis
of clitoris	–n. dorsalis clitoridis	trigeminal (V)	–n. trigeminus
of penis	–n. dorsalis penis	mandibular division (V3)	–n. mandibularis
scapular	–n. dorsalis scapulae	maxillary division (V2)	–n. maxillaris
facial (VII)	–n. facialis	ophthalmic division (V1)	–n. ophthalmicus
in parotid gland	–plexus intraparotideus	trochlear (IV)	–n. trochlearis
femoral	–n. femoralis	ulnar	–n. ulnaris
frontal	–n. frontalis	vagus (X)	–n. vagus
genitofemoral	–n. genitofemoralis	vestibulocochlear (VIII)	–n. vestibulocochlearis
glossopharyngeal (IX)	–n. glossopharyngeus	zygomatic	–n. zygomaticus
gluteal	–n. gluteus	zygomaticofacial	–ramus zygomaticofacialis
hypoglossal (XII)	–n. hypoglossus	zygomaticotemporal	–ramus zygomaticotemporalis
iliohypogastric	–n. iliohypogastricus	nervi erigentes	–nn. pelvici splanchnici
ilioinguinal	–n. ilioinguinalis	nervous system	–system nervosa
intercostal	–nn. intercostales	autonomic	–pars autonomica

ENGLISH	NOMINA ANATOMICA
nervous system (*cont.*)	
parasympathetic	–pars parasympathetica
sympathetic	–pars sympathetica
central	–pars centralis
peripheral	–pars peripherica
neuron	–neuron
nipple	–papilla mammaria
lactiferous duct	–ductus lactiferi
node	
atrioventricular	–nodus atrioventricularis
lymph	–nodus lymphaticus
aortic	–nodi lymphatici aortici
axillary	–nodi lymphatici axillares
cervical	–nodi lymphatici cervicales
iliac	–nodi lymphatici iliaci
inguinal	–nodi lymphatici inguinales
popliteal	–nodi lymphatici popliteales
supraclavicular	–nodi lymphatici supraclaviculares
sinoatrial	–nodus sinuatrialis
nose	–regio nasalis
nostrils	–nares
notch, cardiac of left lung	–incisura cardiaca
nucleus pulposus	–nucleus pulposus

O

ENGLISH	NOMINA ANATOMICA
occipital bone	–os occipitale
olecranon process	–olecranon
omentum	–omentum
bursa	–bursa omentalis
greater	–omentum majus
lesser	–omentum minus
opening	
of diaphragm	
aortic	–hiatus aorticus
caval	–foramen venae cavae
esophageal	–hiatus oesophageus
saphenous	–hiatus saphenus
vaginal	–ostium vaginae
oral cavity	–cavitas oris
orbit	–orbita
eyelids	–palpebrae
lacrimal apparatus	–apparatus lacrimalis
septum	–septum orbitale
orifice	–ostium
of stomach	
cardiac	–ostium cardiacum
pyloric	–ostium pyloricum
ureteric	–ostium ureteris
oropharynx	–pars oralis pharyngis
os, external	–ostium uteri
ovary	–ovarium

P

ENGLISH	NOMINA ANATOMICA
palate	
hard	–palatum durum
soft	–palatum molle
palatine bone	–os palatinum
palm	–palma manus
pancreas	–pancreas
papilla, duodenal	–papilla duodeni
parietal bone	–os parietale
part	–pars
patella	–patella
pedicle, vertebral	–pediculus arcus vertebrae
pelvis	–pelvis
floor (diaphragm)	–diaphragma pelvis
girdle	–cingulum membri inferioris
inlet	–apertura pelvis superior
renal	–pelvis renalis
of ureter	–pelvis renalis
penis	–penis

ENGLISH	NOMINA ANATOMICA
pericardium	–pericardium
fibrous	–pericardium fibrosum
serous	–pericardium serosum
perineum	–perineum
periosteum	–periosteum
peritoneum	–peritoneum
epiploic foramen	–foramen omentale
parietal	–peritoneum parietale
retroperitoneal organ	–organum extraperitoneale
visceral	–peritoneum viscerale
Peyer's patches	–folliculi lymphatici aggregati
phalanges	–ossa digitorum
pharynx	–pharynx
pia mater	–pia mater
pisiform bone	–os pisiforme
plate, cribriform	–lamina cribrosa
pleura	–pleura
cervical	–capula pleurae
mediastinal	–pleura mediastinalis
parietal	–pleura parietalis
visceral	–pleura visceralis
plexus	
nervous	–plexus nervosus
aortic	–plexus aorticus
brachial	–plexus brachialis
cardiac	–plexus cardiacus
celiac	–plexus coeliacus
cervical	–plexus cervicalis
esophageal	–plexus oesophagealis
hypogastric	–plexus hypogastricus
lumbar	–plexus lumbalis
pelvic	–pars pelvica systematis autonomica
pharyngeal	–plexus pharyngeus
pulmonary	–plexus pulmonalis
sacral	–plexus sacralis
venous	–plexus venosus
pampiniform	–plexus pampiniformis
prostatic	–plexus venosus prostaticus
pterygoid	–plexus pterygoideus
uterine	–plexus venosus uterinus
vesical	–plexus venosus vesicalis
plicae circulares	–plicae circulares
pneumatized bone	–os pneumaticum
pole	–extremitas
pons	–pons
porta hepatis	–porta hepatis
pouch	
of Douglas	–excavatio rectouterina
perineal	–spatium perinei
rectouterine	–excavatio rectouterina
rectovesical	–excavatio rectovesicalis
vesicouterine	–excavatio vesicouterina
prepuce	–preputium
process	
articular	–processus articularis
clinoid	–processus clinoideus
coracoid	–processus coracoideus
coronoid	–processus coronoideus
mastoid	–processus mastoideus
odontoid	–dens axis
spinous	–processus spinosus
styloid	–processus styloideus
transverse	–processus transversus
uncinate	–processus uncinatus
xiphoid	–processus xiphoideus
promontory of sacrum	–promontorium basi ossis sacri
protruberance, occipital	–protruberantia occipitalis
pubic bone	–os pubis
pylorus	–pylorus

R

ENGLISH	NOMINA ANATOMICA
radius	–radius

ENGLISH	NOMINA ANATOMICA	ENGLISH	NOMINA ANATOMICA
raphe	–raphe	petrosal	–sinus petrosus
anococcygeal	–ligamentum anococcygeum	sagittal	–sinus sagittalis
pterygomandibular	–raphe pterygomandibularis	sigmoid	–sinus sigmoideus
recess		straight	–sinus rectus
costodiaphragmatic	–recessus costodiaphragmaticus	transverse	–sinus transversus
sphenoethmoidal	–recessus sphenoethmoidalis	skeleton	–skeleton
rectum	–rectum	skin	–cutis
retinaculum		skull	–cranium
extensor, ankle	–retinaculum musculorum extensorum	small intestine	–intestinum tenue
extensor, wrist	–retinaculum extensorum	space	
flexor, ankle	–retinaculum musculorum flexorum	extradural	–spatium epidurale
flexor, wrist	–retinaculum flexorum	intercostal	–spatium intercostale
peroneal	–retinaculum musculorum peroneorum	subarachnoid	–spatium subarachnoideum
rib	–os costale	subhepatic	–recessus subhepatici
false	–costae spuriae	subphrenic	–recessus subphrenici
floating	–costae fluitantes	sphenoid bone	–os sphenoidale
true	–costae verae	sphincter	–musculus sphincter
ridge		anal	–m. sphincter ani
palatoglossal	–arcus palatoglossus	of Oddi	–m. sphincter ampullae hepatopancreat-
palatopharyngeal	–arcus palatopharyngeus	ica	
ring		pupillae	–m. sphincter pupillae
femoral	–annulus femoralis	pyloric	–m. sphincter pyloricus
fibrotendinous	–annulus tendineus communis	urethral, external	–m. sphincter urethrae
inguinal	–annulus inguinalis	spine	–columna vertebralis
root	–radix	cervical	–vertebrae cervicales
of lung	–radix pulmonis	ischial	–spina ischiadica
of mesentery	–radix mesenterii	lumbar	–vertebrae lumbales
of penis	–radix penis	of scapula	–spina scapulae
rugae	–rugae	thoracic	–vertebrae thoracicae
of stomach	–plicae gastrici	spleen	–splen
		sternum	–sternum
S		stomach	–gaster
		cardiac notch	–incisura cardiaca
sac, lesser peritoneal	–bursa omentalis	greater curvature	–curvatura gastrica major
sacrum	–os sacrum	lesser curvature	–curvatura gastrica minor
scaphoid bone	–os scaphoideum	rugae	–plicae gastricae
scapula	–scapula	sulcus	
scrotum	–scrotum	intertubercular	–sulcus intertubercularis
segments, bronchopulmonary	–segmenta bronchopulmonalia	terminalis	–sulcus terminalis
sella turcica	–sella turcica	sustentaculum tali	–sustentaculum tali
septum		sutures	–sutura
interatrial	–septum interatriale	symphysis, pubic	–symphysis pubica
intermuscular	–septum intermusculare		
interventricular	–septum interventriculare	**T**	
nasal	–septum nasi		
orbitale	–septum orbitale	taeniae coli	–taeniae coli
rectovesical	–septum rectovesicale	tail	–cauda
sesamoid bones	–ossa sesamoidea	talus bone	–talus
sheath		tarsal bones	–ossa tarsi
axillary	–fascia axillaris	temporal bone	–os temporali
carotid	–vagina carotica	tendinous intersections	–intersectiones tendineae
fibrous flexor	–vaginae fibrosae digitorum	tendon	
rectus	–vaginae musculi recti abdominis	calcaneus (Achilles)	–tendo calcaneus
synovial	–vaginae synoviales	central, of diaphragm	–centrum tendineum
shoulder joint	–articulatio humeri	conjoint	–falx inguinalis
sinus	–sinus	tentorium cerebelli	–tentorium cerebelli
aortic	–sinus aortae	testis	–testis
cartoid	–sinus caroticus	thigh	–femur
paranasal	–sinus paranasales	thorax	–thorax
ethmoidal	–sinus ethmoidales	bones	–ossa thoracis
frontal	–sinus frontalis	inlet	–apertura thoracis superior
maxillary	–sinus maxillaris	outlet	–apertura thoracis inferior
sphenoidal	–sinus sphenoidalis	thumb	–pollex
pericardial		thymus	–thymus
oblique	–sinus obliquus pericardii	tibia	–tibia
transverse	–sinus transversus pericardii	tissue, connective	–textus connectivus
prostatic	–sinus prostaticus	toe	–digitus pedis
pulmonary	–sinus trunci pulmonalis	great	–hallux
renal	–sinus renalis	tongue	–lingua
venous		muscles	–musculi linguae
coronary	–sinus coronarius	tonsil	–tonsilla
dural	–sinus durae matris	trabeculae carneae	–trabeculae carneae
cavernous	–sinus cavernosus	trachea	–trachea

ENGLISH	NOMINA ANATOMICA	ENGLISH	NOMINA ANATOMICA
tract, iliotibial	–tractus iliotibialis	ileocecal	–valva ileocaecalis
trapezium bone	–os trapezium	vena cava, inferior	–valvula venae cavae inferioris
trapezoid bone	–os trapezoideum	venous	–valvula venosa
tree, bronchial	–arbor bronchialis	vas deferens	–ductus deferens
triangle		vein	–vena
anal	–regio analis	axillary	–v. axillaris
femoral	–trigonum femorale	azygos	–v. azygos
of neck, anterior	–regio cervicalis anterior	basilic	–v. basilica
of neck, posterior	–regio cervicalis lateralis	brachiocephalic	–v. brachiocephalica
urogenital	–regio urogenitalis	cardiac	–vv. cordis
trigone, bladder	–trigonum vesicae	cava	–v. cava
triquetral bone	–os triquetrum	cephalic	–v. cephalica
trochlea	–trochlea	comitantes	–vv. comitantes
trunk		cystic	–v. cystica
brachiocephalic	–truncus brachiocephalicus	deep dorsal of penis	–v. dorsalis profunda penis
costocervical	–truncus costocervicalis	diploic	–vv. diploicae
lumbosacral	–truncus lumbosacralis	epigastric	–v. epigastrica
pulmonary	–truncus pulmonalis	femoral	–v. femoralis
sympathetic	–truncus sympatheticus	gastric	–vv. gastricae
tube		gastroepiploic	–v. gastroomentalis
auditory (Eustachian)	–tuba auditiva	hemiazygos	–v. hemiazygos
uterine	–tuba uterina	accessory	–v. hemiazygos accessoria
intramural part	–pars uterina	hepatic	–vv. hepaticae
tubercle, tuberosity		ileocolic	–v. ileocolica
calcaneal	–tuberculum calcanei	iliac	–v. iliaca
deltoid	–tuberositas deltoidea	intercostal	–vv. intercostales
gluteal	–tuberositas gluteaiis	jugular	–v. jugularis
infraglenoid	–tuberculum infraglenoidale	median cubital	–v. media cubiti
ischial	–tuber ischiadicum	meningeal	–vv. meningeae
pubic	–tuberculum pubicum	mesenteric	–v. mesenterica
radial	–tuberositas radii	musculophrenic	–vv. musculophrenicae
of rib	–tuberculum costae	ophthalmic	–v. ophthalmica
scalene	–tuberculum musculi scaleni anterioris	popliteal	–v. poplitea
supraglenoid	–tuberculum supraglenoidale	portal	–v. portae hepatis
tibial	–tuberositas tibiae	pudendal, external	–vv. pudendae externae
of ulna	–tuberositas ulnae	pulmonary	–vv. pulmonales
tunica		renal	–v. renalis
albuginae	–tunica albuginea	retromandibular	–v. retromandibularis
vaginalis	–tunica vaginalis	sacral	–vv. sacrales
tunnel, carpal	–canalis carpi	saphenous, long	–v. saphena magna
		saphenous, short	–v. saphena parva
		splenic	–v. splenica
U		subclavian	–v. subclavia
ulna	–ulna	suprarenal	–v. suprarenalis
umbilicus	–umbilicus	thoracic, internal	–v. thoracica interna
urachus	–urachus or ligamentum umbilicae medianum	thyroid	–vv. thyroideae
		vertebral	–v. vertebralis
ureter	–ureter	ventricle of heart	–ventriculus cordis
urethra	–urethra	vertebra	–vertebra
female	–urethra feminina	cervical	–vertebrae cervicales
male	–urethra masculina	lumbar	–vertebrae lumbales
crest	–crista urethralis	prominens	–vertebra prominens
membranous	–pars membranacea	sacral	–vertebrae sacrales
prostatic	–pars prostatica	thoracic	–vertebrae thoracicae
spongy	–pars spongiosa	vesicle, seminal	–vesicula seminalis
uterus		vincula vasculosa	–vincula tendinum
surfaces		vomer	–vomer
posterosuperior	–facies intestinalis		
anteroinferior	–facies vesicalis	**W**	
utricle	–utriculus prostaticus	wrist	–carpus
uvula	–uvula		
		X	
V		xiphisternum	–processus xiphoideus
vagina	–vagina		
vaginal opening	–ostium vaginae	**Z**	
valve		zygoma	–os zygomaticum
of heart			
aortic	–valva aortae		
semilunar cusp	–valvula semilunaris		
mitral (bicuspid)	–valva atrioventricularis sinistra		
pulmonary	–valva trunci pulmonalis		
tricuspid	–valva atrioventricularis dextra		

INDEX

A

Abdomen, 454-544
  in anatomic position, 3
  anatomy of
    clinical, 482
    skeletal, 536
    surface, 538
  arterial supply of, 536-537
  case studies of, 539-544
  colon and, 515-521; *see also* Colon
    on CT, 41
  development of, 476-479, 481
    clinical anatomy of, 482
  diaphragm and, 529-531
  esophagus in, 499-501
  fibroids in, 612
  gallbladder and biliary tree in, 488-492
  inguinal canal and descent of testes in,
    464-472
  innervation of, 537-538
  kidneys and, 522-528
  lesser sac in, 503-505
    development of, 476-479, 481
  liver in, 484-489, 493
  lymphatic drainage of, 537
  muscles of, 536
    importance of, 462
  pancreas in, 494-498
  peritoneal membranes and, 473-483
  posterior wall of, 529-535
    abdominal aorta with branches and, 534
    clinical anatomy of, 535
    diaphragm and, 529-531
    general structure of, 529
    lumbar plexus and, 530-534
    venous drainage of, 534-535
  pressure in, in respiration, 68
  quadrants of, 538
  small intestine in, 507-514
  spleen in, 491-494
    symmetry and, 494
  stomach in, 501-505
  suprarenal glands and, 527-528
  systems review and, 536-538
  ultrasound of, 44
  venous drainage of, 537
  viscera of, 390
    tendons and, 390
    in upper abdomen, 56
  wall of; *see* Abdominal wall
  x-ray of, 39
Abdominal aorta, 534, 536

Abdominal aorta—cont'd
  branches of, 534
  distal, thigh and, 658
  lumbar arteries from, 513
Abdominal cavity, apertures of, 531
Abdominal sac; *see* Sac
Abdominal transversalis fascia, 459, 461, 652
Abdominal wall, 457-463
  anterior, 458-459
  bladder and muscles of, 600
  clinical anatomy of, 462
  incisions in, 462
  layers of, 457-462
  muscles of, 654
  neurovascular supply of, 459-461
  posterior, 535
  principles for, 463
  segmentation and, 462
  skeleton of, 458
Abducens nerve (VI), 162, 165, 167, 169
  anterolateral neck and, 210
  brain and, 157, 160
  circle of Willis and, 162
  globe and orbit and, 238, 244-246
  head and neck and, 177, 293
  skull and, 140
  superior orbital fissure and, 238
Abduction, 7
  in glenohumeral joint motion, 322
  of hand and wrist, 370
  of hip, 644-645, 712
  of thumb, 381, 384-385
Abductor digiti minimi muscle
  foot, 715-717
    attachments and innervations of, 719
    on MRI, 709
    superficial fascia of sole of foot and, 708
    on transverse section, 718
  hand, 357, 382-383, 386, 391
    insertion of, 388
    on MRI, 357
Abductor hallucis muscle, 716-719
Abductor muscles of foot, 723
Abductor pollicis brevis muscle, 357, 373,
    382
  hand and, 382-385
  insertion of, 388
  on MRI, 357
Abductor pollicis longus muscle, 361-363,
    375
  tendon of, 357
    on MRI, 357
  wrist and, 375

Abnormalities; *see* Deformities
Abscess
  anal, 520
  psoas, 662
  retropharyngeal, 283
Accessory hemiazygos vein, 71, 121
  mediastinum and, 117-118
  thoracic duct and, 31
Accessory muscles of respiration, 68, 199
Accessory nerve (XI), 165-167, 169
  anterolateral neck and, 210
  in carotid triangle, 210, 213
  cranial origin of, 165, 210
  injury to, 204
  palate and, 267
  in posterior triangle of neck, 199-200, 293,
    296
  shoulder and, 329
  skull and, 140
  spinal origin of, 165, 167, 200-202, 210
    axons in, 213
    injury to, 204
    neck and; *see* Neck, spinal roots and
    palate and, 267
    skull and, 140
    spinal cord and meninges and, 437
Accessory rib, 413
Accessory spleen, 494
Accommodation, 239, 247, 251, 296
Accommodation reflex, 247, 296
Acetabulum, 549-552, 556
  CT scan of, 618
  head of femur in, 641
  hip joint and, 640-641, 643
  labrum of, 640-641
  ligaments of, 643
  notch of, 551
  transverse, 551, 642-643
Achalasia, 500
Achilles tendon, 702, 725
  blood supply to ankle and, 703
  leg muscles and, 689
  popliteal fossa and, 688-689
  posterior compartment of leg and, 692
  posterior view of, 694
  tapping on, 726
Acid–base status, 522
Acoustic meatus, external, 135, 143
Acoustic nerve (VIII), 165, 167, 169
  anterolateral neck and, 210
  brain and, 157
  head and neck and, 293
  otic ganglion and, 195

Acoustic nerve (VIII)—cont'd
  skull and, 140
Acromial artery, 333
Acromioclavicular joint, 61, 313, 317-321, 398
  brachial plexus and, 327
  injury to, 317
  palpation of, 122
Acromioclavicular ligament, 317, 319
  torn, 401, 403
Acromion, 50, 61-62, 312-317, 319
  in anterior view of upper limb, 398
  back and, 449
  surface anatomy and, 398-399
  on x-ray, 312-313
Acronym for scalp layers, 174
Actin, 15
Action potential, 20
Adam's apple, 284-285
Adduction, 7
  of glenohumeral joint, 322
  of hand and wrist, 370
  of hip, 644-645
  of hip joint, 712
  of thumb, 381, 384-385
Adductor brevis muscle, 648-649, 659-661
  attachment of, 657
  on CT, 618
  femoral artery and, 646
Adductor canal, thigh and, 656
Adductor hallucis muscle, 715-719
  on MRI, 709
Adductor hiatus for femoral artery, 646, 660-
    661
Adductor longus muscle, 648-651, 654-661
  anteromedial thigh and, 637, 654-655, 660
    blood supply to, 646
  attachment of, 657
  on CT, 618
  femoral artery and, 646
  lower thigh and, 648
  medial edge of, 651
Adductor magnus muscle, 648-649, 654, 656-
    661
  anteromedial thigh and, 637, 660-661
  attachment of, 657
  on CT, 618
  femoral artery and, 646
  in posterior thigh, 658
    deep view of, 675
    nerves to, 674
Adductor minimus muscle, 661
Adductor muscles, 723
  femoral sheath and, 654
Adductor pollicis muscle, 357, 373, 382-385
  insertion of, 388
  single origin of, 385
Adductor tubercle, 639, 658, 661
Adenitis, mesenteric, 514
Adenohypophysis, 35, 37
Adenoid, 279
Adenoiditis, 283
Adipose tissue, 9
Aditus of middle ear, 227-229
Adrenal gland, 522-523, 527
  abnormalities of, 528
  blood supply to, 526
  as body system, 35, 37

Adrenal gland—cont'd
  clinical anatomy of, 528
  cross-section of, 527
  kidneys and; see Kidney
  steroids and, 528
Adrenal vein, right, 527
Adrenergic innervation of heart, 104-105
Adventitial layer of muscle, 19
Aerodigestive system, 74, 293
Afferent lymphatics, 32
Agonists, 15
Air entering lungs, 68
Air cells
  ethmoidal, 135, 143
  mastoid
    middle ear and, 226
    skull and, 135, 142-143
Air density, x-ray detection of, 36
Air sinuses of skull, 143; see also Paranasal
    sinuses
Airways, 34
  clinical anatomy of, 79
  emergency, 219
  establishing, 290
  obstruction of, 79
  patency of, genioglossus and, 275
Ala
  of ilium, 549
  of nose, 254
Alar cartilage, 253
  greater, 254
  lesser, 254
Alar ligament, 418, 421
Alcock's canal, 568, 589
Allen test, 377
Alpha receptors, 105
ALS; see Amyotrophic lateral sclerosis
Alveolar artery
  entering mandible, 189, 193-194
  maxillary artery and, 192-193
Alveolar disease of lung, 85
Alveolar glands in breast, 54
Alveolar nerve
  anterior, 260
  entering mandible, 189, 193-194
  face and scalp and, 178
  inferior, 194
  posterior, 260
  superior, 245
Alveolar ridge, 268
Alveolar vein, 189, 193-194
Alveoli
  in breast, 54
  of lungs, 29, 34, 80
Ampulla
  of ductus deferens, 614
    on seminal vesiculogram, 615
  of inner ear, 230
  of Vater, 497
    development of, 479
    hepatopancreatic, 487
Amylase, 498
Amyotrophic lateral sclerosis, 151, 447
Anal column, 568, 571
Anal sinus, 571
Anal sphincter, 584
  external, 519, 565, 568-569, 616

Anal sphincter—cont'd
  deep, 568, 571
  description of, 17
  innervation of, 571, 578
  subcutaneous, 568, 571
  superficial, 568, 571
  internal, 519, 568, 571
  innervation of, 571
Anal triangle, 561-562
Anastomoses, 71
  cruciate, 645, 659, 668
  portocaval, 489, 520
  in scalp, 176
  scapular, 329, 397
Anatomic position, 3-4
Anatomic snuff-box, 362, 372, 375
Anatomic terminology, 3-7
Anconeus muscle, 344, 354, 359, 361-363, 398
Android pelvis, 554, 557
Anesthesia
  caudal block, 593
  for childbirth, 628-629, 631
  epidural, 447
  of jaw, 197
  regional
    for abdominal surgery, 539, 542
    pelvis and, 553, 560
  sacral, 553
  spinal, 447
  of upper limb, 403-404
Aneurysm
  of aorta, 119
  of axillary artery, 334
  of circulus arteriosus, 163
  poststenotic, 328
Angina, Ludwig's, 223
Angiotensin, 528
Angle
  costal, 122
  of gaze, 243
  of inclination, of femur, 640
  iridocorneal, 250
  of Louis, 62
  of mandible, 277
  of rib, 60
  of scapula, 62, 398
  sternal, 62, 122
Angular artery, 181-183
Angular incisure of stomach, 501-502
Angular vein, 237, 250
  pterygoid venous plexus and, 195
Anhydrosis, 251
Ankle, 699-703
  in anatomic position, 4
  blood supply to, 703
  clinical anatomy of, 704
  comparison of, to wrist, 723
  injury to, 731
  ligaments of, 699-703
  movements of, 688, 703
  MRI of, 709
  tendons at, 702-703
  x-rays of, 700
Anlage, cartilaginous, 10
Annular bands of hand, 389
Annular ligament, 230, 351-353, 419
  radioulnar joint and, 354

Annular pancreas, 498
Annulus of heart valve, 91, 97-98
Annulus fibrosus, 419, 423
    on MRI, 418
    vertebral column and, 433
Annulus tendineus, 238
Anococcygeal nerve, 583
Anococcygeal raphe, 561-564, 568, 572-574,
        631
Anomalous pulmonary venous
        return, 101
Anorectal canal, 515-517, 519-520, 562; *see*
        also Colon; Rectum
    on CT, 618
    infection in, 520
    levator ani muscle and, 568
    perineal body and, 568
    perineum and, 568-569
    pudendal nerve and, 519
    rectal artery and, 520
    tear in, 584
    thigh and, 648-649
Ansa cervicalis nerve, 168, 200, 202, 215, 217
    anterolateral neck and, 207
    in carotid triangle, 214-216
    hypoglossal nerve and, 214
    upper root of, 214
Ansa hypoglossi, 159
Ansa subclavius nerve
    cranial nerves and, 168
    mediastinum and, 216
    spinal cord and, 444-445
Antagonists, 15
Antebrachial cutaneous nerve, 366
Antecubital vein, 364
Anterior position of structure, 3, 5
Anthropoid pelvis, 554, 557
Antibodies, 254
Antidiuretic hormone, 37
Antihelix, 225
Antitragus, 225
Antrectomy, 501
Antrum of stomach, 501-502, 508
    liver and, 488
Anus, 562, 568-569, 572; *see also* Colon;
        Rectum
    abscess of, 520
    arterial supply of, 569
    canal of; *see* Anorectal canal
    coronal section of, 568
    innervation of, 571
    orifice or opening of, 561, 574
    sphincter of; *see* Anal sphincter
    venous drainage of, 569-571
Aorta
    abdominal, 492, 536
        branches of, 534
        on CT, 41
        distal, thigh and, 658
        lumbar arteries from, 513
    aneurysm of, 119
    anterior view of, 89
    arch of; *see* Aortic arch
    arterial blood in, 25
    ascending
        on CT and MRI, 42-43, 100
        heart and, 89, 91, 98-101

Aorta—cont'd
    mediastinum and, 52
    bifurcation of, peritoneal membranes
        and, 478
    blood flow entering, 102
    clinical anatomy of, 117
    coarctation of, 129
    descending, 81, 100
        branches of, 82, 117
        on CT and MRI, 43
        left edge of, 77
        mediastinum and, 117
        spinal cord and, 445
        in tracheobronchial tree, 80
        on x-ray, 53
    diaphragm and, 530-531
    esophageal branches of, 116
    fibrous pericardium on, 87
    fibrous skeleton of heart and, 91
    gastrointestinal tract and, 477
    iliac artery and, 570
    mediastinum and, 52, 110
    pancreas and, 496-497
    parasympathetic nerves and, 294
    pelvis and, 591, 623
    in pericardial sac, 86
    rectum and, 517
    serous membranes and, 474
    small intestine and, 513
    spinal cord and, 69, 430
    spleen and, 491, 493
    stomach and, 502
    sympathetic plexus on, 591-592
    testis and, 470
    in thoracic blood supply, 121
    thoracic duct and, 117
    ureters and kidneys and, 524-525, 601, 603
    vertebral column and, 428
Aortic arch, 109-111, 172
    carotid artery and, 101, 206
    glossopharyngeal nerve and, 211
    left subclavian artery and, 101
    mediastinum and, 110, 216
    position of, 124
    right-sided, 114
    spinal cord and, 444
    subclavian artery and, 101
    surface projections of, 124
    thyroid gland and, 218
    on x-ray, 53
Aortic bodies, 52, 81
Aortic hiatus of diaphragm, 67, 530, 532
    spinal cord and, 445
Aortic knob or knuckle, 77
    on x-ray, 53
Aortic sac, pharyngeal arches and, 172
Aortic sinus, 101
Aortic sympathetic plexus, 591-592
Aortic valve, 91, 96, 98-99
    blood flow through, 102
    fibrous skeleton of heart and, 91
    position of, 122
    surface anatomy and, 123
    surface projections of, 124
Aortic vestibule, 98
Aorticopulmonary bodies, 52
Aorticorenal nerve, 537

Apex
    of bony orbit, 235, 237
    of fibula, 678
    of heart, 89, 122, 124
    of lungs, 80, 124
    of prostate, 614
Apical ligament of dens, 418
Aponeurosis, 15
    bicipital, 400
    palatine, 263, 265
    palmar, 382
    plantar, 707-708, 716
    of rectus abdominis muscle, 461
    scalp layers and, 175
Appendices epiploica, 516-517
Appendicitis, 540-541, 544
    principles of, 518
Appendicular artery, 513
Appendicular skeleton, 11-12
Appendix, 517
    ileocecal junction and, 511
    McBurney's point and, 538
    small intestine and, 508, 512
    vermiform, 518
Aqueduct of Sylvius, 151, 153
    on MRI, 148
Aqueductal stenosis, 153
Aqueous humor, 239-241
    flow of, 240
Arachnoid granulations, 152, 158, 162-163,
        437
Arachnoid mater, 20
    brain and, 155-156
    cerebrospinal fluid and, 152
    dural sheath lined with, 440
    scalp layers and, 175
    spinal cord and, 434, 437-438
    subarachnoid space and, 439
Arachnoid membrane, 453
Arachnoid villi, 152, 155, 158
Arches
    of aorta; *see* Aortic arch
    of atlas, 135, 148, 415
        first-arch syndromes and, 173
        on MRI, 148
    of azygos vein, 124
    brachial, 134
    of foot, 706-708, 714, 717
        longitudinal, 708
        veins and, 715
    palatal, 264
    palatoglossal, 264, 266, 280
    palatopharyngeal, 264, 266
    palmar; *see* Palmar arch
    pharyngeal; *see* Pharyngeal arch;
        Pharyngeal arches
    of vertebra, 409-411, 414
        in cervical region, 135, 148, 421
    of zygoma, 142, 177, 294, 421
        mastication muscles and, 191
        skull and, 135
Arcuate artery
    kidneys and, 526
    in renal arteriogram, 40
Arcuate ligament
    diaphragm and, 530
    lateral, 529

Arcuate ligament—cont'd
  medial, 529
Arcuate line of ilium, 549-551, 556
  abdominal wall and, 458, 460
  pelvis and, 559
Arcuate popliteal ligament, 681-682
Arcus tendineus, 562-563
Areola of breast, 55
Areolar tissue of scalp, loose, 175
Arm, 309, 342-347
  in anatomic position, 3-4
  brachial vessels of, 346-347
  clinical anatomy of, 346
  compartments of, 342-343
    anterior, 344-346
    formation of, 343
    posterior, 346
  humerus of, 343-344; *see also* Humerus
  medial cutaneous nerve of, brachial
      plexus and, 339
  muscles of, 344-346
  radius of; *see* Radius
  veins of, superficial, 327
Arrector pili muscle, 8, 293, 445
Arteria princeps pollicis, 364
Arteria radicularis magna, 433, 442
Arterial blood gases, 52
Arterial cannulation, alternate site for, 367
Arterial grafts, 593
Arterial pulses at wrist, 377
Arteries; *see also* Blood vessels
  anastomoses between, 71
  of head and neck, 133
    in brain, 158-162
    to scalp, 174-175
    in subarachnoid space, 152
    traversing floor of skull, 140
  of lower limb, 724
    in anterior leg, 696-698
    in anteromedial thigh, 644, 646, 657-658
    in foot, 714-715, 718-719
    in gluteal region, 668
    in hip joint, 644-646
    in knee, 684-685
    in medial thigh, 660-661
    in popliteal fossa, 690, 695
    in posterior leg, 692-696
    in posterior thigh, 674
  of pelvis and perineum, 570, 578, 586-587,
      623
    in anorectal region, 569
    clinical anatomy of, 593
  principles and, 71
  of spinal cord, 439-440, 442
  of thoracic region
    bronchial, 82
    in chest wall, 68-71
    to esophagus, 82, 114, 116
    fetal, 106-107
    to heart, 101-102
    in lungs, 81-85
    to mediastinum, 109-111
  of upper limb
    clinical anatomy of, 328
    to shoulder, 328-329
Arteriography
  celiac, 503

Arteriography—cont'd
  coronary, 93
  femoral, 658
  mesenteric, superior, 513
  popliteal, 685
  pulmonary, 82
  renal, 40, 526
Arterioles, 25, 28
Arteriovenous conduction delay, 104
Arthrodesis, 377
Arthroscopy of knee, 687
Articular capsule, 349
Articular condyle, skull and, 143
Articular disk, 189
  of sternoclavicular joint, 321
  of temporomandibular joint, 189-190
  triangular, 353
Articular facet; *see* Facet, articular
Articular fossa, temporomandibular joint
    and, 190
Articular notch, inferior, 424
Articular surface for rib, 416
Articular tubercle of temporal bone, 135,
    189-190
Articularis genu muscle, 656-657
Articulations between vertebra, 420; *see also*
    Joint
  and ribs, 59-60
Artificial pacing of heart, 105
Aryepiglottic folds, 281-282, 285-286
Aryepiglotticus muscle, 282, 285-286
Arytenoid cartilage, 278, 284-285
Arytenoid muscle
  oblique, 287
    prolongation of, into aryepiglottic fold,
      286
  transverse, 282, 287
ASIS; *see* Iliac spine, anterior superior
Aspiration
  of joint fluid, 669
  of knee joint, 677
  of urine from bladder, 602
Asterion, 134, 137, 140
Asthma, 79
Astigmatism, 237, 251
Atelectasis, 85
Athletic injuries to anteromedial thigh, 662
Atlanto-axial joint, 142, 418
Atlanto-axial membrane, 418
Atlanto-occipital joint, 142, 418
Atlanto-occipital membrane, 412, 418, 421
Atlas, 410, 412-414, 421
  arch of
    anterior, 135, 415
    on MRI, 148, 415
    posterior, 415
  articular facet of, 414
  cranial nerves and, 165
  first-arch syndromes and, 173
  lateral mass of, 142
  ligaments of, 421
    transverse, 418, 433
  muscles and, 426
  spinous process of, 428
    on MRI, 415
  thoracic inlet and, 311
  transverse process of, 142

Atretic follicle, 605
Atria of heart
  appendage of, 94, 97
    on CT, 100
    left, edge of, 77
  on CT and MRI, 42-43, 100
  interior of, 95
  left, 97
    blood flow through, 101-102
    on CT, 100
    edge of, 77
  right, 94-95
    blood flow through, 102
    junction of, with superior vena cava,
      124
  septal defects of, 101
    auscultation of, 124
  sinus venosus junction with, 103
  venous blood into, 101-102
  on x-ray, 53, 77
Atrial septal defect, 101
  auscultation of, 124
Atrial systole or kick, 101
Atrioventricular bundle of His, 95, 103-104
Atrioventricular groove, 89
Atrioventricular nodal artery, 93
Atrioventricular node, 90-91, 103
  atrium and, 95
  conduction system and, 103-104
  position of, 91
Atrioventricular valve of heart, 97-98
Atrium; *see* Atria of heart
Auditory canal, external, 225, 229
  temporomandibular joint and, 190
Auditory cortex, primary, 149
Auditory meatus, 134
  external, 134, 182, 225
    mastication muscles and, 191
    pharyngeal arches and, 172
    skull and, 134, 141
    temporomandibular joint and, 189
  internal, 141
    skull and, 139
Auditory tube, 225, 228-231, 266
  levator veli palatini and, 264
  middle ear and, 225-227
  mucosa of, 211
  orifice of, 266
  otitis and, 232
  skull and, 143
Auerbach's plexus, 520-521
Auricle, 224
Auricular artery, 174-175
  posterior
    anterolateral neck and, 208
    brain and, 159
    as branch of external carotid artery, 209
    face and, 182
    maxillary artery and, 193
    scalp and, 183
Auricular muscle, 178
Auricular nerve, greater
  of cervical plexus, 180, 200
  cervical sympathetic chain and, 215
  face and, 180
  neck and, 202
  parotid gland and, 184

Auricular nerve, greater—cont'd
    pinna of ear and, 225
    sympathetic chain and, 215
Auricular pharyngeal nerve, 211
Auricular vein, posterior
    external jugular vein and, 208-209
    face and, 183
    neck and, 203
    parotid gland and, 185
    pterygoid venous plexus and, 195
    scalp and, 183
Auriculotemporal nerve
    face and scalp and, 178
    otic ganglion and, 194-196
    parotid gland and, 184
    scalp and, 174-175
    temporomandibular joint and, 190
    tympanic membrane and, 225
Auscultation
    of chest, 124
    triangle of, 399
Autodigestion, 480
Autonomic nerves
    ganglia of, 20
    of head and neck, 293
    of lungs and heart, 84
    neurons of, 22, 436
        motor, 22, 26-27
        two-neuron circuit in, 146
    pelvic, 591-593
    spinal cord and, 442-443
    sympathetic division of, 441-446
Autoregulation of blood flow, 133
A-V node; see Atrioventricular node
Avascular necrosis
    of femoral head, 643, 651
    of scaphoid bone, 405
Avulsion fractures at elbow, 352
Axes, rotation around, 7
Axial lines, 16, 18
Axial skeleton, 11-12
Axilla, 330-335
    anatomic position and, 3
    arteries of, 397
        axillary; see Axillary artery
    brachial plexus in, 338-341
    clinical anatomy of, 334
    fascia in, 335
    lymph nodes and, 334-335, 397
    spaces in, 330-333
    veins of, 397
        axillary; see Axillary vein
        superficial, 327
    walls of, 330-331
Axillary artery, 68, 332-334, 397
    aneurysm of, 334
    axilla and, 332
    brachial plexus and, 327
    left, cranial nerves and, 168
Axillary dissection, complete, 334
Axillary fascia, 330
Axillary folds
    anterior, 330, 399
        in anterior view of upper limb, 398
        palpation of, 122
        surface anatomy of, 123
    palpation of, 122

Axillary folds—cont'd
    posterior, 330
        back and, 449
        palpation of, 122
Axillary line, 122
Axillary lymph nodes, 334-335, 397
Axillary nerve, 330, 332, 366, 398
    block of, 334, 403-404
    brachial plexus and, 337-339
    shoulder and, 329
Axillary sheath, 333, 335
    local anesthetic in, 334
Axillary tail of breast, 55, 335
Axillary vein, 55, 327, 329, 334-335, 399
    arm and, 347
Axis, 412-414
    body of, 415
        on MRI, 271, 415
    dens of, 415
    for flexion/extension of elbow joint, 349
    of gaze, 235
    muscles and, 426
    odontoid process of, 135
    of orbit, 235
    spinous process of, 414, 428
        on MRI, 415
    for supination/pronation of elbow joint,
        349
Axon, 20, 23, 145
    afferent
        in central nervous system, 146
        spinal cord and, 435-436
    antidiuretic hormone and, 37
    of brachial plexus, 336
    branchiomotor, 164
    connective tissue and, 24
    of cranial nerves, 164-165, 293
    efferent, 435
    motor, 71, 73
        somatic, 164
        visceral, 164
    with myelin, 21
    oxytocin and, 37
    parasympathetic; see Parasympathetic
        axon
    postganglionic; see Postganglionic axon
    preganglionic; see Preganglionic axon
    sensory, 71, 73
        general, 164
        in heart innervation, 104-106
        special, 164
        visceral, 164
    spinal cord and, 435-436
        of spinal accessory nerve, 213
        synapses in, 442-443
        thoracic, 69
    sympathetic, 25, 71, 164
        otic ganglion and, 196
        in pelvis, 591-592
        postganglionic, 25, 167, 186, 215, 444-
            445, 591-592
        preganglionic, 25, 215, 246, 443, 445-446
    taste, 231
    unmyelinated, 23
Axon hillock, 21
Azygos vein, 71, 121
    arch of, surface projections of, 124

Azygos vein—cont'd
    back and vertebral column and, 430
    bronchus and, 79
    on CT and MRI, 43, 100
    diaphragm and, 531
    esophagus and, 116, 500, 534
    mediastinum and, 117-118
    thoracic duct and, 31, 117
    thoracic spinal cord segment and, 69

B
Babinski reflex, 726
Back and vertebral column, 409-433; see also
        Vertebrae
    anatomy of
        clinical, 431-433
        surface, 449-450
    blood supply of, 427-431
    case studies for, 451-453
    cervical vertebra in, 412-415
    innervation of, 430-431, 449
    lumbar vertebra in, 411, 413-415
    lymphatic drainage of, 449
    muscles of, 423-428, 448
        triangle of, auscultation and, 425
    normal, 409-410
    pain in, 728, 730
        delivery of baby and, 628
    physical examination of, 449-450
    principles for, 419, 423
    sacrum in, 416, 419
    systems review and, 448-449
    thoracic vertebra in, 413, 416-417, 420
    thorax and, 120
    typical vertebra in, 409-413
    vertebral ligaments and articulations in,
        417-424
Baker's cyst, 687
Balance
    organs of, 134
    sensations of, 224
Barium study
    of large intestine, 516
    of small intestine, 509
    of stomach, 502
Baroreceptors, 105
Bartholin's gland, 571, 585
Basal ganglion, 147
    of forebrain, 150
    on MRI, 148
Basal vessels of brain, 157, 160
    oblique view of, 161
Basement membrane in peripheral nervous
        system, 146
Basic terminology, 3-7
Basilar artery, 159, 161
    spinal cord and, 442
Basilar plexus, 157
Basilic vein, 327, 329, 364, 400
    arm and, 347
    axillary vein and, 334
    collection of blood samples and, 367
Basisphenoid, 143
Basivertebral vein, 418
B-cell function, 492
Bell's palsy, 185
Beta receptors, 105

Bicarbonate, pancreatic secretions and, 498
Biceps brachii muscle, 17, 66, 343-344
  anterior compartment and, 344
  in anterior view of upper limb, 398
  long head of, 319-320, 331
    tendon of, 316, 318
  short head of
    axilla and, 331
    on MRI, 323
  tendon of, 318, 354, 400
    on MRI, 323
    radioulnar joint and, 354
    sheath removal from segment of, 320
Biceps femoris brevis muscle; *see* Biceps
     femoris muscle, short head of
Biceps femoris longus muscle, 648
Biceps femoris muscle
  attachment of, 657
  in gluteal region, intermediate layer, 664
  iliotibial band and, 673
  intermuscular septum and, 650
  leg muscles and, 689
  long head of, lower thigh and, 648
  nerves to, 674
  in posterior thigh
    deep view, 675
    superficial view, 673
  posterior view of, 694
  short head of, 657
    lower thigh and, 648
  tendon of, 726
    anterior view of, 697
  thigh and, 648-649
    posterior, 673-674
Bicipital aponeurosis, 400
Bicipital groove, 315, 318
Bicuspid valve; *see* Mitral valve
Bifid rib, 412
Bifid spine, 412-414
  spinal cord and, 438
Bifid ureter, 601
Bifurcate ligament, 707-708
Bifurcation
  of aorta, 478
  of trachea, 52, 77, 87, 109
Bile, 484, 486, 490
Bile duct, 484
  common, 487-488
    liver and, 488
    obstruction of, 543
    peritoneal membranes and, 479
    porta hepatis and, 487
  obstruction of, 490, 543
  principles of, 487
Bile salts, 484
Biliary tree, 488-492
  obstruction of, 490
Bilirubin metabolites in gallstones, 490
Billroth procedures, 506
Bimanual examination of ovary, uterus, and
     nearby structures, 626-627
Biparietal diameter, 556
Bipartite patella, 677
Bipedal locomotion, 423, 714
Bipennate muscle, 17
Birth process; *see* Childbirth
Black eye, 251

Bladder, urinary; *see* Urinary bladder
Blalock-Taussig shunt, 328
Bleeding; *see* Hemorrhage
Blinking of eye, 251
  cornea and, 237
Blood
  in pleural space, 75, 127
  sampling of, 346
  in urine, 541, 544
  volume of, 26
  vomiting of, 541, 544
Blood clots, abdominal wall and, 535
Blood flow
  cerebral; *see* Brain, circulation of
  collateral; *see* Collateral blood flow
  to kidney, factors influencing, 528
  between lungs and heart, 83
  through heart, 101-102
  through liver
    bypassing, 489
    of fetus, 486
    resistance to, 489
Blood gases, 52
Blood pH, carotid body and, 207
Blood pressure, 522
  determinants of, 26
  kidneys and, 528
  location of receptors influencing, 105
  measuring, 346
Blood vessels, 25-29; *see also* Arteries; Veins
  of abdomen, 536-537
  of abdominal wall, 459, 490-461
  of ankle, 703
  of axilla, 332-335
  of back and vertebral column, 427-431,
    448-449
  of breast, 55, 69
  of chest wall, 68-71
  of duodenum, 507-510
  of esophagus, 500
  of eye and orbit, 250
  of face, 175, 181-184
  of femur, 551, 638
    interruption of, 651
  of foot, 714-715, 718-719
    complications of decreased, 721
  of forearm, 363-364
    clinical anatomy of, 367
  of gallbladder, 492
  of hair follicle, 8
  of hand, 391-392
  of head and neck, 292
  of heart, 90-94
  of hip joint, 644-646
  of jejunum and ileum, 511-513
  of kidneys, 524-527
  of knee, 684-685
  of larynx, 289
  of liver, 485, 488-489, 493
  of lower limb, 724
  of lungs, 81-85
    clinical anatomy of, 83
  of mesenteries, development of, 474, 479-
    480
  of orbit, 250
  of palate, 267
  of pancreas, 497-498

Blood vessels—cont'd
  of popliteal fossa, 690, 695
  of rectum, 517
  of scalp, 174-175, 181, 183-184
  of shoulder
    arterial, 326, 328-329
    venous, 327, 329
  smooth muscles of, 19
  of spermatic cord, 469-470
  of spinal cord, 435-436, 439-442, 448-449
  of spleen, 493-494
  of stomach, 501-503
    clinical anatomy of, 506
  supplying nerve, 24
  of testis, 470
  of thigh
    anterior, 644, 646, 654, 657-659
    medial, 660-661
    posterior, 674
  of thorax, 121
  of tongue, 272
  of upper limb, 396-397
  of uterus, 596, 606-607
  of vagina, 596, 606, 608
  of vertebrae, 430, 433, 439-442, 448-449
  of wrist, 372, 375
Blowout fracture, 235
Blurred vision, 300, 304
Bochdalek hernias, 535
Body
  fabric of, 8-20
    bone and cartilage in, 9-11, 13-14
    connective tissue and fascia in, 8-9
    muscles in, 11-20
    skeleton in, 11-14
    skin in, 8
  imaging techniques for, 36-45; *see also*
    Imaging techniques
  planes of, 3-6
  regions of, 3-4
  segmental organization of, 121, 446, 450
  systems of, 20-35
    cardiovascular, 25-30
    endocrine, 35, 37
    gastrointestinal, 30, 35
    lymphatic, 29, 31-33
    nervous, 20-27
    reproductive, 34-36
    respiratory, 29-30, 34
    urinary, 30-35
Bone, 9-11, 13-14
  carpal; *see* Carpal bone
  density of, x-ray detection of, 36
  of foot, 705-707
  growth and maturation of, 10-11
  maturation of, wrist and, 371, 377
  metacarpal, 378-379
  of pelvis, 549-554
  of skull, 136
  tarsal; *see* Tarsal bone
  of upper limb, 309-310
  of wrist; *see* Carpal bone
Bone marrow, 10
  sampling of, from sternum, 63
Bone windows of skull, 142-143
Bony orbit; *see* Orbit, bony
Bony pelvis; *see* Pelvis

Bony rims, 234
Bowleggedness, 640
Brachial arch, 134
Brachial artery, 346-347
    on arteriogram, 345
    from axillary artery, 332-333, 342, 345
    deep, 332, 342, 347, 397
    forearm and, 363
    muscles of arm and, 344
    pulse in, 400
    radioulnar joint and, 354
    surface anatomy of, 397
Brachial nerve, 329, 366
Brachial plexus, 16, 199-201, 336-341
    accessory nerve and, 213
    anatomy of
        clinical, 339
        surface, 397
    in axilla, 330, 337-341
    components of, 336-337
    cords of, 336-338
        lateral, 200, 337, 340-341
        medial, 200, 337, 339-340
    cranial nerves and, 167
    distal branches of, 329, 336-341
    divisions of, 336-337
    embryologic development of, 16
    injury to, 204, 401-402, 404
        upper root, 339
    neck and, 201, 296, 337-338
        posterior triangle of, 199
    nerves of, 337
    organization of neck and, 198
    posterior cords of, 200, 336-339
    prefixed or postfixed, 339
    principles for, 336, 341
    relationship of, to nearby structures, 327
    roots of, 199-202, 336
        cervical sympathetic chain and, 215
        injury to, 339
    structures of, 337
        variations in, 339
    supplying nerves of upper limb, 310
    trunks of, 200, 336-337
Brachial pulse, 400
Brachial vein, 327, 329, 346-347, 354, 364
    arm and, 344, 347
    radioulnar joint and, 354
Brachialis muscle, 17, 318, 343-344, 354
    anterior compartment and, 344-346
    insertion of, 358
Brachiocephalic artery, 101
    aortic arch and, 109-110
    common carotid artery and, 206
Brachiocephalic trunk in MRI, 42
Brachiocephalic vein, 111, 204, 208
    on MRI, 42
    thyroid gland and, 218
Brachioradialis muscle, 344, 359-362, 400
    anterior compartment and, 346
    elbow flexion and, 404
    posterior view of, 399
    surface anatomy of, 398
Brachioradialis reflex, 367
Brain, 145-163
    anatomic features of, 145-147
    central nervous system and, 20

Brain—cont'd
    circulation of
        arterial, 158-162
        clinical anatomy and, 163
        posterior artery in, 160
        regional blood supply in, 147-149
        venous, 154, 157, 160-163
    clinical anatomy of, 151, 163
    critical regions in, 151
    deep structures of forebrain in, 148, 150-153
    fossae or compartments of, 138-140, 149
        anterior, foramen magnum in, 140
        hypophyseal, 160
    functional areas of cerebral cortex in, 149-150
    functional regions of, 151
    gray and white matter in, 147
    herniation of, 155
    lateral view of, 148
    major regions of, 147-149, 154
    meninges and, 145, 152, 154-158
    substance of, subarachnoid space and, 439
    tissue of, scalp and face and, 175
    ultrasound of, 44
    ventricular system of, 145, 150-155
Brain stem, 147-149, 415
    on MRI, 148, 415
    parasympathetic nerves and, 294
    spinal cord and, 442
Brain substance, 152
Branchial arches, 170-173
Branchiomotor axon, 164
Branchiomotor nerve of globe and orbit, 244
Breast, 54-55
    axillary tail of, 55, 335
    cancer of, 56, 126
    clinical anatomy of, 56, 126
    lymphatics of, 56, 121
    physical examination of, 122
    septae of, 54-55
    on x-ray, 53
Breathing, noisy, in newborn, 301
Bregma, 134, 140
Bridging vessels, 170
Broad ligament, 559, 606
Brodmann areas, 149-150
Bronchi
    aorta and, 110
    basal segments of, 100
    on CT and MRI, 42-43, 100
    lobar, 77
    mainstem, 77-79
    mediastinum and, 110
    obstruction of, 79
    at pulmonary hilum, 80
    segments of, 77, 79-80
    on x-ray, 53, 417
Bronchial artery, 81-82, 84, 121
    aortic branches and collaterals of, 500
    posterior mediastinum and, 117
Bronchial vein, 84, 121
Bronchioles, 34
    cranial nerves and, 169
    obstruction of, 79
    terminal, 34
Bronchogenic cyst, 85
Bronchopulmonary segments, 77-79, 100

Bronchoscopy, 85
Buccal branch of facial nerve, 180, 185
Buccal fat pad, 177
Buccal nerve, 193-195
Buccinator muscle, 264, 266, 268-269
    face and scalp and, 178, 180
    parotid gland and, 184
Bucket handle motion in respirations, 66-67
Buck's fascia, 575, 578-579
Bulb
    carotid, 207
    jugular; see Jugular bulb
    of penis; see Penis, bulb of
Bulbar conjunctiva, 250
Bulbocavernosus muscle, 577-578, 615
Bulbospongiosus muscle, 564-565, 577, 580, 615
    innervation of, 578
Bulbourethral gland, 567, 575, 577, 582, 614
Bulla ethmoidalis, 256
Bundle of His, 103
Bundle branch of heart, 95, 104
Bursa, 14
    humerus and, 319-320
    infrapatellar, 679
        on MRI, 418
    olecranon, 351
    omental, 477, 503-505
        development of gut and, 476-479, 481
    prepatellar, 679
        knee and, 677
    subiliac, thigh and, 656
    suprapatellar, 679
        knee and, 677
    of tendon calcaneus, 692
Bursal sac, iliac, 640
Bursitis
    olecranon, 352
    of shoulder joint, 321
Bypass
    of hepatic blood flow, 489
    iliac artery graft and, 593

C

C1; *see* Atlas
C2; *see* Axis
Calcaneal tendon, 702
    blood supply to, 703
    muscles and, 689
    posterior view of, 694
Calcaneocuboid joint, 710
Calcaneocuboid ligament, 707-708
Calcaneofibular ligament, 700, 706
Calcaneonavicular ligament, 707-708, 710
Calcaneus, 700-701, 705-707, 726
    articular surfaces on, 708
    blood supply to, 703
    deltoid ligament and, 702
    ligaments and, 708
    medial view of, 700
    MRI of, 709
    muscles and, 689
    posterior view of, 694
    Pott's fracture and, 704
    sustentaculum tali of, 700-701
    talocalcaneonavicular joint and, 710
    weight bearing and, 712

Calcitonin-secreting cells of thyroid gland, 173
Calcium
  in bones, 9-10
  in gallstones, 490
  kidneys and, 522
Calculi in parotid gland, 185
Calyx of kidneys, 524-525
Camper's fascia, 457
  principles of, 566
Canal
  adductor, thigh and, 656
  Alcock, 568, 589
  anorectal; see Anorectal canal
  auditory, 190, 225, 229
  carotid, 141, 158
  central, 434
  facial, 142-143, 231
  femoral, 558
    femoral sheath and, 653-654
  hypoglossal, 139, 142
  inguinal; see Inguinal canal
  lacrimal, 249
  of Nuck, 472
  optic; see Optic canal
  palatine, 236
  pterygoid, 143
    nerve of, 194, 260-261
  pudendal, 568, 589
  pyloric, 502
  sacral, 416
  semicircular, 226, 228-230, 233
  spinal, 58, 439
    brain and, 150
  subsartorial, 656
  vertebral; see Vertebral canal
  vidian, 143
Cancer
  of breast, 56, 126
  of larynx, 290
  of liver, 489
  pancreatic, 498
  of testis, 469
  uterine, 629, 632
Canine teeth, 188, 267-268
Cannulation
  of femoral vessels, 662, 669
  of vein, 669, 726
Canthus, 241
  lateral, 295
  medial, 249, 295
Capacitance vessels, 26
Capillaries, 25, 28-29
  of alveoli, 34
  in choroid plexus, 152
  in dermis, 8
  pulmonary, 29
Capillary beds, 25, 28-29
Capillary refill time, 400
Capitate, 357, 369-371, 373, 376, 396
  fracture of, 402, 405
  on MRI, 357
  wrist and, 371, 373
Capitellum; see Capitulum of humerus
Capitulum of humerus, 316, 318, 348-350, 394
  elbow movements and, 349
Capsule of kidney, 523

Caput succedaneum, 185
Cardia of stomach, 501-502
Cardiac artery, 444
Cardiac borders, 122-123
Cardiac branches of cervical sympathetic
    ganglia, 113-114
Cardiac catheterization, 328
Cardiac collars, 88
Cardiac conduction system, 103-104
Cardiac cycle, 101-102
  conduction system and, 103
Cardiac impression on lung, 81
Cardiac incisure of stomach, 501-502
Cardiac muscle, 19-20
Cardiac nerve, 84-85, 445
  spinal cord and, 444
Cardiac notch, 81
Cardiac plexus, 97, 104, 109, 114
  lungs and heart and, 84
  mediastinum and, 216
  parasympathetic nerves and, 294
  spinal cord and, 444
Cardiac sphincter, 499
Cardiac surgery, 88
Cardiac transplantation, 105
Cardiac valves; see Heart, valves of
Cardiac vein, 90-94, 121
  anterior, 93
  great, 93
Cardinal ligament, 559, 604, 606
Cardiovascular system, 25-30
Carina, 77
Caroticojugular spine, 143
Carotid artery, 133, 198
  anterolateral neck and, 206-208
  aortic arch and, 101, 110-111
  brain and, 159
  in carotid triangle, 206-207
  common
    aortic arch and, 110-111
    arterial supply to head and neck from,
        133, 292, 296
    ascending aorta and, 101
    bifurcation of, 206-207
    brain and, 159
    branches of external carotid artery and,
        159
    in carotid sheath, 206
    left, 101, 110-111
    subclavian artery and, 203, 326
    thyroid gland and, 218
    vertebral artery and cervical vertebrae
        and, 429
  cranial nerves and, 166
  external, 209, 259
    arterial supply to head and neck from,
        292-293
    branches of, 159, 182, 208
    in carotid sheath, 206
    clinical anatomy of, 215
    maxillary artery and, 193
    parotid gland and, 186
    scalp and, 175, 183
  face and, 182
  internal, 158-159, 162, 208, 259
    arterial supply to head and neck from,
        292-293

Carotid artery—cont'd
    brain and, 157, 160
    maxillary artery and, 192
    middle ear and, 226-228
    on MRI, 271
    orbit and, 250
    skull and, 140
    in wall of cavernous sinus, 259
  middle ear and, 226-228, 233
  special sensory structures in, 206-208
  sympathetic plexus and, 167-168
  thrombosis and embolism in, 215
Carotid bifurcation, 182
  ultrasound images of, 207
Carotid body, 206-208
  anterolateral neck and, 208
  brain and, 159
  glossopharyngeal nerve and, 211
Carotid bulb, 207
Carotid canal, 141, 158
Carotid region, 215
Carotid sheath, 200, 206-207
Carotid sinus, 206
  anterolateral neck and, 208
  brain and, 159
  glossopharyngeal nerve and, 211
Carotid triangle, 198, 201, 206-217
  accessory nerve in, 210, 213
  ansa cervicalis in, 214-216
  carotid arteries in, 206-208
  cervical sympathetic chain in, 215-217
  clinical anatomy of, 215
  glossopharyngeal nerve in, 209-212
  hypoglossal nerve in, 210, 213-214
  jugular vein in, 208-209
  lymphatic drainage in, 209-210
  vagus nerve in, 210-213
Carpal bone, 309, 369-374, 396
  anatomic position of, 3
  anterior view of, 12
  growth and maturation of, 11
Carpal tunnel, 369
  flexor retinaculum and, 371
Carpal tunnel syndrome, 376, 403, 405
  hand and, 392
Carpometacarpal joints, 309, 372, 396
  phalanges and, 378
  of thumb, 370, 380-381
  two to five, 379-380
Carrying angle of forearm, 351
Cartilage, 9-11, 13-14
  costal, 50, 60-61
    anterior view of, 12
  hyaline, 11, 14
  of larynx, 278, 285
  of nose, 177, 253
  in trachea, 77
Cartilaginous anlage, 10
Cartilaginous joint, 10-11, 13
Caruncle, lacrimal, 249
Cataract, 239, 251
Catheter
  bladder, 602
  cardiac, shoulder veins and, 328
  in great vessels, 119
Cauda equina, 416, 439-440, 453
  in dural sac, 423, 430

Cauda equina—cont'd
  lower
    dorsal roots and, 440
    ventral roots and, 440
  on MRI, 418
  sacral anesthesia and, 553
Caudal block, 560, 593
Caudal lumbar thecal sac, 418
Caudate lobe of liver, 485, 487
  of fetus, 486
Caudate nucleus, ultrasound of, 44
Cavernous sinus, 157, 160, 162
  internal carotid artery in wall of, 259
  orbit and, 250
  sphenoid sinuses and, 258
  venous blood into, 292
Cavities
  abdominal, apertures of, 531
  cranial; see Cranial cavity
  joint, for femoral head, 641
  marrow, 10
  of middle ear, 228
    floor of, 229
  nasal; see Nasal cavity; Nose
  oral; see Oral cavity
  orbital, 176
  parietal layer of, 51
  pericardial, 86-88
  pleural, 51, 74-76
    lungs and, 474
    recesses in, 75, 77, 80, 493
    as serous cavities, 49
  serous; see Serous cavities
  in thorax, 49-51
  visceral layer of, 51
Cavum trigeminale, 165
Cecum, 517-518
  anorectal region and, 516-517
  development of, 478
  ileocecal junction and, 511
  peritoneal specialization of, 482-483
  in x-ray, 39
Celiac artery, 479, 494
  abdomen and, 534, 536
  arteriogram of, 503
  clinical anatomy of, 506
  esophagus and, 116
  gastrointestinal tract and, 477
  left gastric branch of, 116
  spinal cord and, 445
  spleen and, 493
  stomach and, 501-502
Celiac axis, 526
Celiac ganglion, 537
  spinal cord and, 445
Celiac plexus, 294
Cell
  of cardiac conduction system, 103
  in connective tissue, 8
  hematopoietic, 10
  of nervous system, 20-24
Cell body of neuron, 20, 146
  spinal cord and, 436
Central nervous system, 20
  axons of, 23
  brain in, 145-163; see also Brain
  clinical anatomy of, 151

Central process of neuron, 20, 146, 436
  short, 435
  spinal nerves and, 164
Central slip of tendon, 384, 390
Central venous catheter, 125, 127
Cephalic vein, 327, 329, 354, 364, 400
  anterior view of, 398
  arm and, 347
  axillary vein and, 334
  collection of blood samples and, 367
Cephalohematoma, 185
Cerebellar artery, 159
  inferior
    anterior, 159, 161
    posterior, 159, 161
    superior, 159, 161
Cerebellar hemisphere, 143
Cerebellar tonsil, 415
  on MRI, 148, 415
Cerebellomedullary cistern, 148
Cerebellum, 147-153, 161
  cranial nerves and, 165
  nodule of, on MRI, 148
  ultrasound of, 44
Cerebral aqueduct, 150-151, 153
Cerebral artery, 159
  anterior, 158-159
  clinical anatomy of, 163; see also Brain,
    circulation of
  middle, 160
  posterior, 159, 161
Cerebral cortex, 145, 147-150
Cerebral hemisphere, 142
Cerebral peduncles of midbrain, 148
Cerebral sinus, 134, 157-158, 162-163, 292; see
    also Ventricles, cerebral
  arachnoid villi in, 152
  confluence of, 139, 154, 157-158, 162
  intercavernous, 157
  meningitis and, 262
  sagittal, 154, 157-158, 161-162
    inferior, 154
    in lower margin of falx, 154
    superior, 154, 161
  sphenoparietal, 157, 162
  straight, 154, 157, 162
  transverse, 134, 139-140, 157-158, 161-
    162
    left, 157
    on MRI, 148
Cerebral vein, 161-163
  clinical anatomy of, 163
  of Galen, 154
  inferior or internal, 151, 157, 162
  middle, 157, 161-162
Cerebral venous sinus; see Cerebral sinus
Cerebral ventricle
  body of, 150
  ultrasound of, 44
Cerebrospinal fluid, 145
  choroid plexus and, 152
  clinical anatomy of, 153
  on MRI, 418
  removal of, 153, 155, 447
  subarachnoid space and, 152
  in ventricular system, 153-155
Ceruminous gland, 225

Cervical artery
  ascending, 429
    spinal cord and, 442
    subclavian artery and, 203, 326
  deep
    back and spinal cord and, 448
    subclavian artery and, 203
  spinal cord and vertebrae and, 440
  subclavian artery and, 203
  superficial, 202-204, 329
  transverse, 204, 329
Cervical branch of facial nerve, 180, 185
Cervical curvature, 409-410
Cervical cyst, 173
Cervical epithelium, 610
Cervical expansion on MRI, 415
Cervical fascia, 198-200
  axilla and, 333
  clinical anatomy of, 215
Cervical ganglion
  cranial nerves and, 168
  inferior, 444
    spinal cord and, 445
    sympathetic chain and, 215
  mediastinum and, 216
  middle, 186, 444
    spinal cord and, 444-445
    sympathetic chain and, 215, 336
  superior, 186, 444
    spinal cord and, 444-445
    sympathetic chain and, 215
Cervical ligament, transverse, 559, 604, 607
Cervical lymph node, 134
  anterior, 210
  tongue and, 272
Cervical muscle, nerves to
  anterior, 202
  sympathetic chain and, 215
Cervical nerves; see also Cervical plexus
  roots of
    cranial; see Cranial nerves
    spinal; see Neck, spinal roots and
    subclavian artery and, 203
  shoulder and, 329
Cervical pleura, 74
Cervical plexus
  ansa cervicalis and, 214
  anterolateral neck and, 215
  auricular nerve of, 180
  motor fibers of, 293
  posterior neck triangle and, 200, 202
  scalp innervation by, 174-175
  surface anatomy of, 296
Cervical region, trauma to, 431
Cervical ribs, 62, 328, 412
Cervical sinus, 172-173
Cervical spinal cord
  body of, 438
  in situ, 438
  on MRI, 148
  segments of, providing head and neck
    innervation, 177
Cervical sympathetic chain, 167-168
  in carotid triangle, 215-217
  ganglia of
    cardiac branches of, 113-114
    middle, 336

Cervical sympathetic chain—cont'd
  lungs and heart and, 84
Cervical vein, deep, 449
Cervical vertebra, 409-415
  anterior view of, 12, 414
  articular facets of, 415
  articulations of, 420
  atlas as; see Atlas
  axis as; see Axis
  body of, 414-415
  C3 to C7, 413, 415
  first, 135, 142
    on MRI, 148
  lateral x-ray of, 415
  longitudinal muscles and, 292
  as movable bones, 133
  on MRI, 415
  posterior neck triangle and, 198
  second, 135
  spinous process of, 412-415, 428
  tubercle of, 415
  on x-ray, 417
Cervicothoracic ganglion, 113
Cervix, uterine, 606-611
  os of, 607
  pregnancy and, 610
  prolapse and, 585
  on ultrasound, 612
Cesarean section, 144, 608
Chalazion, 251
Chambers of eye, 239
  anterior, 239-240, 250
  posterior, 239-240
Charcot joints, 684
Charley-horse, 662
Check ligament, 242
Cheek and constituent parts, 268-269
Cheekbone, 142
Chemoreceptors, 52
Chest
  auscultation of, 124
  cross-sectional imaging of, 100
  wall of; see Chest wall
  x-ray of
    lateral, 53
    posteroanterior, 38, 53
Chest wall, 49-50, 54-73
  anatomy of
    clinical, 72
    surface, 123
  blood vessels of, 68-71
    venous drainage of, 121
  breast and, 54-55
  case studies and, 125, 127
  clavicle and, 59, 61-62
  costal cartilages and, 50, 60-61
  intercostal nerves of, 71-72
  intercostal space of, 65, 72-73
  movement of, 65-68
  muscles of, 64-68
  nerves of, 121-122
  principles and, 68, 71, 73
  respiration and, 65-68
  ribs and, 50, 60-61
  scapula and, 59, 61-62
  sternum and, 62-63
  structure of, 50, 55-59, 61, 66

Chest wall—cont'd
  thoracic vertebrae and, 58-60
Chewing, 177
Child
  cranial vault of, 138
  face of, 138
  fontanelle of, 138
  septal defects in, 101
  skull of, 136, 138
Childbirth
  abdominal musculature and, 462
  anesthesia for, 628-629, 631
  back pain and, 628
  injury in
    brachial plexus, 339, 401-402, 404
    perineal, 620, 630-631
    shoulder, 319
    vaginal, 584
  pelvic diaphragm and, 631
  skull in, 144
Choanae, 253, 279
Cholecystectomy, 490, 492
Cholecystitis, 490
Cholecystostomy, 490
Cholesteatoma, 232
Cholesterol, 484
  in gallstones, 490
Cholinergic receptors, 105
Chondrosternal joint, 449
  synovial, 321
Chorda tympani nerve, 170, 228, 270
  facial nerve and, 171, 231
  malleus and, 230
  middle ear and, 227-229, 232
  parasympathetic nerves and, 294
  in submandibular triangle, 222
  in temporal and infratemporal fossae, 187
  tongue and, 272
Chordae tendineae, 95, 97-99
  false, 98
Chordee of penis, 620
Choroid layer of eye, 235, 238
Choroid plexus, 152
  brain and, 152
  formation of, 155
  ultrasound of, 44
Chylothorax, 75, 114
Ciliaris muscle, 239-240
  head and neck and, 292
  innervation of, 169
Ciliary artery
  long, 237, 250
  short, 250
Ciliary body, 239
  orbit and, 250
  uveal layer of eye and, 238
Ciliary ganglion, 245, 247-248
  in orbit, 169
  otic ganglion in, 195
  parasympathetic nerves and, 294
Ciliary nerve
  long, 245, 247
  short, 245, 248
Ciliary zonule, 238-239
Ciliated epithelium, pseudostratified, 8
Cimetidine, 506
Cingulate gyrus, 148

Circle of Willis, 158-159, 161-162, 292
  clinical anatomy of, 163
Circulation; see Blood vessels
Circulus arteriosus, 158-159, 161-162, 292
  clinical anatomy of, 163
Circumcision, 575, 580
Circumduction
  of thumb, 381, 384-385
  of wrist, 370
Circumflex artery, 92
  femoral
    lateral, 658-659, 668, 684
    medial, 658-659, 668
  humeral
    anterior, 332, 334
    axilla and, 330, 332
    posterior, 330, 332, 334
  obtuse marginal branch of, 93
  scapular, 320, 334
    axilla and, 332
Circumflex vein
  humeral, 330
  thigh and, 653
Circumvallate papilla, 270
Cistern, pontine, 151
Cisterna ambiens, 151
Cisterna chyli, 115, 117, 512
  thoracic duct and, 31
Cisterna magna, 151, 154
  on MRI, 148
Clavicle, 61-62, 331, 394, 398
  anterior view of, 12, 398
  anterolateral neck and, 216
  articular facet of, 62
  articulations of, 61
  axilla and, 330-331
  brachial plexus and, 327
  chest wall and, 59, 61-62
  fracture of, 317
  growth and maturation of, 11
  head of, 216
  joints of, 318-322
  palpation of, 122
  in posterior neck triangle, 199
  shoulder girdle and, 309-311, 313-315, 317, 319
  sternoclavicular joint and, 321
  structural features of, 645
  surface anatomy of, 123, 295
  thoracic cage and, 50, 120
  thoracic inlet and, 59
  on x-ray, 312-313
Clavicular artery, 334
Clavipectoral fascia, 327, 335
  axilla and, 330
  axillary vein and, 334
Claw hand, 339-340, 392
Cleavage lines of Langer, 457
Cleft
  internuclear, on MRI, 418
  pharyngeal, 170-173
Cleft lip, 275
Cleft palate, 173, 275
Clinoid process, 139
  horizontal section through bony orbit and, 237
Clitoris, 571, 574, 577, 609

Clitoris—cont'd
  crus of, 573, 576
  frenulum of, 573, 576
  glans of, 576
  prepuce of, 572-573, 576
Clivus, 135
  on MRI, 148, 415
Cluneal nerve, inferior, 583
Coarctation of aorta, 129
Coccygeal vertebra, 409-410, 552; see also
    Coccyx
  first, 553
Coccygeus muscle, 562-565
  diaphragm and, 532
  gluteal region and, 671
Coccyx; see also Coccygeal vertebra
  bony pelvis and, 549-550, 552-553, 559
  on CT, 618
  in female, 574, 606
  gluteal region and, 663
  sacral anesthesia and, 553
  sacral plexus and, 590
  urogenital and anal triangles and, 562
  views of, 410
Cochlea, 226, 228-230
  inner ear and, 233
Colic artery
  middle, 511
    cecum and, 518
    transverse colon and, 518
  right, 511
    cecum and, 518
  small intestine and, 512-513
Colic flexure of colon
  left
    abdomen and, 492
    anorectal region and, 516
  right, 516
    pancreas and, 496
Colitis, ulcerative, 520
Collagen fibers, 8-9
Collagenous nodule
  in aortic valve, 99
  in pulmonary valve, 97
Collateral artery, superior ulnar, 332
Collateral blood flow, 479
  in posterior triangle, 204
  ribs and, 72
  of shoulder, 328
Collateral ligament
  fibular, 676, 679, 681-682, 691
    musculoskeletal system and, 722
  of interphalangeal joints, 379, 381
  of metacarpophalangeal joint, 379,
    381
  radial, 349, 351, 353, 369, 374
    wrist and, 372, 374
  tibial, 676, 679, 681-682, 691
    musculoskeletal system and, 722
    superior end of tibia and, 680
  ulnar, 349, 351, 353, 369, 374
    bands of, 353
    wrist and, 372, 374
Colles' fascia, 565, 567, 574-575, 619
  principles of, 566
Colles' fracture, 351, 402, 405
Colliculus, seminal, 582

Colon, 515-521
  anorectal canal and; see Anorectal canal
  ascending, 477, 517-518
    anorectal region and, 515-516
    on CT, 41
    ileocecal junction and, 511
    peritoneal membranes and, 478
    small intestine and, 508, 512
    in x-ray, 39
  barium study of, 516
  cecum and, 517-518
  clinical anatomy of, 520
  colic flexure of, 516
  descending, 516, 518-519
    anorectal region and, 516-517
    on CT, 41
    gastrointestinal tract and, 477
    pancreas and, 496
    peritoneal membranes and, 478
    small intestine and, 508, 512
    in x-ray, 39
  form and function of, 515-517
  hepatic flexure of, 516
  innervation of, 520-521
  parasympathetic nerves and, 294, 446
  peritoneal reflections and, 516-517
  peritoneal specialization of, 482-483
  sigmoid, 516-517, 519
    anorectal region and, 516-517
    gastrointestinal tract and, 477
    rectum and, 517
  splenic flexure of, 516
  transverse, 516, 518
    anorectal region and, 515-517
    pancreas and, 496
    peritoneal membranes and, 481
    small intestine and, 512
    vermiform appendix and, 518
Columnar epithelium in trachea, 77
Commissures, 95, 97
  on MRI, 148
Common carotid artery; see Carotid artery,
    common
Communicating artery, 159-160
Communicating hydrocephalus, 155
Communicating rami; see Gray rami
    communicans; Ramus; White rami
    communicans
Compartment
  of anteromedial thigh, 646-650
  of arm; see Arm, compartments of
  of brain, 149
  in femoral sheath, 653
  of knee, 679
  of leg; see Leg, compartments of
  in palm, fascial, 389
  of wrist, 375
Compartment syndrome
  in lower limb, 698, 731
  in upper limb, 343, 351
Compression
  of forearm nerves, 351
  spinal cord, 447
Compression fractures of vertebral bodies,
    431
Computerized tomography
  of chest, 100

Computerized tomography—cont'd
  MRI compared to, 43
  of skull base, 142
  techniques of, 38-39, 41
Conchae, 222, 255
  inferior, 254, 256-257, 265, 281
  middle, 254-257, 265
  superior, 254-255, 257
Conduction system of heart, 103-104
Condylar process
  of mandible, 188-190
  pharynx and, 277
  submandibular triangle and, 220
Condyle
  of femur, 641
    anteromedial thigh and, 637-640
    lateral, 637-641, 676, 678
    medial, 637-640, 676, 678, 683
    posterior leg nerves and, 696
    thigh and knee and, 672
  mandibular, 135, 143
  occipital, 141-142
  of tibia
    lateral, 678, 690
    medial, 678
Cone of light, 225-226
Confluence of sinuses, 139, 154, 157-158, 162
Congenital cysts in neck, 223
Congenital deformities; see Deformities,
    congenital
Congenital diaphragmatic hernia, 535, 544
  principles of, 463
Congenital heart disease, 104
Congenital inguinal hernia, 467
Congenital megacolon, 520
Conjugate diameter, 550, 556
Conjunctiva, 241
  bulbar, 250
  infection and inflammation in, 251
  palpebral, 250
Conjunctival membrane, 239, 250, 295
Connective tissue, 8-9
  of brain cells, 145
  of breast, 54
  in dermis, 8
  neural tissue and, 20, 24
  scalp and face and, 175
  spinal cord and, 434-436
Conoid ligament, 319
Consciousness loss in head trauma, 298, 302-
    303
Constrictor muscle
  inferior, 219, 269, 277-280
  middle, 269, 277, 279-280
    tongue and, 272
  superior, 266, 269, 277, 279-280
Continence, urinary, 598, 600
Contraction of muscle, 15
  heart ventricles and, 101-102
  isometric, 423
Contralateral structure, 6
Conus medullaris, 156, 434, 439
  cauda equina and, 440
  on MRI, 418
Conventional x-ray imaging techniques, 36-
    40
Convergence of eyes, 251

Copula, 171
Coracobrachialis muscle, 318, 343-344
  anterior compartment and, 344-345
  axilla and, 330-331
  on MRI, 323
Coracoclavicular joint, 61
Coracoclavicular ligament, 313-314, 317, 319
  torn, 401, 403
Coracoid fossa, 314
Coracoid process
  of scapula, 398
Coracoid process of scapula, 311-317, 398
  on x-ray, 313
Cornea, 235, 237, 239
  aqueous and vitreous humors and, 240
  ciliary body and, 239
  lubrication of, 185
  refractive errors and, 240, 251
  uveal layer of eye and, 238
Corneal reflex, 247, 251
Corneal ulceration, 185
Corneal-scleral junction, 242
Corniculate cartilage, 278, 286
Corona, 579, 582
Coronal plane, 3, 6
Coronal suture, 134-138
Coronary artery, 90-94, 121
  anterior view of, 91
  aortic sinus origin of, 101
  arteriograms of, 93
  branches of, 92
  clinical anatomy of, 94
  on CT, 100
  diagonal, 93
  interventricular, 89, 93
  left, 92-93
    nodal artery and, 103
  nodal artery and, 103
  posterior view of, 91-92
  right, 90-93
    nodal artery and, 103
Coronary ligament, 486
  knee joint and, 679
  stomach and, 505
Coronary sinus, 92, 94, 121
  atrium and, 95
  valve of, 94
  venous blood into, 101-102
Coronary vein
  anterior view of, 91
  arteriograms of, 93
  branches of, 92
  posterior view of, 91-92
Coronary vessels; *see* Coronary artery;
    Coronary vein
Coronoid fossa, 316, 318, 349
Coronoid process
  of mandible
    pharynx and, 277
    submandibular triangle and, 220
    temporal and infratemporal fossa and,
      188-189
  skull and, 135
  of ulna, 348-349, 354
    on x-ray, 350
Corpora cavernosum, 573, 577-579, 615
Corpus albicans, 605

Corpus callosum, 148, 151
Corpus cavernosum, 565, 567, 573, 576-577,
    579-582
  on CT, 618
Corpus luteum, 605
Corpus spongiosum, 575-577, 579-580, 615,
    619
Corrugator cutis ani muscle, 568
Cortex, 605
  of adrenal glands, 527
  cerebral, 145, 147-150
  renal, 522
    narrowed, 597
Cortical bone, 415
Cortical vein, 157, 161-162
Cortisol, excess, 528
Costal angle, 50, 122-123
Costal cartilage, 50, 60-61, 321
  anterior view of, 12
  first, 61
  second, 62
Costal element of rib, 412
Costal groove, 65, 71-73
Costal margin, 49-50
  abdomen and, 457, 536
Costal pleura, 74
Costal process, 410, 438
Costal surface of lung, 80-81
Costocervical trunk, 68, 202-204, 429
  subclavian artery and, 203, 326
Costochondral joint, 449
Costoclavicular ligament, 321
  clavicle and, 313
Costoclavicular syndrome, 330
Costodiaphragmatic angle, 77
Costodiaphragmatic recess, 75, 77, 80, 493
Costomediastinal recess, 75, 77, 80
Costophrenic angle, 77
Costophrenic recess, 75, 77, 80
Costotransverse facet, 411, 416, 420, 424
Costotransverse joint, 58-59, 423-424
Costovertebral articular surfaces, 60
Costovertebral facet, 411, 420, 424
Costovertebral joint, 59-60, 422, 424
Cowper's gland, 575
Coxa valgum, 640
Coxa varum, 640
Crackling sounds in lungs, 124
Cranial base, 134
Cranial cavity
  arteries in, 158
  floor of, 138-140
  fossae or compartments of, 149
    middle ear and, 226
    orbit and, 234
Cranial dura, 437
Cranial nerves, 145, 164-169
  I; *see* Olfactory nerve (I)
  II; *see* Optic nerve (II)
  III; *see* Oculomotor nerve (III)
  IV; *see* Trochlear nerve (IV)
  V; *see* Trigeminal nerve (V)
  VI; *see* Abducens nerve (VI)
  VII; *see* Facial nerve (VII)
  VIII; *see* Vestibulocochlear nerve (VIII)
  IX; *see* Glossopharyngeal nerve (IX)
  X; *see* Vagus nerve (X)

Cranial nerves—cont'd
  XI; *see* Accessory nerve (XI)
  XII; *see* Hypoglossus nerve (XII)
  components of, 164
  ear and, 231
  functional categories of axons in, 164-165
  head and neck and, 293
    sympathetic innervation of, 167-169
  lower, 210
  parasympathetic outflow from, 294
  pharynx and, 282
  principles of, 169
  reflexes mediated by, 247
  sensory ganglia of, 164-168
Cranial vault, 134-135, 139
  of adult, 138
  bones of, 291
  of child, 138
  foramen of, 134
  inscriptions on, 134
  size ratio of, to face, 136, 138
Craniosacral outflow, 445
Cremaster muscle, 466
  abdomen and, 537
  inguinal canal in male and, 465
Cremasteric reflex, 462, 469, 625, 726
Crests of ilia, 538
Cribriform fascia of thigh, 651
Cribriform plate of ethmoid bone, 139, 141,
    254-256
Cricoarytenoid muscle
  lateral, 282, 285-286
  posterior, 282, 285-286
Cricoid cartilage
  cranial nerves and, 166
  head and neck and, 295
  lamina of, 285
  larynx and, 284-285
  mouth and palate and, 266, 269
  nerve supply of cartilage and, 288
  pharynx and, 277-278
  submandibular gland and, 221
  trachea and, 77
Cricopharyngeus muscle, 116, 269, 277-278,
    280
Cricothyroid membrane, 285
  cranial nerves and, 166
  nerve supply of cartilage and, 288
Cricothyroideus muscle, 269, 277, 285-286
  oblique part of, 285
  thyroid gland and, 218
Crista ampullaris, 233
Crista galli, 255-256
Crista terminalis, 94
Crohn's disease, 514
Cruciate anastomosis, 645, 668
  gluteal region and, 668
  thigh and, 659, 668
Cruciate ligament
  anterior, 676
    knee joint and, 679, 681-682
    rupture of, 730
    superior end of tibia and, 680
  knee joint and, 681
  knee movements and, 682
  musculoskeletal system and, 722
  posterior, 676

Cruciate ligament—cont'd
    knee joint and, 679, 681-682
        superior end of tibia and, 680
    rupture of, 687
    thigh and knee and, 672
Cruciate pulleys, 389
Cruciate retinaculum, superficial view of,
    714
Cruciform ligament, 418, 421
Crura; see Crus
Crus
    of clitoris, 573, 576
    of corpus cavernosum, 573
        on CT, 618
        inguinal canal and, 464
    of diaphragm, 529-530
        pancreas and, 496
        spleen and, 493
    of penis, 576, 582
Cubital fossa, 342, 347, 400
Cubital vein, median, 400
Cuboid bone, 700-701, 705-707
    MRI of, 709
Culdoscopy, 610
Cuneiform bone, 705-707
    cartilage and, 286
    deltoid ligament and, 702
    intermediate
        MRI of, 709
    lateral, 700-701
        MRI of, 709
    medial, 700
        metatarsus adductus and, 720
        MRI of, 709
        talocalcaneonavicular joint and, 710
Cuneonavicular ligament, plantar, 708
Curvatures of stomach, 501-502
Cusps, 267
    of aortic valve, 98-99
    of mitral valve, 97-98
    of pulmonary valve, 97
    of tricuspid valve, 95
Cutaneous branch
    of intercostal arteries, 121
    of intercostal nerves, 121
    of median nerve, palmar, 368
Cutaneous innervation
    of forearm, 367-368
        lateral, 333, 341, 368
        medial, 333, 337, 339, 368
        posterior, 367-368
    of lower limb, 638
        femoral, 557, 589, 671, 725
        in gluteal region, 671
        lateral, 638
        perforating, 671
        in posterior thigh, 674
    of pelvic region, 625
    of upper limb, 398, 400
        antebrachial, 366
        brachial, 366
        in forearm; see Cutaneous innervation,
            of forearm
Cyclist's hand, 377
Cyst
    Baker's, 687
    bronchogenic, 85

Cyst—cont'd
    cervical, 173
        congenital, 223
    pancreatic, 543
    pharyngeal, 173
    salivary duct, 275
    thyroglossal duct, 218
        ectopic thyroid tissue and, 275
Cystic artery, 492
Cystic duct, 488, 490
    liver and, 487-488
    peritoneal membranes and, 479
Cystic remnants, 275
Cystourethrogram, voiding, 617, 620

D

Dacryocystitis, 251
Dartos tunic, 469
Deafness
    otosclerosis in, 230
    stapes and, 232
Deciduous teeth, 267
    eruption of, 269
Deep position of structure, 3
Defecation, 569
Deformities
    of ear and palate, 170
    in foot, 720-721
    in hand, 392
    of vertebral column, 431
Deglutition, 276, 281-282
Delivery; see Childbirth
Deltoid artery, 333
Deltoid ligament
    ankle and, 700, 702
    popliteal fossa and, 691
    stress injury of, 731
    weight bearing and, 712
Deltoid muscle, 343-344, 394, 398-399
    anterior compartment and, 345
    anterior trunk and, 66, 398
    attachments of, to scapula and clavicle, 62
    axilla and, 332
    back musculature and, 326, 425, 449
    brachial plexus and, 338
    clavicle and, 313
    on MRI, 323
    posterior trunk and, 65, 399
    shoulder movement and, 325-326
    veins of arm and axilla and, 327
Deltoid tuberosity, 315, 318, 399
    anterior compartment and, 345
Deltopectoral groove, 327, 329, 399
    anterior view of, 398
Deltopectoral triangle, 329
Demifacet, 60, 416
Dendrite, 20-21
Denonvillier's fascia, 575
Dens, 412, 414-415, 421; see also Odontoid
    ligaments of, 421
    on MRI, 148, 415
    skull and, 135, 142
Denticulate ligament, 156, 437
    spinal cord and, 438
Dentine, 268
Depressor anguli oris muscle, 178
Depressor labii inferioris muscle, 178

Dermatocranium, 136
Dermatomes, 22, 27
    abdominal wall and, 462
    brachial plexus and, 341
    chest wall and, 122
    cutaneous innervation and, 624
    head and neck and, 293
    lower limb and, 638, 725
    in pelvic region, 624-625
    spinal cord and, 447
    upper limb and, 398
Dermis, 8
Descendens cervicalis nerve, 168, 202
    cervical sympathetic chain and, 215
Descendens hypoglossi nerve, 168, 202
    ansa cervicalis nerve and, 215
Descending aorta; see Aorta, descending
Descending artery, anterior, 92
Descending colon; see Colon, descending
Descent
    of ovary in inguinal canal, 472
    of testis, 471-472
Detrusor muscle, 581, 597-598
    of bladder wall, 600
    pelvis and perineum and, 624
    urination and, 600
Dextrocardia, 89
Diabetes mellitus, 498
Diameters, pelvic, 550
Diaphragm
    membranes and
        peritoneal, 481
        serous, 474
    pelvic; see Pelvic diaphragm
    thoracic, 49, 529-530
        abdomen and, 529, 536
        on chest x-ray, 53, 77
        crus of, 492-493, 496, 529-530
        on CT, 41
        fetus in utero and, 611
        inferior view of, 530
        innervation of, 530
        liver and, 485
        mediastinum and, 52
        pancreas and, 496
        pelvic diaphragm compared to, 532
        position of, 115
        in respirations, 66-67
        spleen and, 493
        sternum and, 63, 65
        structures traversing, 530-531
        surface anatomy of, 123
        thoracic duct and, 31
    urogenital; see Urogenital diaphragm
Diaphragma sellae, 157-158
Diaphragmatic crura, 492-493, 496, 529-530
Diaphragmatic hernia, congenital, 535, 544
    principles of, 463
Diaphragmatic pleura, 74
Diaphragmatic surface of lung, 81
Diaphysis, 10
Diastole, 92
    aortic valve in, 98
    cardiac cycle and, 101-102
    pulmonary valve in, 97
Diencephalon, 147
    on MRI, 148

Digastric muscle, 17, 184, 218-221
  anterior belly of, 220
  on MRI, 271
  posterior belly of, 280
  submandibular gland and, 221
  submandibular triangle and, 220
DiGeorge syndrome, 173
Digestion
  cranial nerves and, 169
  pancreatic secretions and, 498
Digestive enzymes, 480
Digestive system; *see also* Gastrointestinal
    tract
  cranial nerves and, 169
  smooth muscles of, 17-19
Digit
  muscle insertions on individual, 387-388
  musculoskeletal system and, 723
Digital artery
  in foot, 715, 718
  in hand, 364, 391-392
Digital bands of sole of foot, 708
Digital nerve, proper, 366
Digital vein, common, 715
Dilator pupillae, 237, 239
  sympathetic nerve to, 246
Diplöe, 135
Diploic vein, 183
Diplopia, 251
Disk
  articular; *see* Articular disk
  intervertebral; *see* Intervertebral disk
Dislocation
  of elbow, 352
  of glenohumeral joint, 317
  of hip, 647, 651, 669
  of lens, 251
  of lunate, 376
  of radial head, 352
  of shoulder, 317
  of temporomandibular joint, 197, 295
Distal position of structure, 3, 5
Diverticulosis, 520
Diverticulum, Meckel's, 542
Dorsal plane, 3-6
Dorsal position of structure, 5
Dorsal spinal nerve root, 24, 164
  cauda equina and, 440
  ganglia in; *see* Ganglia, dorsal root
  neck and, 200, 203-204
  segmentation of body organization and,
    446
Dorsal surface, 6
Dorsalis pedis artery, 715, 724
  dorsum of foot and, 715
  leg and, 698
  pulse in, 726
  transverse section of, 718
Dorsalis penis artery, 579, 582
Dorsalis penis vein, 577, 579
  deep, 577, 579
Dorsum sellae, 135
Double saddle joint, 381
Douglas
  fossa of, 604
  pouch of, 558
Douglas, fossa of, 604

Dub sounds of heart, 104, 124
Duct
  bile; *see* Bile duct
  of bulbourethral gland, 614
  cystic; *see* Cystic duct
  ejaculatory, 613-615
  of gallbladder, 488
  genital, 34
  hepatic; *see* Hepatic duct
  lacrimal, 249, 251
  lactiferous, 54
  of liver, 488
  lymph, subclavian, 335; *see also* Lymphatic
    drainage
  nasolacrimal, 249
  of pancreas; *see* Pancreatic duct
  parotid, 178-179, 183
  prostatic, 613-614, 616
  of reproductive system, 34-35
  salivary, cyst of, 275
  of Santorini, 497
  submandibular, 221-222, 269, 272-273, 296
  thoracic; *see* Thoracic duct
  thyroglossal, 171, 218, 275
  Wharton, 221, 273
  of Wirsung, 496
Ductuli efferenti, 471
Ductus arteriosus, 106
  patent, 104, 106-108
Ductus deferens, 35-36, 613-615
  abdomen and, 459
  autonomic innervation of, 592
  inguinal canal and, 464-465, 471-472
  posterior surface of bladder and, 596
  scrotum and, 471-472
  on seminal vesiculogram, 615
  in spermatic cord, 467
  testis and epididymis and, 468, 471
  umbilical ligaments and, 557
  ureter and, 594
  urogenital diaphragm and, 567
Ductus venosus, 106-107
  closure of, 108
  fetal liver and, 486
Duodenal cap, 502
Duodenal papilla
  greater or major, 487, 494, 497
  lesser or minor, 494, 497
  pancreas and, 495
Duodenum, 30, 477, 507-510
  blood supply to, 507-510
    venous drainage of, 480
  body of, 508
  on CT, 41
  development of, 478-479
  greater curvature of, 508
  kidneys and, 524
  liver and, 488
  obstruction of, 510
  pancreas and, 496
  pathology of, 510
  peritoneal membranes and, 481
  peritoneal specialization of, 482
  small intestine and, 509
  stomach and, 504
  structural deviations of, 507, 509
Dupuytren's contracture, 392

Dura mater, 20
  brain and, 152, 154-158
  displaced inward, 196
  reflections of, 154
  scalp and face and, 175
  sensory axons in, 147
  spinal cord and, 434, 437-438, 453
  subarachnoid space and, 439
Dural sac, cauda equina in, 423, 430
Dural sheath
  on dorsal root ganglion, 438
  lined with arachnoid mater, 440
Dysphagia, 500

E

Ear, 224-233
  clinical anatomy of, 232
  external, 224-226
    malformed, 173
  infections in, 299, 303-304
  inner, 224, 228, 230, 233
    infections of, 232
    perilymph of, 228
  malformation of, 170
  middle, 224-233
    blood supply to, 233
    inflammation in, 232
    lateral wall of cavity of, 228
    lymphatic drainage of, 233
    mucosa of, 211
    ossicles of, 228-230, 291
    promontory of wall of, 226-227, 231
    small bones of, 225-233
    tympanic plexus on promontory of wall
      of, 226-227, 231
  pinna of, 142, 224-225
    innervation of, 225
  popping of, 231, 264
Ear wax, 225
Eardrum, 225-226
Ectoderm, 170-171
Ectopic parathyroid tissue, 218
Ectopic pregnancy, 610, 612
Ectopic thyroid tissue, thyroglossal cysts
    and, 275
Edema of leg, 724
Edentulous person, 268
Efferent axon, 435
Efferent lymphatics, 32
Effusion in elbow joint, 356
Eighth cranial nerve; *see* Vestibulocochlear
    nerve (VIII)
Ejaculation of semen, 616-619
  reflux, 600, 618
Ejaculatory duct, 613-615
  orifices of, 614
  on seminal vesiculogram, 615
Elastic cartilage, 11
Elastic fibers, 8-9
Elbow, 309, 348-353, 396
  anterior capsule of, 353
  clinical anatomy of, 352
  dislocation of, 352
  effusion in, 356
  fractures at, avulsion, 352
  joint capsule of, 353
  ligaments of, 353

Elbow—cont'd
  movements at, 349
Electrolytes
  colon and, 515-516
  disturbances of, brain function and, 151
Eleventh cranial nerve; *see* Accessory nerve
  (XI)
Embolism, carotid artery, 215
Embryology
  axial lines and, 18
  persistence of vessels and, 114
Emergency airway, 219
Emissary foramina of cranial vault, 140-141
  skull and, 137
Emissary vein, 140-141, 163, 183
Enamel, 268
Endochondral ossification, 10
Endocrine cells
  duodenum and, 507
  of pancreas, 497
Endocrine organs, 35, 37, 484
  pancreas as, 494, 497-498
Endoderm, 170-171
Endolymph
  inner ear and, 233
  middle ear and, 228
Endometrium on ultrasound, 612; *see also*
  Heart
Endoneurium, 20, 24
Endopelvic fascia, 558-559, 604
  pelvic interior and, 558
Endoplasmic reticulum, 21
Endoscopy of gallbladder, 490
Enteric nerve, 17, 521
Enteritis, regional, 514
Entropion, 251
Enzymes
  digestive, 480
  renin-angiotensin, 522
Epaxial muscle, 423
Ependyma in brain, 152, 155
Epicanthal fold, 241
Epicardium, 86
  blood vessels of, 90
Epicondylar groove, humeral, 318
  medial, 317, 340
Epicondyle
  of femur
    lateral, 639, 678
    medial, 639, 678
    thigh and knee and, 672
  of humerus, 353
    lateral, 315-316, 394, 399
    medial, 350, 394, 399
    on x-ray, 350
Epicondylitis, lateral, 352, 402, 404-405
Epicranius muscle, 174, 179-180
Epidermis, 8
Epididymis, 471
  testis and, 468
Epidural space, 158, 437
  anesthesia and, 447
  fat filled, on MRI, 418
  hematoma in, 196
Epigastric artery, 118, 587
  inferior, 460-461, 467, 558, 575
    abdomen and, 536

Epigastric artery—cont'd
    diaphragm and, 530
    hernias and, 467
    inguinal canal and, 467
    thigh and, 657
  superficial, 461
  superior, 55, 68, 118, 461
    abdomen and, 536
Epigastric region of abdomen, 538
  pain in, 540
Epigastric vein
  abdomen and, 537
  inferior, 460, 467, 558
    hernias and, 467
    inguinal canal and, 467
  superficial, 461
Epiglottis, 277-278, 281-282, 284-285
Epileptic activity in brain, 151
Epinephrine
  adrenal gland and, 527
  pheochromocytoma and, 528
Epineurium, 20, 24, 439
Epiphyseal line, knee joint and, 678
Epiphyseal plate, 10, 316
  fractures of, 698
Epiphysis, 10
Epiploic foramen of Winslow, 477, 503, 505
Episiotomy, 585
  places for, 584
Epistaxis, 259, 262
Epithelium
  of anal canal, 569
  bladder, 598
  cervical, 610
  of ear canal, 225
  of eyelids, 241
  germinal, 604-605
  middle ear and, 227
  of nose, 253
  olfactory, 254, 258
  pigment, of retina, 237
  pseudostratified ciliated, 8
    in trachea, 77
  of rectum and anus, 519
  in sinuses, 143
  of tongue, 271
Epitympanic recess, 228-229
Erb-Duchenne palsy, 339, 401-402, 404
Erectile tissue of corpus spongiosum, 36, 579
Erection of male penis, 616-619
Erector spinae muscle, 326, 423, 425-426,
    448-449
  abdomen and, 492
  on CT and MRI, 41, 43
  pancreas and, 496
  spinal cord and intercostal space and, 430
Erythrocytes, spleen and, 492
Esophageal artery, 82, 114
Esophageal branches of aorta, 116-117
Esophageal hiatus, 67
  of diaphragm, 67, 530, 532
  surface projections of, 124
Esophageal plexus, 294
Esophageal varices, 116, 500
Esophageal webs, 500
Esophagus, 477
  abnormal innervation of, 116

Esophagus—cont'd
  anterolateral neck and, 219
  aortic arch and, 109
  blood supply to, 500
  clinical anatomy of, 116, 500
  on CT and MRI, 42-43, 100, 415
  diaphragm and, 530-531
  heart imaging and, 116
  liver disease and, 116
  mediastinum and
    posterior, 116
    superior, 114
  nerve supply of, 500
  obstructions of, 500
  peritoneal membranes and, 478-479
  platysma and, 198
  pulmonary artery and, 81
  swallowing and, 281
  in tracheobronchial tree, 80
Esotropia, 251
Estrogen, mild glands and, 55
Ethmoid air cells, 265
Ethmoid artery
  anterior, 250
    meningeal branch of, 139
    nose and, 259
    orbit and, 250
  posterior, 250
Ethmoid bone, 134-136, 138-141
  apertures in, 140-141
  bony orbit and, 236
  cribriform plate of, 139, 254-255
  on CT, 256
  orbit and, 234
  perpendicular plate of, 253-256
Ethmoid sinus, 143, 256-258
Ethmoidal artery, 259
Ethmoidal nerve, anterior, 247, 260
Ethmoidal sinus, 135, 143
  middle, 256
Eustachian tube
  middle ear and, 225, 227
  skull and, 143
Eversion, 7
  of ankle, 703
  of foot, 711
Exocrine gland, 35, 473, 484
  pancreatic secretion of, 498
Exophthalmos, 235
Exotropia, 251
Expiration
  forceful, 68
  muscles of, 120
  thoracic muscles in, 66
Extension, 5, 7
  of ankle, 703
  of elbow, 349
  of foot, 711
  in glenohumeral joint motion, 322
  of hip joint, 644-645, 712
  of knee, 672, 682-684
    patella and, 677
  of thumb, 381, 384-385
Extensor carpi radialis brevis muscle, 360-
    362, 375, 398
  anatomic snuff box and, 372, 375
  tendon of, 357, 373

Extensor carpi radialis brevis muscle—cont'd
  wrist and, 370, 375
Extensor carpi radialis longus muscle, 360-362, 375, 398
  anatomic snuff box and, 372
  anterior compartment and, 346
  tendon of, 357
    on MRI, 357
  wrist and, 370, 375
Extensor carpi ulnaris muscle, 344, 361-362, 375, 398
  tendon of, 357, 373
    on MRI, 357
  wrist and, 375
Extensor digiti minimi muscle, 361-362, 375, 398
  tendon of, 357, 373, 391
    on MRI, 357
  wrist and, 375
Extensor digitorum brevis muscle
  of foot
    anterior compartment and, 696
    anterior view of, 697
    deep view of, 715
    dorsum of foot and, 714
    on MRI, 709
    superficial view of, 714
  of hand, 361-362, 375, 398
    tendon of, 357, 373, 384, 391
    wrist and, 375
Extensor digitorum longus muscle
  of arm, 361-362, 375, 398
    on MRI, 357
    tendon of, 357, 373, 384, 391
    wrist and, 375
  of leg, 693, 695
    ankle tendons and, 702
    anterior view of, 697
    fascial compartments and, 693
    lateral view of, 699
    superficial view of, 714
Extensor expansion in fingers, 375, 384, 390
Extensor hallucis brevis muscle, 714
Extensor hallucis longus muscle, 693, 695
  ankle tendons and, 702
  anterior compartment of leg and, 696-697
  fascial compartments of leg and, 693
  superficial view of, 714
  transverse section of, 718
Extensor indicis muscle, 361-363, 375
  tendons of, 357, 362, 391
    on MRI, 357
  wrist and, 375
Extensor pollicis brevis muscle, 360-363, 375
  anatomic snuff-box and, 372
  tendon of, 357
    on MRI, 357
  wrist and, 375
Extensor pollicis longus muscle, 361-363, 375
  tendon of, 357
    anatomic snuff box and, 372
    on MRI, 357
  wrist and, 375
Extensor retinaculum muscle
  of foot, 714
    inferior, 697, 699, 714

Extensor retinaculum muscle—cont'd
    superior, 697, 699, 714
  of wrist, 360, 372, 375
Extensor sheaths of hand, 361, 384
Extensor synovial compartments, wrist, 375
Extensor tendons
  in foot, 718
  in wrist, 374
External position of structure, 3
External rotation of structure, 5
Extracapsular ligament of knee, 682
Extracellular material, 8
Extraocular muscle, 234, 243, 292
Eye, 134, 234-252
  aqueous and vitreous humors in, 239-241
  blood vessels to, 250
  chambers of, anterior and posterior, 239
  clinical anatomy of, 251-252
  conjunctival membrane and, 250
  cornea of, 237, 239
  eyelids and, 239, 241-242, 249
    muscles of, 246, 248
  flow of tears in, 245, 249-250
  globe of, 235-240
  iris of, 237-239
  lacrimal gland and, 245, 249-250
  lens of, 238-240
  movements of
    brain and, 149
    head and neck and, 295-296
  muscles of globe and orbit and, 237, 243-244
  nerves to globe and orbit and, 238, 244-248
  orbit and; see Orbit, bony
  parasympathetic innervation of, 246
  postoperative movement abnormalities of, 299-300, 304
  principles for, 247
  retina of, 240-241
  smooth muscles of, 19
  sudden onset of pain in, 300, 304
  sympathetic innervation of, 246
  uveal layer of, 238
  visual signal transmission and, 240-241
Eyebrow, lacerations of, 176
Eyelashes, 241
Eyelids, 241-242, 249
  abnormalities of, 251
  head and neck and, 292
  horizontal section of orbit and, 242
  muscles of, 246, 248

F

Fabella, 678, 692
Face, 174-186
  of adult, 138
  anatomy of
    clinical, 185
    surface, 176-177
  blood supply to, 175, 181-184
    venous drainage of, 183
  of child, 138
  cutaneous innervation of, 177-181
  cutaneous vessels of, 180-181, 184
  injury to, 294
  introduction to, 174-177

Face—cont'd
  muscles of; see Facial muscles
  nerves of, 175, 181-184
  parotid gland and, 182-186
  size ratio of cranial vault to, 136, 138
  skeletal components of, 137, 142
  skeletal framework of, 176-177
Facet, articular
  clavicular, 62
  intervertebral, 58
    inferior, 411-413, 415-417, 420
    spinal cord and, 438
    superior, 411-417, 420, 423, 438, 553
    on x-ray, 417
Facial artery, 181-183
  anterolateral neck and, 208
  brain and, 159
  as branch of external carotid artery, 209
  ethmoid perpendicular plate and, 255
  face and, 182
  head and neck and, 181, 296
  parotid gland and, 184
  pharynx and, 280
  superior labial branch of, 259
  transverse, 184
Facial canal, 142-143, 231
Facial muscles
  of expression, 178-181
  head and neck and, 295
  innervation of, 180-181, 184
  view of
    anterior, 179
    lateral, 178
  weakness of, 298, 302
Facial nerve (VII), 165-167, 169
  anterolateral neck and, 210
  brain and, 157
  branches of, 180, 185
  buccinator muscle and, 269
  canal for, 142-143, 231
  chorda tympani of, 171
  ear and, 226-228, 231
  face and, 174
  facial expression and, 180
  head and neck and, 293
  injuries to, 185
  malleus and, 230
  marginal mandibular branch of, 222
  parasympathetic nerves and, 293-294
    postganglionic neurons of, 169
  parotid gland and, 184-185
  pharyngeal arches and, 170-171
  scalp and, 174
  skull and, 140, 143
  tongue and, 270-271
Facial vein
  face and, 183
  neck and, 203
  orbit and, 250
  parotid gland and, 185
  pterygoid venous plexus and, 195
  in submandibular triangle, 222
Falciform ligament, 474, 481, 486-487
  liver and, 487
Fallopian tubes, 558, 575, 605-607
False chordae tendineae, 98
False pelvis, 549

False vocal cords, 285-286
Falx cerebelli, 154, 156
Falx cerebri, 154, 156-157
Falx inguinalis
    abdominal wall and, 460
    inguinal region and, 466
Fascia, 8-9
    axillary, 330, 335
    Buck's, 575, 578-579
    Camper's, 457, 566
    cervical, 198-200
        axilla and, 333
        clinical anatomy of, 215
    clavipectoral, 327, 335
        axilla and, 330
        axillary vein and, 334
    Colles,' 565, 567, 574-575, 619
        principles of, 566
    deep, 9
        of thorax, 54
    Denonvillier's, 575
    Galludet's, 575
    in hand, 381-383
    investing, neck and, 200
    of kidney, 523
    lumbar, 457
    lumbodorsal, 529
    in mid-leg cross-section, 693
    palmar, 356
    in pelvis, 558-560
        of female, 574, 604, 606
        of male, 464, 466, 614
    pharyngobasilar, 279-280
    plantar, 707-708
    pretracheal, 200, 219
    prevertebral, 200, 333
    rectovesical, 575
    renal
        on CT, 41
        pancreas and, 496
    Scarpa's, 457, 566
    spermatic, 464, 466
    submandibular, 223
    superficial, 9, 457
        of thigh, 651
        of thorax, 54
    Tenon's, 242
    of thigh
        anteromedial, 646-647, 650-651
        cribriform, 651
        superficial, 651
    thoracolumbar, 457
    of thorax, 54
    transversalis; see Transversalis fascia
    urogenital diaphragm and, 567
Fascia lata, thigh and, 651
    anteromedial, 646-647, 650
    lateral, 647
    posterior, 673
Fascial compartments
    of leg, 692-699, 703
    in palm, 389
Fascial septa, thigh and, 646, 648-649
Fasciculus, 20
    septomarginal, 103
    transverse, 708
Fasciotomy, 343

Fat
    in anterior mediastinum, 118
    in breast, 54
    on CT, 41
    density of, x-ray detection of, 36
    layer of, 8
    in marrow of clivus on MRI, 148
    pararenal, 523-524
    perineal, 523-524
    perirenal, pancreas and, 496
    in rectal and anal area, 568
    suboccipital, 415
    surrounding synovial membrane of knee
        joint, 679
Fat pads of elbow joint, 349
Fatty lobes of breast, 55
Fatty stools, 543
Fatty tissue, 9
Faucial tonsil, 274
Female
    genitalia of
        external, 571-575
        internal, 558, 606
    pelvis in, 550
        perineal examination and, 626-627
        viscera of; see Pelvic viscera, female
    smooth muscles in reproductive system
        of, 19
Female escutcheon, 626
Feminizing lesions, 528
Femoral artery, 644-646, 648-649, 724
    anteromedial thigh and, 637, 654, 656
    arteriogram of, 658
    branches of, 668
    cannulation of, 662, 669
    circumflex; see Femoral circumflex artery
    common, 658
    course of, 646
    on CT, 618
    deep, 724
        femoral triangle and, 652
        to femur, 644
        lower thigh and, 648
        on posterior view of thigh, 658
        thigh and, 658-659
    femoral canals and, 558
    femoral sheath and, 654
    to femur, 644
    as iliac artery branch, 587
    inferior epigastric vessels and, 467
    inguinal canal in male and, 465
    knee and, 684
    as landmark, 726
    left, 658
    lower, 648
    posterior, 658
    pulse in, 726
    superficial, 648-649, 658
    transversing adductor hiatus, 646
Femoral canal, 558
    femoral sheath and, 653-654
Femoral circumflex artery
    lateral, 644-646, 658-659
        to femur, 644
        gluteal region and, 668
        knee and, 684
    medial, 644-646, 658-659

Femoral circumflex artery—cont'd
    to femur, 644
        gluteal region and, 668
        thigh and, 658
Femoral condyle; see Condyle, of femur
Femoral cutaneous nerve, 555
    gluteal region and, 671
    lateral, 531, 533, 638, 725
        entrapment of, 704
        lumbar and sacral plexus and, 670
        lumbar plexus and, 533
    posterior, 557, 589-590, 638, 725
        lumbar and sacral plexus and, 670
        thigh and, 674
Femoral head; see Femur, head of
Femoral hernia, 662
    principles of, 463
Femoral ligament, 676
Femoral nerve, 638, 725
    hip joints and, 646
    lumbar and sacral plexus and, 670
    medial branches of, 638
    pelvis and, 558, 588, 624
    posterior abdominal wall and diaphragm
        and, 531, 533
    thigh and
        anteromedial, 637, 648-649, 654, 656-
            657, 659
        posterior, 674
Femoral ring, 653-654
Femoral sheath, 652-655
    compartments in, 653
    inguinal canal in male and, 465
    thigh and, 654
Femoral triangle, 637, 644, 651-652, 654
Femoral vein, 467, 558, 652, 724
    cannulation of, 662, 669
    course of, 646
    on CT, 618
    femoral sheath and, 654
    inguinal canal in male and, 465
    thigh and
        anteromedial, 637, 648-649, 653-654, 656
        lower, 648
    x-ray of, 653
Femur, 637-641, 655, 659
    blood supply to, 551, 638
    condyle of; see Condyle, of femur
    distal end of, 672-673
    epicondyle of; see Epicondyle, of femur
    in gluteal region, deep layer, 666
    greater trochanter of; see Trochanter,
        greater
    head of, 639, 641
        in acetabulum, 641
        anteromedial thigh and, 637
        avascular necrosis of, 643, 651
        blood supply to, 643-646, 651
        on CT, 618
        on cystourethrogram, 617
        dislocated hip joint and, 647
        hip joints and, 642, 647
        interruption of blood supply to, 643,
            651
        thigh and knee and, 672
    knee joint and, 674, 678-679
    lesser trochanter of; see Trochanter, lesser

Femur—cont'd
  muscles inserting on, 640
  neck of, 639, 641
    anatomical, 672
    anteromedial thigh and, 640
    on CT, 618
    dislocated hip joint and, 647
    fracture of, 728-730
    thigh and, 648-649
    variations in, 640
  patella and, 677
  in rotation at knee, 683
  shaft of
    anteromedial thigh and, 637, 640
    knee and, 672
  thigh and, 648-649
  valgus and varus deformities and, 686
  view of
    anterior, 12, 639
    medial, 641
    posterior, 639
Fenestra cochleae, 228
Fenestra vestibuli, 228
Fetal circulation, 106-108
  clinical anatomy of, 108
  persistence of, 108
Fetus
  clinical anatomy of, 108
  development of, 18
  ductus venosus in, 107
  in utero, 611
  ligamentum arteriosum in, 106
  liver of, 486
  skull of, 136, 138
  umbilical arteries in, 107
Fibers
  collagen, 8-9
  elastic, 8-9
  transverse, 9
Fibrocartilage, 11
  triangular, 353
Fibroids, 610, 612
Fibrous capsule of acetabulum, 640
Fibrous flexor sheaths of hand, 386, 388-389
Fibrous joints, 10-11, 13
Fibrous pericardial sac, 51
Fibrous pericardium, 88
Fibrous retinaculum of leg, 688
Fibrous skeleton of heart, 89-91
Fibrous tissue, 13
Fibula, 688, 690-691, 693
  ankle and, 700-701
  apex of, 678
  blood supply to knee joint and, 684
  fascial compartments of leg and, 693
  foot and, 706
  head of, 678, 690, 725
    knee and, 676
    lateral view of, 699
    muscles and, 695
    in rotation at knee, 683
  lateral malleolus of, 700-701
  MRI of, 709
  muscles and, 695
  neck of, 690-691
    popliteal fossa and, 690
  nerves and, 696

Fibula—cont'd
  Pott's fracture and, 704
  styloid process of, 690-691
  talocalcaneonavicular joint and, 710
  valgus and varus deformities and, 686
  views of
    anterior, 12, 690
    lateral, 699
    posterior, 690
  weight bearing and, 712
Fibular collateral ligament
  anterior, 676
  knee joint and, 676, 679, 681-682
Fibulocalcaneal ligament, weight bearing
    and, 712
Fifth cranial nerve; see Trigeminal nerve (V)
Filiform papilla, 270
Filum terminale, 156, 438-439
  cauda equina and, 440
Fimbria of oviduct, 36, 558, 605, 612
Finger
  phalanx of middle, 371
  power grip of, 390, 393
  precision grip of, 390, 393
  ring; see Ring finger
First cranial nerve; see Olfactory nerve (I)
First-arch syndromes, 173
Fissures
  of brain, 148-149
  for ligamentum venosum, 492
  of lungs; see Lung, fissures of
  orbital; see Orbital fissure
  palpebral, 241, 295
  of skull
    orbital; see Orbital fissure
    parietooccipital, 148
    petrooccipital, 143
    pterygomaxillary, 143
  of spinal cord, 435
Fistula
  anal, 520
  pharyngeal, clinical anatomy of, 173
  tracheoesophageal, 85
Flail chest, 72
Flexion, 5, 7
  of ankle, 703
  of elbow, 349
  of foot, 711
  in glenohumeral joint motion, 322
  of hip, 644-645, 712
  of knee, 672, 682-684
    patella and, 677
  of thumb, 381, 384-385
Flexor accessorius muscle, 715-716
Flexor carpi radialis muscle, 356, 358-360
  tendon of, 357, 382
  wrist and, 370
Flexor carpi ulnaris muscle, 344, 357-360,
    362, 365
  on MRI, 357
  tendon of, 357, 370
    flexor retinaculum and, 372
    on MRI, 357
  ulnar nerve and, 340
Flexor digiti minimi brevis muscle
  of foot, 715-716, 718-719
    on MRI, 709, 718

Flexor digiti minimi brevis muscle—cont'd
  of hand, 357, 382-383, 386
    insertion of, 388
Flexor digitorum brevis muscle, 716-718
  sole of foot and, 715
Flexor digitorum longus muscle, 693-695
  compartments of leg and, 692-693
  sole of foot and, 715
  tendon of, 702, 716-718
    MRI of, 709
Flexor digitorum profundus muscle, 357-
    360, 373
  insertion of, 388
  on MRI, 357
  tendon of, 373, 382, 384, 386, 389
    on MRI, 357
  ulnar nerve and, 340
Flexor digitorum superficialis muscle, 354,
    357-360, 373
  insertion of, 388
  on MRI, 357
  tendon of, 373, 382, 384, 386, 389
    on MRI, 357
Flexor hallucis brevis muscle, 716-718
  posterior compartment of leg and, 692
  sesamoid bones in, 707
  sole of foot and, 719
Flexor hallucis longus muscle, 693-695, 716-
    718
  ankle tendons and, 702
  posterior compartment of leg and, 692
  sole of foot and, 715
Flexor muscle
  forearm, 358
    deep, 360-362
    superficial, 360, 362
  tendons of
    in foot, 719; see also Flexor digitorum
      longus muscle, tendon of
    in hand, 384, 386, 388
Flexor pollicis brevis muscle, 357, 373, 382-
    385
  insertion of, 388
Flexor pollicis longus muscle, 357-360
  flexor retinaculum and, 371
  insertion of, 388
  on MRI, 357
  tendon of, 373
    on MRI, 357
Flexor retinaculum muscle
  of foot, 700
    leg muscles and, 689
    posterior view of, 694-695
  of hand, 356-357, 370-372, 382, 400
    attachment for, 369
    cross-section of, 374
    on MRI, 357
    palmar fascia and, 382
Flexor sheath, fibrous, 386, 388
Focal point, retina and, 240
Folia, 145
Follicles, 605
  lymphoid, 32
Fontanelles, 136, 138, 295
Foot, 705-721
  in anatomic position, 4
  arches of, 706-708, 714, 717

Foot—cont'd
  arteries of, 714-715, 718-719
  bones of, 705-707
    medial view of, 700
  clinical anatomy of, 721
  decreased circulation of, 721
  deformities of, 720-721
  dorsum of, 705, 714-715
  dynamics of, 712-713
  gait and, 712-713
  injuries to, 721
  joints of
    distal, 711
    subtalar, 708-710
    transverse tarsal, 708, 710
  ligaments of, 707-708
  movements of, 711-712
    musculoskeletal system and, 723
  MRI of, 709
  muscles of, 714-719
  nerves of, 720
  plantar aponeurosis of, 707-708
  plantar surface of, 705
  principles and, 711, 714, 720
  sole of, 715-719
  x-ray of, 707
Foot drop, 690-691
Foramen
  of cranial vault, 134, 137, 140-141
  emissary, 137, 140-141
  epiploic, of Winslow, 477, 503, 505
  greater palatine, 268
  greater sciatic, 555-556, 668
  incisive, 263, 268
  infraorbital; see Infraorbital foramen
  interventricular, 148, 150, 154
  intervertebral; see Intervertebral foramen
  jugular; see Jugular foramen
  of Luschka, 154
  of Magendie, 154
  mandibular, 188-189
  mental; see Mental foramen
  of Monro, 148
  nutrient, 10, 690
  obturator, 549-552, 576
    pelvis and, 559
  in pelvis, 554-557, 559
  pterygopalatine, 236
  sacral; see Sacral foramina
  sciatic, 555-556
    greater, 668
  sphenopalatine, 258
  stylomastoid, 141-142
    middle ear and, 228
  transverse, 412
    spinal cord and, 438
  vertebral, 410
    on CT and MRI, 43
  zygomaticoorbital, 236
Foramen cecum, 270
Foramen lacerum, 141, 158
  skull and, 139, 143
Foramen magnum, 141, 421
  in anterior fossa, 140
  posterior margin of, 415
    on MRI, 415
  skull and, 139, 141

Foramen magnum—cont'd
  spinal cord and, 442
Foramen ovale, 95, 141
  closure of, 107
  mandibular nerve and, 194
  meningeal artery hematoma and, 196
  otic ganglion and, 194
  skull and, 139, 141, 143
Foramen rotundum, 139, 141, 236
Foramen spinosum, 141
  meningeal artery hematoma and, 196
  otic ganglion and, 194
  skull and, 139, 141, 143
Foramen transversarium, 410, 412, 414
Forearm, 309, 348-368
  in anatomic position, 3-4
  blood supply to, 363-364, 367
    venous drainage of, 364-365
  clinical anatomy of, 351-352, 356, 367
  comparison of, to leg, 723
  compression of nerves in, 365
  cutaneous innervation of, 367-368
    brachial plexus and, 339, 341
    lateral, 341, 368
    medial, 339, 368
    posterior, 367
  elbow joint of, 349-353
  extensor muscles of
    deep, 360, 363
    scapula and, 318
    superficial, 360, 362
  force transmission in, 351
  fracture of, 402, 405
  interosseous membrane of, 354-356
  median vein of, 364, 400
  muscles of, 355-363
    anterior, 356-360
    common flexor origin for, anterior
      compartment and, 346
    extensor; see Forearm, extensor muscles
      of
    flexor, 317, 358, 360-362
    hypertrophy of, 351
    posterior, 359-363
  nerves of, 365-368
    compression of, 351
    cutaneous; see Forearm, cutaneous
      innervation of
  radioulnar joints of, 352-355
    movements at, 353
  radius of, 348, 356
  ulna of, 348-349
  venous access in, 367
Forebrain, 147-153
Foregut, 473, 475, 479-480
  development of, 475
Foreskin, 575, 579
  transection of, 580
Fornix, 36, 607
  on MRI, 148
  superior, 249-250
  of uterine cervix, 607
Fossa
  of brain, 138-140, 149
    hypophyseal, 160
  coracoid, 314
  coronoid, 316

Fossa—cont'd
  cranial cavity, 149
    middle ear and, 226
    orbit and, 234
  cubital, 342, 347, 400
  of Douglas, 604
  glenoid; see Glenoid fossa
  hypophyseal, 160
  iliac, 549
    gluteal region and, 663
    pelvic interior and, 558
  infraspinous, 313-315, 317, 334, 399
  infratemporal; see Temporal and
    infratemporal fossae
  intercondylar, 639-640, 672, 678
  intertrochanteric, 637, 639
  ischioanal, 648-649
  ischiorectal, 565-568, 581
    anterior recess of, 566
  lacrimal, 249
  middle cranial, middle ear and, 226
  navicular, 579, 582, 609, 616
  olecranon, 318, 348-350
    on x-ray, 350
  pituitary, 135, 139, 154, 196
  popliteal; see Popliteal fossa
  pterygopalatine, 143, 259-262
  radial, 316, 318
  rectouterine, 558, 574, 604, 609
  of skull; see Skull, fossae of
  for sublingual gland, 188
  for submandibular gland, 188
  subscapular, 314-315, 317
  supraspinous, 313-315, 399
  temporal; see Temporal and infratemporal
    fossae
  transverse septum of, 568
  vesicorectal, 558
  vesicouterine, 574, 604
Fossa ovalis, 95, 650
  atrium and, 95
Fourchettes, 573
Fourth cranial nerve; see Trochlear nerve
  (IV)
Fourth ventricle, 150, 152-155
  on MRI, 148
Fovea capitis, 639, 641, 643
Fovea centralis, 241
Fracture
  of capitate, 402, 405
  of clavicle, 317
  Colles, 351, 402, 405
  of elbow, 352
  of epiphyseal plate, 698
  of femoral neck, 728-730
  of forearm, 402, 405
  greenstick, 310
  of hand, 402, 405
  of hip, 651
  of humerus, 319, 346, 402, 404
  laryngeal, 290
  of leg, 704
  of lunate, 402, 405
  of mandible, 197
  nasal, 262
  of orbit, 235, 294
  pathologic, 346

Fracture—cont'd
    pelvic, 560
    Pott's, 704
    of radius, 351, 402, 405
    of ribs, 72
    of scaphoid, 376, 402, 405
    of skull, 144, 196-197
    of ulna, 351
    of vertebral bodies, compression, 431
    of wrist, 402, 405
Frenulum, 269-270, 281, 295
    of clitoris, 573, 576
    head and neck and, 296
    of lower lip, 264
    of prepuce, 579
    of upper lip, 264
Friction rub, 124
Frontal bone, 134-136, 139, 174, 253
    bony orbit and, 236
    brain and, 154
    failure of, to fuse, 144
    of newborn, 138
    orbit and, 234
    shape of face and, 142
    sinuses in, 143
    skull and, 134, 137
Frontal bossing, 177
Frontal horn, 150, 152
Frontal lobe of brain, 148-149
Frontal nerve, 178, 238, 242, 245, 247
Frontal plane, 3, 6
Frontal process, 135
Frontal sinus, 135, 255-258, 260
    brain and, 148, 154
    face and scalp and, 178
    on MRI, 148
    skull and, 135, 140
Frontal suture, 138, 144
Frontalis muscle
    face and scalp and, 178-179
    scalp and, 174
Fundiform ligament, 580
Fundus, 36, 607
    duodenum and, 508
    of gallbladder, 488
    peritoneal membranes and, 479
    spleen and, 493
    of stomach, 501-502
Fungiform papilla, 270
Funny bone, 317, 340
Fusion of wrist bones, 377

G
Gag reflex, 281-282, 296
Gait, 711-713
    pelvis and, 560
Galea aponeurotica, 174, 178
    clinical anatomy of, 176
Galen, cerebral vein of, 154
Gallbladder, 488-492
    development of, 476, 479, 484
    duodenum and, 508
    fetal liver and, 486
    function of, 480
    liver and, 485, 487
    peritoneal membranes and, 479
    porta hepatis and, 486

Gallstones, 490
Galludet's fascia, 575
Gametes, 35
Ganglia, 20, 24
    basal, 147
        of forebrain, 150
        on MRI, 148
    of brain, 145, 147-148, 150
    celiac, 537
        spinal cord and, 445
    cervical; see Cervical ganglion
    ciliary; see Ciliary ganglion
    dorsal root, 24-25, 164, 435-437
        dural sheath on, 438
        neck and, 200
        segmentation of body organization and, 446
    esophagus and, 500
    geniculate, 166, 231
        middle ear and, 227-228
    of glossopharyngeal nerve, 166, 211
    large intestine and, 521
    otic; see Otic ganglion
    parasympathetic
        otic ganglion in; see Otic ganglion
        in temporal and infratemporal fossae, 187
    prevertebral, 445, 592
    pterygopalatine; see Pterygopalatine ganglion
    sensory, of cranial nerves, 164-168
    spinal; see Ganglia, dorsal root
    stellate, 215, 444
        block of, 328
        mediastinum and, 216
        spinal cord and, 444
    submandibular, 169, 272
        otic ganglion in, 195; see also Otic ganglion
        parasympathetic nerves and, 294
        submandibular and sublingual glands and, 273
        submandibular region and, 222
    superior mesenteric, spinal cord and, 445
    sympathetic, 24, 430, 437, 443-446, 588
        block of, 119
        lumbar and sacral plexus and, 670
        mediastinum and, 112-114, 118
        thoracic spinal cord segment and, 69
    trigeminal; see Trigeminal ganglion
    of vagus nerve, 167
    at wrist, 377
Ganglion impar, 443, 445-446
Gap junctions, 19, 103
Gastric acid
    cranial nerves and, 169
    excess, 499
Gastric artery, 491
    left
        abdomen and, 492
        esophagus and, 500
        liver and, 488
        spleen and, 493
        stomach and, 501-502
    posterior, stomach and, 501-502
    right, duodenum and, 507
    short, 494, 497

Gastric artery—cont'd
    spleen and, 491
    stomach and, 501-503
Gastric development and mesenteries, 505
Gastric hormones, 506
Gastric ulcers, 506
Gastric vein
    esophagus and, 116, 500
    spleen and, 491
Gastrin, 497
    duodenum and, 507
Gastrin-producing cells, 501, 506
Gastrocnemius muscle, 692-695
    compartments of leg and, 692-693
    heads of, 693
        attachment of, 657
    leg muscles and, 689
    medial head of, 675
    popliteal fossa and, 688
    tendon of, 695
    views of
        anterior, 697
        lateral, 699
        posterior, 694
        superficial, 673
Gastroduodenal artery, 492
    clinical anatomy of, 506
    duodenum and, 507
    pancreaticoduodenal branch of, 498
    spleen and, 493
    stomach and, 501-503
Gastroepiploic artery, 481
    duodenum and, 510
    left, 494, 501-503
    right, 501-502
    stomach and, 501-503
Gastroesophageal junction, 499, 501
    surface projections of, 124
Gastroesophageal reflux, 116, 500
Gastroesophageal sphincter, 116
Gastrointestinal tract, 30, 35; see also Digestive system
    development of, 477, 479
    giant glands of, 479
    layers of gut wall in, 35
Gastroschisis, 482
Gastrosplenic ligament, 491, 493, 505
Gaze
    abnormal, 251
    angle of, 243
    axis of, 235
    globe of eye and, 235
G-cells; see Gastrin-producing cells
Gemellus muscle
    hip joints and, 645
    inferior, 664, 666-667, 671
    sciatic nerve origin and, 669
    superior, 664, 666-667, 671
Genial tubercle, 188
Genicular artery, 685
    inferior, 684
    superior, 684
Geniculate ganglion, 166, 231
    middle ear and, 227-228
Geniculate nucleus, lateral, 241
Genioglossus muscle, 271
    airway patency and, 275

Genioglossus muscle—cont'd
  in submandibular triangle, 220
  in submental triangle, 223
  tongue and, 272
Geniohyoid muscle, 168, 218, 220, 272, 281
  nerve to, 202
    ansa cervicalis nerve and, 215
  pharynx and, 276
  in submandibular triangle, 220, 222
  in submental triangle, 223
  tongue and, 272
Geniohyoid nerve, 214
Genital duct, 34
Genital hiatus, 565
Genitalia, 36
  external
    female, 571-575
    male, 575-582
  internal, female, 558, 606
Genitofemoral nerve, 469, 531, 533, 578, 588
  abdomen and, 537
  femoral branch of, 638
  genital branch of, 583
  lumbar and sacral plexus and, 670
  pelvis and perineum and, 625
Genu of corpus callosum, 148
Genu valgum, 686, 729-731
Genu varum, 686
Germinal epithelium, 604-605
Gerota's capsule, 523-524
Giant glands of gastrointestinal tract,
    development of, 479
Gimbernat, lacunar ligament of, 466
Gingiva, inflammation of, 275
Gingival line, 268
Gingivitis, 275
Glabella, 134, 140, 295
Glands
  in breast, 54
  thyroid, 77
Glans
  of clitoris, 572-573, 576
  of penis, 575-576, 579-580, 582, 615
    protective shield for, 580
Glaucoma, 239
Glenohumeral joint, 311, 313-316, 318-320,
    394
  articular capsule of, 320
  dislocation of, 317
  movements of, 322-324
Glenohumeral ligament, 319
Glenoid fossa, 62, 310-311, 314, 316
  axilla and, 331
  brachial plexus and, 327
  dislocated shoulder and, 317
  glenohumeral joint and, 318
  on MRI, 323
  on x-ray, 312-313
Glenoid labrum, 311, 316
  glenohumeral joint and, 318
  on MRI, 323
Glial cells, 20, 145, 434
Glisson's capsule, 484
Globe of eye, 134, 234-240
  horizontal section of orbit and, 242
  muscles of, 235, 237, 243-244
  nerve supply of, 238, 244-248

Globe of eye—cont'd
  skull and, 143
Glomeruli of kidney, 522
Glossoepiglottic space, 281
Glossopharyngeal nerve (IX), 165-167, 169,
    272
  anterolateral neck and, 210
  brain and, 157, 159
  in carotid triangle, 209-212
  ear and, 231
    middle, 227
  head and neck and, 293
  otic ganglion and, 195
  parasympathetic nerves and, 293-294
    postganglionic neurons in, 169
  pharyngeal arches and, 170-171
  pharynx and, 280-281
  sensory ganglia for, 212
  skull and, 140
  submandibular region and, 222
  in submandibular triangle, 222
  tongue and, 270-272
  tympani nerve of, 171
  tympanic membrane and, 226
Glottic region of larynx, 285-286
Glottis, 285-286
  changes in positions of, 285
Glucagon, 497
Glucagonoma, 498
Glucocorticoids
  adrenal gland and, 527
  excess, 528
Gluteal artery, 557, 570, 590
  inferior, 589, 668, 724
    on CT, 618
    hip joints and, 645, 668
    thigh and, 658
  superior, 583, 587, 589, 668, 724
Gluteal fold, 652, 665
Gluteal line, 562, 643
Gluteal nerve, 557, 588-589
  inferior, 555, 588-589, 668, 671, 725
    branch of, 590
    lumbar and sacral plexus and, 670
  superior, 555, 588, 590, 668, 671, 725
    lumbar and sacral plexus and, 670
Gluteal region, 111, 663-671
  anatomy of
    clinical, 669
    skeletal, 663, 666
  layers of
    deep, 666
    intermediate, 665
  muscles of
    large, 663-666
    smaller, 665-669
  sacral plexus and, 668-671
  superficial exposure of, 664
  upper outer quadrant of, 727
  vessels of, 668
Gluteal tuberosity, 637, 639, 641
Gluteal vein, 557, 570
  inferior, 724
    on CT, 618
  superior, 724
Gluteus maximus muscle, 564, 590
  attachment of, 657

Gluteus maximus muscle—cont'd
  on CT, 618
  in gluteal region, 663-665
    intermediate layer, 664
    superficial exposure, 664
  iliotibial band and, 673
  thigh and
    anteromedial, 637
    lateral, 647
    posterior, 673, 675
Gluteus medius muscle, 590
  attachment of, 657
  in gluteal region, 664-665
    intermediate layer, 664
    superficial exposure, 664
    vessels and, 668
  Trendelenburg sign and, 666
Gluteus minimus muscle
  attachment of, 657
  in gluteal region, 664-665
    deep layer, 666
  hip joints and, 645
  Trendelenburg sign and, 666
Goblet cells in trachea, 77
Goiter, 219
Gonad, 34-35, 37
Gonadal artery, 591
  abdomen and, 536-537
  kidneys and, 526
  pelvis and, 623
Gonadal vein, 534-535
Graafian follicle, 605
Gracilis muscle, 654
  adductor magnus muscle and, 661
  attachment of, 657
  femoral artery and, 646
  in gluteal region, intermediate layer, 664
  pes anserinus and, 675
  thigh and, 648-649, 659
    anteromedial, 655, 660
    lower, 648
    posterior, 673-674
Grafts in lower limb, 704
Gray matter, 145, 147, 438
Gray rami communicans, 24, 118, 443-445,
    588
  cranial nerves and, 168
  lumbar and sacral plexus and, 670
  primary
    anterior, 24, 430, 437
    posterior, 430, 436-437
  spinal cord and, 430, 437, 443
  in thoracic and upper lumbar regions, 118
Great cardiac vein, 93
Great saphenous vein; see Saphenous vein,
    great
Great toe, 700, 715
Great vessels, 109-111
  anterior view of, 89
  catheters in, 119
  in pericardial sac, 86
  variations in, 119
Greater abdominal sac, development of, 476-
    479
Greater auricular nerve; see Auricular nerve,
    greater
Greater occipital nerve, 175

Greater omentum; *see* Omentum, greater
Greater palatine artery, 259, 267
Greater palatine foramen, 268
Greater palatine nerve, 260, 267
    pterygopalatine fossa and, 261
Greater petrosal nerve; *see* Petrosal nerve,
    greater
Greater sciatic foramen, 668
Greater sciatic notch; *see* Sciatic notch,
    greater
Greater splanchnic nerve, 118
Greater trochanter; *see* Trochanter,
    greater
Greater vestibular gland; *see* Vestibular
    gland, greater
Greater wing of sphenoid bone; *see*
    Sphenoid bone, greater wing of
Greenstick fractures, 310, 698
Groove
    atrioventricular, 89
    bicipital, 315, 318
    in cerebral cortex, 149
    costal, 65, 71-73
    deltopectoral, 327, 329, 399
        anterior view of, 398
    humeral; *see* Humerus, groove of
    for lacrimal sac, 236
    for middle meningeal vessels, 135, 139
    musculospiral, 315, 318
        injury of, 402, 404
    nasolabial, 295
    patellar
        femur and, 639
        knee and, 676-677
Growth hormone excess, 177
Gut, development of, 473-483
    clinical anatomy of, 482
    fixation and suspension in, 475-479
    giant glands and, 479
    greater and lesser sacs in, 476-479
    growth and rotation in, 475-480
        malrotation and, 482, 514
        of stomach, 476-479
    mesenteries in
        blood supply to, 474, 479-480
        dorsal and ventral, 474-476
        parietal and visceral, 473-474, 476
    omental bursa in, 476-479, 481
    omentum in
        greater, 480-481
        lesser, 479, 481
    organs developing in peritoneal leaflets
        in, 475
    parietal peritoneum in, 480
    principles for, 475, 480
    regions of, 479
    structures in
        intraperitoneal, 478, 483
        peritoneal and retroperitoneal,
            481-483
        retroperitoneal, 476, 483
Gut wall, layers of, 35
Gynecoid pelvis, 557
    principles of, 554
Gynecoid shape of pelvis, 554
Gynecomastia, 54
Gyri in cerebral cortex, 150

H
Hair, 8
    arrector muscles for, 293
    in female mons pubis, 626
    smooth muscles of, 19
    transplants of, 185
Hair cells, inner ear and, 233
Hair follicle, 8
Hamate bone, 357, 369-373, 376
    flexor retinaculum and, 371
    hook of, 371-374
        on MRI, 357
    on MRI, 357
    ulnar artery and, 396, 400
    wrist and, 371-373
Hamstrings, 672-674
    injuries of, 687
    popliteal fossa and, 688
    tendons of, 688
Hamulus, 369
    flexor retinaculum and, 370
    pterygoid; *see* Pterygoid plate, hamulus of
Hand, 309, 378-393
    in anatomic position, 4
    anterior surface of, 368
    blood vessels of, 391-392
    carpometacarpal joints of, 379-381
    central fixed unit of, 393
    clinical anatomy of, 392
    congenital deformities in, 392
    extensor expansions of, 390
    fascial structures in, 381-383
    fibrous flexor sheaths of, 386, 389
    fracture of, 402, 405
    grip of, 390, 393
    infection in, 392
    injury of, 401, 403-404
    loose skin on dorsum of, 9
    metacarpal bones of, 378-379
    metacarpophalangeal joints of, 379, 381
    movements and functions of, 390, 393
    muscles of
        hypothenar, 383, 386
        insertions on individual digits in, 387-
            388
        interosseous and lumbrical, 385-387
        thenar, 382-385
    nerves in, 389, 392-393
    phalanges of, 381-382
    principles of, 391, 393
    thumb opposition in, 384-385, 391, 393
Hard palate, 263-268
    nose and, 253, 256, 260
Hartmann's pouch, 490
Haustra, 516
Head, 130-305
    anatomy of
        skeletal, 291-292
        surface, 293-296
    anterolateral neck and, 206-223; *see also*
        Neck, anterolateral
    arterial blood flow of, 133, 292
    autonomic innervation of, 293
    bony landmarks of, 293-295
    brain and central nervous system and,
        145-163; *see also* Brain; Central
        nervous system

Head—cont'd
    case studies and, 297-305
    cranial nerves and, 164-169; *see also*
        Cranial nerves
    dermatomes of, 27
    ear and, 224-233
    eye and orbit in, 234-252; *see also* Eye;
        Orbit
    of infant, ultrasonography of, 44
    innervation of, 293-294
    larynx and, 284-290
    lymphatic drainage of, 133-134, 292
    mouth and palate and, 263-275; *see also*
        Mouth; Palate
    movements of, 418
        muscles controlling, 426-428
    muscles of, 133, 291-292, 426-428
    nasal cavity and, 253-262
    pharyngeal arches and, 170-173
    pharynx and, 276-283
    physical examination of, 293-296
    position control of, 426, 433
    posterior triangle of neck and, 198-205
    of rib, 59-61
    scalp and face and, 174-186; *see also* Face;
        Scalp
    skull and, 133-144; *see also* Skull
    systems review and, 291-296
    temporal and infratemporal fossa and,
        187-197
    terminology and, 3
    trauma to
        headache and, 298, 302
        loss of consciousness in, 298, 302-303
    venous drainage of, 133, 292
Headache
    head trauma and, 298, 302
    vascular, 197
Hearing
    organs of, 134
    otitis and, 232
Heart, 25, 28, 86-108
    anterior view of, 89
    apex of, 89, 122
        surface projections of, 124
    artificial pacing of, 105
    ascending aorta and, 98-101
    atria of; *see* Atria of heart
    base of, 89
    blood vessels of, 90-94; *see also* Coronary
        artery; Coronary vein
        flow between lungs and, 83
        flow through, 101-102
    borders of, 122-123
    bundle branches of, 95, 104
    case studies and, 126, 128
    clinical anatomy of, 101, 104-105, 126-127
        abnormalities of position in, 89
        coronary arteries in, 94
        fetal, 108
        pericardium in, 88
    conduction system of, 103-104
    cranial nerves and, 169
    fetal circulation and, 106-108
    fibrous skeleton of, 89-91
    imaging of, esophagus and, 116
    innervation of, 84, 104-106, 121

Heart—cont'd
  autonomic, 84
  left side of, 86
  mediastinum and, 52
  muscle fibers of, 90
  myocardial infarction of, 126, 128
  nerves to, 84
  pericardial sac and, 86-88
  position and orientation of, 88-89, 122
    abnormal, 89
  pulmonary artery and, 97
  pulmonary veins and, 97
  receptors in, 105
  rhythmic contraction of, 86
  right side of, 86
  surface anatomy of, 123
  surfaces of, 89
  transplantation of, 105
  transplanted, 105
  valves of
    annulus of, 91, 97-98
    aortic, 91, 96, 98-99
    clinical anatomy of, 101, 104
    congenital atresia of, 104
    fibrous skeleton and, 91
    heart sounds and, 104
    incompetence of, 101
    injury to, 101
    insufficiency of, 101
    leaflets of, 95, 97-99
    left atrioventricular, 97-98
    mitral, 91, 96-99
    prolapse of, 101
    pulmonary, 91, 96-97
    stenosis of, 101
    tricuspid, 91, 95-96
  ventricles of; see Ventricles, of heart
  visceral serous pericardium of, 51
Heart disease, congenital, 104
Heart murmurs, 124
Heart sounds, 104, 124
Heel, 715
Helix, 22
Hematoma
  epidural, 196
  intracranial, 151
Hematopoiesis, 492
Hematopoietic cells, 10
Hematuria, 541, 544
Hemiazygos vein, 71, 121, 500, 534
  accessory, 31
  on CT and MRI, 43
  diaphragm and, 531
  esophagus and, 116
  mediastinum and, 117-118
  spinal cord and, 430
  thoracic duct and, 31
  thoracic spinal cord segment and, 69
Hemidiaphragm, 50
  on x-ray, 53
Hemivertebra, 431
Hemoglobin catabolism, 484
Hemorrhage
  inside skull, 151
  periorbital, 251
  from subclavian artery, 204
Hemorrhoids, 517, 570-571

Hemothorax, 75, 127
Hepatic artery, 485-486
  clinical anatomy of, 506
  common, 488, 492
    spleen and, 493
  liver and, 487
  porta hepatis and, 487
  principles of, 487
  proper, 488
  right and left, 488, 492
  stomach and, 503
Hepatic duct, 487-488, 490
  common, 487
  liver and, 488
  right and left, 487
Hepatic flexure, 515, 518
  of colon, 516
  pancreas and, 496
  transverse colon and, 518
Hepatic vein, 480, 485-486
  abdomen and, 534-535, 537
  fetal liver and, 486
  peritoneal membranes and, 478-479
Hepatoduodenal ligament, 487, 491
  peritoneal membranes and, 478
  spleen and, 491
Hepatopancreatic ampulla, 487, 497
Hepatopancreatic duct, 488
Hernia
  congenital diaphragmatic, 535, 544
    principles of, 463
  femoral, 662
  hiatus, 463, 500, 535
  incarceration of, 539, 542
  inguinal; see Inguinal hernia
  paraesophageal, 500
  principles of, 463
  sliding, 500
Herniated disk, 423, 452, 730
  clinical anatomy of, 482
Herpes zoster, 72, 450
Hiatus
  adductor, femoral artery transversing,
    646, 660-661
  aortic, of diaphragm, 67, 445, 530, 532
  esophageal; see Esophageal hiatus
  genital, 565
  sacral; see Sacral hiatus
Hiatus hernia, 500, 535
  principles of, 463
Hiatus semilunaris, 256
Hilar lymph node, 85
Hilton line, 568
Hilum
  development of gut and, 473
  of kidney, 522, 524
  of lungs, 51, 80, 121
    phrenic nerve and, 112
    visceral pleura and, 74
  of spleen, 493
Hindbrain, 147, 149
Hindgut, 473, 479-480
  development of, 475
Hinge joint, ankle as, 703
Hip, 640-646; see also Gluteal region
  anteroposterior x-ray of, 642
  blood supply to, 644-646

Hip—cont'd
  bones in, 3, 12, 536, 549, 552
    anterior view of, 12
    interior of, 551
  clinical anatomy of, 651
  dislocation of, 647, 651, 669
  fractures of, 651
  gait and, 712
  gluteal region and, 638, 663
  ligaments of, 640-644
  movements of, 644-645, 712
    lateral rotators in, 667
    short rotators in, 667
  on MRI, 649
  muscles and, 324
  musculoskeletal system and, 722
  nerves of, 646
  posterior surfaces of, gluteal region and,
    663, 666
  posterior thigh and, 674
  relations and movements of, 643-645
  surgical replacement of, 651
Hip pointer, 662
His bundle of heart, 95, 104
Histamine blockers, 506
Hook of hamate, 357, 371-374
Hordeolum, 251
Horizontal arches of foot, 707
Horizontal fissures of lungs, 80, 124
Horizontal planes of body, 3, 6
Hormones
  adrenal gland and, 527
  gastric, 506
  imbalance of, brain function and, 151
Horn
  frontal, 150, 152
  of larynx, 278
  of spinal cord, 24
    anterior, 434-435
    dorsal, 24, 434-435, 437
    intermediate, 24, 434-435
    lateral, 434-435
    posterior, 434-435
    ventral, 24, 434-435, 437
Horner's syndrome, 119, 246, 251
Horseshoe kidney, 602-603
Housemaid's knee, 677, 687
Humeral circumflex artery, 320, 397
  anterior, 332, 334
  axilla and, 330, 332
  posterior, 332, 334
    axilla and, 330
Humeral circumflex vein, posterior, 330
Humeral ligament, transverse, 315, 318-319,
  344
Humerus, 314-319, 343-344, 349-350
  anatomy of
    clinical, 319
    skeletal, 394-395
  epicondyles of, 318, 353
    lateral, 318, 350
    medial, 317
    on x-ray, 350
  fracture of, 346, 402, 404
    of humeral head, 319
    midshaft, 319
  glenohumeral joint and, 318

Humerus—cont'd
  groove of
    epicondylar, 317-318, 340
    intertubercular, 312-313, 315, 318, 394, 399
    radial, 318
  growth and maturation of, 11
  head of, 320
    dislocated shoulder and, 317
    on MRI, 323
    on x-ray, 312-313
  movements of, 322-325
    elbow and, 349, 395
  neck of
    anatomic, 312
    surgical, 312, 318
  shaft of, 318, 320
    axilla and, 330
  supracondylar ridges of, 318
  trochlea of; *see* Trochlea, of humerus
  tubercle of, 312-313, 318, 323
  views of
    anterior, 12, 318
    posterior, 318
    on x-ray, 350
Hyaline cartilage, 11, 14
Hyaloid artery, 241
Hydrocephalus, 153, 155
Hydrochloric acid, 506
Hydronephrosis, 524, 597
Hydroureter, 597
5-Hydroxytryptamine, 507
Hymen, 573
Hyoglossus muscle, 168, 214, 271
  lateral view of tongue and, 222
  nerve supply to submandibular region and, 272
Hyoid bone, 265-266, 269, 276-278, 281-282
  brain and, 159
  cranial nerves and, 166
  larynx and, 288
  as movable bone, 133
  neck and, 291, 295
    anterolateral, 208, 216
  submandibular gland and, 221
  submandibular region and, 220-222
  submandibular triangle and, 220
  tongue and, 272
Hypaxial muscle, 423
Hyperacidity, 501
Hyperaldosteronism, 528
Hyperopia, 240
Hypertension
  portal, 116, 489
  pulmonary, 83
Hypobranchial eminence, 171
Hypogastric nerve, 583, 591-592, 624
  inferior, 592
    spinal cord and, 445
  superior, 591-592
  surgical division of, 593
Hypogastric plexus
  parasympathetic nerves and, 294
  pelvic interior and, 558
  in pelvis, 591-592
Hypoglossal canal, 139, 141-142

Hypoglossus nerve (XII), 165, 167-169, 272
  brain and, 159
  in carotid triangle, 210, 213-214
  course and branches of, 215
  neck and, 293
    anterolateral, 210
  skull and, 140
  submandibular region and, 222
  tongue and, 271-272
Hypopharynx, 281-282
Hypophyseal fossa, 160
Hypoplasia
  of lung, 544
  of mandible, 170
Hypospadias, 615, 620
Hypothalamus, 147-148
  capillary network in, 37
  of forebrain, 150
  on MRI, 148
  periventricular nuclei of, 37
  supraoptic nuclei of, 37
Hypothenar eminence, 368, 383, 386
Hypothenar muscle, 372, 383, 386
  insertion of, 388
Hysterosalpingogram, 609

I

IgA; *see* Immunoglobulin A
Ileal artery, 511-513
Ileal branches of superior mesenteric artery, 513
Ileocecal junction, 516
Ileocecal valve, 511, 517-518
  ileocecal junction and, 511
Ileocolic artery, 511
  cecum and, 518
  small intestine and, 513
Ileum, 30, 507, 510-513
  blood supply to, 511-513
  pancreas and, 496
  peritoneal membranes and, 481
  peritoneal specialization of, 482-483
  small intestine and, 508-509, 512
  terminal
    anorectal region and, 516
    ileocecal junction and, 511
Iliac artery, 570, 587
  anorectal region and, 570
  common, 582-583, 586, 594-595, 601
    abdomen and, 534
    right, 477
  external, 467, 557, 583, 586, 595
    to femur, 644
    pelvis and, 623
    thigh and, 657
  internal, 578, 583, 586
    branches of, 589
    colon and, 516
    pelvis and, 623
  rectum and, 517
  small intestine and, 513
Iliac bursal sac, 640
Iliac circumflex artery, deep, 461
  thigh and, 657-658
Iliac crest, 538, 549-552, 555
  abdominal wall and, 458
  on gluteal region superficial exposure, 664

Iliac crest—cont'd
  hip joint ligaments and, 643
  iliotibial band and, 673
  lumbar puncture and, 432
  pelvis and, 559
  position of, back and, 449
Iliac fossa, 549
  gluteal region and, 63
  pelvic interior and, 558
Iliac node, external, 33
Iliac spine, 551
  anterior, 555
  anterior inferior, 550, 552
    hip joint ligaments and, 643
  anterior superior, 550, 552, 562, 631, 650
    femoral sheath and, 654
    hip joint ligaments and, 643
    short rotators of hip joint and, 667
  posterior inferior, 552
    hip joint ligaments and, 643
  posterior superior, 550, 552
    on gluteal region superficial exposure, 664
    hip joint ligaments and, 643
Iliac vein, 570
  anorectal region and, 570
  common, 586, 594
    abdominal wall and, 534
  external, 467, 557, 586
    abdomen and, 459
  internal, 517, 586
    pelvis and, 623
  pelvic interior and, 558
Iliacus muscle, 654
  femoral artery and, 646
  femoral sheath and, 654
  femoral triangle and, 651
  iliopsoas muscle and, 655
  lumbar plexus and, 533
  pelvic interior and, 558
  tendons of, 645
  thigh and, 656
    anterior, 646
Iliococcygeus muscle, 562-565, 631
Iliocostalis muscle, 425-426
Iliofemoral ligament, 642-643, 722
Iliohypogastric nerve, 531, 533, 588
  abdomen and, 537
  lumbar and sacral plexus and, 533, 670
Ilioinguinal nerve, 469, 531, 533, 578, 583, 588
  abdomen and, 537
  inguinal canal in female and, 466
  lower limb views of, 638
  lumbar and sacral plexus and, 533, 670
Iliolumbar artery, 570, 587, 589
Iliolumbar ligament, 556
Iliopsoas muscle, 654
  attachment of, 657
  on CT, 618
  thigh and, 648-649
    anteromedial, 637, 639, 655, 657, 660
Iliopubic eminence, 550-552
Iliotibial band, 650, 654, 669, 726
  fascia lata and, 646-647
  thigh and
    anteromedial, 655

Iliotibial band—cont'd
knee and, 673
lateral, 647
Iliotibial tract
fascia lata and, 646-647
joints and
hip, 645
knee, 673, 681
thigh and, 648-649, 673
Ilium, 549-551
arcuate line of; *see* Arcuate line of ilium
body of, 549
fossa of; *see* Iliac fossa
hip joints and, 642
structural features of, 645
Imaging techniques, 36-45
computerized tomography, 38-39, 41
conventional x-ray, 36-40
magnetic resonance imaging, 39-40, 42-43
ultrasonography, 40-45
Immune response, 254
spleen and, 492
Immunoglobulin A, 254
lymphoid tissue and, 274
Incarceration of hernia, 539, 542
Incision
in abdominal wall, 462
episiotomy, 585
places for, 584
sternotomy, 63
Incisive foramen, 263, 268
Incisors, 267-268
mandible and, 188
Incisure
angular, 501-502
cardiac, 501-502
tentorial, 154
Incontinence, stress, 610
Incus, 225, 228-230
Independent bones, 136
Index finger
extension of, 390
muscle insertions on, 387-388
phalanx of, 371
Indoleamine derivatives, 506
Indomethacin in newborn, 106
Infant
head of, ultrasonography of, 44
spinal cord in, 441
Infarction, myocardial, 126, 128
Infection
in anal canal, 520
conjunctival, 251
in hand, 392
of inner ear, 232
mastoid, 232
in sinuses, 251, 262
Inferior position of structure, 6
Inferior vena cava; *see* Venae cavae, inferior
Inflammation
conjunctival, 251
gallbladder, 490
of gingiva, 275
of inner ear, 232
of maxillary sinus, 262
in middle ear, 232
of palatine tonsils, 283

Inflammation—cont'd
of parotid gland, 185
in pericardial sac, 124
of submandibular lymph nodes, 223
of thoracic cage, 62
Inflow tract, ventricular
left, 98
right, 95
Infraglenoid tubercle, 312, 314, 320
Infrahyoid region, muscles in, 215-217
Inframeniscal compartment, 679
Infraorbital artery, 242
maxillary artery and, 192
pterygopalatine fossa and, 260
Infraorbital foramen, 134, 236
head and neck and, 294
skull and, 134, 137
Infraorbital nerve, 242
face and scalp and, 178, 181
head and neck and, 294
orbit and, 245
pterygopalatine fossa and, 261
Infraorbital vein, 242
Infrapatellar bursa, 679
Infrapubic angle, 550, 557
Infraspinatus muscle
axilla and, 332
back muscles and, 425
chest wall and, 65
on CT and MRI, 43, 100, 323
heart and, 100
posterior compartment and, 346
scapular spine and, 398
shoulder and, 316, 324
Infraspinous fossa, 313-315, 317, 334, 399
Infratemporal fossa; *see* Temporal and
infratemporal fossae
Infratentorial structures, 149, 154, 158
Infratrochlear nerve, 242
Infundibulopelvic ligament, 559, 575, 604-606
Infundibulum, 605-606, 609
brain and, 160
of left ventricle, 98
of oviduct, 575
of pituitary gland, 158
of right ventricle, 97
Inguinal canal, 457, 464-472
abdomen and, 536
arrangement of layers in, 464-467, 471
descent of ovary in, 472
ductus deferens and, 471-472
processus vaginalis in, 472
ring of; *see* Inguinal ring
scrotum in, 468-472
spermatic cord in, 467-470
testis and, 471-472
walls of, 464-466
Inguinal hernia, 539, 542, 662
clinical anatomy of, 469
congenital, 467
epigastric vessels and, 467
principles of, 463
Inguinal ligament, 555-556, 558, 725-726
abdomen and, 457, 538
fascia of upper thigh and, 650
femoral artery and, 646

Inguinal ligament—cont'd
femoral sheath and, 654
femoral triangle and, 651
of Poupart, 466
thigh and, 654, 658
anteromedial, 637, 654
Inguinal lymph node, 33, 582, 724-725
Inguinal region of abdomen, 538
clinical anatomy of, 469
Inguinal ring, 458-459, 464-465, 467, 538
deep, 459, 557, 575
external, 650
superficial, 458, 531
superior, 650
Inion, 140
Injection, intramuscular, 726-727
gluteal region and, 669
Injuries
to acromioclavicular joint, 317
to ankle, 731
to anterolateral compartment of leg, 698
to brachial plexus, 204, 339, 401-402, 404
to breast, 55
to facial nerve, 185
to foot, 721
to hamstrings, 687
to hand, 401, 403-404
to knee, 687
to median nerve
sensory loss from, 340
at wrist, 392
to musculospiral groove, 402, 404
to orbit, 251
to radial nerve, 402, 404
to recurrent laryngeal nerve, 290
to rotator cuff, 321
to scalp, 185
to shoulder joints, 401, 403
to ulnar nerve, 392
to vertebral column, 431-433
to wrist, 401, 403-404
Inner ear; *see* Ear, inner
Innervation; *see* Nerves
Innominate artery, 206
Innominate bone, 549, 552
Inspiration
forceful, 68
muscles of, 120
quiet, 68
thoracic muscles in, 66-68
Insulin, 497
Intercalated disks, 19
Intercavernous sinus, 157
Intercondylar area, tibial, 679
Intercondylar eminence, 690
tubercles of, 678
Intercondylar fossa, 639-640
knee and, 672, 678
thigh and, 672
Intercostal artery, 460-461
anterior, 68, 118
to breast, 55
to chest wall and, 68-69, 121
costal groove and, 73
cutaneous branches of, 73
deep cervical, 204
diaphragm and, 530
first, 117

Intercostal artery—cont'd
  cervical vertebrae and, 429
    subclavian artery and, 326
  lower, abdomen and, 536
  posterior, 68, 117
    back and spinal cord and, 442, 448
    posterior mediastinum and, 117
  second, 117
    cervical vertebrae and, 429
    subclavian artery and, 326
  spinal cord and vertebrae and, 440
  superior, 68, 117, 204
    cervical vertebrae and, 429
    subclavian artery and, 203, 326
  thoracic spinal cord segment and, 69
  upper, 68, 70
Intercostal membrane, anterior, 64
Intercostal muscle, 64-65
  external, 64
  in respiration, 68
Intercostal nerve, 55, 71-72, 121
  abdomen and, 537
    wall of, 461
  blocks of, 72
  costal groove and, 72-73
  cutaneous branches of, 72-73, 121
  diaphragm and, 529
  first, 337
  muscular branches of, 73
Intercostal space, 65, 72-73
  herpes zoster and, 72
  spinal cord and, 430
Intercostal vein
  abdomen and, 537
    wall of, 460-461
  accessory hemiazygos vein and, 118
  aortic arch and, 109
  azygos vein and, 117
  breast and, 55
  chest wall and, 68-71, 121
  costal groove and, 73
  cutaneous branches of, 73
  first, 70
    accessory hemiazygos vein and, 118
    azygos vein and, 117
  hemiazygos vein and, 117
  posterior
    accessory hemiazygos vein and, 118
    azygos vein and, 117
    back and spinal cord and, 449
    hemiazygos vein and, 117
  right, 70
    azygos vein and, 117
  superior, 70-71, 109
    accessory hemiazygos vein and, 117
    azygos vein and, 117
Intercostobrachial nerve, 329, 334, 337, 366
Interdigitating processes, brain and, 146
Interlobar artery, 526
  in renal arteriogram, 40
Intermuscular septum
  lateral
    arm and, 343-344
    thigh and, 646, 648-649
  medial
    arm and, 343-344
    thigh and, 648, 650

Intermuscular septum—cont'd
  posterior, 650
    thigh and, 648
Internal position of structure, 3
Internal rotation of structure, 5
Interneuron, 20, 444
Internuclear cleft on MRI, 418
Interosseous artery
  anterior, 345, 355, 363
    on arteriogram, 345
    wrist and, 372
  common, 345, 363
    on arteriogram, 345
  posterior, 345, 355, 363
    on arteriogram, 345
    wrist and, 372
Interosseous membrane
  of forearm, 349, 354-356, 394
  of leg, 691
    fascial compartments and, 693
    muscles and, 695
    posterior nerves and, 696
    Pott's fracture and, 704
    tibiofibular articulations and, 692
Interosseous muscle
  palmar, 382, 384-387, 390
    dorsal, 357, 373, 387, 390
    dual origin of, 385
    extrinsic extensor tendons and, 391
    first, 382
    fourth, insertion of, 388
    on MRI, 357
    single origin of, 385
    ventral, 357, 373
  plantar, 719
    deep view of, 715
    dorsal, 709
    MRI of, 709
Interosseous nerve, posterior, 359, 365
Interosseous tendon of hand, 388
Interosseous vein of hand, 355
Interpeduncular cistern, 151
  oculomotor nerve in, 148
Interphalangeal joint, 381, 396, 400
Interspinous distance, 550
Interspinous ligament, 420, 422, 453
  on MRI, 418
Intertransverse ligament, 422
Intertrochanteric crest, 637, 639
Intertrochanteric fossa, 637, 639
Intertrochanteric ridge, 648-649
Intertubercular groove, 312-313, 315, 318, 394, 399
Interureteric crest, 598
Interventricular coronary artery, 89, 92
  anterior, 89, 93
  posterior, 92
Interventricular foramen, 148, 150, 154
Interventricular septal artery, 93
Interventricular septum, 103
Interventricular sulci, 89
Intervertebral articular facets, 413, 415, 417, 420
Intervertebral disk, 411, 419
  body of, 422
    costovertebral and costotransverse joints and, 424

Intervertebral disk—cont'd
  herniation of, 423, 452, 482, 730
  longitudinal ligaments and, 422
  normal vertebral column and, 409
  nucleus pulposus of; see Nucleus pulposus
  thoracic vertebrae and, 58-59, 416
Intervertebral facet; see Facet, articular, intervertebral
Intervertebral foramen, 410-411
  exiting nerve root in, 411
  skeletal anatomy and, 448
  spinal cord and
    intercostal space and, 430
    spinal nerves and, 436
    vertebral canal and, 439
  thoracic vertebrae and, 416
Intervertebral space, lumbar puncture and, 432
Intestine, 30
  large; see Colon
  layers of wall of, 510
  lymphatic drainage of, 480
  small; see Small intestine
Intraabdominal pressure in respiration, 68
Intracapsular ligament, knee joint and, 681
Intracranial hematoma, 151
Intracranial pressure, 133
  increase in, 252
Intracranial venous sinus, 233
Intramembranous ossification, 10
Intramural fibroid, 612
Intramuscular injections, 726-727
  gluteal region and, 669
Intraperitoneal structures, 474, 477
  development of, 478, 483
Intrapulmonary shunting, 79, 83
Intrauterine devices, 626
Intravenous pyelogram, 525
Intrinsic factor, 506
Intrinsic hand muscle, 385-387
Intrinsic vertebral muscle, 200
Introitus, vaginal, 576
Intussusception, 514
Inversion, 7
  of ankle, 703
  of foot, 711
Investing fascia, 200
IP joints; see Interphalangeal joint
Ipsilateral structure, 6
Iridocorneal angle, 239, 250
Iris, 237-239, 295
  aqueous and vitreous humors and, 240
  pathology of, 246, 251
  uveal layer of eye and, 238
Ischial ramus, 559
Ischial spine, 550-552, 562
  on CT, 618
  gluteal region and, 663
Ischial tuberosity, 550-552, 562, 568, 631
  in gluteal region, 663-664
    intermediate layer, 664
  hip joint ligaments and, 642-643
  pelvis and, 559
  perineum and, 561
  sacral plexus and, 590
  thigh and, 648-649

Ischial tuberosity—cont'd
    posterior, 658, 675
Ischioanal fossa, 648-649
Ischiocavernosus muscle, 564-565, 572-573, 577-578, 580
    innervation of, 578
Ischiofemoral ligament, 642-643, 722
Ischiopubic ramus, 550-552, 561, 565, 573
Ischiorectal fossa, 565-568, 581
    anterior recess of, 566
Ischium, 549-551, 581
    on CT, 618
Islets of Langerhans, 35, 498
Isometric contraction, 15-16, 423
    of heart ventricles, 101
Isotonic contraction, 15
    of heart ventricles, 101
Isthmus, 605-606
    of oviduct, 558, 605

J
Jaundice, 489, 540, 543
Jaw
    asymmetric movements of, 197
    upper and lower, 177
Jejunal artery, 511-513
Jejunum, 30, 507, 510-513
    anorectal region and, 517
    blood supply to, 511-513
    pancreas and, 495
    peritoneal membranes and, 481
    peritoneal specialization of, 482-483
    small intestine and, 508-509
    spleen and, 493
Joint, 11
    cartilaginous, 10-11, 13
    of clavicle and scapula, 320
    fibrous, 10-11, 13
    of foot
        distal, 711
        subtalar, MRI of, 708-710
        transverse tarsal, 708, 710
    of forearm, 349-355
    of hand, 379-381
    of knee, 676-682
    patellofemoral, 676-679
    of pelvis, 550, 553-557
    of shoulder, 309-315, 318-322
        clinical anatomy of, 321
    sternochondral, 50, 60
    of sternum, 50, 60, 321
    striated muscle of, 25
    synovial, 11, 13-14
    tibiofibular, 691-692
    of upper limb, 396
    of upper vertebral column, 421, 433
    in vertebra, 417-424
    between vertebrae and ribs, 59-60
    of wrist, 370, 374
Joint capsule, 14, 353
    carpometacarpal joint and, 379-380
    of elbow, 349, 353
    glenohumeral joint and, 318
Joint cavity for femoral head, 641
Joint fluid, aspiration of, 669
Jugular bulb, 162, 208
    brain and, 157

Jugular bulb—cont'd
    skull and, 140
Jugular foramen, 141
    anterolateral neck and, 210
    cranial nerves and, 167
    skull and, 139, 143
Jugular fossa, 142
Jugular notch, 62, 122
Jugular tubercle, 142
Jugular vein, 133, 198
    catheters in, 119
    external, 183, 208-209, 292
        parotid gland and, 185
        posterior triangle and, 204
    internal, 157, 183, 208, 292, 296
        anterolateral neck and, 207
        in carotid sheath, 206
        catheters in, 119
        middle ear and, 226-227
        on MRI, 271
        parotid gland and, 186
        posterior triangle and, 204
    neck and, 203
    pterygoid venous plexus and, 195

K
Keratotomy, radial, 251
Kidney, 30-35, 522-528, 582
    anatomy of
        clinical, 528
        surface, 538
    blood pressure and, 528
    blood supply to, 524-528
    collecting system of, 524-525
    on CT, 41
    function of, 522
    horseshoe, 602-603
    left, 595
        adrenal glands and, 526
    normal, 597
    pancreas and, 497
    peritoneal membranes and, 478
    position and structural features of, 522-524
    rotation of stomach and, 476
    serous membranes and, 474
    stabbed, 541, 544
    suprarenal glands and, 527-528
    testis and, 470
    thoracic duct and, 31
    ureteropelvic junction of, 524-525
    urinary collection in, 525
    on x-ray, 39
Klumpke's paralysis, 339
Knee, 672, 674-686
    anterior view of, 12
    arthroscopy of, 687
    articular surface for compartments of, 679
    blood supply to, 684-685
    center of gravity and, 672
    clinical anatomy of, 687
    flexion and extension of, 5, 672, 682-684
        patella and, 677
    injuries to, 687
    interior of, 676, 679-682
    ligaments of, 676, 679-682
        in flexion and extension, 682-684

Knee—cont'd
    transverse, 680-681
    movements of, 682-684
    musculoskeletal system and, 722-723
    neurovascular supply of, 684-685
    patellofemoral joint of, 676-679
    rotation at, 682-683
    valgus or varus deformity at, 686-687
    x-rays of, 678
Knock-knees, 640, 729-731
Kyphosis, 409

L
L1-5; *see* Lumbar vertebra
Labia majora and minora, 571-572, 574, 576, 609
    inguinal canal and, 466, 468
Labial artery
    face and, 182
    inferior, 183
    superior, 183, 259
Labial nerve, posterior, 583
Labial vein, superior, 195
Labrum
    acetabular, 640-641
    glenoid, 311, 316, 318, 323
Labyrinth, membranous, 233
Labyrinthine artery, 161
Laceration
    of eyebrow, 176
    scalp, 185
    of wrist, 377
Lacertus fibrosus, 400
Lacrimal artery, 242, 250
    orbit and, 250
Lacrimal bone, 236
    orbit and, 234
Lacrimal caruncle, 249
Lacrimal duct, 249
    abnormalities of flow of, 251
Lacrimal fossa, 249
Lacrimal gland, 245, 249-250
    face and scalp and, 178
    innervation of, 168
    parasympathetic nerves and, 294
Lacrimal nerve, 168, 238, 242, 247, 250
    face and scalp and, 178
    orbit and, 245
    pterygopalatine fossa and, 261
Lacrimal punctum, 239, 249
Lacrimal sac, 249
    groove for, 236
Lactiferous duct, 54
Lactiferous sinus, 54-55
Lacunar ligament, 555
    femoral sheath and, 653-654
    of Gimbernat, 466
Lambda, 134, 137, 140
Lambdoidal suture, 135-138, 141
Lamellae of eye, 248
Lamina of vertebra, 58, 409-411, 414, 416, 423
Lamina papyracea, 234
Lamina terminalis, 148
Langerhans, islets of, 498
Language areas of brain, 149
Large intestine; *see* Colon
Laryngeal artery, 289

Laryngeal nerve, 84, 109, 111-112, 116
  compression of, 119
  cranial nerves and, 166
  glossopharyngeal nerve and, 211
  recurrent, 288
    aortic arch and, 109
    injury to, 290
    larynx and, 287-289
    left, 109, 111-112, 213
    right, 211-213, 288-289
    thyroid gland and, 218
  superior, 288-289
    external branch of, 288
    injury to, 290
    internal branch of, 288
    thyroid gland and, 218
    vagus nerve and, 211
Laryngeal prominence, 284-285
Laryngeal vein, 289
Laryngeal ventricle, 285-286
Laryngectomy, 290
Laryngopharynx, 281-282
Laryngoscopy, 290
Larynx, 284-290, 292
  blood supply to, 289
  cancer of, 290
  cartilage of, 278, 284-285
  clinical anatomy of, 290
  fracture of, 290
  glottic region of, 285-286
  horns of, 285
  inlet of, 285-286
  innervation of, 287-289
  maturational changes in, 290
  muscles of, 282, 285-287
  principles and, 287
  surgical risk to, 290
  thyroid gland and, 290
  trauma to, 290
  viewing of, 290
Latarjet, nerve of, 503-504
Lateral position of structure, 3, 5
Lateral rotation of structure, 5-6
Lateral slip, 384
Latissimus dorsi muscle
  abdomen and, 492
  anatomy of
    musculoskeletal, 394
    surface, 398
  anterior compartment and, 345
  axilla and, 330-331
  back and vertebral column and, 423, 425
  on CT and MRI, 43, 100
  posterior trunk and, 65
  in respiration, 68
  shoulder movement and, 325-326
  tendon of, 331
Leaflets of heart valves, 95, 97-99
Left dominance, 92
Leg, 688-699
  in anatomic position, 3-4
  anterior
    arteries of, 696-698
    muscles of, 696-697
    nerves of, 696-698
  clinical anatomy of, 698
  comparison of, to forearm, 723

Leg—cont'd
  compartments of, 692-699, 703
    anterior, 696-698
    anterolateral, injuries to, 698
    fascial, 692-699, 703
    injuries to, 698
    lateral, 697, 699
    posterior, 692-696, 703
  cross-section through, 693
  edema of, 724
  fibula and, 690-691
  fracture of, 704
  lateral, muscles of, 699
  localized swelling in, 729
  on MRI, 693
  musculoskeletal system and, 723
  popliteal fossa and, 688-690, 694-696
  posterior
    arteries of, 692-696
    lymphatic drainage of, 696
    nerves of, 696
  tibia and, 690-691
  tibiofibular articulations and, 691-692
Lens, 234, 238-240
  aqueous and vitreous humors and, 240
  ciliary body and, 239
  clinical anatomy of, 251
  dislocation of, 251
  horizontal section of orbit and, 242
  shape of, cranial nerves and, 169
  skull and, 143
  uveal layer of eye and, 238
Lesser occipital nerve; see Occipital nerve,
    lesser
Lesser omentum; see Omentum, lesser
Lesser palatine artery, 267
Lesser palatine nerve, 260, 267
Lesser pelvis, 549
Lesser petrosal nerve, 227
  parasympathetic nerves and, 294
Lesser sac; see Omentum, lesser
Lesser sciatic notch; see Sciatic notch, lesser
Lesser splanchnic nerve, 118
Lesser trochanter; see Trochanter, lesser
Lesser wing of sphenoid bone, 139, 236
  horizontal section through bony orbit
    and, 237
Levator ani muscle, 562-566, 568-571
  abdomen and, 459
  anal canal and, 568
  attached to arcus tendineus, 565
  bladder neck in female and, 581
  diaphragm and, 532
  female internal genitalia and, 606
  ligamentous supports of bladder and
    rectum and, 599
  nerve to, 671
  perineum and, 573
  pudendal artery and, 590
  thigh and, 648-649
  umbilical ligaments and, 557
Levator labii superioris alaeque nasi muscle,
    178-180
Levator palatini muscle, 269
Levator palpebrae superioris muscle, 180,
    237, 243, 248
  optic canal and, 249

Levator prostatae, 563-565
Levator scapulae muscle, 425
  innervation of, 329
  shoulder movement and, 325-326
  vertebral column and, 423
Levator veli palatini muscle, 264, 266
  swallowing and, 282
Levatores costarum, 64
Lidocaine, 542
Lienorenal ligament, 483, 491, 493
Ligaments, 9, 14
  of ankle, 699-703
  of carpometacarpal joints, 379-381
  of elbow joint, 353
  of foot, 707-708
  of hip joint, 640-644
  of knee, 676, 679-682
  of mediastinum, 118
  of ovary, 36
  of pelvis, 550, 553-557
  of pericardium, 88
  of shoulder, 319
  of spleen, 491, 493-494
  of Treitz, 507-508
  of vertebrae, 417-424
  of wrist, 369, 372
Ligamentum arteriosum, 81, 97
  aortic arch and, 109
  formation of, 106
  mediastinum and, 216
  spinal cord and, 444
Ligamentum capitis femoris, 642-643
Ligamentum flavum, 420-422, 453
Ligamentum nuchae, 422
Ligamentum teres
  abdomen and, 459
  artery of, 645
  femur and, 641
  hip joints and, 642-643
  liver and, 484-485, 487
  porta hepatis and, 486
Ligamentum venosum
  abdomen and, 492
  liver and, 487
  porta hepatis and, 486
Light reflex, 237-238, 251
Light transmission of globe of eye, 235
Limb
  growth of, dermatomes and, 27
  lower; see Lower limb
  upper; see Upper limb
Limbus fossa ovalis, 95
Line
  arcuate, of ilium; see Arcuate line of ilium
  axial, 16, 18
  axillary, 122
  cleavage, of Langer, 457
  epiphyseal, knee joint and, 678
  gingival, 268
  gluteal, 562, 643
  Hilton, 568
  intertrochanteric, 639
  Langer, 457, 462
  midaxillary, 122
  midclavicular, 122-123
  midsagittal, 123
  milk, 55

Line—cont'd
  mylohyoid, 187-188
  pectinate, 556, 568-569, 571, 639
    pelvis and, 559
  supracondylar, 637, 639
  trapezoid, 314
  white, of rectum, 568-569, 571
Linea alba, 63, 457, 459-462, 538, 575
Linea aspera
  anteromedial thigh and, 637, 639
  thigh and, 659, 672
Linea semilunaris, 460, 462, 538
Lingual artery, 159, 272
  as branch of external carotid artery, 209
  face and, 182
  pharynx and, 280
  submandibular region and, 222
  tongue and, 272
Lingual nerve, 170, 222, 231, 270, 272
  face and scalp and, 178
  mandibular nerve and, 194
  submandibular region and, 222
  tongue and, 272
Lingual septum on MRI, 271
Lingual swelling, pharyngeal arches and,
    171
Lingual thyroid, 275
Lingual tonsil, 270
Lingual vein, 272, 296
  submandibular region and, 222
  tongue and, 272
Lingula, 189
  mandible and, 188
Lip
  cleft, 275
  lower, 264
  upper, frenulum of, 264
Lipases
  deficiency of, 543
  pancreatic secretions and, 498
Lips, 177
Lister's tubercle, 361-362
Lithiasis, 602
Little finger
  extension of, 390
  muscle insertions on, 387-388
Liver, 477, 484-489, 493, 611
  blood supply to, 485, 488-489, 493
    bypassing, 489
    resistance to, 489
    venous drainage for, 480
  clinical anatomy of, 489
  common bile ducts and, 487-488; see also
      Bile duct
  development of, 476, 479, 484
    peritoneal specialization in, 482-483
  disease of, esophagus and, 116
  ducts of, 488
  fetal, 486
  function of, 480
  functional reserve in, 489
  greater omentum and, 504
  hepatic duct and, 487-488; see also Hepatic
      duct
  kidneys and, 524
  lobes of, 484-486
    pancreas and, 496

Liver—cont'd
  metastatic cancer and, 489
  pancreas and, 497
  parasympathetic nerves and, 294
  peritoneal membranes and, 481
  peritoneal reflections and, 485-486
  porta hepatis and, 486-487
  principles of, 487-488
  rotation of stomach and, 476
  serous membranes and, 474
  spleen and, 491
  stomach and, 505
  transplantation of, 489
Lobar artery, 526
  in renal arteriogram, 40
Lobar bronchi, 77
Lobes
  of abdomen, 492
  of fetal liver, 486
  of liver, 485, 487
  of pancreas, 496
Lobules
  in breast, 54
  of kidney, 524
  of testis, 471
Local anesthesia of jaw, 197
Locomotion, 711, 714
Long finger
  extension of, 390
  muscle insertions on, 387-388
Long rotator muscle, 427
Longissimus muscle of head, 265, 425-426
  spinal cord and, 445
  vertebral column and, 433
Longitudinal arches of foot, 708
Longitudinal arterial vessel, 427
Longitudinal ligament, anterior and
    posterior, 411, 418-423
  on MRI, 415, 418
  triangular extension of, 422
Longitudinal muscles of vertebra, 425
  cervical, 292
  external, 598
Longus colli muscle, 168
  spinal cord and, 445
Loose areolar tissue of scalp and face, 175
Lordosis, 409
Loss of consciousness in head trauma, 298,
    302-303
Lower limb, 634-731
  anatomic position and, 3
  anterior and posterior views of, 638
  blood supply to, 724
    superficial veins and, 652
    venous drainage of, 652, 724
  case studies and, 728-731
  in fetus, 18
  foot in, 705-721; see also Foot
  gluteal region of, 663-671
  innervation of, 725
  knee in, 672-687; see also Knee
  leg and ankle joint in, 688-704; see also
      Ankle; Leg
  lymphatics of, 724-725
    thoracic duct and, 31
  pelvic girdle in, 310-311
  physical examination of, 725-727

Lower limb—cont'd
  surface anatomy of, 722-727
  systems review of, 722-727
  thigh in
    anteromedial, 637-662; see also Thigh,
        anteromedial
    posterior, 672-674
    vascular grafts in, 704
Lower limb buds, 18
Lower limb girdle, comparison of, to upper
    limb girdle, 723
Lower lip, 264
Lower respiratory tract, 74
Lub sounds of heart, 104, 124
Ludwig's angina, 223
Lumbar artery, 428, 460
  abdomen and, 513, 536
  back and spinal cord and, 440, 442, 448
Lumbar chains, ascending, 33
Lumbar curvature, 409-410
Lumbar fascia, 457
Lumbar hernia, 463
Lumbar nerve, abdominal wall and, 461
Lumbar plexus, 530-534, 586
  gluteal region and, 670-671
  pelvis and perineum and, 624
Lumbar puncture, 153, 155, 431-432, 447, 449
Lumbar ribs, 62, 412
Lumbar vein, 460
  abdomen and, 534, 537
  ascending, 428
  back and spinal cord and, 449
Lumbar vertebra, 409-415
  abdomen and, 536
  articular surface for, 553
  lumbar puncture and, 153, 155, 431-432,
      447, 449
  MRI of, 418
  pelvic ligaments and, 556
  surface for articulation with, 419
  x-ray of, 417
Lumbodorsal fascia, 529
Lumbosacral angle, 409-410
Lumbosacral joint, 556
Lumbosacral ligament, 556
Lumbosacral plexus, 16, 586
  pelvic interior and, 558
Lumbosacral trunk, 531-533, 588
Lumbrical muscles
  foot and, 715-716, 719
  hand and, 357, 373, 384-387
    extensor expansions and, 390-391
    extrinsic extensor tendons and, 391
Lumen, 607
Lumpectomy, 127
Lunate, 357, 369-374, 376, 396
  dislocation of, 376
  fracture of, 402, 405
  on MRI, 357
  radiocarpal joint and, 370
  wrist and, 371, 373-374
Lung, 28-29, 34, 80-85
  air entering, 68
  alveoli of, 80
  anatomy of
    clinical, 83, 85, 126, 128
    radiographic, 77

Lung—cont'd
  surface, 123
  apex of, 80, 124
    surface projections of, 124
  auscultation of, 124
  blood supply to, 81-85
    blood flow between heart and, 83
    clinical anatomy of, 83
    vascular shunting in, 79, 83
  case studies and, 126, 128
  on CT and MRI, 43, 100
  dome or cupola of, 205
  fissures of, 80, 124
    horizontal or minor, 123
    oblique or major, 80, 100, 123-124
    plane of, 100
  hilum of, 51, 80, 121
    phrenic nerve and, 112
    visceral pleura and, 74
  hypoplastic, 544
  innervation of, 84-85, 122
    autonomic, 84
    cranial nerves and, 169
    parasympathetic nerves and, 294
    phrenic nerve and, 112
  left, 76, 80-81
  lymphatics of, 81-85
  malignancy of, 126, 128
  pleural spaces of, 74-76
  position of, 124
  principles for, 68
  receptors in, 105
  right, 76, 80
    surface anatomy of, 123
  surfaces of, 80-81
  views of
    anterior, 75
    lateral and medial, 76
Lung bud
  pharyngeal arches and, 171
  tracheal, pharyngeal arches and, 172
Luschka foramen, 154
Lymph duct, subclavian, 335
Lymph node, 29, 32; see also Lymphatic
    drainage
  in anterior mediastinum, 118
  axillary, 334-335, 397
  hilar, 85
  inguinal, 724-725
  of neck, 134, 198
    anterior, 210
  occipital, 210
  preauricular, 210
  submandibular, 210, 222
    clinical anatomy of, 223
  submental, 210
  supraclavicular, 210
  of thorax, 121
  venous and arterial vessels to, 32
Lymphangiography, 33, 721
Lymphatic drainage, 29, 31-33; see also
    Lymph node
  of abdomen, 537
    from lower limb, 115
  afferent, 32
  of axilla, 334-335, 337
  of back and spinal cord, 449

Lymphatic drainage—cont'd
  of breast, 56, 121
    cancer and, 56
  in carotid triangle, 209-210
  efferent, 32
  of head and neck, 133-134, 292
  interruption of, 114
  of intestine, 480
  of larynx, 289
  of lower limb, 115, 724-725
  of lungs, 84-85
  of mediastinum, 114, 117
  of pelvis, 623
  of penis and scrotum, 578, 581
  of perineum, 578, 582, 623
  of posterior leg, 696
  of small intestine, 512
  of thorax, 29, 31, 114-115, 117, 121; see also
    Thoracic duct
  of tongue, 272-273
  of upper limb, 397
Lymphoid follicles, 32
Lymphoid tissue, ring of, 279
Lysosome, 21

M

Macula, 241
Magendie foramen, 154
Magnetic resonance imaging
  of chest, 100
  CT compared to, 43
  of foot and ankle, 709
  of leg, 693
  techniques of, 39-40, 42-43
Male
  external genitalia of, 575-582
  pelvic and perineal examination in, 624-
    626
  pelvic viscera of; see Pelvic viscera, male
  pelvis in, 550
    floor of, 565
    imaging, 618, 620
  reproductive system of, smooth muscles
    of, 19
  urethra in, traumatic injury to, 619-621
  urogenital diaphragm in, 564
Malformation; see Deformities
Malignancy
  lymph nodes and, submandibular, 223
  in oral cavity, 275
Malleolus
  ankle and, 700
  lateral, 690-691, 725-726
    ankle tendons and, 702
    blood supply to ankle and, 703
    of fibula, 700-701
    fibula and, 691
    leg muscles and, 695
    MRI of, 709
    posterior leg nerves and, 696
    Pott's fracture and, 704
  ligaments connecting, to tarsal bones, 707
  medial, 652, 690-691, 725-726
    ankle tendons and, 702
    blood supply to ankle and, 703
    deltoid ligament and, 702
    leg muscles and, 695

Malleolus—cont'd
    medial view of, 700
    MRI of, 709
    popliteal fossa and, 691
    posterior leg nerves and, 696
    Pott's fracture and, 704
    of tibia, 700-701
Malleus, 225-230
  head of, 226, 228
Malrotation of gut, 482, 514
Mamillary body
  cranial nerves and, 165
  on MRI, 148
Mammography, 56-57
Mandible, 174, 187-194
  alveolar vessels and nerves entering, 189,
    193-194
  anterior view of, 12
  attachment of, 291
  body of, 187-188
  chewing apparatus and, 192
  condyle of, 135, 143, 189-190
  coronoid of, 188-189
  developmental changes of, 197
  external surface of, 187-188
  fibrous joints and, 13
  foramen of, 188-189
  fossa of, 143
  fractures of, 197
  hypoplasia of, 170
  internal surface of, 187-189, 193
  loss of teeth and, 268
  as movable bone, 133
  pharynx and, 277
  ramus of, 135, 137, 187-189
  in skeletal framework of face, 177, 291
  skull and, 134-135, 137
  sublingual gland and submandibular duct
    and, 273
  submandibular region and, 220, 222, 273
  submandibular triangle and, 220
  surface anatomy of, 295
  temporomandibular joint and, 189
  tongue and, 272
Mandibular branches, 195
  of facial nerve, 178, 180, 185
  of trigeminal nerve (V3), 165-166, 178-180,
    193-195
Mandibular nerve, 193-195
  branches of; see Mandibular branches
  to face and scalp, 178
  mastication and, 190
  pharyngeal arches and, 171
  posterior trunk of, 194
  skull and, 140
  tensor veli palatini and, 267
  trunks of, 194
Maneuvers, Valsalva, 120
Manubriosternal joint, 62
Manubrium of sternum, 50, 61-63, 168, 321,
    398, 429
  anterolateral neck and, 216
  clavicle and, 313, 317
  on MRI, 42
  subclavian artery and, 203, 326
  thoracic inlet and, 311
Marfan's syndrome, 251

Marginal artery
    abdomen and, 537
    cecum and, 518
    left, 92
    right, 92
Marginal sinus, 157
Marginal vein on foot, 715
Marrow of bone, 10
    sampling of, from sternum, 63
Marrow cavity, 10
Massa intermedia, 148
Masseter muscle, 133, 178-183, 295
    mastication and, 190-192
    parotid gland and, 184
Masseteric nerve, 181
Mastectomy, 127
    modified radical, 127
    winging of scapula and, 324
Mastication, 177, 269
    muscles of, 190-192, 292
        in temporal and infratemporal fossae,
            187
    structures of, 134
Mastoid air cells
    middle ear and, 226
    skull and, 135, 142-143
Mastoid infection, 232
Mastoid process
    face and, 182
    mandibular nerve and, 194
    mastication muscles and, 191
    skull and, 134, 141
    temporomandibular joint and, 190
Matrix
    in connective tissue, 8
    proteoglycan, in bones, 9
Maxilla
    bony orbit and, 234, 236
    hard palate and, 268
    mastication muscles and, 191
    nose and, 253
    processes of
        maxillary, 135
        palatine, 135, 255
    recession of, 170
    sinuses in, 143
    skeletal framework of face and, 13, 134,
        141-142, 174, 177-178
    surface anatomy of, 294
    temporomandibular joint and, 189
    tooth socket in, 13
    views of
        frontal, 137
        posterior, 137
        on x-ray, 417
Maxillary artery, 259
    anterolateral neck and, 208
    brain and, 159
    as branch of external carotid artery, 209
    ethmoid perpendicular plate and, 255
    face and, 182
    fossae and
        pterygopalatine, 260-261
        temporal and infratemporal, 187, 192-
            193
    middle ear and, 233
    nose and, 259

Maxillary artery—cont'd
    otic ganglion and, 194
    parotid gland and, 186
    pharyngeal arches and, 171
    pharynx and, 280-281
Maxillary branch of trigeminal nerve (V2),
        165-166, 179-180
Maxillary nerve (VII), 162, 178-179
    nose and, 259
    orbit and, 245
    pterygopalatine fossa and, 260-261
    skull and, 140
Maxillary sinus, 135, 178, 256-258
    inflammation of, 262
    orbit and, 234-235
Maxillary vein, 195
McBurney's point, 538
Meatus, nasal
    inferior, 249, 256-258
    middle, 256, 258
    superior, 256-258
Meckel's diverticulum, 542
Medial position of structure, 3, 5
Medial rotation of structure, 5-6
Median nerve, 365-366, 398, 400
    in arm, 344
    axilla and, 333
    brachial plexus and, 337, 339, 341
    compression of, 376
    constant pressure on, 403, 405
    in forearm, 356, 366
    in hand, 392-393
    injury to, 340
        high and low lesions to, 367
        sensory loss from, 340
        at wrist, 392
    on MRI, 357
    palmar cutaneous branch of, 368
    radioulnar joint and, 354
    in wrist, 374
Median sagittal plane, 3, 6
Median sternotomy incision, 63
Median vein
    collection of blood samples and, 367
    in forearm, 364
Mediastinal pleura, 74
Mediastinal surface of lungs, 80
Mediastinoscopy, 119
Mediastinum, 52-53, 109-119
    anterior, 52, 118
    boundaries of, 52, 110
    case studies of, 126, 128
    clinical anatomy of, 114, 119
    heart and great vessels and, 89
    inferior, 52, 109, 114-118
    innervation of, 122, 216
    lateral surface of
        left, 113
        right, 112
    lung attachment to, 51
    middle, 52, 86, 109
    palpation of, 122
    posterior, 52, 114-118
    principles and, 111
    referred pain to, 119
    superior, 52, 109-114
        palpation of, 122

Mediastinum—cont'd
    surgical approaches to, 119
    trauma to, 114
    visual inspection of, 119
Medulla
    of adrenal gland, 527
        abnormalities of, 528
    of brain, 147-149, 161
        on MRI, 148
    cranial nerves and, 165
    of kidney, 522
Medullary velum, superior, 148
Megacolon, congenital, 520
Meibomian gland, 241
Meissner's corpuscle, 8
Meissner's plexus, 520-521
Membranes
    conjunctival, 250
    intercostal, 64
    interosseous, 356
    peritoneal; see Peritoneal membrane
    pleural, 30
    serous, 51, 474
    tympanic, 225-226, 228
Membranous labyrinth, 230, 233
Membranous urethra, 609, 616, 619
    on CT, 618
    on cystourethrogram, 617
    with external urethral sphincter, 616
Meniere's disease, 232
Meningeal artery, 134
    middle, 134, 196
        groove for, 135, 139
        maxillary artery and, 192-193
        otic ganglion and, 194
        skull and, 139-140
    middle ear and, 233
    orbit and, 250
Meningeal nerve, 193-195
    recurrent, 449
Meningeal vein, 135
Meninges, 155-158
    choroid plexus and, 152
    clinical anatomy of, 155
    as component of central nervous system,
        20, 145
    spinal cord and, 435-440
Meningiomas, 155
Meningitis, 153, 155
    sinuses and, 262
Meningoencephalitis, 155
Meniscofemoral ligament, posterior, 676,
        679, 681
    superior end of tibia and, 680
Meniscus, 679
    injuries to, 687
    lateral and medial, 676, 681
        superior end of tibia and, 680
    transverse ligament of, 679
Mental foramen, 134, 187-188
    head and neck and, 295
    mandible and, 188
    mastication muscles and, 191
    mental nerve exiting, 194
    skull and, 134, 137
Mental nerve
    exiting mental foramen, 194

Mental nerve—cont'd
    face and, 181
    head and neck and, 295
Mental status, sudden change in, 297, 301-302
Mental symphysis, 187-188, 295
Mental tubercle, 187-188
Mesencephalon, 147-148
    on MRI, 148
Mesenchyme, 480
Mesenteric adenitis, 514
Mesenteric arteriogram, superior, 513
Mesenteric artery
    inferior, 477, 479, 591, 603
        abdomen and, 534, 536-537
        colon and, 516, 519
        rectum and anus and, 517, 519
    kidneys and, 526
    small intestine and, 512
    superior, 476-477, 479
        abdomen and, 534, 536-537
        arteriogram of, 513
        colon and, 516
        duodenum and, 508
        jejunal and ileal branches of, 511-512
        kidneys and, 526
        pancreas and, 496, 498
        spinal cord and, 445
        spleen and, 493
        stomach and, 502
Mesenteric ganglion, 445
Mesenteric nerve, 537
Mesenteric sling, 35
Mesenteric vein
    inferior, 479
        rectum and, 517
    peritoneal membranes and, 479
    superior, 479
        abdomen and, 537
        duodenum and, 508, 510
        liver and, 488
        pancreas and, 496
        spleen and, 494
        stomach and, 480
Mesentery
    anorectal region and, 517
    development of, 474-481, 505
        dorsal, 474-476, 480-481
            greater omentum and, 480-481
            lesser omentum and, 481
        parietal, 473-474, 476
        ventral, 474-476, 481
        visceral, 473-474, 476
    omentum and
        greater, 480-481, 504
        lesser, 481
    principles of, 475
    root of, peritoneal membranes and, 478
    of spleen, 491, 493-494
Mesocolon
    principles of, 475
    transverse, stomach and, 504
Mesoderm, 170-171
Mesoduodenum, 475
Mesogastrium
    greater omentum and, 504
    principles of, 475

Mesometrium, 559, 604, 606
Mesosalpinx, 559, 604, 606
Mesosigmoid, peritoneal membranes and, 478
Mesotendon, 49
    serous membranes and, 474
    visceral and parietal, 390
Mesovarium, 559, 604, 606
Metabolism
    adrenal gland and, 527
    kidneys and, 522
Metacarpal, 378-379, 384, 396, 400
    anterior view of, 12
    carpal bones and, 370
    carpometacarpal joint and, 372, 379-380
    damage to, 402, 405
    fifth
        base of, 357, 371, 373
        head of, 371
        shaft of, 371
    first, base of, 357
    fourth, base of, 357, 373
    growth and maturation of, 11
    head of, 376
    ligament of
        deep transverse, 381, 390
        superficial transverse, 382
    on MRI, 357
    second
        base of, 357, 373
        on x-ray, 371
    shaft of, 357
    skeletal anatomy of, 309-310
    third, base of, 357, 373
    of thumb, 370, 372, 378, 393
        base of, 376
        on x-ray, 371
    wrist and, 372
    on x-ray, 371
Metacarpophalangeal joint, 378-379, 381, 386, 396, 400
Metaphysis, 10
Metastatic cancer, liver and, 489
Metatarsal, 706-708
    great toe, 707
    metatarsus adductus and, 720
    on MRI, 709
    transverse section of, 718
    tuberosity of, 700-701
    views of
        anterior, 12
        lateral, 699
        medial, 700
Metatarsus adductus, 720
Metopic suture, 138, 144
Micrognathia, 173
Micturition, 600
    spinal cord injuries and, 592, 602
Midaxillary line, 122
Midbrain, 147-150
    MRI of, 148
Midclavicular line, 122-123
Middle ear; see Ear, middle
Middle ear cavity, floor of, 229
Midgut, development of, 473, 475-476, 479-480
Midpalmar space, 389

Midsagittal line, 123
Midsagittal plane, 3
Milk letdown, 55
Milk line, 55
Mineral density, x-ray detection of, 36
Mineralocorticoids, 527
Miosis, 251
Mitochondrion, 21
Mitral heart valve, 91, 96-99
    blood flow through, 102
    position of, 122
    prolapse of, 101
    surface anatomy of, 123
    surface projections of, 124
Mitral valve annulus, 91
Moderator band, 95, 103-104
Molars, 267-268
    mandible and, 188
Monro, foramen of, 148
Mons pubis, 571-572, 626; see also Symphysis pubis
Morgagni hernias, 535
Motor axon, 71, 73
    visceral, 164
Motor control of speech, 149
Motor cortex, 149
Motor neuron, 20, 22
    autonomic, 22, 26-27
    peripheral, in brain, 146
    somatic, 20-22, 25, 436
    spinal, diseases of, 447
Motor root of mandibular branch of trigeminal nerve, 165
Mouth, 30, 177, 263-267; see also Palate
    borders of oral cavity in, 263-264
    cheek of, 268-269
    clinical anatomy of, 275
    floor of, 292
    palate of, 263-268
        hard, 263, 265, 268
        palatine tonsil of, 266, 274
        soft, 263
    sublingual glands of, 272-274
    submandibular glands of, 272-274
    teeth in, 267-269
    tongue of, 269-273
Movement
    of ankle joint, 703
    of chest wall, 65-68
    at elbow, 349
    of eye, postoperative abnormalities in, 299-300, 304
    of foot, 711-712
    of glenohumeral joint, 322-324
    of hand, 390, 393
    of head, 418
        muscles controlling, 426-428
    of hip joint, 643-645
    of humerus, 324
    of knee, 682-684
    of radioulnar joints, 353
    of scapula, 313, 316
    sensations of, 224
    of shoulder, 316, 322-327
    terms describing, 6-7
    of thumb, 380-381, 384-385
    of upper limb, 7

Movement—cont'd
    of vertebral column, 427, 448
MS; see Multiple sclerosis
Mucopolysaccharide, 8
Mucosa, 19
    of gastrointestinal system, 30, 499
        in gut wall, 35, 510
    of middle ear and auditory tube, 211
    of nose, 254
    of rectum and anus, 519
Mucus, 506
    cells secreting, in duodenum, 507
    cranial nerves and, 169
    obstruction to flow of, 262
Muller, tarsal muscle of, 248
Multifidus muscle, 426-427
Multiple rib fractures, 72
Multiple sclerosis, 151
Multipolar neuron, 20-22
Mumps, 185
Murmurs of heart, 124
Muscle, 11-20
    of arm, 344-346
    of back and vertebral column, 423-428
    cardiac, 19-20
    of chest wall, 64-68
    classification of, 16
    contraction of, 15
    disturbance of normal conduction
        between neuron and, 151
    of expiration, 120
    of face, 174
        expression and, 178-181
        innervation of, 180-181, 184
    of fetus, 18
    of foot
        dorsal, 714-715
        in sole, 715-719
    of forearm, 355-363
        hypertrophy of, 351
    of gluteal region
        large, 663-666
        smaller, 665-669
    of gut wall, 35
    of hand, 382-388
    of head and neck, 133
        anterior, 216
        controlling movement, 426-428
    of heart, 89-90
    in infrahyoid region, 215-217
    innervation of, 16
        mesodermal origin and, 398
        spinal nerve, 341
        of upper limb, 397
    inserting on femur, 640
    of inspiration, 120
    of larynx, 285-287
    of leg
        anterior, 696-697
        lateral, 699
        posterior compartment, 692, 694-695
    of mastication, 187, 190-192, 292
    mesodermal origin of, 398
    of pelvic diaphragm, 564
    of pelvis and perineum, 622-623
    popliteal fossa and, 688-689, 694
    of shoulder, 322-327

Muscle—cont'd
    clinical anatomy of, 324
    skeletal, 11-18
    smooth, 16-19
        of soft palate, 263-266
    striated, 11-18
        shapes of, 17
    synovial joints and, 14
    of thigh
        anterior, 638, 646, 653-657, 660
        anteromedial, compartments for, 646-
            650
        medial, 655, 657-661
        posterior, 673-674
    of trachea, 77
    of vertebral column
        extrinsic, 423-425
        intrinsic, 425-427
    voluntary, 11-18
Muscle spindles, 17
Muscle wasting
    in carpal tunnel syndrome, 392
    median nerve injury and, 405
Muscular triangle of neck, 198, 201
    anterolateral, 211, 215-219
Musculocutaneous nerve, 398
    arm and, 344
    axilla and, 333
    brachial plexus and, 337, 341
    forearm and, 368
    spinal cord segments in, 400
Musculophrenic artery, 68, 118, 461, 536
Musculoskeletal anatomy review
    of abdomen, 536
    of back and spinal cord, 448
    of head and neck, 291-292
    of lower limb, 722-724
    of pelvis and perineum, 622-623
    of thorax, 120-121
    of upper limb, 394-395
Musculospiral groove, 315, 318
    injury of, 402, 404
Myasthenia gravis, 119
Mydriasis, 251
Myelin, 20, 23, 145-146
    axon with, 21
    deterioration of, 151
    neurons and, 146
    spinal cord and, 436
Myelin lamellae, 146
Myelin sheath, 146
Myenteric plexus, 35
Mylohyoid line, 187-188
Mylohyoid muscle, 218-220, 272-273
    nerve to, 194
    pharynx and, 276
    submandibular gland and, 221
    submandibular region and, 220-222
    submandibular triangle and, 220
    in submental triangle, 223
Myocardial infarction, 126, 128
Myocardial muscle, 89
Myocytes, cardiac, 103
Myometrium on ultrasound, 612; see also
    Heart
Myopia, 240
Myosin, 15

Myotome, 24, 26
    brachial plexus and, 341
Myringotomy, 232

N

Nares, 176-177, 253-254
Nasal apertures, 134
    posterior, 279
Nasal artery
    dorsal, 242
        orbit and, 250
    external, 259
    internal, 259
    lateral, 183
Nasal bone, 236, 253-254, 294
    scalp and face and, 174, 177
    skull and, 134, 137, 142
Nasal cartilage, 254
Nasal cavity, 176-177, 253-262; see also Nose
    anatomy of, 253-254, 257
        clinical, 262
    blood supply to, 259
    innervation of nose in, 259-260
    lateral nasal wall in, 254-256
        spaces in, 255-258
    nasal septum and, 253-255
    olfactory epithelium and, 254, 258
    olfactory nerve and, 254, 258
    orbit and, 235
    pterygopalatine fossa in, 259-261
Nasal conchae; see Conchae
Nasal flaring, 180
Nasal nerve
    external, 247, 260
    internal, 260
Nasal process, brain and, 154
Nasal septum, 253-255
    brain and, 160
    skull and, 143
Nasal wall, lateral, 254-256
    spaces in, 255-258
Nasalis muscle, 180-181
Nasion, 134, 140
Nasociliary nerve, 238, 247
    orbit and, 245
Nasolabial groove, 295
Nasolacrimal duct, 249
Nasolacrimal nerve, 178
Nasopalatine nerve, 259, 267
Nasopharynx, 265, 278-279, 281
    on MRI, 148
Navicular bone
    ankle and, 700-701
    articular surface on, 708
    deltoid ligament and, 702
    foot and, 705-707
    medial view of, 700
    metatarsus adductus and, 720
    MRI of, 709
    talocalcaneonavicular joint and, 710
Navicular fossa, 579, 582, 609, 616
Neck
    anatomy of
        musculoskeletal, 291-292
        surface, 293-296
    anterolateral, 206-223
        carotid triangle in, 206-217; see also Neck

Neck—cont'd
    Carotid triangle
        clinical anatomy of, 215, 219
        muscular triangle in, 211, 215-219
        submandibular triangle in, 210, 218-223
        submental triangle in, 223
    autonomic innervation of, 293
    blood flow to, 292
        arterial, 133
        venous drainage of, 133, 203-204, 292
    bony landmarks of, 293-295
    case studies and, 297-305
    cysts in, 223
    dermatomes of, 27
    head and, 130-305; see also Head
    innervation of, 199-202, 293-294; see also
        Neck, spinal roots and
        brachial plexus and, 337-338; see also
        Brachial plexus
    lateral masses of, 173
    lymphatic drainage of, 133-134, 292
    muscles of, 133, 291-292
    organization of, 198
    physical examination of, 293-296
    spinal roots and, 200, 203-204, 293, 296
        anterolateral, 210
        in posterior triangle, 199
        spinal cord and, 439, 445
        subclavian artery and, 203
        transverse cervical plexus and, 200
        transverse head and neck and, 177
        vertebral canal and, 439
    systems review and, 291-296
    triangles of; see Neck triangles
Neck triangles
    anterior, 198, 201
    carotid, 206-217; see also Carotid triangle
    posterior, 198-205
        clinical anatomy of, 204
        floor of, 199, 202
Neoplasm, pancreatic, 498
Nerve blocks, intercostal, 72
Nerve endings in dermis, 8
Nerves
    to abdomen, 537-538
    to abdominal wall, 459, 490-461
    to anorectal region, 571
    to back and vertebral column, 430-431,
        449
    blood vessels supplying, 24
    to colon, 520-521
    cranial; see Cranial nerves
    to diaphragm, 530
    entrapments of, 704
    to esophagus, 500
    to face, 180-181, 184
        cutaneous, 177-181
    to foot, 720
    to forearm, 365-368
        clinical anatomy of, 367
    to hair follicle, 8
    to hand, 389, 392-393
    to head, 293-294
    to heart, 84, 104-106
    to hip joint, 646
    intercostal, 71-72
    to knee, 684-685

Nerves—cont'd
    to larynx, 287-289
    of Latarjet, 503-504
    leg
        anterior, 696-698
        lateral, 699
        posterior, 696
    to lower limb, 725
    to lungs, 84-85
    to neck, 199-202, 293-294
    to palate, 267
    to pancreas, 498
    parasympathetic; see Parasympathetic
        nervous system
    to pelvis, 555, 586-593, 623-624
        clinical anatomy of, 593
    to perineum, 623-624
        autonomic, 578-584
        somatic, 578
    peripheral, 20, 23-24
    to pharynx, 281-282
    to pleurae, 85
    to popliteal fossa, 689-690, 696
    to scalp, 174-175
        cutaneous, 177-181
    to shoulder, 327-329
        clinical anatomy of, 328
    to spermatic cord, 469
    spinal; see Spinal nerves
    to stomach, 503
    to submandibular triangle, 222
    sympathetic; see Sympathetic nervous
        system
    to temporomandibular joint, 190
    to thigh
        anterior, 648, 654, 659
        medial, 660-661
        posterior, 674
    to tongue, 271-272
    traversing floor of skull, 140
    to upper limb, 397-398, 400
    to wrist, 372, 375
Nervi erigentes; see Pelvic nerve
Nervous system, 20-27
    cellular components of, 20-24
    central; see Central nervous system
    enteric, 17
    functional groups of neurons in, 20-22, 25
    organization of, 22-25, 27
    peripheral; see Peripheral nervous system
Neural arch of vertebra, 409-411
Neural retina, 237-238, 250
Neurectomy, presacral, 593
Neurocranium, 136
Neurogenic bladder, 601
Neurolemma, Schwann cell, 146
Neurons, 20
    autonomic, 22, 436
    of brain, 145-146
    cell bodies of, 434-437
    central process of; see Central process of
        neuron
    cluster of, 21
    disturbance of normal conduction
        between muscle and, 151
    functional groups of, 20-22, 25-27
    internal structure of, 21

Neurons—cont'd
    motor, 22
        somatic, 436
    parasympathetic, 26, 445
        in bladder wall, 25
    postganglionic; see Postganglionic neuron
    preganglionic; see Preganglionic neuron
    pseudounipolar, 20
    sensory, 20-22, 146, 436
    spinal cord and, 436, 443
    spinal motor, diseases of, 447
    sympathetic, 26
        postganglionic, 443
        preganglionic, 186, 434, 437
    varieties of, 22
Neurovascular pedicle of muscle, 328
Neurovascular supply; see Blood vessels;
        Nerves
Newborn
    fontanelle of, 138
    frontal bone of, 138
    head of, ultrasonography of, 44
    parietal bone of, 138
    unusual appearance in, 298, 302
    urinary abnormality in, 629, 632
Ninth cranial nerve; see Glossopharyngeal
        nerve (IX)
Nipple, 55
Nodal artery, 92, 103
Nodal cells, 103
Node
    in brain
        with interdigitating processes, 146
        on MRI, 148
    collagenous
        in aortic valve, 99
        in pulmonary valve, 97
    of heart, 90, 94
        conduction system and, 103
    lymph; see Lymph node
    of Ranvier, 146
    of thorax, 121
Noisy breathing in newborn, 301
Noncoronary leaflet, 98
Nonneuronal tissues of spinal cord, 434-436
Nonprecision grip of hand, 393
Norepinephrine, 528
Nose, 292; see also Nasal cavity
    blood supply to, 259
    bridge of, 254
    fractures of, 262
    innervation of, 259-260
    internal anatomy of, 253-254, 257
    mucosa of, 254
Nosebleed, 255, 259, 262
Nostrils, 176-177, 253-254
Notch
    acetabular, 551
    articular, inferior, 424
    cardiac, 81
    jugular, 62, 122
    radial, 348-350, 352, 354, 356
    rib, 72
    scapular, 313
    sciatic; see Sciatic notch
    of skull bone, 134
    spinoglenoid, 313-314

Notch—cont'd
  sternal, 62, 122-123
  supraorbital, 134, 238
    skull and, 134, 137
  suprascapular, 312, 314, 319
  tentorial, 154-155, 158
  trochlear, 348-349
    interosseous membrane and, 356
    on x-ray, 350
  ulnar, 348-350, 356, 371
    on MRI, 357
  vertebral, 410, 416
    on x-ray, 417
Notochord, 419
Nuchal ligament, 200
Nuck, canal of, 472
Nucleus, 21
  in brain, 145
Nucleus pulposus, 419, 423
  herniation of, 423, 452
  on MRI, 415, 418
  vertebral column and, 433
Nutrient foramen, 10, 690
Nystagmus, 251

O

Oblique aponeurosis in inguinal canal,
    external
  in female, 466
  in male, 465
Oblique diameter, 550
Oblique muscle
  external abdominal, 457-461
    on CT, 41
    hernias and, 467
    inguinal canal and, 464, 466
    sternum and, 63
  inferior
    of eyeball, 237, 243-244, 248, 271
    of head, 427-428
  internal abdominal, 460
    on CT, 41
    inguinal region and, 465-466
    rectus abdominis muscle and, 461
    sternum and, 63
    testis and, 468
  superior
    of eyeball, 235-237, 243-245
    of head, 427-428
Oblique pericardial sinus, 87-88
Oblique popliteal ligament, 676
Obliquus capitis inferior muscle, 427-428
Obliquus capitis superior muscle, 427-428
Obstetrical conjugate, 550
Obstetrics, pelvic outlet and, 550, 556-557
Obstruction
  of airways, 79
  of bile ducts, 543
  biliary, intrahepatic and extrahepatic, 490
  of duodenum, 510
  of esophagus, 500
  to mucus flow, 262
Obturator artery, 570, 587, 589, 724
  anteromedial thigh and, 637, 654
  on CT, 618
  to femur, 644
  hip joint and, 645

Obturator foramen, 549-552, 576
  pelvis and, 559
Obturator membrane, 555
Obturator muscle, 581, 645
  external, 565, 573, 648-649
    anteromedial thigh and, 655, 660
    in gluteal region, 664, 667-668
    as short rotator of hip joint, 667
  internal, 531, 562-566, 573, 648-649
    on CT, 618
    diaphragm and, 532
    in gluteal region, 664, 666-667, 671
    nerve to, 557, 671
    sciatic nerve origin and, 669
    as short rotator of hip joint, 667
Obturator nerve, 531, 588, 638, 725
  accessory, 661
  adductor magnus muscle and, 661
  gluteal region and, 668
  hip joints and, 646
  lumbar and sacral plexus and, 670
  lumbar plexus and, 533
  pelvis and perineum and, 624
  posterior thigh and, 674
  targets of, 661
  thigh and, 656, 661
    anteromedial, 637, 654, 660
Obturator vein, 570
  anteromedial thigh and, 637, 654
  on CT, 618
Occipital artery
  anterolateral neck and, 208
  back and vertebral column and, 429
  brain and, 159
  as branch of external carotid artery, 209
  face and, 182
  middle ear and, 233
  scalp and, 174-175, 183
Occipital bone, 134-136, 138-141, 415, 421
  apertures in, 140-141
  mastication muscles and, 191
  on MRI, 415
  os incae of, 136
  posterior view of, 137
Occipital condyle, 141-142, 421
Occipital horn, 150, 152
Occipital lobe, 148-149
Occipital lymph node, 210
Occipital neck triangles, 198, 201
Occipital nerve
  greater, 175
  lesser, 175, 202
    cervical plexus and, 200
    cervical sympathetic chain and, 215
    neck and, 202
Occipital protuberance, skull and, 137
Occipital sinus, 154, 157, 162
Occipital triangle of neck, 201
Occipital vein, 183
Occipitalis muscle, 174, 178
Occipitofrontalis muscle, 179, 295
Occlusion, dental, 267
Oculocephalic reflex, 247
Oculomotor nerve (III), 162, 165, 167, 169
  brain and, 157, 160
  globe and orbit and, 238, 244-246
  in interpeduncular cistern, MRI of, 148

Oculomotor nerve (III)—cont'd
  mastication and, 190
  mental branch of, 187-188
  neck and, 293
    anterolateral, 210
  orbit and, 245
  parasympathetic nerves and, 293-294
    postganglionic neurons of, 169
  root of
    inferior, 237, 245-246
    superior, 238, 244-246
  skull and, 140
  temporomandibular joint and, 190
Oculovestibular reflex, 247
Oddi, sphincter of, 487, 497
Odontoid process, 412, 414; see also Dens
    of axis, 135
  ligaments of, 421
  on MRI, 148
  skull and, 142
Olecranon, 348-349, 353-354, 363
  posterior view of, 399
  radioulnar joint and, 354
  on x-ray, 350
Olecranon bursa, 351-352, 354
Olecranon bursitis, 352
Olecranon fossa, 318, 348-350
  on x-ray, 350
Olecranon process of ulna
  elbow movements and, 349
  interosseous membrane and, 356
Olfactory bulb, 254, 260
  left, 159
  skull and, 140
Olfactory epithelium, 253-254, 258
Olfactory fila, 254
Olfactory nerve (I), 165, 169, 254, 258, 260
  head and neck and, 293
  nose and, 259-260
Olfactory tract, 159, 254
Oligodendrocyte, 23
Oligodendroglial membranes, 146
Omental bursa, 477, 503-505
  development of gut and, 476-479, 481
  peritoneal membranes and, 481
Omental sac; see Omental bursa
Omentum
  greater, 504-505
    development of gut and, 480-481
    stomach and, 505
    transverse colon and, 518
  lesser, 477, 486-487, 491, 503-505
    development of gut and, 476-479, 481
    liver and, 487
    peritoneal membranes and, 479, 481
    stomach and, 504-505
Omohyoid muscle
  brain and, 159
  neck and, 200
    ansa cervicalis in, 214
    anterolateral, 208, 216-217
    in posterior triangle, 199
  pharynx and, 276
Omphalocele, 482
Oocytes, 604
  primary, 605
Oogonia, primary, 604

Ophthalmic artery, 158, 250
  branches of, 238
  face and, 181
  horizontal section through bony orbit
      and, 237
  nose and, 259
  scalp and, 183
  skull and, 140
  superior orbital fissure and, 238, 248
  sympathetic axons and, 168
Ophthalmic branch of trigeminal nerve (V1),
      165-166, 179-180
Ophthalmic nerve (VI), 162
  to eye and orbit, 245, 247-248
  nose and, 259-260
  skull and, 140
Ophthalmic vein, 157, 162, 250
  brain and, 157
  branches of, 238
  head and neck and, 292
Opponens digiti minimi muscle, 357, 382-
      383, 386
  insertion of, 388
  MRI of, 709
Opponens pollicis muscle, 357, 373, 382-385
  insertion of, 388
  on MRI, 357
Opposition of thumb, 384-385, 391, 393
Optic canal, 141, 235-236, 238, 248
  horizontal section through bony orbit
      and, 237
  levator palpebrae superioris muscle and,
      249
  rectus muscle and, 248
  skull and, 139
Optic chiasma, 151, 241
  in suprasellar cistern, 148
  tumor of, 151
Optic disc, 241
Optic nerve (II), 165, 167, 169
  abnormal swelling of, 252
  bony orbit and, 237, 241
      horizontal section of, 237, 242
      superior orbital fissure in, 238, 248
  brain and, 157
  circle of Willis and, 162
  nasal branches of, 260
  neck and, 293
      anterolateral, 210
  skull and, 140
  surgery and, 262
  uveal layer of eye and, 238
Optic papilla, 241
Optic tract, 167
  anterolateral neck and, 210
Oral apertures, 134
Oral cavity, 177
  borders of, 263-264
  floor of, 263
  inspection of, 296
  malignancy in, 275
  muscles of, 295
  roof of, 263-264
Orbicularis oculi muscle, 242
  face and scalp and, 178-180
  head and neck and, 295
  parotid gland and, 184

Orbicularis oculi muscle—cont'd
  segments of, 180
Orbicularis oris muscle, 178-179, 181
Orbit, bony, 234-238, 292; *see also* Eye
  apex of, 235, 237
  axis of, 234-235
  blood supply to, 250
  bony walls of, 236
  ciliary ganglion in, 169
  clinical anatomy of, 235
  connective tissue in, 242-243
  fascia in, 242-243
  fracture of, 294
  fractures of, 235
  muscles of, 237, 243-244
  nerve supply to, 238, 244-248
      parasympathetic, 246
      sympathetic, 246
  optic canal and, 238, 248-249
  rims of, 176
  septum of, 241-242, 249
  superior orbital fissure and, 238, 248-249
  trauma of, 251
  walls of, 234-238, 242
Orbital branch of facial nerve, 180
Orbital cavities, 176
Orbital fissure
  inferior, 235-236, 256
  superior, 137, 139, 141, 235-238, 248-249
      abducens nerve (VI) and, 238
      horizontal section through bony orbit
          and, 237
      ophthalmic artery and, 238, 248
      optic nerve in, 238, 248
      trochlear nerve in, 238
Orbital lobe, 249
Orbital rims, 176
Orbital septum, 241-242, 249
Orbital wall, 234-238, 242
Organs, sense, 133-134
Oropharynx, 280-281
  on MRI, 271
Os of cervix, 607
Os incae of occipital bone, 136
Osgood-Schlatter disease, 687
Ossicles of middle ear, 228-230, 291; *see also*
      Incus; Malleus; Stapes
  as movable bones, 133
Ossification, 10
Otic ganglion, 169, 186, 193-196
  connections and relations of, 194
  parasympathetic nerves and, 294
  in temporal and infratemporal fossae, 187
Otitis, 232
Otosclerosis, 230, 232
Outflow tract, ventricular
  left, 98
  right, 97
Oval window, 227-228, 230
Ovarian artery, 537, 558, 591, 605-606
  oviduct and, 607
Ovarian ligament, 36, 558, 575, 604-606
Ovarian vein, 605
Ovary, 34-37, 558-559, 604-605
  blood supply to, 606
  descent of, in inguinal canal, 472
  views of

Ovary—cont'd
  midsagittal, 574
  parasagittal, 606
  superior, 575
Oviduct, 35-36, 558-559, 605-607
  ectopic pregnancy in, 612
  fimbria of, 558, 605
  on hysterosalpingogram, 609
  infundibulum of, 575
  isthmus of, 558
  and sexually transmitted disease, 610
  sympathetic nerves in pelvis and, 591
  views of
      midsagittal, 574
      parasagittal, 606
      superior, 575
Ovum, 35
Oxytocin, 37, 55
  axons conveying, 37

P

Pacemaker, artificial, 105
Pacinian corpuscle, 8
Pain
  abdominal, 539-540, 542
  back, 728, 730
      childbirth and, 628
  in eye, sudden, 300, 304
  referred, 447, 544, 624
      to mediastinum, 119
  principles of, 518
Palatal process of maxilla; *see* Palatine bone,
      process of
Palate, 263-267; *see also* Mouth
  blood supply to, 267
  cleft, 275
  clinical anatomy of, 275
  elevation of, 264
  hard, 263-268
      nose and, 253, 256, 260
  malformation of, 170
  nerve supply of, 267
  soft; *see* Soft palate
Palatine aponeurosis, 263-265
Palatine artery
  greater, 259, 267
  lesser, 267
Palatine bone, 236
  orbit and, 234
  process of
      horizontal, 141
      maxillary, 135, 141
      palatal, 255
  skull and, 141
Palatine canal, 236
Palatine foramen, greater, 255-256, 268
Palatine nerve, 178
  greater, 260, 267
      pterygopalatine fossa and, 261
  lesser, 260, 267
Palatine process of maxilla; *see* Palatine
      bone, process of
Palatine tonsil, 264, 266, 274, 280
  arches and
      palatal, 264
      pharyngeal, 172-173
  dorsal view of tongue and, 270

Palatine tonsil—cont'd
  inflammation of, 283
  soft palate and, 280
  swallowing and, 281
Palatine vein, external, 274
Palatoglossal arch, 264, 266, 280
Palatoglossus muscle, 264-265, 271
  swallowing and, 282
Palatopharyngeal arch, 264, 266
Palatopharyngeal incompetency, 275
Palatopharyngeus muscle, 264, 266, 278-280
  swallowing and, 282
Palm, fascial compartments in, 389
Palmar arch
  deep, 363-364, 391
    on MRI, 357
  superficial, 357, 363-364, 391, 397
Palmar cutaneous branch of median nerve,
    368
Palmar fascia, 356, 382
Palmar interosseous muscle, 382-385
  insertion of, 388
Palmar ligament of interphalangeal joints,
    381
Palmar plate of interphalangeal joints, 381
Palmar radiocarpal ligament, 369
Palmar septum, 382
Palmar surface, 6
Palmaris brevis muscle, 374, 383, 386
Palmaris longus muscle, 356, 358-360
  palmar fascia and, 382
  tendon of, 357
    flexor retinaculum and, 372
    on MRI, 357
Palpebrae, 241
Palpebral artery, 242
Palpebral conjunctiva, 250
Palpebral fissure, 241, 295
Palpebral ligament, 242, 249
Palpebral lobe, 249
Palpebral muscle, 242
Palpebral nerve, 242
Palpebral vein, 242
Palsy
  Bell's, 185
  Erb-Duchenne, 339, 401-402, 404
Pampiniform plexus, 469-470
Pancreas, 37, 494-498
  anatomy of
    clinical, 498
    developmental, 494-497
  annular, 498
  blood supply to, 497-498
  cysts of, 543
  development of, 476, 479, 484
    anatomy and, 494-497
  duct of; see Pancreatic duct
  duodenum and, 508
  endocrine, 497-498
  exocrine, 498
  function of, 480
  islets of, 35, 494
  kidneys and, 524
  neoplasms of, 498
  nerves to, 498
    parasympathetic, 294
  peritoneal membranes and, 478, 481-483

Pancreas—cont'd
  regions of, 494-496
  spleen and, 493
  splenectomy and, 498
  stomach and, 504
  stones in, 498
  tumor in, 543
  uncinate process of head of, 496, 508
Pancreatic artery, 503
Pancreatic duct, 488, 495-497
  accessory, 497
  liver and, 488
  main, 497
  peritoneal membranes and, 479
Pancreatic polypeptide, 497
Pancreaticoduodenal artery, 497
  abdomen and, 537
  duodenum and, 510
  jejunum and ileum and, 511
  small intestine and, 513
  stomach and, 503
Pap smear, 610
Papilla
  duodenal; see Duodenal papilla
  optic, 241
  renal, 524-525, 597
  of sublingual gland, 221, 269-270, 273
  of tongue, 221, 269, 273, 296
    circumvallate, 270
    on dorsum, 266
    filiform, 270
    fungiform, 270
    valate, 270
Papillary muscle, 95, 98, 104
Papilledema, 252
Paraaortic node, 582
Paraaortic sympathetic ganglion, 600
Paracentesis, 482
Paracolic gutters, 482
Paraesophageal hernia, 500
Paralysis, Klumpke's, 339
Paranasal sinuses, 256-257, 291
  on CT, 142
  ethmoid, 143, 256-258
  frontal; see Frontal sinus
  growth of, 136
  infection in, 251, 262
  maxillary; see Maxillary sinus
  nasal cavity and, 253
  sphenoid; see Sphenoid sinus
  on x-ray, 135
Pararenal fat, 523-524
  on CT, 41
Parasagittal plane, 3
Parasympathetic axon, 164
  of cranial nerves, 293
  eye and orbit and, 246
  otic ganglion and, 194
  postganglionic, 194
  preganglionic
    back and spinal cord and, 446
    eye and orbit and, 246
    femoral cutaneous nerve and, 589
    head and neck and, 169
    pelvis and perineum and, 589, 592-593
  sacral, 587
  of ureter, 594

Parasympathetic nervous system, 17, 293-
    294
  to abdomen, 538
  axon of; see Parasympathetic axon
  cardiac muscle and, 19, 104, 121
  to eye and orbit, 237, 246
  ganglia of, 20
    otic ganglion in, 193
    in temporal and infratemporal fossae,
        187
  to head and neck, 293-294
    cranial nerves and, 169
  of large intestine, 520-521
  to lungs and pleurae, 85
  neurons of, 25-26, 445
  outflow from, 592
  to pelvis and perineum, 584, 624
  spinal cord and, 445-446
  to stomach, 503-504
  to urinary bladder, 600
Parasympathetic neuron, 26, 445
  in bladder wall, 25
Parathormone, 218
Parathyroid gland, 35, 37, 198, 218-219
  clinical anatomy of, 173
  ectopic tissue of, 218
  pharyngeal arches and, 172-173
  surgery and, 219
Paraurethral gland, 574, 608-609
Parietal bone, 134-135, 137, 139, 141
  mastication muscles and, 191
  of newborn, 138
Parietal layer of cavity, 51
Parietal lobe of brain, 148-149
Parietal mesenteries, development of, 473-
    474, 476
Parietal peritoneum, development of, 480
Parietal pleura, 49, 74
  on CT and MRI, 43
Parietal serous pericardium, 51
Parietooccipital fissure, 148
Parotid duct, 178-179, 182-184, 295-296
Parotid gland, 178-179
  clinical anatomy of, 185
  face and, 181-186
  horizontal section through, 184
  on MRI, 271
  otic ganglion and, 194
  parasympathetic nerves and, 294
  submandibular and sublingual glands
      and, 274
Parotid lymph node, middle ear and, 233
Pars flaccida, 225-226
Pars tensa, 225
Patella, 676, 679, 725-726
  anteromedial thigh and, 654-655
  bipartite, 677
  femoral artery and, 646
  knee and, 674, 676-679
  lateral view of, 699
  pes anserinus and, 675
Patellar groove
  femur and, 639
  knee and, 676-677
Patellar ligament, 681
Patellar retinaculum, 676-677, 682
  pes anserinus and, 675

Patellar tendon, 14, 676, 679, 725
  knee joint and, 682
  tests of, 726
Patellofemoral joint, 676-679
Patent ductus arteriosus, 104, 106, 108
Patent ductus venosus, 106
Pathologic fractures, 346
Pecten pubis, 460
Pectinate line, 568-569, 571
Pectineal ligament, 555
  femoral sheath and, 654
Pectineal line, 556, 639
  pelvis and, 559
Pectineal muscle, 94, 97, 654
  attachment of, 657
  on CT, 618
  femoral artery and, 646
  femoral sheath and, 654
  femoral triangle and, 651
  hip joints and, 645
  thigh and, 648-649, 655-656, 658-661
    anteromedial, 655, 660
    posterior, 658
Pectoral artery, 121, 334
Pectoral axillary lymph node, 397
Pectoral girdle; see Shoulder girdle
Pectoral nerve
  lateral, 337, 340
    brachial plexus and, 339
  medial, 337
    brachial plexus and, 339
Pectoralis major muscle, 17, 394, 399
  abdomen and, 458, 461
  anterior compartment and, 345
  anterior view of, 66, 398
  axilla and, 330-331
  clavicle and, 62, 313, 327
  on CT, 100
  female breast and, 55
  on MRI, 323
  in respiration, 68
  shoulder movement and, 325-326
  sternum and, 63, 327
Pectoralis minor muscle
  anterior view of, 66
  axilla and, 330, 332
  clavicle and, 62, 313
  female breast and, 55
  on MRI, 323
  in respiration, 68
  shoulder movement and, 325-326
  sternum and, 63
Pectus carinatum, 63
Pectus excavatum, 63
Pedicle of vertebra, 58, 409-411, 416
  at thoracic level, on x-ray, 417
Pelvic diaphragm, 531-532, 549, 561-565
  abdomen and, 536
  childbirth and, 631
  muscles of, 564
Pelvic examination, 624-627
Pelvic girdle, 310-311
  musculoskeletal system and, 722
  structural features of, 645
Pelvic inflammatory disease, 610
Pelvic nerve, 587-588, 592-593
  lumbar and sacral plexus and, 670

Pelvic nerve—cont'd
  parasympathetic nerves and, 294, 584
    sacral, 538
  pelvic plexus and, 583
  pelvis and perineum and, 624
  spinal cord and, 445-446
Pelvic plexus, 583
Pelvic vein, 586
  thrombophlebitis of, 593
Pelvic viscera, 558-560
  fascial structures in, 574, 604, 606
  female, 604-612; see also Pelvic viscera,
      female
    clinical anatomy of, 610-612
    imaging of, 610, 612
    ovaries in, 558, 575, 604-605
    oviducts in, 558, 575, 605-607
    uterus in, 558, 574, 606-608
    vagina in, 558, 573-574, 608
  male, 613-621; see also Pelvic viscera, male
    clinical anatomy of, 620-621
    ductus deferens and, 613-615
    erection and ejaculation and, 616-619
    penis and, 564-565, 580-581, 615-619
    prostate gland and, 613-614
    seminal vesicles and, 613-615, 619
    urethra and, 580, 582, 614-616
  peritoneal structures in, 574, 604, 606
  urethra in, 574, 608-609
Pelvis, 549-560
  anterior view of, 12
  anteroposterior x-ray of, 559-560
  arteries of, 570, 586-587, 623
    clinical anatomy of, 593
  bones of, 549-554
  case studies of, 628-633
  dermatomes of, 624-625
  diameters of, 550
  examination of, 624-627
  fascia in, 558-560
  floor of, surgery on, 593
  foramina in, 559
    greater, 554-557
    lesser, 554-557
  fracture of, 560
  greater, 549
  inlet of, 549-550
  interior of, 553, 556-558
  joints of, 550, 553-557
  ligaments of, 550, 553-557
  lymphatic drainage of, 623
  male
    floor of, 565
    imaging, 618, 620
  muscles of, 622-623
  nerves to, 555, 586-593, 623-624
    autonomic, 591-593
    clinical anatomy of, 593
  outlet of, 549-550, 561
    dimensions of, 556-557
  peritoneum and, 558-560
  physical examination of, 624-627
  posterior surfaces of, gluteal region and,
      663, 666
  principles for, 554
  renal, dilated, 597
  shape of, 554

Pelvis—cont'd
    sexual dimorphism in, 550, 554, 557
  skeleton and, 622
  surface anatomy of, 622-627
  sympathetic nerves in, 583, 591-593
  systems review of, 622-627
  urinary system and; see Urinary
      system
  veins of, 570, 586, 614, 623
    clinical anatomy of, 593
  venous plexus of, 583, 623
  viscera of; see Pelvic viscera
  x-ray of, 559-560
Penile artery, dorsal, 590
Penile urethra, 609, 616, 619
  on cystourethrogram, 617
  rupture of, 566
Penis, 564-565, 575-577, 580-581, 615
  bulb of, 561, 564, 567, 578-579, 614-615
    on CT, 618
    urethra in, on cystourethrogram, 617
  chordee of, 620
  crus of, 576, 582
  dorsal artery of, 579, 582
  dorsal vein of, 579
    deep, 577, 579
  erectile bodies and structure of, 579
  glans of, 576, 580, 582
    protective shield for, 580
  lymphatic drainage of, 578, 581
  phimosis of, 620
  prepuce of, 582
  shaft of, 567
  structure of, 580
  urethra in bulb of, on cystourethrogram,
      617
Pepsinogen, 506
Peptic ulcer, 499, 510
Percussion of thorax, 122
Perforating artery
  hip joints and, 645
  from peroneal artery, 692, 698
  of profunda femoris, 668, 674
  of thigh, 658, 661
Perforating cutaneous nerve, 671
Pericardiacophrenic artery, 87-88, 118
Pericardiacophrenic vein, 87
Pericardial cavity, 86-88
Pericardial recess on CT and MRI, 43
Pericardial sac, 86-88
  fibrous, 51
  inflammation in, 124
  tamponade and, 88
Pericardial sinus, 87-88
Pericardiocentesis, 88
Pericarditis, 88
Pericardium, 49-51
  branches of aorta to, 117
  clinical anatomy of, 88
  on CT and MRI, 43
  fibrous, 87-88
  serous, 49, 87
    parietal, 51
    visceral, 51
Perikaryon, 20
Perilymph of inner ear, 228, 233
Perineal artery, 572, 590

Perineal body, 631
  anus and anal canal and, 568
  boundaries of perineum and, 561-564
  clinical anatomy of, 585
  external genitalia and
    female, 572-574
    male, 577-578
Perineal fat, 523-524
Perineal injury during childbirth, 620, 630-631
Perineal membrane, 565, 572, 574, 614
  urogenital diaphragm and, 567
Perineal muscle, transverse, 564
  deep, 567, 574
  superficial, 564, 567, 573, 577-578, 631
Perineal nerve, 572, 583
Perineal pouch, 577, 581
  deep, 565, 574, 581
  superficial, 565, 574, 581, 619
Perineal vein, 572
Perineum, 561-585; see also Pelvis
  anatomy of
    clinical, 585
    surface, 622-627
  anus and anal canal and, 568-569
  blood supply to, 578
    arteries in, 569, 623
    veins in, 569-571, 623
  boundaries of, 561-564
  case studies of, 628-633
  external genitalia and
    female, 571-575
    male, 575-582
  innervation of
    anorectal region and, 571
    autonomic, 578-584
    somatic, 578
  ischiorectal fossa and, 565-568
  lymphatics of, 578, 582, 623
  muscles of, 622-623
  nerves of, 623-624
  pelvic diaphragm and, 562-565
  physical examination of, 624-627
  principles for, 566
  prolapse and, 585
  systems review of, 622-627
  trauma to, 629, 633
  urinary system and; see Urinary system
  urogenital diaphragm and, 564-566
    in female, 573-575
    in male, 577-578
Perineurium, 20, 24
Periodontitis, 275
Periorbital area, 242
  bleeding in, 251
Periosteum, 175
Peripheral motor neuron in brain, 146
Peripheral nervous system, 20, 23-24
  axons of, 23
  branches of, 73
  categorization of, 73
Peripheral process of neuron, 20, 146, 436
Peripheral sensory neuron in brain, 146
Perirenal fat
  on CT, 41
  pancreas and, 496

Peristalsis
  cranial nerves and, 169
  esophagus and, 500
  of large intestine, 520
  of pharynx, 276
Peritoneal cavity
  serous membranes and, 474
  special regions within, 482
Peritoneal leaflets, organs developing in, 475
Peritoneal membrane, 473-483, 585
  clinical anatomy of, 482
  greater and lesser sacs and, 476-479
    fixation versus suspension of, 479
    giant glands of gastrointestinal tract and, 479
  gut in
    fixation and suspension of, 475-478
    regions of developing, 479
  mesenteries and
    blood supply to, 474, 479-480
    dorsal and ventral, 474-476
    parietal and visceral, 473-474, 476
  omentum and
    greater, 480-481
    lesser, 479, 481
  organs developing in peritoneal leaflets and, 475
  parietal peritoneum and, 480
  principles for, 475, 480
  retroperitoneal structures and, 476, 483
  rotation of stomach and, 476-479
  structures and
    intraperitoneal, 478, 483
    peritoneal and retroperitoneal, 481-483
  uterine prolapse and, 585
Peritoneal reflections, 516-517
  liver and, 485-486
Peritoneum, 460, 565, 600
  abdomen and, 459, 461
  bladder neck and, 581
  inguinal region and, 466
  innervation of, 537
  jejunum and ileum and, 510
  layers of, 481
  parietal, development of, 480
  pelvis and, 558-560
    interior, 558
  as serous cavity, 49
  serous membranes and, 474
  stomach and, 505
  structures of
    development of, 481-483
    female pelvic viscera and, 574, 604, 606
  testis and, 468
Peritonitis, 490
Periventricular nuclei of hypothalamus, 37
Permanent teeth, 267, 269
Peroneal artery
  ankle and, 703
  knee and, 684-685
  leg and
    lateral, 699
    muscles of, 695
    posterior compartment of, 692, 703
  perforating branch of, 692, 698
Peroneal muscle of leg, 695

Peroneal nerve
  common, 587-588, 668-669, 671
    deep branch of, 697-698
    entrapment of, 704
    leg and, 696, 698-699
    popliteal fossa and, 689
    in posterior thigh, 675
    sciatic nerve origin and, 669
  deep, 638, 693, 725
    anterior compartment of leg and, 696
    entrapment of, 704
    popliteal fossa and, 689
    tibiofibular articulations and, 692
  superficial, 638, 725
    lateral compartment of leg and, 699
    popliteal fossa and, 689-690
Peroneal portion of sciatic nerve, common, 674
Peroneal retinaculum muscle
  inferior
    dorsum of foot and, 714
    lateral view of, 699
  leg muscles and, 689
  posterior view of, 694-695
  superior
    dorsum of foot and, 714
    lateral view of, 699
Peroneus brevis muscle, 693
  leg compartments and, 693, 697, 699
  tendon of
    ankle tendons and, 702
    MRI of, 709
  views of
    anterior, 697
    lateral, 699
Peroneus longus muscle, 693
  foot and, 708
  leg compartments of
    anterior, 697
    fascial, 693
    lateral, 699
  tendon of, 717, 726
    ankle tendons and, 702
    foot ligaments and, 708
    MRI of, 709
    sole of foot and, 719
  views of
    anterior, 697
    lateral, 699
Peroneus tertius muscle
  ankle tendons and, 702
  anterior compartment of leg and, 696
  views of
    anterior, 697
    lateral, 699
    superficial, 714
Perpendicular plate of ethmoid bone, 253-256
Persistence
  of embryonic vessel, 114
  of fetal circulation, 108
  of left superior vena cava, 114
Pes anserinus, 674-675
  insertion of, 697
  knee joint and, 682
  tendons of, popliteal fossa and, 691
Petrooccipital fissure, 143

Petrosal nerve
  deep, 260
    pterygopalatine fossa and, 261
  greater, 227, 231-232, 260
    pterygopalatine fossa and, 261
  lesser, 186, 212, 227, 231-232
    otic ganglion and, 195
    parasympathetic nerves and, 294
Petrosal sinus, 157-158, 162
Petrous ridge temporal bone, 139
pH, blood, 207
Phagocytosis, 492
Phalanx, 309-310, 378-379
  anterior view of, 12
  of foot, 707
    distal, 707
      great toe, medial view of, 700
      metatarsus adductus and, 720
    middle, 707
    proximal, 707, 709, 720
  growth and maturation of, 11
  of hand, 381-382
    damage to, 405
    distal, 357, 376, 379
    index finger, 371
    intermediate, 379
    middle finger, 357, 371, 376
    on MRI, 357
    proximal, 357, 371, 376, 379
    ring finger, 371
    serous membranes and, 474
    shaft of, 357, 373
    thumb, 371
Phantom limb pain, 447, 518
Pharyngeal arches, 134, 136, 170-173
  clinical anatomy of, 173
  components of, 170-172
  development of, 475
  dorsal, 172
  innervation and, 185
  palatine tonsil and, 172-173
  pouches and clefts and, 171-173
  principles for, 173
  structure and position of, 170-171
Pharyngeal artery
  ascending
    as branch of external carotid artery, 209
    face and, 182
    middle ear and, 233
    pharynx and, 280-281
    pterygopalatine fossa and, 261
Pharyngeal cysts, 173
Pharyngeal muscle, intrinsic, 277-280
Pharyngeal nerve, auricular, 211
Pharyngeal plexus, 281
  motor branches of, 267
  tongue and, 272
Pharyngeal pouches and clefts, 171-173
Pharyngeal recess, 279
Pharyngeal tonsil, 279
Pharyngobasilar fascia, 279-280
Pharynx, 30, 276-283, 292
  clinical anatomy of, 173, 283
  deglutition and, 281-282
  external muscles forming and acting on, 278-280
  fistulas of, 173

Pharynx—cont'd
  innervation of, 281-282
  intrinsic pharyngeal muscles of, 277-280
  laryngopharynx and, 281-282
  muscles of, 279
  nasopharynx and, 278-279, 281
  oropharynx and, 280-281
  posterior, 219
  posterior wall of, 266
  principles for, 282
  skeletal structures of, 276-278
Pheochromocytoma, 528
Philtrum, 295
Phimosis of penis, 620
Phrenic artery, 116
  inferior, 116, 500, 526
    abdomen and, 536
    adrenal gland and, 527
    with branch to suprarenal gland, 526
    diaphragm and, 530
  stomach and, 503
  superior, 116
Phrenic nerve, 87, 109, 121
  abdomen and, 537
  brachial plexus and, 327
  cardiac surgery and, 88
  diaphragm and, 529-531
  head and neck and, 200, 202, 296
    in posterior triangle, 199
  left, 109
  mediastinum and, 110-112
  pericardial sac and, 88
Phrenic vein, 534-535
Phrenicocolic ligament, 518
Pia mater
  brain and, 152, 155-156
  cerebrospinal fluid space and, 152
  scalp and face and, 175
  spinal cord and, 434, 436, 438
  subarachnoid space and, 439
Pierre Robin syndrome, 173
Pigment epithelium of retina, 237
Pinna of ear, 142, 224-225
  innervation of, 225
Piriform recess, 281, 286
Piriformis muscle, 557, 562, 570, 590
  attachment of, 657
  in gluteal region, 663-667
    deep layer, 666
    intermediate layer, 664
    nerves and, 671
    vessels and, 668
  sciatic nerve origin and, 669
  as short rotator of hip joint, 667
Pisiform, 369-374, 376, 396
  flexor retinaculum and, 370
  on MRI, 357
Pisohamate ligament, 369-370
Pisometacarpal ligament, 369
Pituitary fossa, 135, 139
  brain and, 154
  meningeal artery hematoma and, 196
  skull and, 135, 139
Pituitary gland, 35, 37
  anterior, 37
    capillary network in, 37

Pituitary gland—cont'd
  axons conveying oxytocin and antidiuretic hormone to, 37
  brain and, 148, 151, 157, 160
  horizontal section through bony orbit and, 237
  infundibulum or stalk of, 158
  portal system in, 488
  posterior lobe of, 37
  surgery and, 262
Pituitary stalk, cranial nerves and, 165
Pixels, 38
Plane of body, 3-6
  anterior, 3, 6
  posterior, 3-6
Plantar aponeurosis, 707-708, 716
Plantar artery, 724
  foot and, 718-719
Plantar calcaneocuboid ligament, 708
Plantar calcaneonavicular ligament, 707-708, 710
Plantar cuneonavicular ligament, 708
Plantar ligament, long, 706-708
Plantar nerve, 638, 725
  foot and, 720
Plantar surface, 6
Plantaris muscle
  attachment of, 657
  popliteal fossa and, 688
  posterior leg and, 694-695
Plantaris tendon, 693, 695
  rupture of, 698
Plate
  cribriform, 139, 141, 254-256
  epiphyseal, 10, 316
    fractures of, 698
  palmar, of interphalangeal joints, 381
  perpendicular, of ethmoid bone, 253-256
  pterygoid; see Pterygoid plate
  quadrigeminal, of midbrain, 148
  tarsal, 241-242
Platelets, spleen and, 492
Platypelloid pelvis, 554, 557
Platysma muscle, 198, 200
  face and scalp and, 178
  neck and, 200
Pleurae, 49-51, 74-76
  anterior, junction of, 100
  clinical anatomy of, 85
  innervation of, 85
  parietal, 49
    on CT and MRI, 43
  pulmonary ligament extending down from, 76
Pleural cavity, 51, 74-76
  lungs and, 474
  recesses in, 75, 77, 80, 493
  as serous cavities, 49
Pleural membrane, 30
Pleural rub, 75
Pleural sac, 30
  anterior views of, 75
  heart and, 87
  medial borders of
    mediastinum and, 52, 75, 110
    pericardial sac and, 87
Pleural spaces, 74-76

Pleural spaces—cont'd
  blood in, 75, 127
  case studies and, 125, 127
  clinical anatomy of, 75, 125
  removing fluid or air from, 72
  substances abnormally filling, 75
Pleuritis, 75
Plexus, 16
  Auerbach, 520-521
  basilar, 157
  brachial; *see* Brachial plexus
  cardiac; *see* Cardiac plexus
  celiac, 294
  cervical; *see* Cervical plexus
  choroid, 44, 152, 155
  esophageal, 294
  hypogastric
    parasympathetic nerves and, 294
    pelvic interior and, 558
    in pelvis, 591-592
  lumbar; *see* Lumbar plexus
  lumbosacral, 16, 586
    pelvic interior and, 558
  Meissner, 520-521
  myenteric, 35
  pampiniform, 469-470
  pelvic, 583
  pharyngeal, 267, 272, 281
  prostatic, 599, 614
  pterygoid; *see* Pterygoid venous plexus
  pulmonary; *see* Pulmonary plexus
  of Purkinje fibers, 104
  sacral; *see* Sacral plexus
  submucus, 35, 520
  sympathetic
    aortic, 591-592
    on carotid, 260
  tympanic, 212, 226-228, 231
  venous; *see* Venous plexus
  vesical, 570, 599
Plicae circulares, 507, 509
PMI; *see* Point of maximal impulse
Pneumonia, 85
Pneumopericardium, 88
Pneumothorax, 72, 75
Point of maximal impulse, 124
Polar artery, 524
Pollicis longus muscle, tendon of, 382
Pons, 147-148, 159
  cranial nerves and, 165
  on MRI, 148
Pontine artery, 159
Pontine cistern, 151
Popliteal artery, 724
  arteriogram of, 685
  knee and, 684
  leg muscles and, 695
  popliteal fossa and, 690
  pulse in, 726
  thigh and, 656, 674
    posterior view of, 658
Popliteal fossa, 688-690, 694-696
  muscles and, 688-689, 694-695
  nerves of, 689-690, 696
  posterior view of, 694
    deep, 675, 695
    superficial, 673

Popliteal fossa—cont'd
  vessels of, 690, 695
Popliteal ligament
  arcuate, 681-682
  oblique, 676, 681-682
Popliteal vein, 652, 724
  popliteal fossa and, 690
  thigh and, 656, 674
Popliteus muscle, 690
  fascial compartments and, 693
  knee and, 672, 676
  popliteal fossa and, 689
  posterior leg and, 694-695
  tendon of, 676, 681
    popliteal fossa and, 691
  thigh and, 672
Popping of ears, 231, 264
Porta hepatis, 485-487
Portal hypertension, 116, 489
Portal system, 489; *see also* Portal vein
  anorectal region and, 570
  principles for, 488
  rectum and anus and, 517, 519
  spleen and, 494
Portal triad, 487
Portal vein, 479-480, 485-486; *see also* Portal
    system
  abdomen and, 37, 492
  duodenum and, 510
  liver and, 487-489
    abdomen and, 537
  pancreas and, 497
  porta hepatis and, 487
  principles for, 487
Portocaval shunt, 489, 520
Position
  anatomic, 3-4
  of structure, anterior or posterior, 3, 5
Postaxial muscle, 18
Posterior position of structure, 3, 5
Posterior thigh; *see* Thigh, posterior
Posterior wall of abdomen; *see* Abdomen,
    posterior wall of
Postganglionic axon, 25
  eye and orbit and, 246
  otic ganglion and, 194-195
  in pelvis, 591-593
  sympathetic, 25
    back and spinal cord and, 444-445
    head and neck and, 167, 186, 215
    in pelvis, 591-592
Postganglionic element, 442-443
Postganglionic neuron, 22
  brain and central nervous system and, 146
  cell bodies of, 146
  large intestine and, 520
  spinal cord and, 436, 443
  thorax and, 104, 118
Posture, foot and, 711
Pott's fracture, 704
Pouch, 170-171
  of Douglas, 558
  Hartmann's, 490
  perineal; *see* Perineal pouch
  pharyngeal, 171-173
  vesicouterine, 606
Poupart, inguinal ligament of, 466

Power grip of hand, 390, 393
Preauricular lymph node, 210
Preaxial muscle, 18
Precapillary arterioles, 25-26
Precision grip of hand, 390, 393
Preganglionic axon, 25
  eye and orbit and, 246
  femoral cutaneous nerve and, 589
  neurons and, 146
  otic ganglion and, 195
  parasympathetic
    eye and orbit and, 246
    femoral cutaneous nerve and, 589
    head and neck and, 169
    of pelvis, 592-593
    spinal cord and, 446
  of pelvis, 592-593
  in peripheral nervous system, 146
  spinal cord and, 436, 442-443, 446
  in splanchnics, 593
  sympathetic, 25
    back and spinal cord and, 442-443, 445-
      446
    eye and orbit and, 246
    head and neck and, 215
    spinal cord and, 443
    thorax and, 118
  synapses of, 442-443
Preganglionic element, 442-443
Preganglionic neuron
  cell bodies of
    neurons and, 146
    sympathetic, 434, 437
  large intestine and, 520-521
  spinal cord and, 436, 443
  sympathetic, 22, 104, 118, 186
    cell bodies of, 434, 437
    spinal cord and, 443
Pregnancy
  cervix of uterus and, 610
  ectopic, 610, 612
    site for, 612
  uterus in, 610-611
  wrist immobility and, 403, 405
Premature closure of skull sutures, 136
Premature infant, inguinal hernias in, 469
Premolars, 267-268
  mandible and, 188
Prepatellar bursa, 677, 679
Prepontine cistern, 148
Preprostatic sphincter, 600
Prepuce, 575
  of clitoris, 572-573, 576
  frenulum of, 579
  of penis, 582
Presacral neurectomy, 593
Presbyopia, 239
Pretracheal fascia, 200, 219
Prevertebral fascia, 200, 333
Prevertebral ganglion, 445, 592
Priapism, 620
Probe-patent foramen ovale, 108
Procerus muscle, 178
Process
  central, 436
    short, 435
  clinoid, 139, 237

Process—cont'd
  condylar
    of mandible, 188-190
    pharynx and, 277
    submandibular triangle and, 220
  coracoid, 311-317, 398
    on x-ray, 313
  coronoid; see Coronoid process
  costal, 410
    spinal cord and, 438
  frontal, skull and, 135
  interdigitating, of brain, 146
  mastoid; see Mastoid process
  maxillary, 135, 255
  nasal, 154
  odontoid; see Odontoid process
  olecranon, of ulna, 349, 356
  palatine, 135
  peripheral, 436
  skull and, 134-135, 139, 141
  spinal cord and, 435-436
  of spinal nerve, lateral, 164
  spinous; see Spinous process
  styloid; see Styloid process
  transverse; see Transverse process of
    vertebra
  uncinate, 496, 508
  vocal, 285
  xiphoid; see Xiphoid
  zygomatic, of temporal bone, 141
Processus vaginalis, 466, 472
  remnants of, 468
Profunda brachii artery, 332
  arm and, 342, 347
  axilla and, 332
Profunda femoris artery
  on CT, 618
  femoral triangle and, 652
  perforating branches of, 668, 674
  thigh and, 658, 674
Projectile vomiting, 540, 543
Prolactin, 55
Prolapse
  of mitral heart valve, 101
  of uterus, perineum and, 585
Promontory of wall of middle ear, 226-227,
    231
Pronation, 5, 7
  daily activities and, 356
  muscles mediating, 355
  radioulnar joint and, 352
Pronator quadratus muscle, 355, 357-360,
    373, 375
  on MRI, 357
Pronator teres muscle, 344, 355-356, 358-360,
    365
  anterior compartment and, 346
  radial fracture and, 351
Prone position of structure, 3, 5
Proper digital artery, 391, 718
Proper digital nerve, 366
Prostaglandin E¹ in newborn, 106
Prostate gland, 36, 613-614, 616, 619-620
  abdomen and, 459
  anterolateral view of, 597
  apex of, 614
  autonomic innervation and, 592

Prostate gland—cont'd
  bladder and, 596, 598-599
  floor of pelvis and, 565
  palpation of, 616
  pelvic plexus and, 583
  thigh and, 648-649
  umbilical ligaments and, 557
  urethra and, 582, 599, 609, 616, 619
    on cystourethrogram, 617
    reflux ejaculation into, 618
  urogenital diaphragm and, 567
Prostatic duct, 613-614, 616
Prostatic plexus, 599, 614
Prostatic sinus, 582, 614, 616
Prostatic urethra; see Prostate gland, urethra
    and
Prostatic utricle, 614, 616
Proteoglycan matrix in bones, 9
Proteoglycan molecules, 8
Proximal position of structure, 3, 5
Pseudostratified ciliated epithelium, 8
  in trachea, 77
Pseudounipolar neuron, 20
Psoas major muscle, 654
  abdominal wall and, 529
  abscess of, 662
  on CT, 41
  diaphragm and, 530
  femoral artery and, 646
  iliopsoas muscle and, 655
  pancreas and, 496
  pelvic interior and, 558
  tendons of, 645
    femoral triangle and, 651
  thigh and, 656
  ureter and, 594
  on x-ray, 39
Pterion, 134, 140
Pterygoid canal, 143
  nerve of, 194, 260-261
Pterygoid muscle
  lateral
    maxillary artery and, 192
    temporomandibular joint and, 189-190
  mastication and, 191
  medial, 280
Pterygoid plate
  hamulus of, 188, 264, 266
    face and scalp and, 178
    pharynx and, 276
    skull and, 137, 141
  infratemporal fossa and, 188
  lateral, 141, 245
    face and scalp and, 178
    mastication and, 190-192
    skull and, 141
  medial
    hamulus of, 264, 266
    mastication and, 190-192
    nerve to, 193-195
    of sphenoidal bone, 255
Pterygoid venous plexus, 183, 195-196, 233,
    267
  orbit and, 250
Pterygomandibular raphe, 188, 220, 268-269
  pharynx and, 276
Pterygomandibular septae, 189

Pterygomaxillary fissure, 143
Pterygopalatine foramen, 236
Pterygopalatine fossa, 143, 259-262
Pterygopalatine ganglion, 169, 178, 260, 294
  otic ganglion in, 195
  pterygopalatine fossa and, 260-261
  salivary glands and, 263
PTH; see Parathormone
Ptosis, 248, 251
Pubic ramus
  inferior, 551
    hip joint ligaments and, 641
  superior, 551
    sacral anesthesia and, 553
Pubis, 549, 609
  crest of, 551-552
    abdominal wall and, 458
  femur and, 641
    blood supply to, 644
  hip joints and, 642
    ligaments of, 643
  ramus of; see Pubic ramus
  symphysis of; see Symphysis pubis
  tubercle of, 550-552, 555-557, 725
    abdominal wall and, 458
    anteromedial thigh and, 655
    femoral sheath and, 654
    pelvis and, 559
Pubococcygeus muscle, 562-565
Pubofemoral ligament
  hip joints and, 642-643
  musculoskeletal system and, 722
Puboprostatic ligament, 599
Puborectalis muscle, 519, 562-565, 568-569,
    599
Pubovaginalis muscle, 562-565, 631
Pubovesical ligament, 599, 606-607
Pudendal artery, 557, 568, 578
  internal, 568, 570, 572-573, 587, 589-590
    colon and, 516
    pelvis and, 623
    rectum and, 517, 573
Pudendal canal, 568, 589
Pudendal nerve, 555, 557, 568-569, 588-589
  anesthesia and, 631
  anorectal canal and, 519
  block of, 610
  cutaneous branch of, 583
  gluteal region and, 671
  internal, 572-573
  lumbar and sacral plexus and, 670
  perineum and, 578
  rectum and, 571, 573
  urinary flow and, 601
Pudendal vein, 557, 568
  internal, 517, 568, 570, 572-573
Pulleys of hand, 389
Pulmonary artery, 25, 79-85, 121
  anterior view of, 89
  aorta and, 110
  on arteriogram, 82
  bifurcation of, surface projections of, 124
  blood in, 29, 34, 102
  branches of, 81
  on CT and MRI, 42-43, 100
  in fetus and newborn, 106
  fibrous pericardium on, 87

Pulmonary artery—cont'd
  heart and, 97
    fibrous skeleton of, 90-91
  to lung lobes
    left, 80-82, 97
    middle, 81-82
    right, 77, 79, 81-82, 97
  mediastinum and, 110, 216
  in pericardial sac, 86
  pressure in, 83
  at pulmonary hilum, 80
  serous membranes and, 474
  spinal cord and, 444
  on x-ray, 53, 55
Pulmonary capillaries, 29
Pulmonary hypertension, 83
Pulmonary ligament, 75-76
Pulmonary lymphatics, 84-85
Pulmonary plexus, 85, 213
  lungs and heart and, 84
  mediastinum and, 216
  parasympathetic nerves and, 294
  spinal cord and, 444
Pulmonary sequestration, 85
Pulmonary trunk, 79
  on CT, 100
  lateral margin of, 77
  on x-ray, 53
Pulmonary valve, 91, 96-97
  blood exiting heart through, 102
  congenital stenosis of, 104
  fibrous skeleton of heart and, 91
  position of, 122
  surface anatomy of, 123-124
Pulmonary vein, 83-84, 121
  anomalous return of blood from, 101
  on CT and MRI, 43, 100
  heart and, 96-97, 101-102
  in pericardial sac, 86
  pressure in, 83
  at pulmonary hilum, 80
  serous membranes and, 474
Pulp, 268
Pulses, 400
  in lower limb, 726
Puncta, lacrimal, 239, 249
Pupil, 292, 295
  constriction and dilation of, 239, 246, 296
  dilator muscle of, 239
    innervation to, 169, 246
  pathology of, 246, 251
  sphincter of, 239
Pupillary reflex, 247
Purkinje fibers, 103-104
Pyelogram, intravenous, 525
Pyloric canal, 502
Pyloric vein, 501
Pylorus
  antrum of, 501-502, 508
    liver and, 488
  liver and, 488
  sphincter of, 501-502
    cranial nerves and, 169
  stenosis of, 540, 543
  stomach and, 501-502
Pyramid, middle ear and, 227-228
Pyramidal lobe of thyroid gland, 218

Pyramidalis muscle, abdomen and, 461

Q

Quadrangular muscle, 17
Quadrangular space, 330, 332
Quadrants of abdomen, 538
Quadrate lobe of liver, 485, 487
  in fetus, 486
Quadratus femoris muscle, 17, 648-649, 667
  attachment of, 657
  on CT, 618
  layers of
    deep, 666
    intermediate, 664
  nerves to, 557, 646, 671
  vessels to, 668
Quadratus lumborum muscle, 588
  abdominal wall and, 529
  on CT, 41
  diaphragm and, 530
  iliopsoas muscle and, 655
  lumbar and sacral plexus and, 533, 670
Quadratus plantae muscle, 715-717, 719
Quadriceps muscles, 653
  attachment of, 657
  iliotibial band and, 673
  patella and, 676
  pes anserinus and, 675
  tendons of, 646, 679, 726
    anteromedial thigh and, 655
    femoral artery and, 646
    lateral view of, 699
Quadrigeminal cistern, 148
Quadrigeminal plate of midbrain, 148
Quadrilateral space, 330
Quadripedal muscle, 423

R

Raccoon's eyes, 251
RAD; see Reactive airways disease
Radial artery, 363-364, 397, 400
  arm and, 342, 345, 347
  on arteriogram, 345
  axilla and, 332
  for blood sampling and/or placement of
    indwelling catheter, 377
  branches of
    deep, 391
    deep vena comitantes and, 364
    superficial, 363-364, 391
  forearm and, 363
  on MRI, 357
  pulses in, 377
  tear in, 351
  wrist and, 372, 374
Radial collateral artery, superior, 332
Radial collateral ligament, 353, 374
Radial fossa, 316, 318
Radial keratotomy, 251
Radial nerve, 332, 338, 354, 365, 398
  arm and, 344
  axilla and, 332
  brachial plexus and, 337-339
  branches of
    deep, 365
    superficial, 365-368
  elbow flexion and, 404

Radial nerve—cont'd
  forearm and, 365, 368
  in hand, 392-393
  injury to, 340, 402, 404
  musculospiral groove for, 318
  radioulnar joint and, 354
Radial recurrent artery, 345
Radial tuberosity; see Radius, tuberosity of
Radial vein, 364
Radical mastectomy, 127
Radicular artery, 427-429, 440, 448
  and vertebral column, 428
Radicular vein, 428, 430
  spinal cord and, 441
Radiocarpal joint, 370, 374, 396
Radiocarpal ligament, palmar, 369
Radioulnar joint, 348, 352-355
Radius, 348, 350, 353, 356-357
  anatomic snuff box and, 372
  anatomy of
    skeletal, 309-310, 394
    surface, 400
  anterior view of, 12
  carpal bones and, 370
  deviation of, 370
  epicondyles of, 353, 363, 365
  fracture of, 351, 402, 405
  growth and maturation of, 11
  head of, 348-350, 354
    dislocation of, 352
    elbow movements and, 349
    interosseous membrane and, 356
    on x-ray, 350
  interosseous membrane and, 356
  joints and
    radiocarpal, 370, 374, 396
    radioulnar, 348, 352-355
  ligaments of, 353
    annular, 353-354
    collateral, 353
  longitudinal axis of, 349
  on MRI, 357, 373
  neck of, 348-350
  notch of, 348-349, 352, 354
    ulnar, 357, 371
  styloid process of, 348, 371, 400
    interosseous membrane and, 356
  tuberosity of, 348-349, 353
    dorsal, 357, 373
    elbow movements and, 349
    interosseous membrane and, 356
    ligaments and, 353
  on x-ray, 350
Radix; see Root
Rales, 124
Rami communicantes
  gray; see Gray rami communicans
  white; see White rami communicans
Ramus
  ischial, 559
  ischiopubic, 550-552, 565, 573
  of mandible, 135, 137, 187-189
  pubic
    on CT, 618
    inferior, 618, 648-649
    sacral anesthesia and, 553
    superior, 551, 618

Ramus—cont'd
  of spinal nerves, 118, 416, 437, 449
    dorsal primary, 293
    gray; *see* Gray rami communicans
    lumbar plexus and, 530-531
    thoracic spinal cord segment and, 69
    white; *see* White rami communicans
Ranitidine, 506
Ranula, 275
Ranvier node, 146
Raphe
  anococcygeal, 561-564, 568, 572-574, 631
  diaphragm and, 532
  at mylohyoid muscle, 219
  pterygomandibular, 188, 220, 268-269
    pharynx and, 276
  soft palate and, 280
  submental triangle and, 219, 223
Reactive airways disease, 79
Receptors, blood pressure and, 105
Recess
  costodiaphragmatic, 493
  costomediastinal, 75, 77, 80
  costophrenic, 75, 77, 80
  epitympanic, 228-229
  of ischiorectal fossa, 566
  pericardial, on CT and MRI, 43
  pharyngeal, 279
  piriform, 281, 286
  in pleural cavities, 75, 77, 80
  in serous cavities and pleural spaces, 75,
    77, 80
  sphenoethmoidal, 255-258
  vesicouterine, 558
Recession of maxilla, 170
Rectal artery
  inferior, 568-569, 590-591
    anorectal canal and, 520
  middle, 569-570, 587, 589
    anorectal canal and, 520
  superior, 517, 569
    sigmoid colon and, 519
Rectal canal, tear in, 584; *see also* Anorectal
    canal; Rectum
Rectal nerve, inferior, 568, 571, 583
Rectal vein
  inferior, 517, 520, 568, 623
  middle, 517, 520
  superior, 520, 623
Rectal venous plexus, 569-570
Rectosigmoid artery, 519
Rectouterine fossa, 558, 574, 604, 609
Rectouterine ligament, 606
Rectovaginal examination, 627
Rectovesical fascia, 575
Rectovesical ligament, 599
Rectum, 30, 36, 516-517, 519-520, 568-569; *see
    also* Anus; Colon
  bleeding from, painless, 539-540, 542
  blood supply to, 517, 587, 591
    arteries in, 569
    venous drainage of, 569-571
  coronal section of, 568
  on CT, 618
  examination of, 520, 625-626
    bimanual, 616
    in prostatic examination, 616

Rectum—cont'd
  in female, 575, 606, 609
    pelvic plexus and, 583
    in pregnancy, 611
  fibromuscular layer of, 568
  gastrointestinal tract and, 477
  innervation of, 571
  ligaments of, 599
  muscles of
    circular, 568
    longitudinal, 568
  pelvic diaphragms and, 532
  pelvic floor and, 565
  peritoneal membranes and, 478
  peritoneal specialization of, 482
  tear in, 584
  uterine prolapse and, 585
  wall of, 584
Rectus abdominis muscle, 17, 460-461, 575
  abdomen and, 458-459, 492, 538
  on CT, 41
  lateral edge of, 557
  sternum and, 63
Rectus capitis muscle, 427-428
  on MRI, 271
Rectus diastasis hernia, principles of, 463
Rectus femoris muscle, 654
  abdomen and, 538
  on CT, 618
  hip joints and, 645
  lumbar plexus and, 533
  thigh and, 648-649, 653, 656
    anteromedial, 655
    lower, 648
Rectus muscle of eye, 237, 243-244
  inferior, 243
    bony orbit and, 237
  lateral, 235, 243
    bony orbit and, 237
    horizontal section of orbit and, 242
  medial, 235, 243
    bony orbit and, 237
    horizontal section of orbit and, 242
  optic canal and, 248
  superior, 243
    bony orbit and, 237
  tendinous ring and, 249
Rectus sheath, 460
Recurrent laryngeal nerve, 109
  aortic arch and, 109
  compression of, 119
  injury to, 290
  in innervation of heart and lungs, 84
  left, 213, 287-289
  mediastinum and, 109
    posterior, 116
    superior, 111-112
  right, 211-213, 288-289
Recurrent meningeal nerve, 449
Red blood cell production, 522
Referred pain; *see* Pain, referred
Reflex
  accommodation, 247, 296
  Babinski, 726
  brachioradialis, 367
  corneal, 247, 251
  cranial nerves and, 247

Reflex—cont'd
  cremasteric, 462, 469, 625, 726
  deep tendon, 400
  eye and, 237-238, 247, 251, 296
  gag, 281-282, 296
  light, 237-238, 251
  oculocephalic, 247
  oculovestibular, 247
  pupillary, 247, 296
  testing of muscular, in lower limb, 726
Reflex bladder emptying mechanism, 601
Reflux, gastroesophageal, 116, 500
Reflux ejaculation, 600, 618
Refractive errors, 240, 251
Regional anesthesia for abdominal surgery,
    539, 542
Regional enteritis, 514
Regions of body, 3-4
Remnant thymic tissue, 119
Remnant thyroid tissue, 218
Renal arteriogram, 40, 526
Renal artery, 524, 526
  abdomen and, 536
  adrenal gland and, 526-527
  kidneys and, 525-526
  in renal arteriogram, 40
  spinal cord and, 445
Renal cortex, narrowed, 597
Renal fascia
  on CT, 41
  pancreas and, 496
Renal papilla, 524-525, 597
Renal pelvis, 522
  dilated, 597
  kidneys and, 525
Renal vein, 527
  abdominal wall and, 534-535
  jejunum and ileum and, 511
  ovaries and, 605
  pancreas and, 496
Renin, 528
Renin-angiotensin enzymes, 522
Reproductive system, 34-36; *see also* Female;
    Male
  genitalia of, 36
  smooth muscles of, 19
Resistance to blood flow through liver, 489
Respirations
  accessory muscles of, 68, 199
  chest wall and, 65-68
  obstruction of, 259
  principles for, 68
  ribs, sternum, and vertebral column and,
    56, 67
Respiratory congestion, 259
Respiratory diaphragm; *see* Diaphragm,
    thoracic
Respiratory system, 29-30, 34
  diaphragm in; *see* Diaphragm, thoracic
  lower, 74
  smooth muscles of, 19
  upper, 74
Retina, 234-237, 240-241
  central artery of, 158, 238, 241, 250
  central depression of, 241
  central vein of, 157, 162, 241
  neural, 237-238, 240-241, 250

Retina—cont'd
  pathology of, 252
  pigment epithelium of, 237
Retinaculum muscle, 688, 699, 714
Retractions in respiratory distress, 122
Retromandibular vein, 185, 203
  external jugular vein and, 208
  face and, 183
  on MRI, 271
  pterygoid venous plexus and, 195
Retroperitoneal structures, development of,
    474, 476-478, 481-483
Retropharyngeal abscess, 283
Retropharyngeal lymph node, 233
Retzius, space of, 600, 602
Rhomboid major muscle, 65, 326, 394, 425
  on CT and MRI, 43, 100
  shoulder movement and, 325-326
  vertebral column and, 423
Rhomboid minor muscle, 65, 326, 394, 425
  shoulder movement and, 325-326
  vertebral column and, 423
Rib, 12, 50, 54-55, 60-61, 120
  abdomen and, 536
    wall of, 458
  accessory, 413
  anatomy of
    clinical, 62
    surface, 123
  anterior view of, 12
  articular surface of, 416
  articulations of, 422-424
  atypical, 60
  axilla and, 331
  bifid, 412
  cervical, 62, 328, 412
  collateral blood flow and, 72
  costal element of, 412
  costal margin of, 458
  costovertebral and costotransverse joints
    and, 424
  demi-facets for head of, 416
  first, 331
    axilla and, 330
    brachial plexus and, 327
    cranial nerves and, 168
    neck and, 201
    spinal cord and, 445
    thoracic inlet and, 311
    on x-ray, 417
  fracture of, 72
    spleen and, 494
  heads of, 59-61
  inferior, 72
  lumbar, 62, 412
  lungs and pleural sacs and, 75
  neck of, 60-61
  notching of, 72
  posterior angle of, 60
  in respirations, 66-67
  second, 168, 399
  superior, 72
  supernumerary, 60, 62
  tenth, on x-ray, 417
  tubercles of, 60-61, 422-423
  twelfth, 588
    back and, 449

Rib—cont'd
    lumbar and sacral plexus and, 670
  typical, 60
  variation in structure of, 412
Rib cage, 331
Ribosomes, endoplasmic reticulum with, 21
Ridge
  alveolar, 268
  intertrochanteric, 648-649
  petrous, of temporal bone, 139
  supraciliary, 177
  supracondylar, 315, 318, 399, 639, 672
  supraorbital, 295
Right dominance, 92
Ring
  femoral, 653-654
  of inguinal canal; see Inguinal ring
  of lymphoid tissue, 279
  subendocardial fibrous, 97
  tendinous, of eye, 248-249
  tracheal; see Tracheal ring
  Waldeyer's, 274, 279
Ring finger, 371
  extension of, 390
  muscle insertions on, 387-388
  ulnar nerve and, 368
Risorius muscle, 178
Root
  of ansa cervicalis nerve, 214
  of brachial plexus, 199-202, 336
    cervical sympathetic chain and, 215
    injury to, 339
  of cranial nerves; see Cranial nerves
  of mesentery, peritoneal membranes and,
    478
  of spinal nerves
    accessory nerve and; see Accessory
      nerve (XI), spinal origin of
    dorsal; see Dorsal spinal nerve root
    exiting intervertebral foramen, 411
    on MRI, 418
    ventral; see Ventral spinal nerve root
  of tooth, 267
Rotation
  around axes, 7
  of hip joint, 712
Rotator cuff
  dislocated shoulder and, 317
  injuries to, 321
  muscles of, 316, 318, 324-325, 394
  tendons of, 320
Rotator muscles, 426-427
Rough zone of valve leaflet, 95, 97
Round ligament, 36, 558, 605
  descent of ovary and, 472
  labia majora and, 571
  migration of, 464, 468, 559
  porta hepatis and, 486
  superior view of, 575
  sympathetic nerves and, 591
Round window, 227-228, 230
Roux-en-Y procedure, 506
Rugae of stomach, 501-502
Rupture
  of cruciate ligament, 687, 730
  of plantaris tendon, 698
  of thoracic duct, 114

Rupture—cont'd
  of urethra, 566
    traumatic, 619

S

S1; see Sacral vertebra; Sacrum
SA node; see Sinoatrial node
Sac
  greater, development of, 476-479
  lesser
    development of, 481
    stomach and, 504
  omental; see Omental bursa
Sacculations, 516
Saccule, 233
Saccus vaginalis, 468
Sacral artery, lateral, 570, 589
Sacral canal, 416
Sacral foramina, 550, 552-553
  anterior, 416, 419
    pelvis and, 559
  posterior, 416, 419
Sacral hiatus, 416, 419, 552-553
  caudal block and, 593
Sacral nerve, 583
Sacral plexus, 533, 587-589, 668-671
  branches of, 555, 587-591
  gluteal region and, 670-671
  lumbar plexus and, 533
  parasympathetic outflow and, 294, 587
  pelvis and perineum and, 623-624
  rectum and, 571
Sacral vein, 570
Sacral vertebra, 409-410, 553; see also Sacrum
  anesthesia and, 553
  curvature of, 409-410
  spinous process of, 416, 419, 553
Sacroiliac facet, 419
Sacroiliac joint, 416, 554, 556
  articular surface of, 551-552
  hip joints and, 642
  pelvis and, 559
Sacroiliac ligament, 554-556
  gluteal region and, 663
Sacrospinous ligament, 555-556, 562
  on CT, 618
  gluteal region and, 663
Sacrotuberous ligament, 555-556, 561-562,
    573, 590
  in gluteal region, 663
    deep layer, 666
    intermediate layer, 664
    vessels and, 668
Sacrum, 416, 419, 552-553; see also Sacral
    vertebra
  abdomen and, 536
  anterior and lateral views of, 410
  articular surface of, 557
  gluteal region and, 663
  hip joints and, 642
  lumbar puncture and, 432
  pelvis and, 549
    female internal genitalia in, 606
    interior of, 557-558
    pelvic diaphragm in, 532, 562
  promontory of, 416, 419, 550, 553
    on MRI, 418

Sacrum—cont'd
pelvis and, 559
Sagittal plane, 3, 6
Sagittal sinus; *see* Cerebral sinus, sagittal
Sagittal suture, 136-138, 295
Saliva, 186
cranial nerves and, 169
drainage of, 275
submandibular and sublingual glands and, 273
swallowing and, 282
Salivary duct cyst, 275
Salivary gland, 263, 272-274
cystic swellings in duct from, 275
minor, 274
sublingual, 188, 274
submandibular, 219, 274
Salpingopharyngeus muscle, 231, 264, 266, 278-280
swallowing and, 282
Salpinx, 231
Sampling of blood, 346
Santorini, duct of, 497
Saphenous nerve, 638, 648, 656, 659
Saphenous vein
great, 648-653, 662, 695, 724
fascial compartments and, 693
foot and, 715
as landmark, 726
long, 648-649
fascial compartments and, 693
small, 652, 693, 695, 724
fascial compartments and, 693, 696
x-ray of, 653
Sarcomere, 15
Sartorius muscle, 650, 654
anteromedial thigh and, 655
on CT, 618
femoral artery and, 646
femoral sheath and, 654
lumbar plexus and, 533
medial edge of, 651
pes anserinus and, 675
thigh and, 648-649, 656
anterior, 646
lower, 648
posterior, 674
Satellite cells, 20
Scalene muscle, 200-201, 292
anterior, 111, 199, 201, 326-327, 429
accessory nerve and, 213
cranial nerves and, 167
spinal cord and, 445
subclavian artery and, 203, 326
cranial nerves and, 168
medial, 167, 327
spinal cord and, 445
in respiration, 68
Scalp, 174-186
anastomoses in, 176
blood supply to, 174-175, 181, 183-184
venous drainage of, 183
clinical anatomy of, 176
injuries to, 185
innervation of, 174-175, 293
cutaneous, 177-181
layers of, 174-175

Scalp—cont'd
palpation of, 295
parotid gland and, 182-186
Scalping, 176
Scaphocephaly, 144
Scaphoid bone, 357, 369-371, 373-374, 376, 396
avascular necrosis of, 405
fracture of, 376, 402, 405
on MRI, 357
radiocarpal joint and, 370
tubercle of, 374, 400
flexor retinaculum and, 370
wrist and, 371, 373-374
Scapula, 61-62, 120, 309-314
anastomosis around, 329, 397
angle of
inferior or superior, 62
vertebral border and, 398
axilla and, 330-331
chest wall structure and, 55
coracoid process of, 398
growth and maturation of, 11
joints of, 61, 315, 318-322
ligaments and, 319
movements of, 313, 316
on MRI, 323
musculoskeletal anatomy of, 394
neck of, 62
notch of, 313
serratus anterior muscle and, 331
spine of, 312-315, 317, 326
ligaments and, 319
position of, back and, 449
surface anatomy of, 398-399
structural features of, 645
thoracic inlet and, 59, 311
view of
anterior, 12
posterior, 320
winging of, 324
on x-ray, 312-313
Scapular artery
circumflex, 334
axilla and, 332
dorsal, 70, 204, 320, 329, 397
cervical vertebrae and, 429
subclavian artery branches and, 326
Scapular ligament, transverse, 312, 319
Scapular nerve, dorsal, 337
Scapulohumeral rhythm, 322
Scarpa's fascia, 457
principles of, 566
Schwann cell, 20, 23, 435-436
neurolemma of, 146
spinal cord and, 436
Sciatic foramen, 555-556
greater, 668
Sciatic nerve, 534, 555, 557, 587-588, 725
common peroneal branch of, 668-669, 671, 674
on CT, 618
gluteal region and, 663, 668-671
lumbar and sacral plexus and, 670
origin of, 669
pelvis and perineum and, 624
popliteal fossa and, 689

Sciatic nerve—cont'd
posterior leg and, 696
sacral plexus and, 590
thigh and, 648-649
posterior, 674-675
tibial portion of, 674
Sciatic notch
greater, 552, 643, 663
lesser, 551-552, 556, 663
gluteal region and, 663
lower thigh and, 648
Sciatic notch, greater and lesser, 551-552, 556-557, 643
gluteal region and, 663
Sclera, 235, 295
Scleral venous sinus, 239
Scoliosis, 409, 450
Scrotum, 468, 577, 615
in inguinal canal, 468-472
lymphatic drainage of, 578, 581
Sebaceous gland, 8
Second cranial nerve; *see* Optic nerve (II)
Section, cesarean, 144, 608
Segmental bronchi, 77
Segmental cutaneous innervation, 624
Segmental organization of body, 121, 450
principles of, 446
Seizures, functional regions of brain and, 151
Self-examination, testicular, 625
Sella turcica, 135
Semen, reflux ejaculation of, 600, 618
Semicircular canals, 226, 228-230, 233
Semimembranous muscle, 690
attachment of, 657
leg muscles and, 689
pes anserinus and, 675
tendon of
knee joint and, 676
popliteal fossa and, 691
thigh and, 648-649
lower, 648
nerves to posterior, 674
posterior, 673-675
Seminal colliculus, 582, 614, 616
on cystourethrogram, 617
on seminal vesiculogram, 615
Seminal vesicle, 613-615, 619, 621
abdomen and, 459
bladder and
autonomic innervation of, 592
posterior surface of, 596
on CT, 618
umbilical ligaments and, 557
vesiculogram of, 615
Semispinalis muscle, 425-426, 433
of head, 426
on MRI, 271
Semitendinous muscle
attachment of, 657
on CT, 618
in gluteal region, 664
leg muscles and, 689
pes anserinus and, 675
posterior view of, 694
thigh and, 648-649
lower, 648

Semitendinous muscle—cont'd
  posterior, 673-675
Sensation
  of movement and balance, 224
  of sound, 224
Sense organs, 133-134
Sensory axons; see Axon, sensory
Sensory cortex, primary, 149
Sensory ganglion of cranial nerve, 164-168
Sensory neuron, 20-22, 436
  peripheral, in brain, 146
Separated shoulder, 317, 401, 403
Septae of breast, 54-55
Septal artery, 93, 104
  posterior, 104, 259
Septal cartilage, 253, 255
Septal defects, 101
  auscultation of, 124
  congenital, 104
Septal leaflet of tricuspid valve, 95
Septal wall of right atrium, 94-95
Septomarginal fasciculus, 95, 103-104
Septum, nasal, 253-255
Septum primum, 107
Septum secundum, 95, 107
Serosa of gut wall, 35, 499, 510
Serous cavities, 49, 51
  case studies of, 125
Serous cavities in thorax, 49-51
  case studies and, 125, 127
  formation of, 51
Serous membranes and spaces, 51, 474
Serratus anterior muscle, 64-66, 100, 325,
    331, 394
  abdomen and, 458
  axilla and, 330-331
  on CT and MRI, 43, 323
  winging of scapula and, 324
Serratus posterior muscle, 64-65, 326, 425
Sesamoid bone, 369, 371
  flexor hallucis brevis and, 707
Seventh cranial nerve; see Facial nerve (VII)
Sex hormones, 527
  abnormal levels of, 528
Sexual dimorphism in pelvic shape, 550,
    554, 557
Sexually transmitted disease, 610
Shin splints, 698
Shingles, 72, 450
Short rotator muscle, 427
Shoulder, 309-329
  in anatomic position, 4
  anteroposterior x-ray of, 312
  blood supply to
    arterial, 326, 328-329
    clinical anatomy of, 328
    venous drainage in, 327, 329
  clavicle in; see Clavicle
  clinical anatomy of, 317, 319, 321, 324-325,
      328
  dislocation of, 317
  humerus in, 314-318
    clinical anatomy of, 319
  injury of, 401, 403
  joints of, 318-322, 396
    clinical anatomy of, 321
  ligaments of, 319

Shoulder—cont'd
  movements of, 322-327
  on MRI, 323
  muscles of, 322-327
    clinical anatomy of, 324
  nerve supply to, 327, 329
    clinical anatomy of, 328
  principles for, 310, 316, 324
  scapula in; see Scapula
  separation of, 317, 401, 403
  shoulder girdle and; see Shoulder girdle
Shoulder girdle, 309-314, 394
  joints of, 315-322
  movements of, 316
  structural features of, 645
  superior and inferior views of, 317
  thorax and, 55, 61-62, 120
Shunt, vascular, 28-29
  Blalock-Taussig, 328
  iliac arteries and, 593
  lungs and, 79, 83
  portocaval, 489, 520
Sigmoid arterial arcade, 519
Sigmoid colon, 516-517, 519
  anorectal region and, 516-517
  gastrointestinal tract and, 477
  rectum and, 517
  on ultrasound, 612
Sigmoid sinus, 134, 139-140, 157-158, 162
Signal transmission, visual, 240-241
Simple elongated muscle, 17
Sinoatrial node, 90, 94, 103
Sinus
  air, of skull, 143; see also Paranasal
      sinuses
  anal, 571
  aortic, 101
  carotid; see Carotid sinus
  cavernous; see Cavernous sinus
  cerebral; see Cerebral sinus
  cervical, 172-173
  coronary; see Coronary sinus
  epithelium in, 143
  lactiferous, 54-55
  marginal, 157
  occipital, 154, 157, 162
  paranasal; see Paranasal sinuses
  pericardial, 87-88
  petrosal, 157-158, 162
  prostatic, 582, 614, 616
  of pulmonary valve, 97
  sagittal; see Cerebral sinus, sagittal
  scleral, 239
  sigmoid, 134, 139-140, 157-158, 162
  of skull, air, 143; see also Paranasal sinuses
  sphenoid, 135, 154, 160, 255-259
    meningeal artery hematoma and, 196
    on MRI, 148
  sphenoparietal, 157
  straight, 154, 157, 162
  tarsal, 709
  toothache and, 262
  transverse, 139-140, 148, 157, 161
    on MRI, 148
Sinus venarum, 94
Sinus venosus, 103
Situs inversus, 89

Sixth cranial nerve; see Abducens
    nerve (VI)
Skeletal framework of face, 176-177
Skeletal muscle, 11-18
Skeleton, 11-14
  anterior view of, 12
  appendicular, 11-12
  axial, 11-12
  fibrous, of heart, 89-90
  of head and neck, 291
  pelvis and, 622
  thoracic, 120-121
Skene's gland, 574
Skin, 8
  hernias and, 467
  incised, 9
  loose, on dorsum of hand, 9
  scalp and face and, 175
  of testis, 468
Skull, 133-144
  air sinus of; see Paranasal sinuses
  anatomy of
    introduction to, 133-134
    surface, 134-141
  apertures of, 139-141, 291
  base of, 141-143, 421, 428
    bony prominences of, 141-143
    CT of, 142
    muscles and, 426
  bones of, 133-136, 139
    synchondroses of, 133
    union of, 10, 13
  of child, 136, 138
  childbirth and, 144
  cranial vault and, 134-135, 139
  fissures of; see Fissures, of skull; Orbital
      fissure
  floor of, 136, 138-140
  fossae of, 139
    jugular, 142
    mandibular, 143
    middle, 139
    pituitary, 135, 139, 154, 196
    posterior, 142
    pterygopalatine, 143, 259-262
  fractures of, 144, 196-197
  growth disturbance of, 297, 301
  hemorrhage inside, 151
  palpation of, 295
  shape variations in shape of, 144
  sutures of, 134-137
  vertebral column and
    attachments to, 418, 421
    ligaments of, 421
  views of
    anterior or frontal, 12, 137
    basal, 141
    lateral, 135
    posterior, 137
    x-rays of, 144
Sliding hernia, 500
Slip of tendon, central, 390
Slipped disk, 423
Small cardiac vein, 93
Small intestine, 507-514
  antimesenteric side of, 512
  barium study of, 509

Small intestine—cont'd
  clinical anatomy of, 514
  displaced upward, 611
Small intestine—cont'd
  duodenum in, 507-510
  gastrointestinal tract and, 477
  herniating, 463
  ileum in, 510-513
  jejunum in, 510-513
  lymphatic drainage of, 512
  parasympathetic nerves and, 294
  peritoneal membranes and, 481
  superior mesenteric arteriogram of, 513
Small saphenous vein, 652, 693, 695, 724
  fascial compartments of leg and, 693
Smell, 254
Smooth muscle, 16-19, 292
  in bladder neck, 600
  of bronchiole, 34
  of intestinal tract, 499, 510
  sphincters of, 25-26
  in uterine wall, 607
    tumors of, 610
  in vessel wall, 25
Snuff-box, anatomic, 362, 372, 375
Soft palate, 253, 260, 263-266, 281
  abnormalities of, 275
  muscles of, 263-266
  palatine tonsil and, 280
  surface anatomy of, 296
Soft spots on infant skull, 136, 138
Sole of foot, 715-719
Soleus muscle, 692-693, 695
  fascial compartments of leg and, 692-693
  popliteal fossa and, 688-689
  posterior leg nerves and, 696
  views of
    anterior, 697
    posterior, 694-695
Somatic motor nerve, 442, 446
  axon of, 164
  of globe and orbit, 244
  neuron of, 20-22, 25, 436
  spinal cord and, 442-443
Somatostatin, 497, 506
  duodenum and, 507
Sound
  movement of tympanic membrane in
    response to, 226
  sensation of, 224
Space
  in axilla, 330-333
  epidural; see Epidural space
  glossoepiglottic, 281
  intercostal; see Intercostal space
  intervertebral, lumbar puncture and, 432
  midpalmar, 389
  in nasal cavity wall, 255-258
  pleural; see Pleural spaces
  quadrangular, 330, 332
  quadrilateral, 330
  of Retzius, 600, 602
  serous, 51, 474
  subarachnoid; see Subarachnoid space
  subdural, 158
  supracolic, 482
  synovial, 14; see also Synovial cavity

Space—cont'd
  thenar, 389
  triangular, 330, 332
Speech, 287
  motor control of, 149
Sperm, 35
  reflux ejaculation and, 600, 618
Spermatic cord, 464, 466-470
  blood vessels in, 469-470
  contents of, 468-469
  on CT, 618
  epigastric vessels and, 467
  hernias and, 467
  inguinal canal and, 465
  nerves in, 469
  thigh and, 648-649
Spermatic fascia
  external, 464
  internal, 466
Sphenoethmoidal recess, 255-258
Sphenoid bone, 134-136, 138-141, 255
  apertures in, 140-141
  greater wing of, 236
    infratemporal fossa and, 188
    skull and, 134-135, 141
    temporomandibular joint and, 189
  lesser wing of, 139, 236
    horizontal section through bony orbit
      and, 237
  medial pterygoid plate of, 255
  orbit and, 234
  otic ganglion and, 194
  sinuses in; see Sphenoid sinus
  skull and, 139
  surgery and, 262
Sphenoid sinus, 135, 143, 255-260
  cross-section of, 160
  falx cerebri and, 154
  meningeal artery hematoma and, 196
  on MRI, 148
  skull and, 135
Sphenomandibular ligament, 189, 277
Sphenopalatine artery, 258-259
  maxillary artery and, 193
  pterygopalatine fossa and, 261
Sphenopalatine foramen, 258
Sphenoparietal sinus, 157, 162
Sphincter, 17
  anal; see Anal sphincter
  gastroesophageal, 116
  of Oddi, 487, 497
  of pupil, 237, 239
    parasympathetic nerves and, 294
  pyloric, 501-502
    cranial nerves and, 169
  urethral; see Urethra, sphincter of
Spina bifida, 431, 449
Spinal accessory nerve (XI); see Accessory
    nerve (XI), spinal origin of
Spinal anesthesia, 447
Spinal artery
  anterior, 159, 161, 429, 440
    brain and, 159
    formation of, 429
    spinal cord and, 442
  posterior, 429, 440
    spinal cord and, 442

Spinal canal, 58, 439
  brain and, 150
Spinal cord, 20, 24, 434-447
  anatomy of
    clinical, 447
    musculoskeletal, 448
    surface, 449-450
  arachnoid mater and, 438
  blood supply to, 439-442, 448-449
    arteries in, 439-440, 442
    veins from, 441
  case studies for, 451-453
  compression of, 447
  dorsal column of, 435
  dorsal horn of, 24, 434-435, 437
  dorsal roots and, 435, 437-438; see also
    Dorsal spinal nerve root
  gray and white matter in, 147, 438
  in infant, 441
  injuries to, urination and, 592, 601-602
  innervation and, 449
  intercostal nerves and, 69, 71
  intercostal space and, 430
  intermediate horn and, 437, 443
  lateral column of, 435
  lateral horn of, 435
  lumbar puncture and, 153, 155, 431-432,
    447, 449
  lymphatic drainage of, 449
  mediastinum and, 118
  meninges and, 436-440
  on MRI, 415
  musculocutaneous nerve and, 400
  parasympathetic nerves and, 294, 445-446
  peripheral process and, 20, 146, 436
  physical examination and, 449-450
  pia mater covering, 438
  principles for, 446
  segments of
    cervical, 148
    S2-S4, 592
    thoracic, 69, 118
  somatic and autonomic nerves in, 442-443
  spinal nerves and, 435-436
    typical, 446
  structure of, 434-435, 437
  subarachnoid space and, 439
  sympathetic nervous system and, 441-446
  systems review and, 448-449
  ventral column of, 435
  ventral horn of, 24, 434-435, 437
  vertebral canal and, 439-441
Spinal motor neuron, diseases of, 447
Spinal nerves, 20, 24, 435-436
  back and spinal cord and, 449
  brachial plexus and, 341
  central process of neuron and, 164
  cervical, 293
  cranial nerves and, 164-165
  cutaneous branches of, 295
  of dorsal primary rami, 293
  first, 167
    anterolateral neck and, 210
  herniation of intervertebral disk and, 423
  lateral process of, 164
  mediastinum and, 118
  roots of

Spinal nerves—cont'd
　accessory nerve and, 165, 167, 202, 210,
　　213, 437
　dorsal; see Dorsal spinal nerve root
　exiting intervertebral foramen, 411
　on MRI, 418
　ventral; see Ventral spinal nerve root
　sympathetic chain connections to, 444-445
　true, 437
　typical, 446
Spinal reflex bladder emptying mechanism,
　601
Spinal tap, 153, 155, 431-432, 447, 449
Spinal vein, 441
Spinalis muscle, 425-426
Spine; see also Vertebrae
　anterior superior, 725
　　pelvis and, 559
　bifid, 414
　scapular, 312, 314, 326
　of vertebra, 411
Spinoglenoid notch, 313-314
Spinous process, 58, 410-420, 422-423, 448-
　　449
　in atlas, 415, 428
　in axis, 414-415, 428
　in cervical region, 412-415, 428
　in lumbar region, 415, 417-418
　on MRI, 418
　in sacral region, 416, 419, 553
　spinal cord and, 430
　in thoracic region, 413, 416-417
　transverse, 410-417, 422, 424, 448
　　of atlas, 142
　　spinal cord and, 438
　　on x-ray, 417
Splanchnic nerve, 445
　abdomen and, 537
　adrenal gland and, 527
　diaphragm and, 531
　greater, 118
　lesser, 118
　pelvic, 584, 587, 671
　spinal cord and, 443, 445
Spleen, 491-494
　abdominal symmetry and, 494
　accessory, 494
　anatomy of
　　clinical, 494
　　surface, 538
　blood supply to, 493-494
　　venous drainage of, 480
　consequences of being without, 494
　function of, 484
　gastrointestinal tract and, 477
　hilum of, 493
　ligaments and, 491, 493-494
　mesenteries and, 491, 493-494
　　development of, 476
　parasympathetic nerves and, 294
　peritoneal membranes and, 478
　relations and position of, 491, 493
　rib fracture and, 494
　stomach and, 502, 505
Splenectomy, 483
　approach for, 494
　pancreas and, 498

Splenic artery, 491, 494
　liver and, 488
　pancreas and, 497
　peritoneal membranes and, 479
　spleen and, 491, 493
　stomach and, 501-503
Splenic flexure, 515
　anorectal region and, 516
　transverse colon and, 518
Splenic vein, 479-480, 494
　abdomen and, 537
　liver and, 488
　pancreas and, 497
　peritoneal membranes and, 479
　spleen and, 491
Splenius capitis muscle, 65, 425-427
　on MRI, 271
Splenius cervicis muscle, 326
Spondylolisthesis, 433, 452, 628, 630
Spondylolysis, 431, 628, 630
Spongiose urethra, 616
Spontaneous depolarization-repolarization,
　103
Spring ligament, 707, 710
Squamosal suture, 134, 136
Squamous temporal bone, 188-189
Stalk of pituitary gland, 158
Stapedial artery, 171
Stapedius muscle, 133, 225, 227-228, 231
Stapes, 225, 227-230
　deafness and, 232
STDs; see Sexually transmitted disease
Stellate ganglion, 113, 215, 444
　block of, 119, 328
　mediastinum and, 216
　spinal cord and, 444
Stenosis
　aqueductal, 153
　heart valve, 101
　　congenital, 104
　pyloric, 540, 543
Stereotaxic surgery, 144
Sterilization by tubal ligation, 610
Sternal angle, 62, 122, 399
　subclavian artery and, 203
Sternal notch, 62, 122-123
Sternebrae, 62
Sternochondral joint, 50, 60
Sternoclavicular joint, 63, 310, 318, 321-322,
　　394, 398
Sternoclavicular ligament, 321
Sternocleidomastoid muscle, 62, 292
　abdomen and, 458
　accessory nerve and, 213
　anterior trunk and, 66
　brain and, 159
　cervical sympathetic chain and, 215
　clavicle and, 313
　cranial nerves and, 167
　on MRI, 271
　neck and, 296
　　anterolateral, 207-208, 216
　　posterior triangle of, 199-200, 202
　in respiration, 68
　shoulder movement and, 325-326
　submandibular gland and, 221
　surface anatomy of, 295-296

Sternohyoid muscle, 17, 62
　ansa cervicalis and, 214
　neck and
　　anterolateral, 216, 271
　　posterior triangle of, 200
　pharynx and, 276
Sternopericardial ligament, 88
　in anterior mediastinum, 118
Sternothyroid muscle
　ansa cervicalis and, 214
　neck and
　　anterolateral, 216-217
　　posterior triangle of, 200
Sternotomy, 63, 119
Sternum, 62-63, 120
　anatomy of
　　clinical, 63
　　surface, 123
　anomalies of, 63
　anterior view of, 12
　body of, 62, 321
　bone marrow sampling from, 63
　brachial plexus and, 327
　chest wall and, 54-55
　on CT and MRI, 43, 100
　joints of, 321
　lungs and pleural sacs and, 75
　manubrium of; see Manubrium of
　　sternum
　mediastinum and, 52
　neck and, 201, 216
　palpation of, 122
　shoulder girdle and, 317
　thoracic cage and, 50
　xiphoid process of; see Xiphoid
　on x-ray, 53, 77
Steroids, adrenal, 527-528
Stethoscope, 124
Stomach, 477, 501-505
　abnormal emptying of, 506
　barium contrast study of, 502
　bed of, 505
　blood supply to, 501-503
　　clinical anatomy of, 506
　　venous drainage of, 480
　body of, 492, 501-502
　clinical anatomy of, 506
　curvature of, 492, 502
　development of, 505
　greater omentum and, 504
　innervation of, 503
　　parasympathetic nerves in, 294
　pancreas and, 495, 497
　peritoneal membranes and, 481
　peritoneal specialization of, 482-483
　pyloric sphincter and pyloric antrum of,
　　501-502
　rotation of, 476
　　development of gut and, 476-479
　secretions of, 506
　serous membranes and, 474
　small intestine and, 509
　spleen and, 491
　on x-ray, 39
Stones
　pancreatic, 498
　in parotid gland, 185

Stones—cont'd
   salivary gland, 275
   in urinary system, 602
Strabismus, 251
Straight sinus, 154, 157, 162
Strap muscle, 17, 217, 292
Stratum corneum, 8
Stress incontinence, 610
Striate artery, 160
Striated muscle, 11-18
   extraocular, 243
   of joint, 25
   shapes of, 17
   in sphincter urethrae, 600
   superficial, in scalp and face, 292
Stroke, 151
Structures
   anterior position of, 3, 5
   posterior position of, 3, 5
   relationship of, 3, 5
Sty, 251
Styloglossus muscle, 269, 271-272
   swallowing and, 282
   tongue and, 272
Stylohyoid ligament, 269, 276-277
   in submandibular triangle, 222
   tongue and, 272
Stylohyoid muscle, 218, 220, 222, 272, 280
   pharynx and, 276
   tongue and, 272
Styloid process
   of fibula, 690-691
   infratemporal fossa and, 188
   mandibular nerve and, 194
   mastication muscles and, 191
   pharyngeal structures and, 269, 277
   of radius, 348, 356, 371, 400
   skull and, 134, 137, 141-142, 421
   submandibular region and, 222
   tensor veli palatini muscle and, 266
   tongue and, 272
   triangular fibrocartilage and, 353
   of ulna; see Ulna, styloid process of
Stylomandibular ligament, 189, 220-221
Stylomastoid foramen, 141-142
   middle ear and, 228
Stylopharyngeus muscle, 184, 269, 278-280
   swallowing and, 282
Stylopharyngeus nerve, 280
Subacromial bursa, 320
Subarachnoid septum, 156, 437
   spinal cord and, 438
Subarachnoid space, 151-154, 158, 437-439
   cerebrospinal fluid in, 415
     on MRI, 415
   scalp and face and, 175
Subclavian artery, 326-330, 332-333, 396-397
   aortic arch and, 101, 110-111
   brachial plexus and, 327
   branches of, 203, 326
   cervical rib and, 328
   cervical vertebrae and, 429
   chest wall and, 68
   costocervical trunk and, 202-204
   cranial nerves and, 168
   divisions of, 202-204
   head and neck and, 292

Subclavian artery—cont'd
   hemorrhage from, 204
   in posterior neck triangle, 199
   spinal cord and, 442, 445
   thyroid gland and, 218
Subclavian lymph duct, 335
Subclavian triangle, 198, 201
Subclavian vein, 333, 398
   aortic arch and, 110
   axilla and, 330, 333
   axillary vein and, 334
   catheters in, 119
   cervical rib and, 328
   cervical vertebrae and, 429
   posterior triangle and, 204
   subclavian artery branches and, 326
   thoracic duct and, 117
   thyroid gland and, 218
Subclavius muscle, 62, 64
   axilla and, 330
   clavicle and, 313
   on MRI, 323
   nerve to, 337-338
Subcostal artery, 68
Subcostal muscle, 64
Subcostal nerve, 71
Subcutaneous tissue, 9
Subdural space, 158
Subendocardial fibrous rings, 97
Subendocardial Purkinje fibers, 103-104
Subiliac bursa, 656
Sublingual gland, 188, 272-274
   duct from, 273
     submandibular triangle and, 220
   fossa for, 188
   papilla of, 221, 269-270, 273, 296
   parasympathetic nerves and, 294
   submandibular gland and, 221
   submandibular region and, 220-222
   submandibular triangle and, 220
   tongue and, 272
Submandibular ganglion, 169, 272-273
   otic ganglion in, 195
   parasympathetic nerves and, 294
   submandibular and sublingual glands
     and, 273
   submandibular region and, 222, 273
Submandibular gland, 188, 219-222, 272-274
   duct from, 221-222, 269, 272-273, 296
     tongue and, 272
   fossa for, 188
   parasympathetic nerves and, 294
   position of, 221
   structures related to, 221
   submandibular region and, 222
   surface anatomy of, 296
   tongue and, 272
Submandibular lymph node, 210, 222
   inflammation of, 223
   and malignancy, 223
Submandibular region, 218-223
   clinical anatomy of, 223
   nervous supply to, 222
Submandibular triangle, 198, 201, 210, 218-
   223
   nerves in, 222
   vascular structures near, 210, 222-223

Submental node, 210, 292
   tongue and, 272
Submental region, clinical anatomy of, 223
Submental triangle, 198, 201
   in anterolateral neck, 223
Submucosa of intestinal tract, 8, 35, 499, 510
Submucous venous plexus, 35, 520
Suboccipital fat, 415
Suboccipital muscle, 426
Suboccipital triangle, 428
Subsartorial canal, 656
Subscapular artery, 70, 121, 397
   axilla and, 332, 334
Subscapular axillary lymph node, 397
Subscapular bursa, 316
Subscapular fossa, 314-315, 317
Subscapular nerve, 337-338
   brachial plexus and, 338
Subscapularis muscle, 100, 316, 324, 398
   anterior compartment and, 345
   axilla and, 330-331
   on CT and MRI, 43, 100, 323
Subtalar joints of foot, 708-710
Sulcus
   of atrium, 94, 270
   of calcaneus, 705
   in cerebral cortex, 150
   interventricular, 89
   vaginal tear and, 584
Sulcus terminalis, 94, 270
Superficial position of structure, 3
Superior position of structure, 6
Superior vena cava syndrome, 114; see also
     Venae cavae, superior
Supernumerary ribs, 60, 62
Supination, 5, 7
   daily activities and, 356
   muscles mediating, 355
   radioulnar joint and, 352
Supinator muscle, 355, 359, 361-363, 398
   head of, 365
Supine position of structure, 3, 5
Supraciliary ridge, 177
Supraclavicular lymph node, 210
Supraclavicular nerve, 177, 202, 366
   cervical plexus and, 200
   cervical sympathetic chain and, 215
   shoulder and, 329
Supracolic space, 482
Supracondylar lines, 637, 639
Supracondylar ridge, 315, 318, 399, 639, 672
Supraglenoid tubercle, 312, 314, 320
Suprahyoid muscle, 218-220
Suprameniscal compartment, 679
Supraoptic nuclei of hypothalamus, 37
Supraorbital artery, 174-175, 242
   face and, 181
   orbit and, 250
   scalp and, 175, 183
Supraorbital nerve, 174-175, 247
   face and, 178, 181
   scalp and, 175, 178
Supraorbital notch, 134, 137, 238
Supraorbital ridge, 295
Supraorbital vein, 242
   pterygoid venous plexus and, 195
   scalp and, 183

Suprapatellar bursa, 677, 679
Suprapleural membrane, 205
Suprapubic region, 538
Suprarenal artery, 526, 536
Suprarenal gland, 527; *see also* Adrenal
        gland
    anterior view of, 523
    clinical anatomy of, 528
    inferior phrenic artery with branch to, 526
    kidneys and; *see* Kidney
    pancreas and, 497
    renal artery with branch to, 526
    testis and, 470
Suprarenal vein, 535
Suprascapular artery, 320, 328-329, 397
    axilla and, 332
    back and spinal cord and, 429
    on MRI, 323
    posterior triangle of neck and, 202-204
    subclavian artery branches and, 326
Suprascapular nerve, 332, 337-338
Suprascapular notch, 312, 314, 319
Suprascapular vein, 332
Suprasellar cistern, 148
Supraspinatus muscle, 100, 316, 324, 326, 398
    axilla and, 332
    tendon of, 345
Supraspinous fossa, 313-315, 399
Supraspinous ligament, 420, 422, 453
Supratentorial structures, 149, 154, 158
Supratrochlear artery
    orbit and, 250
    scalp and, 174-175, 183
Supratrochlear nerve
    orbit and, 242, 247
    scalp and face and, 174-175, 178, 181
Supratrochlear vein
    pterygoid venous plexus and, 195
    scalp and, 183
Supraventricular crest, 97
Sural nerve, 638, 693, 725
    fascial compartments of leg and, 696
    popliteal fossa and, 689-690
    tibial nerve branch to, 689
Surface, anterior or posterior, 6
Surfactant, 85
Suspensory ligament, 574, 576
Suspensory sling of orbit, 243
Sustentaculum tali, 700-701, 706-707
    medial view of, 700
    MRI of, 709
Suture of skull, 11, 13, 134-137, 291
    coronal, 134-135
    lambdoid, 135, 141
    sagittal, 295
Swallowing, 281-282
Sweat gland, 8, 445
    sympathetic axons and, 293
Sylvius, aqueduct of, 151, 153
    on MRI, 148
Sympathetic axon
    intercostal nerves and, 71
    otic ganglion and, 196
    postganglionic, 25, 443-446
        anterolateral neck and, 215
        head and neck and, 167
        in pelvis, 591-592

Sympathetic axon—cont'd
    scalp and face and, 186
    preganglionic, 25, 443-446
        anterolateral neck and, 215
        eye and orbit and, 246
    spinal nerves and, 164
Sympathetic branch of phrenic nerve to
        heart, 109
Sympathetic chain, 24, 588, 591
    cervical, 215-217
    cranial nerves and, 168
    diaphragm and, 531
    ganglia of; *see* Sympathetic ganglion
    kidneys and, 524
    lumbar and sacral plexus and, 670
    mediastinum and, 216
        posterior, 118
        superior, 112-114
    in orbit, 246
    pelvic interior and, 558
    spinal cord and, 437, 443-446
    spinal nerve connections and, 444-445
Sympathetic ganglion, 20, 24, 443-446, 588
    cardiac branches of cervical, 113-114
    connectives of, 118
    paraaortic, 600
    spinal cord and, 430, 443
        cervical, 336
        lumbar and sacral plexus and, 670
        thoracic, 69
Sympathetic nervous system, 17
    abdomen and, 537-538
    cardiac muscle and, 19, 104, 121
    eye and orbit and, 246
        postganglionic axons to, 246
    head and neck and, 293
        cranial nerves to, 167-169
    Horner's syndrome and, 119
    large intestine and, 520-521
    lungs and pleurae and, 85
    mediastinum and, 112-114, 118
    orbit and, 246
    pelvis and perineum and, 578-584, 591-
        593, 624
    principles of, 336
    pupil of eye and, 237, 246
    spinal cord and, 441-446
    stomach and, 503-504
    urinary bladder and, 600
Sympathetic neuron, 26
    postganglionic, spinal cord and, 443
    preganglionic, 186, 434, 437
        cell bodies of, 434, 437
        spinal cord and, 443
Sympathetic plexus
    aortic, 591-592
    on carotid, 260
Sympathetic splanchnics, 592
Sympathetic trunk, 592
    in chest wall, 68
Symphysis mentalis, 187-188
Symphysis pubis, 36, 550-551, 556-557
    abdomen and, 538
    anterior superior spines and, 552
    articular surface of, 551
    bimanual examination of, 627
    on CT, 618

Symphysis pubis—cont'd
    in female, 550, 574
        uterine prolapse and, 585
    innominate bone and, 552
    ligaments of bladder and rectum and, 599
    in male, 550, 576
    medial end of, pelvis and, 559
    on MRI, 559
    pelvic ligaments and, 556
    pelvic plexus and, 583
    perineum and, 561
    prostate gland and, 616
    ramus of
        inferior, 648-649
        superior, 618
    sacral anesthesia and, 553
    thigh and, 648-649
    in ultrasound, 44
    union of bones of, 10, 13
    urogenital and anal triangles and, 562
    urogenital diaphragm and, 567
Synapses, spinal cord and, 436, 442-443
Synchondroses of skull bones, 133
    on MRI, 415
Synovial cavity, 14
    carpometacarpal joint and, 379-380
    of interphalangeal joints, 381
    of patella, 679
Synovial compartments of wrist, 375
Synovial joints, 11, 13-14
    chondrosternal, 321
    of wrist, 369, 372
Synovial membrane
    of acetabulum, 640
    of elbow joint, 349
    of glenohumeral joint, 320
    humerus and, 319
    of knee joint, 677
Synovial sheaths, 389
Synovial space, 14; *see also* Synovial cavity
Systemic venous blood to heart, 101-102
Systole, 92
    aortic valve in, 98
    cardiac cycle and, 101-102
    tricuspid valve in, 95

T

Taenia coli, 508, 516
Talocalcaneal joint, 708-710
Talocalcaneonavicular joint, 708-710
Talocrural joint, 705
Talofibular ligament, 700, 706
Talonavicular joint, 710
Talonavicular ligament, 706, 708
Talus, 691
    ankle and, 700-701
        blood supply to, 703
    foot and, 705-707
    head of
        ankle and, 700-701
        MRI of, 709
    medial view of, 700
    MRI of, 709
    Pott's fracture and, 704
    talocalcaneonavicular joint and, 710
    tubercle of, 700-701
        MRI of, 709

Talus—cont'd
  weight bearing and, 712
Tamponade, pericardial, 88
Tarsal bone, 3, 705
  anterior view of, 12
  movements in, 712
Tarsal gland, 241
Tarsal muscle, 180
  of Muller, superior, 246, 248
Tarsal plate, 241-242
Tarsal sinus, 709
Tarsal tunnel, 700
Tarsal tunnel syndrome, 704
Tarsometatarsal ligament, 706
Taste
  disturbance of, 185
  otitis and, 232
Taste axon, 231-232
Taste buds, 263, 270
T-cell function, 492
Tears, flow of, 245, 249-250
Tectorial membrane, 418-419, 421
Teeth, 267-269
  deciduous, 267
    eruption of, 269
  permanent, 267, 269
Tegmen tympani, 227, 229
Tegmentum of pons, 148
Telencephalon, 147-148
Temporal and infratemporal fossae, 187-197
  articular, 190
  clinical anatomy of, 197
  mandible and, 187-189, 193-194
  mandibular branch of trigeminal nerve in, 193-195
  maxillary artery and, 192-193
  meningeal artery hematoma and, 196
  muscles of mastication and, 190-192
  orbit and, 235
  otic ganglion and, 193-196
  principles and, 192
  pterygoid venous plexus and, 195-196
  skull and, 137, 139; see also Skull, fossae of
  for sublingual gland, 188
  for submandibular gland, 188
  temporomandibular joint and, 189-190
Temporal artery, superficial, 174-175, 182
  anterolateral neck and, 208
  brain and, 159
  as branch of external carotid artery, 209
  face and, 181-182
  maxillary artery and, 192-193
  parotid gland and, 186
  scalp and, 183
Temporal bone, 134-141, 421
  apertures in, 140-141
  articular tubercle of, 189
  levator veli palatini and, 264
  middle ear cavity in, 226
  petrous ridge of, 139
  shape of face and, 142
  skull and, 134, 137, 141
  squamous
    infratemporal fossa and, 188
    skull and, 139
    temporomandibular joint and, 189
Temporal branch of facial nerve, 180, 185

Temporal horn, 150, 152
Temporal lobe of brain, 148-149, 159
  on MRI, 148
Temporal vein, superficial
  face and scalp and, 183
  head and neck and, 203, 292
  pterygoid venous plexus and, 195
Temporalis muscle
  face and scalp and, 178-179, 182
  head and neck and, 295
  mastication and, 190-192
Temporary pacemaker, 105
Temporomandibular joint, 189-190, 291, 295
  articular disk of, 189-190
  articular tubercle for, 135
  chewing apparatus and, 192
  coronoid and condylar processes and, 189
  dislocation or laxity in, 197, 295
  mechanisms of, 190
  muscles of mastication and, 191
  nerve supply of, 190
  passive and forced opening of, 190
Temporomandibular ligament, 189, 191
Tendinous inscription, 458
Tendinous muscle, 17
Tendinous ring, common, 248-249
Tendo calcaneus, 702-703
  popliteal fossa and, 688-689
  posterior compartment of leg and, 692
Tendon, 15
  and abdominal viscera, 390
  at ankle, 688-689, 692, 702-703
  central, of diaphragm, 530, 532
  central slip of, 384, 390
  in hand, 390
  insertion of, into bones, 14
  patellar, 14
  serous membranes and, 474
Tendon reflexes, deep, 400
Tennis elbow, 352, 402, 404-405
Tenon's fascia, 242
Tenosynovitis, 376
Tensor fascia lata muscle, 650, 654
  on CT, 618
  femoral artery and, 646
  in gluteal region, 664-665
  iliotibial band and, 673
  lumbar plexus and, 533
  thigh and
    anteromedial, 646, 655
    lateral, 647
    posterior, 673
Tensor tympani muscle, 225, 227-229, 231
  nerves to, 193-195
Tensor veli palatini muscle, 263-264, 266, 269, 280
  nerves to, 193-195
  swallowing and, 282
Tenth cranial nerve; see Vagus nerve (X)
Tentorial incisure, 154-155, 158
Tentorial notch, 154-155, 158
Tentorium cerebelli, 142, 149, 151, 154, 156-157
  on MRI, 148
Teres major muscle, 398, 425
  anterior compartment and, 344-345
  axilla and, 330-332

Teres major muscle—cont'd
  brachial plexus and, 338
  on CT, 100
  shoulder movement and, 325-326
  tendon of, 331
Teres minor muscle, 398
  arm and, 344
  axilla and, 330, 332
  on CT, 100
  on MRI, 323
  posterior compartment and, 346
  shoulder movement and, 316, 324
Terminal bronchiole, 34
Terminal ileum
  anorectal region and, 516
  ileocecal junction and, 511
Terminology, 3-7
Testicular artery, 469-470, 537
  inguinal canal and, 465
Testicular self-examination, 625
Testicular vein, 469-470
  inguinal canal and, 465
Testing of muscular reflexes in lower limb, 726
Testis, 35-37, 464, 468
  blood supply to, 470
  cancer of, 469
  descent of, 471-472
  in inguinal canal, 471-472
  perineum and, 582
  self-examination of, 625
  urogenital diaphragm and, 567
Thalamostriate artery, 160
Thalamus, 147-148
  of forebrain, 150
  on MRI, 148
  olfactory epithelium and, 254
  ultrasound of, 44
Thenar eminence, 368, 383
Thenar muscle, 382-385
  flexor retinaculum and, 372
  insertion of, 388
Thenar space, 389
Thigh
  in anatomic position, 3-4
  anterior, 644, 646, 650-660
    blood supply to, 644, 646, 657-658
    clinical anatomy of, 651, 662
    femoral nerve in, 648, 654, 659
    femoral sheath in, 652-655
    femoral triangle in, 644, 651-652, 654
    muscles of, 638, 646, 653-657, 660
    superficial fascia in, 651
  anteromedial, 637-662
    anteromedial thigh in, 644, 646, 650-660; see also Thigh, anterior
    athletic injuries to, 662
    clinical anatomy of, 662
    fascia lata in, 646-647, 650
    femur in, 637-641, 655, 659
    hip joint in, 640-646
    medial thigh in, 655, 657-661
    muscle compartments of, 646-650
    principles and, 645
  axis of rotation for, 641
  cross-section through, 648
  deep fascia of, 646-647, 650

Thigh—cont'd
  medial, 655, 657-661
    clinical anatomy of, 662
    muscles of, 655, 657-661
    neurovascular supply of, 660-661
    rotation of, 659, 661
  MRI of, 649
  posterior, 658, 672-675
    distal end of femur and, 672-673
    muscles of, 673-674
    neurovascular supply of, 674
Third cranial nerve; see Oculomotor nerve
    (III)
Third ventricle, 150-155
  on MRI, 148
Thoracentesis, 72, 127
Thoracic artery, 55, 68-70
  in anterior mediastinum, 118
  on CT and MRI, 43
  intercostal branches of, 118
  internal, 55, 68-69, 121, 202-204
    abdomen and, 536
    in anterior mediastinum, 118
    cervical vertebrae and, 429
    diaphragm and, 530
    subclavian artery and, 203, 326
  lateral, 55, 70, 121, 332-333
  superior, 333
  supreme, 332
Thoracic cage, 49-50, 54
  inflammation of, 62
  surface anatomy of, 538
Thoracic curvature, 409-410
Thoracic diaphragm; see Diaphragm,
    thoracic
Thoracic duct, 29, 31, 115
  aortic arch and, 109
  area draining to, 115
  diaphragm and, 531
  mediastinum and
    posterior, 117
    superior, 114-115
  rupture of, 114
  small intestine and, 512
  of upper limb, 397
Thoracic inlet, 58-59, 109, 309, 311
  arteries and veins in, 309
Thoracic nerve, long, 337
Thoracic outlet, 58
Thoracic spinal cord segment, 69
Thoracic vein
  in anterior mediastinum, 118
  on CT and MRI, 43
Thoracic vertebra, 409-410, 413, 416-417
  articulations of, 420
  on MRI, 415
  thorax and, 54, 58-60
    inlet of, 311
  vertebral canal and, 416
  on x-ray, 53, 417
Thoracic viscera, 49, 121
Thoracic wall, 49-50, 54-73; see also Chest
    wall
Thoracoacromial artery, 55, 397
Thoracoacromial trunk, 332-333
  subclavian artery and, 203
Thoracodorsal nerve, 337-338

Thoracolumbar fascia, 457
Thorax, 3, 46-128
  blood supply to, 121
  case studies of, 125-129
  cavities of, 49-51, 74-76
    surface anatomy of, 538
  heart in, 86-108; see also Heart
  introduction to, 49-53
  landmarks of, 124
  lungs in, 80-85
  mediastinum in, 52-53, 109-119
  MRI of, 42-43
    CT compared to, 43
  nerves of, 121-122
  pericardium in, 49-51
  physical examination of, 122-124
  pleurae of, 49-51, 74-76
  principles and, 51
  segmental nature of, 121
  surface anatomy of, 122-124
  systems review and, 120-122
  trachea in, 77-80
  tracheobronchial tree in, 77-80
  wall of, 49-50, 54-73; see also Chest wall
Thrombophlebitis, 704
  of pelvic veins, 593
Thrombosis, carotid artery, 215
Thumb, 372
  abduction or adduction of, 381, 384-385
  carpometacarpal joints of, 380-381
  circumduction of, 381, 384-385
  flexion or extension of, 381, 384-385
  metacarpals of, 372, 393
    base of, 376
    hand and, 378
  movements of, 380-381, 384-385
  muscle insertions on, 387-388
  opposition of, 384-385, 391, 393
  phalanges of, 371
Thymus, 198
  impression for, on lung, 81
  migration of, 173
  myasthenia gravis and, 119
  pharyngeal arches and, 172-173
  tissue remnants of, 119
Thyroarytenoideus muscle, 285-286
Thyrocervical trunk, 202-204, 332
  axilla and, 332
  branches of, 202-204
    inferior thyroid, 218
Thyroepiglotticus muscle, 285
Thyroglossal duct
  cysts of, 218
    ectopic thyroid tissue and, 275
  pharyngeal arches and, 171
Thyrohyoid membrane, 269, 278, 282, 288
  submandibular gland and, 221
Thyrohyoid muscle, 217
  anterolateral neck and, 216
  pharynx and, 276
Thyrohyoid nerve, 214
Thyroid artery, 116
  inferior, 116, 289, 429, 500
    subclavian artery branches and, 326
    thyroid gland and, 217-218
  superior
    anterolateral neck and, 208

Thyroid artery—cont'd
  brain and, 159
  as branch of external carotid artery, 209
  face and, 182
  thyroid gland and, 217-218
Thyroid cartilage, 276-278, 284-285
  cranial nerves and, 166
  fascial layers of neck and, 200
  laryngeal prominence of, 266, 295
  mediastinum and, 216
  nerve supply of, 288
  pharyngeal muscles and, 269
  spinal cord and, 444
  submandibular gland and, 221
Thyroid gland, 35, 37, 217-219, 296
  calcitonin-secreting cells of, 173
  isthmus of, 217-218
    laryngeal blood supply and, 289
  larynx and, 290
  lateral lobes of, 217-218
    laryngeal blood supply and, 289
  on MRI, 42
  organization of neck and, 198
  pyramidal lobe of, 218
  right lobe of, 207
  surgery on; see Thyroidectomy
  tissue of
    ectopic, thyroglossal cysts and, 275
    remnant, 218
  tongue and, 270
  trachea and, 77
Thyroid membrane, 277-278
  cranial nerves and, 166
Thyroid vein, 116
  inferior, 218, 289
    esophagus and, 500
  middle, 218
  superior, 218
Thyroidea ima branch of brachiocephalic
    artery, 110
Thyroidectomy, 219, 290
  complications of, 299, 303
Tibia, 690-691, 693
  ankle and, 700-701
  anterior, 12, 690, 697, 726
  condyles of, 678, 690
  distal end of femur and, 672
  intercondylar area of, 679
  knee and, 674, 676, 679
  leg and, 688
    fascial compartments of, 693
    muscles of, 695
    posterior nerves of, 696
  malleolus of, 700-701
  on MRI, 709
  plateau of, 672, 690
  posterior views of, 690
  Pott's fracture and, 704
  in rotation at knee, 683
  superior end of, 680
  talocalcaneonavicular joint and, 710
  torsion of, 698
  tuberosity of, 678, 725
    fascial compartments and, 693
    pes anserinus and, 675
    popliteal fossa and, 691
    superior end of tibia and, 680

Tibia—cont'd
  valgus and varus deformities and, 686
  weight bearing and, 712
Tibial artery
  anterior, 693
    dorsum of foot and, 715
    fascial compartments and, 693
    knee and, 684-685
    leg and, 692-693, 698
    muscular branches of, 685
    posterior compartment and, 692
    tibiofibular articulations and, 692
  knee joint and, 684
  posterior, 693, 695, 724
    to ankle, 703
    fascial compartments and, 693
    knee and, 684-685
    leg muscles and, 695
    posterior compartment and, 692, 695
    pulse in, 726
    sole of foot and, 718-719
Tibial collateral ligament, 676, 679, 681-682
Tibial nerve, 587-588, 693, 695, 725
  adductor magnus muscle and, 661
  calcaneal branch of, 638
  entrapment of, 704
  fascial compartments and, 696
  in gluteal region, 669, 671
  popliteal fossa and, 689
  posterior leg and, 696
  posterior thigh and, 674
    deep view, 675
  sciatic nerve origin and, 669
Tibial vein, 692-693, 695
Tibialis anterior muscle, 693, 695
  ankle tendons and, 702
  compartments and
    anterior, 696
    fascial, 693
  foot and, 708
  tendon of, on MRI, 709
  transverse section of, 718
  views of
    anterior, 697
    lateral, 699
    superficial, 714
Tibialis posterior muscle, 693, 695
  ankle tendons and, 702
  compartments of leg and
    fascial, 693
    posterior, 692
  posterior leg and, 692, 694-695
  tendon of
    inserting on navicular/cuneiform, 710
    sole of foot and, 719
Tibiocalcaneal ligament
  ankle and, 700
  deltoid ligament and, 702
  stress injury of, 731
Tibiofibular joint, 690-692, 700-701
Tibiofibular ligament, 700, 706
Tibionavicular ligament, 700, 702
Tibiotalar ligament, 700, 702
Tietze's syndrome, 62
Tinnitus, 232
Tissue density, x-ray detection of, 36
TMJ; see Temporomandibular joint

Toe
  fifth, ball region at base of, 715
  great, 715
    phalanges of, 700
Tongue, 257, 265-266, 269-273
  anatomic relationships and, 272
  base of, 269
  blood supply to, 272
  deviation of, 296
  dorsum of, 269-271
  floor of, 292
  innervation of, 271-272
  lateral view of, 272
  lymphatic drainage of, 272-273
  mobility of, 275, 296
  on MRI, 271
  muscles of, 269, 271
  papilla of; see Papilla, of tongue
  soft palate and palatine tonsil and, 280
  strength of, 296
  submandibular region and, 222
  swallowing and, 282
  tumors in tip of, 223
  ventral surface of, 269
Tonsil
  cerebellar, on MRI, 148, 415
  lingual, 270
  palatine, 264, 266, 274
    pharyngeal arches and, 172-173
Tonsillar artery, 274
Tonsillar pillar, 264-265, 274
Tonsillectomy, 275
Tonsillitis, 300-301, 305
  palatine, 283
Tooth
  roots of, 267
  in socket, 13
Toothache, 262
Torus tubarius, 279
Trabeculae, 599
  bladder, 597
  subarachnoid space with, 439
Trabeculae carneae, 95
Trachea, 77-81, 198, 269
  anterolateral neck and, 207, 219
  aortic arch and, 109
  bifurcation of, 52, 77, 87, 109-110
    aortic arch and, 109
    surface projections of, 124
  on lung radiography, 77
  mediastinum and, 114, 216
  on MRI, 415
  obstruction of, 79
  spinal cord and, 444
  submandibular gland and, 221
  on x-ray, 53, 417
Tracheal lung bud, 172
Tracheal ring, 278, 288
  first, 284
  nerve supply of cartilage and, 288
Trachealis muscle, 77
Tracheobronchial node, 85
Tracheobronchial tree, 29, 77-80
  case studies and, 126, 128
  clinical anatomy of, 83, 85
  principles and, 83
Tracheoesophageal fistula, 85

Tracheostomy, 217, 290
Tracheotomy, 79, 290
Tragus, 225
Transitional cells, 103
Transmission
  of force in forearm, 351
  of light, eye and, 235
Transplant
  corneal, 251
  hair, 185
  heart, 105
  liver, 489
Transvenous pacemaker, 105
Transversalis fascia, 460-461
  abdomen and, 459, 461, 652
  hernias and, 467
  inguinal region and, 466
  testis and, 468
Transverse cervical artery, 203
Transverse cervical nerve, 177
Transverse colon, 516, 518
  anorectal region and, 515-517
  pancreas and, 496
  small intestine and, 512
Transverse diameter, 550
Transverse facial artery, 184
Transverse fasciculi, 708
Transverse fibers, 9
Transverse foramina, 412
  spinal cord and, 438
Transverse ligament
  of atlas, 418, 433
  of knee, 676
Transverse mesocolon, 504
Transverse pericardial sinus, 87-88
Transverse plane, 3, 6
Transverse process of vertebra, 410-414, 416,
    422-424, 448
  in cervical region, 414, 416, 423
    atlas and, 142
    spinal cord and, 438
  on x-ray, 417
Transverse septum of fossa, 568
Transverse sinus; see Cerebral sinus,
    transverse
Transversospinal muscles, 423, 425-427, 448
Transversus abdominis muscle, 459-461
  abdomen and, 459, 461
  on CT, 41
  hernias and, 467
  inguinal region and, 465-466
  testis and, 468
Transversus thoracis muscle, 63-64
Trapezium bone, 357, 369-374, 376, 396
  on MRI, 357
  tubercles of, flexor retinaculum and, 370
Trapezius muscle, 62, 65-66, 292, 326
  accessory nerve and, 213
  back and, 449
  brain and, 159
  clavicle and, 313
  on CT and MRI, 43, 100
  innervation of, 329
    cranial nerves and, 167
  neck and, 200
    anterolateral, 208
    in posterior triangle, 199

Trapezius muscle—cont'd
  shoulder movement and, 325-326
  superficial muscles of back and, 425
  surface anatomy of, 399
Trapezoid bone, 357, 370-371, 373, 396
  on MRI, 357
Trapezoid ligament, 314, 319
Trapezoid line, 314
Trauma
  facial, 294
  hip fracture in, 651
  to larynx, 290
  to mediastinum, 114
  to perineum, 629, 633
Treacher Collins syndrome, 173
Treitz, ligament of, 507-508
Trendelenburg sign, 588
  gluteal region and, 666
Triangle
  of back muscles, auscultation and, 399,
    425
  neck, posterior, 198-205
    fasciae in, 198-200
    nerve supply to, 199-202
    organization of neck and, 198
    root of spinal nerve in, 200, 203-204
    scalenus anterior muscle in, 199, 201
    subclavian artery divisions in, 202-204
    suprapleural membrane in, 205
    venous drainage of, 203-204
Triangular articular disk, 353
Triangular fibrocartilage, 348-349, 353-354,
    372, 374
  radiocarpal joint and, 370
Triangular interval, 330
Triangular ligament, 485-486
Triangular muscle, 17
Triangular space, 330, 332
Triceps brachii muscle, 326, 343-344, 398,
    400
  axilla and, 330, 332
  head of
    lateral, 318, 332
    long, 316, 330, 332, 344
    medial, 318
  posterior compartment and, 346
  posterior view of, 399
Triceps surae muscle, 692
Tricuspid valve
  blood flow through, 102
  of heart, 91, 95-96
    congenital atresia of, 104
    position of, 122
    septal leaflet of, 95
    surface anatomy of, 123-124
Tricuspid valve annulus, 91
Trigeminal ganglion, 165, 245
  brain and, 157
  face and scalp and, 178
  mandibular nerve and, 194
  otic ganglion and, 194
  position of, 139
Trigeminal nerve (V), 165-167, 169
  branches of, 245, 247-248, 293
    mandibular (V3), 165-166, 178-180, 193-
      195
    maxillary (V2), 165-166

Trigeminal nerve (V)—cont'd
  ophthalmic (V1), 165-166, 179-180
  divisions of, 166, 178
  face and, 174
  motor root of, 165
  neck and, 177, 293
    anterolateral, 210
  pinna of ear and, 225
  postganglionic sympathetic axons and,
    168
  scalp and, 174-175
  in temporal and infratemporal fossae, 187
  tongue and, 271
Trigone of bladder, 35, 565, 582, 597-599
  urination and, 600
Triquetrum bone, 357, 369-371, 373-374, 396
  on MRI, 357
  radiocarpal joint and, 370
Trisomy 21, 431
Trochanter
  greater, 639, 641-642, 725-726
    anteromedial thigh and, 637
    center of, 642
    on CT, 618
    dislocation of, 647
    ligaments and, 642
    thigh and knee and, 672
    unclosed epiphysis of, 642
  lesser, 618, 639, 641
    anteromedial thigh and, 637
    center of, 642
    on CT, 618
    femur and, 639, 641
    hip joints and, 642, 667
    short rotators and, 667
    thigh and knee and, 672
Trochlea
  ankle and, 700
  of humerus, 237, 245, 316, 318, 349-350,
    394
    articulation of, 349
    elbow movements and, 349
    on x-ray, 350
  knee and, 676
Trochlear nerve (IV)
  brain and central nervous system and,
    160, 162, 165, 167, 169
  globe and orbit and, 237-238, 244-246
  neck and, 293
    anterolateral, 210
  skull and, 140
Trochlear notch, 348-350, 354
  interosseous membrane and, 356
  on x-ray, 350
True pelvis, 549
  entrance to, 559
True vocal cords, 285-286
Truncus arteriosus, 104
Trunk, 3
  anterior and posterior, 587
    muscles of, 65-66
Trypsin, 498
Tubal elevation, 231
Tubal ligation, 610
Tubercle; see also Tuberosity
  adductor, 639, 658, 661
  anterior, of zygoma, 189

Tubercle—cont'd
  articular, temporomandibular joint and,
    135, 189-190
  of cervical vertebra, 415
  genial, 188
  of humerus, 312-313, 318, 323
  infraglenoid, 312, 314, 320
  of intercondylar eminence, 678
  jugular, 142
  Lister's, 361-362
  mental, 187-188
  pubic; see Pubis, tubercle of
  of ribs, 60-61, 422-423
  scaphoid, 374, 400
    flexor retinaculum and, 370
  supraglenoid, 312, 314, 320
  of talus, 700-701
    MRI of, 709
  tibial; see Tibia, tuberosity of
  of trapezium, 370
  of vertebra, posterior, 414
Tuberculum impar, 171
Tuberosity; see also Tubercle
  deltoid, 315, 318, 345, 399
  gluteal, 637, 639, 641
  ischial; see Ischial tuberosity
  of metatarsal base, 700-701
  radial; see Radius, tuberosity of
Tubules of kidney, 522
Tubuloalveolar gland in breast, 54
Tumor
  of optic chiasma, 151
  pancreatic, 543
Tunica albuginea, 471, 575, 577-579, 604-605
Tunica vaginalis, 471
Turbinates, 255
Turner syndrome, 352
Twelfth cranial nerve; see Hypoglossus
    nerve (XII)
Tympanic membrane, 225-226, 228-229
  openings in, 232
  pharyngeal arches and, 173
Tympanic nerve
  glossopharyngeal nerve and, 212
  otic ganglion and, 195
  pharyngeal arches and, 170-171
Tympanic plexus, 212, 226-228, 231

U
Ulcer
  corneal, 185
  of duodenum, 510
  gastric, 506
Ulcerative colitis, 520
Ulna, 309-310, 348-350, 353, 373, 394
  carpal bones and, 370
  deviation of, 370
  elbow movements and, 349
  fracture of, 351
  growth and maturation of, 11
  head of, 371
  interosseous membrane and, 356
  ligaments and, 353
  on MRI, 357
  processes of
    coronoid, 350
    olecranon, 349, 353, 356

Ulna—cont'd
  styloid; *see* Ulna, styloid process of
  shaft of, 349
  styloid process of, 349, 370-371, 373, 400
    interosseous membrane and, 356
    on MRI, 357
  views of
    anterior, 12
    posterior, 399
  on x-ray, 350
Ulnar artery, 397, 400
  arm and, 342, 345, 347
  on arteriogram, 345
  axilla and, 332
  deep branch of, 391
  deep vena comitantes of, 364
  forearm and, 363-364
  hand and, 391-392
  on MRI, 357
  pulses in, 377
  wrist and, 372, 374
Ulnar collateral artery, 332, 347
Ulnar collateral ligament, 353, 374
Ulnar nerve, 398, 400
  arm and, 344
  axilla and, 333
  brachial plexus and, 337, 339
  branches of
    deep, 367, 391
    dorsal, 368
    superficial, 367, 391-392
  forearm and, 354, 365-367
  in hand, 392-393
  high and low lesions in, 392
  humerus and, 317
  injury to, 340
  radioulnar joint and, 354
  ring finger and, 368
  in wrist, 374
Ulnar notch, 348-349, 353-354
  on MRI, 357
Ulnar recurrent artery on arteriogram, 345
Ulnar vein, 364
Ultimobranchial body, 173
Ultrasound
  of female bladder and uterus, 612
  gallbladder and, 490
  techniques of, 40-45
Umbilical artery, 106-107, 558, 593
Umbilical hernia, 463
Umbilical ligament, 557
  abdomen and, 459
  lateral, 557-558
  medial, 557-558, 596, 599
Umbilical vein, 106-107, 558
  fetal liver and, 486
Umbo, 225
Uncinate process of pancreas, 496
  duodenum and, 508
Unmyelinated axon, 23
Upper limb, 3, 306-405
  anesthesia of, 403-404
  arm in, 342-347
  axilla in, 330-335
  blood supply to, 396-397
  brachial plexus in; *see* Brachial plexus
  case studies of, 401-405

Upper limb—cont'd
  comparison of lower limb girdle to, 723
  dermatomes of, 27
  in fetus, 18
  forearm in, 348-368; *see also* Forearm
  hand in, 378-393; *see also* Hand
  innervation of, 397-398
    cutaneous, 398, 400
    major nerves in, 400
    muscle origins and, 398
  lymphatic drainage of, 397
  movements of, 7
    joint, 396
    muscle origins and, 398
    musculoskeletal anatomy of, 394-395
  physical examination of, 399-400
  shoulder in, 309-329; *see also* Shoulder
  surface anatomy of, 399-400
  systems review of, 394-400
  wrist in, 369-377
Upper limb buds, 18
Upper lip frenulum, 264
Upper respiratory tract, 74
Urachus, 462, 558, 596
Ureter, 30-35, 522-524, 594-598
  anomalies of, 601-602
  bifid, 601
  bony pelvis and, 558
  cross-section of, 595
  on CT scan, 41
  descent of, into pelvis, 595
  developmental errors in, 601-602
  in female, 606
  left, 603
  in male, 614
  perineum and, 565
  right, 603
Ureteropelvic junction, 524-525, 594, 597
Urethra, 30-36, 598-599
  clitoris and, 576
  corpus spongiosum with, 577
  on cystourethrogram, 617
  diaphragm and, 532
  in female, 571-574, 576, 581, 608-609
  lumen of, with glands, 582
  in male, 582, 613-617, 619
    traumatic injury to, 619-621
  membranous, 609, 616, 619
    on CT, 618
    on cystourethrogram, 617
    with external urethral sphincter, 616
  orifice of
    in female, 571-572, 574, 576, 581
    in male, 582
    pelvic diaphragm and, 563
  penile, 582, 609, 616, 619
    on cystourethrogram, 617
    rupture of, 566
  perineum and, 562, 567, 573, 577-580, 582
  prostatic, 599, 609, 616, 619
    on cystourethrogram, 617
    reflux ejaculation into, 618
  sperm and, 35
  sphincter of, 562, 574, 599
    on cystourethrogram, 617
    external, 599, 617
    innervation of, 578

Urethra—cont'd
  internal, 582, 598, 600
    preprostatic, 600
    striated muscles in, 600-601
    vesical, smooth muscle, 600
  spongiose, 616
  traumatic rupture of, 619
  urogenital diaphragm and, 567
  valves of, posterior, 620
Urinary bladder, 30-36, 595-596, 599-601
  abdominal wall and, 459
  anterolateral view of, 597
  aspiration of urine from, 602
  base of, 596
  catheterization of, 602
  cluster of neurons in, 21
  on CT, 618
  epithelium of, 598
  in female, 606, 609, 611
  in male, 582, 611
    inguinal canal and, 465
  neck of, 581
    on cystourethrogram, 617
  neurogenic, 601
  neurovascular supply of, 570, 583, 587,
    591-592, 598-600
  perineum and, 565, 567, 573-574, 582-583
  peritoneal membranes and, 478
  structures of, 581, 597-599, 614
  surfaces and position of, 557, 595-597
  trabeculae of, 597
  on ultrasound, 44, 612
  umbilical ligaments and, 557
  ureter and, 594
  urinary, 459, 606
  urine in, 598
  uterine prolapse and, 585
  wall of, 598, 614
    parasympathetic neurons in, 25
    Waldeyer's sheath in, 598
Urinary continence, 598, 600
Urinary system, 30-35, 594-603
  abnormality of, in newborn, 629, 632
  bladder of; *see* Urinary bladder
  clinical anatomy of, 601-603
  functional regulation in, 600-601
  principles for, 601
  smooth muscles of, 19
  stones in, 602
  ureter of, 594-597
Urination, 600
  spinal cord injuries and, 592, 602
Urine
  in bladder, 598
    aspiration of, 602
  blood in, 541, 544
  collection of, in kidney, 525
  principles of, 601
Urogenital diaphragm, 549, 565-566
  abdomen and, 459
  in female, 573-575
  inferior view of, 564
  layers of, 567
  in male, 564, 577-578, 582, 614, 619
  pelvic diaphragm and, 563
  prostate gland and, 614
  umbilical ligaments and, 557

Urogenital diaphragm—cont'd
  urogenital triangle and, 562
Urogenital membrane, 616
Urogenital triangle, 561-562
Uterine artery, 558, 587, 589, 596, 606
  oviduct and, 607
  ureter and, 594
  uterus and, 596, 607
  vagina and, 596, 608
Uterosacral ligament, 559, 604, 606-607
Uterus, 35-36, 606-609
  bimanual examination of, 627
  blood supply to, 606
  body of, 607, 609
  cancer of, 629, 632
  descent of ureter into pelvis and, 595
  normal position of, 585
  pelvic floor and, 574
  positions of, 607-608
  posterior surface of bladder and, 596
  pregnant, 610-611
  prolapse of, 585
  round ligament of, 605
  smooth muscle tumors of, 610, 612
  structures lateral to, 558
  sympathetic nerves and, 591
  views of
    midsagittal, 574
    parasagittal, 606
    superior, 575
Utricle
  of ear, 233
  prostatic, 614, 616
Uvea, 235, 238
Uvula, 263-266, 280, 296
  on MRI, 148, 271
  muscle of, 265-266

V

Vagal branch of phrenic nerve, 109
Vagal trunk, anterior and posterior, 116
Vagina, 36, 606-609, 611
  blood supply to, 596, 606, 608
  boundaries of perineum and, 561-562, 574
  childbirth and, 144
    tears from, 584
  diaphragm and, 532
  dilated, 631
  in dissection, 572-573
  iliac artery and, 587
  orifice of, 563, 572
  outlet of, 571
  tear in wall of, 584
  on ultrasound, 612
Vaginal artery, 578, 596
Vaginal introitus or vestibule, 574, 576, 626
Vagotomy, 504, 506, 543
Vagus nerve (X), 84-85, 121-122, 165-167, 169
  to abdomen, 538
  anterolateral neck and, 207, 210
  aortic arch and, 109
  brain and, 157, 159
  branches of, 211
  in carotid sheath, 206
  in carotid triangle, 210-213
  diaphragm and, 531
  ear and, 231

Vagus nerve (X)—cont'd
  esophagus and, 499-500
  gastric ulcers and, 506
  glossopharyngeal nerve and, 211
  head and neck and, 293
  larynx and, 287-288
  left, 109
  lungs and heart and, 84
  mediastinum and
    posterior, 116
    superior, 111-112
  nerve supply of cartilage and, 288
  nuclei of, 104
  palate and, 267
  pancreas and, 498
  parasympathetic nerves and, 294
    axons of, 293
    postganglionic neurons of, 169
  pharynx and, 281
  pinna of ear and, 225
  sensory ganglia of, 212
  skull and, 140
  of stomach, 503-504
  tongue and, 270-271
  trachea and, 77
  tympanic membrane and, 226
Valate papilla, 270
Valgus
  at femoral neck, 640
  at knee, 686-687
Vallecula, 281
Valsalva maneuver, 120, 290, 569
Valve
  of coronary sinus, 94
  heart; see Heart, valves of
  of inferior vena cava, 94
  in veins, 26, 30
Varices, esophageal, 116, 500
Varicocele, 469-470
  pelvis and perineum and, 625
Varicose vein, 724
Varus
  at femoral neck, 640
  at knee, 686-687
Vas deferens, 467
  on seminal vesiculogram, 615
Vascular grafts in lower limb, 704
Vascular headaches, 197
Vascular shunt; see Shunt, vascular
Vascular supply; see Blood vessels
Vascular system
  capacity of, 26
  receptors in, 105
Vasectomy, 620
Vasoactive intestinal peptide, 506-507
Vasomotor tone, mediastinum and, 122
Vastus intermedialis muscle
  attachment of, 657
  on CT, 618
  thigh and, 648-649, 653, 656
    anteromedial, 655
    lower, 648
Vastus lateralis muscle, 654
  attachment of, 657
  on CT, 618
  femoral artery and, 646
  intermuscular septum and, 650

Vastus lateralis muscle—cont'd
  lumbar plexus and, 533
  thigh and, 646, 648-649, 653, 656
    anteromedial, 655
    lower, 648
Vastus medialis muscle, 17, 654
  attachment of, 657
  patella and, 676
  thigh and, 653, 656
    anteromedial, 655
    lower, 648
Vater, ampulla of, 497
  development of, 479
  hepatopancreatic, 487
Veins, 26, 30; see also Blood vessels
  of anorectal region, 569-571
  of brain, 154, 157, 160-163
  of chest wall, 121
  of esophagus, 116
  of face, 183
  fetal, 106
  of foot, 714-715, 718-719
  of forearm, 364-365
    access to, 367
  of gluteal region, 668
  of head and neck, 133
  to heart, 101-102
  of hip joint, 644-646
  of knee, 684-685
  of lower limb, 724
    superficial, 652
  of pelvis, 570, 586, 614, 623
    clinical anatomy of, 593
  of perineum, 578, 623
  of popliteal fossa, 690, 695
  of posterior wall of abdomen, 534-535
  of scalp, 183
  of shoulder, 329
    clinical anatomy of, 328
  to spinal cord, 441
  superficial, 400
  of thigh
    anteromedial, 644, 646, 657-658
    medial, 660-661
    posterior, 674
  traversing floor of skull, 140
  valves in, 26, 30
    thigh and, 653
  and varicoceles, 469-470
Vena comitantes, 335, 364
  arm and, 347
Venae cavae
  aortic arch and, 109
  inferior, 480, 586, 591, 603, 611
    abdomen and, 492
    abdominal wall and, 534
    adrenal gland and, 527
    anorectal region and, 570
    aperture for, 530
    blood entering heart from, 102
    on CT scan, 41
    diaphragm and, 67, 124, 530-532
    ductus venosus and, 107
    entering atrium, 95
    esophagus and, 500
    hepatic veins and, 537
    kidneys and, 524, 527

Venae cavae—cont'd
  liver and, 485, 487
  ovaries and, 605
  pancreas and, 496-497
  pelvis and, 558, 623
  peritoneal membranes and, 478
  porta hepatis and, 486
  rectum and, 517
  serous membranes and, 474
  spleen and, 491
  testis and, 470
  tributaries of, 534-535
  vertebral column and, 428, 430
  in pericardial sac, 86
  position of, 124
  superior, 109, 204
    anterior view of, 89
    azygos vein and, 117
    blood entering heart from, 102
    on CT and MRI, 43
    entering atrium, 124
    on lung radiography, 77
    mediastinum and, 111
    persistence of, 114
    position of, 124
    serous membranes and, 474
    thoracic duct and, 31
    thyroid gland and, 218
    on x-ray, 53
Venae comitantes, 724
Venae cordis minimae, 94
Venous arch on foot, 715
Venous plexus, 213
  pelvic, 583, 623
  posterior compartment of leg and, 692
  pterygoid; see Pterygoid venous plexus
  rectal, 569-570
  submucous, 35, 520
  vertebral; see Vertebral venous plexus
Venous sinus
  cerebral; see Cerebral sinus
  scleral, 239
Ventral plane, 3
Ventral position of structure, 5
Ventral spinal nerve root, 24, 164, 435-438
  anterolateral neck and, 210
  axons from, 435
  cauda equina and, 440
  segmentation of body organization and, 446
  spinal accessory nerve and, 167
Ventricles
  cerebral, 145, 150-155; see also Cerebral sinus
    clinical anatomy of, 153
    ependymal lining of, 152
    fourth, 148, 150, 152
    interior of, 151
    lateral, 148, 150-155
    on MRI, 148
    third, 148, 150-152
    ultrasound of, 44
  of heart
    blood entering, 102
    contraction of, 101-102
    coronary arteries to, 93
    on CT and MRI, 43

Ventricles—cont'd
  left, 77, 93, 96, 98, 102
  myocytes of, 103
  outflow tracts of, 97-98
  posterior vein of, 93
  right, 95-97
  septal defects of, 101, 104, 124
  on x-ray, 53, 77
  laryngeal, 285
Ventriculoperitoneal shunt, 153
Venule, 26, 28
Vermiform appendix, 518
Vertebrae
  abdomen and, 538
    wall of, 529
  articulations of, 420, 422-424
  attachments of
    to each other, 418-423
    to skull, 418, 421
  blood supply to, 430, 433, 439-442, 448-449
  body of, 58-59, 409-411, 416
    compression fractures of, 431
    costovertebral and costotransverse
      joints and, 424
    on MRI, 42, 415
  cervical; see Cervical vertebra
  clinical anatomy of, 431-433
  coccygeal, 552
    first, 553
  congenital abnormalities of, 431
  curvatures of, 409-410
  diaphragm and, 530
  inferior notch of, 411
  injury to, 431-433
  lamina of, 58, 409-411, 414, 416, 423
  ligaments and articulations in, 417-424
  ligaments of skull and, 421
  lumbar, 411, 413-415
    abdomen and, 536
    on MRI, 418
  midsagittal section through, 422
  as movable bones, 133
  movements of, 427, 448
  muscles to
    extrinsic, 423-425
    intrinsic, 200, 425-427
  sacral, 416, 419, 553
  spinous processes of; see Spinous process
  thoracic, 54-55, 58-60, 413, 416-417, 420
    on CT and MRI, 43
    on x-ray, 53
  transverse process of; see Transverse
    process of vertebra
  tubercle of, 414
  typical, 409-413
  upper, joints of, 421, 433
Vertebral artery, 133, 161, 202-204, 413
  back and spinal cord and, 448
  brain and, 157, 159
  cervical vertebrae and, 429
  head and neck and, 292
  spinal cord and, 442
  subclavian artery and, 203, 326
Vertebral body; see Vertebrae, body of
Vertebral canal, 416
  intervertebral foramen and, 439
  spinal cord and, 439-441

Vertebral canal—cont'd
  thoracic vertebra and, 416
Vertebral column; see Back and vertebral
    column; Vertebrae
Vertebral foramen, 410
  on CT and MRI, 43
Vertebral notch, 410, 416
  on x-ray, 417
Vertebral spine; see Spinous process
Vertebral vein, 133, 412-413
Vertebral venous plexus, 412, 433
  back and spinal cord and, 449
  external, 429-430
    spinal cord and, 430
  internal, 429-430, 453
    spinal cord and, 430
Vertebral-basilar artery, 160
Vertex, 134, 140
Vertigo, 232
Verumontanum, 614, 616
  on cystourethrogram, 617
Vesical artery, 570, 587, 589, 599
Vesical plexus, 570, 599
Vesical sphincter, 598
  smooth muscle of, 600
Vesicorectal fossa, 558
Vesicouterine fossa, 574, 604
Vesicouterine pouch, 606
Vesicouterine recess, 558
Vestibular bulb, 575, 577-578
Vestibular fold, 285-286
Vestibular gland, greater, 571, 576, 585
  orifice of, 572-573, 576
Vestibule, 571
  aortic, 98
  bulb of, 573, 576
    anterior extensions of, 581
  inner ear and, 233
  of larynx, 285
  of middle ear, 226, 228-230
  of nose, 253-254
  of oral cavity, 263
  teeth and, 268
  vaginal, 576
Vestibulocochlear nerve (VIII), 165-167,
    169
  anterolateral neck and, 210
  brain and, 157, 159
  head and neck and, 293
  otic ganglion and, 195
  parasympathetic nervous system and
    axons of, 293
    postganglionic neurons in, 169
  pharyngeal arches and, 170
  pharynx and, 280-281
  sensory ganglia for, 212
  skull and, 140
  submandibular region and, 222
  tongue and, 271-272
  tympanic membrane and, 226
Vibrissa, 253
Vidian canal, 143
Villi, arachnoid, 155, 158
Vincula, 384, 390, 474
VIP-like substance, 497
Virilizing lesions, 528
Viscera

Viscera—cont'd
  abdominal; *see also* Abdomen
    principles of, 390
    tendons and, 390
  development of, 473-483
  layers of, in cavities, 51
  in pelvis; *see* Pelvic viscera
  pericardium and, 51
  pleura and, 49, 74
  thoracic, 49, 121; *see also* Thorax
Visceral layer of cavity, 51
Visceral mesenteries, development of, 473-474, 476
Visceral motor axon, 164
Visceral peritoneum, serous membranes and, 474
Visceral pleura, 49, 74
Visceral sensory axon, 164
Visceral serous pericardium, 51
Visceral skeleton of skull, 136
Vision
  blurred, 300, 304
  disturbances of, cornea and, 237
  refractive errors in, 240
Visual axis of gaze, 234-235
Visual cortex, primary, 149
Visual signal transmission, 240-241
Vitreous humor, 239-241
  flow of, 240
Vocal cords, 287
  false, 285-286
  maturational changes in, 290
  positions of, 288
  true, 285-286
Vocal folds, 285-286
Vocal ligament, 282, 284-285
Vocal process, 285
Vocalis muscle, 282, 285-286
Voice, 254
Voiding cystourethrogram, 617, 620
Volar surface, 6
Voluntary muscle, 11-18
Volvulus, 514, 520, 542
Vomer, 253-255
Vomeronasal nerve, 254

Vomiting
  of blood, 541, 544
  projectile, 540, 543
Vorticose vein, 238
VP shunt; *see* Ventriculoperitoneal shunt
Vulva, 571

W

Waldeyer's ring, 274, 279
Waldeyer's sheath in bladder wall, 598
Web
  of duodenum, 510
  esophageal, 500
Werdnig-Hoffman disease, 447
Wharton's duct, 221, 273
Wheezing, 124
Whiplash injury, 402, 431
White line of rectum, 568-569, 571
White matter, 145, 147, 434
  diseases of, 151
White rami communicans, 24, 118, 443-444, 588
  lumbar and sacral plexus and, 670
White rami communicans—cont'd
  primary
    anterior, 24, 430, 436-437
    posterior, 24, 436
  spinal cord and, 430, 437, 443
  in thoracic and upper lumbar regions, 118
Willis, circle of, 158-159, 161-162, 292
  clinical anatomy of, 163
Winslow, epiploic foramen of, 477, 503, 505
Wirsung, duct of, 496
Wisdom tooth, 267
Wormian bone, 136
Wrist, 309, 369-377, 396
  in anatomic position, 4
  anatomic snuff-box in, 372, 375
  arterial pulses at, 377
  blood vessels and nerves of, 372, 375
  clinical anatomy of, 376-377
  comparison of, to ankle bones, 723
  cross-section of, 374
  extensor synovial compartments in, 375
  fusion of bones in, 377

Wrist—cont'd
  ganglia at, 377
  injury of, 401, 403-404
    fracture in, 402, 405
    laceration in, 377
    median nerve in, 392
  joint at, 348
    radiocarpal, 370, 374
  maturation of, 371, 377
  retinaculum in
    extensor, 372, 375
    flexor, 370-372, 374
Wrist drop, 319, 340

X

Xiphoid, 62-63, 122, 536
  abdominal wall and, 457-458
  diaphragm and, 532
X-ray imaging; *see also* specific study
  of chest, 38, 53
  conventional, 36-40
  CT in, 38-39, 41
  MRI in, 39-40, 42-43
  of pelvis, 559-560
  of skull, 144
  ultrasonography in, 40-45

Z

Zygoma, 134, 177
  arch of, 142, 177, 294, 421
    mastication muscles and, 191
  lacrimal gland and, 249
  maxillary artery and, 193
  orbit and, 234
  skull and, 134-135, 137, 141
  temporomandibular joint and, 189
Zygomatic bone, 174
  orbit and, 234
Zygomatic nerve, 180-181, 185
Zygomatic process of temporal bone, 141
Zygomaticofacial nerve, 242
Zygomaticoorbital foramen, 236
Zygomaticotemporal artery, 242
Zygomaticotemporal nerve, 174-175
Zygomaticus muscle, 178-180

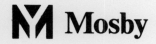 **Mosby**

Dedicated to Publishing Excellence   **WE WANT TO HEAR FROM YOU!**

To help us publish the most useful materials for students, we would appreciate your comments on this book. Please take a few moments to complete the form below, and then tear it out and mail to us. Thank you for your input.

C.L.A.S.S.: *CLINICAL ANATOMY ATLAS*

1. What courses are you using this book for?

___medical school   ___1st year
___pharmacy school   ___2nd year
___physician assistant program   ___3rd year
___nursing school   ___4th year
___dental school   ___other
___osteopathic school
___undergrad
___other _____

2. Was this book useful for your course? Why or why not?

___yes ___no _____
_____
_____

3. What features of textbooks are important to you? (*check all that apply*)

___color figures
___summary tables and boxes
___summaries
___self-assessment questions
___price
___other _____
_____

4. What influenced your decision to buy this text? (*check all that apply*)

___required/recommended by insructor
___recommendation by student
___bookstore display
___other _____

5. What other instructional materials did/would you find useful in this course?

___computer-assisted instruction
___lab time   ___slides
___case studies book
___other _____

Are you interested in doing in-depth reviews of our basic science textbooks? If so please fill out the information below.

NAME:_____

ADDRESS:_____

_____

TELEPHONE:_____

THANK YOU!

A Times Mirror Company

BUSINESS REPLY MAIL

FIRST CLASS MAIL   PERMIT No. 135   St. Louis, MO.

POSTAGE WILL BE PAID BY ADDRESSEE

CHRIS REID
MEDICAL EDITORIAL
MOSBY–YEAR BOOK, INC.
11830 WESTLINE INDUSTRIAL DRIVE
ST.LOUIS, MO 63146-9987

NO POSTAGE
NECESSARY
IF MAILED
IN THE
UNITED STATES

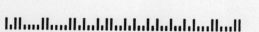